CONGENITAL HEART DEFECTS

From Origin to Treatment

Edited by

DIEGO F. WYSZYNSKI

Amgen, Inc.
Thousand Oaks, California

ADOLFO CORREA-VILLASEÑOR

Centers for Disease Control and Prevention
Atlanta, Georgia

THOMAS P. GRAHAM

Vanderbilt University Medical Center
Nashville, Tennessee

OXFORD
UNIVERSITY PRESS
2010

OXFORD
UNIVERSITY PRESS

Oxford University Press, Inc., publishes works that further
Oxford University's objective of excellence
in research, scholarship, and education.

Oxford New York
Auckland Cape Town Dar es Salaam Hong Kong Karachi
Kuala Lumpur Madrid Melbourne Mexico City Nairobi
New Delhi Shanghai Taipei Toronto
With offices in
Argentina Austria Brazil Chile Czech Republic France Greece
Guatemala Hungary Italy Japan Poland Portugal Singapore
South Korea Switzerland Thailand Turkey Ukraine Vietnam

Copyright © 2010 by Oxford University Press, Inc.

Published by Oxford University Press, Inc.
198 Madison Avenue, New York, New York 10016
www.oup.com

Oxford is a registered trademark of Oxford University Press.

1006084063

Library of Congress Cataloging-in-Publication Data
Congenital heart defects / [edited by] Diego F. Wyszynski, Adolfo Correa-Villaseñor,
Thomas P. Graham.
p. ; cm.
Includes bibliographical references.
ISBN 978-0-19-537388-2
1. Congenital heart disease. I. Wyszynski, Diego F. II. Correa-Villaseñor, Adolfo.
III. Graham, Thomas P.
[DNLM: 1. Heart Defects, Congenital. WG 220 C7485 2009]
RC687.C654 2009
616.1'2043—dc22
2008056037

1 3 5 7 9 8 6 4 2
Printed in the United States of America
on acid-free paper.

Foreword

Pediatric Cardiology arose suddenly and dramatically as a medical discipline. This in spite of the gloomy assessment of cardiovascular malformations by Sir William Osler:

> These congenital afflictions of the heart have only limited interest as in a large proportion of the cases the condition is not compatible with life and in others nothing can be done to remedy the defect or even to relieve the symptoms. (1892)

Who could then have imagined that half a century later a new specialty would arise to give hope and longevity to many of these patients?!

REFLECTIONS

The relief of hypoxia by a subclavian–pulmonary artery shunt operation "turned a blue baby pink" in the Johns Hopkins Hospital in Baltimore, MD, on November 29, 1944. The excitement reverberated around the world:

> For the first time miserable and squatting little children became pink, could run and play and join the human race

wrote Alexander Nadas in remembrance of that time.

A stream of patients came to Hopkins seeking help, as did physicians eager to make the advances their own. Young pediatricians and surgeons found themselves in a new and compelling career. I was one of those pediatricians, deeply inspired and driven to contribute to the care of the children, to expand knowledge and help to create ways to improve diagnosis, and in time, to follow-up with adolescent and adult patients. We became the first "certified" Pediatric Cardiologists.

It was truly a magical time, but also an insight into the hardships of the families who came from all over the world, often at great personal and financial sacrifice, to have their child seen by Dr. Helen Taussig and operated by Dr. Alfred Blalock. Their comments inadvertently revealed their anxieties: The mother of a deeply cyanotic toddler exclaimed in surprise when she entered the waiting room "There are other blue children here—I thought Eddie was the only one!"

We shared their grief when operation was not feasible or was not successful, but we also shared the joy of many whose child did well. We remember a little boy and his moving surprise: "How come I can walk so far??" And a young girl a year after operation: "You can't recognize me; look at my clear skin and shiny hair!"

Training programs expanded worldwide, and within a few years treatment centers of excellence arose in medical institutions all over the developed world. Regrettably, thousands of children remain without help even today!!

Clinical practice changed rapidly and continuously. In the early days at the Johns Hopkins Hospital we saw mostly patients with tetralogy of Fallot, the classic "blue baby" malformation that permitted survival into childhood and even adult life. The diagnostic work-up was history and physical examination, chest X-ray and fluoroscopy, electrocardiogram, and blood counts. A decision to operate could then be made in most cases. Those with unusual findings required cardiac catheterization in Dr. Richard Bing's laboratory, and sometimes angiocardiography in the X-ray department in an adjacent building.

Surgical interventions multiplied. The Blalock–Taussig shunt was the first operation for cyanotic children. It was soon followed by the Potts shunt and by the Brock procedure for pulmonary stenosis. Extracorporeal circulation permitted intracardiac surgery with a great expansion of palliative and curative procedures. New operations and revisions of "old" procedures followed one another in rapid succession, bringing new hopes in life-outlook for many. Others, however, suffered deep disappointments as they ran out of surgical improvements. These patients faced insurmountable barriers in complex structural anomalies and in the late postoperative complications of these anomalies. For these patients cardiac transplantation has become the last resort, although, in the words of Dr. Helen Taussig "a procedure which requires the death of a healthy child cannot, fundamentally, be the final answer."

NEW TECHNOLOGIES

The technologic revolution, which affects all aspects of our lives, is rapidly changing our understanding of biology and human health and disease. We now have better diagnostic methods to define the anatomic abnormalities of the heart, diagnoses are established early, and even in fetal life there are new approaches in surgical interventions applied to newborn infants and contemplated also for near-term fetuses. Most important, there are stronger links to other disciplines, most notably Genetics and Teratology, in searching for clues to heritable and nonheritable factors of origin.

It is somewhat daring to create a new textbook in this time of rapidly changing knowledge, but it is also very important. Medical texts are the stepping stones to the future as they condense past experiences and introduce new horizons of thoughts. This new textbook fulfills these requirements well in a comprehensive approach, adding new topics to the usual diagnostic and surgical discussions including molecular embryology, epidemiologic issues, and challenges for personal care and public health activities.

Molecular embryology is the new way of understanding growth and development in terms of the nature and interaction of developmental genes and gene products that direct tissue growth and changes. There will be thousands of these compounds that play a part in transforming primitive embryonic cells into functional tissues and organs. Variations may be endless, but a new image of stem cells and development will in time be created. A concept of these changes can be found in James J Nora's writings (1993):

> Although we have opened many doors to learn about the causes of congenital heart disease, we have found that the doors lead to new corridors flanked by many more doors.

Molecular embryology is surely one of these corridors. A "genetic" origin of birth defects, which, at first, had only a vague meaning, is now developing into more concrete knowledge. Heritable abnormalities and chromosome disorders are already defined for many forms of heart defects.

EPIDEMIOLOGY

Epidemiologic studies of congenital heart defects are essential in the search for causes and the evaluation of treatments. They need to be well focused and greatly expanded. Their value will depend on careful consideration of each aspect of a study. The conduct of a good epidemiologic study is expensive, but the investment in expertise and methods served us well over the decade of our regional collaborative investigation, the Baltimore-Washington Infant Study (1981–1989). The analyses of this study revealed many important observations on case and control differences that represent many important targets for further intensive efforts.

- Child health and survival: Infants with severe cardiac defects and associated non-cardiac anomalies were of low birth weight, which compromised their survival; the existing data could be searched for risk factors for the fetal growth retardation and the increased mortality of this patient group.
- Parental congenital heart disease: Adults with congenital heart disease are at increased risk of a recurrence of the cardiac abnormality in their offspring. This risk varies with the type of defect and the associated noncardiac anomalies, some of which may be of genetic origin. Careful attention to detailed family relationships may reveal important genetic and nongenetic factors.
- Maternal diabetes: Prepregnancy diabetes was the major risk factor for nonchromosomal cases with severe cardiac defects. The similarity in the spectrum of these malformations to those with autosomal trisomies suggests some common steps in the cardiac origins of these severe defects. Early diagnosis of diabetes and conscientious control of maternal blood glucose should be evaluated for their effect on the prevention and reduction of the excess mortality of these vulnerable infants.
- Major coagulation defects: The occurrence of hemophilia and von Willebrand's disease in case parents but not in control parents has gained increasing emphasis by recent advances in vascular biology. It is now well established that coagulation affects vasculogenesis and angiogenesis and may also affect the development of the heart. Joint studies in hematology, cardiology, and vascular biology should elucidate these associations and also determine the frequency and types of congenital heart disease in families affected with the hemophilias in comparison to unaffected families.
- Parents' use of medications and recreational drugs, and medical, home, and occupational exposures to toxicants were associated with the occurrence of certain cardiac defects. These findings, together with those of many investigators obligate a great responsibility to verify the findings and, if confirmed, to institute preventive measures to protect vulnerable individuals.

THE ADULT WORLD

It took many years to overcome the separation of "pediatric" and "adult" cardiology to achieve a joint understanding of the many needs of young persons with congenital heart disease. Beyond the serious problems of complex malformations and repeated attempts at surgical amelioration, we did not understand the fears and stresses experienced by the growing boys and girls who so much wanted to be like their peers. So many failed to find the many legislated and community support services that might have improved their lives.

Today, many infants born with congenital heart disease can expect to reach adulthood. With continued and future advances in cardiac surgery and medical care the number of adults with congenital heart disease in the population will increase. Because treatment of congenital heart disease is rarely curative many of these adults will be at increased risk for reoperation, dysrhythmias, and other serious complications for which specialized and intensive medical follow-up is needed. Because the centralized, expert medical and surgical treatment currently available to children with heart defects is not readily available to many adults there is no orderly transition of care as adolescents with congenital heart disease become adults. As a result many adults will be medically underserved and at risk of premature death, disabilities, and complications that are costly to the individual, family, the health care system, and society, deserving increased attention from the clinical, population research and policy-making communities.

In the United States an amazing range of service is mandated to keep all persons with disabilities in the "mainstream" of society, but it is necessary for patients and their families to be aware of these programs and to know how to gain access to them. Today, the wide range of information available on the Internet should help to better inform our patients. We still hope to achieve the goal so well summarized in the motto of the 1940 White House Conference on Children:

> No child should incur any disability that human ingenuity can prevent, nor suffer from one that intelligent care can remove or cancel.

The multidisciplinary contributors to this new textbook take a great step in expanding the disciplinary horizons relating to congenital heart disease, which were not previously included in textbooks on Pediatric Cardiology. This will help our expanding patient population toward a better future.

CHARLOTTE FERENCZ, M.D., M.P.H.
Professor Emeritus
Departments of Epidemiology and
Preventive Medicine and Pediatrics
University of Maryland School of Medicine
Baltimore, Maryland

REFERENCES

1. Osler W. Congenital Affections of the Heart. In: *The Principles and Practice of Medicine.* New York and London: D Appleton Century Company; 1892.
2. Blalock A, HB Taussig. The surgical treatment of malformations of the heart in which there is pulmonary stenosis or pulmonary atresia. *JAMA.* 1945;128:189–202.
3. Nadas A, RJ Bing. Congenital Heart Disease. In: *Cardiology. The Evaluation of the Science and the Art*: R J Bing, Editor, 2nd Ed. New Brunswick, NJ :Rutgers University Press; 1999.
4. Nora JJ. Causes of congenital heart diseases: old and new modes, mechanisms and models. *Am Heart J.* 1993;125:1409–1419.

Preface

Congenital heart defects, or CHDs, are the most frequently occurring birth defect. In the United States alone, over 25,000 babies are born each year with a CHD. That translates to 1 out of every 115 to 150 births. In the last two decades a vast proportion of children's heart abnormalities have been successfully treated, dramatically decreasing their mortality rate. Moreover, much research is continuing to provide a better understanding of the medical and societal needs of heart defect patients in their adult years.

This book is intended to present detailed descriptions of the many aspects related to CHDs, closely following the aims and structure of its "distant relatives", *Cleft Lip and Palate: From Origin to Treatment* (Oxford University Press, 2002) and *Neural Tube Defects: From Origin to Treatment* (Oxford University Press, 2006). The book is organized with a wide readership in mind; virtually everyone interested in CHDs, be it casual readers, research workers, clinicians, epidemiologists, or any others concerned with heart abnormalities. Many of the chapters will be especially informative to parents, siblings, and affected individuals.

The book includes a broad range of theoretical, experimental, and clinical topics written by experts in the fields of development, epidemiology, genetics, treatment, and public health. The text is divided into six parts: I. Clinical and Molecular Embryology of the Cardiovascular System, II. Diagnosis and Management of CHDs, III. Special Management Issues, IV. Epidemiology of CHDs, V. Genetics of CHDs, and VI. Public Health Issues.

Part I, *Clinical and Molecular Embryology of the Cardiovascular System*, is essential reading for those who need to update their knowledge of the embryology, physiology, and anatomy of the fetal heart.

Part II, *Diagnosis and Management of CHDs*, includes chapters describing the technologies that diagnose CHDs, followed by a series of detailed descriptions of the most common CHDs. For each condition, these chapters include morphological and embryological considerations, hemodynamic characteristics, clinical features, differential diagnoses, and principles of treatment and management.

Part III, *Special Management Issues*, is devoted to topics that are less known to the wider readership, such as CHDs in adulthood and in pregnancy, neurodevelopment and psychological aspects of CHDs, and current trends in meeting the needs of children, adolescents, and parents with CHDs.

Part IV, *Epidemiology of CHDs*, includes chapters that describe the difficulties of collecting meaningful population data, the geographical frequency distribution of CHDs, and the environmental factors suspected to be involved in the etiology of CHDs. These topics will be of greater interest to scientists, researchers, and clinicians.

Part V, *Genetics of CHDs*, discusses the role genes, alone or in interaction with environmental factors, play in the susceptibility to CHDs. A chapter on genetic counseling translates those concepts to the clinical setting.

Finally, Part VI, *Public Health Issues*, presents new areas of emerging interest to the public, such as strategies for the prevention of CHDs, the costs for treatment of CHDs, coverage of health care needs, and the ethics of end of life in pediatric cardiac care.

Although there is a large amount of information available on CHDs—from scientific journals, popular magazines, newsletters, and books to television shows and Web pages—it is difficult to sift through it all and know what is current and accurate. *Congenital Heart Defects: From Origin to Treatment* provides invaluable state-of-the-art information to graduate students, researchers, practitioners, and family members interested in these conditions. It is written with the collective knowledge garnered from more than 60 experts in the field in the hopes that it will help readers better understand the possibilities of prevention, diagnosis, and treatment of congenital heart defects.

DIEGO F. WYSZYNSKI
ADOLFO CORREA-VILLASEÑOR
THOMAS P. GRAHAM

Acknowledgments

As the editors of this book, we wish to acknowledge with gratitude the contributors' investment of time and knowledge in the face of numerous competing demands for their attention. Drafts of each chapter were presented for formal review and comments to at least two anonymous experts in the respective field. We are grateful to the following individuals for engaging the contributors in challenging and incisive discussions and for supplying them with detailed comments about their work:

Aidan Bolgers, Cynthia H. Cassell, Tiffany Colarusso, Vernat Exil, Uta Francke, Jennifer Garbarini, Vidu Garg, Daniel Garros, Caren Goldberg, Mark Hill, Dana Janssen, Kathy Jenkins, James Johns, Prince Kannankeril, Ann Kavanaugh-McHugh, Rae-Ellen Kavey, Francois Lacour-Gayet, Mike Liske, Christopher Loffredo, Leena Mildh, Joe Mulinare, Dan Murphy, Jane Newberger, Dita Obler, David Parra, Gail D. Pearson, Paul Riley, Geoffrey Rosenthal, Annika Rydberg, David J. Sahn, Ulrike Salzer, Michael Simons, Matthew Strickland, Norman Talner, Elizabeth Tong, Elisabeth Utens, Karen Uzark, Gary Webb, Jo Wray, and Katherine E. Yutzey.

Our involvement in the field of birth defects and this book are fruits of the warm support we received from many people and many organizations. However, the latter part of our lives, including the period while editing this book, have been especially touched by the love, affection, and understanding of those who are our most important companions, our dear wives: Carolien Panhuysen, Ana I. Alfaro-Correa, and Carol Ann Graham. To them we sincerely dedicate this book.

Contents

Contributors

MICHAEL J. ACKERMAN, M.D., PH.D.
Departments of Medicine, Pediatrics, and Molecular Pharmacology & Experimental Therapeutics/Divisions of Cardiovascular Diseases and Pediatric Cardiology
Mayo Clinic
Rochester, Minnesota

H. SCOTT BALDWIN, M.D.
Department of Pediatrics, Division of Pediatric Cardiology
Vanderbilt University School of Medicine
Nashville, Tennessee

JOHN W. BELMONT, M.D., PH.D., FACMG
Departments of Molecular and Human Genetics and Pediatrics
Baylor College of Medicine
Houston, Texas

DAVID BICHELL, M.D.
Department of Surgery, Division of Pediatric Cardiac Surgery
Vanderbilt University School of Medicine
Nashville, Tennessee

LORENZO D. BOTTO, M.D.
Division of Medical Genetics, Department of Pediatrics
University of Utah
Salt Lake City, Utah

SHEREE L. BOULET, DR.P.H., M.P.H.
Centers for Disease Control and Prevention
National Center on Birth Defects and Developmental Disabilities
Atlanta, Georgia
and
Oak Ridge Institute for Science and Education
Oak Ridge, Tennessee

MARY M. CANOBBIO, R.N., M.N., FAAN, FAHA
Ahmanson/UCLA Adult Congenital Heart Disease Center
University of California School of Nursing
Los Angeles, California

FRANK CETTA, M.D.
Department of Pediatrics
Mayo Clinic Transplant Center
Rochester, Minnesota

RUEY-KANG CHANG, M.D.
Department of Pediatrics
Harbor-UCLA Medical Center
Torrance, California

REEMA CHUGH, M.D., F.A.C.C.
Department of Cardiology
Kaiser Foundation Hospitals
Panorama City, California

ANNE J. L. CHUN, M.D.
Pediatric Cardiology Program and Department of Pediatrics
New York University School of Medicine
New York, New York

MARIO A. CLEVES, PH.D.
Department of Pediatrics
UAMS College of Medicine
Arkansas Center for Birth Defects Research and Prevention
Little Rock, Arkansas

JEAN ANNE CONNOR, D.N.SC., R.N., CPNP
Cardiovascular Program
Children's Hospital Boston
Boston, Massachusetts

ADOLFO CORREA-VILLASEÑOR, M.D., PH.D.
National Center on Birth Defects and Developmental Disabilities
Centers for Disease Control and Prevention
Atlanta, Georgia

PETER N. COX, M.B., CH.B., D.C.H., F.F.A.R.C.S. (U.K.), F.R.C.P. (C)
Department of Critical Care Medicine
Hospital for Sick Children
and
Departments of Anaesthesia, Critical Care and Paediatrics
University of Toronto
Toronto, Canada

BRUNO DALLAPICCOLA, M.D.
Ospedale CSS
San Giovannni Rotondo and CSS-Mendel Institute
Rome, Italy

JOSEPH A. DEARANI, M.D.
Department of Pediatrics
Mayo Clinic Transplant Center
Rochester, Minnesota

ELLEN DEES, M.D.
Department of Pediatrics
Division of Pediatric Cardiology
Vanderbilt University School of Medicine
Nashville, Tennessee

MARIA CRISTINA DIGILIO, M.D.
Medical Genetics
Bambino Gesù Pediatric Hospital
Rome, Italy

DEBRA A. DODD, M.D.
Pediatric Heart Transplant Program
Division of Pediatric Cardiology
Vanderbilt Children's Hospital
Nashville, Tennessee

THOMAS DOYLE, M.D.
Department of Pediatrics, Division of Pediatric Cardiology
Vanderbilt University School of Medicine
Nashville, Tennessee

WELTON M. GERSONY, M.D.
New York Presbyterian Hospital
and
Columbia University College of Physicians & Surgeons
New York, New York

ADRIANA C. GITTENBERGER-DE GROOT, PH.D.
Department of Anatomy & Embryology
Leiden University Medical Center
Leiden, The Netherlands

THOMAS P. GRAHAM, M.D.
Department of Pediatrics, Division of Pediatric Cardiology
Vanderbilt University School of Medicine
Nashville, Tennessee

SCOTT D. GROSSE, PH.D.
Centers for Disease Control and Prevention
National Center on Birth Defects and Developmental Disabilities
Atlanta, Georgia

KIYOSHI HASHIGAMI-SHINN, M.D.
Pediatric Cardiology Program and Department of Pediatrics
New York University School of Medicine
New York, New York

CHARLOTTE A. HOBBS, M.D., PH.D.
Arkansas Center for Birth Defects Research and Prevention
Arkansas Children's Hospital Research Institute
and
Department of Pediatrics
University of Arkansas for Medical Sciences/College of Medicine
Little Rock, Arkansas

MARGARET A. HONEIN, PH.D., M.P.H.
National Center on Birth Defects and Developmental Disabilities
Centers for Disease Control and Prevention
Atlanta, Georgia

LISA K. HORNBERGER, M.D.
Fetal & Neonatal Cardiology Program
Department of Pediatrics, Division of Cardiology
Department of Obstetrics & Gynecology
University of Alberta
Edmonton, Canada

KATHY J. JENKINS, M.D., M.P.H.
Department of Cardiology
Children's Hospital Boston
Boston, Massachusetts

RUIPING JI, M.D., PH.D.
Pediatric Cardiology Program and Department of Pediatrics
New York University School of Medicine
New York, New York

HENRI JUSTINO, M.D., C.M.,
F.R.C.P.C., F.A.C.C., F.S.C.A.I.
*CE Mullins Cardiac Catheterization
Laboratories,*
Texas Children's Hospital
and
Baylor College of Medicine
Houston, Texas

LYNNE KENDALL M.C.S.P.,
GRADDIPPHYS, M.SC.
*Departments of Pediatric Cardiology and
Physiotherapy*
Leeds General Infirmary
Leeds, United Kingdom

THOMAS S. KLITZNER, M.D.,
PH.D.
Department of Pediatrics
David Geffen School of Medicine
University of California
Los Angeles, California

ROBERT I. KOPPEL, M.D.
Department of Pediatrics
Schneider Children's Hospital
New York, New York

ADRIENNE H. KOVACS, PH.D.,
C.PSYCH.
Peter Munk Cardiac Centre
University Health Network
The University of Toronto
Toronto, Canada

KAREN S. KUEHL, M.D., M.P.H.
Children's National Medical Center
*Center for Clinical and Community
Research (CCCR)*
and
*George Washington University School of
Medicine and Health Sciences*
Washington, DC

MICHAEL J. LANDZBERG, M.D.
Department of Cardiology
Children's Hospital Boston
and
Brigham & Women's Hospital
Harvard Medical School
Boston, Massachusetts

ANGELA E. LIN, M.D., F.A.A.P,
F.A.C.M.G.
Harvard Medical School
and
*Genetics Unit, MassGeneral Hospital for
Children*
Boston, Massachusetts

WILLIAM T. MAHLE, M.D.
Sibley Heart Center
Children's Healthcare of Atlanta
and
Department of Pediatrics
Emory University School of Medicine
Atlanta, Georgia

BRUNO MARINO, M.D.
Pediatric Cardiology
Department of Pediatrics
University La Sapienza
Rome, Italy

JEFFERY MEADOWS, M.D.
Children's Hospital
Boston, Massachusetts

STEPHEN G. MILLER, M.D.
Pediatric Cardiology
Duke University Medical Center
Durham, North Carolina
and
Duke Children's Cardiology of Fayetteville
Fayetteville, North Carolina

ANITA J. MOON-GRADY, M.D.
Department of Pediatrics
*University of California Davis Medical
School*
Sacramento, California

PHILLIP MOORE, M.D.
*Pediatric Cardiac Catheterization
Laboratory*
University of California at San Francisco
Children's Hospital
San Francisco, California

SHARON E. O'BRIEN, M.D.
Department of Pediatrics
Boston University School of Medicine
and
Children's Hospital
Boston, Massachusetts

PATRICK W. O'LEARY, M.D.
Department of Pediatrics
Mayo Clinic Transplant Center
Rochester, Minnesota

MARK D. PARRISH, M.D., M.P.H.
Department of Pediatrics
*University of California Davis Medical
School*
Sacramento, California

JOSEPH K. PERLOFF, M.D.
Ahmanson/UCLA Adult Congenital Heart Disease Center
Geffen School of Medicine, UCLA
Los Angeles, California

COLIN K.L. PHOON, M.PHIL., M.D.
Pediatric Cardiology Program and Department of Pediatrics
New York University School of Medicine
New York, New York

MARY ELLA PIERPONT, M.D., PH.D, A.F.A.C.C., F.A.C.M.G.
University of Minnesota
Children's Hospital of Minnesota
St. Paul, Minnesota

ROBERT E. POELMANN, PH.D.
Department of Anatomy & Embryology
Leiden University Medical Center
Leiden, The Netherlands

SONJA A. RASMUSSEN, M.D., M.S.
National Center on Birth Defects and Developmental Disabilities
Centers for Disease Control and Prevention
Atlanta, Goergia

GRAHAM J. REID, PH.D., C.PSYCH.
Departments of Psychology, Family Medicine, and Paediatrics
The University of Western Ontario
and
Children's Health Research Institute
London, Canada

TIFFANY RIEHLE-COLARUSSO, M.D.
Centers for Disease Control and Prevention
National Center on Birth Defects and Developmental Disabilities
Atlanta, Georgia

CRAIG A. SABLE, M.D.
Children's National Medical Center
and
George Washington University Medical School
Washington, DC

ANNA SARKOZY, M.D.
Ospedale CSS
San Giovannni Rotondo and CSS-Mendel Institute
Rome, Italy

R. SCOTT SIMPSON, M.B., B.S., D.A. (U.K.) , F.A.N.Z.C.A., F.F.P.M.A.N.Z.C.A., F.J.F.I.C.M.
The Townsville Hospital, Royal Children's Hospital and Mater Children's Hospital
North Queensland, Australia

MONVADI B. SRICHAI, M.D.
Department of Radiology and Department of Medicine
New York University School of Medicine
New York, New York

MATTHEW A. STUDER, M.D.
Department of Pediatrics Uniformed Services University of the Health Sciences,
Bethesda, Maryland Tripler Army Medical Center,
Honolulu, HI

ROBERT J. TOMANEK, PH.D.
Department of Anatomy and Cell Biology and the Cardiovascular Center
University of Iowa Carver College of Medicine
Iowa City, Iowa

ELISABETH M.W.J. UTENS, PH.D.
Department of Child and Adolescent Psychiatry
Erasmus MC - Sophia Children's Hospital
Rotterdam, The Netherlands

ELISABETH H.M. VAN RIJEN, PH.D.
Institute of Psychology
Erasmus University Rotterdam
Rotterdam, The Netherlands

AMY VERSTAPPEN
Adult Congenital Heart Association
Philadelphia, Pennsylvania

FRED M. WU, M.D.
Department of Cardiology
Children's Hospital Boston
and
Brigham & Women's Hospital
Harvard Medical School
Boston, Massachusetts

DIEGO F. WYSZYNSKI, M.D., M.H.S., PH.D.
Maternal and Pediatric Safety
Global Regulatory Affairs and Safety
Amgen, Inc.
Thousand Oaks, California

I

Clinical and Molecular Embryology of the Cardiovascular System

1

Molecular Developmental Biology of the Cardiovascular System

ADRIANA C. GITTENBERGER-DE GROOT
ROBERT E. POELMANN

GENERAL INTRODUCTION

During development of the human embryo, it is essential to construct a system for delivering nutrients to the growing organ systems. A cardiovascular network is laid down with the heart as a central pump. This pumping organ is already functional at 3 weeks of human development although it is far from fully formed. Several major processes like looping, addition of myocardium, septation, valve formation, and finally coronary vasculogenesis are necessary for the development of heart in its complex mature form. During this process that takes about 8 weeks in human development, many genetic and epigenetic (environmental) factors are involved and if disturbed, can also lead to cardiac malformations. Recent advances in mouse transgenic technology revealed that the heart is crucial as about 50% of embryo lethality is due to a cardiovascular anomaly (Conway et al., 2003). If this finding is extrapolated to humans, it is to be expected that many spontaneous abortions within the first 8 weeks of pregnancy have a cardiac anomaly background. The general belief that a heart malformation in utero is not lethal is therefore not true. We are only seeing the "mild end" of the spectrum after pregnancy has been confirmed by standard tests.

In this chapter, the major processes of cardiac development will be addressed and links to congenital malformations will be presented where appropriate.

CARDIOGENIC PRIMORDIA AND LOOPING

In the embryo, a mesodermal layer develops between the ectoderm and the endoderm. The mesoderm becomes separated in a splanchnic and a somatic layer by the developing coelomic cavity. In the rostral area of the splanchnic mesoderm, bilateral cardiogenic differentiation (Figure 1–1A) is observed and followed by midline fusion (DeRuiter et al., 1992). This area expresses procardiogenic markers such as GATA4 (Laverriere et al., 1994) and Nkx2.5 (Harvey, 1996). Craniocaudal bending of the embryo brings the cardiac primordium in its definitive thoracic position just cranial of the developing transverse septum (the future diaphragm). This cardiogenic mesoderm develops into a small heart tube with a connection to the omphalomesenteric veins (venous pole) and the pharyngeal arch arteries (arterial pole) (Figure 1–1B) (Gittenberger-de Groot et al., 2005). Until recently, this primary heart tube was considered to contain most elementary segments of the future heart. In many textbooks, segments and transitional zones were described to indicate these elements. Elegant and meticulous single-cell tracing studies have shown that the primary heart tube in fact consists of a small atrial part, the atrioventricular canal, the primitive left ventricle, and a short but yet undetermined part of the outflow tract (OFT) (Figure 1–1C). During development, addition of myocardium from the so-called second heart field defined by Isl1 expression

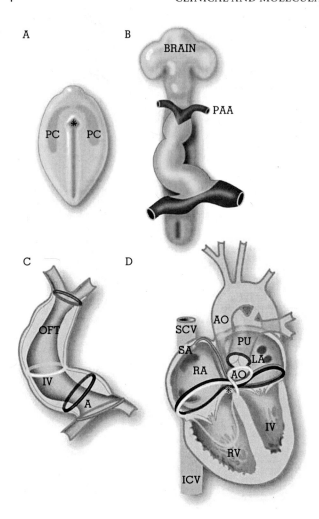

FIGURE 1-1. Schematic representation of heart development. A: Dorsal view of the embryo indicating the precardiogenic plates (PC) flanking the primitive streak and the primitive node (*). B: After rightward looping, the primary heart tube takes up a ventral position with blood entering at the venous pole and leaving at the arterial pole into the pharyngeal arch arteries (PAA). C: Internal view of the heart tube depicted in B showing the outer myocardial layer lined on the inside by cardiac jelly and endocardium. The transitional zones are indicated by rings and at this stage a primitive atrium (A), a primitive left ventricle (LV), and an outflow tract (OFT) can be distinguished. D: Fully septated four-chambered heart in which the rings of the transitional zones are still visible. *Abbreviations*: AO, aorta; ICV, inferior caval vein; LA, left atrium; LV, left ventricle; PU, pulmonary trunk; RA, right atrium; RV, right ventricle; SA, sinoatrial node; SCV, superior caval vein. Note: * Atrioventricular node. (Modified after Fetal Cardiology 2nd edition, ed Yagel, Silverman and Gembruch, 2009.)

(Cai et al., 2003) to both arterial and venous poles will result in the formation of all cardiac segments. When this takes place, the heart tube is already in the process of genetically determined looping, which is usually to the right-hand side (Figures 1–1C, 1–2A and 1–2B)

due to the involvement of the Nodal–Lefty–Pitx2 axis (Levin and Palmer, 2007).

FIRST AND SECOND HEART FIELDS

Although the formation of the heart is an ongoing process, if the distinction between first and second heart fields is assumed to be artificial, several factors allow the description of these heart fields separately. The heart tube, derived from the first heart field, consists of primary myocardium (Figure 1–3). Through differentiation and an intricate cascade of Tbx signaling, part of this primary myocardium will differentiate into working myocardium in a process referred to as ballooning of the ventricular and atrial cavities. The persisting primary myocardium forms the transitional zones or interchamber connections as well as the future atrioventricular conduction system. In this process, left–right determination or actually ventral–dorsal differentiation is guided by Pitx2 expression (Franco and Campione, 2003). When this concept was presented, the notion of addition of myocardium to the venous (inflow tract) and arterial (outflow tract) poles had not emerged yet.

The recent emphasis on second heart field addition (Cai et al., 2003; Gittenberger-de Groot et al., 2007; Kelly, 2005) shows that at least the major part of the right ventricle, including the semilunar valve area, are secondary structures. Nomenclature is confusing as this has been introduced as anterior (Mjaatvedt et al., 2001) and secondary (Waldo et al., 2005) heart field, whereas they only refer to the addition of contiguous parts of the OFT (Figure 1–3). Studies of splanchnic mesoderm-expressed genes like *Isl1* (Cai et al., 2003) show that the precardiac mesoderm in fact runs parallel to the dorsal axis of the developing heart, from the outflow to the inflow tract. This whole region is referred to as the second heart field (Figure 1–3). Recent studies (Gittenberger-de Groot et al., 2007; Meilhac et al., 2004) have shown that the area at the venous entry of the heart (so-called posterior heart field [PHF]) is important for the formation of the main body of the atria as well as the sinoatrial node (SAN) and the pulmonary vein myocardium. It is intriguing that the PHF-derived myocardium, distinguished by the transcription factor Tbx18 and the cardiac myosin light chain marker (MLC2a), does initially not express the early cardiogenic marker Nkx2.5 (Christoffels et al., 2006; Gittenberger-de Groot et al., 2007).

EXTRACARDIAC CELLULAR CONTRIBUTION

In addition to the above described cardiogenic precursors from the splanchnic mesoderm, two cell

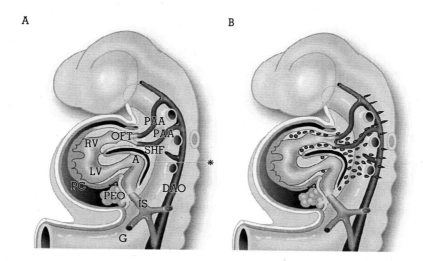

FIGURE 1–2. Lateral view of the looped heart tube in the embryo. A: The tube shows an inflow at the venous pole (IS) continuing in the primitive atrium (A), the primitive left (LV), and right ventricle (RV). The outflow tract (OFT) connects at the arterial pole, at this stage, to two pharyngeal arch arteries (PAA). The heart tube is embedded in the pericardial cavity (PC). At the venous pole, the proepicardial organ, the source of epicardium, is visible. Posterior to the heart tube the splanchnic mesoderm, ventral of the gut (G) is designated as the second heart field (SHF) that contributes myocardium (light colored) to both the outflow and inflow tract. B: The addition of neural crest cells (black droplets) to both outflow and to a lesser extent inflow tract is indicated. Note: * Atrioventricular node. (Modified after Fetal Cardiology 2nd edition, ed Yagel, Silverman and Gembruch, 2009.)

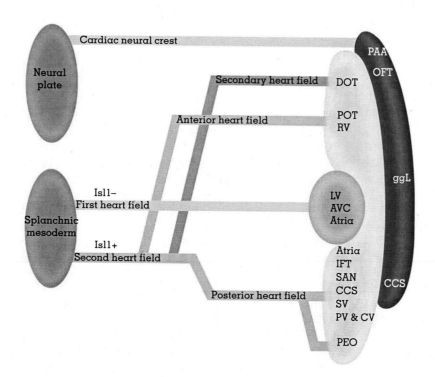

FIGURE 1–3. Schematic representation of the contribution of the different heart fields and their nomenclature. *Abbreviations*: AVC, atrioventricular canal; CCS, cardiac conduction system; CV, myocardium cardinal veins; DOT, distal outflow tract; ggl, nervous ganglia; IFT, inflow tract; LV, left ventricle; OFT, outflow tract; POT, proximal outflow tract; PV, myocardium pulmonary veins; PAA, pharyngeal arch arteries; PEO, proepicardial organ; RV, right ventricle; SAN, sinoatrial node; SV, sinus venosus myocardium. (Modified after Fetal Cardiology 2nd edition, ed Yagel, Silverman and Gembruch, 2009.)

populations deserve special attention. They are (1) the cardiac neural crest and (2) the epicardium.

Cardiac Neural Crest

During looping and septation of the cardiac tube, cells migrate from the dorsal rims of the neural tube into the mesoderm. These so-called ectomesenchymal or neural crest cells migrate through the embryo. At the thoracic level, they remain within their segmental boundaries. At the cephalic level, from the otic placode to the third somite, the neural crest region is referred to as cardiac neural crest and these cells intermingle to some extent in the area of the developing pharyngeal arches (I to VI in mammals including human development, but lacking the V arch) (Bergwerff et al., 1998; Molin et al., 2002).

Migration and homing of neural crest cells could be followed by several techniques including quail chicken chimera (Kirby and Waldo, 1995), avian retroviral LacZ tracing (Bergwerff et al., 1998; Poelmann et al., 1998), and more recently mouse neural crest reporter models (Jiang et al., 2000; Molin et al., 2004a; Poelmann et al., 2004; Waldo et al., 1999b). These neural crest cells have various destinations and differentiation fates. For cardiac development it is important that they differentiate into smooth muscle cells of the pharyngeal arch arteries, the aortic sac (Gittenberger-de Groot et al., 1999), and possibly the proximal part of the coronary arteries (Jiang et al., 2000). They also form the cells of the sympathetic and parasympathetic innervation of the heart and coronary vascular system (Kirby and Stewart, 1984; Verberne et al., 2000b). Part of the neural crest cells migrate into the intracardiac cushion mesenchyme lining the OFT (Poelmann et al., 1998; Waldo et al., 1998), where their eventual fate is apoptosis. We have postulated a signaling role for this process in activating growth factors like TGFβ2 to induce myocardialization of the OFT septum. A disputed, but recently confirmed, population of neural crest cells enters the venous pole of the heart (Poelmann and Gittenberger-de Groot, 1999) where these cells take up positions surrounding the cardiac conduction system. These cells also undergo apoptosis and are considered to have a role in induction of the differentiation and/or isolation of atrioventricular conduction system (Gurjarpadhye et al., 2007; Poelmann et al., 2004).

The intensive searches for the regulatory role of neural crest cells have provided new insights into the development of cardiac malformations. The group of Kirby in the early 1980s (Kirby and Bockman, 1984; Waldo et al., 1999a) found that ablation of the cardiac neural crest leads to cardiac malformations of the OFT resembling specific human malformations. Part of such malformations was connected to the genetic mutation

of chromosome 22. The syndrome related to this deletion has various phenotypes and names but in the cardiac form it is referred to as the DiGeorge syndrome. Eventually the crucial missing gene in this 22q11 deletion complex turned out to be Tbx1 (Lindsay et al., 2001). Tbx1, however, was not expressed in the cardiac neural crest cell population itself but in the surrounding splanchnic mesoderm through which the neural crest cells migrate before entering the heart, referred to as secondary or anterior heart field (Kelly, 2005). This mesoderm, as already described, is responsible for the addition of new myocardium to the OFT, explaining why this population deserves special attention in the continuum of cardiac formation. It needs further investigation whether neural crest cell–cardiogenic mesoderm interaction abnormalities also lead to inflow tract malformations (Poelmann and Gittenberger-de Groot, 1999).

It has to be kept in mind that neural crest cells are neurogenic in origin. An important derivative is also the autonomous nervous system. The vagal nerve and the cardiac neural crest have an overlapping ancestry. During development both neural and mesenchymal daughter cells derive from the same progenitor (Dupin and Le Douarin, 1995; Teillet et al., 1987). It is interesting, however, that complete removal of the cardiac neural crest by manual or laser ablation did not result in a complete aneuronal heart (Kirby and Stewart, 1984), suggesting existence of yet another source for neural cells or compensation by neighbor neural tube origins (Couly et al., 1996). Most of the neuronal cells aggregate into small ganglia that are found finally in the subepicardial space of the atrioventricular groove (Hierck et al., 2004). These ganglia are positive for NPY, tyrosine hydroxylase, SNAP25, neurofilament, and HNK1 (Verberne et al., 2000a), and give rise to thin fibers that are spread among the cardiomyocytes and along the coronary arteries to regulate probably the tone of the smooth muscle cells (Verberne et al., 2000a; Waldo et al., 1999a). A separate innervation that provides the SAN while a specific innervation of the AV node did not receive much attention. Furthermore, a large cluster of neuronal cells that are positioned surrounding the entrance of the pulmonary veins seem important (Poelmann et al., 2004). A proper evaluation of this area is needed.

Epicardium

The primary heart tube is positioned inside the developing coelomic cavity and initially consists of an outer myocardial layer and an inner lining of endocardium with cardiac jelly in between (Gittenberger-de Groot et al., 2005) (Figure 1–1C). At the venous pole, a dual anlage of a proepicardial protrusion develops (Manner et al., 2001) and the right side of this protrusion persists (mouse and chick the same) to form a cauliflower-like proepicardial organ (PEO) (Lie-Venema et al., 2007; Winter and Gittenberger-de Groot, 2007). From this PEO (Figure 1–2A), epicardial cells spread as a single layer over the myocardium, eventually covering the complete primary heart tube (Vrancken Peeters et al., 1995). It is still unresolved whether there is also primary contribution of epicardial cells to the OFT, as in case of PEO ablation, a mesothelium-covered OFT region is seen (Gittenberger-de Groot et al., 2000), which has special characteristics (Perez-Pomares et al., 2003).

Tracing experiments by chicken-quail chimeras (Männer et al., 2001; Poelmann et al., 1993; Vrancken Peeters et al., 1999) as well as retroviral LacZ marking (Dettman et al., 1998) have shown that epicardial cells undergo a process of epithelium-to-mesenchymal transformation to form epicardium-derived cells (EPDCs). These cells differentiate into the cardiac fibroblasts, smooth muscle cells, and adventitial fibroblasts of the coronary vasculature (Figure 1–4). They have an inductive role in Purkinje fiber differentiation (Eralp et al., 2006; Gittenberger-de Groot et al., 1998). The origin of the endothelial cells of the coronary vasculature remains a matter of debate, but our in vivo experiments indicate an origin from the sinusoids of the adjacent developing liver region (Poelmann et al., 1993). This has recently been supported by a GATA5 epicardial reporter mouse model (Lie-Venema et al.,

2007). Several indications point toward the PEO as also being derived from the PHF (Gittenberger-de Groot et al., 2007). An intricate signaling mechanism involving TGFβ, FGFs, and BMPs in the PHF is responsible for either a myocardial or an epicardial differentiation (Kruithof et al., 2006).

The essential role for EPDCs in cardiac development is exemplified by studies in which the PEO is completely or partially ablated (Eralp et al., 2005) or in which EMT is genetically inhibited (Lie-Venema et al., 2003). In the most dramatic cases involving complete destruction of the PEO, formation of the compact myocardium is severely deficient, ventricular septation does not take place, and endocardial cushions are hypoplastic (Gittenberger-de Groot et al., 2000) leading to embryo lethality. Partial inhibition of PEO outgrowth and ensuing EMT, in the longer surviving embryos, still results in coronary vascular abnormalities and diminished Purkinje fiber differentiation (Eralp et al., 2005, 2006).

INTRODUCTION INTO MORPHOGENESIS

In the previous section, we have introduced the building blocks essential for cardiac development. In this section, we will follow heart development using the sequential segmental analysis. This method is used in many (pediatric) cardiac centers when describing and analyzing the normal heart as well as heart malformations. The

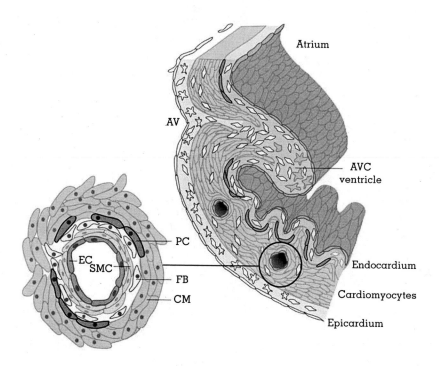

FIGURE 1–4. Schematic representation of the atrial and ventricular cardiac wall. The epicardium-derived cells (white spindle-shaped and stellate cells) enter from the atrioventricular sulcus (AV) the subepicardial space, the atrioventricular cushions (AVC), as well as the myocardium (CM). The detail of the coronary artery (enlarged circle) shows the epicardium-derived cells that form the smooth muscle cells (SMC) and the adventitial fibroblasts (FB). The Purkinje cells (PC) differentiate from the myocardium by inductive influences of the epicardium derived cells. The endothelial cells (EC) have a separate origin. (Modified after Fetal Cardiology 2nd edition, ed Yagel, Silverman and Gembruch, 2009.)

course of the blood flow from venous to arterial pole is followed.

Atrial and Pulmonary Vein Development

The cardiac atria develop at the venous pole of the heart. The right and left appendages are most probably derived from ballooning of the primary heart tube. This process is regulated by a balance of Tbx2 and 3 expression (Hoogaars et al., 2007). The atrial appendages are trabeculated and have a blunt-end morphology on the right side while a slender fingerlike morphology is seen on the left side. The left–right determination is regulated by genetic pathways including Pitx2 (Franco and Campione, 2003; Poelmann et al., 2008). The smooth walled posterior part of both right and left atria are derived from the sinus venosus myocardium of the PHF (Figures 1–1A and 1–2). At the venous pole the heart tube is still connected to the PHF by a persisting dorsal mesocardium that penetrates deeply into the septating atria as the atrial spine.

The origin of the primary atrial septum is most probably from PHF origin. In this septum, fenestrations develop and allow for a foramen (foramen secundum) between the right and left atrium. Late during development an infolding of the atrial wall and roof occurs, leading to formation of a second atrial septal component, the so-called septum secundum in mammals. Between these septal components, a patent foramen ovale is present before birth. During addition of sinus venosus myocardium to the atria, the systemic cardiac veins are incorporated with their ostia into the smooth walled part of the right atrium. They are flanked by embryonic venous valves referred to as the right venous valve, the left venous valve, and the anteriorly located fusion of these valves, the so-called septum spurium (Blom et al., 1999).

Embedded in the dorsal mesocardium and the PHF, the anlage of the pulmonary veins becomes connected to the smooth posterior wall of the left atrium, flanking the primary atrial septum. There is much debate whether the pulmonary veins are part of the sinus venosus that incorporate the right and left cardinal veins or whether they have a separate central dorsal mesocardium-derived origin. Current consensus is achieved for findings that sinus venosus myocardium and the venous tributaries are all derived from the PHF (or venous pole part of the second heart field) and locally have their own differentiation characteristics. Recent studies on the incorporation of the common pulmonary vein into the left atrium have shown that the inner lining of the mature left atrium is actually formed by pulmonary venous wall up to the boundary of the left atrial appendage (Douglas et al., 2006).

Congenital Malformations. Our main source of information derives mostly from mouse models with a disturbed situs of the atrial appendages as observed in, for example, the iv/iv mouse, the inversus mouse, and the Pitx2 knockout mouse (Franco and Campione, 2003; Tessari et al., 2008). It is yet to be investigated in what way the PHF is also affected by genes involved in these malformations. The recent discoveries of the importance of addition of the PHF will provide novel "insight" into the role of the Tbx transcription factors, where Tbx5 was already known to play an important role, also in human malformations (Bruneau et al., 2001). Details on the role of Nkx2.5 mutations (Benson et al., 1999) have to be revised as the PHF myocardium is initially negative for this procardiogenic marker (Gittenberger-de Groot et al., 2007). Recently it was shown that in knock out mice for podoplanin, normally expressed in the PHF, there is an abnormal development of the pulmonary veins (Douglas et al., 2009). As the second heart field myocardium links developmental mechanisms of the OFT with those of the inflow tract, a better understanding is to be expected of complex heart malformations that combine, for example, abnormal pulmonary venous return and OFT malformations. Up till now, the neural crest–derived cells could not be considered to be playing a role in such malformations.

Development of the Atrioventricular Connection and Atrioventricular Valves

The atrioventricular canal is formed from primary myocardium and is already present in the primary heart tube. During development, this transitional segment is lined by so-called endocardial cushions developing during an interactive process between myocardium and endocardium. Through endocardium-to-mesenchyme transformation (EMT), cells are deposited into the cardiac jelly. Many transcription factors, growth factors, and extracellular matrix molecules are involved in endocardial cushion differentiation (Eisenberg and Markwald, 1995). Recently, also a role for hemodynamics and ensuing shear stress-responsive gene pathways has been distinguished (Groenendijk et al., 2007). The atrioventricular endocardial cushions have a dual role during embryonic development. They function as primitive atrioventricular valves and also act as a "glue" between the muscular ventricular septum and the primary atrial septum.

A complicated process of inner curvature remodeling is necessary to position the right part of the atrioventricular canal above the right ventricular inlet part that developed shortly before (Jongbloed et al., 2005). Initially, the complete atrioventricular canal is positioned above the primitive left ventricle, belonging to the primary heart tube. There is ample evidence that

Greenfield Medical Library - Issue Receipt

Customer name: Onuwe, Toluwalope

Title: Congenital heart defects : from origin to treatment / edited by Diego F. Wyszynski, Adolfo Correa-Vi

ID: 1006084063
Due: 30 Jun 2017 23:59

Total items: 1
22/02/2017 18:18

All items must be returned before the due date and time.

The Loan period may be shortened if the item is requested.

www.nottingham.ac.uk/library

the formation of most of the right ventricle derives from second heart field myocardium (Kelly, 2007). The main cavities of the right and left ventricles are also formed in a ballooning process comparable to the atrial appendages (Moorman and Christoffels, 2003). During ballooning, the muscular ventricular septum is formed and as such is not an actual structure growing into a main unseptated ventricular cavity. The resulting right and left ventricular inflows harbor thus a left-sided mitral valve with two leaflets and a right-sided tricuspid valve with three leaflets. These valves and their chordae tendinae differentiate from the endocardial cushion tissue (Oosthoek et al., 1998). The cellular contribution to the cushions consists of endocardium-derived cells as has recently been reconfirmed by Tie2 reporter mouse studies. The epicardium-derived cells (Winter and Gittenberger-de Groot, 2007) also contribute and there is still discussion on a possible minor contribution of neural crest cells (Poelmann and Gittenberger-de Groot, 1999; Poelmann et al., 2004) as well as transformed myocardial cells.

The complicated processes underlying the remodeling and repositioning of the atrioventricular canal, the ventricular inlet septations, and valve differentiation make an understanding of the background of congenital malformations in this area rather challenging. It is evident that septation and valve anomalies are linked because they are part of one mechanistic system.

Congenital Malformations. Insufficient repositioning of the right side of the atrioventricular canal can lead to straddling tricuspid valve and, in extreme cases, to tricuspid atresia (Ottenkamp et al., 1984). In these cases, the inlet part of the right ventricle is not well developed or even absent, resulting in a hypoplastic right ventricle. This phenomenon is often combined with incomplete ventricular septations, leading to perimembranous inlet ventricular septal defects.

In cases of aberrant fusion of the atrioventricular cushions, a defect may persist at the central connection of atria and ventricles, the so-called atrioventricular septal defect (AVSD). This may result from deficient endocardial cushion development based on abnormal contribution of the cellular or extracellular components. Several mechanisms can be held responsible for AVSDs, which are often seen in human trisomy 21, having the trisomy 16 mouse as animal model counterpart. Studies show an essential role for the EPDCs. Cases in which EPDCs are not normally differentiating are often associated with an AVSD or common AV valve like in Sp3-/- embryos (Van Loo et al., 2007) and podoplanin knockout mouse (Mahtab et al., 2008). The TGFβ2 mutant mouse shows a combination of EPDCs and endocardium-related disturbed EMT (Bartram et al., 2001). This process is probably linked to a different

expression of periostin (Lie-Venema et al., 2008), a protein that is important for the induction of collagen I (Norris et al., 2007).

Development of Ventriculoarterial Connections and Semilunar Valves

The differentiation of the primary heart tube into a fully developed four-chamber heart is incomplete without formation of right (subpulmonary) and left (subaortic) OFTs.

The myocardium at the arterial pole of the heart tube connects to a yet unseptated aortic sac. An extensive addition of myocardium contributes to the formation of the trabeculated part of the right ventricle as well as to the proximal and distal OFT (Kelly, 2007). As in the atrioventricular canal, the complete OFT (Gittenberger-de Groot et al., 2005) is lined by endocardial cushions that also expand through an EMT process. Cellular contribution of EPDCs is absent or minimal in the OFT whereas neural crest cells are massively present within these cushions (Poelmann et al., 1998; Waldo et al., 1999a). It is necessary to distinguish the proximal OFT cushions as they will myocardialize and form an OFT septum (Gittenberger-de Groot et al., 2005), separating the long right ventricular (subpulmonary) from the short left ventricular (subaortic) ouflow tract. The distal OFT cushions will produce the semilunar valves of both the aortic and pulmonary orifices. The proximal OFT cushions merge with the atrioventricular cushions to ensure complete septation of the ventricles. The remnant of the fused cushions results in the membranous part of the ventricular septum or the septum membranaceum.

Genes proven to be essential for OFT formation are linked to the arterial pole-related second heart field and include versican (Mjaatvedt et al., 2001), Tbx1 (Lindsay et al., 2001), and neural crest-related genes such as Cx43 (Waldo et al., 1999b) and Pax3 (Conway et al., 1997). Furthermore, many genes that are relevant for inner curvature remodeling are essential in repositioning the OFT in such a way that the pulmonary orifice remains connected to the right ventricle, whereas the aorta becomes connected to the left ventricle.

Congential Malformations of the Outflow Tract. Outflow tract malformations form the major part of all congenital heart defects. It is clear that many developmental processes converge in this area. The extensive research on the 22q11 deletion syndrome that typically presents with OFT malformations has revealed many facts. Human genetics research has proven that Tbx1 mutations explain at least part of the 22q11 deletion syndrome malformations (Lindsay et al., 2001). Tbx1 is specifically expressed in the

OFT–related second heart field and its interaction with FGF8 and FGF10 is obvious (Waldo et al., 2005). Most probably, the influence of neural crest cells is secondary after their interaction with defective splanchnic mesoderm of the second heart field. This hypothesis needs to be explored to incorporate also the often concurrently seen facial anomalies that are likewise influenced by Tbx1.

If second heart field cells are not properly added to the OFT, a shortening of the outflow region is shown, for example, in diabetic rat embryos (Molin et al., 2004b) as well as in several other animal models with OFT abnormalities. In the most severe form complete OFT septation is absent, leading to a common arterial trunk. When the obligatory OFT septation and myocardialization has not taken place, there is always a ventricular septal defect. If the OFT does not become correctly repositioned, a double outlet right ventricle (DORV) might develop with a malaligned outlet septum. There is again the obligatory ventricular septal defect. For unknown reasons, DORV is the most common anomaly seen in mouse models, whereas in human fetuses, an isolated ventricular septal defect (VSD) is far more common.

Tetralogy of Fallot is a common human malformation with only few relevant animal models. We have shown a role for vascular endothelial growth factor (VEGF) isoforms as well as abnormalities in the Jagged/Notch pathway (van den Akker et al., 2007). Gene mutations in human neonates showing the disease support the relevance of correlating human and mouse developmental data.

The prevalence of semilunar valve abnormalities, including the often not detected bicuspid aortic valve, has hardly been linked to a genetic defect. Recently, Notch1 mutations were found in human patients with bicuspid aortic valve. We have strong evidence that hemodynamic remodeling and shear stress responsive gene interactions might play a far more prominent role in development of specifically semilunar valve abnormalities (Hogers et al., 1999).

Differentiation of the Cardiac Conduction System

The cardiac conduction system differentiates and develops from myocardial cells (Gourdie et al., 2003) not from neural crest cells as was once postulated (Poelmann and Gittenberger-de Groot, 1999). Recent evidence demonstrates that second heart field–derived structures are important (Gittenberger-de Groot et al., 2007; Jongbloed et al., 2008) apart from the primary heart tube, which contributes to the atrioventricular node and common bundle.

The primitive sinoatrial conduction system derives from the PHF-derived myocardium, which originates initially on the left side and then extends to encircle the right-sided sinus venosus structures. This myocardium is Nkx2.5-negative and podoplanin-positive (Gittenberger-de Groot et al., 2007). Other genes have also been specifically linked to this myocardium such as Tbx18 and HCN4 (Christoffels et al., 2006). This sinus venosus myocardium is incorporated in the posterior wall of the right and left atrium and forms the myocardium of the venous valves and surrounds the pulmonary vein. It is described in human embryos by the expression of HNK1 (Blom et al., 1999) and tachycardia can be by, for example, CCS LacZ (Jongbloed et al., 2004). Functionally, the sinus venosus myocardium only remains as the future right-sided SAN. Interestingly, it was already described in the early 1980s that pacemaker activity started in the developing heart on the left side of the atria (Kamino et al., 1981).

An important inductive role has been attributed to neural crest cells for the atrioventricular conduction system (Gurjarpadhye et al., 2007; Poelmann et al., 2004). These neural crest cells undergo apoptosis and probably the emitted growth factors are important for compaction of the conduction system. EPDCs are important for proper differentiation of the Purkinje fibers (Eralp et al., 2006) (Figure 1–4).

Congenital Abnormalities. Little is known about a possible link between development of the cardiac conduction system and arrhythmias in the adult. The recent findings of the more extensive anlage of the primitive conduction system and the emerging data on origin sites of cardiac arrhythmias make it very likely that embryonic remnants might be the source of rhythm disturbances in the adult. These can be linked to abnormal pacemaking activity in the terminal crest around the pulmonary veins and coronary sinus (Jongbloed et al., 2004). Likewise Mahaim tachycardia can be explained on the basis of cardiac developmental abnormalities (Jongbloed et al., 2005). Studies on the formation and differentiation of the fibrous anomalies, separating atria from ventricles, can be linked to delayed apex to basis conduction as seen in some late human fetal pregnancies as well as in symptoms of Wolff-Parkinson-White (WPW) syndrome (Kolditz et al., 2007; Kolditz et al., 2008). Mouse models on PHF-expressed genes such as Shox2 (Blaschke et al., 2007) and podoplanin (Mahtab et al., 2009) show sinoatrial nodehypoplasia and possibly functional defects.

For the human situation, second heart field–expressed genes such as Tbx5 (Bruneau et al., 2001) have been linked to conduction system abnormalities. It is interesting that Nkx2.5 heterozygotes do show AVN abnormalities but lack pacemaking problems. This can now be understood as the SAN does not express Nkx2.5 during development (Blaschke et al., 2007).

This approach of linking developmental data to adult cardiac disease has already been explored for cardiomyopathies and studies will be continued for detailed study in future.

Coronary Vascular Development

The developing myocardial wall thickens and grows, needing an independent nutrition. This is provided by the formation of a coronary vascular network. This network is not formed from budding of the endocardial cells lining the trabeculae of the ventricles but from a network of endothelial progenitor cells that derive from the embryonic liver sinusoids at the venous pole (Poelmann et al., 1993). Before this network can expand, a covering layer of epicardium (Figure 1–4) is needed that develops from the PEO spreading over the heart (Vrancken Peeters et al., 1995). These epicardial cells undergo EMT and provide eventually the smooth muscle cells and fibroblasts of the coronary arteries (Winter and Gittenberger-de Groot, 2007). For the formation of a mature coronary vascular system of arteries, capillaries, and veins, VEGF and platelet-derived growth factor (PDGF) are essential (van den Akker et al., 2005; van den Akker et al., 2008a; van den Akker et al., 2008b). Also Tbx1- and neural crest–related genes that are essential for the innervation of the main stems of the coronary arteries might be important.

Congenital Anomalies. It is not easy to distinguish congenital anomalies and variations of normal patterning because they will be classified as pathological only if they present clinical problems.

Our studies have produced a number of relevant findings to understand coronary vascular malformations. It is essential that the coronary vascular network connects to the aorta (Bogers et al., 1989) as well as to the right atrium (Vrancken Peeters et al., 1997). If epicardial outgrowth is mechanically or genetically inhibited, coronary ostia are small or even absent (Eralp et al., 2005; Lie-Venema et al., 2003). In such a case, ventriculoarterial coronary connections (VACC) are found to supply the coronary vascular bed. Our studies thus show that embryonic connections between ventricles and coronary arteries are not normal and only develop as a pathological phenomenon. This had interesting implications for understanding of pulmonary atresia without VSD with and without VACC (Gittenberger-de Groot et al., 1988, 2001).

A role for neural crest cells (Gittenberger-de Groot et al., 2004) and possibly Tbx1-derived SHF might play a role in the coronary vascular variations seen in common arterial trunk (Bogers et al., 1993; Gittenberger-de Groot et al., 2002).

In the adult, it is important to realize that the primitive coronary network will develop into arteries and veins connected by capillaries. These formations can also persist as potential arteriovenous connections and can be relumenized upon demand by a pathological condition. Like in the reoccurrence of electrical capacities of cardiac cells, these potential arteriovenous connections will highly vary between individuals.

CLOSING COMMENTS

The above description of linking new and more mature data on cardiac development to congenital disease only provides an overview. The literature cited is not complete and does not credit all authors who are active in the field. Specific literature searches will guide the interested reader in further exploring this field linking cardiac development and (congenital) cardiac disease.

REFERENCES

Bartram U, Molin DGM, Wisse LJ, et al. 2001. Double-outlet right ventricle and overriding tricuspid valve reflect disturbances of looping, myocardialization, endocardial cushion differentiation, and apoptosis in TGFß2-knockout mice. *Circulation.* 2001;103:2745–2752.

Benson DW, Silberbach GM, Kavanaugh-McHugh A, et al. Mutations in the cardiac transcription factor NKX2.5 affect diverse cardiac developmental pathways. *J Clin Invest.* 1999;104:1567–1573.

Bergwerff M, Verberne ME, DeRuiter MC, Poelmann RE, Gittenberger-de Groot AC. Neural crest cell contribution to the developing circulatory system. Implications for vascular morphology? *Circ Res.* 1998;82:221–231.

Blaschke RJ, Hahurij ND, Kuijper S, et al. Targeted mutation reveals essential functions of the homeodomain transcription factor Shox2 in sinoatrial and pacemaking development. *Circulation.* 2007;115:1830–1838.

Blom NA, Gittenberger-de Groot AC, DeRuiter MC, Poelmann RE, Mentink MM, Ottenkamp J. Development of the cardiac conduction tissue in human embryos using HNK-1 antigen expression: possible relevance for understanding of abnormal atrial automaticity. *Circulation.* 1999;99:800–806.

Bogers AJJC, Bartelings MM, Bökenkamp R, et al. Common arterial trunk, uncommon coronary arterial anatomy. *J Thorac Cardiovasc Surg.* 1993;106:1133–1137.

Bogers AJJC, Gittenberger-de Groot AC, Poelmann RE, Péault BM, Huysmans HA. Development of the origin of the coronary arteries, a matter of ingrowth or outgrowth? *Anat Embryol.* 1989;180:437–441.

Bruneau BG, Nemer G, Schmitt JP, et al. A murine model of Holt-Oram syndrome defines roles of the T-box transcription factor Tbx5 in cardiogeensis and disease. *Cell* 2001;106:709–721.

Cai CL, Liang X, Shi Y, Chu PH, Pfaff SL, Chen J, Evans S. Isl1 identifies a cardiac progenitor population that proliferates prior to differentiation and contributes a majority of cells to the heart. *Dev Cell.* 2003;5:877–889.

Christoffels VM, Mommersteeg MT, Trowe MO, et al. Formation of the venous pole of the heart from an Nkx2–5-negative precursor population requires Tbx18. *Circ Res.* 2006;98:1555–1563.

Conway SJ, Henderson DJ, Copp AJ. Pax3 is required for cardiac neural crest migration in the mouse: evidence from the splotch (Sp2H) mutant. *Development*. 1997;124:505–514.

Conway SJ, Kruzynska-Frejtag A, Kneer PL, Machnicki M, Koushik SV. What cardiovascular defect does my prenatal mouse mutant have, and why? *Genesis*. 2003;35:1–21.

Couly G, Grapin-Botton A, Coltey P, Le Douarin NM. The regeneration of the cephalic neural crest, a problem revisited: the regenerating cells originate from the contralateral or from the anterior and posterior neural fold. *Development*. 1996;122:3393–3407.

DeRuiter MC, Poelmann RE, VanderPlas-de Vries I, Mentink MMT, Gittenberger-de Groot AC. The development of the myocardium and endocardium in mouse embryos. Fusion of two heart tubes? *Anat Embryol*. 1992;185:461–473.

Dettman RW, Denetclaw W, Ordahl CP, Bristow J. Common epicardial origin of coronary vascular smooth muscle, perivascular fibroblasts, and intermyocardial fibroblasts in the avian heart. *Dev Biol*. 1998;193:169–181.

Douglas YL, Jongbloed MR, Gittenberger-de Groot AC, et al. Histology of vascular myocardial wall of left atrial body after pulmonary venous incorporation. *Am J Cardiol*. 2006;97:662–670.

Douglas YL, Mahtab EAF, Jongbloed MR, et al. Pulmonary vein, dorsal atrial wall and atrial septum abnormalities in podoplanin knock out mice with disturbed posterior heart field contribution. *Ped Res*. 2009; 65:27–32.

Dupin E, Le Douarin NM. Retinoic acid promotes the differentiation of adrenergic cells and melanocytes in quail neural crest cultures. *Dev Biol*. 1995;168:529–548.

Eisenberg LM, Markwald RR. Molecular regulation of atrioventricular valvuloseptal morphogenesis. *Circ Res*. 1995;77:1–6.

Eralp I, Lie-Venema H, Bax NAM, et al. Epicardium-derived cells are important for correct development of the Purkinje fibers in the avian heart. *Anat Rec*. 2006;288A:1272–1280.

Eralp I, Lie-Venema H, DeRuiter MC, et al. Coronary artery and orifice development is associated with proper timing of epicardial outgrowth and correlated Fas ligand associated apoptosis patterns. *Circ Res*. 2005;96:526–534.

Franco D, Campione M. The role of Pitx2 during cardiac development. Linking left-right signaling and congenital heart diseases. *Trends Cardiovasc Med*. 2003;13:157–163.

Gittenberger-de Groot AC, Bartelings MM, Bogers AJJC, Boot MJ, Poelmann RE. The embryology of the common arterial trunk. *Progr Pediatr Cardiol*. 2002;15:1–8.

Gittenberger-de Groot AC, Bartelings MM, DeRuiter MC, Poelmann RE. Basics of cardiac development for the understanding of congenital heart malformations. *Pediatr Res*. 2005;57:169–176.

Gittenberger-de Groot AC, DeRuiter MC, Bergwerff M, Poelmann RE. Smooth muscle cell origin and its relation to heterogeneity in development and disease. *Arterioscler Thromb Vasc Biol*. 1999;19:1589–1594.

Gittenberger-de Groot AC, Eralp I, Lie-Venema H, Bartelings MM, Poelmann RE. Development of the coronary vasculature and its implications for coronary abnormalities in general and specifically in pulmonary atresia without ventricular septal defect. *Acta Paediatr Suppl*. 2004;93:13–19.

Gittenberger-de Groot AC, Sauer U, Bindl L, Babic R, Essed CE, Buhlmeyer K. Competition of coronary arteries and ventriculo-coronary arterial communications in pulmonary atresia with intact ventricular septum. *Int J Cardiol*. 1988;18:243–258.

Gittenberger-de Groot AC, Tennstedt C, Chaoui R, Lie-Venema H, Sauer U, Poelmann RE. Ventriculo coronary arterial communications (VCAC) and myocardial sinusoids in hearts with pulmonary atresia with intact ventricular septum: two different diseases. *Progr Pediatr Cardiol*. 2001;13:157–164.

Gittenberger-de Groot AC, Vrancken Peeters M-PFM, Bergwerff M, Mentink MMT, Poelmann RE. Epicardial outgrowth inhibition leads to compensatory mesothelial outflow tract collar and abnormal cardiac septation and coronary formation. *Circ Res*. 2000;87:969–971.

Gittenberger-de Groot AC, Vrancken Peeters M-PFM, Mentink MMT, Gourdie RG, Poelmann RE. Epicardium-derived cells contribute a novel population to the myocardial wall and the atrioventricular cushions. *Circ Res*. 1998;82:1043–1052.

Gittenberger-de Groot AC, Mathab EAF, Hahurij ND, et al. Nkx2.5 negative myocardium of the posterior heart field and its correlation with podoplanin expression in cells from the developing cardiac pacemaking and conduction system. *Anat Rec*. 2007;290:115–122.

Gourdie RG, Harris BS, Bond J, et al. Development of the cardiac pacemaking and conduction system. *Birth Defects Res*. 2003;69:46–57.

Groenendijk BCW, Van der Heiden K, Hierck BP, Poelmann RE. The role of shear stress on ET-1, KLF2, and NOS-3 expression in the developing cardiovascular system of chicken embryos in a venous ligation model. *Physiology*. 2007;22:380–389.

Gurjarpadhye A, Hewett KW, Justus C, et al. Cardiac neural crest ablation inhibits compaction and electrical function of conduction system bundles. *Am J Physiol Heart Circ Physiol*. 2007;292:H1291–H1300.

Harvey RP. NK-2 homeobox genes and heart development. *Dev Biol*. 1996;178:203–216.

Hierck BP, Molin DGM, Boot MJ, Poelmann RE, Gittenberger-de Groot AC. A chicken model for DGCR6 as a modifier gene in the DIGeorge critical region. *Ped Res*. 2004;56:440–448.

Hogers B, DeRuiter MC, Gittenberger-de Groot AC, Poelmann RE. Extraembryonic venous obstructions lead to cardiovascular malformations and can be embryolethal. *Card Res*. 1999;41:87–99.

Hoogaars WM, Barnett P, Moorman AF, Christoffels VM. T-box factors determine cardiac design. *Cell Mol Life Sci*. 2007;64:646–660.

Jiang X, Rowitch DH, Soriano P, McMahon AP, Sucov HM. Fate of the mammalian cardiac neural crest. *Development*. 2000;127:1607–1616.

Jongbloed MR, Mahtab EA, Blom NA, et al. Development of the cardiac conduction system and possible relation to predilection sites of arrhythmogenesis. *ScientificWorldJournal*. 2008;3:239–269.

Jongbloed MR, Wijffels MC, Schalij MJ, et al. Development of the right ventricular inflow tract and moderator band: a possible morphological and functional explanation for Mahaim tachycardia. *Circ Res*. 2005;96:776–783.

Jongbloed MRM, Schalij MJ, Poelmann RE, et al. Embryonic conduction tissue: a spatial correlation with adult arrhythmogenic areas? Transgenic CCS/lacZ expression in the cardiac conduction system of murine embryos. *J Cardiovasc Electrophysiol*. 2004;15:349–355.

Kamino K, Hirota A, Fujii S. Localization of pacemaking activity in early embryonic heart monitored using voltage-sensitive dye. *Nature*. 1981;290:595–597.

Kelly RG. Molecular inroads into the anterior heart field. *Trends Cardiovasc Med*. 2005;15:51–56.

Kelly RG. Building the right ventricle. *Circ Res*. 2007;100:943–945.

Kirby M, Bockman DE. Neural crest and normal development:a new perspective. *Anat Rec*. 1984;209:1–6.

Kirby ML, Stewart D. Adrenergic innervation of the developing chick heart: neural crest ablations to produce sympathetically aneural hearts. *Am J Anat*. 1984;171:295–305.

Kirby ML, Waldo KL. Neural crest and cardiovascular patterning. *Circ Res*. 1995;77:211–215.

Kolditz DP, Wijffels MCEF, Blom NA, et al. Epicardium-derived-cells (EPDCs) in annulus fibrosis development and persistence of accessory pathways. *Circulation.* 2008;117:1508–1517.

Kolditz DP, Wijffels MCEF, Blom NA, et al. Persistence of functional atrioventricular accessory pathways in post-septated embryonic avian hearts: implications for morphogenesis and functional maturation of the cardiac conduction system. *Circulation.* 2007;115:17–26.

Kruithof BP, van Wijk B, Somi S, et al. BMP and FGF regulate the differentiation of multipotential pericardial mesoderm into the myocardial or epicardial lineage. *Dev Biol.* 2006;295:507–522.

Laverriere AC, Macniell C, Mueller C, Poelmann RE, Burch JBE, Evans T. GATA-4/5/6, a subfamily of three transcription factors transcribed in developing heart and gut. *J Biol Chem.* 1994;269:23177–23184.

Levin M, Palmer AR. Left-right patterning from the inside out: widespread evidence for intracellular control. *Bioessays.* 2007;29:271–287.

Lie-Venema H, Eralp I, Markwald RR, et al. Periostin expression by epicardium-derived cells (EPDCs) is involved in the development of the atrioventricular valves and fibrous heart skeleton. *Differentiation.* 2008;1432–1436.

Lie-Venema H, Gittenberger-de Groot AC, van Empel LJP, et al. Ets-1 and Ets-2 transcription factors are essential for normal coronary and myocardial development in chicken embryos. *Circ Res.* 2003;92:749–756.

Lie-Venema H, van den Akker NMS, Bax NAM, et al. Origin, fate, and function of epicardium-derived cells (EPCDs) in normal and abnormal cardiac development. *ScientificWorldJournal.* 2007;7:1777–1798.

Lindsay EA, Vitelli F, Su H, et al. Tbx1 haploinsufficieny in the DiGeorge syndrome region causes aortic arch defects in mice. *Nature.* 2001;410:97–101.

Mahtab EAF, Vicente-Steijn R, Hahurij ND, et al. Podoplanin deficiënt mice show a RhoA-related hypoplasia of the sinus venosus myocardium including the sinoatrial node. *Dev Dyn.* 2009;238:183–1193.

Mahtab EAF, Wijffels MCEF, van den Akker NMS, et al. Cardiac malformations and myocardial abnormalities in podoplanin knockout mouse embryos: correlation with abnormal epicardial development. *Dev Dyn.* 2008;237:847–857.

Männer J, Perez-Pomares JM, Macias D, Munoz-Chapuli R. The origin, formation and developmental significance of the epicardium: a review. *Cells Tissues Organs.* 2001;169:89–103.

Meilhac SM, Esner M, Kelly RG, Nicolas JF, Buckingham ME. The clonal origin of myocardial cells in different regions of the embryonic mouse heart. *Dev Cell.* 2004;6:685–698.

Mjaatvedt CH, Nakaoka T, Moreno-Rodriguez R, et al. The out-flow tract of the heart is recruited from a novel heart-forming field. *Dev Biol.* 2001;238:97–109.

Molin DGM, DeRuiter MC, Wisse LJ, et al. Altered apoptosis pattern during pharyngeal arch artery remodelling is associated with aortic arch malformations in Tgf beta 2 knock-out mice. *Card Res.* 2002;56:312–322.

Molin DGM, Poelmann RE, DeRuiter MC, Azhar M, Doetschman T, Gittenberger-de Groot AC. Transforming growth factor beta-SMAD2 signaling regulates aortic arch innervation and development. *Circ Res.* 2004a;95:1109–1117.

Molin DGM, Roest PA, Nordstrand H, et al. Disturbed morpho-genesis of cardiac outflow tract and increased rate of aortic arch anomalies in the offspring of diabetic rats. *Birth Defects Res A Clin Mol Teratol.* 2004b;70:927–938.

Moorman AFM, Christoffels VM. Cardiac chamber for-mation: development, genes and evolution. *Physiol Rev.* 2003;83:1223–1267.

Norris RA, Damon B, Mironov V, et al. Periostin regulates collagen fibrillogenesis and the biomechanical properties of connective tissues. *J Cell Biochem.* 2007;101:695–711.

Oosthoek PW, Wenink ACG, Vrolijk BCM, et al. Development of the atrioventricular valve tension apparatus in the human heart. *Anat Embryol.* 1998;198:317–329.

Ottenkamp J, Wenink ACG, Rohmer J, Gittenberger-de Groot AC. Tricuspid atresia with overriding imperforate tricuspid mem-brane: an anatomic variant. *Int J Cardiol.* 1984;6:599–609.

Perez-Pomares JM, Phelps A, Sedmerova M, Wessels A. Epicardial-like cells on the distal arterial end of the cardiac outflow tract do not derive from the proepicardium but are derivatives of the cephalic pericardium. *Dev Dyn.* 2003;227:56–68.

Poelmann RE, Gittenberger-de Groot AC. A subpopulation of apoptosis-prone cardiac neural crest cells targets to the venous pole: multiple functions in heart development? *Dev Biol.* 1999;207:271–286.

Poelmann RE, Gittenberger-de Groot AC, Mentink MMT, Bökenkamp R, Hogers B. Development of the cardiac coronary vascular endothelium, studied with antiendothelial antibodies, in chicken-quail chimeras. *Circ Res.* 1993;73:559–568.

Poelmann RE, Jongbloed MRM, Gittenberger-de Groot AC. Pitx2, a challenging teenager. Invited editorial. *Circ Res.* 2008;102:749–751.

Poelmann RE, Jongbloed MRM, Molin DGM, et al. The neu-ral crest is contiguous with the cardiac conduction system in the mouse embryo: a role in induction? *Anat Embryol.* 2004;208:389–393.

Poelmann RE, Mikawa T, Gittenberger-de Groot AC. Neural crest cells in outflow tract septation of the embryonic chicken heart: differentiation and apoptosis. *Dev Dyn.* 1998;212:373–384.

Teillet MA, Kalcheim C, Le Douarin NM. Formation of the dor-sal root ganglia in the avian embryo: segmental origin and migratory behavior of neural crest progenitor cells. *Dev Biol.* 1987;120:329–347.

Tessari A, Pietrobon M, Notte A, et al. Myocardial Pitx2 Differentially Regulates the Left Atrial Identity and Ventricular Asymmetric Remodeling Programs. *Circ Res.* 2008;102:813–822.

van den Akker NMS, Caolo V, Wisse LJ, et al. Developmental coronary maturation is disturbed by aberrant cardiac VEGF-expression and Notch signaling. *Card Res.* 2008a;78:366–375.

van den Akker NMS, Lie-Venema H, Maas S, et al. Platelet-derived growth factors in the developing avian heart and maturing coronary vasculature. *Dev Dyn.* 2005;233:1579–1588.

van den Akker NMS, Molin DGM, Peters PPWM, et al. Tetralogy of Fallot and alterations in VEGF- and Notch-signalling in mouse embryos solely expressing the VEGF120 isoform. *Circ Res.* 2007;100:842–849.

van den Akker NMS, Winkel LCJ, Nisancioglu MH, et al. PDGF-B signaling is important for murine cardiac development; role in developing atrioventricular valves, coronaries and cardiac inner-vation. *Dev Dyn.* 2008b;237:494–503.

Van Loo PF, Mahtab EA, Wisse LJ, et al. Transcription Factor Sp3 knockout mice display serious cardiac malformations. *Mol Cell Biol.* 2007;27:8571–8582.

Verberne ME, Gittenberger-de Groot AC, Poelmann RE. Distribution of antigen epitopes shared by nerves and the myo-cardium of the embryonic chick heart using different neuronal markers. *Anat Rec.* 2000a;260:335–350.

Verberne ME, Gittenberger-de Groot AC, VanIperen L, Poelmann RE. Distribution of different regions of cardiac neural crest in the extrinsic and the intrinsic cardiac nervous system. *Dev Dyn.* 2000b;217:191–204.

Vrancken Peeters M-PFM, Gittenberger-de Groot AC, Mentink MMT, Hungerford JE, Little CD, Poelmann RE. Differences in development of coronary arteries and veins. *Cardiovasc Res.* 1997;36:101–110.

Vrancken Peeters M-PFM, Gittenberger-de Groot AC, Mentink MMT, Poelmann RE. Smooth muscle cells and fibroblasts of the coronary arteries derive from epithelial-mesenchymal transformation of the epicardium. *Anat Embryol.* 1999;199: 367–378.

Vrancken Peeters M-PFM, Mentink MMT, Poelmann RE, Gittenberger-de Groot AC. Cytokeratins as a marker for epicardial formation in the quail embryo. *Anat Embryol.* 1995;191:503–508.

Waldo K, Zdanowicz M, Burch J, et al. A novel role for cardiac neural crest in heart development. *J Clin Invest.* 1999a;103:1499–1507.

Waldo K, Miyagawa-Tomita S, Kumiski D, Kirby ML. Cardiac neural crest cells provide new insight into septation of the cardiac outflow tract: aortic sac to ventricular septal closure. *Dev Biol.* 1998;196:129–144.

Waldo KL, Hutson MR, Ward CC, et al. Secondary heart field contributes myocardium and smooth muscle to the arterial pole of the developing heart. *Dev Biol.* 2005;281:78–90.

Waldo KL, Lo CW, Kirby ML. Connexin 43 expression reflects neural crest patterns during cardiovascular development. *Dev Biol.* 1999b;208:307–323.

Winter EM, Gittenberger-de Groot AC. Cardiovascular development: towards biomedical applicability: epicardium-derived cells in cardiogenesis and cardiac regeneration. *Cell Mol Life Sci.* 2007;64:692–703.

2

Developmental Cardiovascular Physiology

KIYOSHI HASHIGAMI-SHINN

RUIPING JI

COLIN K.L. PHOON

INTRODUCTION

Congenital heart disease (CHD) is the most common of all birth defects, occurring in approximately 1% of live births (Hoffman and Kaplan, 2002). There are now over 1 million adults living with CHD in the United States, a figure that is increasing at a rate of about 5% per year (Hoffman and Kaplan, 2002). These numbers underestimate the "true" incidence of CHD, however, because the prenatal incidence of CHD is some 10-fold higher, and the great majority of these defects result in intrauterine demise (Hoffman, 1995).

Like many other birth defects, congenital heart defects are considered to be the result of little-understood developmental processes gone awry (Garg, 2006; Gruber and Epstein, 2004). Especially over the past decade, many genetic pathways have been elucidated to define critical steps in early cardiogenesis, such as cardiomyocyte specification, heart tube formation, valve formation, and chamber specification. Early cardiogenic pathways are well-conserved throughout the vertebrate phyla (Olson, 2006; Srivastava, 2006), and several genes have now been directly implicated in several forms of human CHD (Garg, 2006; Gruber and Epstein, 2004). A discussion of these genetic pathways is beyond the scope of this chapter, and the reader is referred to several excellent reviews on this subject (Bruneau, 2002; Garg, 2006; Gruber and Epstein, 2004; Olson, 2006; Srivastava, 2006). In addition to underlying genomics, epigenetic mechanisms influence normal as well as abnormal development (Hove et al., 2003; Phoon, 2001). We now believe that in the early developing heart, there occurs an evolution of morphology during abnormal development, intertwined with changes in function, before arriving at the "final" phenotype. Cardiovascular growth and development are thus likely to benefit from early correction or mitigation of hemodynamic aberrations, and indeed, this rationale drives prenatal therapies, which are postulated to slow progression to, or even prevent, severe congenital heart defects (Tworetzky et al., 2004; Makikallio et al., 2006).

By understanding the structure–function relationships influencing cardiac development, we can gain better insights into the origins of human CHD and ultimately into potential therapeutic targets. Despite the profound advances in molecular cardiology, there has been a notable lag in defining the physiology of the developing cardiovascular system. The expanded availability and versatility of animal model systems (Table 2–1), particularly the mouse (Yutzey and Robbins, 2007), coupled with technological advances (Table 2–2; see also Dickinson, 2006 for recent overview; and Figure 2–1) have only recently allowed for the detailed characterization of embryonic hemodynamic parameters. Compiling data from both animal and human studies and with the recognition that there are likely to be differences between species, this chapter will describe many of the known physiological changes in embryonic and fetal cardiovascular functioning, relating them briefly to changes in cellular and organ architecture throughout development. We will then discuss the effects of altered hemodynamic forces on the morphology of the developing heart.

TABLE 2–1. *Summary of Commonly Used and Representative Animal Systems in Embryonic Cardiovascular Physiology*

Animal Model	Advantages	Disadvantages	Genome Known?
Mouse (*Mus musculus*)	- Mammalian system - Short lifespan - Rapid reproductive rate - Genetic manipulation possible	- Develops in utero; thus manipulation is difficult	Yes Dietrich, 1996
Chick (*Gallus gallus*)	- Embryo develops in egg - Easily accessible for surgical manipulation with minimal invasiveness - Allows for direct observation of developing cardiovascular system	- Avian system - Lack of gene-targeted models	Yes Wallis et al., 2004
Zebrafish (*Danio rerio*)	- Embryo is optically clear, allowing for direct longitudinal observation - Short lifespan - Rapid reproductive rate - Genetic manipulation possible	- Poikilothermic animal system; difficult to extrapolate physiological data to mammalian system - Two-chambered heart	Yes Woods et al., 2000
Frog (*Xenopus laevis*)	- Embryo is large, and develops outside of mother	- Amphibian; difficult to extrapolate physiological data to mammalian system - Three-chambered heart	Yes Klein, 2006

Adapted from Burggren, 2004; Clark and Hu, 1982; Hu et al., 1991; Hove, 2004; Keller, 1997; Lohr and Yost, 2000; Mohun et al., 2000; Sedmera et al., 1999, 2002, 2003; Stainier, 1993; Warkman and Krieg, 2006; Wessels and Sedmera, 2003; Yutzey and Robbins, 2007.

HEART BEAT/HEART RATE

Initiation of the Embryonic Heartbeat and Pacing

Heart rate (HR) is the simplest and most reproducible parameter to ascertain. Zebrafish hearts beat with a nearly regular rhythm by 26–28 hours postfertilization (hpf), when the heart is a single tube consisting of endocardial and myocardial layers separated by cardiac jelly (Liebling et al., 2006). In the chick, cardiac contractions begin after heart tube fusion (approximately HH stage 9), with propagation of contractile waves seen at HH stages 10–11 (Taber, 1998). Using high-frequency UBM-Doppler to image the in utero early mouse heart, Ji et al. (2003) reported initial detection of heart rates shortly after linear heart tube fusion and prior to cardiac looping, at the 5-somite stage or approximately embryonic day (postconceptional day, E)8.25. In exteriorized mouse embryos imaged by video recordings, others have noted the earliest heartbeat even prior to complete fusion of the primitive heart tube at the 3-somite stage (Nishii and Shibata, 2006). By about E9, the murine heart has been observed to have regular, more powerful contractions (Ji et al., 2003; Myers and Fishman, 2003; Phoon, 2001). Taken together, these data indicate that vertebrate hearts begin to beat very close to the time when the primitive paired cardiac

tubes fuse into a single straight heart tube. In the early human fetus, onset of cardiac contractile activity has been detected by clinical ultrasound as early as the fifth week of gestation (Makikallio et al., 1999); in in vitro fertilized embryos, cardiac activity has been detected at 25 days postfollicle aspiration (postovulation) (Schats et al., 1990). Although these timelines represent when the early human heartbeat is *detected*, it is generally accepted that the first rhythmic contractions of the human heart *occur* at approximately day 21 (Gourdie et al., 2003; Hirschy et al., 2006; Nishii and Shibata, 2006).

In the embryonic chick heart, the sinus venosus is the dominant pacemaker, and the HR is approximately 60 beats per minute (bpm) close to its discernible onset (HH stage 10–11). The pacemaker cells of the sinoatrial segment are located on the posterior-most segment of the heart tube, and the unidirectional flow of blood marks the start of circulatory function. Evidence points to the importance of both the hyperpolarization-activated cyclic nucleotide-gated family of ion channel subunits and the sodium–calcium exchanger in embryonic pacemaker activity (Koushik et al., 2001; Gourdie et al., 2003), and perhaps the L-type calcium channel as well (Wakimoto et al., 2000). Notably, data suggest that normal calcium handling, and its normal maturation, influence the structural development of the embryonic cardiomyocyte. For example, mutations

TABLE 2–2. *Commonly Employed Phenotyping Techniques, and Specific Advantages and Disadvantages of Each System (Also Reviewed in Dickinson, 2006); Not All Permit Study of Cardiovascular Physiology*

Phenotyping Technique	Resolution	Penetration Depth	Advantages	Disadvantages
Histology	Optical resolution (submicron)	N/A	1. Can provide detailed anatomic descriptions through development	1. Limited to postmortem tissue 2. Tissue fixation can distort anatomical structures 3. Unable to study dynamic in vivo systems
Episcopic fluorescence image capture (EFIC) Rosenthal et al., 2004	Optical resolution (submicron)	N/A	1. Accurate 3-D reconstruction 2. Ability to digitally resection specimen 3. Combining with fluorescence allows gene or protein expression mapping	1. Limited to postmortem tissue 2. Unable to study dynamic in vivo systesms
Magnetic resonance imaging; microMRI Schneider et al., 2003, 2004; Schneider and Bhattacharya, 2004	25 µm	Centimeters	1. Superb in anatomical soft tissue imaging; excellent tissue contrast 2. Nondestructive 3. Allows for collection of 3-D datasets	1. Long acquisition times 2. Unsuitable for accurate in vivo imaging 3. High resolution systems require magnet strengths not widely available
40–50 MHz ultrasound biomicroscopy (UBM) Phoon and Turnbull, 2003; Phoon, 2006; Ji and Phoon, 2005; Ji et al., 2003	30–40 µm (axial resolution)	5–15 mm	1. Noninvasive, allowing study of in vivo hemodynamic parameters under physiologic conditions 2. Serial imaging possible	1. Persistent difficulty in assessment of low-flow vessels, such as veins 2. Anesthesia needed 3. Images limited by gas, bone 4. Relatively poor tissue contrast
Clinical ultrasound systems (13–15 MHz) Spurney et al., 2004, 2006; Phoon 2006	440 µm (axial resolution)	10–30 mm	1. Noninvasive, allowing in vivo imaging 2. Color Doppler flow mapping 3. Serial imaging possible	1. Poor spatial resolution for embryonic imaging 2. Other limitations of ultrasound similar to UBM
Optical coherence tomography (OCT) Yelbuz et al., 2002, Low et al., 2005	Near-optical resolution, 1–16 µm	2–3 mm	1. Allows for optical resolution 2. Can image in vivo systems	1. Penetration depth only 2–3 mm, which is not enough to image embryonic mouse systems
Optical projection tomography (OPT) Sharpe, 2004	Optical resolution	N/A	1. Maximum resolution of 5–10 µm 2. OPT can be combined with fluorescent protein labeling to map gene expression patterns	1. Cannot be used currently for in vivo imaging
Confocal/multiphoton laser-scanning microscopy Megason and Fraser, 2003, Lucitti and Dickinson, 2006	Cellular resolution, approx. 1 micron	200–500 microns	1. Combined with fluorescent protein (GFP) labeling, can track individually labeled cells through development 2. Allows 3-D and 4-D dataset collection	1. Older sampling speeds insufficient for fast movements, such as the contracting heart, although temporal resolution recently improved (Liebling et al., 2006) 2. Tissue transparency needed
Digital particle imaging velocimetry (DPIV) Hove, 2004, 2006	Optical resolution	Low (requires tissue transparency)	1. Provides information on fluid displacement vectors, providing intravital flow pattern maps	1. Requires invasive injection of tracer particles into circulatory system 2. Results can be confounded by selection of inappropriate particles 3. Requires tissue transparency for particle visualization and tracking

in the sodium–calcium exchanger have been associated with myofibrillar disarray, both in mice without calcium overload (Koushik et al., 2001) and in zebrafish with calcium overload (Ebert, 2005), and L-type calcium channel blockade disrupts cardiac looping, gene expression, and chamber development (Porter et al., 2003). During these early stages of cardiac development, the heart is yet to be innervated, and there is little HR variability (Stekelenburg-de Vos et al., 2003). In the mouse, shortly before heart tube completion, slow peristaltic contractions are observed along the tube; this timing represents postconception day 21 in human embryos (Nishii and Shibata, 2006). New data in zebrafish derived from high-speed in vivo video confocal microscopy indicates that the early tubular embryonic heart is not a peristaltic pump as is traditionally believed, but is rather a hydroelastic impedance pump acting as a dynamic suction pump (Forouhar, 2006). The advantage of this relatively simple system is that only a single activation site is required, rather

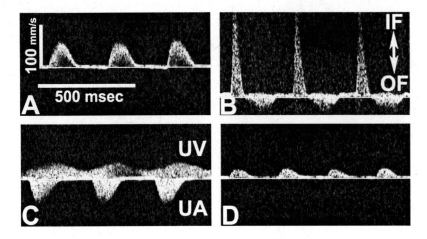

FIGURE 2–1. Ultrasound biomicroscopy-Doppler can interrogate multiple sites in mouse embryos (here, E12.5). A: dorsal aorta; B: inflow (IF) (—note the absence of an E-wave at this early developmental stage) and outflow (OF); C: umbilical artery (UA) and vein (UV); D: vitelline artery. The velocity (100 mm/s) and time (500 ms) scales are equivalent for all panels. (From Phoon, 2006. Copyright © Lippincott Williams & Wilkins, 2006, used with permission.)

than complete synchrony throughout the heart tube (Forouhar, 2006).

The initiation of a murine heartbeat at E8.25 coincides with an appearance of erythroblasts within the embryo (Ji et al., 2003; McGrath et al., 2003), representing approximately the earliest onset of a circulation capable of hemoglobin-mediated oxygen transport. The need for a heartbeat first to initiate and then to maintain erythrocyte circulation is strongly suggested in mouse models that lack a heartbeat (Wakimoto et al., 2000). These results established the early timing of the initiation of the heartbeat and circulation in the mouse, and indicate that early development of the circulation follows a tightly coordinated program that brings together maturing red blood cells, an intact vascular network, and cardiac function over a 48-hour period (approximately E8–E10) to permit continued embryonic growth (Ji et al., 2003).

Atrioventricular Conduction

Effective cardiac contraction relies not only on an intact pacemaking system, but also on the highly coordinated atrioventricular conduction of electrical impulses through the heart that improves the efficiency of cardiac contraction. Many types of CHD exhibit conduction abnormalities, and conduction and rhythm abnormalities in turn may adversely impact the hemodynamics of the developing organism. Thus, the developing organism's cardiac rhythm, atrioventricular conduction, developmental physiology, and cardiac morphology are all likely to be intertwined. Indeed, artificial pacing that eliminates normal atrioventricular conduction significantly compromises circulatory output (MacLennan and Keller, 1999). The initiation of the heartbeat and development of the sinoatrial pacemaker is followed by the development of other

two main structural and functional elements of the cardiac pacemaking and conduction system, the atrioventricular conduction delay generator and then the His-Purkinje conduction system (Gourdie et al., 2003).

As the heart in the embryonic chick begins to receive parasympathetic innervation at HH 24, HR shows progressive variation. The sinoatrial (SA) node in the chick starts to form in the right atrium at HH 27–28, while the atrioventricular (AV) node and the AV bundle begins to form at HH 28 (Stekelenburg-de Vos et al., 2003). In the chick, delay at the atrioventricular canal becomes evident from around 42 h of development, corresponding to approximately E8 in the mouse and 25 days in the human embryo (Gourdie et al., 2003). Full functionality of the cardiac autonomic nervous system in chick is not achieved until HH 41 (Stekelenburg-de Vos et al., 2003). The development of the fast conduction system, the His-Purkinje system, in the chick is marked by an apparent reversal in the sequence of ventricular activation, from an immature base-to-apex direction, to a mature apex-to-base direction; the mature activation pattern coincides with completion of ventricular septation (reviewed in Gourdie et al., 2003).

During cardiac morphogenesis in both mouse and human species, the differentiation of each of these three elements follows a conserved and repeatable sequence, respectively emerging during the formation of the heart tube, looping, and septation of the cardiac chambers (Gourdie et al., 2003). In the mouse, the initial peristaltic contractions are only transient, as sequential contractions of the primitive cardiac chambers are observed at E9, after rudimentary looping has occurred (Myers and Fishman, 2003). At this stage of development, the AV canal acts as the embryonic AV node to delay impulse propagation to the ventricular conduction pathways (Myers and Fishman, 2003). Using *lacZ* reporter gene expression and optical mapping with voltage-sensitive dyes, investigators have shown that electrical epicardial activation of the ventricles is accomplished at early stages in a base-to-apex direction. In the E9.5 mouse, impulse propagation proceeds through the atrioventricular canal, along the dorsal wall of the ventricle, which is the putative site of conduction system development; the excitatory wave reaches the apex, then spreads along the ventral surface from the apex toward the base and outflow tract (Myers and Fishman, 2003; Rentschler et al., 2001). In short, the direction of electrical propagation follows the direction of blood flow (Sedmera et al., 2004). The fast conduction system of the heart, the His-Purkinje conduction system, is the last element to differentiate. At E10.5, apical activation first becomes evident, and most hearts will exhibit a "breakthrough" at the apex (that is, initial apical activation) by E11.5; by E12.5, all hearts show two "breakthrough" regions, corresponding to the maturing His-Purkinje bundles (Myers and Fishman, 2003; Rentschler et al., 2001). In the mouse, the maturation of the His-Purkinje conduction system corresponds to cardiac chamber septation; heart morphogenesis and conduction system maturation are thus linked (Gourdie et al., 2003; Sedmera et al., 2004). Recent data in the rabbit, however, show that the mature apex-to-base activation pattern is present even before completion of cardiac septation, and the appearance of the atrioventricular interval, or delay, coincides with the presence of collagen in the atrioventricular junction (Rothenberg et al., 2005).

Notably, hemodynamics may play an important role in the patterning of the conduction system. In chick embryos, periarterial Purkinje fibers are only found next to coronary arteries and never associated with low-tension vessels such as capillary networks and veins (Gourdie et al., 2003; Takebayashi-Suzuki, 2001). The timing of periarterial Purkinje fibers also has a conspicuous association with the onset of sequential cardiac contractions (Gourdie et al., 2003). In experiments in which cultured chick myocytes were exposed to endothelin-1, a shear stress-modulated circulatory factor, there were changes in myocyte gene expression consistent with Purkinje fiber differentiation (Gourdie et al., 1998). Altered ventricular loading conditions have also been shown to change conduction system maturational patterns in the mouse ventricle. In mouse ventricles experiencing increased loading conditions due to conotruncal banding, Reckova et al. (2001) observed precocious maturation of the His-Purkinje system. In the contrary scenario in which ventricular load was reduced via left atrial ligation, there was a delay in His-Purkinje maturation (Reckova, 2001). These results provided support for the critical role of epigenetic factors in the development of the conduction system.

Heart Rate Progression

In the chick and mouse embryo, HRs steadily increase throughout gestation, providing necessary increases in cardiac output to meet the rising metabolic demands (Hu et al., 1991; Kamino, 1991; Phoon, 2001). In the HH 12 chick, HR is approximately 100 bpm and increases to ~230 bpm by HH 35 (Hu et al., 1991; Phoon, 2001). In the mouse, different methods of HR determination have yielded significantly variable data throughout embryonic development. Invasive observation methods in E10–15.5 mouse embryos have shown HR to increase from ~130 to ~240 bpm. However, with noninvasive ultrasound biomicroscopy (UBM) technology, HR at E10 was ~190 bpm, increasing to ~260 bpm by E14.5 (Phoon et al., 2000; Phoon, 2001). The initial reported bradycardia may have been induced by decreases in temperature and/or by surgical manipulation (Nakazawa et al., 1988; Nishii and Shibata, 2006; Phoon, 2001) (Figure 2–2).

It is important to obtain physiologic intrinsic HR in the study of the embryonic cardiovascular system. Most hemodynamic parameters are heavily influenced by HR, including Doppler indices of cardiac function. Cardiac output is optimized when normal atrioventricular synchrony is preserved at or near the embryonic intrinsic heart rate (Casillas et al., 1994; MacLennan and Keller, 1999; Phoon, 2001). In earlier studies in fetal sheep, Anderson et al. concluded that rate-dependent alterations in LV output were determined in large part by LV filling, as reflected in end-diastolic dimension (Anderson et al., 1986; Casillas et al., 1994). Similar observations have been noted in mouse embryos,

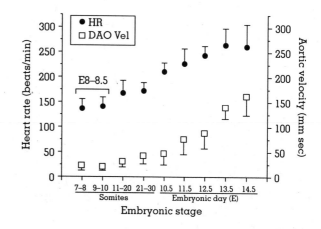

FIGURE 2–2. Aggregate heart rate (HR) and dorsal aortic (DAO) velocity data (mean ±SD) from mouse embryos imaged with 40 MHz UBM-Doppler in utero, from close to the initiation of the heartbeat (7–8 somite stage, ~E8.25) through completion of cardiogenesis (E14.5). (Data adapted from Phoon et al., 2000 and Ji et al., 2003.)

showing that the developing mammalian cardiovascular system and placenta have rate-dependent features for providing effective circulation (MacLennan and Keller, 1999).

In humans, there is a distinct difference in HR progression when compared to the development of avian and murine hearts. After fetal HR is first detected in the fifth week of gestation at a rate of ~110 bpm, it gradually increases until the eighth week, at which time a plateau is reached at about 150–170 bpm (Makikallio et al., 1999, 2005). This rate is maintained until birth of the newborn without significant change. This interspecies difference in HR progression may provide insight into differences in cardiac development among vertebrate species.

Is the Initiation of Circulation Critical for Organism Survival?

In both scientific and lay communities, it has long been believed that a beating heart is always required to sustain life in organisms. However, as a result of recent investigations, this dogma has come into debate and the question now is: When the heart starts to beat, is it truly necessary for organism survival? If not, what purpose does the embryonic heartbeat serve?

There are several lines of research to suggest that an organism in its early embryonic stages does not require a fully functioning cardiovascular system in order to survive. Although many genetically manipulated animal models die in utero, the early embryo can survive for some time without a fully functioning unidirectional circulation. Several examples follow. The *Nkx2.5 -/-* zebrafish mutant displays an acardic phenotype throughout development. Despite this, they can survive and even swim for approximately 2 weeks after hatching (Lohr and Yost, 2000). Lacking the sodium–calcium exchanger, *Ncx1 -/-* mouse embryos have a complete absence of a heartbeat after heat tube formation, but survive until around E10.5–11.5 (Conway et al., 2003; Koushik et al., 2001; Wakimoto et al., 2000). This model also provided the first genetic evidence to support the finding that heartbeat is not required for normal early heart morphogenesis (Conway et al., 2003; Koushik et al., 2001). *MEF2c* null mutant mice generate a fused heart tube that does not progress to looping (Lin et al., 1997). The cardiac tube in these mutants shows slower, less rhythmic contractions when compared to wild-type animals. However, despite the observed contractile and hemodynamic dysfunction, these embryos can survive until ~E10.5 (Conway et al., 2003), a full 2 days after the first observed cardiac contractions in wild-type mice (Ji et al., 2003; Nishii and Shibata, 2006). Mouse embryos deficient in *c-kit* develop severe anemia by late gestation (Chui, 1978).

In a different mouse knockout model, lack of erythropoietin receptor signaling leads to a severe decrease in erythrocyte numbers by E11.5, but the mice are able to survive until approximately E13.5 (Lin et al., 1996). Several investigators have described experimental models in which embryos were stripped of nutrient and oxygen delivery via convective flow, for example, with carbon monoxide exposure in zebrafish, frog, and chick embryos. In each of these cases, cessation of hemoglobin-mediated oxygen transport did not result in immediate deleterious effects to the developing embryo system (Burggren et al., 2000; Cirotto and Arangi, 1989; Pelster and Burggren, 1996; Territo and Altimiras, 2001). Instead, deleterious effects on growth were seen later, when the nutrient demands of the growing embryo could no longer be supplied by diffusion alone (Burggren, 2004).

Experimental evidence also shows clearly that for approximately the first 36 hours following the initiation of the circulation in the mouse, a fully functional and rigorous circulation is established in a step-wise pattern, such that the number, density, and distribution of red blood cells increases to populate the embryo proper at an "equilibrium" level by approximately E10.5 (McGrath et al., 2003). The above described experiments and animal models lend support to the "prosynchronotropy" theory coined by Burggren et al. This theory proposes that the initiation of a unidirectional circulation is not necessary for oxygen delivery to the developing embryo, but rather plays a more important role in the morphological determination of the cardiovascular system (Burggren et al., 2004).

SYSTOLIC FUNCTION

Systems- and Organ-Level Systolic Cardiac Function

Overall cardiac systolic function must and does increase as the embryo grows. For example, between E10.5 and E18.5 in the mouse, embryonic weight increases exponentially, by approximately 75-fold (Mu and Adamson, 2006). The pioneering work of Clark and his colleagues demonstrated that stroke volume and cardiac work increase geometrically to parallel embryonic growth (Clark and Hu, 1982; Hu and Clark, 1989; Keller et al., 1994). Ejection fraction in the embryonic ventricle probably is in the range of 30%–50%, although the methods by which this is measured leave a substantial margin for error (Keller et al., 1994; Tanaka et al., 1997); a recent determination using BODPIY-ceramide fluorescence labeled blood cells showed an ejection fraction of approximately 60% in the embryonic 4.5 days postfertilization (dpf) zebrafish (Hove et al., 2003). Studies in HH18, 24, and 29 chick embryos have revealed the presence of length–tension relations, such that experimentally increased loading conditions induced linear increases in stroke volume (Wagman et al., 1990). Still, the Frank–Starling mechanism in the embryo appears limited in its ability to increase cardiac output when compared to the mature ventricle (Keller et al., 1994; Wagman et al., 1990). The embryonic ventricle does appear to have a significant contractile reserve, unmasked when ventricular–vascular interaction is uncoupled by conotruncal occlusion (Keller et al., 1997). The limited ability of the embryonic myocardium to increase stroke volume in response to increasing preload can likely be attributed to an immature cardiomyocyte architecture (see below). An intriguing alternative explanation is that put forth by Grant et al., who suggested that fetal stroke volume was limited by ventricular constraint due to extrinsic compression of the fetal heart by surrounding structures (Grant, 1999; Grant et al., 1992). Relief of this constraint at birth, with aeration of the lungs, may be the key mechanism responsible for the acutely increased LV preload stroke volume observed in the newborn infant (Grant, 1999; Grant et al., 1992).

Intracardiac and intra-arterial pressures also increase as the embryo grows. In HH12–29 chick, ventricular systolic pressure rises from approximately 1–4 mmHg, diastolic pressure from approximately 0.2–0.8 mmHg, arterial systolic pressure from 0.3–2 mmHg, and arterial diastolic pressure from approximately 0.2–1.2 mmHg (Clark and Hu, 1990, 1982; Clark et al., 1986; Hu et al., 2000; Keller et al., 1994; Nakazawa et al., 1988). Similar increases have been noted in similarly staged rat and zebrafish models. Ventricular pressure is directly related to cardiac mass (Clark and Hu, 1990). More recently, human fetal intracardiac pressures have been determined as early as gestation at 16 weeks, when intraventricular pressures are approximately 16/3 mmHg, increasing to approximately 35–40 mmHg systolic/10 mmHg diastolic by 28 weeks of gestational age (Johnson et al., 2000). Both ventricular systolic and end diastolic pressures increase throughout fetal development, without any noticeable difference between left and right ventricles (Johnson et al., 2000). Interestingly, pressure waveforms in both animal models and human fetuses throughout gestation closely resemble those of the mature organism (Clark and Hu, 1990; Clark et al., 1986; Hu and Clark, 1989; Ishiwata et al., 2003; Johnson et al., 2000; Zahka et al., 1989).

More recent studies, especially those employing Doppler ultrasound, have shown consistently that flow velocities in different animal models also increase throughout the circulation as gestation progresses (Broekhuizen et al., 1999; Clark et al., 1990, 1982;

1986; Gui et al., 1996; Keller et al., 1996; MacLennan and Keller, 1999; Phoon et al., 2000). Cardiac output and stroke work increase dramatically from even the earliest stages of cardiac functioning, around E8.25 (Ji et al., 2003). Combining high-frequency 40 MHz ultrasound biomicroscopy–Doppler data and biophysical modeling in the mid-gestation (E13.5–14.5) mouse, Phoon and colleagues (2002) corroborated estimates of stroke volume data in the similarly sized and staged chick obtained earlier by Clark and his colleagues (1982) and in the mid-gestation mouse embryo by Keller and colleagues (1996), in the range of 0.50–0.60 µL. Studies in human fetuses have recently revealed a similar increase in mean outflow velocity between 6–8 weeks of gestation, and increases in mean umbilical artery velocity between 7–10 weeks of gestation (Makikallio et al., 2005). During the second half of pregnancy, similar increases in peak systolic blood flow velocities have been reported. However, researchers have noted a slight decrease in umbilical arterial flow velocities in fetuses as they progressed from 22 to 38 weeks of gestation (from approximately 52.5 to 46.2 cm/s), concomitant with a decrease in umbilical artery resistance index (Da Costa et al., 2005).

In zebrafish, investigators were able to approximate intracardiac shear forces in normal embryos using individual erythrocyte velocities and vessel diameter: with a Reynolds number of 0.02, shear would be greater than 75 dyn/cm (Hove et al., 2003). Importantly, these calculated shear forces appear to be of sufficient magnitude, which in other experiments could elicit a response from cultured vascular endothelial cells (Hove et al., 2003; Pelster and Burggren, 1996); thus, the data provided strong evidence for the interaction between mechanical fluid forces and gene expression.

Cardiac output and work, circulatory pressures, and flow velocity may increase through any combination of increased contractility, increased preload, or changes in peripheral impedance. Cardiac work may also simply increase if ventricular myocardial mass increases. Ventricular weight decreases as a proportion of the total embryonic body weight, yet the heart achieves progressively more work and output (Clark and Hu, 1990; Clark et al., 1986; Hu et al., 2000). This finding suggests that the embryonic cardiovascular system improves its effectiveness as gestation progresses (Clark and Hu, 1990). It is clear that blood volume (reflected as preload) increases, while impedance decreases (see below). However, a complete picture of how myocardial contractility increases remains incompletely answered. We do expect contractility to increase, given the known changes in cardiomyocyte architecture and intracellular calcium handling (Anderson, 1996; Anderson et al., 1984; Artman et al., 2000; Clark et al., 1986; Hirschy et al., 2006;

Navaratnam et al., 1986; Sedmera et al., 1997); moreover, there exists an emerging response to humoral factors such as catecholamines, acetylcholine, and adenosine during cardiogenesis (Porter et al., 2001). There is some evidence of increasing contractility: increasing ventricular dP/dt (Clark and Hu, 1990; Clark et al., 1986), increasing peak flow acceleration (Clark et al., 1986; Broekhuizen et al., 1993), and increasing end-systolic myocardial stiffness (Tobita and Keller, 2000a). Also, peak velocity of circumferential shortening remains constant in early chick gestation, consistent with a matched increase in preload and contractile states (Keller et al., 1994). Tobita et al., after studying end-systolic stress–strain relations in HH 24 chick embryos, demonstrated end-systolic myocardial stiffness to be a measure of myocardial contractility, unaffected by changes in loading and HR conditions (1999). This same group later noted linear decreases in stress–strain relations when comparing chicks at HH17, 21, and 24, suggesting that the embryonic ventricle increases contractility throughout development (Tobita and Keller, 2000a). Furthermore, from E10.5 to E19.5 in the mouse embryo, the Ca^{2+}-activated isometric force has been shown to increase fivefold when normalized to cross-sectional area (Siedner, 2003). From E10.5 until 6–8 weeks after birth, this factor has been shown to increase 20-fold (Siedner, 2003). This is in agreement with previous studies in embryonic chick and fetal sheep hearts (Anderson et al., 1984; Godt, 1991). In the E13.5–19.5 mouse embryo, the ratio of myosin heavy chain (MHC) to total protein appeared to be relatively stable, but there is a twofold increase in myofiber density within the ventricular walls during this time (McLean et al., 1989). This correlates with the observed increase in contractile force. Ca^{2+} sensitivity of contraction actually decreases slightly during embryonic, fetal, and prenatal stages in the mouse, due in part to troponin isoform switching, so that this cannot be responsible for the observed increases in contractile force seen through gestation (Siedner, 2003). These discoveries have led to the conclusion that structural organization of myofilaments is a key factor governing cardiac contractile force generation throughout development (Navaratnam et al., 1986; Siedner, 2003). Although not well-studied at early stages of embryonic development, the maturation of calcium handling also undoubtedly plays a major role in the increases in contractility seen as well; these include the increasing role of the sarcoplasmic reticulum and the propagation of the T-tubule system (Artman et al., 2000). In first trimester human fetuses, isovolumic contraction time, an index of myocardial contractile function, decreased between 7 and 10 weeks of gestation, suggesting an increase in contractile function (Makikallio et al., 2005). Area-shortening fraction, an ejection phase index of contractile function that is load-dependent, does not change significantly between 14 and 28 weeks of gestational age in human fetuses (Goldinfeld, 2004), similar to animal models (Phoon et al., 2004). In contrast to the above studies, Phoon et al. (2000) found no change in acceleration time, a touted load-independent index of contractility (Van Bel et al., 1991), in the mouse from E9.5 to E14.5, although acceleration time decreased significantly from E8.25 at the start of cardiac contractions through to about E10.5 in a study of the earliest stages of cardiac functioning (Ji et al., 2003). One should interpret such Doppler data with caution, however, since ejection-phase flow velocity indices of cardiac function are typically influenced by loading conditions. Still, it is notable that even the earliest Doppler waveforms in the unseptated embryonic mouse heart bear a striking resemblance to those in the mature organism; this finding suggests relative strength and velocity of contraction that belie the seemingly disorganized myofibrils in these early hearts (Navaratnam et al., 1986).

Ventricular Cardiomyocyte Growth and Changes in Cytoarchitecture

The ability of the myocardium to support a progressively increasing mechanical load during development is partly derived from the developmental increase in ventricular mass (Ishiwata et al., 2003). This increase in mass can be largely attributed to cardiomyocyte hyperplasia. However, the cytoarchitecture of the individual cardiomyocyte undergoes developmental changes as well, and more recent data argue against a clear-cut "prenatal-hyperplasia" and "postnatal-hypertrophy" distinctions in myocardial growth (Hirschy, 2006; Perriard et al., 2003). The earliest cardiomyocytes are round in shape, and these cells elongate as embryonic development progresses. Notably, while cell width does not change appreciably, cell length grows at a rate similar to that of myofibrillar length. The growth and location of the myofibrils are initially constrained by a large nucleus; this constraint is obviated as the cell elongates. At birth, isolated heart cells are characterized by a spindle shape (Leu et al., 2001), and gradually elongate during development to eventually assume the rodlike shape of the adult cardiomyocyte (Perriard et al., 2003).

In addition to the contributions of cell size and number to a heart's contractile function, the contractile ability per unit volume of a cardiomyocyte also changes during development; that is, the cellular contractile apparatus undergoes a maturational process. In considering the contractile ability of the developing cardiomyocyte, one must consider two critical cell elements, myofibrils and intercalated discs. *Myofibrils* are crucial in the generation of force by the heart cell, achieved by the shortening of the sarcomeres (see Hirschy et al., 2006). There is a progressive maturation in myofibril organization during development, from a sparse disorganized pattern in the early embryo to a densely packed parallel orientation in the mature cardiomyocyte (Hirschy et al., 2006; Perriard et al., 2003). It is also notable that while myofibril in-plane number and organization in the ventricular wall are generally poor prior to E12 in the mouse, many fibers can be observed in the numerous trabeculae throughout gestation (McLean et al., 1989). Myofibrillar development is characterized by a sequential expression of sarcomeric elements, which are rapidly organized into functional sarcomeres (Ehler, 1999, 2004; Hirschy et al., 2006). *Intercalated disks*, found at cell–cell contact sites, translate sarcomere shortening into cellular contractions (Hirschy et al., 2006). The intercalated disk is defined by the presence of three types of junctions: the adherens junction, the desmosome junction, and the gap junction. The adherens junction is a complex of proteins that links the actin cytoskeleton to the cell membrane, while the desmosome junction links the intermediate filaments to the cell membrane (Hirschy et al., 2006). The adherens junction and desmosome junction thus provide the mechanical coupling of the individual cardiomyocyte to generate the contractile force of the heart. In the early mouse embryo (E8.5–9.5), both the adherens junction and desmosome junction are expressed in a circumferential distribution around the cardiomyocyte. As the heart cell matures and assumes its rodlike shape, both adherens and desmosome junctions become restricted to the bipolar ends of the cell, allowing efficient contraction of the cell along one axis (Hirschy et al., 2006). The gap junction plays an essential role in the maintenance of an ionic gradient in the cardiomyocyte, thereby electrically coupling individual cells (Hirschy et al., 2006). The main embryonic connexin isoforms expressed in the heart are connexin 40 and 45, but these are replaced by connexin 43 during development (Alcolea, 1999; Delorme, 1997; Hirschy et al., 2006). Thus, the maturation of the intercalated disk, as reflected in the maturational patterns of these three different junctions, appears to play an important role in increasing force development as gestation progresses.

It has long been believed that hemodynamic forces play a significant role in the determination of cardiac morphology, due in part to its influence on cardiomyocyte growth regulation. However, it has been difficult to identify cellular and molecular responses to mechanical strain. In order to specifically observe the effects of mechanical strain on myocyte hyperplasia, Miller et al. studied an in vitro cell culture model of HH stage 31 chick embryo cardiomyocytes. In response to cyclical strain imposed onto cell cultures,

investigators observed a 37% increase in cell number as compared to controls (Miller et al., 2000), which is consistent with previous studies (Sedmera et al., 1999). In postnatal cardiomyocytes, similar stretching manipulations result in hypertrophy as compared to proliferation. Data in immature neonatal cardiomyocytes also suggest that both the degree and direction of stretch regulate myofibrillar organization, as well as metabolism and rate of turnover of the contractile proteins (Simpson, 1999).

Changes in Organ Myoarchitecture

Beyond the ultrastructural changes that occur at the cellular level, the developing myocardium also undergoes specific maturational patterns in organ architecture that likely contribute to its increasing systolic function (see Sedmera, 2005; Tobita et al., 2005). In the early tube-like heart, the myocardium is one- or two-cells thick, but there is already some anisotropic arrangement of the myocytes. As the heart matures, the inner trabecular myocardium develops, initially in a radial pattern and with only some indication of spiraling during systole. The compact layer at these stages is not yet well developed and is quite thin. Finally, with the development of the coronary circulation, the trabecular layer forms the compact myocardium. At this time and through the remainder of fetal development, the heart matures into the typical three-layered structure, with innermost longitudinal, middle circular, and subepicardial oblique preferential orientation (Sedmera, 2005). Throughout this process, the transmural myofiber angle distribution in the compact layer of the left ventricle shifts gradually in orientation from circumferential (endocardium) to longitudinal (epicardium). It is believed that this nonuniform transmural myofiber distribution allows the left ventricle its characteristic twist during systolic contraction (Tobita et al., 2005). The importance of the formation of the compact layer in the maturation of cardiac function is seen in the failure of compaction in animal models, as well as in patients with isolated noncompaction of the left ventricle (Sedmera, 2005).

DIASTOLIC FUNCTION

Diastolic filling of the ventricles improves throughout early morphogenesis and development. Preload increases as the total blood volume and flow increase in the growing embryo (Phoon et al., 2000; Phoon, 2001). The embryonic heart requires normal preloading for normal structural and functional development (Tobita and Keller, 2000; Broekhuizen et al., 1999; Sedmera et al., 1999). Even in the embryo, diastolic suction plays an important role in filling the immature ventricle (Braunstein et al., 1994; Hu et al., 2000; Keller et al., 1991; Phelan et al., 1995). However, characterizing ventricular diastolic properties and ventricular relaxation in the developing embryo has been very challenging, underscored by disparate results of different experiments and their interpretations.

Embryonic chick ventricular end-diastolic pressure doubles from stage 12 through 27, from approximately 0.24 to 0.55 mmHg (Clark et al., 1986; Hu et al., 1991; Hu and Clark, 1989). As measured by the servo-null pressure technique, as passive ventricular filling decreases with gestation, the active atrial contractile contribution to ventricular filling increases (Campbell et al., 1992; Hu et al., 1991; Phelan et al., 1995). Increasing end-diastolic ventricular volumes or ventricular pressures also have been observed in other studies of chick, rat, and mouse embryos (see Phoon, 2001), and in the mid-gestation to late-gestation human fetus (Johnson et al., 2000). End-diastolic pressure and volume are heavily load-dependent, and increasing preload likely explains the increasing ventricular end-diastolic pressure. However, the relative contributions of passive and active filling are influenced by cycle length (Keller, 1997, 1996, 1994; Nakazawa et al., 1988; Tanaka et al., 1997). The heart rate dependence of filling parameters therefore further confounds the data.

Other experimental data indicate that the early embryonic ventricle is very stiff when compared with the mature myocardium (Gui et al., 1996; Keller et al., 1994; Nakazawa et al., 1995). Recent data from high-speed confocal 3-D microimaging in zebrafish confirm that the early vertebrate ventricle fills only during atrial contraction through 128 hpf, but from 148 hpf onward, increasing passive ventricular filling occurs before the atrial contribution (Liebling et al., 2006). These zebrafish data corroborate longstanding data from the early chick embryo, in which pressure–volume loop analysis reveals increasing ventricular compliance as gestation progresses, providing further evidence for improved diastolic function of the developing ventricle (Keller, 1997, 1994, 1991; Stekelenburg-de Vos et al., 2005; Ursem et al., 2004). Using noninvasive Doppler measures of diastolic filling—which are admittedly load and heart rate dependent—Gui et al. (1996) described the maturation of atrioventricular inflow in mouse embryos, from a monophasic waveform at E11 to a biphasic (separate E and A waves) pattern by E15, and with increased E/A ratios by E17. Using UBM-Doppler imaging, Zhou et al. (2003) recently reported the measurements of E/A wave ratios in embryonic mouse hearts, studying atrioventricular flow velocities from E14.5 through the neonatal period. Their results were consistent with previous data, showing an increasing E/A ratio paralleling gestation (Phoon, 2001), and also showed that ventricular diastolic function matured fully approximately 3 weeks after birth (Zhou et al., 2003). Thus, passive filling, not active filling, seems to be increasingly prominent as gestation advanced.

Human fetal Doppler studies have shown similar results. A monophasic atrioventricular waveform is observed initially at 6+ to 8+ weeks of gestation, but becomes biphasic at 9–10 weeks (Leiva et al., 1999; Makikallio et al., 2005; Van Splunder et al., 1996). The gestational age-dependent progression in atrioventricular inflow may be caused by increasing ventricular compliance, faster ventricular relaxation, or a combination of both. This trend is observed throughout human gestation (Wladimiroff et al., 1992). These results suggested an increasing ventricular compliance, paralleling the increasing volume flow across the atrioventricular orifice (Gui et al., 1996). Makikallio et al. (2005) have speculated that the improvement in diastolic function is important for the fetal heart to adapt to an increased blood flow volume.

The known changes in embryonic diastolic filling have recently been correlated with changing trabeculation and compaction patterns of the developing ventricular myocardium, as well as myocardial mass (Hu et al., 1991, 2000). Utilizing left atrial ligation and conotruncal banding manipulations, Tobita et al. (2002) proposed that ventricular active relaxation is the result of compact myocardium proliferation, whereas the proliferation of trabecular myocardium correlates with ventricular passive compliance. At the tissue and cellular levels, the embryonic chick heart exhibits a maturing pattern in the distribution and extent of elastic matrix proteins, such as elastin, fibrillin, and type VI collagen (Hurle et al., 1994). Ishiwata et al. (2003) showed that between E9.5–E19 in the mouse, the peak velocity A wave correlated significantly with the area of trabecular myocardium in both ventricles, while the peak velocity E wave correlated with the area of compact myocardium in the ventricles. These results have led to the conclusion that during embryogenesis, the development of compact myocardium heavily influences the known changes in ventricular compliance (Ishiwata et al., 2003).

Ventricular relaxation, an active and energy-dependent process, has been difficult to characterize. The relaxation time constant tau (τ) decreases from HH17 to 27 in the chick, a finding that suggests faster ventricular relaxation with gestation (Cheanvechai, 1992). However, τ is also influenced by cycle length, and because decreases in cycle length change τ in the same direction as advances in gestation do, it is difficult to separate the confounding influence of cycle length (Braunstein et al., 1994; Cheanvechai, 1992).

Determination of τ also requires certain assumptions about isovolumic relaxation time (IRT) (Braunstein et al., 1994; Cheanchevai, 1992), but the data on IRT have been inconsistent. Absolute IRT remained constant throughout early development in some studies, but the reported values demonstrated great variability, ranging from 58 to 120 ms (Keller et al., 1994, 1991). The dependence of IRT on cycle length has been variable as well (Casillas et al., 1994; Naheed et al., 1996). Still other studies demonstrated a proportionately constant IRT, constituting 16%–20% of the cardiac cycle (Gui et al., 1996; Leiva et al., 1999); because heart rate increased, absolute IRT increased as well. A very recent study, however, found that IRT as a proportion of the cardiac cycle decreased steadily through the first trimester (Makikallio et al., 2005).

Taken together, the data indicate that diastolic function of the embryonic and fetal ventricle improves as gestation progresses. Understanding of the precise contribution of various components to diastolic function, including such physiological processes as calcium sequestration and extrusion, and ultrastructural properties of the developing cardiomyocyte, awaits further research.

PERIPHERAL CIRCULATORY PHYSIOLOGY AND VENTRICULO-VASCULAR INTERACTIONS

The term "afterload" is frequently applied to the peripheral resistance (or even more correctly, impedance) into which the ventricle must eject, and this dynamic resistance affects ventricular morphologic development (Clark and Hu, 1990; Sedmera et al., 1999). In chick and mouse embryos, indices of peripheral resistance or impedance have been shown to decrease progressively throughout gestation (Clark and Hu, 1982; Hu and Clark, 1989; 2000; Phoon et al., 2000; Phoon, 2001; Nakazawa et al., 1988), concurrent with the increasing surface area of intraembryonic and extraembryonic vascular beds. However, since afterload is the load against which a muscle contracts, a more accurate representation of afterload would be systolic myocardial wall stress (Colan et al., 1992), which incorporates ventricular pressure, myocardial wall thickness, and peripheral resistance (Phoon, 2001). Indeed, given the many factors playing into ventricular cyclical load, including regional differences in biomechanical load (Ling et al., 2002), defining the contributions of "afterload" in shaping the developing heart is a very complex task. In this section, we will focus on the growth of the peripheral vascular bed and, briefly, on the complex interplay between the embryonic ventricle and the vascular bed (ventriculovascular interaction).

Blood Vessel Formation and Arteriovenous Differentiation

The processes of vasculogenesis and angiogenesis have been well-described elsewhere (Eichmann et al., 2005; Isogai et al., 2003; Le Noble et al., 2005). In order for the developing organism to receive an adequate oxygen and nutrient supply, the vascular system in any organ and tissue must be established early in development (Eichmann et al., 2005), and indeed, the establishment of an intact, closed vascular circuit is coordinated precisely with the appearance of embryonic erythroblasts and the onset of the heartbeat (Ji et al., 2003; McGrath et al., 2003). Even before the onset of perfusion, vasculogenesis occurs with the in situ differentiation of endothelial cells from the mesoderm and their coalescence into tubes of a primary capillary plexus, leading to the formation of the major embryonic vessels, including the dorsal aorta and the primary capillary plexus of the yolk sac (Eichmann et al., 2005). We now know that the role of hemodynamics in the continued development of an organized, oxygen-carrying vascular network is proving to be as important as it is in the morphological development of the heart.

Blood pressure, shear stress, and flow dynamics have been implicated in the formation of arterial and venous plexi in the developing embryo for over 100 years, first suggested by Thoma in 1893 (cited in Eichmann et al., 2005). The interactions between genetic patterning and hemodynamic forces are just now starting to be elucidated. Although there are much data to indicate that embryonic arterial and venous differentiation is genetically predetermined, more recent work has shown considerable plasticity of the endothelial cell population. After the formation of the vitelline artery and initiation of flow, it has been shown that the vitelline veins are produced from former branches of the artery that have now disconnected (Eichmann et al., 2005). It was proposed that high blood flow velocities in arterial side-branches cause vessels to increase their diameter to accommodate cardiac output and that this process secondarily obstructs the lumens of small arterial side branches. These side branches subsequently anastomose with one another to form a secondary venous system parallel to the arterial system (Eichmann et al., 2005). The work of Le Noble et al. (2003) demonstrated that flow arrest via vitelline artery ligation (VAL) causes a morphological transformation of the artery into a vein at sites distal to ligation. The same manipulation caused venous differentiation into arteries, shown by the arteriolization of the contralateral vitelline vein following VAL. Not only is morphological differentiation a plastic process, but also is expression of genetic markers of arteriolization and venularization plastic; manipulation of flow patterns can both morphologically and genetically transform arteries into veins (Eichmann et al., 2005 review). Moreover, even the embryonic dorsal aorta appears to be sensitive to increased arterial load: VAL-induced increases in wall stress, without significant changes in strain or intraluminal pressure, led to changes in the distribution of smooth muscle α-actin and cell shape and increased collagen type I and III content (Lucitti et al., 2006). Furthermore, other studies have shown that in the absence of a heartbeat, angiogenesis is inhibited (Koushik et al., 2001; Wakimoto et al., 2000). These results demonstrate that arterial remodeling and angiogenesis can be regulated by flow-driven hemodynamic parameters, and not solely by genetic predetermination as previously believed (Le Noble et al., 2003).

The process of blood vessel formation, like cardiac morphogenesis, has elemental molecular signaling pathways that have been highly conserved amongst vertebrate species. Although these molecular signaling pathways are an area of current vigorous research, it is beyond the scope of this chapter, and the reader is referred to other reviews on the subject (Eichmann et al., 2002; Ferguson et al., 2005).

Yolk Sac and Placental Blood Flow: Vitelline and Chorioallantoic Circulations

An understanding of the extraembryonic circulation is necessary for an understanding of the developing cardiovascular system as a whole. The yolk sac is the initial organ of hematopoiesis and primordial germ cells (Palis et al., 1999; Palis and Yoder, 2001; Tavian and Péault, 2005). The mammalian yolk sac, including that in humans, is also capable of synthesizing a variety of proteins, and has also been implicated in transient nutritive effects for the early embryo. The placenta becomes necessary when the embryo begins to require oxygen and nutrients that can no longer be derived from diffusion alone, and the chorioallantoic circulation becomes a major part of the extraembryonic circulation from early on (see Kurjak and Kupesic, 1998; Mu and Adamson, 2006). Yolk sac dysfunction has been associated with a number of congenital malformations and embryonic lethality in rats, chicks, and humans, whereas placental dysfunction is associated with such important human conditions as preeclampsia and intrauterine growth retardation (Mu and Adamson, 2006).

Scant data exist on yolk sac hemodynamics, in experimental models such as the mouse as well as in human studies. Vitelline arterial flow in the mouse can be detected first at the onset of the circulation, approximately E8.25–8.5 (Ji et al., 2003; Mu and Adamson, 2006), and increases steadily until E13.5, when the flow velocities plateau (Mu and Adamson, 2006). As might be expected, vitelline arterial flow velocities are lower than those in the umbilical artery (see below), with peak Doppler velocities averaging ~15 mm/s at E9.5, ~20–25 mm/s at E11.5, and ~35 mm/s at E13.5 (Mu and Adamson, 2006). The human secondary yolk sac can be visualized by Doppler color flow mapping in all normally developing pregnancies between 6 and 12 weeks of gestation. Highest visualization rates are obtained between 7 and 9 weeks, but visualization of yolk sac vascularity decreases from about 9 weeks gestation onward, which indicates progressive loss of functional capacity concomitant with the increase in placental intervillous blood flow velocity (Kurjak and Kupesic, 1998). Using transvaginal ultrasonography, Makikallio et al. (1999) showed that arterial flow velocity signals in human yolk sac increased between the fifth and seventh week of gestation, and disappeared between the eighth and tenth weeks, as placental circulation increased. That human vitelline flow appears only transiently during the first trimester contrasts with the situation in the mouse, where vitelline arterial flow velocities increase during organogenesis and then remain constant until term.

More data are available on umbilical and placental hemodynamics. As the mammalian embryo grows, it depends increasingly on placental blood flow for blood oxygenation and nutrition (Cross et al., 1994), and the placenta increases its volume, fetal capillary bed, and oxygen diffusion capacity through much of gestation to accommodate such increasing demands (Coan, 2004). In the mouse embryo, studies consistently have demonstrated steady increases in both systolic and end-diastolic flow velocities and in blood flow volume (MacLennan and Keller, 1999; Mu and Adamson, 2006; Phoon et al., 2000; Shah, 2004) from early stages onward. Peak systolic flow velocities in the umbilical artery increase in roughly linear fashion, averaging ~20 mm/s at E9.5, ~50–60 mm/s at E11.5–12.5, and ~90–100 mm/s at E14.5 (Mu and Adamson, 2006; Phoon et al., 2000), while blood flow volume increases in a geometric fashion (MacLennan and Keller, 1999). End-diastolic forward flow in the umbilical artery is absent through stages of cardiogenesis and into early fetal life, approximately until E16 (MacLennan and Keller, 1999; Mu and Adamson, 2006; Phoon et al., 2000), which suggests high placental impedance. Notably, the appearance of nonzero end-diastolic umbilical blood flow occurs shortly after the end of organogenesis in both mice and human beings (Mu and Adamson, 2006). Our laboratory first suggested that this Doppler parameter of absent end-diastolic flow was insensitive to the decreases in placental impedance occurring in the normally developing embryo (Phoon et al., 2000; Phoon, 2001). However, the presence of antegrade end-diastolic flow in the umbilical artery may be attributed not only to increasing placental vascularity (and decreasing impedance) but perhaps also to increasing aortic capacitance (Mu and Adamson, 2006) (Figure 2–3). In human embryos, umbilical arterial flow increases from 5+ weeks onward (Makikallio et al., 1999, 2005) and intervillous arterial flow velocities increase steadily (Kurjak and Kupesic, 1998). Moreover, the placental vascular impedance decreases steadily as gestation progresses, as evidenced by increasing, nonzero, forward end-diastolic flow that first becomes evident at 13–17 weeks of gestational age (Guzman et al., 1990); reductions in or elimination of the end-diastolic flow velocity in the umbilical artery has been clearly correlated with placental pathology and increased placental impedance (Adamson, 1999).

Umbilical venous flow is pulsatile in the mouse embryo and fetus through stages encompassing cardiogenesis and even through term (Mu and Adamson, 2006; Phoon et al., 2000), in contrast to human fetuses, which exhibit a mostly flat, nonpulsatile flow

profile by approximately 23 weeks of gestation. While in human fetal echocardiography such pulsations are attributed to retrograde waves caused by cardiac contractions (Mu and Adamson, 2006) and are often seen with right heart failure (Hofstaetter, 2006; Huhta, 2005), we have speculated that umbilical venous pulsatility may be related to higher placental impedance, especially the capacitance component, which permits transmission of the umbilical arterial pulsation to the umbilical vein (Phoon et al., 2000).

Peripheral resistance or impedance will also be influenced by the distribution of the cardiac output between the embryo and extraembryonic circulation, although little work has been done in this area. Hu et al. (1996) found that the proportion of the cardiac output distributed to the extraembryonic beds in the chick, namely the vitelline circulation, decreases with gestation. In our laboratory, we also found a decreasing proportion of the cardiac flow volume in the dorsal aorta coursing to the placenta as gestation advanced from E12.5–E14.5 in the normal mouse (Phoon et al., 2004).

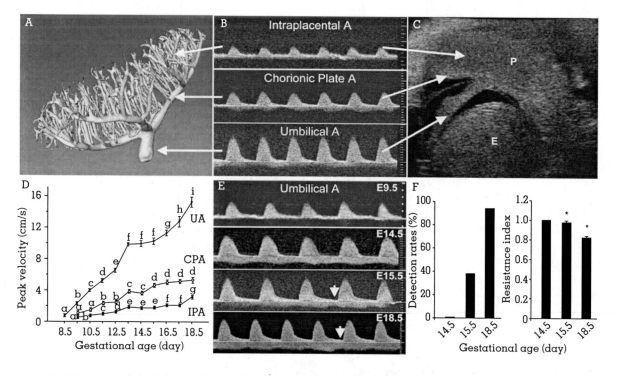

FIGURE 2–3. Umbilicoplacental circulation. A: Image of arterial vasculature (>20 µm diameter) supplied by the umbilical artery was obtained by microcomputed tomography. Umbilical cord has a single umbilical artery (UA) that gives rise to branches known as chorionic plate arteries (CPA) that run along the surface of the chorionic plate. Intraplacental arteries (IPA) are perpendicular branches that penetrate deeply into the placental labyrinth. B: Doppler velocity waveforms recorded from UA, CPA, and IPA. Positive-velocity waveforms were arterial, whereas negative-velocity waveforms were caused by venous flow within Doppler sample volume. C: Example of UBM image of embryonic placental circulation from pregnant mouse in vivo. D: Peak systolic velocity in UA, CPA, and IPA increased significantly with gestational age. E, embryo; P, placenta. Different letters indicate significant changes with gestational age (P <0.05). E: umbilical arterial end-diastolic velocity (arrow) was not observed in velocity waveforms at E9.5 and E14.5 but progressively appeared toward term. F: detection rate for end-diastolic velocity increased and resistance index decreased with gestational age (*P <0.001 vs. E14.5). (From Mu and Adamson, 2006. Copyright © The American Physiological Society, 2006, used with permission.)

Alterations in hemodynamics, such as occurs with pacing (MacLennan and Keller, 1999) and in abnormal models with outflow tract regurgitation (Phoon et al., 2004; Shah, 2004), and increased placental impedance (Dubiel et al., 2003), appear to alter the distribution of flow between the placenta and embryo proper, and would likely have global effects on the impedance seen by the embryonic heart.

Afterload

The afterload "seen" by the ventricles increases as gestation progresses, because ventricular wall stress increases (Lin and Taber, 1995). As noted above, however, peripheral vascular resistance decreases as the peripheral vascular bed expands. In the developing chick, as pulse pressure increases, vascular resistance decreases geometrically from approximately 25 peripheral resistance units at HH12 to less than 1 unit at HH29 (Clark and Hu, 1982; Hu and Clark, 1989; Hu et al., 2000; Keller et al., 1991; Nakazawa et al., 1988; Zahka et al., 1989). The dynamic characteristics of the vascular bed also change: changes in impedance moduli in the dorsal aorta indicate shifts in wave reflection sites that reflect compliance of the vascular bed (Zahka et al., 1989).

The questions of how myocardial wall stress and regional strain influence cardiac development have been the purview of the relatively nascent field of cardiac biomechanics. Here, investigators try to characterize precisely the loads (stress, strain) on the heart and vasculature that govern morphogenesis and developmental adaptation, and viscoelastic properties of the developing myocardium (Ling et al., 2002; Miller, 1997a, 1997b; Taber, 1998; Taber et al., 1992; Taber and Miller, 1995). Wall stress and strain depend on the interaction of ventricular (or vessel) geometry, loading conditions, and material properties (Taber et al., 1992). Most of the work in this area has been performed in the embryonic chick model.

As an approximation, the HH16 chick ventricle can be modeled as a thick-walled, pseudoelastic cylindrical shell composed of three isotropic layers undergoing large deformation. Embryonic myocardium exhibits such properties as material nonlinearity, viscoelastic and poroelastic behavior, residual strain, and muscle activation (Ling et al., 2002; Taber et al., 1992). In passive stress–strain experiments, in vitro excised embryonic myocardium displayed preconditioning, hysteresis, and nonlinearity, which are properties of mature myocardium (Miller, 1997b). A model of stress-induced growth based on highly idealized diastolic behavior of embryonic myocardium was found to fit experimental data to a good first approximation (Lin and Taber, 1995). Regional wall strain data

suggest that myocardial shortening is maintained within a relatively narrow range, despite dramatic maturation in cardiomyocyte architecture, loading conditions, and cycle length (Taber and Miller, 1995; Taber et al., 1994), consistent with more global estimates of ejection fraction mentioned above. Therefore, normal cardiac growth in the early embryo may be biomechanically similar to volume overload hypertrophy, otherwise termed concentric hypertrophy; here, cavity volume increases in proportion to myocardial wall thickness so that the same ejection fraction results in a greater stroke volume as the heart increases in size (Taber et al., 1992). Still, patterns of ventricular deformation apparently change from globally isotropic to chamber-specific anisotropic during early morphogenesis (Tobita, 2000b).

Despite the high peripheral resistance in the young embryo, the very early ventricle, with lower pressures and a smaller cavity, would be subjected to wall stresses—and therefore actual ventricular afterload—far lower than in the older animal. Nevertheless, even small regional variations in mechanical forces, ventral bending and torsion in particular, appear to be important in such morphogenetic events as cardiac looping (Ramasubramanian et al., 2006). While ventral bending is driven mainly by active myocardial cell-shape changes (Ramasubramanian et al., 2006), torsion is exerted by external forces by structures such as the splanchnopleure (Nerurkar et al., 2006). Wall stress increases steadily during development (Lin and Taber, 1995). However, there appears to be significant regional differences in wall stress within the embryonic ventricle. Studies in HH18 chick have shown the passive stiffness of the dorsal ventricular wall to be greater than that of the ventral wall, and it was suggested that these changes likely influence the function and morphogenesis of the developing embryonic heart (Chabert and Taber, 2002). Computational fluid dynamics also predicts that intracardiac variations in shear are likely to influence morphogenesis (DeGroff et al., 2003).

Ventriculo-Vascular Interaction

The complex interplay between the embryonic ventricle and the vascular bed, or ventriculovascular interaction, appears to contribute to both cardiac growth and vascular expansion. The work performed by a ventricle can be differentiated into oscillatory and steady-state power components. Data suggest that oscillatory power comprises a larger proportion of total hydraulic power in the early embryo than in the mature circulation, and imply that the ventricle "wastes" more power on producing pulsatility; investigators have speculated that such oscillatory power may contribute to the distension needed to promote growth of the vascular bed (Yoshigi et al., 1996; Zahka et al., 1989). The observation that oscillatory power appears to be maintained even during circulatory derangements suggests that energy efficiency for vascular growth is tightly controlled (Yoshigi et al., 1996). In embryonic chick, wave propagation velocity increases with gestation and parallels changes in stroke volume and mean aortic pressure, findings that further indicate that pulsatile ventriculovascular interactions are tightly controlled throughout early development (Zahka et al., 1989).

Several experiments in the conotruncal banded chick embryo have demonstrated an adaptive response of the developing myocardium to chronically altered loads (Miller et al., 2003; Tobita et al., 2002; Tobita et al., 2005). For example, the left ventricle is able to normalize stress and strain chronically after conotruncal banding (Tobita et al., 2002), although in another study, stress–strain relationships were significantly stiffer (Miller et al., 2003). Three-dimensional myofiber architecture matured precociously following conotruncal banding (Tobita et al., 2005). What is not known is how such adaptive responses by the developing myocardium protect either normal cardiac morphogenesis or normal angiogenesis, if at all.

The preinnervated embryo appears to be capable of regulating peripheral vascular tone, although mechanisms are as yet undefined (Casillas et al., 1994; Yoshigi et al., 1996). For example, in response to volume depletion, chick embryos increase peripheral vascular resistance and maintain blood pressure at the expense of blood volumetric flow without significant changes in either proximal (aortic) resistance or oscillatory power as a proportion of total power (Yoshigi et al., 1996). In more recent experiments, chick embryos, which had undergone ligation of the vitelline artery, continued to maintain arterial pressure at the expense of changes in flow and arterial resistance (Lucitti et al., 2005). These results are somewhat surprising, in light of the influence of shear forces on both cardiac and vascular development, but the complexity of the interplay between wall stress and cyclical strain, pulsatility, and shear is evident. In any case, the embryonic cardiovascular system appears to be able to optimize ventriculovascular coupling by altering peripheral vascular tone in response to alterations in loading conditions (Keller et al., 1994; Lucitti et al., 2005; Yoshigi et al., 1996).

VALVE FUNCTION

The embryonic heart is able to function without anatomic valves for some time in early gestation. Most studies have demonstrated that the atrioventricular inflow orifice does not regurgitate during systole (Campbell et al., 1992; Gui et al., 1996; Hu et al., 2000), and data have long supported the concept of dynamic closure of the endocardial cushions, which then function as rudimentary valves (Patten et al., 1948). The outflow tract also does not regurgitate before the proper development of the semilunar valves, and recent data indicate a valve-like function of the outflow tract endocardial cushions as well, even before the development of the valves proper, in the mouse (Phoon et al., 2006a). This is illustrated by the lack of retrograde diastolic flow in the dorsal aorta in the chick (Clark et al., 1986; Hu and Clark, 1989), and mouse (Ji et al., 2003; Phoon et al., 2000, 2004). However, both insensitivity of instrumentation and the embryonic stages studied may have contributed to this traditional view of unidirectional flow throughout embryogenesis. New data employing high-speed, high-resolution video microscopy have now shown that the circulation is not in fact unidirectional from the earliest stages of cardiovascular functioning. In the mouse, Nishii et al. (2006) discovered consistent "to–fro" immature flow across the atrioventricular orifice during early peristaltic contractions in the pre-15-somite embryo. Unidirectional flow was established only at approximately the 20-somite stage, correlating with the development of the endocardial cushions, and when the entire ventricle began to exhibit true, almost simultaneous contractions that probably marked the development of the emerging conduction system (Nishii and Shibata, 2006). Liebling et al. (2006) found even more intriguing results in the zebrafish. At 26–28 hpf, close to the initiation of the heartbeat, unidirectional flow was present even in the absence of any valve tissue or valve-like structure; recall, however, that blood is being propelled not by peristaltic contractions exactly, but by the action of a suction pump (Forouhar, 2006; Liebling et al., 2006). From 33 hpf through to about 72–96 hpf, bidirectional flow predominated, even when thickening of the atrioventricular and ventriculobulbar boundaries became evident at 48 hpf and 60 hpf, respectively, and dynamic expansion and closure of the endocardial rings was observed. Unidirectional, nonregurgitant, flow was established in all zebrafish embryos only at 111 hpf, accompanied by developing endocardial cushions (Liebling et al., 2006).

A pressure gradient between the ventricle and the arterial system, whether in the aorta or vitelline artery (Clark et al., 1986; Hu and Clark, 1989; Hu et al., 2000; Nakazawa et al., 1995), suggests the presence of dynamic obstruction at the conotruncal level (Gui et al., 1996; Keller et al., 1996), or in the aortic arches (Clark et al., 1986; Hu et al., 2000). Prior to true valve formation at approximately E13 in the mouse (Hurle et al., 1980; Phoon et al., 2004; Viragh and Chalice,

1981), the outflow tract endocardial cushions appose dynamically in a valve-like fashion, likely accounting for the observed ventriculoarterial pressure gradient described in embryo systems (Clark et al., 1986; Hu and Clark, 1989, 2000). Pressure gradients in the aortic arches are also speculated to play an important role in aortic arch selection (Clark et al., 1986). The presence of flow streams in the aorta may also be implicated in the modeling and normal development of the aortic arches (Kosaki et al., 1997).

Valves, or valve-like functioning of the endocardial cushions, is necessary not only for efficient unidirectional blood flow, but also to maintain the arterial diastolic pressures that generate a coronary artery perfusion head. The acute intrauterine deaths of *NFATc1-/-* mouse embryos lacking outflow tract valves at E13.5–15.5 raise the speculation of whether this is indeed the stage at which the coronary arterial supply to the embryonic myocardium becomes absolutely necessary (Phoon et al., 2004).

BLOOD

A review of the developing functional circulatory system would not be complete without the consideration of developing blood cells, and in particular the red blood cells that carry oxygen throughout the body (Baron, 2003; McGrath and Palis, 2005; McGrath et al., 2003; Palis et al., 1999; Tavian and Péault, 2005). The extraembryonic yolk sac is the earliest and only source of hematopoietic progenitors in the early vertebrate and mammalian embryo. Primitive erythroid progenitors originate from the mesodermal cells of the yolk sac before establishment of circulation in the embryo proper. These progenitors then give rise to maturing erythroblasts within the yolk sac blood islands, which begin to form at ~E7.5 in the mouse, or between the second to third week of human gestation. There is also accumulating evidence of hemogenic endothelium as a source of hematopoietic stem cells (see McGrath and Palis, 2005; Tavian and Péault, 2005). The close apposition of mesoderm and visceral endoderm in the gastrulating embryo and mature yolk sac, along with experimental evidence, suggests that interactions between primitive endoderm and mesoderm might play roles in the initiation of both embryonic hematopoiesis and vasculogenesis (Baron, 2003).

At E8.25 in the mouse, the heart begins its first discernible contractions and propels primitive erythroblasts into the circulation (Ji et al., 2003). Depending somewhat on the study quoted, erythroblasts are detected in the embryo proper between the 3- and 5-somite stages (Ji et al., 2003; McGrath et al., 2003;

Tavian and Péault, 2005), or at 21 days of human gestation (Tavian and Péault, 2005) (Figure 2–4).

Shortly after colonization by hematopoietic elements, the liver emerges as a hematopoietic organ at ~E10 and soon becomes the site of definitive erythroid maturation in the embryo, followed later by the spleen and bone marrow (McGrath and Palis, 2005; Tavian and Péault, 2005). It is notable that the initial wave of erythroblasts from yolk sac to embryo proper are considered primitive, and these mature in the embryonic bloodstream; this sequence of events occurs most likely because of the need in the mammalian embryo for the rapid establishment of a functional cardiovascular system that includes oxygen-carrying media (Copp, 1995; McGrath and Palis, 2005). Definitive erythrocytes are first noted in the bloodstream at ~E11.5–12.5 (Kingsley, 2004; McGrath and Palis, 2005). Morphologically, the erythrocytes exhibit marked changes over gestation: as a generalization, earlier and more primitive erythrocytes are larger and contain larger nuclei than later, more mature erythrocytes; such changes appear to be responsible for the changes in ultrasound backscatter seen throughout gestation (Le Floc'h et al., 2004).

The data on oxygen-carrying capacity—specifically the red cell mass and hematocrit—in the developing embryo are rather scant. Published erythrocyte counts in normal mouse embryos are approximately 4×10^5 per mm^3 at E12, and $6–10 \times 10^5$ mm^3 at E14, compared with $4–5 \times 10^6$ per mm^3 in the early newborn mouse; from these numbers, Phoon et al. (2002) estimated the hematocrit at E11.5–14.5 to be in the range of 5%–10%, yielding a kinematic viscosity of 0.016–0.017 stokes, which is 1.2–1.3 times that of plasma. Using confocal line scanning, investigators have recently found the hematocrit to increase slightly from approximately 15% at E8.5 to ~20% of total intravascular volume at E10.5 (Jones et al., 2004); it should be noted that unless the erythrocytes are spherical, this method may overestimate the hematocrit. Le Floc'h et al. (2004) measured hematocrit from blood samples taken from the umbilical cord in mouse embryos, increasing from 12% at E13.5 to 29% at E15.5, with little further change to E17.5. As one other measure of red cell mass within the mouse embryo proper, McGrath et al. (2003) determined the density of red blood cells as a percentage of the total cells in the embryo: after E9, there was a sharp increase in the density of red cells in the embryo, reaching an equilibrium, or plateau, of 40% at approximately E10. This increase in red cell density corresponded tightly with the development of the vascular bed and functional cardiac parameters (McGrath et al., 2003). The data suggest that by approximately E10.5, the embryonic

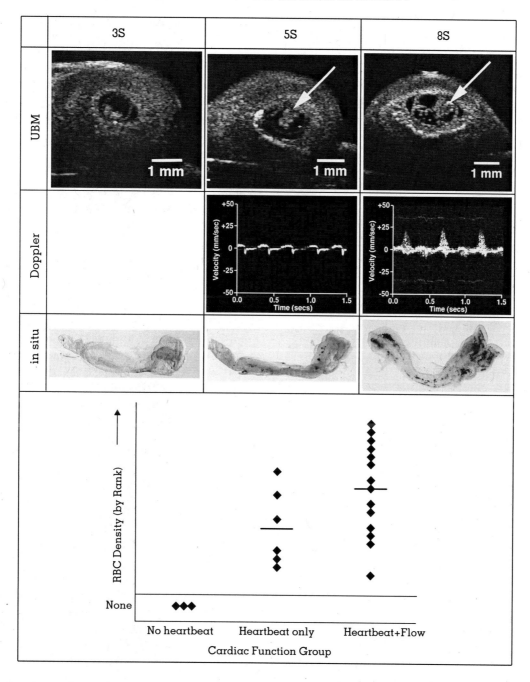

FIGURE 2–4. Correlation of UBM-Doppler cardiac functional parameters with whole-mount in situ hybridization in the early mouse embryo. Representative data at the 3-somite (3S), 5-somite (5S), and 8-somite (8S) stages are shown. Arrows show the embryonic heart. At 3S, neither a heartbeat nor Doppler flow was detectable. At 5S, only a heartbeat was present by UBM; the panel shows maternal respirations, distinct from embryonic Doppler blood flow. At 3S, when there is no heartbeat, no erythroblasts (RBCs) are seen within the embryo; at 5S, with a heartbeat, few RBCs; and at 8S, with Doppler flow, many RBCs. In the bottom panel, UBM-Doppler functional category is plotted against RBC density ranking (bars show mean rank). No embryos lacking a heartbeat showed any cells, whereas maturation of cardiac function as characterized by UBM-Doppler correlated with RBC density ranking. (From Ji et al., 2003. Copyright © Lippincott Williams & Wilkins, 2003, used with permission.)

circulation has been established for rigorous support of the growing embryo. However, it is not at this time clear how to associate these results with the somewhat discrepant estimates of embryonic hematocrit above.

In addition, erythrocyte oxygen-carrying capacity also depends on the evolution of different hemoglobin forms produced by the cell, which is beyond the scope of this chapter.

HUMAN MODELS OF ABNORMAL HEMODYNAMICS LEADING TO CARDIAC MALFORMATIONS

Hemodynamics have been implicated in the etiology and progression of human fetal heart disease (for review, see Gardiner, 2005). We will briefly discuss two illustrative examples in which abnormal hemodynamics can lead to human congenital heart malformations, hypoplastic left heart syndrome (HLHS), and twin-to-twin transfusion syndrome (TTTS).

Hypoplastic Left Heart Syndrome

HLHS is a heterogeneous group of CHD characterized by a small or absent LV with an underdeveloped aortic valve and usually mitral valve. Without treatment, there is a 95% mortality rate in the first month of life (Rosenthal, 1996), and HLHS accounts for approximately half of CHD-related mortality in the first week of life (Khoshnood et al., 2005). Although familial occurrence of HLHS occurring in families with associated left-sided cardiac disease indicate a contributory genetic component, it is well-established that aortic stenosis (AS) in the midgestation fetus without LV abnormalities can progress to HLHS at birth, due to aberrations in blood flow through the left heart (Gruber and Epstein, 2004; Tworetzky et al., 2004). Hemodynamics have been postulated to play a major role in the development of HLHS (Grossfeld, 1999; Sedmera et al., 2005), and for some time, in utero intervention has been postulated to prevent the progression of congenital aortic stenosis into HLHS by improving left heart hemodynamics (Kohl et al., 2000; Sedmera et al., 2005), but only recently have advances in fetal medicine made fetal intervention truly feasible, with hopeful early results. Tworetzky et al. (2004) demonstrated that, in fetuses likely to progress to HLHS, balloon aortic valvuloplasty improved aortic and mitral valve growth in all who survived the procedure, although only a small number achieved biventricular repair postnatally. More recently, Makikallio et al. (2006) detailed several physiological markers in midgestation that may predict evolution of AS into HLHS: (1) the presence of reversed flow in the transverse aortic arch, (2) monophasic flow across the mitral valve, (3) left-to-right flow across the foramen ovale, and (4) LV dysfunction. All of these physiological markers reduce blood flow in and out of the left ventricle and into the aortic arch. It is therefore clearly logical that such abnormal physiological features should contribute to the definition of a "final" morphology of HLHS. However, an important question remains of when a left ventricle can no longer recover despite improvement of hemodynamics with fetal aortic balloon valvuloplasty (Makikallio et al., 2006).

Twin-to-Twin Transfusion Syndrome

In TTTS, it is believed that deep intraplacental vascular connections cause an unstable equilibrium, causing a shift of blood flow from the donor to recipient twin. Most of the cardiovascular compromise occurs in the recipient twin, and mortality is high. In addition to the volume load imposed on the recipient twin, there is mounting evidence that alterations in the renin–angiotensin system, as well as hypertensive mediators such as endothelin-1, are associated with the pathophysiology of TTTS. Recipient twins can develop a progressive cardiomyopathy, in which hypertrophy dominates over dilatation, with suprasystemic right ventricular pressures and atrioventricular valve regurgitation that may lead to hydrops and intrauterine demise (see Harkness and Crombleholme, 2005; Pedra et al., 2002; Rychik, 2004).

In a subset of patients, the right ventricular hypertrophic cardiomyopathy can evolve to such a degree as to cause infundibular pulmonary stenosis and leads even to pulmonary atresia (Harkness and Crombleholme, 2005; Lougheed et al., 2001; Marton et al., 2001; Nizard et al., 2001; Karatza et al., 2002; Rychik, 2004). This phenomenon can best be described as an "acquired" form of CHD and supports the notion that certain forms of CHD may be the consequence of altered cardiac hemodynamics in utero (Rychik, 2004). Further supporting the concept that altered hemodynamics are responsible for the CHD in TTTS, a recently published series demonstrated that selective laser ablation of placental anastomoses improved biventricular systolic and diastolic function, and even resolved two cases of functional pulmonary atresia; postnatally, neither progressive myocardial hypertrophy nor anatomical right ventricular outflow tract obstruction was found (Barrea et al., 2006). On the other hand, another recent series found an incidence of pulmonary outflow obstruction of 7.8%, with a total incidence of CHD of 11.2%, despite treatment with intrauterine laser coagulation of placental anastomoses with resolution of TTTS (Herberg, 2006). Thus, we still do not fully understand the precise hemodynamic contributions found in TTTS to CHD.

ANIMAL MODELS OF ABNORMAL HEMODYNAMICS LEADING TO CARDIAC MALFORMATIONS

Studies in the zebrafish, chick, and mouse embryo have thus far provided invaluable insight into the role of hemodynamics in cardiovascular morphogenesis using genetic and surgical manipulation techniques. Mechanical load is one of the major epigenetic factors regulating embryonic cardiovascular function and structure during morphogenesis. Developing cardiovascular systems operate at a pressure of approximately 0.1–1 mmHg, and even minor perturbations in hemodynamics can cause profound changes on morphologic development. Most such experiments have examined the role of reduced load on cardiogenesis, given the clinical importance of HLHS. It should be noted that a relative lack of "pure" abnormal physiological models makes extrapolation to human CHD difficult.

Preload has been manipulated in genetic models through the targeting of atrial functioning and mechanically, via left atrial ligation, vitelline vein ligation, and bead occlusion of cardiac inflow. Taken together, the data strongly indicate that reductions in ventricular load appear to alter both hemodynamic parameters and material properties of the embryonic myocardium that may play critical roles in proper cardiac morphogenesis.

To lend support to the notion that early atrial function and ventricular filling influence ventricular morphogenesis, one can look at the *weak-atrium* (*wea*) zebrafish model described by Berdougo et al. (2003). Defects are observed in both cardiac chambers in the zebrafish: contractility defects in the atrium as well as morphological defects in the ventricle. Mutant mice deficient in atrial myosin heavy chain protein (*Amhc -/-*) have deficient atrial contractions beginning at the first heart beat (a consequence of disrupted atrial sarcomere assembly), but their ventricular heart rate remains unchanged (similar to the MLC2a mouse [Huang et al., 2003; see below]). Despite some circulation, a characteristic blood pool forms caudal to the atrium, indicating an inefficient blood flow relative to wild-type controls. At 48 hpf, the ventricle becomes more compacted and thick-walled compared to wild-type controls, although sarcomere assembly proceeds normally. Notably, the increased ventricular wall thickness does not appear to be caused by excess cellular proliferation, although clearly some sort of reorganization occurs. Because expression of *atrial myosin heavy chain (ahmc)* is restricted to the atrium, the ventricular phenotype, including defects in chamber circumference, wall thickness, lumen size, and gene expression, are felt to be an epigenetic response of the ventricle to atrial dysfunction. In their discussion and comparison with other zebrafish mutants, Berdougo et al. (2003) suggest that reduced blood flow alone is not necessarily sufficient to provoke the ventricular phenotypes observed in *wea* mutants.

Huang et al. (2003) developed mice deficient in myosin light chain (MLC) 2a, one of two major myosin isoforms in cardiac muscle, to evaluate the influences of early atrial function on cardiac morphogenesis. With growth retardation evident by E9.0–9.25, mice with the inactivated *Mlc2a* gene exhibited uniform embryonic lethality at E10.5–11.5 from cardiovascular

insufficiency, as evidenced by severe chest edema (Huang et al., 2003). Compared to wild-type littermates, these mutants started to show differences in morphogenesis as early as E8.5 (8–10 somite stage), shortly after the time of initiation of the heartbeat observed by other researchers (Ji et al., 2003; Nishii and Shibata, 2006). The mutant heart tubes at this stage were enlarged, without clear distinctions between the bulbus arteriosus and the future ventricles. Cardiac looping was observed in null embryos, but with aberrance in the distribution of cardiac segments among all studied embryos. The atria and outflow tracts were enlarged. Also observed were distinct differences in the ventricular myocyte architecture, with mutant embryos displaying thin-walled, dilated ventricles with underdeveloped trabeculations (Huang et al., 2003). Interestingly, there was little difference in ventricular function, as judged by the rate of ventricular beating, although true hemodynamic studies were not performed; in any case, myofibrillar development and organization in the ventricular myocardium appeared normal. In addition, there was a lack of activated endocardial cell migration into the cardiac jelly, which has been shown to be important for the development of atrioventricular valves. These embryos did not survive long enough to determine whether the formation of atrioventricular valves occurred in the absence of cardiac jelly seeding (Huang et al., 2003). Finally, MLC2a-deficient embryos displayed defects in formation of intraembryonic and yolk sac vasculature. Huang's above study showed that atrial function plays key roles in the progression of ventricular myocyte architecture, looping mechanics, and possibly atrioventricular valve formation. They postulated that the morphologic abnormalities seen in *Mlc2a -/-* mice, both in cardiogenesis and in angiogenesis, resulted from altered hemodynamics in the developing heart.

It is notable that in the *wea* zebrafish mutant and the *Mlc2a* mouse mutant, despite what should be similar defects in atrial functioning, ventricular dysmorphogenesis is in fact somewhat different. Whereas the *Mlc2a* mouse mutant displays a dilated and thin-walled ventricle, the *wea* zebrafish mutant exhibits a thick-walled, compacted ventricle. Nevertheless, the data strongly argue for normal preloading of the embryonic ventricle to permit normal ventricular morphogenesis; proposed mechanisms of the problems seen include mechanical (hemodynamic) fluid forces (pressure, shear) or oxygen/nutrient delivery (Berdougo et al., 2003; Huang et al., 2003).

Techniques to induce mechanical obstruction of blood flow have been most extensively implemented in the chick. Sedmera et al. (2002) showed that a reduction in LV volume load via LAL in the chick embryo resulted in structural phenotypes similar to that seen in HLHS. At the cellular level, decreased cellular proliferation, levels of myosin, and growth factors were evident, suggesting that changes in cardiomyocyte proliferation play a significant role in the pathogenesis of HLHS (Figure 2–5).

Tobita et al. (2005) studied changes in timing and organization of myofiber architecture in chick embryos HH stage 21–36 after left atrial ligation (LAL). During normal development, transmural myofiber distribution in LV compact myocardium changes from a uniform circumferential orientation to a more differentiated pattern wherein the endocardium shows a more circumferential organization than the epicardium. When LV load was reduced via LAL, investigators found an association with immature transmural patterns of myofiber orientation.

Changes in microtubule content and distribution in response to altered mechanical load have been shown to affect cardiomyocyte structure and function. Schroder et al. (2002) studied microtubule involvement in developing chick myocardium in response to altered mechanical hemodynamics and found an increase in microtubule density after decreasing LV load via LAL. This may partially explain the increased passive stiffness observed in the LV of the LAL model; for the low-pressure embryonic cardiovascular system, changes in diastolic function may be a critical regulatory pathway during cardiac morphogenesis.

In the vitelline vein ligation (VVL) chick model, extra-embryonic blood flow is manipulated without direct mechanical interference with the heart. VVL causes a detour of venous inflow to the heart, altering intracardiac blood flow patterns (Hogers, 1999). Common malformations thought to be derived from these VVL-induced flow changes include ventricular septal defect, semilunar valve anomalies, AV anomalies, and pharyngeal arch artery malformations (Stekelenburg-de Vos et al., 2003). Stekelenburg-de Vos et al. (2003) studied the instantaneous hemodynamic effects of VVL in HH 17 chick embryos, following HR, blood flow velocities, acceleration, and stroke volume. They noted acute decreases in all hemodynamic parameters measured. Later pressure–volume loop analyses in the VVL chick showed decreased contractility of the ventricle one day after venous clipping that may have accounted for the hemodynamic derangements (Stekelenburg-de Vos et al., 2005). Moreover, diastolic properties of the embryonic myocardium appear to be altered by VVL, specifically with reduced passive ventricular filling (Ursem et al., 2004).

The studies cited so far have demonstrated mechanical influences primarily on gross morphological and functional changes. Mechanical occlusion of the cardiac flow using a surgically placed bead has yielded additional insights into some of the fluid forces present in the developing embryo and their possible relationship to gene expression in zebrafish (Hove et al., 2003). One

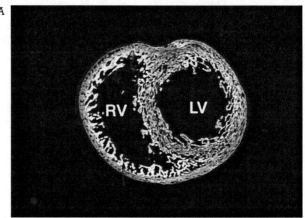

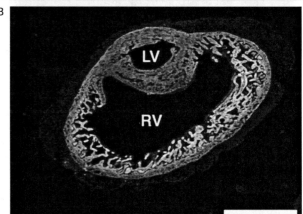

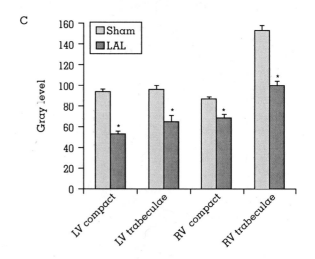

FIGURE 2–5. Myosin expression in the stage 34 chick embryo. Example of antimyosin staining in A: sham and B: LAL hearts. C: Quantification of immunostaining shows a significant decrease in LAL hearts. (From Sedmera et al., 2002. Copyright © Wiley-Liss, Inc., 2002. Reprinted with permission of Wiley-Liss, Inc., a subsidiary of John Wiley & Sons, Inc.).

would expect increased intracardiac pressure after outflow tract occlusion and decreased pressures following inflow occlusion. Interestingly, investigators noted that both experimental models showed similar resultant cardiac phenotypes, with an abnormal third chamber (bulbus), abnormal heart looping, and fusion of inflow/outflow tracts (Hove et al., 2003). Based on these findings, it was suggested that the reduction in mechanical shear forces, and not changes in intracardiac pressure, was responsible for the generation of the observed phenotype; it was estimated that shear forces were reduced approximately 10-fold (Hove et al., 2003). Since the normal shear forces appear to be more than adequate in inducing gene expression, such a dramatic reduction in fluid forces may have important implications in cardiac development (Hove et al., 2003).

The VVL chick model has also provided clues to the link between hemodynamic forces and alterations in gene expression. KLF-2 (Krüppel-like factor), NOS-3 (nitric oxide synthase), and ET-1 (endothelin-1) are all factors expressed in specific regions of the developing myocardium and their expression is thought to be mediated by flow-induced shear forces (Dekker et al., 2002; Malek and Izumo, 1995). Dysregulated expression of these factors has been implicated in a wide variety of congenital malformations, including atrioventricular septal defects, pharyngeal arch abnormalities, and craniofacial deformities (Groenendijk et al., 2005). VVL studies have revealed upregulation of KLF-2 and NOS-3 expression in regions experiencing high shear stress and decreased ET-1 expression in low shear stress regions (Groenendijk et al., 2005). From these data, it was postulated that acute hemodynamic changes induced by VVL may cause changes in shear-stress-related gene expression, which in turn would lead to the formation of cardiac malformations observed in this model.

CONCLUSIONS AND FUTURE DIRECTIONS

We are currently at a nascent stage of intrauterine treatment for CHD (Makikallio et al., 2006; Tworetzky et al., 2004). Although it is clear that medical and surgical advances have greatly improved both life expectancy and quality of life for patients with CHD, it is also clear that much progress needs to be made, if we are to ultimately cure, and possibly even prevent, most CHDs. One of the tenets of pediatric cardiac care is that early therapy improves outcomes; that is, cardiovascular growth and development benefit from early correction or mitigation of hemodynamic aberrations. Therefore, a thorough understanding of cardiovascular biology in the immature organism, and of the specific relationships of structure to function, is needed to appropriately treat and manage CHD, even in the developing embryo and fetus.

The field of embryonic cardiovascular physiology is still a nascent one, but as summarized in this chapter,

progress has been marked by remarkable research advances over even the past half decade (see Phoon, 2001). Developmental cardiovascular physiology comprises researchers from many fields, including pediatric cardiology, molecular biology, developmental physiology, developmental zoology, and imaging physics, as well as vascular biology and developmental hematology. Animal models have proliferated, allowing for the study of abnormal hemodynamics, and its epigenetic influence on morphologic and functional cardiac development. New imaging and phenotyping approaches now permit detailed study of many aspects of cardiovascular physiology in the embryonic heart in such models.

Although much of CHD has genetic underpinnings, viable gene therapy is still many years into the future. As evident in this chapter, the manipulation of embryonic and fetal physiology and pharmacology may ultimately be an important epigenetic tool with which to mitigate or even prevent congenital heart defects.

REFERENCES

Adamson SL. Arterial pressure, vascular input impedance, and resistance as determinants of pulsatile blood flow in the umbilical artery. *Eur J Obstet Gynecol Reprod Biol.* 1999;84:119–125.

Alcolea S, Theveniau-Ruissy M, Jarry-Guichard T, et al. Downregulation of connexin 45 gene products during mouse heart development. *Circ Res.* 1999;80: 88–94.

Anderson PA. The heart and development. *Semin Perinatol.* 1996;20:482–509.

Anderson PA, Glick KL, Killam AP, Mainwaring RD. The effect of heart rate on in utero left ventricular output in the fetal sheep. *J Physiol.* 1986;372:557–573.

Anderson PA, Glick KL, Manring A, Crenshaw C. Developmental changes in cardiac contractility in fetal and postnatal sheep: in vitro and in vivo. *Am J Physiol Heart Circ Physiol.* 1984;247:371–379.

Artman M, Henry G, Coetzee WA. Cellular basis for age-related differences in cardiac excitation-contraction coupling. *Prog Pediatr Cardiol.* 2000;11:185–194.

Baron MH. Embryonic origins of mammalian hematopoiesis. *Exp Hematol.* 2003;31:1160–1169.

Barrea C, Hornberger LK, Alkazaleh F, et al. Impact of selective laser ablation of placental anastomoses on the cardiovascular pathology of the recipient twin in severe twin-twin transfusion syndrome. *Am J Obstet Gynecol.* 2006;195:1388–1395.

Berdougo E, Coleman H, Lee DH, Stainier DY, Yelon D. Mutation of weak atrium/atrial myosin heavy chain disrupts atrial function and influences ventricular morphogenesis in zebrafish. *Development.* 2003;130:6121–6129.

Braunstein JB, Donovan M, Hughes S. Assessment of ventricular relaxation in the embryo using a monoexponential model. *Am J Physiol.* 1994;267:H631–H635.

Broekhuizen ML, Mast F, Strujik PC. Hemodynamic parameters of stage 20 to stage 35 chick embryo. *Pediatr Res.* 1993;34:44–46.

Broekhuizen ML, Hogers B, DeRuiter MC. Altered hemodynamics in chick embryos after extraembryonic venous obstruction. *Pediatr Res.* 1999;13:437–445.

Bruneau BG. Transcriptional regulation of vertebrate cardiac morphogenesis. *Circ Res.* 2002;90:509–519.

Burggren WW. What is the purpose of the embryonic heartbeat? Or how facts can ultimately prevail over physiological dogma. *Physiol Biochem Zool.* 2004;77:333–345.

Burggren WW, Warburton SJ, Slivkoff MD. Interruption of cardiac output does not affect short-term growth and metabolic rate in day 3 and 4 chick embryos. *J Exp Biol.* 2000;203:3831–3838.

Campbell KA, Hu N, Clark EB. Analysis of dynamic atrial dimension and function during early cardiac development in the chick embryo. *Pediatr Res.* 1992;32:333–337.

Casillas CB, Tinney JP, Keller BB. Influence of alterations in cycle length on ventricular function in chick embryos. *Am J Physiol.* 1994;267:H905–H911.

Chabert S, Taber LA. Intramyocardial pressure measurements in the stage 18 embryonic chick heart. *Am J Physiol Heart Circ Physiol.* 2002;282:H1248–H1254.

Cheanchevai V, Hughes SF, Benson DW. Relation between cardiac cycle length and ventricular relaxation rate in the chick embryo. *Pediatr Res.* 1992;13:480–482.

Chui DHK, Liao S, Walker K. Foetal erythropoiesis in Steel mutant mice. *Blood.* 1978;51:539–547.

Cirotto C, Arangi I. Chick embryo survival under acute carbon monoxide challenges. *Comp Biochem Physiol A.* 1989;94:117–123.

Clark EB, Hu N. Developmental hemodynamic changes in the chick embryo from stage 18 to 27. *Circ Res.* 1982;51:810–815.

Clark EB, Hu N. Hemodynamics of the developing cardiovascular system. *Ann NY Acad Sci.* 1990;588:41–47.

Clark EB, Hu N, Dummett JL. Ventricular function and morphology in chick embryo from stage 18 to 29. *Am J Physiol.* 1986;250:407–413.

Coan PM, Ferguson-Smith AC, Burton GJ. Developmental dynamics of the definitive mouse placenta assessed by stereology. *Biol Reprod.* 2004;70:1806–1813.

Colan SD, Parness IA, Spevak PJ, Sanders SP. Developmental modulation of myocardial mechanics: age- and growth-related alterations in afterload and contractility. *J Am Coll Cardiol.* 1992;19:619–629.

Conway SJ, Agnieska KF, Kneer PL, Machnicki M, Koushik SV. What cardiovascular defect does my mouse have, and why? *Genesis.* 2003;35:1–21.

Copp AJ. Death before birth: clues from gene knockouts and mutations. *Trends Genet.* 1995;11:87–93.

Cross JC, Werb Z, Fisher SJ. Implantation and the placenta: key pieces of the development puzzle. *Science.* 1994;266:1508–1518.

Da Costa G, Filho MF, Spara P, Barreto GE, Netto VS. Fetal hemodynamics evaluated by Doppler velocimetry in the second half of pregnancy. *Ultrasound Med Biol.* 2005;31:1023–1030.

DeGroff CG, Thronburg BL, Pentecost JO, Gharib M, Sahn DJ, Baptista A. Flow in the early embryonic human heart: a numerical study. *Pediatr Cardiol.* 2003;24:375–380.

Dekker RJ, Van Soest S, Fontijn RD, et al. Prolonged fluid shear stress induces a distinct set of endothelial cell genes, most specifically lung Kruppel-like factor (KLF-2). *Blood.* 2002;100:1689–1698.

Delorme B, Dahl E, Jarry-Guichard T, Briand JP, Willecke K, Gros D, Theveniau-Ruissy M. Expression pattern of connexin gene products at the early developmental stages of the mouse cardiovascular system. *Circ Res.* 1997;81:423–437.

Dickinson ME. Multimodal imaging of mouse development: tools for the postgenomic era. *Dev Dyn.* 2006;235:2386–2400.

Dietrich WF, Miller J, Steen R, et al. A comprehensive genetic map of the mouse genome. *Nature.* 1996;380:149–152.

Dubiel M, Breborowicz GH, Gudmundsson S. Evaluation of fetal circulation redistribution in pregnancies with absent or reversed diastolic flow in the umbilical artery. *Early Hum Dev.* 2003;71:149–156.

Ebert AM, Hume GL, Warren KS, et al. Calcium extrusion is critical for cardiac morphogenesis and rhythm in embryonic zebrafish hearts. *Proc Natl Acad Sci.* 2005;102:17705–17710.

Ehler E, Fowler VM, Perriard JC. Myofibrillogenesis in the developing chicken heart: role of actin isoforms and of the pointed end actin capping protein tropomodulin during thin filament assembly. *Dev Dyn.* 2004;229:745–755.

Ehler E, Rothen BM, Hammerle SP, Komiyama M, Perriard JC. Myofibrillogenesis in the developing chicken heart: assembly of Z-disk, M-line and thick filaments. *J Cell Sci.* 1999;112:1529–1539.

Eichmann A, Pardanaud L, Yuan L, Moyon D. Vasculogenesis and the search for the hemangioblast. *J Hematother Stem Cell Res.* 2002;11:207–214.

Eichmann A, Yuan L, Moyon D, LeNoble F, Pardanaud L, Breant C. Vascular development: from precursor cells to branched arterial and venous networks. *Int J Dev Biol.* 2005;49:259–267.

Forouhar AS, Leibling M, Hickerson A, Nasiraei-Moghaddam A, Tsai H-J, Hove JR, Fraser SE, Dickinson ME, Gharib M. The embryonic vertebrate heart tube is a dynamic suction pump. *Science.* 2006;312:751–753.

Ferguson JE III, Kelley RW, Patterson C. Mechanisms of endothelial differentiation in embryonic vasculogenesis. *Arterioscler Thromb Vasc Biol.* 2005;25:2246–2254.

Gardiner HM. Progression of fetal hart disease and rationale for fetal intracardiac interventions. *Semin Fetal Neonat Med.* 2005;10:578–585.

Garg V. Insights into the genetic basis of congenital heart disease. *Cell Mol Life Sci.* 2006;63:1141–1148.

Godt RE, Fogaca RT, Nosek TM. Changes in force and calcium sensitivity in the developing avian heart. *Can J Physiol Pharmacol.* 1991;69:1692–1697.

Goldinfeld M, Weiner E, Peleg D, Shalev E, Ben-Ami M. Evaluation of fetal cardiac contractility by two-dimensional ultrasonography. *Prenat Diagn.* 2004;24:799–803.

Gourdie RG, Harris BS, Bond J, et al. Development of the cardiac pacemaking and conduction system. *Birth Defects Res C.* 2003;69:46–57.

Gourdie RG, Wei Y, Kim D, Klatt SC, Mikawa T. Endothelin-induced conversion of embryonic heart muscle cells into impulse-conducting Purkinje fibers. *Proc Natl Acad Sci.* 1998;95:6815–6818.

Grant DA. Ventricular constraint in the fetus and newborn. *Can J Cardiol.* 1999;15:95–104.

Grant DA, Maloney JE, Tyberg JV, Walker AM. Effects of external constraint on the fetal left ventricular function curve. *Am Heart J.* 1992;123:1601–1609.

Groenendijk BC, Hierck BP, Vrolijk J, et al. Changes in shear stress-related gene expression after experimentally altered venous return in the chicken embryo. *Circ Res.* 2005;96:1291–1298.

Grossfeld PD. The genetics of hypoplastic left heart syndrome. *Cardiol Young.* 1999;9:627–632.

Gruber PJ, Epstein JA. Development gone awry: congenital heart disease. *Circ Res.* 2004;94:273–283.

Gui YH, Linask KK, Khowsathit P, Huhta JC. Doppler echocardiography of normal and abnormal embryonic mouse heart. *Pediatr Res.* 1996;40:633–642.

Guzman ER, Schulman H, Karmel B, Higgins P. Umbilical artery Doppler velocimetry in pregnancies of less than 21 weeks' duration. *J Ultrasound Med.* 1990;9:655–659.

Harkness UF, Crombleholme TM. Twin-twin transfusion syndrome: where do we go from here? *Semin Perinatol.* 2005;29:296–304.

Herberg U, Gross W, Bartmann P, Banek CS, Breuer J. Long term cardiac follow up of severe twin to twin transfusion syndrome after laser coagulation. *Heart.* 2006;92:95–100.

Hirschy A, Schatzmann F, Ehler E, Perriard JC. Establishment of cardiac cytoarchitecture in the developing mouse heart. *Dev Biol.* 2006;289:430–441.

Hoffman JIE. Incidence of congenital heart disease: II. Prenatal incidence. *Pediatr Cardiol.* 1995;16:155–165.

Hoffman JIE, Kaplan S. The incidence of congenital heart disease. *J Am Coll Cardiol.* 2002;39:1890–1900.

Hofstaetter C, Hansmann M, Eik-Nes SH, Huhta JC, Luther SL. A cardiovascular profile score in the surveillance of fetal hydrops. *J Matern Fetal Neonatal Med.* 2006;19:407–413.

Hogers B, DeRuiter MC, Gittenberger-de Groot AC, Poelmann RE. Extraembryonic venous obstructions lead to cardiovascular malformations and can be embryolethal. *Cardiovasc Res.* 1999;41:87–99.

Hove JR. In vivo biofluid dynamic imaging in the developing zebrafish. *Birth Defects Res C Embryo Today.* 2004;72:277–289.

Hove JR. Quantifying cardiovascular flow dynamics during early development. *Pediatr Res.* 2006;60:6–13.

Hove JR, Köster RW, Forouhar AS, Acevedo-Bolton G, Fraser SE, Gharib M. Intracardiac fluid forces are an essential epigenetic factor for embryonic cardiogenesis. *Nature.* 2003;421:172–177.

Hu N, Clark EB. Hemodynamics in stage 12 to stage 29 chick embryo. *Circ Res.* 1989;65:1665–1670.

Hu N, Connuck DM, Keller BB. Diastolic filling characteristics in the stage 12 to 27 chick embryo ventricle. *Pediatr Res.* 1991;29:334–337.

Hu N, Ngo T, Clark EB. Distribution of blood flow between embryo and vitelline bed in the stage 18, 21 and 24 chick embryo. *Cardiovasc Res.* 1996;31:E127–E131.

Hu N, Sedmera D, Yost, HJ. Structure and function of the developing zebrafish heart. *Anat Rec.* 2000;260:148–157.

Huang C, Sheikh F, Hollander M, et al. Embryonic atrial function is essential for mouse embryogenesis, cardiac morphogenesis and angiogenesis. *Development.* 2003;130:6111–6119.

Huhta JC. Fetal congestive heart failure. *Semin Fetal Neonatal Med.* 2005;10:542–552.

Hurle JM, Colveé E, Blacno AM. Development of mouse semilunar vavles. *Anat Embryol.* 1980;160:83–91.

Hurle JM, Kitten GT, Sakai LY, Volpin D, Solursh M. Elastic extracellular matrix of the embryonic chick heart: an immuno-histological study using laser confocal microscopy. *Dev Dyn.* 1994;200:321–332.

Isogai S, Lawson ND, Torrealday S, Horiguchi M, Weinstein BM. Angiogenic network formation in the developing vertebrate trunk. *Development.* 2003;130:5281–5290.

Ishiwata T, Nakazawa M, Pu WT, Tevosian SG, Izumo S. Developmental changes in ventricular diastolic function correlate with changes in ventricular myoarchitecture in normal mouse embryos. *Circ Res.* 2003;93:857–865.

Ji RP, Phoon CKL. Noninvasive localization of Nuclear Factor of Activated T cells c1-/- mouse embryos by ultrasound biomicroscopy–Doppler allows genotype–phenotype correlation. *J Am Soc Echocardiogr.* 2005;18:1415–1421.

Ji RP, Phoon CKL, Aristizábal O, McGratch KE, Palis J, Turnbull DH. Onset of cardiac function during early mouse embryogenesis coincides with entry of primitive erythroblasts into the embryo proper. *Circ Res.* 2003;92:133–135.

Johnson P, Maxwell DJ, Tynan MJ, Allan LD. Intracardiac pressures in the human fetus. *Heart.* 2000;84:59–63.

Jones EAV, Baron MH, Fraser SE, Dickinson ME. Measuring hemodynamic changes during mammalian development. *Am J Physiol Heart Circ Physiol.* 2004;287:H1561–H1569.

Kamino K. Optical approaches to ontogeny of electrical activity and relate functional organization during early heart development. *Physiol Rev.* 1991;71:53–91.

Karatza AA, Wolfenden JL, Taylor MJO, Wee L, Fisk NM, Gardiner HM. Influence of twin-twin transfusion syndrome on fetal cardiovascular structure and function: prospective case-control study of 136 monochorionic twin pregnancies. *Heart.* 2002;88:271–277.

Keller BB. Embryonic cardiovascular function, coupling and maturation: a species view. In: Burggren WW, Keller BB, eds. *Development of Cardiovascular Systems: Molecules to Organisms.* Cambridge, UK: Cambridge University Press; 1997:65–87.

Keller BB, Hu N, Serrino PJ, Clark EB. Ventricular pressure-area loop characteristics in the stage 16 to 24 chick embryo. *Circ Res.* 1991;68:226–231.

Keller BB, MacLennan MJ, Tinney JP. In vivo assessment of embryonic cardiovascular dimension and function in day 10.5 to 14.5 mouse embryos. *Circ Res.* 1996;79:247–255.

Keller BB, Tinney JP, Hu N. Embryonic ventricular diastolic and systolic pressure-volume relations. *Cardiol Young.* 1994;4:19–27.

Keller BB, Yoshigi M, Tinney JP. Ventricular-vascular uncoupling by acute conotruncal occlusion in the stage 21 chick embryo. *Am J Physiol Heart Circ Physiol.* 1997;273:2861–2866.

Khoshnood B, De Vigan C, Vodovar V, et al. Trends in prenatal diagnosis, pregnancy termination, and perinatal mortality of newborns with congenital heart disease in France, 1983–2000: a population-based evaluation. *Pediatrics.* 2005;115:95–101.

Kingsley PD, Malik J, Fantauzzo KA, Palis J. Yolk sac-derived primitive erythroblasts enucleate during mammalian embryogenesis. *Blood.* 2004;104:19–25.

Klein SL, Gerhard DS, Wagner L, et al. Resources for genetic and genomic studies of Xenopus. *Methods Mol Biol.* 2006;322:1–16.

Kohl T, Sharland G, Allan LD, et al. World experience of percutaneous ultrasound-guided balloon valvuloplasty in human fetuses with severe aortic valve obstruction. *Am J Cardiol.* 2000;85:1230–1233.

Kosaki K, Suzuki H, Schmid-Schonbein GW, Nelson TR, Jones KL. Parametric imaging of the chick embryonic cardiovascular system: a novel functional measure. *Pediatr Res.* 1997;41:451–456.

Koushik SV, Wang J, Rogers R, et al. Targeted inactivation of the sodium-calcium exchanger (Ncx1) results in the lack of a heartbeat and abnormal myofibrillar organization. *FASEB J.* 2001;15:1209–1211.

Kurjak A, Kupesic S. Parallel Doppler assessment of yolk sac and intervillous circulation in normal pregnancy and missed abortion. *Placenta.* 1998;19:619–623.

Le Floc'h J, Chérin E, Zhang MY, et al. Developmental changes in integrated ultrasound backscatter from embryonic blood *in vivo* in mice at high US frequency. *Ultrasound Med Biol.* 2004;30:1307–1319.

Leiva MC, Tolosa JE, Binotto BS. Fetal cardiac development and hemodynamics in the first trimester. *Pediatr Res.* 1999;14:169–174.

Le Noble F, Fleury V, Pries A, Corvol P, Eichmann A, Renerman RS. Control of arterial branching morphogenesis in embryogenesis: go with the flow. *Cardiovasc Res.* 2005;65:619–628.

Le Noble F, Moyon D, Pardanaud L, et al. A. Flow regulates arterial-venous differentiation in the chick embryo yolk sac. *Development.* 2003;131:361–375.

Leu M. Ehler E, Perriard JC. Characterisation of postnatal growth of the murine heart. *Anat Embryol.* 2001;204:217–224.

Liebling M, Forouhar AS, Wolleschensky R, et al. Rapid three-dimensional imaging and analysis of the beating embryonic heart reveals functional changes during development. *Dev Dyn.* 2006;235:2940–2948.

Lin C-S, Lim S-K, D'Agati D, Constantini F. Differential effects of an erythropoietin receptor gene disruption on primitive and definitive erythropoiesis. *Genes Dev.* 1996;10:154–164.

Lin IE, Taber LA. A model for stress-induced growth in the developing heart. *J Biomech Eng.* 1995;116:343–349.

Lin Q, Schwarz J, Bucana C, Olson EN. Control of mouse cardiac morphogenesis by transcription factor MEF2C. *Science.* 1997;276:1404–1407.

Ling P, Taber LA, Humphrey JD. Approach to quantify the mechanical behavior of the intact embryonic chick heart. *Ann Biomed Eng.* 2002;30:636–645.

Lohr JL, Yost HJ. Vertebrate model systems in the study of early heart development: *Xenopus* and zebrafish. *Am J Med Genet.* 2000;97:248–257.

Lougheed J, Sinclair BG, Fung KFK, et al. Acquired right ventricular outflow tract obstruction in the recipient twin in twin-twin transfusion syndrome. *J Am Coll Cardiol.* 2001;38:1533–1538.

Low AF, Tearney GJ, Bouma BE, Jang IK. Technology insight: optical coherence tomography—current status and future development. *Nat Clin Pract Cardiovasc Med.* 2005;3:154–162.

Lucitti JL, Tobita K, Keller BB. Arterial hemodynamics and mechanical properties after circulatory intervention in the chick embryo. *J Exp Biol.* 2005;208:1877–1885.

Lucitti JL, Dickinson ME. Moving toward the light: using new technology to answer old questions. *Pediatr Res.* 2006;60:1–5.

Lucitti JL, Visconti R, Novak J, Keller BB. Increased arterial load alters structural and functional properties during embryogenesis. *Am J Physiol Heart Circ Physiol.* 2006;291:H1919–H1926.

MacLennan MJ, Keller BB. Umbilical arterial flow in the mouse embryo during development and following acutely increased heart rate. *Ultrasound Med Biol.* 1999;25:361–370.

Mäkikallio K, Jouppila P, Rasanen J. Human fetal cardiac function during the first trimester of pregnancy. *Heart.* 2005;91:334–338.

Mäkikallio K, McElhinney DB, Levine JC, et al. Fetal aortic valve stenosis and the evolution of hypoplastic left heart syndrome: patient selection for fetal intervention. *Circulation.* 2006;113:1401–1405.

Mäkikallio K, Tekay A, Jouppila P. Yolk sac and umbilicoplacental hemodynamics during early human embryonic development. *Pediatr Res.* 1999;14:175–179.

Malek AM, Izumo S. Control of endothelial cell gene expression by flow. *J Biomechanics.* 1995;28:1515–1528.

Marton T, Hajdu J, Papp C, Patkos P, Hruby E, Papp Z. Pulmonary stenosis and reactive right ventricular hypertrophy in the recipient fetus as a consequence of twin-twin transfusion. *Prenat Diagn.* 2001;21:452–456.

McGrath KE, Koniski AD, Malik J, Palis J. Circulation is established in a stepwise pattern in the mammalian embryo. *Blood.* 2003;101:1669–1676.

McGrath KE, Palis J. Hematopoiesis in the yolk sac: more than meets the eye. *Exp Hematol.* 2005;33:1021–1028.

McLean M, Ross MA, Prothero J. Three-dimensional reconstruction of the myofiber pattern in the fetal and neonatal mouse heart. *Anat Rec.* 1989;224:392–406.

Megason SG, Fraser SE. Digitizing life at the level of the cell: high-performance laser-scanning microscopy and image analysis for in toto imaging of development. *Mech Dev.* 2003;120:1407–1420.

Miller CE, Donlon KJ, Toia L, Wong CL, Chess PR. Cyclic strain induces proliferation of cultured embryonic heart cells. *In Vitro Cell Dev Biol.* 2000;36:633–639.

Miller CE, Vanni MA, Keller BB. Characterization of passive embryonic myocardium by quasi-linear viscoelastic theory. *J Biomech.* 1997a;30:985–988.

Miller CE, Vanni MA, Taber LA. Passive stress-strain measurements in the stage-16 and stage-18 chick heart. *J Biomech Eng.* 1997b;119:445–451.

Miller CE, Wong CL, Sedmera D. Pressure overload alters stress-strain properties of the developing chick heart. *Am J Physiol Heart Circ Physiol.* 2003;285:H1849–H1856.

Mohun TJ, Leong LM, Weninger WJ, Sparrow DB. The morphology of heart development in *Xenopus laevis. Dev Biol.* 2000;218:74–88.

Mu J, Adamson SL. Developmental changes in hemodynamics of uterine artery, utero- and umbilicoplacental, and vitelline circulations in mouse throughout gestation. *Am J Physiol Heart Circ Physiol.* 2006;291:H1421–1428.

Myers DC, Fishman GI. Molecular and functional maturation of the murine cardiac conduction system. *Trends Cardiovascs Med.* 2003;13:289–295.

Naheed ZJ, Lahoti A, Hughes SF. Ventricular relaxation in the stage 24 chick embryo following changes in volume and blockade of Na+ and Ca2+ channels. *Cardiovasc Res.* 1996;31:E139–E144.

Nakazawa M, Miyagawa S, Ohno T. Developmental and hemodynamic changes in rat embryos at 11 to 15 days of gestation: normal data of blood pressure and the effect of caffeine compared with data from chick embryo. *Pediatr Res.* 1988;23:200–205.

Nakazawa M. Morishima M, Tomita H. Hemodynamics and ventricular function in the day-12 rat embryo: basic characteristics and the responses to cardiovascular drugs. *Pediatr Res.* 1995;37:117–123.

Navaratnam V, Kaufman MH, Skepper JN, Barton S, Guttridge KM. Differentiation of the myocardial rudiment of mouse embryos: an ultrastructural study including freeze-fracture replication. *J Anat.* 1986;146:65–85.

Nerurkar NL, Ramasubramanian A, Taber LA. Morphogenetic adaptation of the looping embryonic heart to altered mechanical loads. *Dev Dyn.* 2006;235:1822–1829.

Nishii K, Shibata Y. Mode and determination of the initial contraction stage in the mouse embryo heart. *Anat Embryol.* 2006;211:95–100.

Nizard J, Bonnet D, Fermont L, Ville Y. Acquired right heart outflow tract anomaly without systemic hypertension in recipient twins in twin-twin transfusion syndrome. *Pediatr Res.* 2001;18:669–672.

Olson EN. Gene regulatory networks in the evolution and development of the heart. *Science.* 2006;313:1922–1927.

Palis J, Robertson S, Kennedy M, Wall C, Keller G. Development of erythroid and myeloid progenitors in the yolk sac and embryo proper of the mouse. *Development.* 1999;126:5073–5084.

Palis J, Yoder MC. Yolk-sac hematopoiesis: the first blood cells of mouse and man. *Exp Hematol.* 2001;29:927–936.

Patten BM, Kramer TC, Barry A. Valvular action in the embryonic chick heart by localized apposition of endocardial masses. *Anat Rec.* 1948;102:299–311.

Pedra SRFF, Smallhorn JF, Ryan G, et al. Fetal cardiomyopathies: pathogenic mechanisms, hemodynamic findings, and clinical outcomes. *Circulation.* 2002;106:585–591.

Pelster B, Burggren WW. Disruption of hemoglobin oxygen transport does not impact oxygen-dependent physiological processes in developing embryos of zebra fish (*Danio rerio*). *Circ Res.* 1996;79:358–362.

Perriard JC, Hirschy A, Ehler E. Dilated cardiomyopathy: a disease of the intercalated disc? *Trends Cardiovasc Med.* 2003;13:30–38.

Phelan CM, Hughes SF, Benson DW Jr. Heart rate-dependent characteristics of diastolic ventricular filling in the developing chick embryo. *Pediatr Res.* 1995;37:289–293.

Phoon CKL. Circulatory physiology in the developing embryo. *Curr Opin Pediatr.* 2001;13:456–464.

Phoon CKL. Imaging tools for the developmental biologist: ultrasound biomicroscopy of mouse embryonic development. *Pediatr Res.* 2006;60:1–8.

Phoon CKL, Aristizábal O, Turnbull DH. 40 MHz Doppler characterization of umbilical and dorsal aortic blood flow in the early mouse embryo. *Ultrasound Med Biol.* 2000;26:1275–1283.

Phoon CKL, Aristizábal O, Turnbull DH. Spatial velocity profile in mouse embryonic aorta and Doppler-derived volumetric flow: a preliminary model. *Am J Physiol Heart Circ Physiol.* 2002;283:H908–H916.

Phoon CKL, Ji RP, Aristizábal O, et al. Embryonic heart failure in *NFATc1-/-* mice: novel mechanistic insights from in utero ultrasound biomicroscopy. *Circ Res.* 2004;95:92–99.

Phoon CKL, Kitabayashi A, Mishina Y. Outflow tract regurgitation and arrhythmias contribute to in utero demise in early P0-Alk3 knockout embryos as defined in vivo by 40 MHz ultrasound biomicroscopy-Doppler. (abstract) *Circulation.* 2006a;114(suppl S18):196.

Phoon CKL, Turnbull DH. Ultrasound biomicroscopy-Doppler in mouse cardiovascular development. *Physiol Genomics.* 2003;14:3–15.

Porter GA Jr, Rivkees SA. Ontogeny of humoral heart rate regulation in the embryonic mouse. *Am J Physiol Regul Integ Comp Physiol.* 2001;281:R401–R407.

Porter GA Jr, Makuck RF, Rivkees SA. Intracellular calcium plays an essential role in cardiac development. *Dev Dyn.* 2003;227:280–290.

Ramasubramanian A, Latacha KS, Benjamin JM, Voronov DA, Ravi A, Taber LA. Computational model for early cardiac looping. *Ann Biomed Eng.* 2006;34:1655–1669.

Reckova M, Rosengarten C, deAlmeida A, et al. Hemodynamics is a key epigenetic factor in development of the cardiac conduction system. *Circ Res.* 2001, 93:77–85.

Rentschler S, Vaidya DM, Tamaddon H, et al. Visualization and functional characterization of the developing murine cardiac conduction system. *Development.* 2001;128:1785–1792.

Rosenthal A. Physiology, diagnosis, and clinical profile of the hypoplastic left heart syndrome. *Prog Pediatr Cardiol.* 1996;5:19–28.

Rosenthal J, Mangal V, Walker D, Bennett M, Mohun TJ, Lo CW. Rapid high resolution three dimensional reconstruction of embryos with episcopic fluorescence image capture. *Birth Defects Res C Embryo Today.* 2004;72:213–223.

Rothenberg F, Nikolski VP, Watanabe M, Efimov IR. Electrophysiology and anatomy of embryonic rabbit hearts before and after septation. *Am J Physiol Heart Circ Physiol.* 2005;288:H344–H351.

Rychik J. Fetal cardiovascular physiology. *Pediatr Cardiol.* 2004;25:201–209.

Schats R, Jansen CA, Wladimiroff JW. Embryonic heart activity: appearance and development in early human pregnancy. *Br J Obstet Gynaecol.* 1990;97:989–994.

Schneider JE, Bhattacharya S. Making the mouse embryo transparent: identifying developmental malformations using magnetic resonance imaging. *Birth Defects Res C Embryo Today.* 2004;72:241–249.

Schneider JE, Bamforth SD, Farthing CR, Clarke K, Neubauer S, Bhattacharya S. Rapid identification and 3D reconstruction of complex cardiac malformations in transgenic mouse embryos using fast gradient echo sequence magnetic resonance imaging. *J Mol Cell Cardiol.* 2003;35:217–222.

Schneider JE, Bose J, Bamforth SD, et al. Identification of cardiac malformations in mice lacking Ptdsr using a new high-throughput magnetic resonance imaging technique. *BMC Dev Biol.* 2004;4:16.

Schroder EA, Tobita K, Tinney JP, Foldes JK, Keller BB. Microtubule involvement in the adaptation to altered mechanical load in developing chick myocardium. *Circ Res.* 2002;91:353–359.

Sedmera D. Form follows function: developmental and physiological view on ventricular myocardial architecture. *Eur J Cardiothorac Surg.* 2005;28:526–528.

Sedmera D, Cook AC, Shirali G, McQuinn TC. Current issues and perspectives in hypoplasia of the left heart. *Cardiol Young.* 2005;15:56–72.

Sedmera D, Hu N, Weiss KM, Keller BB, Denslow S, Thompson RP. Cellular changes in experimental left heart hypoplasia. *Anat Rec.* 2002;267:137–145.

Sedmera D, Pexieder T, Hu N, Clark EB. Developmental changes in the myocardial architecture of the chick. *Anat Rec.* 1997;248:421–432.

Sedmera D, Pexieder T, Rychterova V. Remodeling of chick embryonic ventricular myoarchitecture under experimentally changed loading conditions. *Anat Rec.* 1999;254:238–252.

Sedmera D, Reckova M, Bigelow MR, et al. Developmental transitions in electrical activation patterns in chick embryonic heart. *Anat Rec* Part A. 2004;208A:1001–1009.

Sedmera D, Reckova M, deAlmeida A, et al. Functional and morphological evidence for a ventricular conduction system in zebrafish and Xenopus hearts. *Am J Physiol Heart Circ Physiol.* 2003;284:H1152–H1160.

Shah AM, Ji RP, Phoon CKL. 40 MHz ultrasound biomicroscopy (UBM)-Doppler of umbilical-placental blood flow: validation of a technique with early insights into the *NFATc1-/-* mutant. (abstract) *Pediatr Cardiol.* 2004;25:579.

Sharpe J. Optical projection tomography. *Ann Rev Biomed Eng.* 2004;6:209–228.

Siedner S, Kruger M, Schroeter M, et al. Developmental changes in contractility and sarcomeric proteins from the early embryonic to the adult stage in the mouse heart. *J Physiol.* 2003;548:493–505.

Simpson DG, Majeski M, Borg TK, Terracio L. Regulation of cardiac myocyte protein turnover and myofibrillar structure in vivo by specific directions of stretch. *Circ Res.* 1999;85:e59-e69.

Spurney CF, Leatherbury L, Lo CW. High-frequency ultrasound database profiling growth, development, and cardiovascular function in C57BL/6J mouse fetuses. *J Am Soc Echocardiogr.* 2004;17:893–900.

Spurney CF, Lo XW, Leatherbury L. Fetal mouse imaging using echocardiography: a review of current technology. *Echocardiography.* 2006;23:891–899.

Srivastava D. Making or breaking the heart: from lineage determination to morphogenesis. *Cell.* 2006;126:1037–1048.

Stainier DY, Lee RK, Fishman MC. Cardiovascular development in the zebrafish. *Development.* 1993;119:31–40.

Stekelenburg-de Vos S, Steenduk P, Ursem NT, Wladimiroff JW, Delfos R, Poelmann RE. Systolic and diastolic ventricular function assessed by pressure-volume loops in the stage 21 venous clipped embryo. *Pediatr Res.* 2005;57:16–21.

Stekelenburg-de Vos S, Ursem NT, Hop WC, Wladimiroff JW, Gittenberger-de Groot AC, Poelmann RE. Acutely altered hemodynamics following venous obstruction in the early chick embryo. *J Exp Biol.* 2003;206:2051–2057.

Taber LA. Mechanical aspects of cardiac development. *Prog Biophys Mol Biol.* 1998;69:237–255.

Taber LA, Keller BB, Clark EB. Cardiac mechanics in the stage-16 chick embryo. *J Biomech Eng.* 1992;114:427–434.

Taber LA, Miller CE. Overview: biomechanics of cardiac development. In: Clark EB, Markwald RR, Takao A eds. *Developmental Mechanisms of Heart Disease.* Armonk, NY: Futura Publishing; 1995:387–419.

Taber LA, Sun H, Clark EB. Epicardial strains in embryonic chick ventricle at stages 16 through 24. *Circ Res.* 1994;75:896–903.

Takebayashi-Suzuki K, Pauliks LB, Eltsefon Y, Mikawa T. Purkinje fibers of the avian heart express a myogenic transcription factor program distinct from cardiac and skeletal muscle. *Dev Biol.* 2001;234:390–401.

Tanaka N, Mao L, Delano FA. Left ventricular volumes and function in the embryonic mouse heart. *Am J Physiol.* 1997;273:H1368–H1376.

Tavian M, Péault B. Embryonic development of the human hematopoietic system. *Int J Dev Biol.* 2005;49:243–250.

Territo PR, Altimiras J. Morphometry and estimated bulk oxygen diffusion in larvae of *Xenopus laevis* under chronic carbon monoxide exposure. *J Comp Physiol B.* 2001;171:145–153.

Tobita K, Garrison JR, Liu LJ, Tinney JP, Keller BB. Three-dimensional myofiber architecture of the embryonic left ventricle during normal development and altered mechanical loads. *Anat Rec Part A.* 2005;283A:193–201.

Tobita K, Keller BB. Maturation of end-systolic stress-strain relations in chick embryonic myocardium. *Am J Physiol Heart Circ Physiol.* 2000a;279:H216–H224.

Tobita K, Keller BB. Right and left ventricular wall deformation patterns in normal and left heart hypoplasia in chick embryos. *Am J Physiol Heart Circ Physiol.* 2000b;279:H959–H969.

Tobita K, Keller BB. End-systolic myocardial stiffness is a load-independent index of contractility in stage 24 chick embryonic heart. *Am J Physiol Heart Circ Physiol.* 1999;276:H2102–H2108.

Tobita K, Schroder EA, Tinney JP, Garrison JB, Keller BB. Regional passive ventricular stress-strain relations during development of altered loads in chick embryo. *Am J Physiol Heart Circ Physiol.* 2002;282:H2386–H2396.

Tworetzky W, Wilkins-Haug L, Jennings RW, et al. Balloon dilation of severe aortic stenosis in the fetus: potential for prevention of hypoplastic left heart syndrome: candidate selection, technique, and results of successful intervention. *Circulation.* 2004;110:2125–2131.

Ursem NT, Stekelenburg-de Vos S, Wladimiroff JW, Poelmann RE, Gittenberger-de Groot AC, Clark EB. Ventricular diastolic filling characteristics in stage-24 chick embryos after extraembryonic venous obstruction. *J Exp Biol.* 2004;207:1487–1490.

Van Bel F, Schipper IB, Klautz RJ. Acceleration of blood flow velocity in the carotid artery and myocardial contractility in the newborn lamb. *Pediatr Res.* 1991;30:375–380.

Van Splunder P, Stijnen T, Wladimiroff JW. Fetal atrioventricular flow-velocity waveforms and their relation to arterial and venous flow-velocity waveforms at 8 to 20 weeks of gestation. *Circulation.* 1996;94:1372–1378.

Virágh S, Chalice CE. The origin of the epicardium and the embryonic myocardial circulation in the mouse. *Anat Rec.* 1981;201:157–168.

Wagman AJ, Hu N, Clark EB. Effect of changes in circulating blood volume on cardiac output and arterial and ventricular blood pressure in the stage 18, 24, and 29 chick embryo. *Circ Res.* 1990;67:187–192.

Wakimoto K, Kobayashi K, Kuro-o M, et al. Targeted disruption of Na$^+$/Ca^{2+} exchanger gene leads to cardiomyocyte apoptosis and defects in heartbeat. *J Biol Chem.* 2000;275:36991–36998.

Wallis JW, Aerts J, Groenen MA, et al. A physical map of the chicken genome. *Nature.* 2004;432:679–680.

Warkman AS, Krieg PA. *Xenopus* as a model system for vertebrate heart development. *Semin Cell Dev Biol.* 2006 Nov 24;[Epub ahead of print]

Wessels A, Sedmera D. Developmental anatomy of the heart: a tale of mice and man. *Physiol Genomics.* 2003;15:165–176.

Wladimiroff JW, Stewart PA, Brurhouwt MT. Normal fetal cardiac flow velocity waveforms between 11 and 16 weeks of gestation. *Am J Obstet Gynecol.* 1992;167:736–739.

Woods IG, Kelly PD, Chu F, et al. A comparative map of the zebrafish genome. *Genome Res.* 2000;10:1903–1914.

Yelbuz TM, Choma MA, Thrane L, Kirby ML, Izatt JA. Optical coherence tomography. a new high-resolution imaging technology to study cardiac development in chick embryos. *Circulation.* 2002;106:2771–2774.

Yoshigi M, Hu N, Keller BB. Dorsal aortic impedance in stage 24 chick embryo following acute changes in circulating blood volume. *Am J Physiol Heart Circ Physiol.* 1996;270:H1597–H1606.

Yutzey KE, Robbins J. Principles of genetic murine models for cardiac disease. *Circulation.* 2007;115:792–799.

Zahka KG, Hu N, Brin KP. Aortic impedance and hydraulic power in the staeg 18 to 29 chick embryo. *Circ Res.* 1989;64:1091–1095.

Zhou Y, Foster FS, Parkes R, Adamson SL. Developmental changes in left and right ventricular diastolic filling patterns in mice. *Am J Physiol Heart Circ Physiol.* 2003;285:H1563–H1575.

3

Vascularization of the Developing Heart: Implications for Congenital and Acquired Disease

ROBERT J. TOMANEK

JOSEPH K. PERLOFF

INTRODUCTION

The early embryonic heart is avascular. The bulk of the myocardium is trabecular, a feature that facilitates O_2 diffusion from blood passing through its chambers. Vascular tubes form (Figure 3–1) as the compact regions of the ventricles thicken and O_2 diffusion from the ventricular lumens becomes inadequate. Signals from the myocardium, for example hypoxia-inducible factor (HIF), stimulate the differentiation and migration of cells from the epicardium, including endothelial cells, pericytes, smooth muscle cells, and fibroblasts. Endothelial-lined channels form throughout the myocardium and strands of these tubes ultimately encircle the aortic root and selectively penetrate the aorta to form the ostia of the left and right main coronary arteries. Smooth muscle cells are recruited to form coronary arteries and their branches. The larger venous channels subsequently acquire smooth muscle.

An understanding of formation of the coronary vasculature was very limited before the 1990's, when it was documented that two main coronary artery stems form by ingrowth rather than outgrowth into the aorta (Bogers et al., 1989; Waldo et al., 1990). Details regarding formation of the coronary vasculature are the subjects of recent reviews (Majesky, 2004; Tomanek, 2005). Studies establishing cell lineages and regulation by transcription and growth factors are even more recent (reviewed in Tomanek, 2005). One reason why we know relatively little about the relationship of coronary angiogenesis to congenital heart disease (CHD)

is because this area of investigation has lagged considerably behind that of heart development. This chapter reviews the formation of the coronary vasculature and examines the possibilities that faulty coronary vascularization contributes to or is a consequence of congenital and acquired heart disease.

CORONARY PROGENITOR CELLS

Progenitor cells for coronary vessels migrate from the mesothelial proepicardium located near the dorsal sinoatrium, which is in proximity to the liver primordium. The progenitor cells form the epicardium and are dependent on transcription factor GATA-4 (Watt et al., 2004) and bone morphogenic protein (Schlueter et al., 2006). Cx43 plays a key role in the coupling of these cells to form the epicardial layer (Li et al., 2002), a process that is also dependent upon erythropoietin (Wu et al., 1999), as well as the adhesion molecule VCAM-1 (vascular cell adhesion molecule-1) and its α4 integrin (Kwee et al., 1995; Yang et al., 1995). Epicardial cells undergo epithelial-mesenchymal transformation, and then delaminate from the epicardium and differentiate into vascular cells (Figure 3–2). These events are regulated by a number of molecules reviewed by Olivey et al. (2004), Wessels and Perez-Pomares (2004), Lie-Venema et al. (2007), and Ratajska et al. (2008). One key gene in is Wilm's Tumor-1, which is expressed in proepicardial, epicardial, and subepicardial cells and is required for mesothelial development, connection

Tubulogenesis in the embryonic heart

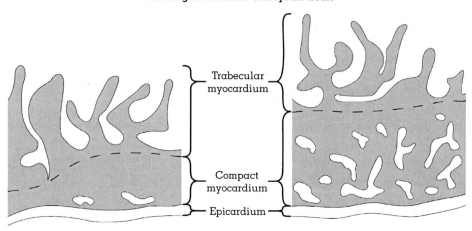

FIGURE 3–1. The embryonic heart is initially avascular, and the myocardium is largely trabecular, which facilitates O_2 diffusion. As the compact region of the ventricular myocardium thickens endothelial cells form tubes which become perfused when the coronary ostia form.

of epidermal cells, and formation of coronary vessels (Kreidberg et al., 1993; Moore et al., 1999). Epithelial mesenchymal transformation is also regulated by several growth factors, as shown by experiments in both mammalian and avian models. FGF-1, FGF-2, and FGF-3; vascular endothelial growth factor (VEGF); and epidermal growth factor (EGF) stimulate this transformation, while TGFβ-1, TGFβ-2, and TGFβ-3 inhibit the process (Morabito et al., 2001; Wada et al., 2003; Holifield et. al., 2004). The appropriate levels of growth factors are likely to play critical roles in epicardial/mesenchymal transformation, as demonstrated by the finding that over-expression of angiopoietin-1 causes defective formation of the epicardium (Ward

et al., 2004). A recent study has documented a key role of thymosin β4 in the induction of epicardial progenitor cell mobilization and vascularization (Smart et al., 2007).

The discovery that vascular progenitor cells populate the epicardium and subepicardium and differentiate into endothelial cells, smooth muscle cells, and fibroblasts was first documented by Mikawa and Fischman (1992), who employed retroviral cell tagging in the embryonic quail (Mikawa and Fischman, 1992). Poelmann and colleagues (1993) provided proof that the entire coronary endothelium had extra cardiac origins. Subsequently, Mikawa and Gourdie (1996) demonstrated that the precursors for each of the cells

Coronary progenitor cells

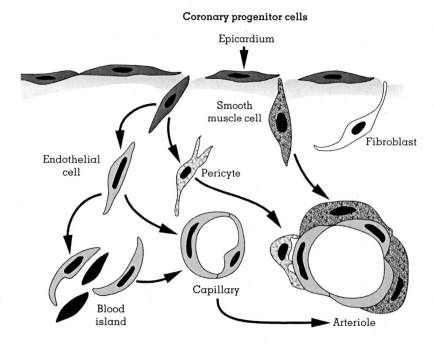

FIGURE 3–2. Coronary progenitor cells migrate from a proepicardium to the epicardium and differentiate into vascular cells: endothelial, pericytes, smooth muscle cells and fibroblasts. Blood islands also play a key role in vascular development in the heart.

comprising the coronary vasculature were indeed derived from the proepicardium, a cell mass located on the septum transversum in mammals and on the sinus venosus in birds. Other studies have also documented the proepicardium as the source of all cells comprising the coronary vasculature (Dettman et al., 1998; Nahirney et al., 2003; Vrancken Peters et al., 1999). The link between the proepicardium and heart has been shown to be a heparin sulfate and fibronectin bridge that enables proepicardial cells to move to the epicardial surface (Nahirney et al., 2003). A novel cell adhesion molecule—blood vessel epicardial substance (bves)—was later shown to play a key role in both epicardial cell formation and migration (Wada et al., 2001).

TUBULOGENESIS: CREATING THE VASCULAR NETWORK

Vascular tube formation in the myocardium depends on the proliferation, migration, differentiation, and assembly of vascular progenitor cells, a cascade of events that requires a primary stimulus and temporal and spatial regulation by multiple growth factors. Hypoxia is considered to be a key stimulus for vasculogenesis (the formation of vascular tubes from angioblasts). An endothelial PAS protein, which is a transcription factor that facilitates the cell's response to hypoxia, coincides with vascular endothelial growth factor receptor-1 (VEGFR-1) and Tie-2 expression in embryos (Favier et al., 2001). We have shown that both of these receptors are important in coronary tubulogenesis in vivo and in vitro (Tomanek, 2002, 2006) and have documented the role of hypoxia on embryonic heart vasculogenesis/angiogenesis (Yue and Tomanek, 1999). Further support for the hypoxia hypothesis comes from two observations, namely, that the endothelial cell protein and hypoxia-inducible factor-1 α (HIF-1α) are often co-localized (Favier et al., 2001), and that VEGF expression, which is stimulated by hypoxia, is highest in the epicardial region, which is farthest from the O$_2$ supply in the embryonic heart (Tomanek et al., 1999). Tubulogenesis first appears in this myoepicardial region of the ventricles. Endothelial precursor cells migrate, differentiate, and form vascular tubes (vasculogenesis).

The establishment of an endothelial cell-lined tubular network is important, not only for a capillary network, but also as a template for larger vessels. One critical consideration with regard to the tubular plexus that surrounds the base of the aorta is that appropriate signals are received to assure penetration of the aortic wall, thus forming the coronary ostia. In addition to the growth factors that are necessary for tubulogenesis

(see above) inhibitors also play an important role in preventing vascular overgrowth. For example, TGF-β inhibits tube formation in explanted embryonic quail hearts even in the presence of vasculogenic/angiogenic growth factors VEGF-A and fibroblast growth factor (FGF-2) (Holifield et al., 2004). Moreover, TGF-β inhibits epicardial-mesenchymal transformation, as well (Morabito et al., 2001).

A recent study has documented that Hedgehog (HH) signaling is necessary for coronary vascular development (Lavine et al., 2006). Their data show that HH is activated by myocardial FGF-9 signaling to cardiomyocytes via a redundant function of FGFR-1 and FGFR-2. They found that HH signaling is essential for the expression of key angiogenic growth factors, namely VEGFs A, B, and C, and angiopoietin 2.

CREATION OF THE CORONARY OSTIA

Penetration of the aortic wall by endothelial strands and tubes is followed by the formation of channels at the left and right cusps (Figure 3–3). Although multiple strands and tubes partially penetrate the aortic wall, the fusion of these structures is normally limited to sites at the left and right cusps (Ando et al., 2004; Ratajska and Fiejka, 1999; Tomanek et al., 2006b). The remaining strands then disappear, consistent with apoptosis in this region (Velkey and Bernanke, 2001). Smooth muscle cells identified by smooth muscle α-actin are recruited in a base-apex pattern (Hood and Rosenquist, 1992) to the sites of the coronary ostia, as illustrated in the quail (Ando et al., 2004) and rat (Tomanek et al., 1999). Data from human embryos illustrate a similar pattern, that is, the capillary plexus at the aortic root, which is followed by smooth muscle cell recruitment (Boucek et al., 1984; Hutchins et al., 1988). The diameters of the main coronaries increase dramatically as flow is established. In the rat, diameter increases fourfold during the three days before birth (Ratajska et al., 2000). The role of mechanical forces associated with flow in the embryo is able to influence gene expression (Jones et al., 2006). These forces affect the specification of arterial and venous identity.

Discovering the mechanisms that direct the endothelial invasion of the aortic wall is challenging. Using the quail as a model, we documented a role for VEGF in this important event. First, VEGF expression is especially high in selective cells at the aortic root (Tomanek et al., 2006a). Second, transcripts for the VEGF receptor Flk-1 are especially dense at the sites of the forming coronary ostia (Tomanek et al., 2002). Finally, inhibition of VEGF-B with neutralizing antibodies prevents formation of the coronary ostia (Tomanek et al., 2006b). A role for neural crest cells is also suggested

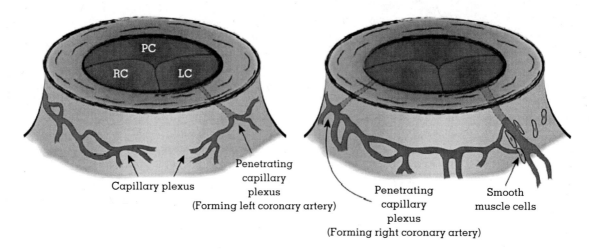

FIGURE 3–3. Formation of the coronary ostia gives rise to the left and right main coronary arteries. A tubular (capillary) plexus surrounds the aortic root, from which some endothelial cells penetrate the aortic wall to form an opening initiating a coronary circulation. The left main coronary artery is almost always formed first, quickly followed by the right main coronary artery. As soon as the coronary ostia are patent smooth muscle cells are recruited to form the tunica media of the coronary arteries. Muscularization of the coronary arteries proceeds in a base to apex direction.

because their ablation was found to result in a single coronary artery and ectopic origins of a second coronary artery (Hood and Rosenquist, 1992). These cells also penetrate the aortic tunica media and contribute to parasympathetic nerves and ganglia, which precede the formation of the coronary artery roots (Waldo et al., 1994). The proteoglycan perlecan, found in basal laminae, may also provide signals for endothelial cell penetration of the aorta. A perlecan mutation in mice is associated with anomalous origins of coronary arteries, that is, right and left coronary arteries arising from the dorsal and ventral sinuses of Valsalva, respectively (Gonzalez-Iriarte et al., 2003). This mutation causes a misdirection of capillary plexus formation at the base of the heart, that is, the plexus forms at the pulmonary trunk rather than at the aorta. Since the precursors of the cells that comprise the coronary vessels migrate from the epicardium, proper development of the epicardium is requisite for coronary artery formation. Consistent with this postulate are data that reveal anomalous origins (Li et al., 2002) and reduced branching (Walker et al., 2004) of coronary arteries. Moreover, the outgrowth of the epicardial-derived cells must occur within a time frame, because delay can lead to the formation of only a single coronary artery (Gittenberger-De Groot et al., 2004).

FORMATION AND REMODELING OF CORONARY ARTERIES

Formation of a tunica media, as documented in a number of species, begins at the roots of the left and right coronary arteries and progresses from the base to the apex of the heart (Hood and Rosenquist, 1992; Ratajska and Fiejka, 1999; Ratajska et al., 2001). Smooth muscle cells arise as epicardial-derived mesenchymal cells initially express smooth muscle α-actin and serum response factor, and subsequently express calponin, smooth muscle 22-α, and smooth muscle γ-actin (Landerholm et al., 1999). This process involves several genes and transcription factors, for example, myocardin, GATA factors, Rho A-Rho K (reviewed in Majesky, 2004). Cytoskeletal reorganization required for differentiation and migration of smooth muscle cells is mediated by rho A/p160 Rho K-dependent pathway that is stimulated by PDGF-BB (Lu et al., 2001). Experiments on quail embryos have documented a role for VEGFs, especially VEGF-B, FGF-2, and PDGF in the formation of coronary ostia and arteries (Tomanek et al., 2006a, 2008).

With formation of the coronary ostia, flow through the coronary vasculature commences, an event that plays a role in remodeling of the arterial tree as reflected in the fourfold increase in diameter of the main coronary arteries in the rat during a 4-day period in late gestation (Ratajska et al., 2001) (see above). The role of flow in the absence of hypoxemia has been shown to increase maximal coronary conductance (flow adjusted for pressure) in fetal lambs (Wothe et al., 2002). The increased capacity for maximal flow occurred by the fourth day after chronic adenosine infusion. The number of terminal coronary arterioles increases substantially during the perinatal period (Kurosawa et al., 1986) in parallel to rapid growth of the myocardium. FGF-2, a growth factor protein that peaks in the neonatal rat (Tomanek et al., 1996), plays a key role in coronary arterial development, as indicated experimentally; its inhibition during the early postnatal period attenuates arteriolar growth (Tomanek, et al., 2001, 2008). Precocious expression of FGF-2 in prehatched chicks leads to abnormal coronary vessel branching (Mikawa, 1995). FGF-1 also contributes to arteriolar growth in the heart, as indicated by studies in mice in which this growth factor is over-expressed, resulting in increased numbers of arteriolar branches (Fernandez et al., 2000). Mechanical factors (enhanced shear stress, stretch) and hypoxia are both believed to act as primary stimuli for myocardial vascularization during postnatal development (reviewed in Hudlicka and Brown, 1996; Tomanek et al., 2002, 2003). HIFs have been shown to play a role in early embryonic vasculogenesis and angiogenesis. I was unaware that hypoxia played a role in *angiogenesis*. For example, deletion of HIF-β subunit ARNT inhibits both of these processes (Ramirez-Bergeron et al., 2006). Arnt $^{-/-}$ embryos have lower VEGF protein levels and enhanced numbers of apoptotic hematopoietic cells.

SIGNIFICANCE OF CORONARY ANOMALIES

There are numerous coronary anomalies, some of which are of clinical significance (Burch and Sahn, 2001; Cademartiri et al., 2006). Many coronary anomalies are undetected until announced by a serious cardiac event (Swinbourne and Bezaquen, 2004). In a study of 1950 angiograms that included patients with (66%) and without (33%) coronary artery disease, coronary anomalies were found in 5.6% of this population (Angelini et al., 1999). The incidence of coronary anomalies in young victims of sudden death was higher (15% vs. 4%) than in adults at necropsy. A review of the clinicopathologic records of 242 patients with isolated coronary artery anomalies revealed that of the 142 patients who died, 78 (45%) died suddenly (Taylor et al., 1992). Of the sudden deaths, 64% were exercise related. A study that reviewed 1101 cases of sudden deaths reported in athletes under the age of 35 (Bille et al., 2006) found that CHD, or cardiomyopathy, was present in 50% of these cases. Athletes under the age of 16 years accounted for 33% of the deaths. There is believed to be an interplay between coronary morphogenesis and congenital heart defects, but little is known about how that interplay expresses itself (Mawson, 2002; Hauser, 2006). The classification of congenital anomalies of the coronary circulation employed herein is found in Table 3–1.

Because of the importance of temporal and spatial expressions of signaling molecules, coronary artery ostia can develop at "inappropriate" sites in the aorta

TABLE 3-I. *A Classification of Congenital Anomalies of the Coronary Circulation*

Congenital Anomalies Of Coronary Arteries *Unassociated* With Congenital Heart Disease.
Anomalous aortic origin
Anomalous proximal course
Anomalous distal connection
Anomalous origin from the pulmonary trunk
Anomalies of size—atresia, hypoplasia, ectasia, aneurismal

Congenital Anomalies Of Coronary Arteries *Associated* With Congenital Heart Disease.
Tetralogy of Fallot
Transposition of great arteries
Univentricular heart
Congenital Anomalies of the Coronary Sinus:

Anomalies Of Coronary Arteries Secondary To Congenital Heart Disease.
Cyanotic congenital heart disease
Coronary atresia and stenosis
Pulmonary atresia
Truncus arteriosus

Adapted from Perloff JK. Clinical Recognition of Congenital Heart Disease, 5th Edition. Philadelphia: WB Saunders, Elsevier Publishers; 2003.

or at an ectopic site, for example the pulmonary artery. Neural crest cells appear to guide endothelial cell penetration of the aorta to form the coronary ostia, as noted earlier. Moreover, previous work on VEGF receptors in embryonic quail hearts documented a selective density of VEGFR-2 receptor transcripts, which are the sites of the two coronary ostia (Tomanek et al., 2002). Thus, the positioning of factors that regulate formation of the ostia is critical in determining their normal location in the aorta.

VENTRICULAR NONCOMPACTION AND MICROCIRCULATORY ABNORMALITIES

As illustrated in Figure 3–1, the early myocardium (before the 5th week of embryonic life in humans) is primarily trabecular. This arrangement is necessary to minimize O_2 diffusion distances from the ventricular lumen since the coronary circulation has not yet been established. Gradual compaction of the myocardium results in a decrease in the trabecular component and an increase in the thickness of the compact myocardium. It is during this period that a vascular tubular network develops, followed by establishment of the coronary ostia and coronary circulation.

Myocardial noncompaction is a congenital anomaly characterized by areas with a thin, compact, and excessive spongy myocardium (reviewed by Bartram et al., 2007). Transmural perfusion defects in the zones on noncompacted myocardium have been reported, and postmortem analysis has documented ischemic lesions

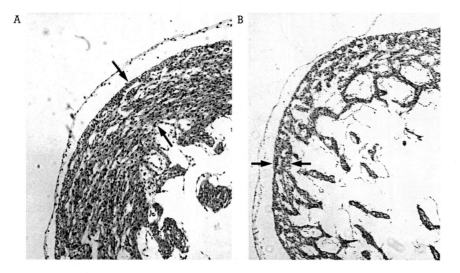

FIGURE 3–4. Micrographs of ventricular cross-sections of embryonic day 10 quail hearts. A. control (nontreated heart) and B. heart from an embryo treated 3 days earlier with anti-FGF-2 neutralizing antibody. Note the limited thickness of the compact region of the ventricle (between arrows) of the heart from the treated embryo.

and fibrosis in these regions. It is not clear whether the persistence of the embryonic (trabeculated) myocardium is secondary to developmental failures of the coronary circulation or whether a stunted growth of the compact region lacked stimuli for vascularization.

Recent data (Tomanek, 2008) indicates that limited compaction with excessive trabeculation is characteristic of embryonic quail treated with neutralizing antibodies to PDGF, FGF-2, or VEGF (Figure 3–4). We also noted that vascular density is compromised in these hearts. Since these neutralizing antibodies also inhibit the in vitro formation of vascular tubes, a direct effect on the vascular system is implied. Further insight into cardiac morphogenesis and coronary vessel development comes from a study on the retinoid X receptor α (RxRα). Epicardial-restricted RxRα mutants lack a myocardial compaction and display defective coronary arteriogenesis (Merki et al., 2005).

Left ventricular noncompaction commonly leads to progressive dysfunction, tachyarythmias, and a risk for cardioembolic events (Blessing et al., 2005; Chin et al., 1990). Heart failure and both systolic and diastolic ventricular dysfunction may occur with noncompaction, along with thromboembolic complications (Bartram et al., 2007).

ANOMALIES OF THE CORONARY ARTERIES SECONDARY TO CONGENITAL HEART DISEASE

Coronary Artery Anomalies and Atherosclerosis

An NIH Multicenter Coronary Artery Study examined data from 24,959 patients, 73 of whom had a detectable coronary anomaly (Click et al., 1989). Sixty percent of the patients had a coronary anomaly that involved the left circumflex artery, that is origin adjacent to the

right coronary ostium, origin from the right coronary artery, or from a branch of the right coronary artery. Anomalous circumflex coronary arteries had a significantly greater prevalence of stenosis compared to nonanomalous arteries in sex- and age-matched controls. A relationship between coronary artery anomalies and atherosclerosis is suggested by subsequent studies (von Ludinghausen, 2003). Consistent with this premise, Ikari and colleagues (1999) pointed out that intimal masses develop in the proximal left anterior descending coronary artery beginning in the peripartum or postpartum period. Neonatal intimal formation occurs in the human LAD at about 30 weeks of gestation, and by the third postnatal month, all hearts examined revealed an intimal mass. The finding that all 3-month postnatal hearts had these intimal masses indicates that they are probably natural occurrences of coronary artery development. However, formation of intimal masses may predispose to atherosclerosis in later life.

Cyanotic Congenital Heart Disease and Atherogenesis

Hypoxemic erythrocytotic residents acclimatized to high altitude are hypocholesterolemic, with a negligible incidence of clinical coronary artery disease, and no coronary atherosclerosis as revealed in 300 necropsies done in Cerro de Pasco in the Peruvian Andes (Arias-Stella and Topilsky, 1971; Mortimer, 1977). A study in New Mexico revealed a lower age-adjusted mortality from atherosclerotic heart disease in men living at high altitudes than in men living at lower altitudes, but in women, there was no difference in high and low altitude mortality (Mortimer, 1977). Because hypoxemic erythrocytic adults with cyanotic congenital heart disease (CCHD) might be analogous to hypoxemic erythrocytotic residents of high altitude, four CHD categories were studied: *Group A*—143 unoperated inherently cyanotic patients aged 18–69 years with systemic arterial oxygen saturations 57%–73%; *Group B*—47 inherently cyanotic patients who were rendered acyanotic by surgery between ages 22 and 69 years, mean postoperative follow-up being 16.9 years; *Group C*—41 unoperated inherently acyanotic patients aged 22–75 years; and *Group D*—48 patients who were acyanotic both before and after operation, mean postoperative follow-up being 15 years (Fyfe, 2005). No patient was taking or had ever taken a cholesterol-lowering medication. All were born and raised at sea level.

In the general population, fatty streaks and raised lesions are present at age 15–34 years, but inherently cyanotic Group A and B patients who ranged in age from the fourth to the sixth decade were devoid of both angiographic and necropsy evidence of coronary atherosclerosis (Fyfe, 2005). Inherently cyanotic unoperated Group A patients and inherently cyanotic Group B patients who had been rendered acyanotic by operation had significantly lower total cholesterol levels than inherently acyanotic unoperated or acyanotic operated Group C and D patients. Low total cholesterol levels defined as <160 mg/dL, which was the cutoff level in the Framingham Study (Kannel, 1971), occurred in 58% of inherently cyanotic unoperated Group A patients, and persisted after surgical elimination of cyanosis in 52 % of Group B patients. Only 11% of cyanotic patients who were hypocholesterolemic before surgery experienced a postoperative rise in total cholesterol levels to >160 mg/dL. Hypocholesterolemia primarily reflected reductions in LDL cholesterol with lesser reductions in VLDL cholesterol.

Three variables associated with CCHD might account for hypocholesterolemia: cyanosis/hypoxemia, erythrocytosis, and genetic determinants. Cyanosis and hypoxemia are obligatory, but insufficient causes need not be present at birth, which is consistent with the observation that within two years after sea level residents ascend to high altitude, their total cholesterol, LDL cholesterol, and HDL cholesterol levels are the same as levels of indigenous high altitude residents (Arias-Stella and Topilsky, 1971; Moerimer, 1977). Hypocholesterolemia tends to persist after surgical elimination of cyanosis and hypoxemia in patients with CCHD, but whether high altitude hypocholesterolemia persists after hypoxemia is eliminated by descent to sea level is not known. Persistence of hypocholesterolemia after surgical elimination of hypoxemia and erythrocytosis implies that once the gene(s) that influence cholesterol levels are expressed, their effects apparently persist despite elimination of the initiating stimulus (Fyfe, 2005). Lack of a relationship between cholesterol levels and age at surgical repair, and the

failure of the levels to normalize decades after surgical elimination of hypoxemia and erythrocytosis suggest a developmental genetic program that maintains childhood levels and profiles of cholesterol, and does not permit emergence of adult lipoprotein characteristics (Fyfe, 2005).

In addition to hypocholesterolemia, four coexisting but independent variables contribute to the low incidence of coronary atherosclerosis in CCHD, namely, hypoxemia, upregulated nitric oxide, hyperbilirubinemia, and low platelet counts (Fyfe, 2005). Hypoxemia is associated with a reduction in oxidized plasma LDL and a reduction in atherogenic intimal oxidized LDL (Fyfe, 2005). Nitric oxide, a ubiquitous signaling molecule synthesized from L-arginine and oxygen, is upregulated in CCHD because endothelial shear stress of the viscous erythrocytotic perfusate is a major factor in nitric oxide elaboration and eNOS gene expression (Adimoolam and Cooke, 1999) (see earlier). Nitric oxide is an antiatherogenic molecule because it opposes platelet aggregation, stimulates disaggregation of preformed platelet aggregates, inhibits monocyte adherence and infiltration, and turns off transcription of intercellular adhesion molecule-1 that governs the endothelial adhesion of monocytes and inhibits smooth muscle proliferation (Adimoolam and Cooke, 1999). Unconjugated bilirubin is an endogenous antioxidant that inhibits LDL oxidation and reduces atherosclerotic risk (Madhavan et al., 1997). Gilbert's syndrome, a benign disorder of bilirubin metabolism, is accompanied by elevated levels of unconjugated bilirubin and a reported immunity from coronary atherosclerosis (Madhavan et al., 1997). Bilirubin is formed from the breakdown of heme, a process that is excessive in CCHD because an increase in red cell mass coincides with an increase in uncongugated bilirubin (Niwa, 1999). Low platelet counts are antiatherogenic, and platelet counts are typically low or thrombocytopenic in CCHD (Lill 2006).

The Coronary Circulation in Cyanotic Congenital Heart Disease

The extramural coronary arteries in CCHD are typically dilated and tortuous, sometimes ecstatic (Perloff, 2006). Flow-mediated shear stress at the luminal surface results in elaboration of vasodilator nitric oxide and prostaglandins (Han et al., 2007). Increased shear stress of the viscous erythrocytotic perfusate in CCHD is responsible for initiating dilatation, but the dilatation often reaches proportions far in excess of responses that could be expected from vasodilator substances alone. Coronary arterial dilation in response to elaboration of endothelial vasodilator substances is coupled with mural attenuation caused by abnormalities of the media (Chugh, 2004) that recall the medial abnormalities associated with disproportionate dilatation of great arterial walls in CHD (Niwa, 2001).

In an attempt to elucidate the structural adaptations of the coronary microcirculation that underlie the preservation of flow reserve in CCHD, we studied necropsy specimens in patients with Eisenmenger syndrome (Dedkov et al., 2006). Histological sections were analyzed from the hypoxic, but not hypertrophic, left ventricles of the Eisenmenger group and compared with data from structurally normal and abnormal hearts with ventricular hypertrophy, and from normal nonhypertrophic hearts. Thus, we were able to contrast hypoxemic, nonhypertrophied left ventricles (Eisenmenger) with nonhypoxemic left ventricles with and without hypertrophy. Our data revealed that the hypoxemic hearts from Eisenmenger patients had lower arteriolar length densities, but larger mean arteriolar diameters than the other groups. Arteriolar volume density was similar to the other groups. These results indicate that the arteriolar bed in patients with CCHD remodels to increase its capacity and preserve normal myocardial perfusion. Patients with CCHD have reduced bioavailability of nitric oxide and impaired endothelial-dependent vasodilation (Oechslin et al., 2005). The relative sparsity of terminal arterioles in hearts from Eisenmenger patients may be the consequence of reduced VEGF-mediated angiogenesis, which is nitric oxide dependent. Basal flow per arteriole would therefore increase and result in the increase in arteriolar diameter via remodeling.

Prenatal Environment as a Determinant of Adult Coronary Disease

Genetics and the prenatal environment may explain why some otherwise healthy individuals are at cardiovascular risk. A recent review (Louey and Thornburg, 2005) identified several intrauterine stressors that affect organ development, for example diet, hypoxemia, and hormonal changes. Of particular relevance to the coronary circulation is endothelial dysfunction and its relationship to coronary disease (Han, 2006). Poor nutrition generally related to protein restriction or placental insufficiency has been shown in experimental animals to alter endothelial-dependent vasodilation (Brawley et al., 2003; Payne et al., 2003; Ozaki et al., 2000), and prehatching hypoxia in chickens has resulted in a similar alteration (Ruijtenbeek et al., 2003). Endothelial dysfunction may predispose coronary arteries to plaque formation and compromised flow (Louey and Thornburg, 2005). A "developmental" model for coronary heart disease suggests an association between low birth weights and coronary heart disease (Barker et al., 1998, 2004; Osmond,

et al., 1993), although adverse environmental factors in childhood and adult life are among many confounding variables (Barker, 2004). An example of the sensitivity of the embryonic coronary vasculature to toxic chemicals has been documented in a study on 2, 3, 7, 8-tetrachlorodibenzo-p-dioxin (TCDD). Chicken eggs treated with TCDD manifested dose-dependent reductions in the number of coronary arteries and in the number and lengths of vascular tubes, effects that were associated with a reduction in VEGF-A (Ivitski-Steele et al., 2005). These limitations in coronary vascular growth were not secondary to limitations of myocardial growth, because left ventricular wall thickness and cavity size were not different from controls.

Coronary Atresia and Stenosis

There are occasional reports of absent, atretic, or stenosed coronary arteries in hearts that are otherwise considered normal (Angelini et al., 1999; Perloff, 2003). The right coronary artery occasionally arises normally from the right aortic sinus, and the circumflex and left anterior coronary arteries arise by separate orifices from the left aortic sinus, an arrangement that has been called "absent left main coronary artery" (Perloff, 2003). In atresia of the left main coronary artery, the ostium is represented by an imperforate dimple, and the proximal course is reduced to a fibrous strand (Perloff, 2003). A large conus branch from the right coronary artery supplies the left anterior descending and circumflex arteries (Musiani, 1997; Perloff, 2003). If this arrangement occurs after formation of the distal coronary tree, obstruction would more likely reflect limited increase in diameter of the segment rather than faulty endothelial cell penetration of the aorta or malformation of the coronary ostium (Angelini, 1999). Coronary artery stenosis is discussed in the next section.

Pulmonary Atresia with Intact Ventricular Septum and Small Right Ventricle

Anomalies of the coronary vascular bed accompanying this malformation are secondary to the hemodynamic derangements. Suprasystemic systolic pressure drives blood from the small, isovolumetrically contracting right ventricle through primitive vascular channels that connect the right ventricular cavity to epicardial coronary arteries (Freedom et al., 2005; Perloff 2003). Myocardial ischemia is an important sequel of these ventriculo-coronary arterial connections. Intramyocardial channels that end blindly punctuate the endocardium of the thick walled right ventricle, creating the appearance of a highly trabeculated muscular wall.

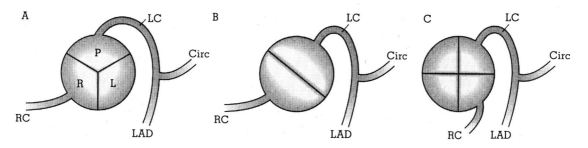

FIGURE 3–5. Origins of the coronary arteries in truncus arteriosus. These anomalous origins are related to the number of leaflets of the truncal valve: A: trileaf; B: bicuspid; and C: quadricuspid. In all situations the left coronary artery (LC) has an acute angle of takeoff. Reproduced with permission, from Dedkoff, 2003.

Truncus Arteriosus

A failure of septation of the fetal truncus arteriosus results in a common truncal valve, which may be quadricuspid, tricuspid, or bicuspid (Perloff, 2003). Coronary artery malformations were found in 64% of 44 postmortem specimens with a common arterial trunk (Bogers et al., 1993), which were believed to have had clinical consequences in all but one specimen. The origins of the coronary arteries vary according to the type of truncal valve (quadricuspid, tricuspid, or bicuspid), illustrated in Figure 3–5. In all types of truncal valves, the left coronary artery originates from a posterior cusp and turns anteriorly with an acute angle that may be the cause of sudden death in truncus arteriosus (Lenox et al., 1992). A detailed study of 30 pathological specimens with truncus arteriosus disclosed coronary ostia that were either small or slit like in the majority of specimens, even if the angle of takeoff was not acute.

Retinoic Acid: A Model of Cardiac and Coronary Malformations

Retinoic acid-induced embryonic heart malformations were proposed as a model for coronary artery abnormalities by Ratajska and colleagues (2005). Retinoic acid affects outflow tract malformations that include double outlet right ventricle, transposition of the great arteries, and truncus arteriosus. The position of the aorta was a determinant of the coronary abnormalities because the signal for capillary penetration of the aorta was altered. In transposition of the great arteries with the pulmonary artery positioned side by side and with the aorta to the right, the peritruncal capillary plexus penetrated the posterior cusp to form the left coronary artery. The left ventricular myocardium was devoid of an arterial supply, but a capillary bed was retained. In truncus arteriosus, the position of the peritruncal capillary plexus was normal and penetrated the aorta at the normal sites. Absence of a septal artery was attributed to the obligatory malaligned ventricular septal defect. In double outlet of right ventricle, a dilated capillary plexus contributed to a dorsal coronary artery. When subpulmonary or subaortic ventricular defects were present, a single coronary artery arose from the anterior aortic sinus and coursed to the right, leaving the left ventricular myocardium devoid of coronary artery branches.

CONGENITAL ANOMALIES OF THE CORONARY ARTERIES UNASSOCIATED WITH CONGENITAL HEART DISEASE

Anomalous Aortic Origin

Coronary arteries that originate from normally located ostia arise from the aortic wall at right angles, whereas coronary arteries that originate from ectopic ostia arise at acute angles and run tangentially, often resulting in a slit-like stenotic orifice that can compress or collapse during aortic root systolic expansion (Perloff, 2003). It has been proposed that expansion of the aortic root and pulmonary trunk during exercise is responsible for increasing an already acute angulation of an ectopic coronary artery and for flap-like closure of its slit-like ostium (Perloff, 2003). The course taken by anomalous coronary arteries and their branches is far more important than the ectopic origin. Intramyocardial tunneling incurs little or no risk but angina pectoris, myocardial infarction, and sudden death are, with few exceptions, reserved for anomalous coronary arteries that course between the aorta and the right ventricular outflow tract, or originate from a slit-like ostium caused by acute angulation (see above) (Perloff, 2003; Roberts,

1982; Taylor, 1992). The high percentage (64%) of sudden deaths noted earlier in individuals with coronary artery anomalies underscores the significance of these anomalies.

Anomalous origins of ostia suggest a miscommunication of signaling at the aortic root where endothelial cell penetration and ostial formation occur. Absence of a main coronary artery represents failure of endothelial cells surrounding the aortic root to penetrate the aorta and form a coronary ostium during the late embryonic period. An "ostial dimple", that is, an aortic wall depression in an aortic sinus that lacks a coronary artery, has been noted in cases of single coronary artery (Angelini et al., 1999) (see above). Anomalous origins or absence of a coronary artery have been achieved experimentally. As noted earlier, neural crest cells play a regulatory role in formation of the coronary stems (Hood and Resenquist, 1992). Ablation of neural crest cells in chick embryos resulted in single coronary arteries originating from the subclavian artery, the right coronary cusp, or a persistent truncus arteriosus. Connexin-43, a component of gap junctions, which plays a role in regulating cell proliferation, differentiation, and embryonic development, is also considered important for coronary artery patterning (Li et al., 2002). Connexin-43 homozygous and heterozygous knockout mice display a variety of coronary artery perturbations, including a single main coronary artery, small accessory coronary arteries, and origin of the septal coronary artery directly from the left cusp.

Origin from the Pulmonary Artery

Anomalous origin of the left coronary artery from the pulmonary trunk is the most common major congenital malformation of the coronary circulation (Perloff, 2003; Schwerzmann, 2004) (Table 3–1). Physiologic, pathologic, and clinical derangements arise from ischemic consequences of the malformation during the transition from antegrade perfusion of the anomalous left coronary artery, to flow through the right coronary artery into the low resistance intercoronary anastomoses and then into the pulmonary trunk (Perloff, 2003). Eighty to ninety percent of patients with anomalous origin of the left coronary artery from the pulmonary trunk die in their first year, but the clinical course is a continuum ranging from death in infancy to asymptomatic adult survival (Perloff, 2003).

Coronary Arterial Fistula

Coronary arterial fistulas are the most frequent hemodynamically significant congenital malformations of the coronary circulation (Perloff, 2003) (Table 3–1). Right and left coronary arteries arise from their appropriate aortic sinuses, but a fistulous branch of one or more than one of the two coronary arteries drains into a cardiac chamber or into the pulmonary trunk, coronary sinus, vena cava, or a pulmonary vein. The drainage site is more important than the site of origin, and consists of either single or multiple vascular channels or a maze of fine channels that form a diffuse network or plexus. More than 90% of coronary arterial fistulas drain into the right side of the heart and are therefore arteriovenous. The coronary artery that gives rise to the fistula is characteristically dilated, elongated, and tortuous. The physiologic responses to coronary arterial fistulas reflect the volume of blood flowing through the fistula, the chamber, or vascular bed into which the fistula drains, and the myocardial ischemia that may result from a coronary steal caused by low resistance vascular channels.

CONGENITAL ANOMALIES OF THE CORONARY ARTERIES THAT COEXIST WITH CONGENITAL HEART DISEASE

Tetralogy of Fallot

This malformation is associated with anomalies of origin, course, and distribution of coronary arteries in 19%–36% of cases (Perloff, 2003). Most common are anomalous origin of a conus artery from the right coronary artery or from the right aortic sinus, origin of a circumflex coronary artery from the right coronary artery or origin of the left anterior descending artery from the right aortic sinus, and origin of a single coronary artery from the right aortic sinus (Dabizzi, 1980; Perloff, 2003). The physiologic consequences of these anomalies are unimportant, but the surgical risk incurred when an anomalous coronary artery crosses the right ventricular outflow tract is most important.

Complete Transposition and Congenitally Corrected Transposition of the Great Arteries

Coronary artery morphology and ventricular morphology are concordant. In complete transposition of the great arteries, a morphologic right coronary artery is assigned to the morphologic subaortic right ventricle, and a morphologic left coronary artery is assigned to the morphologic subpulmonary left ventricle. In congenitally corrected transposition of the great arteries, morphologic right and morphologic left coronary arteries are concordant with the morphologic right and morphologic left ventricles.

The Univentricular Heart

In univentricular hearts with left ventricular morphology, the aortic sinus from which the right or left coronary artery originates is determined by inversion or noninversion of the outlet chamber (Perloff, 2003). When the outlet chamber is inverted, the aortic sinus from which each coronary artery originates is the same as in congenitally corrected transposition of the great arteries with a biventricular heart (see above).

Congenital Anomalies Involving the Coronary Sinus

The coronary sinus is associated with a variety of congenital anomalies, namely, partial or complete absence, stenosis, hypoplasia, atresia, and drainage of a left superior vena cava, or total anomalous pulmonary venous connection (Perloff, 2003).

ACQUIRED DISEASE OF THE CORONARY ARTERIES IN CHILDREN: KAWASAKI DISEASE (MUCOCUTANEOUS LYMPH NODE SYNDROME)

This inflammatory vasculitis has a predilection for coronary arteries, and is the commonest cause of acquired heart disease in children (Burgner and Harnden, 2005). Eighty percent of patients are younger than 5 years of age. The vasculitis is believed to be caused by infectious agent(s) that provokes an abnormal immunological response in susceptible individuals (Burgner and Harnden, 2005). Because Kawasaki disease is most prevalent in children younger than 5 years, it has been proposed that a genetic predisposition during coronary artery formation and growth may underlie the susceptibility.

SUMMARY

Vascularization of the developing heart requires precise temporal and spatial expression of signaling molecules. The process begins with epithelial-mesenchymal transformation of epicardial cells and their migration and differentiation into endothelial and smooth muscle cells, pericytes, and fibroblasts. Following the formation of a tubular, endothelium-lined network, coronary ostia are formed when strands and/or tubes of endothelial cells penetrate the aorta. These events must be precisely regulated and coordinated in order to form a coronary circulation that provides adequate myocardial perfusion. Not surprisingly, anomalies and malformations of the coronary vasculature occur when the necessary cascade of events is interrupted. Coronary artery anomalies may or may not be associated with CHD, or may be a consequence of the prenatal diet or hypoxemia. Formation of an intimal mass in the coronary arteries of fetuses may predispose to atherosclerosis. Although we have detailed many coronary artery anomalies, the basis of their origins remains to be established.

REFERENCES

Adimoolam S, Cooke JP. Endothelial-derived nitric oxide: an anti-atherogenic molecule. In: Panza JA, Camnon RO, eds. *Endothelium, NO, and Atherosclerosis.* Armonk, New York: Futura Publishing; 1999:257–267.

Ando K, Nakajima Y, Yamagishi T, Yamamoto S, Nakamura H. Development of proximal coronary arteries in quail embryonic heart: multiple capillaries penetrating the aortic sinus fuse to form main coronary trunk. *Circ Res.* 2004;94:346–352.

Angelini P, Villason S, Chan AV, Diez JG. Normal and anomalous coronary arteries in humans. In: Angelini P, ed. *Coronary Artery Anomalies. A Comprehensive Approach.* Philadelphia: Lippincott, Williams and Wilkins; 1999:27–79.

Arias-Stella J, Topilsky M. *Anatomy of the Coronary Artery Circulation at High Altitude. High Altitude Physiology.* Edinburgh: Churchill Livingstone Publishers; 1971:149–157.

Barker DJ. The fetal origins of coronary heart disease. *Acta Paediatr Suppl.* 1997;422:78–82.

Barker DJ. The developmental origins of chronic adult disease. *Acta Paediatr Suppl.* 2004;93:26–33.

Barker DJ, Winter PD, Osmond C, Margetts B, Simmonds SJ. Weight in infancy and death from ischaemic heart disease. *Lancet.* 1989;2:577–580.

Bartram U, Bauer J, Schranz D. Primary noncompaction of the ventricular myocardium from the morphogenetic standpoint. *Pediatr Cardiol.* 2007;28:325–332.

Bille K, Figueiras D, Schamasch P, et al. Sudden cardiac death in athletes: the Lausanne Recommendations. *Eur J Cardiovasc Prev Rehabil.* 2006;13(6):859–875.

Blessing WW. Clozapine increases cutaneous blood flow and reduces sympathetic cutaneous vasomotor alerting responses (SCVARs) in rats: comparison with effects of haloperidol. *Psychopharmacology (Berl).* 2005;181:518–528.

Bogers AJ, Bartelings MM, Bokenkamp R, Stijnen T, van Suylen RJ, Poelmann RE, Gittenberger-de Groot AC. Common arterial trunk, uncommon coronary arterial anatomy. *J Thorac Cardiovasc Surg.* 1993;106(6):1133–1137.

Bogers AJ, Gittenberger-de Groot AC, Poelmann RE, Peault BM, Huysmans HA. Development of the origin of the coronary arteries, a matter of ingrowth or outgrowth? *Anat Embryol (Berl).* 1989;180:437–441.

Boucek RJ, Morales AR, Romanelli R, Judkins MP. Embryology and congenital anomalies of the coronary arteries. In: Boucek RJ, Morales AR, Romanelli R, Judkins MP, eds. *Coronary Artery Disease, Pathologic and Clinical Assessment.* Baltimore: Williams and Wilkins; 1984:38–65.

Brawley L, Itoh S, Torrens C, et al. Dietary protein restriction in pregnancy induces hypertension and vascular defects in rat male offspring. *Pediatr Res.* 2003;54:83–90.

Burch GH, Sahn DJ. Congenital coronary artery anomalies: the pediatric perspective. *Coron Artery Dis.* 2001;12:605–616.

Burgner D, Harnden A. Kawasaki disease: what is the epidemiology telling us about the etiology? *Int J Infect Dis.* 2005;9:185–194.

Cademartiri F, Runza G, Luccichenti G, et al. Coronary artery anomalies: incidence, pathophysiology, clinical relevance and role of diagnostic imaging. *Radiol Med (Torino)* 2006;111:376–391.

Chin TK, Perloff JK, Williams RG, Jue K, Morhmann R. Isolated non-compaction of left ventricular myocardium. *Circ.* 1990;82:507.

Chugh R, Perloff JK, Fishbein M, Child JS. Extramural coronary arteries in adults with cyanotic congenital heart disease. *Am J Cardiol.* 2004;94(10):1355–1357.

Click RL, Holmes DR Jr., Vlietstra RE, Kosinski AS, Kronmal RA. Anomalous coronary arteries: location, degree of atherosclerosis and effect on survival—a report from the coronary artery surgery study. *J Am Coll Cardiol.* 1989;13:531–537.

Dabizzi RP, Caprioli G, Aiazzi L, et al. Distribution and anomalies of coronary arteries in tetralogy of fallot. *Circulation.* 1980;61:95–102.

Dedkov EI, Christensen LP, Weiss RM, Tomanek RJ. Reduction of heart rate by chronic beta1-adrenoceptor blockade promotes growth of arterioles and preserves coronary perfusion reserve in postinfarcted heart. *Am J Physiol Heart Circ Physiol.* 2005;288:H2684–H2693.

Dedkov EI, Perloff JK, Tomanek RJ, Fishbein MC, Gutterman DD. The coronary microcirculation in cyanotic congenital heart disease. *Circulation.* 2006;114(3):196–200.

Dettman RW, Denetclaw W, Jr., Ordahl CP, Bristow J. Common epicardial origin of coronary vascular smooth muscle, perivascular fibroblasts, and intermyocardial fibroblasts in the avian heart. *Dev Biol.* 1998;193:169–181.

Espanion G, Franz WM, Niemann H, Doevendans PA, Schaper W, Zimmermann R. Transgenic myocardial overexpression of fibroblast growth factor-1 increases coronary artery density and branching. *Circ Res.* 2000;87:207–213.

Favier J, Kempf H, Corvol P, Gasc JM. Coexpression of endothelial PAS protein 1 with essential angiogenic factors suggests its involvement in human vascular development. *Dev Dyn.* 2001;222:377–388.

Fernandez B, Buehler A, Wolfram S, et al. Coexpression of endothelial PAS protein 1.

Freedom RM, Anderson RH, Perrin D. The significance of ventriculo-coronary arterial connections in the setting of pulmonary atresia with an intact ventricular septum. *Cardiol Young.* 2005;15:447–468.

Fyfe A, Perloff JK, Niwa K. Cyanotic congenital heart disease and coronary atherogenesis. *Am J Cardiol.* 2005;96:283–290.

Gittenberger-de Groot AC, Erlap I, Lie-Venema H, Bartelings MM, Poelmann RE. *Acta Paediatrica.* 2004;(suppl. 446):13–19.

Gonzalez-Iriarte M, Carmona R, Perez-Pomares JM, Macias D, Costell M, Munoz-Chapuli R. Development of the coronary arteries in a murine model of transposition of great arteries. *J Mol Cell Cardiol.* 2003;35:795–802.

Han SH, Ahn TH, Kang WC, et al. The favorable clinical and angiographic outcomes of a high-dose dexamethasone-eluting stent: randomized controlled prospective study. *Am Heart J.* 2006, 152(5):887.e1–e7.

Han T, Perloff JK, Liao JC. Nitric oxide metabolism in adults with cyanotic congenital heart disease. *Am J Cardiol.* 2007;99:691–695.

Hauser M. Congenital anomalies of the coronary arteries. *Heart.* 2005;91:1240–1245.

Holifield JS, Arlen AM, Runyan RB, Tomanek RJ. TGF-beta(1), -beta(2) and -beta(3) Cooperate to Facilitate Tubulogenesis in the Explanted Quail Heart. *J Vasc Res.* 2004;41:491–498.

Hood LC, Rosenquist TH. Coronary artery development in the chick: origin and deployment of smooth muscle cells, and the effects of neural crest ablation. *Anat Rec.* 1992;234:291–300.

Hudlicka O, Brown MD. Postnatal growth of the heart and its blood vessels. *J Vasc Res.* 1996;33:266–287.

Hutchins GM, Kessler-Hanna A, Moore GW. Development of the coronary arteries in the embryonic human heart. *Circulation.* 1988;77:1250–1257.

Ikari Y, McManus BM, Kenyon J, Schwartz SM. Neonatal intima formation in the human coronary artery. *Arterioscler Thromb Vasc Biol.* 1999;19(9):2036–2040.

Ivnitski-Steele ID, Walker MK. Vascular endothelial growth factor rescues 2,3,7,8-tetrachlorodibenzo-p-dioxin inhibition of coronary vasculogenesis. *Birth Defects Res A Clin Mol Teratol.* 2003;67(7):496–503.

Jones EA, le Noble F, Eichmann A. What determines blood vessel structure? Genetic prespecification vs. hemodynamics. *Physiology (Bethesda).* 2006;21:388–395.

Kannel WB, Castelli WP, Gordon T, McNamara PM. Serum cholesterol, lipoproteins, and the risk of coronary heart disease. The Framingham Study. *Ann Int Med.* 1971;74: 1–12.

Kreidberg JA, Sariola H, Loring JM, et al. WT-1 is required for early kidney development. *Cell.* 1993;74:679–691.

Kurosawa S, Kurosawa H, Becker AE. The coronary arterioles in newborns, infants and children. A morphometric study of normal hearts and hearts with aortic atresia and complete transposition. *Int J Cardiol.* 1986;10:43–56.

Kwee L, Baldwin HS, Shen HM, et al. Defective development of the embryonic and extraembryonic circulatory systems in vascular cell adhesion molecule (VCAM-1) deficient mice. *Development.* 1995;121:489–503.

Landerholm TE, Dong XR, Lu J, Belaguli NS, Schwartz RJ, Majesky MW. A role for serum response factor in coronary smooth muscle differentiation from proepicardial cells. *Development.* 1999;126:2053–2062.

Lavine KJ, White AC, Park C, et al. Fibroblast growth factor signals regulate a wave of Hedgehog activation that is essential for coronary vascular development. *Genes Dev.* 2006;20:1651–1666.

Lenox CC, Debich DE, Zuberbuhler JR. The role of coronary artery abnormalities in the prognosis of truncus arteriosus. *J Thorac Cardiovasc Surg.* 1992;104(6):1728–1742.

Li WE, Waldo K, Linask KL, et al. An essential role for connexin43 gap junctions in mouse coronary artery development. *Development* 2002;129:2031–2042.

Lie-Venema H, van den Akker NM, Bax NA, et al. Origin, fate, and function of epicardium-derived cells (EPDCs) in normal and abnormal cardiac development. *ScientificWorldJournal.* 2007;7:1777–1798.

Lill M, Perloff JK, Child JS. Pathogenesis of thrombocytopenia in cyanotic congenital heart disease. *Am J Cardiol.* 2006; 98:254–258.

Louey S, Thornburg KL. The prenatal environment and later cardiovascular disease. *Early Hum Dev.* 2005;81:745–751.

Lu J, Landerholm TE, Wei JS, et al. Coronary smooth muscle differentiation from proepicardial cells requires rhoA-mediated actin reorganization and p160 rho-kinase activity. *Dev Biol.* 2001;240:404–418.

Madhavan PN, Wu LL, Hunt DC. Serum bilirubin distribution and its relationship to cardiovascular risks in children and young adults. *Atherosclerosis.* 1997;131:107–113.

Majesky MW. Development of coronary vessels. *Curr Top Dev Biol.* 2004;62:225–259.

Mawson J B. Congenital heart defects and coronary anatomy. *Tex Heart Inst J.* 2002;29:279–289.

Merki E, Zamora M, Raya A, et al. Epicardial retinoid X receptor alpha is required for myocardial growth and coronary artery formation. *Proc Natl Acad Sci U S A.* 2005;102(51): 18455–18460.

Mikawa T. Retroviral targeting of FGF and FGFR in cardiomyocytes and coronary vascular cells during heart development. *Ann N Y Acad Sci.* 1995;752:506–516.

Mikawa T, Fischman DA. Retroviral analysis of cardiac morphogenesis: discontinuous formation of coronary vessels. *Proc Natl Acad Sci U S A.* 1992;89:9504–9508.

Mikawa T, Gourdie RG. Pericardial mesoderm generates a population of coronary smooth muscle cells migrating into the heart along with ingrowth of the epicardial organ. *Dev Biol.* 1996;174:221–232.

Moore AW, McInnes L, Kreidberg J, Hastie ND, Schedl A. YAC complementation shows a requirement for Wt1 in the development of epicardium, adrenal gland and throughout nephrogenesis. *Development.* 1999;126:1845–1857.

Morabito CJ, Dettman RW, Kattan J, Collier JM, Bristow J. Positive and negative regulation of epicardial-mesenchymal transformation during avian heart development. *Dev Biol.* 2001;234:204–215.

Mortimer EA, Monson RR, Mahon B. Reduction in mortality from coronary heart disease in men residing at high altitude. *N Eng J Med.* 1977;296:581–585.

Musiani A, Cernigliaro C, Sansa M, Maselli D, De Gasperis C. Left main coronary artery atresia: literature review and therapeutical considerations. *Eur J Cardiothorac Surg.* 1997;11(3):505–514.

Nahirney PC, Mikawa T, Fischman DA. Evidence for an extracellular matrix bridge guiding proepicardial cell migration to the myocardium of chick embryos. *Dev Dyn.* 2003;227:511–523.

Niwa K, Perloff JK, Kaplan S, Child JS, Miner PD. Eisenmenger syndrome in adults: ventricular septal defect, truncus arteriosus, univentricular heart. *J Am Coll cardiol.* 1999;34:223–3219.

Niwa K, Perloff JK, Bhuta S, et al. Structural abnormalities of great arterial walls in congenital heart disease. Light and electron microscopic analyses. *Circulation.* 2001;103:393.

Oechslin E, Kiowski W, Schindler R, Bernheim A, Julius B, Brunner-La Rocca HP. Systemic endothelial dysfunction in adults with cyanotic congenital heart disease. *Circulation.* 2005;112(8):1106–1112.

Olivey HE, Compton LA, Barnett JV. Coronary vessel development: the epicardium delivers. *Trends Cardiovasc Med.* 2004;14:247–251.

Osmond C, Barker DJ, Winter PD, Fall CH, Simmonds SJ. Early growth and death from cardiovascular disease in women. *BMJ.* 1993;307:1519–1524.

Ozaki T, Hawkins P, Nishina H, Steyn C, Poston L, Hanson MA. Effects of undernutrition in early pregnancy on systemic small artery function in late-gestation fetal sheep. *Am J Obstet Gynecol.* 2000;183:1301–1307.

Payne JA, Alexander BT, Khalil RA. Reduced endothelial vascular relaxation in growth-restricted offspring of pregnant rats with reduced uterine perfusion. *Hypertension.* 2003;42:768–774.

Perloff JK. Congenital anomalies of the coronary circulation. In: Perloff JK, ed. Clinical recognition of congenital heart disease. 5th ed. Philadelphia: WB Saunders Elsevier Publishers; 2003.

Poelmann RE, Gittenberger-de Groot AC, Mentink MM, Bokenkamp R, Hogers B. Development of the cardiac coronary vascular endothelium, studied with antiendothelial antibodies, in chicken-quail chimeras. *Circ Res.* 1993;73:559–568.

Ramirez-Bergeron DL, Runge A, Adelman DM, Gohil M, Simon MC. HIF-dependent hematopoietic factors regulate the development of the embryonic vasculature. *Dev Cell.* 2006;11:81–92.

Ratajska A, Fiejka E. Prenatal development of coronary arteries in the rat: morphologic patterns. *Anat Embryol (Berl).* 1999;200:533–540.

Ratajska A, Fiejka E, Sieminska J. Prenatal development of coronary arteries in the rat: morphometric patterns. *Folia Morphol (Warsz).* 2000;59:297–306.

Ratajska A, Zarska M, Quensel C, Kramer J. Differentiation of the smooth muscle cell phenotypes during embryonic development of coronary vessels in the rat. *Histochem Cell Biol.* 2001;116:79–87.

Ratajska A, Zlotorowicz R, Blazejczyk M, Wasiutynski A. Coronary artery embryogenesis in cardiac defects induced by retinoic acid in mice. *Birth Defects Res A Clin Mol Teratol.* 2005;73:966–979.

Ratajska A, Czarnowska E, Ciszek B. Embryonic development of the proepicardium and coronary vessels. *Int J Dev Biol.* 2008;52:229–236.

Roberts WC, Waller BF, Roberts CS. Fatal atherosclerotic narrowing of the right main coronary artery: origin of the left anterior descending or left circumflex coronary artery from the right (the true "left-main equivalent"). *Am Heart J.* 1982;104:638–641.

Ruijtenbeek K, Kessels LC, De Mey JG, Blanco CE. Chronic moderate hypoxia and protein malnutrition both induce growth retardation, but have distinct effects on arterial endothelium-dependent reactivity in the chicken embryo. *Pediatr Res.* 2003;53:573–579.

Schlueter J, Manner J, Brand T. BMP is an important regulator of proepicardial identity in the chick embryo. *Dev Biol.* 2006;295:546–558.

Schwerzmann M, Salehian O, Elliot T, Merchant N, Siu SC, Webb GD. Images in cardiovascular medicine. Anomalous origin of the left coronary artery from the main pulmonary artery in adults: coronary collateralization at its best. *Circulation.* 2004;110:e511–e513.

Shirani J, Roberts WC. Coronary ostial dimple (in the posterior aortic sinus) in the absence of other coronary arterial abnormalities. *Am J Cardiol.* 1993;72:118–119.

Smart N, Risebro CA, Melville AA, et al. Thymosin beta4 induces adult epicardial progenitor mobilization and neovascularization. *Nature.* 2007;445:177–182.

Swinburne JL, Benzaquen BS. Congenital anomalies of the coronary circulation. *Can J Cardiol.* 2004;20:353–356.

Taylor AJ, Rogan KM, Virmani R. Sudden cardiac death associated with isolated congenital coronary artery anomalies. *J Am Coll Cardiol.* 1992;20:640–647.

Tomanek RJ. Formation of the coronary vasculature during development. *Angiogenesis.* 2005;8:273–284.

Tomanek RJ, Hansen HK, Christensen LP. Temporally expressed PDGF and FGF-2 regulate embryonic coronary artery formation and growth. *Arterioscler Thromb Vasc Biol.* 2008.

Tomanek RJ, Hansen HK, Dedkov EI. Vascular patterning of the quail coronary system during development. *Anatomical Record.* 2006a;288A:989–999.

Tomanek RJ, Haung L, Suvarna PR, O'Brien LC, Ratajska A, Sandra A. Coronary vascularization during development in the rat and its relationship to basic fibroblast growth factor. *Cardiovasc Res.* 1996;31 Spec No:E116–E126.

Tomanek RJ, Holifield JS, Reiter RS, Sandra A, Lin JJ. Role of VEGF family members and receptors in coronary vessel formation. *Dev Dyn.* 2002;225:233–240.

Tomanek RJ, Ishii Y, Holifield JS, Sjogren CL, Hansen HK, Mikawa T. VEGF family members regulate myocardial tubulogenesis and coronary artery formation in the embryo. *Circ Res.* 2006b;98:947–953.

Tomanek RJ, Lund DD, Yue X. *Hypotic Induction of Myocardial Vascularization during Development.* New York: Kluwer Academic/Plenum Publishing; 2003.

Tomanek RJ, Ratajska A, Kitten GT, Yue X, Sandra A. Vascular endothelial growth factor expression coincides with coronary vasculogenesis and angiogenesis. *Dev Dyn.* 1999;215:54–61.

Tomanek RJ, Sandra A, Zheng W, Brock T, Bjercke RJ, Holifield JS. Vascular endothelial growth factor and basic fibroblast growth factor differentially modulate early postnatal coronary angiogenesis. *Circ Res*. 2001;88:1135–1141.

Tomanek RJ, Zheng W, Peters KG, Lin P, Holifield JS, Suvarna PR. Multiple growth factors regulate coronary embryonic vasculogenesis. *Dev Dyn*. 2001;221(3):265–273.

Velkey JM, Bernanke DH. Apoptosis during coronary artery orifice development in the chick embryo. *Anat Rec*. 2001;262:310–317.

von Lüdinghausen M. *The Clinical Anatomy of Coronary Arteries. (Advances in Anatomy, Embryology and Cell Biology, vol. 167)*. Berlin: Springer; 2003.

Vrancken Peeters M-PFM, Gittenberger-de Groot AC, Mentink MMT PR. Smooth muscle cells and fibroblasts of the coronary arteries derive from epithelial-mesenchymal transformation of the epicardium. *Anat Embryol (Berl)*. 1999;199:367–378.

Wada AM, Reese DE, Bader DM. Bves: prototype of a new class of cell adhesion molecules expressed during coronary artery development. *Development* 2001;128:2085–2093.

Wada AM, Smith TK, Osler ME, Reese DE, Bader DM. Epicardial/Mesothelial cell line retains vasculogenic potential of embryonic epicardium. *Circ Res*. 2003;92:525–531.

Waldo KL, Kumiski DH, Kirby ML. Association of the cardiac neural crest with development of the coronary arteries in the chick embryo. *Anat Rec*. 1994;239:315–331.

Waldo KL, Willner W, Kirby ML. Origin of the proximal coronary artery stems and a review of ventricular vascularization in the chick embryo. *Am J Anat*. 1990;188:109–120.

Walker DL, Vacha SJ, Kirby ML. An essential role for connexin 43 in coronary vasculogenesis. *Mol Biol Cell*. 2004;15(suppl): 312.

Ward NL, Van Slyke P, Sturk C, Cruz M, Dumont DJ. Angiopoietin 1 expression levels in the myocardium direct coronary vessel development. *Dev Dyn*. 2004;229:500–509.

Watt AJ, Battle MA, Li J, Duncan SA. GATA4 is essential for formation of the proepicardium and regulates cardiogenesis. *Proc Natl Acad Sci U S A*. 2004;101:12573–12578.

Wessels A, Perez-Pomares JM. The epicardium and epicardially derived cells (EPDCs) as cardiac stem cells. *Anat Rec*. 2004;276A:43–57.

Wothe D, Hohimer A, Morton M, Thornburg K, Giraud G, Davis L. Increased coronary blood flow signals growth of coronary resistance vessels in near-term ovine fetuses. *Am J Physiol Regul Integr Comp Physiol*. 2002;282:R295–R302.

Wu H, Lee SH, Gao J, Liu X, Iruela-Arispe ML. Inactivation of erythropoietin leads to defects in cardiac morphogenesis. *Development*. 1999;126:3597–3605.

Yang JT, Rayburn H, Hynes RO. Cell adhesion events mediated by alpha 4 integrins are essential in placental and cardiac development. *Development*. 1995;121:549–560.

II

Diagnosis and Management
of Congenital Heart Defects

4

Noninvasive Imaging of Congenital Heart Defects

COLIN K.L. PHOON

ANNE J.L. CHUN

MONVADI B. SRICHAI

Noninvasive imaging has become the cornerstone of the diagnosis of congenital cardiac malformations. The era of diagnostic pediatric cardiology truly began with the clinical observations of Dr. Helen Taussig in the 1930s and 1940s, combined with the use of fluoroscopy (Taussig, 1947). The introduction of cardiac catheterization and its application to children greatly augmented the accuracy of diagnosis especially prior to surgical intervention (Noonan, 2004), but clinical examination along with chest roentgenograms and electrocardiography remained the mainstays of diagnostic evaluation—usually along with "tincture of time." In 1954, Edler and Hertz first reported recordings of ultrasound reflections from the heart (Edler and Hertz, 1954), but it was the 1970s that witnessed widespread application of first M-mode and shortly thereafter, two-dimensional (2-D) echocardiography, which revolutionized diagnostic capabilities in pediatric cardiology. The rapid refinement of ultrasound technology in the 1980s, including the additions of spectral Doppler and color Doppler flow mapping, and the introduction of transesophageal and fetal echocardiography, vaulted ultrasound imaging to its current position as the primary diagnostic and imaging modality in both children and adults with known or suspected heart disease (Feigenbaum, 1996; Grech, 1999; Gutgesell et al., 2000; Gowda et al., 2004; Noonan, 2004; Silverman, 1996).

Starting in the 1990s and capable of not only anatomical but also functional analyses in both 2-D and 3-D, cardiac magnetic resonance imaging (MRI) has made tremendous advances and now complements echocardiography as an important imaging technique (see Pignatelli et al., 2003; Russell et al., 2000). Because of its spatial resolution and ability to acquire images rapidly, cardiac computed tomography (CT) has recently also emerged as a valuable adjunct in noninvasive imaging (see Goo et al., 2005; Russell et al., 2000). Together, echocardiography, MRI, and CT comprise the vast majority of noninvasive studies for the diagnosis and management of congenital cardiac malformations. In addition to the myocardium, chambers, and valvular structures, noninvasive imaging also evaluates the outflow tracts, coronary arteries, great arteries, aortic arch(es), systemic arteries, and systemic and pulmonary veins. Structures and relationships, both to one another and tructures in the chest and to the viscera, and the cardiac function, are also examined.

Their noninvasive nature and the concomitant ability to follow patients longitudinally with precise measurements have made these imaging modalities critical to the initial diagnosis of congenital heart defects and the ongoing management thereof. Because all diagnostic approaches carry intrinsic strengths and limitations, optimal care of the patient with congenital heart disease (CHD) requires facility with and an understanding of noninvasive imaging approaches; still, use of such technology must be tempered with clinical acumen as part of a complete and comprehensive approach to patient care (Phoon et al., 1999). With a specific emphasis on congenital cardiac malformations, the goals of this chapter are to review (1) basic underlying physical principles used to generate ultrasound, MRI, and CT images, as well as aspects of biosafety;

(2) common indications and specific questions to ask of each noninvasive imaging modality; (3) laboratory requirements for equipment and staffing; (4) common and widely used approaches for morphological and functional analyses; (5) briefly, newer advances within each imaging modality.

ECHOCARDIOGRAPHY

General Physical and Technical Principles

General Overview. Echocardiography is the ultrasound examination (ultrasonography) of the heart and related vascular structures. Because echocardiography is the cornerstone of both diagnosis and management, outstanding echocardiography begins with generation of the best possible images and ends with highly skilled interpretation based on training, knowledge, experience, and ongoing and continual self-improvement. An understanding of the basic physics underlying clinical ultrasound, including image generation, allows an appreciation of the power and the pitfalls of echocardiography. The purpose of this section is to provide the reader with an essential understanding of ultrasound physics in order to optimize imaging quality; for further details, the reader is referred to several excellent and thorough reviews (Danford and Murphy, 1998; DeGroff, 2002; Geva, 1998; Shandas, 1999).

Ultrasound energy comprises sound waves whose frequencies are >20 kHz (20,000 Hertz [Hz]). In a beam generated by piezoelectric crystals housed within the imaging transducers, clinical ultrasound is typically in the range of 2–12 MHz (2–12 million Hz), corresponding to wavelengths of approximately 0.80–0.13 mm, and allows subsurface imaging through the property of backscatter. Sound travels through tissue at approximately 1540 m/s. Sound energy is reflected at the boundaries between two materials of different acoustical properties (specifically, acoustical impedance)—blood and myocardium, or inhomogeneities within myocardial tissue, for example. Some of the reflected ultrasound will then be detected by the transducer, some of the sound energy continues to the next layer of tissue, and some of the energy will be scattered elsewhere or absorbed by the tissue. As the ultrasound wave passes into deeper and deeper tissue, therefore, there is invariably energy loss, with concomitant degradation of imaging quality.

Frequency and wavelength are important because they govern the spatial resolution and depth of penetration of the ultrasound beam. Spatial resolution is the smallest distance that can be discerned between two objects; the higher the frequency and shorter the wavelength, the better the spatial resolution. Because

at higher frequencies, energy absorption (and thus losses) and reflected energy at near fields are all greater, depth of penetration is poorer. One therefore trades off spatial resolution for penetration. It should be noted that spatial resolution is further categorized into axial and lateral resolution (see McElhinney et al., 2000). In addition to transducer frequency, lateral resolution is also related to depth of structure and size of the transducer; therefore, all else given equal, deeper structures are imaged with less resolution. As a general rule, high-frequency transducers (8–12 MHz) are used for newborns and young infants, medium-frequency transducers (5–8 MHz) for children and young adolescents, and low-frequency transducers (2–5 MHz) for older adolescents and adults.

The nature of the surface and tissue, and the angle relative to the ultrasound beam may also impact the image quality. Certain interfaces produce such dense acoustical boundaries that most of the ultrasound energy is reflected, and deeper objects are obscured. Bone, air (lung, gastrointestinal), dense scar tissue, and prosthetic material (metal, dense plastic) will severely degrade imaging quality.

Physical laws also dictate other limitations to image production. If an ultrasound beam is simply directed into tissue in one direction to generate a 1-D image (an "ice pick" view: M-mode), then the time required for the transducer to emit the beam pulse and "listen" over a specified time period, then generate a display of dots based on distance plotted against time (M-mode), is quite short, and this can be done approximately 1000 times/s. The temporal resolution, or the time interval between ultrasound beam pulses, is high. To generate a 2-D image, the ultrasound beam must be "swept" in a fan-shaped sector by the transducer. Although in the past, this was achieved mechanically using a rotating transducer head, in modern echocardiography systems, this is achieved with phased-array transducers that generate "sweeps" electronically. Nevertheless, the system must still "wait" for one beam to be sent out, and according to the parameters specified by the operator, must then "listen" for a certain time period to determine the reflections arriving back at the transducer. By "listening" for a specified time interval, the system can translate time into distance and display the reflected echoes as a function of distance, in near-real time. The ultrasound system must then transmit and receive the beam to the next part of the sector, then the next, and so forth, in order to generate the familiar fan-shaped image sector. How fast the system can accomplish this depends on the speed of sound in the medium, the depth of penetration chosen, the size of the sector, and the density of the scan lines. Still, because a sector must now be scanned, the temporal resolution is considerably lower. The operator can optimize the image quality by setting the depth of penetration appropriately (the region of interest should mostly fill the sector), narrow the sector wedge to what is required, and specify the scan line density according to needs (trading off spatial for temporal resolution). However, the "bottleneck" to all of this is the speed of sound, which of course cannot be altered by the operator.

Doppler echocardiography relies on reflected ultrasound energy from moving objects, namely red blood cells or, as in the case of tissue Doppler, contracting and relaxing myocardium. It is based on the Doppler principle: the frequency of the transmitted ultrasound beam changes, or shifts, when the sound energy is reflected off the moving target(s) (see Quinones et al., 2002). The degree of Doppler shift is proportional to the speed of the blood flow and the cosine of the Doppler incident angle (see below). This Doppler shift is processed and converted by the ultrasound system to a spectral display of blood flow, with flow velocity plotted against time. In practical usage, if the red blood cells interrogated by the ultrasound beam are mostly moving within a narrow range of velocities (as is the case with laminar flow in a large vessel), then the Doppler flow wave envelope will exhibit a "clean" envelope with a narrow spectral spread; conversely, the many red blood cells interrogated by the ultrasound beam may be moving at widely varying velocities, which will generate a "noisy" Doppler flow wave envelope. Doppler is generally divided into pulsed-wave (PW) Doppler and continuous-wave (CW) Doppler. In CW Doppler, the echocardiography system is essentially "listening" continuously while transmitting the ultrasound beam; thus, the reflected shifted ultrasound frequencies arrive from anywhere along the path of the beam, and one cannot tell where the velocities are increased. There is thus no "range specificity," although in theory, the maximal velocities that can be interrogated are infinite, since in theory the system is sampling the reflected echoes at an infinite rate. In PW Doppler, an ultrasound beam is transmitted from the imaging transducer, and the echocardiography system waits for a defined period of time before listening to the reflected (and shifted) ultrasound; in this way, the system "knows" exactly what distance the shift occurred at, and so there is "range specificity." However, sampling theory dictates when one seeks range specificity, a maximal flow velocity is imposed before aliasing; this is known as the Nyquist limit. Color Doppler flow mapping is essentially the information from spectral PW Doppler converted from individual points to an amalgamated "color map." Within this map, velocity is encoded into colors: shades of red represent the spectrum of velocities coming toward the imaging transducer, while shades of blue represent the spectrum of velocities moving away from the imaging transducer.

TABLE 4-1. *Optimizing Your Echocardiographic Image by Considering Physics of Ultrasound*

Use the highest frequency transducer that can accomplish imaging
Adjust the sector depth and width to your region of interest
Especially in patients with limited or difficult acoustical windows, move around the chest or subxyphoid regions to obtain the best windows
Use PW, CW, or HPRF (high-pulsed repetition frequency) Doppler appropriately
Reduce the size of your color Doppler flow map to the region of interest
Adjust systems gains appropriately to optimize spatial resolution

Because now entire jets of flow can be visualized, color Doppler flow mapping revolutionized the detection of shunt or regurgitant jets, as well as the evaluation of blood flow across valves and through blood vessels. It should be clear that the general limitations of ultrasound imaging also apply to Doppler echocardiography. In particular, the frequency of the transmitted Doppler beam, the nature of the objects scanned, and the speed of sound all create certain immutable limitations.

Table 4-1 provides suggestions for optimizing image quality based on the physical considerations that go into the generation of an ultrasound beam.

In summary, physical laws dictate certain inherent operator-independent limitations of all ultrasound imaging. Because of the presence of air, dense tissue, or prosthetic material, as well as the need for increased depth of penetration at the expense of spatial resolution, patients with respiratory distress or chest deformities, postoperative patients, and large patients may all exhibit suboptimal imaging. Operator-dependent parameters include proper adjustment of gains, sector size, and choice of transducer and Doppler mode. The goal always is to produce the most beautiful images possible within a logical story, in order to limit the amount of interpretation and/or speculation the pediatric echocardiographer must make.

M-mode. M-mode echocardiography is a 1-D "ice pick" view of the heart and vascular structures (see Figure 4-8). No longer used for anatomical delineation of congenital defects since the advent of 2-D imaging, it nevertheless remains useful for defining valvular motion and ventricular function and certain structures. Because there is no sweep of the ultrasound beam, the ultrasound beam is pulsed frequently, and the temporal resolution (frame rate) is high. The echocardiographer must remember that to make accurate measurements of cross-sectional dimensions (for example, internal vessel diameters or endocardial borders); the M-mode beam must be perpendicular to the structure in question; this is a common technical error that would increase dimensions artificially.

Two-Dimensional Echocardiography. Two-dimensional echocardiography is the mainstay of anatomical diagnosis (see section Segmental Analysis). Because an ultrasound beam must be swept across a fan-shaped sector in order to generate the image, the frame rate and, therefore, temporal resolution of 2-D echo is considerably lower than M-mode echo. Still, with newer technologies, the frame rates achieved on state-of-the-art systems are now adequate for analysis of most of the cardiac motions. The pulsed repetition frequency depends on the sector width, depth, and transducer frequency. Therefore, the smaller the patient and the smaller the region of interest defined by the sector, the higher the spatial and temporal resolution.

The primary disadvantage of 2-D echo is that the interpreter must reconstruct 2-D images back into their native 3-D configurations. While this can be accomplished as a matter of course for most congenital heart defects with the help of multiple planes of imaging during transthoracic echocardiography, it becomes a more challenging task with complex disease and relationships (De Castro et al., 2006; Seliem et al., 2006), and with techniques such as transesophageal echocardiography.

Three-Dimensional Echocardiography. The next logical step up from 2-D echocardiography is the 3-D echocardiography: the ability to acquire, process, and render ultrasound data from a complex 3-D, beating object that is the heart, into a 3-D dataset that permits optimal surgical and anatomic views, and accurate determination of volumes. Conceptually, 3-D echo is simply 2-D echo, now swept through a third orthogonal plane of imaging; processing provides for volume and surface rendering to achieve a "3-D" effect on a 2-D projection screen. Until recently, however, the technology underlying the transducers and computer processing needed to generate and render the images was not adequate for either the spatial or temporal resolution needed, and the process of image generation too time-consuming, for routine clinical use (De Castro et al., 2006a; Marx and Sherwood, 2002; Nanda et al., 2004; van den Bosch et al., 2006). Current technology now permits "real time" 3-D echo, utilizing advanced transducer technology that essentially houses multiple 2-D transducers across a third axis of imaging; modern 3-D "matrix array" transducers typically hold 3000-element arrays. To date, frequencies permitted by modern 3-D transducer technology has been in the 2–4 MHz range (De Castro et al., 2006; Hlavacek et al., 2006; Seliem et al., 2006; van den Bosch et al., 2006a, 2006b), such that high-resolution imaging in the small patient has not been optimal; however, higher-frequency transducers are on the horizon.

After almost three decades of routine 2-D echo use, the clinical utility of 3-D echo is being investigated with great enthusiasm. The complex anatomy of septal defects, valves, and volume calculations all seem to be better imaged using 3-D echocardiography (De Castro et al., 2006; Hlavacek et al., 2006; Seliem et al., 2006; van den Bosch et al., 2006a, 2006b). The ideal goal is to generate images from a "surgeon's point of view," theoretically resulting in improved preoperative preparation and planning (De Castro et al., 2006; Marx and Sherwood, 2002). Moreover, real-time 3-D echocardiography may facilitate transcatheter interventions such as device closure of atrial septal defects, since the definition of anatomy is better than that of 2-D transthoracic and transesophageal imaging (McKendrick and Owada, 2005). The introduction of this new technology and imaging modality has led to the development of early examination protocols, the better to effectively describe and understand 3-D echocardiographic images (Nanda et al., 2004).

Doppler Ultrasound

General Considerations. Doppler ultrasound has proven invaluable to noninvasive imaging, playing a central role in the elucidation of cardiovascular hemodynamics in the patient with CHD. Velocity (of blood, tissue) is derived from the Doppler equation:

$$\text{Velocity} = [c\,(F_r - F_0)]/[2F_0(\cos\theta)]$$

where c is the average speed of ultrasound in soft tissue (1540 m/s); F_r and F_0 are the reflected and emitted ultrasound frequencies, respectively (so that their difference is the frequency shift); and θ is the angle between the path of the ultrasound beam and that of the blood flow or moving tissue (Pellett and Kerut, 2004; Quinones et al., 2002). Although the choice of transducer frequency will make some difference in one's ability to obtain accurate velocities (McElhinney et al., 2000), the most important source of error is the Doppler incident angle θ. It is important to remember that blood flow jets and tissue motion occur in three dimensions, while the image projected onto the screen is 2-D; therefore, the echocardiographer must scan from multiple planes in order to achieve the smallest Doppler incident angle and thus, the most accurate velocity. In practice, if the angle is 20 degree or less, the error is acceptable, since the cosine of 20 degree is 0.94; there is thus a maximal error of 6%. Because of the cosine term, velocities can only be underestimated; therefore, the highest velocities obtained from multiple views are considered the most accurate.

A second important general Doppler equation allows calculation of volumetric flow (DeGroff, 2002; Quinones et al., 2002). When blood flow is laminar, there is narrow spectral spread of the Doppler flow envelope, which is displayed as velocity plotted against time. Two standard Doppler measures are the velocity time integral (VTI) and the time-averaged velocity (TAV). VTI is the area under spectral velocity–time curve, while TAV is the VTI divided by the duration of the cardiac cycle. Most frequently, volumetric flow Q is calculated as:

$$Q = \text{VTI} \times \text{CSA (where } Q \text{ is in units of volume), or}$$
$$Q = \text{TAV} \times \text{CSA (where } Q \text{ is in units of volume per unit time)}$$

where CSA is the cross-sectional area of the region of interest. This equation assumes a steady flow, a non-varying circular cross-sectional area, and uniform velocities across the entire cross-sectional area. Despite the limitations and errors imposed by these assumptions, these equations remain widely used and indeed are helpful in determining stroke volume, cardiac output, and the magnitude of intracardiac shunts such as the ratio Qp:Qs (DeGroff, 2002) (see Quantitative Methods section). Other methods of determining volumetric flow are being investigated but are not in widespread use (DeGroff, 2002).

The various Doppler modes used include PW, CW, and HPRF Doppler, all of which interrogate the flow of blood; color Doppler flow mapping, which is a specialized projection of PW Doppler data onto a broad sector of interest; and tissue Doppler imaging (TDI), which through different frequency filters, interrogates the lower-velocity motion of the myocardium itself (Quinones et al., 2002).

Pulse-Wave Doppler. Given its range specificity but limited by maximal velocities that can be interrogated, PW Doppler is best used to determine laminar volumetric flow, sites of obstruction (but not necessarily pressure gradients at those sites), and very mild obstructions. Specific flow situations where PW Doppler is useful include volumetric flow in normal vessels or across normal valves, including Qp:Qs; determining where flow accelerates further in multiple left-sided outflow obstruction or in a patient with tetralogy of Fallot; and pulmonary regurgitation jet velocities, if these are not elevated.

Continuous-Wave Doppler. CW Doppler is most useful in determining the significant pressure gradients across vessels, valves, and septal defects where there are high velocities. One must remember that since the reflected–shifted ultrasound frequencies arrive from anywhere along the path of the beam, one cannot tell where the velocities are highest; therefore, in situations of multiple-level obstruction, the pressure gradient obtained is the maximal gradient from somewhere along the path. One must also be careful that

the maximal velocities interrogated are in the region of interest, and not arising from elsewhere in the heart or a different blood vessel; for example, flow acceleration across the proximal left pulmonary artery may in a small infant be mistaken for aortic coarctation, since the signals could arise very closely.

Because the velocities represented within the Doppler spectral display arise from anywhere along the Doppler beam, the envelope is in general not used to calculate volumetric flow.

High Pulse Repetition Frequency Doppler. Modern ultrasound systems are able to offer a "compromise" between PW and CW Doppler. Simplistically, by "listening" more frequently (i.e., before the pulse returns to the transducer), the system is able to interrogate more than one sample volume. More frequent sampling allows for higher Nyquist limits, but maintains some degree of range specificity. HPRF Doppler is useful when one would like range specificity (e.g., in multiple-level obstruction), but requires Nyquist limits that permit accurate determination of pressure gradients. Because the Nyquist limit is still not as high as with CW Doppler, mild to moderately elevated velocities are best ascertained with this method.

Color Doppler Flow Mapping. Because the color Doppler flow map is essentially the information from spectral PW Doppler converted from individual points to an amalgamated "color map," it is subject to the general limitations of Doppler echocardiography, including the angle dependency of data accuracy. It should also be remembered that the processing used to generate the color flow map does not translate points of PW Doppler precisely into accurate flow velocities, which requires too much time and processing power. Therefore, technical considerations include optimizing the Doppler incident angle, and refining one's imaging sector to the region of interest. The Nyquist limit of the color flow map should be adjusted to approximately the flow velocity of interest: for most applications, this should be set as high as possible, although one would deliberately set a lower Nyquist limit in order to detect flow in venous structures and coronary vessels. Finally, it should be remembered that the color map represents a map of flow velocities, not flow itself—this is particularly relevant when assessing severity of regurgitant jets (see below).

The marriage of color Doppler mapping with M-mode echocardiography provides information on left ventricular diastolic function, namely relaxation. Briefly, in early diastole, there exists an intraventricular pressure gradient from base (mitral orifice) to apex that generates an apically-directed "velocity propagation" wavefront; the spatiotemporal distribution of the blood-column velocities contained within the entire scanline is reflected in the color Doppler flow map contained within the distance–time domain of the M-mode strip (see Border et al., 2003; De Boeck et al., 2005). Although promising as a relatively load-independent index of left ventricular relaxation, the technique is technically challenging and difficult to interpret, and data are scant in children (Border et al., 2003; Bess et al., 2006; De Boeck et al., 2005; Gomez et al., 2005).

Tissue Doppler Imaging. When special low-pass filters are incorporated, signals from higher-velocity blood flow are attenuated, permitting display of myocardial tissue motion. TDI has assumed importance in the assessment of diastolic function (see below), as well as regional wall motion abnormalities. Like all Doppler modalities, it is subject to the weaknesses of Doppler physics, most notably the angle dependence of the returning ultrasound signal. Relative ease of use and reproducibility appear to be strengths of this imaging technique (Bess et al., 2006).

Contrast Echocardiography. The physical basis of contrast echocardiography lies in the volume pulsations and output signals generated by microbubbles excited by the fundamental ultrasound beam; these microbubbles produce enhanced echo reflections. Contrast echocardiography has proven useful in the delineation of congenital heart defects and associated problems (see Van Hare and Silverman, 1989). Much of contrast echocardiography in children uses simple saline contrast (Van Hare and Silverman, 1989). In CHD, most contrast/microbubble use has been limited to detection of right-to-left shunts at the atrial or ventricular levels; patch leaks and baffle leaks in Senning/Mustard operations and Glenns and Fontans; fistulas and pulmonary AVMs; systemic venous connections to the atria in complex heart disease; and improved border delineation—of vessels and of endocardium (Bernstein et al., 1995; Chang, 1999; Larsson, 2001; Van Hare and Silverman, 1989). One problem with saline contrast is that it does not cross the pulmonary capillary bed. Newer commercially available contrast agents with more stable shells, combined with harmonic imaging, allow improved delineation of left ventricular endocardial borders and, therefore, left ventricular function including during stress testing, while appearing to be safe (McMahon et al., 2005; Zilberman et al., 2003). Myocardial contrast echocardiography permits the assessment of the myocardial microcirculation (Lepper 2004), and in limited studies, may be useful in children with myocardial perfusion abnormalities (Ishii et al., 2002; Sheil et al., 2003).

Harmonic Imaging. In our experience and in that of others, tissue harmonic imaging may aid in the image quality of the pediatric patient with poor windows (McMahon et al., 2001). Harmonics are additional vibrations generated by the tissue superimposed on the fundamental frequency and thereby distorting the fundamental sine-wave pattern, resulting in indistinct tissue–tissue and tissue–blood interfaces. Tissue harmonic imaging transmits at a fundamental frequency and receives at the second harmonic (twice the fundamental frequency) to reduce the ultrasound artifacts that distort and muddy the tissue interfaces. The net result is an improvement in endocardial border detection, albeit at the expense of spatial resolution (Turner and Monaghan, 2006)—the image produced is considerably grainier than fundamental frequency imaging.

Miscellaneous Technologies. The backscatter of ultrasound signals may be processed in sophisticated ways to allow definition of the physical state of the muscle itself. Thus, tissue characterization may be a way to assess abnormal myocardium, such as that found in ischemia or chronic fibrosis. Work in children has been limited, but shows some promise in defining cardiomyopathies and myocardial changes with chronic CHDs, perhaps even prior to the onset of overt systolic or diastolic dysfunction (Goens et al., 1996; Giglio et al., 2003; Hopkins et al., 1994).

Speckle tracking is another promising new technology that enables determination of the strain rate, without the angle dependence of tissue Doppler imaging, and so may be useful in the definition of both systolic and diastolic functions, in both the right and left ventricles under a variety of disease states (Amundsen, 2006; Pirat et al., 2006; Takeuchi et al., 2006).

Biosafety Considerations. Diagnostic ultrasound and echocardiography have a long record of safety, but there are potential issues with which the pediatric echocardiographer and sonographer ought to be familiar (Carstensen et al, 1992; Skorton et al., 1988). Ultrasound energy can be converted into thermal energy (heat), generate acoustic cavitation, and produce acoustical forces, torques, and flows, at high enough power (Nyborg, 2001). Guidelines have therefore been developed by the appropriate organizations and oversight bodies on the proper use and monitoring of ultrasound. The echocardiographer should be aware that the PW Doppler uses longer pulse lengths, higher frequency repetition, and focuses on a single site for a longer period of time, and, therefore, carries a greater potential for damage (Danford and Murphy, 1998). Local heating is more likely with intracavitary or intraluminal probes such as those used in transesophageal echocardiography (TEE) and intracardiac echocardiography (ICE) (Danford and Murphy, 1998). It is likely that fetal tissue is more susceptible to injury (see the chapter on Fetal Cardiology). In short, the echocardiographer should be cognizant of the potential biosafety aspects of diagnostic medical ultrasound and scan as safely with the minimum power necessary to generate images to answer the questions posed.

Common Indications for and Objectives of Pediatric Echocardiography

Its noninvasive nature, unparalleled safety profile, and ability to collect important anatomical and hemodynamic information rapidly make echocardiography central to diagnostic pediatric cardiology, but opens up the possibility of overuse and suboptimal use, particularly in an era of cost-containment and cost-benefit analyses. Therefore, indications for its use and specific questions to be answered must always be considered before performing a study (Cheitlin et al., 1997; Geva, 1998; Phoon et al., 1999); asking specific questions that best help to round out the clinical evaluation is especially important in the patient with suboptimal imaging windows. This is simply good medicine. It should be noted that heart murmurs, chest pain, and syncope are relatively common presenting complaints during childhood, and are frequently normal or noncardiac in origin. As stated in the ACC/AHA Guidelines for the Clinical Application of Echocardiography (Cheitlin et al., 1997), history and physical examination by a skilled observer are usually sufficient to distinguish functional-, from pathological murmurs and are more cost-effective than referral for an echocardiogram. However, in the presence of "ambiguous clinical findings," echocardiography may be useful to determine the presence of pathology. In particular, certain clinical scenarios and patient populations may not be as reliably assessed by clinical means alone, and echocardiography will play an important role in determining or ruling out heart disease—for example, newborns and young infants (Danford, 1997, 2002; Du et al., 1997; Azhar and Habib, 2006). The "story" told by the echocardiogram ultimately should make sense when weaved into the clinical context.

Echocardiography also affords the clinician the opportunity to confirm or corroborate clinical findings, and the opportunity to hone clinical skills (Phoon, 2001). Thus, when an echocardiogram is done, the correlation of echo-Doppler data with the clinical picture helps one rapidly gather experience and clinical acumen, because of the immediate feedback (Phoon, 2000).

The ACC/AHA Guidelines for the Clinical Application of Echocardiography, most recently promulgated in 1997 and updated in 2003, provide guidelines for the indications and use of echocardiography in both adults and children, as well as in fetal echocardiography. Common indications, with a particular

TABLE 4–2. *Common Indications for Echocardiography*

Heart murmurs or other exam findings suggestive of congenital/ structural heart disease
Monitoring for late postoperative complications and/or subclinical evolution thereof
Primary or secondary pulmonary hypertension, monitoring for progression thereof
Cardiomyopathies (primary or secondary)
Pericardial disease, including effusions, intrapericardial tumors, and congenital absence of the pericardium
Cardiac masses and tumors
Structural and functional heart disease associated with arrhythmias and palpitations
Persistent pulmonary hypertension of the newborn
Genetic syndromes and familial heart disease; multiple congenital anomalies
Arteriovenous malformations with high-output state
Chest pain
Syncope
Cerebrovascular accident
Diagnosis and management of acquired pediatric heart disease, including:
  – Kawasaki disease
  – Rheumatic heart disease
  – Endocarditis
  – Secondary cardiomyopathies: postchemotherapeutic, tachycardia-induced, HIV, etc.
  – Cardiac and aortic trauma

emphasis on congenital heart defects, are listed in Table 4–2 (Cheitlin et al., 1997, 2003; Geva and van der Velde, 2006; Phoon et al., 1999).

Pediatric echocardiography has evolved to the level where in the majority of cases, surgery can be undertaken with echocardiography as the sole diagnostic imaging modality, with high accuracy and an excellent patient safety record, in centers around the world; only rarely is there an error significant enough to prompt important changes in management of the disease (Lopes et al., 2005; Marek et al., 1995; Pfammatter et al., 2000; Tworetzky et al., 1999). Our philosophy is that the echocardiogram should be taken within the complete clinical context of the patient; however, additional imaging or testing should be considered when important questions are not yet answered. The high diagnostic accuracy of preoperative transthoracic echocardiography as the sole preoperative imaging modality and the safety of this approach may also be attributed in part to the now-routine use of comprehensive TEE prebypass to confirm and refine diagnoses, and to establish baseline echocardiographic parameters for comparison with postbypass imaging (Ayres et al., 2005; Phoon et al., 1999).

People, Equipment, and Technology in the Pediatric Echocardiography Laboratory

The pediatric echocardiography laboratory is the central facility among a pediatric cardiovascular center's noninvasive diagnostic elements. Most pediatric cardiology programs will have dedicated pediatric echocardiography labs (AAP, 2002). The echo laboratory must have physicians and sonographers staff trained in pediatric echocardiography and CHD, and state-of-the-art equipment and facilities suitable for children (AAP, 2002). Appropriate ongoing experience with a broad clinical spectrum is also necessary for maintenance and continual improvement of skills (AAP, 2002). Finally, optimal imaging is generated only if our young patients can cooperate adequately for the examination.

Staffing, Training, and Qualifications.
The pediatric cardiologist–echocardiographer must understand the anatomical and hemodynamic bases of congenital and pediatric heart disease, and their natural and "unnatural" histories, as well as complications of management. Training in CHD, acquired pediatric heart disease, and pediatric cardiology is therefore essential to competent imaging in an echocardiography laboratory, and training guidelines have been promulgated recently (Sanders et al., 2005). In addition, the sonographer staff must also be well-versed in congenital and pediatric heart disease. Both cognitive and technical skills are needed for outstanding pediatric cardiovascular imaging, and guidelines reflect the scope—both breadth and depth—needed for adequate training (Cheitlin et al., 1997; Sanders et al., 2005).

The issue of training and competence in pediatric echocardiography is not a trivial one. Studies of pediatric echocardiograms performed in adult echocardiography laboratories and interpreted by adult cardiologists now have demonstrated a high error rate, including both overdiagnoses (such as labeling a normal heart as abnormal) and underdiagnoses (of all spectrum of congenital heart defects); major and life-threatening errors as well as delays in diagnosis and treatment have occurred (Hurwitz and Caldwell, 1998; Stanger et al., 1999). Another study confirmed that the diagnostic accuracy of pediatric echocardiograms interpreted by nonpediatric cardiologists—radiologists, neonatologists, and adult cardiologists—was unacceptably poor (Ward and Purdie, 2001). All three studies showed that errors could be attributed to both technical and interpretive errors. Specific factors resulting in poor diagnostic accuracy also seemed to be related to a failure to acknowledge or recognize relevant clinical information, and failure to complete a structured and complete pediatric echocardiogram (Ward and Purdie, 2001). The data therefore not only point to the importance of the proper training background of individuals imaging children but also the importance of the clinical context in which the echocardiogram is performed.

Equipment

Basic Equipment and Setup. Equipment and ultrasound systems in the pediatric echo laboratory should be appropriate for use in the wide range of ages encountered, including for fetal echocardiography. The modern pediatric laboratory will have transducers that cover 2–12 MHz, including multiband/broadband transducers, allowing for optimal imaging in both the smallest patients (as well as coronary arteries, etc.) and the largest patients. M-mode and 2-D echocardiography, PW and CW Doppler, and color flow Doppler mapping are used routinely. Additional imaging modes include harmonic imaging, TDI, and strain rate analysis, found on more current ultrasound systems. 3-D echo is now being used at several centers, but is not considered routine by the broader community yet. Ultrasound systems should include processing and software packages for pediatric/congenital heart work, and must be initially set up by individuals knowledgeable in pediatric applications. Methods of storage include videotape (ideally S-VHS tape, which is higher resolution than standard VHS mode) or digital archiving (see below). A strip chart recorder is useful for M-mode echo, and electrocardiogram (EKG) on the echo study is useful for determining timing within the cardiac cycle and for certain echocardiographic time interval measurements.

Weight and height determination allow for calculation of body surface area, and at a minimum, weight allows for indexing to obtain Z scores of various measurements. An echocardiographic study is often best interpreted in the context of basic clinical information such as heart rate, blood pressure, and pulsoximetry oxygen saturation, which ideally is recorded in the echo report along with the other echo data. The echo request should contain a brief clinical history and the clinical question.

Digital Echocardiography and Telemedicine. Over the past decade, the digital pediatric echocardiography laboratory has become a reality. Advances in computer technology have moved us into an era of rapid processing and inexpensive electronic storage that permits the acquisition, reading, and storage of pediatric echocardiograms. Primary advantages of digital echo are listed in Table 4–3 (from Hansen et al., 2004; Mathewson et al., 2000, 2002; Sable, 2002).

Although digital streaming technology allows the capture of long video streams much as videotape does, the advantages of a digital echo laboratory are best realized with data capture via time- or beat-defined loops and still frames. Many laboratories have adopted single-beat loops for most of their image data capture, although for more complex disease, longer sweeps may be useful (Frommelt et al., 2002; Hansen, 2004;

TABLE 4–3. *Primary Advantages of a Digital Echocardiography Laboratory*

Reproduction of high-quality images without degradation
Ability to transmit date across great distances nearly
  instantaneously, without image degradation
Rapid review of "loops" of data; reduced review time
Electronic archiving and retrieval: no more searching for tapes!
  – Ability to compare side-by-side with previous studies
  – Ability to review where there is a networked workstation,
    onsite or offsite
  – Facilitation of research and education
  – Reduced long-term storage space requirements
Easy copying of studies onto digital media for transport/transmis-
  sion to other laboratories

Mathewson et al., 2000, 2002; Sable, 2002). JPEG-compression ratios of approximately 20:1 or better will result in image quality superior to that of videotape, while keeping file sizes manageable at on average 20–30 MB (Frommelt et al., 2002; Mathewson et al., 2000; Sable, 2002). Importantly, the use of loops—as opposed to "free" video streaming—mandates a defined imaging protocol to ensure complete data capture for complete segmental and functional analyses (see Frommelt et al., 2002; Hansen 2004; Mathewson et al., 2002; Sable, 2002). It should be noted that because of the complex nature of CHD, the number of loops and the file sizes for a single patient can be enormous. Because one can no longer freely tape and hope to capture the relevant information in a "catch as catch can" manner, sedation may assume a more important role than in the traditional videotape echo laboratory (Frommelt et al., 2002—see below).

While many have enthusiastically embraced the digital echocardiography laboratory, issues related to setting up a digital pediatric echocardiography laboratory include reservations about industry DICOM standards and compatibility among various vendors (Sable, 2002), the expense of setting up a digital laboratory (Frommelt et al., 2002), and future compatibility issues and system obsolescence as well as issues related to rapid recovery and data backup (Hanson, 2004). The use of digital loops and still frames in often-moving children too causes consternation in some. Still, the transition to a digital laboratory is typically not difficult (Mathewson et al., 2000), although it requires careful planning based on a thorough analysis of one's own echocardiography laboratory practice, as well as support from the hospital information technology group (Hansen, 2004; Sable, 2002).

Tele-echocardiography uses digital technology to transmit image data from remote sites; large networks can be covered. Given the alternative of having a currier send a videotape to the echo laboratory, telemedicine has proven very useful, especially in areas with problems of access to care (Cloutier and Finley, 2004; Sable, 2002; Sable et al., 2002; Widmer et al., 2003; Woodson et al., 2004). Tele-echocardiography has exhibited high-diagnostic accuracy and cost-effectiveness (Cloutier and Finley, 2004; Widmer et al., 2003; Woodson et al., 2004). Practical issues to consider include store-and-forward approaches versus real-time review of studies (and inherently the broadband lines and bandwidth needed [Milazzo et al., 2002; Sable et al., 2002; Woodson et al., 2004]), and quality of the imaging performed at the outlying site (Sable, 2002; Widmer et al., 2003). In particular, diagnostic inaccuracies appear to be related especially to sonographer inexperience and lack of a proper or accurate clinical context (Widmer et al., 2003). Because protected health information is being transmitted electronically, legal issues related to telemedicine include security (unless the data are transmitted over a dedicated line) and confidentiality (Widmer et al., 2003).

Portable Hand-Carried Echocardiography Units: "Point of Service" Care. Portable handheld, "point of service" echocardiography units have garnered much recent attention as the next primary diagnostic tool, touted as an extension of the physical examination (Mondillo et al., 2000; Seward et al., 2002). It is generally acknowledged that the image quality is not as good as on full-featured ultrasound imaging systems (Li et al., 2003; Seward et al., 2002). However, very limited data in infants and children suggest that screening for CHD is quite feasible (Li et al., 2003). Moreover, it may have clinical utility in pediatric critical-care units by noncardiologists to rapidly and reliably diagnose pericardial effusions, ventricular dysfunction, and left ventricular enlargement (Spurney et al., 2005). Hand-carried units may assume an important role in the diagnosis and management of significant CHD particularly in remote and underserved areas (Li et al., 2003). Although advances in technology will improve their ability to diagnose CHD, parallel advances will concomitantly improve full-featured systems as well. Therefore, the question of the role of hand-carried echo when full-featured systems are available remains an open one.

Sedation. In many echo laboratories, conscious sedation is an important technique to facilitate optimal imaging quality, and in certain cases, to mimic consciousness levels in the cardiac catheterization laboratory for proper comparison of hemodynamic data. Krauss and Green (2006) have stated that "the ideal sedation endpoint is one at which the procedure can be successfully accomplished with as little distress to the patient as possible and with cardiopulmonary stability and retention of protective airway reflexes." Because many children, especially under the age of 3 years, do not cooperate for an echocardiogram, moderate to deep sedation may be required.

By far, the most widely used agent is the sedative-hypnotic chloral hydrate, which carries a documented track record of efficacy and safety (Heistein et al., 2006; Napoli et al., 1996; Malviya et al., 2004; Wheeler et al., 2001). In general, the dose used is 75–100 mg/kg orally (maximum dose, 1–2 g), although doses as low as 25 mg/kg have also been used. Lower doses may be used in conjunction with other agents, such as diphenhydramine or midazolam (Heistein et al., 2006). Its onset of action is approximately 30 minutes, with recovery taking some 1–2 hours; it is most reliable in children under 3 years of age (Krauss and Green, 2006), the group most likely to benefit from sedation in the pediatric echocardiography laboratory. Side effects with chloral hydrate are uncommon, but include apnea, airway obstruction, hypoxemia, hypercarbia, vomiting, prolonged sedation, and in rare cases, hypotension (Heistein et al., 2006).

Others have used the benzodiazepine midazolam successfully, which may have a shorter recovery time, but produces a less-deep sedation than chloral hydrate (Wheeler et al., 2001). Midazolam has anxiolytic, amnestic, sedative-hypnotic, muscle relaxant, and anticonvulsant properties, is reversible, and can be administered orally, intranasally, or rectally. It carries an excellent safety profile when used alone, but as with all sedatives, respiratory depression may be an issue. The onset of action after oral intake is approximately 15–30 minutes, with a duration of 60–90 minutes (Krauss and Green, 2006). Limited data on other sedative agents, such as rectal thiopental (Okutan et al., 2000), also exist.

Guidelines for pediatric sedation are extensively reviewed elsewhere (see Krauss and Green, 2006). A presedation history and examination are necessary to determine the level of risk. Equipment for airway protection and maintenance, and cardiopulmonary resuscitation are required to be on hand. The child should be NPO prior to the administration of sedation, although the minimum time required is a matter of some debate (Ghaffar et al., 2002). Vital signs and hemodynamic parameters that need to be monitored either continuously or frequently include heart rate, respiratory rate, pulsoximetry oxygen saturation, and blood pressure; and level of consciousness, rhythm, and end-tidal CO_2 (capnography) may be desirable as well. Since continuous observation by a healthcare provider is needed in addition to the individual performing the echocardiogram, typically a physician and a nurse/respiratory therapist will be present. A postprocedural assessment is made after the study is done, and the

child may be discharged from the echocardiography laboratory when a "presedation level of responsiveness or a level as close as possible to the normal level for that individual should be achieved [before discharge]" (Malviya et al., 2004). It is clear that routine sedation in a pediatric echocardiography laboratory will require additional resources and personnel, along with a longer stay in the laboratory for the family (Bezold and Ayres, 1998; Malviya et al., 2004).

Many pediatric centers now routinely sedate young children and infants (Ghaffar et al., 2002). Although we use sedation when necessary, we do not adhere to the philosophy of routine sedation in any age group. We find that complete echocardiograms of excellent quality can be achieved in most babies and children when they are distracted with a bottle, toy, or video (Phoon et al., 1999; Stevenson et al., 1990; Silverman, 1993). Other factors that help to a great extent in dealing with the fussy child are a child-friendly environment, allowing a child to sit up or in a parent's lap, and patience. In our experience, when echocardiographic data are taken in the context of the complete clinical picture, the conundrum of unsedated echo data and how they might translate into cardiac-catheterization data arises only uncommonly.

The Echocardiographic Examination: Nomenclature and Segmental Analysis

The "fun" of pediatric cardiology lies in the myriad structural anomalies that may be present. However, without a systematic approach to the CHD, describing and understanding the morphology and hemodynamics behind some of the most complex lesions can be nearly impossible. We will discuss a systematic, segmental approach to using the echocardiogram in understanding the CHD, based on determination of segments (systemic and pulmonary veins, atria, ventricles, and great arteries) and their junctions/connections (venoatrial, atrioventricular, and ventriculo-arterial). Given that the heart is a 3-D structure, the challenge in the development of echocardiography is how to translate 3-D relationships into single or 2-D representations. In this section, we will review the various "views" one uses in the complete examination. Although chronologically, M-mode echocardiography was developed before 2-D echocardiography, for practical purposes, we will review the 2-D views first. This sequential, segmental approach has enjoyed great success in delineating the complexities of the CHD, and permits a standardized, logical imaging approach to pediatric echocardiography (see Gutgesell et al., 1985; Gerlis et al., 1999; Garg et al., 2003; Lai et al., 2006; Pasquini et al., 1988).

Below is a suggested order of the various views. All of the views listed are standard views; however the order may vary depending on the individual laboratory as well as patient cooperation. Furthermore, it is important to recognize that for complex lesions, the skilled echocardiographer must obtain "nonstandard" views for complete delineation of morphology.

Two-Dimension Examination. Multiple views have been developed as part of the complete transthoracic study offering perspectives on the superior–inferior, anterior–posterior, right–left relationships of various intracardiac and extracardiac structures. The following summary of the various views highlights the best structures imaged from various locations. In general, "long axis" refers to views that parallel the long or major axis of the heart. "Short axis" is the orthogonal view that parallels the short or minor axis of the heart. Images are displayed on the screen as if the patient was facing the imager with the patient's right on the left side of the screen and vice versa. Furthermore, and different from adult imaging protocols, the image is presented "upright" (the image sector as an upright "V") in the subcostal and apical views, whereas in the parasternal and suprasternal views, the image is "inverted" (the image sector as an upside down "V").

Subcostal Long Axis/Coronal. This view is obtained by placing the transducer just distal to the xiphoid process. Its advantage lies in the minimal lung interference with the images. It has limited utility in older adolescents and adults in whom there is increased abdominal muscle tone or increased girth. Bending the knees can help minimize some of the abdominal tone, as well as using slow, steady pressure. It establishes the superior–inferior and right–left relationships of the structures, with posterior–anterior sweeps. This view helps to establish abdominal and atrial situs and veno-atrial connections, in addition to the atrioventricular and ventriculo-arterial relationships (Figure 4–1). The atrial septum is perpendicular to the plane of imaging and thus, this view is good for assessing various types of atrial septal defects. Images from this view also help establish the presence of a pericardial effusion in the inferior aspect, which may be amenable to pericardiocentesis.

Pleural effusions can also be noted on this view. As tempting as it may be to quantify the effusions, echocardiographic assessment is inaccurate.

Subcostal Short Axis/Sagittal. This view establishes systemic venous anatomy and connections, including the presence of a persistent left superior vena cava and the superior and inferior sinus venosus anatomy (Figure 4–2). An intact inferior vena cava should be documented. In addition, the right upper pulmonary vein can be defined coursing in between the right superior vena cava and the right pulmonary artery. This

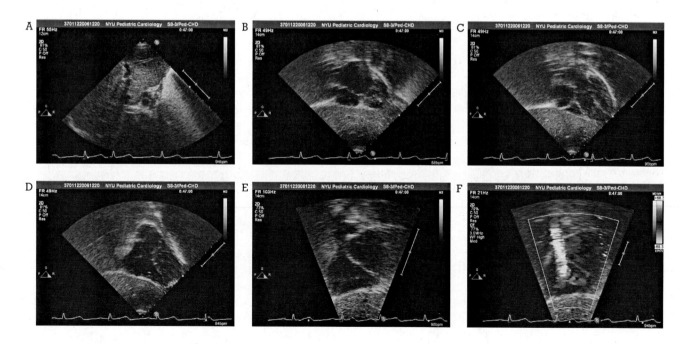

FIGURE 4–1. Subcostal coronal plane imaging. A: Imaging starts generally with establishing the abdominal and veno-atrial situs. B: As the transducer is angled anteriorly, the right and left atria come into view, along with the interatrial septum. C and D: Further anterior angulation brings the right and left ventricles (C) into view, then the right ventricular outflow tract (D). E and F: Zoomed-in view of the interatrial septum, by 2-D/cross-sectional imaging (E) and with color Doppler flow mapping to rule out interatrial shunts (F).

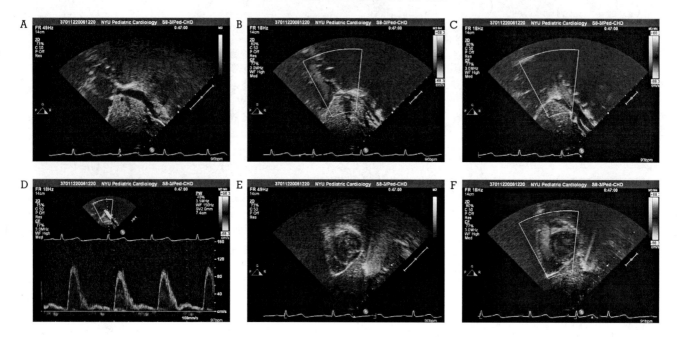

FIGURE 4–2. Subcostal sagittal plane imaging. A: SVC, IVC, and interatrial septum are imaged. B: Color Doppler flow mapping is used to detect interatrial shunting. C: With leftward angulation, the descending aorta comes into view. D: Pulsed-wave Doppler interrogation of the descending aorta. E: Subcostal short-axis imaging of the ventricles. F: Color Doppler flow mapping of the ventricles and their outflow tracts.

view also gives the orthogonal view of the atrial septum and the dimensions of atrial communications should include measurements from both the short and long axis view. As one sweeps leftward from the atria, this is a good view to define the right ventricular outflow tract. The left ventricular outflow tract and left ventricle come into view with further leftward imaging, and the left ventricle is seen in younger children beautifully in its short axis.

Lastly, the thoracic/abdominal descending aorta can be visualized parallel to this plane. Obtaining a PW-Doppler signal of the descending aorta can suggest any run-off lesions, such as a patent ductus arteriosus or aortopulmonary window, or can give information about a possible coarctation lesion. The subcostal short axis gives the superior–inferior and anterior–posterior relationships, with right–left sweeps.

The echocardiographer should recognize that these two subcostal sweeps, which can be performed in a newborn expeditiously, can very quickly establish the presence or absence of significant CHD.

Apical Four-Chamber. The transducer is held over the cardiac apex and offers perspective of right and left chamber sizes. The standard view displays the heart in a direct up–down relationship such that the atrioventricular valves are perpendicular to the transducer beam (Figure 4–3). This view defines superior–inferior and right–left relationships, with posterior–anterior sweeps. To minimize lung interference,

a left lateral decubitus position is advisable. This view offers the optimal line-up to obtain PW Doppler signals of the tricuspid and mitral valve inflows, as well as a right pulmonary vein. Posterior angulation of the transducer brings the coronary sinus into view, while anterior angulation of the transducer affords imaging of the left ventricular outflow tract, although the even more anterior right ventricular outflow tract is usually less well-seen. Defining atrial communications from this view is least optimal due to the parallel position to the transducer beam with resultant dropout artifact.

The apical view is also well suited to defining the systolic function of the apical segments of both ventricles.

Parasternal Long Axis. The transducer is aligned with the long axis of the heart at the left mid-sternal border such that the apex of the heart is on the left side of the screen and the base on the right side. Images from this view offer superior–inferior and poster–anterior relationships, with right–left sweeps (Figure 4–4). As noted in the apical four-chamber view, there can be considerable interference of the images due to air-filled lungs overlying the heart. To optimize imaging in the parasternal views, a left lateral decubitus position is again advisable. Standard imaging begins with establishing the left ventricular inflow and outflow tracts, and aortic-mitral annular continuity; this is an excellent view for imaging of the mitral valve and the left

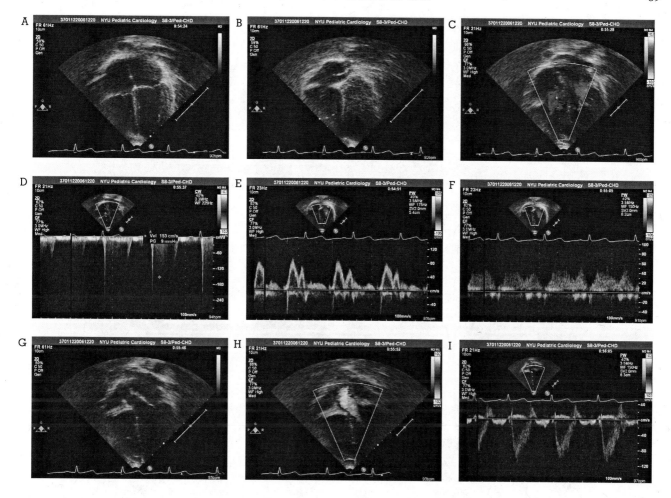

FIGURE 4-3. Apical four chamber view. A: Right and left atria, tricuspid, and mitral valves, and right and left ventricles are seen in this view. B: Posterior angulation of the transducer will show the more posterior aspects of the interventricular septum, as well as the coronary sinus. C: Color Doppler flow mapping at the level of the atrioventricular valves gauges AV valve regurgitation as well as guides placement of the Doppler sample volume for interrogation of AV inflow. D: Continuous-wave Doppler interrogation of mild tricuspid regurgitation to estimate pulmonary artery pressures. E: Pulsed-wave Doppler interrogation of the mitral inflow pattern, demonstrating the dominant E wave and the A wave. F: Pulsed-wave Doppler interrogation of the right pulmonary venous flow, demonstrating the S and D waves, as well as physiological "a" reversal. G: From the four chamber view, anterior angulation opens up the left ventricular outflow tract and the aortic outflow. H: Color Doppler flow mapping of the left ventricular and aortic outflow tract. I: Pulsed-wave Doppler interrogation of the aortic outflow.

ventricular outflow tract. Sweeps then proceed rightward/posteriorly to examine the tricuspid valve, and then leftward/anteriorly to the right ventricular outflow tract and main pulmonary artery. The branch pulmonary arteries can be partially seen in this view, but this is not the optimal view.

Parasternal Short Axis. This view offers posterior–anterior and right–left relationships, with right/superior–left/inferior sweeps (Figure 4–5). Starting from the base of the heart, the right side of the heart can be seen wrapping around clockwise starting with the right atrium at the left lower part of the screen going into the right ventricle as the most anterior structure, then going out to the main pulmonary artery and the

proximal branch pulmonary arteries. The ductus can be seen in this view as well, though optimal imaging of the length of the ductus requires rotating the transducer to a position nearly halfway between a long axis and a short axis cut, that is, the "ductal view." The coronary anatomy and aortic valve anatomy can be defined by visualizing the base of the heart in the parasternal short axis view. Scanning towards the apex defines the mitral valve papillary muscles and qualitative assessment of the left ventricular function, including segmental wall motion analysis. Quantitative evaluation of the left ventricular systolic function can be obtained with an M-mode scan of the left ventricle in this view just distal to the mitral valve leaflet tips.

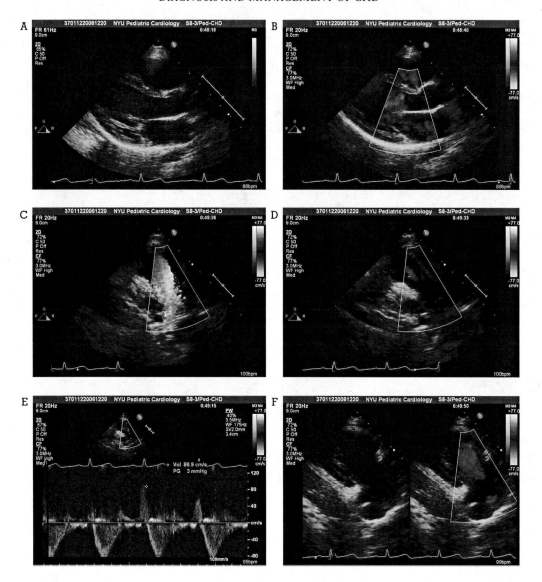

FIGURE 4–4. Parasternal long axis view. A (2-D) and B (color Doppler flow mapping): LV, mitral valve, and aortic outflow are seen. C and D: With leftward tilt of the transducer, the pulmonary outflow is brought into view, with color Doppler flow mapping demonstrating normal forward flow in the main pulmonary artery (C) and normal mild pulmonary regurgitation (D). E. Pulsed-wave Doppler interrogation of normal flow in the main pulmonary artery. F. With rightward transducer tilt, the right ventricle and tricuspid valve are brought into view.

Suprasternal Long Axis. This is known as the "candy cane" or the "arch view." As can be deduced from the nicknames, this view offers the best view of the aortic arch with the head and neck vessels (Figure 4–6). The suprasternal views are obtained by placing the transducer in the patient's suprasternal notch, with the long axis plane being anterior–posterior with slight clockwise rotation for a normal left-sided aortic arch; the imaging plane is more vertical in orientation with a right arch. In young infants, the view is usually best achieved from an area between the right infraclavicular region and the suprasternal notch, with the transducer tilted slightly back rightward toward the patient's midline. This view offers imaging of the anterior–posterior and superior–inferior axes with right–left sweeps. One can examine the aortic arch from the ascending to the thoracic descending portion. It is a useful view for delineating the source of the run-off lesions, localizing coarctation, and determining arch-sidedness. Arch-sidedness can be determined by the directionality of the branching of the first head and neck vessel as the transducer pivots to the patient's right; alternatively, if the transducer is in a completely horizontal plane, the innominate artery as the first brachiocephalic vessel will course rightward and branch into two, the right common carotid artery and the right subclavian artery. This view can also be used to examine the proximal left pulmonary artery, left innominate veins, and proximal portion of the right superior vena cava.

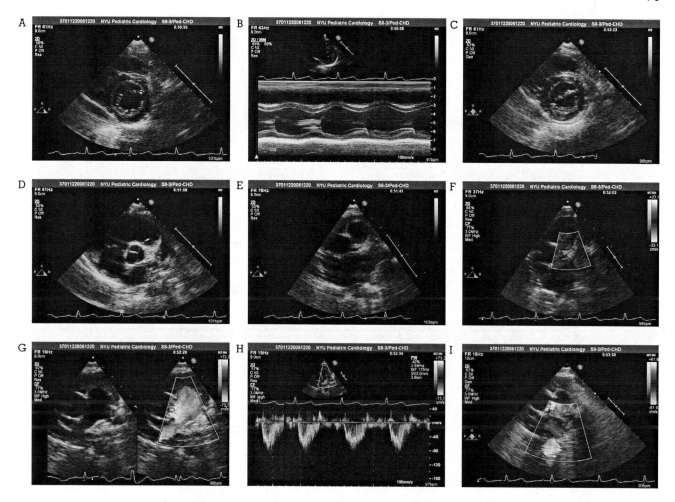

FIGURE 4–5. Parasternal short axis view. A: Left and right ventricles in short axis. B: M-mode of the left ventricle. C: As one scans toward the base of the heart, the mitral valve is brought into view en face. D: Further scanning toward the base brings the aortic valve into view. E and F: Coronary artery imaging by 2-D/cross-sectional imaging (E) and with color Doppler flow mapping (F). G: Further cranial angulation beyond the aortic root brings the pulmonary outflow and pulmonary arteries into view, with and without color Doppler flow mapping. H: Pulsed-wave Doppler interrogation of the main pulmonary artery flow. I: From the high parasternal short axis view, generally the pulmonary veins may be imaged.

Suprasternal Short Axis. By turning the transducer 90 degrees clockwise such that the transducer is in a horizontal imaging plane, the short axis or "crab" view comes into position. This view demonstrates the right–left and superior–anterior axes. Sweeps can be performed in the anterior–posterior direction. The standard beginning view is that of the left innominate vein at the most superior position, with the transverse arch in the cross-section underneath, then the proximal right pulmonary artery coursing leftward on the screen visualizing the first branching point of the right pulmonary artery, and finally the left atrium with the pulmonary veins ("the crab") at the most inferior part of the image. Sweeping more anteriorly brings the proximal branch pulmonary arteries into view offering a clear image of the branch points. This view can also

demonstrate the upper systemic venous drainage pattern very well.

Within each view, typically a complete 2-D scan is performed to define the anatomy and relationships of structures with one another, and to qualitatively assess ventricular function with pertinent measurements. The long axis sweeps are in the anterior–posterior plane using the coronary sinus as the most posterior landmark, and the right ventricular outflow and main pulmonary artery as the most anterior landmarks. This is then followed by a color flow Doppler sweep, a PW and/or CW Doppler analyses of inflows, outflows, and defects.

A complete and thorough pediatric echocardiogram can be time-consuming. In our laboratory, a complete study is generally mandated for every new patient, but

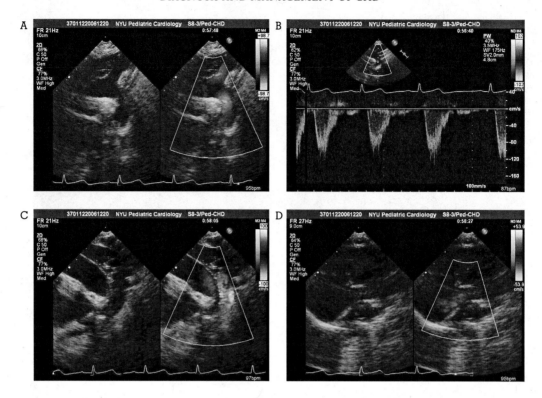

FIGURE 4–6. Suprasternal notch imaging. A: The "candy cane" view, by 2-D and color Doppler flow imaging, demonstrating a normally patent aortic arch. B: Pulsed-wave Doppler interrogation of the proximal descending (thoracic) aorta. C: Slight counterclockwise rotation of the transducer into a "vertical" imaging plane orientation leads to the "ductal" view, allowing imaging of the main pulmonary artery and the proximal descending aorta; patent arterial ducts are best seen in this imaging plane. D: Right parasternal imaging of the SVC-RA junction and interatrial septum.

we encourage the use of an initial "3-minute screen" for newborns suspected of having CHD. This initial screening echocardiogram, which is immediately followed by a complete study, provides rapid identification of significant CHD, particularly in the sick and unstable baby. Should the performance of the complete study be interrupted by hemodynamic instability, or the need for intravenous line placement or other procedures, then at least the echocardiographer has already obtained essential information for initial management decisions. The "3-minute screen" can generally be accomplished using steady sweeps from the subcostal, apical, and suprasternal notch views. We establish whether there are four chambers and four valves, normal atrioventricular and ventriculo-arterial relationships (e.g., are there two normal outflow tracts that criss-cross normally?), the normal drainage of at least two pulmonary veins, and the presence of an intact aortic arch and, qualitatively, the biventricular function and presence of a significant pericardial effusion.

Quantitative Morphometric Analysis

Excellent spatial and temporal resolution on modern ultrasound systems permits precise measurement of linear dimensions, areas, and volumes, and can provide important quantitative information relevant to disease processes and progression (Lang et al., 2006; Lai et al., 2006). Because children grow, and because disease conditions often exhibit abnormally sized vessels, valves, and chambers, there must be methods for either normalizing measurements to body size, or comparing measurements to known normative data. Measurements in children are commonly indexed to body surface area (BSA). However, it does not make sense for linear, area, and volume measurements all to be indexed to BSA, and it is known that different structures may grow at different, even nonlinear, rates. Indeed, such indexing yields less than satisfactory results (see Geva, 1998; Nidorf et al., 1992). Also available are tables that graphically depict normative data across weights or BSA (see for examples, Lang et al., 2006; Silverman, 1993; Snider et al., 1997; Roman et al., 1989).

The concept of a Z-score has proven to be very useful. Simplistically, the Z-score is the number of standard deviations from the expected mean (Daubeney et al., 1999; Geva, 1998). Thus, an aortic root whose diameter exhibits a Z score of –2.0 in a patient with a certain BSA is one whose diameter is 2 standard deviations below the mean for that BSA, whereas a root whose diameter shows a Z score of +3.1 is 3.1 standard deviations above the mean for that BSA.

Longitudinal monitoring of the growth of structures is only as good as the measurements that are made. The echocardiographer must optimize image quality as discussed above, especially transducer frequencies and system gains. Importantly, if one is to measure diameters, measurements should be made in a plane orthogonal to the walls; oblique measurements will overestimate diameters. Finally, one should keep in mind that calculations of areas and volumes require even more careful measurements, since any errors may be squared or cubed, respectively (Lang et al., 2006; Lai et al., 2006).

Quantitative Functional Analysis

In addition to the anatomical evaluation of the heart, echocardiography is the primary imaging modality used to determine systolic and diastolic cardiac function. The appeal of echocardiography is obvious in the noninvasive nature of the examination, and ability to perform longitudinal measurements. Its other benefits include relative ease of use and portability. The role that echocardiography has in quantitating cardiac function is particularly important because cardiac dysfunction, both global and regional, is often a sequela of intrinsic heart disease (e.g., cardiomyopathy), or of intervention (e.g., postsurgical or postheart transplant) (Lang et al., 2006; Lai et al., 2006).

Systolic Function. Systolic function is composed of four independent factors: contractility, afterload, preload, and end-diastolic myocardial length (Katz, 2001). Contractility is an inherent characteristic of the myocardium that is difficult to assess independent of afterload and preload conditions. Ideally, echocardiography would be able to determine or gauge myocardial contractility noninvasively in the context of loading conditions, although as we shall see, measuring contractility per se remains largely elusive; most measurements of systolic function cannot be made without the influence of preload and/or afterload conditions. Recommendations for chamber quantification, including quantification of ventricular function, have recently been updated (Lang et al., 2006).

The most often used parameters of systolic function in echocardiography are ejection fraction (EF) and shortening fraction (SF). In pediatric cardiology, SF of the left ventricle, as measured by M-mode, is more commonly used as it avoids many errors in the assumptions that go into the calculation of EF, as well as being simpler to determine. The SF is the difference between the left ventricular end-systolic and end-diastolic dimensions divided by the left ventricular end-diastolic dimension:

$$SF = (LVEDD - LVESD)/LVEDD$$

SF = shortening fraction
LVEDD = left ventricular end-diastolic dimension
LVESD = left ventricular end-systolic dimension

The LVEDD and LVESD are derived from the M-mode measurement in the parasternal short axis with the image at the level of the posterior leaflet of the mitral valve. Alternatively, one can measure dimensions from the 2-D images, but because the frame rate is far lower than that of M-mode, one may risk not obtaining the exact end-diastolic and end-systolic dimensions. Under the newest recommendations, end-diastolic and end-systolic dimension is defined as the largest and smallest dimensions, respectively—not by electrocardiographic timing or motion of the mitral valve, as in the past (Lang et al., 2006). By the "ice pick" nature of the M-mode measurements, this evaluation of the left ventricular function is limited to the particular septal and left ventricular free wall regions that the M-mode is looking at, making the calculated SF of limited value in those patients with left ventricular regional wall motion abnormalities. However, of all the echocardiographic techniques of assessing ventricular function, SF is by far the most simple to use. Normal values are from 28 to 44%.

Ejection fraction, on the other hand, is a 3-D assessment of ventricular function. Normal EF, in adults, is ≥55% (Lang et al., 2006). EF is calculated from tracing areas of the left ventricle in different dimensions at end-diastole and end-systole:

$$EF (\%) = (LVEDV - LVESV)/LVEDV \times 100$$

EF = ejection fraction (in percent)
LVEDV = left ventricular end-diastolic volume
LVESV = left ventricular end-systolic volume

A multitude of geometric models have been developed, but most are time-consuming and prone to error. The most accurate and widely used is the modified Simpson's rule as it is relatively independent of the left ventricle geometry (Lang et al., 2006). The modified Simpson's rule is based on the areas of orthogonal planes of the left ventricle as seen on apical four-chamber and apical two-chamber. The left ventricle is treated as a stack of discs, and the volume calculated by summating the volumes of the individual disks. This method has been validated against volume measurements obtained by angiography, but requires meticulous technique in obtaining a true apical view with well-defined endocardial borders; otherwise, the left ventricle will be foreshortened and volumes underestimated.

Left ventricular volumes may also be estimated by the method of the prolate ellipsoid. This is also known as the "bullet" formula or the "area-length method"; however, this assumes that the left ventricle is shaped like a bullet, or prolate ellipsoid (Lang et al., 2006). The "bullet formula" is given by:

$$LV \text{ volume} = 5/6 \times (\text{area})(\text{length})$$

Area = mid-LV cross-sectional area planimetered in the parasternal short axis view

Length = length of the LV taken from the mid-point of the mitral annulus to the LV apex in the apical four-chamber view

The precise determination of regional wall motion abnormalities is an important facet of adult echocardiography, less so in pediatric echocardiography. Although mostly used to define the amount of ischemic or infarcted myocardium, it should be remembered that regional wall motion abnormalities may occur in the absence of coronary artery disease. Standards for assessing wall motion abnormalities include analysis of the 16-segment model, which provides insights into the coronary perfusion. Segments are analyzed according to the following scoring system: 1 = normal or hyperkinetic, 2 = hypokinetic, 3 = akinetic (negligible thickening), 4 = dyskinetic (paradoxical systolic motion), and 5 = aneurysmal (diastolic deformation) (Lang et al., 2006).

The normal right ventricle is a complex, crescent-shaped chamber that is normally wrapped around the left ventricle. CHD and postoperative sequelae further compound right ventricular geometric complexity in pediatric cardiology, through right ventricular hypertrophy and/or dilatation. Accurate assessment of the right ventricle requires integrative imaging from multiple planes. In clinical practice, and certainly in pediatric cardiology, 2-D assessment of right ventricular structure and function remains mostly qualitative (Bleeker et al., 2006; Lang et al., 2006). Although some have attempted to quantify systolic right ventricular function using 2-D methods such as the fractional area shortening (see Boucek and Martinez, 2005), such methods are not widely used in clinical practice (Friedberg and Rosenthal, 2005). Other techniques, including Doppler echocardiography and strain-rate imaging, are discussed below.

With the advent of real-time 3-D echocardiography (see above), there are promising data that suggest that ventricular volumes, both right and left, will be more accurately measured than by standard current techniques, and without the geometric assumptions necessary for most of the current measurements (Lang et al., 2006).

Doppler echocardiography can also be useful in the assessment of ventricular function. It is a technique free from the limitations of situations in which there is regional wall motion abnormality and is geometry-independent, providing a measure of global ventricular systolic function. CW Doppler signal of a mitral or tricuspid regurgitant jet can be used to measure mean dP/dt. By measuring the time interval between 1 m/s and 3 m/s in the upstroke of the regurgitant jet envelope, the dP/dt can be calculated, which offers an index of ventricular function. Because the difference in pressure (dP) between 3 m/s and 1 m/s is 36 minus 4, or 32 mm Hg, dP/dt can be derived from:

$$dP/dt \text{ (mmHg/sec)} = 32/dt \times 1000 \text{ ms/s}$$

dt = time difference between the 3 m/s and 1 m/s marks, in milliseconds.

Normal value for the left ventricle is > 1200 mmHg/s. Assumption is made that the atrial pressure remains unchanged between those two points in time. Also, one must be aware that the value may be depressed in the setting of significant downstream obstruction.

2-D echocardiography by itself or in combination with Doppler echocardiography may be used to determine stroke volume and cardiac output. As in the cardiac catheterization laboratory, normal cardiac output is 2.5 L/min/m² or above. Commonly used formulas are summarized in the Table 4–4.

When the SF or the EF is divided by the ejection time, then one obtains a rate of shortening known as the velocity of circumferential shortening (VCF), which is felt to be relatively insensitive to preload (Katz, 2001). Since ejection time depends on the heart rate, VCF is corrected (VCFc) by:

$$VCFc = VCF/\sqrt{R\text{–}R} \text{ interval (seconds)}$$

In some centers around the country, the VCFc is plotted against left ventricular end-systolic wall stress to

TABLE 4–4. *Systolic Function: Commonly Used Formulas in Echocardiography*

Parameter	Equation(s)	Comments
Stroke volume	End-diastolic volume – end-systolic volume	Volumes may be calculated by modified Simpson's rule or area-length rule [= (5/6)(area)(length)]
Stroke volume	SV = VTI × vessel cross-sectional area	Velocity-time integral (VTI) should be traced through the mode of the be traced through the mode of the spectral Doppler envelope
Cardiac output	CO = SV × heart rate	

obtain a VCFc–wall stress relationship (Colan et al., 1984). Since wall stress is theoretically the afterload that the left ventricle "sees," both preload and afterload are accounted for in the plot; the slope of this relationship is felt to represent the myocardial contractility. This approach is rather labor-intensive, and some investigators have questioned its validity as a single-beat index of contractility (Banerjee et al., 1994). Nonetheless, this measure of contractility appears to be the best one available, and has been used in a number of pediatric studies (Colan et al., 1992; Lipshutz et al., 2000).

Diastolic Function. Diastolic function refers to the ability of the ventricles to relax and receive blood volume from the atria by both passive flow in early diastole and late diastolic atrial contraction. The importance of assessment of diastolic function has been important in the management of patients with cardiomyopathies, the CHD postrepair (e.g., tetralogy of Fallot), and status postorthotopic heart transplantation. Identification of parameters which accurately measure this has been a recent area of research interest. Frommelt recently summarized much of the research into diastology in children with CHD, as well as acquired pediatric heart disease (Frommelt, 2006). Basic parameters include PW Doppler signals of pulmonary and systemic venous structures, as well as analysis of the inflow signals of the atrioventricular valves. Newer techniques involve measurements of TDI as well as other methods (Frommelt, 2006; Khouri et al., 2004; Lai et al., 2006). As more work is being done to evaluate the clinical utility of these various indices of diastolic function, more tools will become available to the clinician taking care of children with both congenital and acquired cardiac disease to help guide therapies.

Pulsed-wave Doppler. Pulsed-wave Doppler of the atrioventricular valves give characteristic wave forms that can be interpreted in varying degree of diastolic function (DeGroff, 2002; Quinones et al., 2002). There is a characteristic E wave and A wave, which mark early and late diastole, respectively. From the apical four-chamber view, the cursor is placed parallel to the ventricular inflows to minimize the angle of incidence with the gate just distal to the valve leaflets in diastole. In the neonate, due to decreased ventricular compliance, the A wave is the predominant wave in both the tricuspid and mitral valve inflow patterns. Over the first 3 months of life, the ventricular compliance improves and the inflow patterns become E-wave predominant, and this pattern remains the normal pattern into adulthood (Schmitz et al., 2004). With age, the velocities change such that the E-wave velocity and early diastolic filling fraction increase with age in early childhood (Harada et al., 1998).

Other indices include the left ventricular isovolumic relaxation time, deceleration time, ratio of the peak E and A velocities.

Systemic and pulmonary venous pulsed Doppler signals can also be used to obtain additional information regarding left and right ventricular diastolic function, respectively. The normal pulmonary venous flow pattern is a low-velocity continuous flow pattern with an anterograde systolic wave (S), followed by a higher velocity anterograde early diastolic filling phase (D), then a brief low velocity retrograde late diastolic wave (A). Specifically, the pulmonary venous flow pattern can differentiate between normal diastolic function and "pseudonormalization." Pseudonormalization refers to abnormal diastolic states that still display a "normal" E-wave predominant mitral valve inflow pattern, due to cardiac compensation by increased left atrial pressures. The relationship between the A-wave of the pulmonary venous Doppler signal and that of the mitral valve inflow has been well studied (O'Leary et al., 1998). O'Leary et al found that both the ratio of and difference between the pulmonary venous A wave duration and the mitral valve A-wave duration was highly sensitive to identify those children with elevated end-diastolic pressures (O'Leary et al., 1998). They used a cutoff a ratio of greater than or equal to 1.2, and a difference of greater than or equal to 29 ms.

Because the mitral inflow and pulmonary venous flow indices are influenced by many physiological factors, especially by changes in filling pressures, the data from these indices may sometimes be inconclusive (Khouri et al., 2004). Therefore, echocardiographers, including pediatric echocardiographers, have incorporated other indices of diastolic function into their overall assessment, as discussed below.

Tissue Doppler. Tissue Doppler refers to low-velocity, large Doppler signals generated by myocardial movement. The values of interest include the systolic descent value (S'), the diastolic ascent velocity (D'), and a late diastolic velocity (A'). Values are directly related to age and are inversely related to heart rate. Normal values have been developed depending on the view used. Views used are mainly the apical four-chamber view and the parasternal short axis. One of the more comprehensive and largest pediatric studies to establish normal values is that by Eidem et al. (2004) which evaluated normal tissue Doppler velocities in 325 healthy children who had been referred for murmur, chest pain, syncope, cardiomegaly, or an abnormal electrocardiogram (ECG). Velocities were measured with the beam parallel to the respective ventricular walls. Nyquist was set to 10–30 cm/s, lowest-wall filter and minimal gain, a sample volume size of <5 mm, sweep speed of at least 100 mm/s. It should be noted that the variances from the mean are quite large, and TDI data should be taken in the context of other indices of diastolic function as well as the clinical status of the patient.

Miscellaneous Indices of Ventricular Function

Global Left or Right Ventricular Function: The Tei or Myocardial Performance Index. The Tei index, otherwise known as the myocardial performance index (MPI), is the sum of the isovolumic relaxation time and isovolumic contraction time divided by the ejection time. The time durations can be derived from a simultaneous PW Doppler signal from the left ventricular inflow and outflow, and the MPI may also be used for the right ventricle. It is a parameter that assesses both systolic and diastolic function, independent of heart rate and blood pressure. The number inversely correlates with function. Ishii examined 150 normal children of ages between 30 days and 18 years and compared their Tei indices with those of kids with atrial septal defects (right ventricular volume overload) and kids who are status post Senning operation (right ventricular pressure overload). There was no significant difference between the normal cohort and the *atrial septal defect* (ASD) cohort, but the Senning group had a Tei index of twice that of the other two groups (Ishii et al., 2000).

New Modalities. Strain rate imaging is one of the newest modalities available to the pediatric cardiologist, and has become more feasible with the introduction of strain-rate imaging packages on the newest ultrasound imaging systems (Sutherland et al., 2004; Weidemann et al., 2002). Traditionally, regional myocardial wall motion has been defined by combining visual analysis of wall motion with the measurement of wall thickening and thinning. The measurement of regional velocity or strain (ε) or strain rate (SR) indices by color Doppler myocardial imaging represents an alternative to these traditional indices, and may gauge both systolic and diastolic myocardial function. Changes in both segmental systolic velocities and deformation are closely linked with changes in contractility, but local deformation, like more global indices of shortening, remain dependent on load and myocardial stiffness. Strain rate imaging may be particularly helpful in assessing right ventricular function in children (see Sutherland et al., 2004; Weidemann et al., 2002).

Color M-mode Doppler measures the propagation of flow in early systole across the mitral valve. It was first described by Brun et al. (1997) as a useful tool for assessing left ventricular early relaxation. The propagation velocity of early flow into the left ventricle (v_p) not only correlates well with τ (tau), the time constant of isovolumic pressure decay, a catheterization-derived index of early relaxation, but also is preload- and heart-rate independent (Garcia et al., 2000; Khouri et al., 2004; Stugaard et al., 1993, 1994). Color

M-mode is determined by obtaining an M-mode image with color Doppler displayed and the cursor in line with the mitral valve inflow. At a sweep speed of 100 mm/s, the flow propagation velocity is measured by measuring the slope of the first 50% isovelocity contour line.

Valvular and Vascular Stenoses. One of the most important equations used in Doppler echocardiography is the modified Bernoulli equation, which allows calculation of pressure gradients, based on the physical principle that flow in a tube that narrows must accelerate to higher velocities across the narrowed region. For pulsatile viscous flow, pressure gradient ΔP is derived from the general Bernoulli equation:

$$\Delta P = [\rho/2 \times (V_2^2 - V_1^2)] + [\rho\textstyle\int_1^2 \partial Vs/\partial t\ ds] + [R(V)]$$

convective	flow	viscous
acceleration	acceleration	friction

Convective acceleration refers to a particle being pushed into a region of higher or lower velocity; flow acceleration applies only during the onset and offset of flow; and viscous friction is applicable primarily in low-flow states, or in long-segment narrowing or in situations with multiple-level obstruction (Danford and Murphy, 1998; DeGroff, 2002; Yoganathan et al., 1988). In most clinical situations, the pressure gradient is measured at the peak of systole, when flow acceleration is assumed to be zero; at a discrete stenosis, where viscous friction is negligible; and with a low proximal velocity V_1 such that this term can be ignored. Therefore, the convective acceleration term is the most important and can be simplified to:

$$\Delta P = 4V_2^2 = 4V^2$$

where V is the maximal velocity across the stenosis

Important errors produced by using the modified Bernoulli equation arise especially when the proximal velocity V_1 is nonnegligible (greater than approximately 1.5 m/s); and when viscous forces are nonnegligible, such as in long-segment stenoses or multiple-level obstruction. In the latter cases, since the modified Bernoulli equation ignores viscous forces, the pressure gradient will be underestimated.

For many years, echocardiographers have attempted to reconcile gradients determined noninvasively using Doppler with those obtained at cardiac catheterization, since many of the natural history studies have utilized cardiac catheterization data. In most cases, the peak gradient obtained with Doppler echocardiography "overestimates" the pressure gradients across valves or vessels obtained at cardiac catheterization (see Aldousany, 1989; Bengur et al., 1989; DeGroff, 2002;

Frank et al., 2002; Lemler et al., 1999; Seifert et al., 1999; Silvilairat et al., 2005; Weyman and Scherrer-Crosbie, 2005), while in other situations, Doppler echocardiography will underestimate the pressure gradients, for example, across Blalock–Taussig shunts (Tacy et al., 1998). But fundamentally, one is measuring different "pressure gradients" with these two methods, and an understanding of the differences will help the pediatric echocardiographer interpret values and measurements obtained noninvasively.

It is first necessary to appreciate the hydrodynamic principles underlying flow across a stenosis. In any closed system, the law of conservation of mass dictates that the volume flow be constant at all points. Since flow is equal to the product of mean velocity and vessel cross-sectional area, the flow velocity must increase as the vessel (or valve) area decreases at the site of stenosis. As the flow exits the stenotic orifice, the streamlines converge to form a minimum jet width at the vena contracta; it is at this point that the pressure in the system is lowest. Notably, the vena contracta is smaller than the actual anatomic stenotic orifice. Further downstream from the stenosis and vena contracta, the pressure will increase again, although not to prestenosis levels, a phenomenon known as pressure recovery. Pressure recovery is not complete because there is energy loss in the system, as heat, from flow turbulence generated beyond the vena contracta. Pressure recovery has been demonstrated to be an important reason why Doppler methods typically "underestimate" pressure gradients when compared to those obtained at cardiac catheterization (Baumgartner et al., 1999; DeGroff, 2002; Levine et al., 1989; Lemler et al., 1999; Villavicencio et al., 2003; Weyman and Scherrer-Crosbie, 2005). Pressure recovery is influenced by several factors germane to pediatrics, including jet eccentricity, orifice geometry, the size of the stenotic orifice relative to the size of the remainder of the vessel, and flow rates (Villavicencio et al., 2003; Weyman and Scherrer-Crosbie, 2005). Aortic stenosis has been the most-studied stenotic lesion and, clinically, pressure recovery is most relevant in patients with moderate aortic stenosis, small aortas, and high flow rates (Weyman and Scherrer-Crosbie, 2005)—all typical of the small child. The estimation of aortic stenosis may also be confounded by the presence of aortic regurgitation (Wright et al., 1996).

The echocardiographer should understand that Doppler echocardiography measures different hemodynamic quantities, at different places, in different times, and often under different awake states especially in children, than does the cardiac catheterization. Evaluation of stenosis depends on measurements of transvalvular pressure gradients and valve area (Weyman and Scherrer-Crosbie, 2005). Cardiac catheterization relies on the measurement of peak-to-peak

pressure differences, with catheters placed proximal to, and also usually several centimeters distal to, the stenosis. In children, measurements are usually performed under sedation. It is very difficult to maintain a catheter within the vena contracta, and the pressure measurement at the distal site is typically distal to the vena contracta, in the zone of pressure recovery. Therefore, the distal pressure measured by cardiac catheterization is usually higher than the pressure in the vena contracta.

Doppler echocardiography gauges the highest velocity across the stenotic orifice. From the hydrodynamic principles outlined above, it is clear that the highest flow velocities must occur within the vena contracta, where the pressures are lowest. Moreover, Doppler ultrasound measures instantaneous differences across the stenosis: this is known as the peak instantaneous pressure gradient. Peak instantaneous pressure gradients are typically higher than peak-to-peak gradients measured at cardiac catheterization. Echocardiography is also often performed in the awake child; perhaps in a child who is somewhat agitated, in whom the higher cardiac output will increase the pressure gradient further. Finally, the modified Bernoulli equation ignores the proximal velocity. If this is significant (greater than approximately 1.5 m/s), then the Doppler peak gradient is artifactually increased since this term is not subtracted out.

Confounding factors that may artifactually increase the pressure gradient include any condition that increases cardiac output across the stenotic orifice, such as fever, anemia, and valvular regurgitation. Conversely, poor ventricular function may cause the pressure gradients obtained by Doppler principles to underestimate the severity of the stenosis.

The determination of valve area by Doppler echocardiography relies on the principle of conservation of mass. Determining stenotic orifice area appears desirable, since the area is independent of the flow. Since volume flow across the stenotic orifice must be the same as the volume flow proximal to and distal to the orifice, as velocity increases the CSA proportionately decreases according to:

$$Q_1 \text{ (proximal to stenosis)} = Q_2 \text{ (at stenosis)}$$
$$= CSA_1 \times V_1 = CSA_2 \times V_2$$

and

$$CSA_2 \text{ (at stenosis)} = (CSA_1 \times V_1)/V_2$$

In reality, the highest velocities measured by Doppler occur at the vena contracta, which is in fact smaller than the true stenotic orifice. Therefore, this method tends to underestimate stenotic orifice areas.

TABLE 4–5. *Assessment of Pressure Gradients: A Comparison of Doppler Echocardiography Versus Cardiac Catheterization*

Parameter	Cardiac Catheterization	Doppler Echo	Effect
Consciousness	Usually sedated	Often unsedated	Increases Doppler gradient
Gradient (discrete stenosis)	Peak-to-peak gradient	Peak instantaneous PG but ignores viscous friction term	Doppler > catheterization
Gradient gradient (long-segment or multiple stenosis)	Peak-to-peak gradient	Peak instantaneous PG but ignores viscous friction term	Doppler underestimates gradient
Gradient gradient (modified Bernoulli equation)	Peak-to-peak gradient	Peak instantaneous PG, but ignores proximal velocity	Doppler underestimates gradient
Gradient (pressure recovery effect)	Proximal—distal pressure difference; distal pressure outside of vena contracta	Instantaneous velocity; highest velocity in vena contracta	Doppler > catheterization
Valve area	Gorlin formula → based on continuity and Bernoulli equations, has correction factor	Conservation of mass → diameter of vena contracta	Doppler underestimates area

The general comparison between Doppler and cardiac catheterization is shown in the Table 4–5.

Other Uses of the Bernoulli Equation. Use of the modified Bernoulli equation to calculate the pressure gradients, is not limited to simply gauging the severity of stenoses. Commonly, pediatric echocardiographers estimate the pressure difference between left and right ventricles (and therefore, systolic pulmonary arterial pressures) by determining the pressure gradient across ventricular septal defects. From the jet of an inter-atrial communication with left-to-right shunting, one can estimate left atrial pressures using assumed central venous pressures. From the blood pressure and the end-diastolic pressure gradient from the aortic regurgitation jet, diastolic left ventricular pressure can be estimated.

Because of its important association with CHD, the estimation of pulmonary arterial (PA) pressures deserves some detailed discussion. In addition to systolic PA pressure, diastolic and mean PA pressure can be important to estimate, especially since the working definition of pulmonary hypertension is a mean PA pressure of 25 mmHg (see Bossone et al., 2005). Although several methods exist to estimate systolic PA pressure, by far the method most widely used utilizes the tricuspid regurgitant jet velocity to determine the right ventricle-to-right atrium pressure gradient. One can assume a right atrial v-wave pressure of approximately 5 mm Hg in children to derive a rather precise numerical value for systolic right ventricular pressure; others do not "correct" for right atrial pressure, since this number is small. This method, with and without the right atrial "correction" factor, has been shown in numerous studies to agree and correlate very well with invasively confirmed systolic PA pressures at cardiac catheterization (Bossone et al., 2005; Chan et al., 1987; DeGroff, 2002; Friedberg et al., 2006; Lanzarini et al., 2002; Stevenson, 1989; Quinones, 2002). Other echocardiographic findings to corroborate significant pulmonary hypertension should include the presence of right ventricular hypertrophy, flattening or even right-to-left systolic bowing of the interventricular septum, and diastolic pulmonary hypertension. Most commonly, the pulmonary regurgitation jet is used to estimate diastolic PA pressure by assessing the pressure gradient at end-diastole between the pulmonary artery and the right ventricle; again, one must assume a certain value for diastolic right ventricular pressure, such as 5 mmHg. A newer method relies on the concept that the right ventricular pressure at the time of pulmonary valve opening is the same as the diastolic PA pressure (Lanzarini et al., 2002). By using the time interval from the beginning of the QRS complex on electrocardiography to the opening of the pulmonary valve, and applying this time interval to the velocity spectrum of the tricuspid regurgitation jet envelope, one knows at what right ventricular pressure the pulmonary valve opens—this is the diastolic PA pressure. The agreement with catheterization-derived diastolic PA pressures is good, but not as good as the estimation of systolic PA pressures from the tricuspid regurgitation jet (Lanzarini et al., 2002). Another recent and novel approach takes advantage of the fact that diastolic PA pressure is 69% of the systolic PA pressure, and mean PA pressure is 49% of the systolic PA pressure; diastolic and mean PA pressures predicted solely from the tricuspid regurgitation-derived systolic PA pressure showed very good agreement with catheterization-derived PA pressures (Friedberg et al., 2006).

Valvular Regurgitation. Improvements in the outcomes of heart surgery, as well as residua of certain congenital heart operations, have mandated the need for reliable and quantitative methods to assess valvular regurgitation. The advent of spectral Doppler and especially color Doppler flow mapping made the assessment of valvular regurgitation more "direct" and convenient in clinical practice. Both semiquantitative and quantitative methods are currently being applied to determine the severity of valvular regurgitation. The echocardiographer is also responsible for determining the underlying etiology of the regurgitation as well as its secondary effects on cardiac size and function. Thus, a careful inspection of valve leaflet morphology and dynamic motion, and characterization of ventricular function should accompany assessment of the degree of regurgitation (Irvine et al., 2002).

When one wishes to know the degree of valvular regurgitation, what one really wants to know is the regurgitant volume relative to the stroke volume, or the regurgitant fraction; it is this abnormal volume load that leads to chronic (or acute) overloading of the ventricle that may demand intervention. The Doppler assessment of valvular regurgitation most commonly relies on indices related to flow velocity (e.g., Doppler color map) and flow volume (e.g., flow convergence method). It should be recalled that the Doppler flow color map is a display of flow velocities and not flow volumes, and is therefore not the equivalent of the angiographic regurgitant jet (Irvine et al., 2002; Thomas, 2002). The Doppler velocity map is prone to error because several factors determine the color-jet area, including jet momentum (dependence especially on jet velocity and therefore proximal and distal pressures); chamber constraint (jets are then not ideal "free" jets and cannot entrain blood from all sides and expand properly); physiological variables (pressures proximal and distal to the regurgitant jet, dynamic orificemotion, cardiac function); other patient variables (poorimaging windows); and imaging-system settings (e.g., transducer frequency, gains, Nyquist scale of the color Doppler map) (Irvine et al., 2002; Khanna et al., 2005; Thomas, 2002). Nonetheless, the flow convergence method (as discussed below) is not necessarily optimal for assessing every type of valvular regurgitation. Several commonly used approaches are discussed for each specific type of valvular regurgitation.

Mitral and Tricuspid Valve Regurgitation. Because of the importance and prevalence of mitral valve disease in both the pediatric and adult populations, the echocardiographic assessment of mitral regurgitation has been the most studied among all valves. As with any valvular regurgitation, the experienced echocardiographer will analyze several parameters to gauge mild-, moderate-, or severe-mitral regurgitation. Seen in a substantial proportion of normal children, trace "physiological" mitral regurgitation is considered a normal variation; in our laboratory, we define this as nonholosystolic, with a very narrow or tiny flow jet by color Doppler mapping, similar to other definitions (Minich et al., 1997).

Most commonly, pediatric echocardiographers grade severity of mitral regurgitation semiquantitatively using the Doppler color flow jet area in the left atrium (Irvine et al., 2002; Thomas, 2002). Many echocardiographers simply gauge the jet area by the "eyeball" method in a number of views (Khanna et al., 2005). In our laboratory, we qualitatively couple the jet area and length in the left atrium with the width of the jet at the valve coaptation point, to arrive at a semiquantitative assessment. The advantages of such a semiquantitative approach are that it is rapid and sufficient for most clinical purposes, especially in children (Irvine et al., 2002; Khanna et al., 2005). Others calculate specific jet areas as a percentage of the left atrial area, which shows good correlation with angiographic regurgitation: < 20%–30%, 20%–30% to 40%–50%, and >40%–50% for mild, moderate, and severe mitral regurgitation, respectively (see DeGroff, 2002; Irvine et al., 2002).

Truly quantitative methods include calculations of regurgitant volume, regurgitant flow rate, regurgitant fraction, and regurgitant orifice area or effective regurgitant orifice area (EROA) (Thomas, 2002). Regurgitant volumes methods rely on calculations that subtract forward or left ventricular outflow tract stroke volume (determined by aortic CSA and VTI), from total left ventricular stroke volume (or stroke volume across the mitral valve in diastole) (determined by various methods, including biplane Simpson's method, or Doppler evaluation of stroke volume across the mitral valve). The regurgitant fraction can then be calculated as the ratio of the regurgitant volume to total transmitral stroke volume. However, these methods are timeconsuming, requiring multiple calculations, and are prone to error (Khanna et al., 2005; Thomas, 2002). The proximal flow convergence method, or proximal isovelocity surface acceleration (PISA) method to calculate the EROA has gained favor in recent years. This is a more direct approach to assessing mitral regurgitation, since it establishes the size of the regurgitant orifice. Conceptually, as flow converges on an orifice, it accelerates along a series of streamlines whose velocities form a series of concentric hemispheric shells. These velocities increase as they converge toward the orifice, where they reach a maximal velocity at the orifice or just beyond at the vena contracta. That is, when one is close to the orifice, at any given radius from the orifice along a hemispheric shell, the velocity of blood flow is the same. Because blood is incompressible, the flow moving across any concentric hemisphere shell must be the same, and therefore, we can measure flow through any one of these shells to obtain instantaneous flow through the regurgitant orifice itself. In practice, one can visualize the concentric shells by lowering the Nyquist limit on the color flow Doppler map to approximately 40 cm/s, so that the isovelocity shell where the flow aliases is the radius from the orifice used in the calculations. Under ideal conditions, once the flow rate Q is known, then the EROA $= Q/V_{max}$ through the orifice (DeGroff, 2002; Irvine et al., 2002; Khanna et al., 2005; Thomas, 2002).

Theoretically, the flow convergence/EROA technique can assess mitral regurgitation severity quantitatively, and the method is reasonably rapid. For some, this is the method of choice for quantitating mitral regurgitation (Thomas, 2002). However, its limitations include an assumption of constant orifice area; dependence on orifice geometry, especially true with congenitally malformed valves, since an orifice which is not round may not yield concentric hemispheric shells; and the radius from the orifice to the shell may not be easily visualized. Also, if there is more than one regurgitant jet, there may be limitations to calculating EROA and defining the vena contracta (Khanna et al., 2005).

In general, mild mitral regurgitation (angiographic grade 1) corresponds to a regurgitant fraction of < 30%; moderate mitral regurgitation (angiographic grade 2–3) to 30%–50%; and severe mitral regurgitation (angiographic grade 4) to >50%. In adults, the EROA for mild mitral regurgitation is <20 mm^2; moderate mitral regurgitation, 20–40 mm^2; and severe mitral regurgitation, >40 mm^2.

Vena contracta width has also been used, since theoretically, the width of the vena contracta jet corresponds directly to the EROA. However, since the mitral regurgitation jet is a 3-D entity, one must image the 1-D jet in different planes to best appreciate the extent of the vena contracta. Limitations include issues of axial and lateral resolution that contribute to errors in width measurement (Irvine et al., 2002; Khanna et al., 2005). Our laboratory combines this method with the left atrial jet area most commonly in our assessment of mitral regurgitation severity.

The various methods for the assessment of mitral regurgitation severity have been recently reviewed in an extensive article that provided methods, advantages, limitations, optimal utilization, comparison with angiography, and comparison with other echocardiographic methods (Khanna et al., 2005).

The effects of mitral regurgitation on cardiac structure and function can also yield indirect measures of its severity, especially left ventricular size and function, left atrial size, and pulmonary artery pressures. Assessment of pulmonary venous flow can be helpful, since moderate to severe mitral regurgitation typically results in systolic reversal of flow in the pulmonary veins. In addition, it is common for significant regurgitation to result in a higher transmitral E-wave velocity (Irvine et al., 2002; Khanna et al., 2005; Thomas, 2002). Stress echocardiography can be used to gauge ventricular contractile reserve (see below) (Irvine et al., 2002). 3-D echocardiography and 3-D color Doppler flow mapping may ultimately aid in the quantitative assessment of mitral regurgitation as well (Khanna et al., 2005).

In our laboratory and others, tricuspid regurgitation is mostly assessed semi-quantitatively by "eyeball" methods, incorporating vena contracta jet width at the valve annulus with the jet area and width in the right atrium. Far less has been published on tricuspid regurgitation, probably because of the low incidence of clinically significant tricuspid regurgitation; most "trace" and "mild" tricuspid regurgitation is considered a normal variation. However, in pediatric cardiology, one must be able to determine and follow severity in such conditions as Ebstein anomaly and in postoperative patients, particularly those with atrioventricular septal defects and hypoplastic left heart syndrome. Methods include measuring jet area and length in the right atrium, and the ratio of jet area to right atrial area (see DeGroff, 2002; Mahle et al., 2003). There is some variability in the definitions used in the literature. Echocardiographers have defined mild tricuspid regurgitation as a jet area 30%–33% of right atrial area; moderate tricuspid regurgitation as 30%–33% to 50%–66% of right atrial area; and severe tricuspid regurgitation as greater than 50%–66% of right atrial area (Groundstroem et al., 1999; Mahle et al., 2003). The presence of significant or abnormal backflow in the inferior vena cava and/or hepatic veins suggests at least moderate tricuspid regurgitation (DeGroff, 2002). On occasion, the flow convergence/PISA method is also used (DeGroff, 2002). As with mitral regurgitation, it is important to gauge the secondary effects of tricuspid regurgitation, such as right atrial and right ventricular dimensions and function.

Aortic and Pulmonary Valve Regurgitation. In the assessment of aortic regurgitation, echocardiography allows for the assessment of the aortic leaflets and root, severity of aortic regurgitation, and characterization of left ventricular size and function (Bekeredjian and Grayburn, 2005). Published studies in children are scant. Tani et al. (1997) correlated echocardiographic aortic regurgitation with angiographic severity and found the best correlations for normalized narrowest jet width (jet width/left ventricular outflow tract [LVOT] width, or jet width/BSA), and for jet area in the short axis view at the level of the aortic valve. For AR/LVOT ratio, groups could be separated distinctly according to the following categories: no or 1+ aortic regurgitation, 0–0.26; 2+ aortic regurgitation, 0.27–0.50; 3+ aortic regurgitation, 0.51–0.70; and

4+ aortic regurgitation, >0.71. These values compare favorably with those reported in the adult literature: mild aortic regurgitation, <0.25; moderate (2+) aortic regurgitation, 0.25–0.45, and moderate (3+) aortic regurgitation, 0.46–0.64; and severe (4+) aortic regurgitation, >0.65 (see Maurer, 2006; Zoghbi et al., 2003). In adults, absolute measurements are used: mild aortic regurgitation, <3 mm, and severe aortic regurgitation, > 6 mm (Maurer, 2006; Zoghbi et al., 2003). With eccentric jets, the use of jet widths is less reliable (Maurer, 2006). Other limitations occur when the regurgitant orifice is not round in shape (Bekeredjian and Grayburn, 2005) and a dependence on system settings that influence the size of the Doppler color map (Tani et al., 1997).

Other quantifiable parameters and techniques include the aortic regurgitation pressure half-time slope (measured as pressure half-time, in milliseconds), and the flow convergence/PISA method of regurgitant volume quantitation. The latter technique is much less commonly used than for mitral regurgitation. The pressure half-time is a reasonably common method, and relies on the concept that greater degrees of aortic regurgitation lead to faster equilibration of diastolic aortic and left ventricular pressures, with a steeper slope of the Doppler envelope. Guidelines suggest mild aortic regurgitation, >500 ms; moderate aortic regurgitation, 200–500 ms; and severe aortic regurgitation, <200 ms (Zoghbi et al., 2003). Because diastolic aortic and left ventricular pressures may vary even with the same degree of aortic regurgitation, the pressure half-time method is confounded by changes in systemic vascular resistance, loading conditions, and left ventricular compliance (DeGroff, 2002).

In our laboratory, we combine the jet width/LVOT ratio (in reality, this is the jet width to aortic valve annulus ratio, since the narrowest portion of the jet is at the valve coaptation point) with jet length (generally categorized as confined to the LVOT, coursing through the LVOT, the mid-left ventricle, and to the left ventricular apex), along with the pressure half-time slope. We also gauge the degree of diastolic retrograde flow in the descending aorta. However, it should be noted that Tani et al. (1997) found a low correlation of angiographic aortic regurgitation severity with degree of retrograde aortic flow; still, holodiastolic flow reversal in the abdominal aorta usually signaled the presence of at least moderate aortic regurgitation (Tani, 1997).

2-D echocardiography provides additional and important data on secondary effects on left ventricular size and function (Zoghbi et al., 2003).

Despite the importance of pulmonary regurgitation in the pediatric population, especially the patient following repair of tetralogy of Fallot (Frigiola et al., 2004), very little has been published on how to gauge severity. As with tricuspid regurgitation, "trace" or "mild" pulmonary regurgitation with a narrow jet is considered to be a normal variation. For more severe pulmonary regurgitation, pediatric echocardiographers are assessing qualitatively the jet width and area, and slope of the deceleration phase of the pulmonary regurgitation Doppler waveform (DeGroff, 2002). In a study of children, Williams et al. (2002) correlated 1+ to 3+ angiographic pulmonary regurgitation with the ratio of the color Doppler flow jet width to annular width, and obtained reasonably good separation between categories of severity as follows: 0+ angiographic pulmonary regurgitation, 0.0–0.1; 1+, 0.1–0.4; 2+, 0.4–0.7; and 3+, >0.7. An important finding was that the branch pulmonary arteries demonstrated diastolic flow reversal in most patients with at least 2+ angiographic pulmonary regurgitation, whereas none had such flow reversal when the pulmonary regurgitation was 1+ or less (Williams et al., 2002). Others have also used the presence of retrograde flow to gauge pulmonary regurgitation severity: mild, no retrograde diastolic flow in the pulmonary trunk despite a clear regurgitant jet; moderate, retrograde diastolic flow in the main pulmonary artery; and severe, retrograde diastolic flow in the branch pulmonary arteries (Frigiola et al., 2004). In the end, however, pulmonary regurgitation has perhaps been less well-studied because pediatric cardiologists are more interested in its secondary effects on right ventricular size and function, and use these endpoints to decide on intervention (see Frigiola et al., 2004).

Specialized Echocardiographic Techniques

Although surface echocardiographic imaging by transthoracic echocardiography provides the most versatile and multifaceted approach to the diagnosis of the CHD, other ultrasound modalities are sometimes used, either (1) when standard transthoracic echo cannot provide adequate imaging windows or (2) in conjunction with interventions such as during surgery or therapeutic cardiac catheterization.

Transesophageal Echocardiography. Although not the cornerstone of diagnosis and certainly not routinely used for serial follow-up of patients, TEE may be useful when standard transthoracic imaging windows are poor. Its primary utility, however, is in the operating room and the cardiac catheterization laboratory, where anatomy and hemodynamics can be well-delineated just prior to and following a procedure or intervention (Ayres et al., 2005; Kavanaugh-McHugh et al., 2000; Phoon, 1999). On occasion, TEE may be performed outside of the operating room or catheterization laboratory, in the PICU or on an outpatient, using sedation or anesthesia (see Marcus et al., 1993; Phoon, 1999). Although TEE is somewhat limited by a single-vantage point—the esophagus—the versatility of TEE has been aided by the development of multiplane, steerable probes for both adults and children, including infants as small as approximately 3 kg. TEE is also limited by its semiinvasive nature, and the need for sedation or more commonly, anesthesia especially in younger children (Phoon, 1999; Kavanaugh-McHugh et al., 2000).

Much of cardiac anatomy can be visualized. Standard imaging planes along with minor deviations (given commonly rotation of the heart with congenital defects and chamber dilatation) permit good imaging of the four chambers, interatrial and interventricular septa, atrioventricular inflow and great arterial outflow, the great veins, and function. Limitations include poorer ability to image the transverse aortic arch and aortic isthmus particularly in younger children and infants; collateral pulmonary vessels; and anomalous pulmonary veins that drain relatively far from the heart (Ayres et al., 2005; Phoon, 1999). With experience, structures that have been historically difficult to image, such as coronary arteries and the left pulmonary artery, can be imaged reasonably well (Phoon, 1999).

Recently, the Task Force of the Pediatric Council of the American Society of Echocardiography confirmed that given the limitations of TEE, a preoperative transthoracic echocardiography (TTE) be performed in every patient undergoing TEE during congenital heart surgery, and that the findings be reviewed by the echocardiographer before the TEE is performed. In this fashion, not only can a "baseline" TEE prebypass be done, but also specific questions that had been unanswered by TTE may be addressed. Some of the indications for TEE are listed in Table 4–6 (Ayres et al., 2005; Cheitlin et al., 2003).

Complications related to TEE are uncommon, but may occur in up to 1%–3% of pediatric patients (Ayres et al., 2005). Risks include trauma to the oropharynx, hypopharynx, esophagus, and stomach, including esophageal perforation and thermal injury. Complications can also include arrhythmias, pulmonary complications (bronchospasm, hypoxemia, and laryngospasm), and circulatory compromise. Airway obstruction may occur, particularly in small infants (Phoon and Bhardwaj, 1999). Contraindications are listed in the Table 4–7 (from Ayres et al., 2005).

Because of the specialized skills necessary for the proper, safe, and optimal use of TEE, task forces have recommended certain minimal levels of training, skills, and knowledge that differ from those required for adult TTE and TEE, most notably training in and knowledge of the CHD (Ayres et al., 2005). Of note, however, although standardized imaging planes have been established for adult TEE (Shanewise et al., 1999), there is currently no uniform consensus on standardized views and planes to be used for TEE examination in the pediatric patient (Ayres et al., 2005). Nevertheless, the Task Force of the Pediatric Council of the American Society of Echocardiography encourages the use of a careful, detailed, and consistent systematic approach to each and every TEE performed. Our laboratory follows the philosophy that "[regardless] of the particular indication, a TEE study should always examine all the regions of the heart and the great vessels that can be imaged" (Daniel and Mugge, 1995) (see Figures 4–7, 4–8, and 4–9 for our approach).

Intracardiac Echocardiography. Intracardiac imaging is assuming an increasing role in the cardiac catheterization laboratory during interventions for CHD. Intracardiac imaging—for our purposes, intracardiac echocardiography (ICE)—is defined as imaging from within the cardiac chambers and major blood vessels (Kort, 2006). Utilize phased-array transducers with electronic steering and Doppler capabilities, and produce a sector of 90 degree, similar to that produced by

TABLE 4–6. *Common Indications for Transesophageal Echocardiography in Children*

Intraoperative imaging of CHD requiring cardiopulmonary bypass for repair or palliation
Transcatheter interventions such as:
  – ASD or VSD occlusion device placement- Blade or balloon atrial septostomy
  – Catheter tip valve perforation and balloon dilation
  – Radiofrequency ablation procedures
Certain diagnostic indications, such as:
  – Suspected CHD with nondiagnostic transthoracic echocardiogram
  – Evaluation for PFO in a patient with stroke or patient undergoing pacemaker placement
  – Evaluation of intra- or extracardiac baffles (Senning/Mustard procedures, Fontan circuits)
  – Aortic dissection
  – Evaluation of intracardiac thrombus or vegetation.

TABLE 4–7. *Contraindications for Pediatric Transesophageal Echocardiography*

Absolute Contraindications	Relative Contraindications
Unrepaired tracheoesophageal fistula	History prior esophageal surgery
Esophageal obstruction or stricture	Esophageal varices or diverticulum
Perforated hollow viscus	Gastric or esophageal bleeding
Poor airway control	Vascular ring, aortic arch anomaly with or without airway compromise
Severe respiratory depression	Oropharyngeal pathology
Uncooperative, unsedated patient	Severe coagulopathy
	Cervical spine injury or anomaly

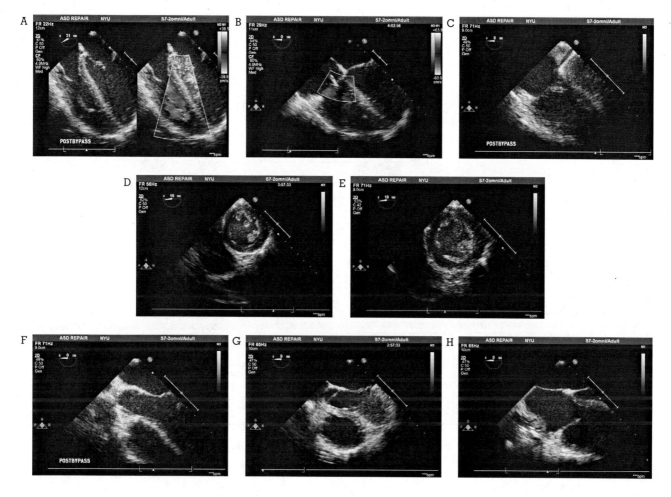

FIGURE 4–7. Representative images from a complete TEE examination. A: "Four-chamber view" in a horizontal or zero-degree plane. B: Four-chamber view with color Doppler flow mapping showing mild tricuspid regurgitation. C: Further insertion of the TEE probe yields more inferior and posterior structures; here, the coronary sinus is seen well. D and E: With further insertion of the TEE probe and some flexion of the tip, a modified short axis view of the left ventricle can be achieved; this is useful for gauging ventricular function. The mitral valve chordal and papillary muscle apparatus can also be seen (E). F: As one pulls the TEE probe out slightly from the four chamber view, more superior and anterior structures can be seen; the left ventricular outflow tract is seen. G: Further superior positioning of the probe yields the aortic valve in the horizontal or zero-degree plane. H: Rightward rotation of the probe from the four chamber view yields the interatrial septum.

TTE or TEE probes, catheters are currently available in 8F and 10F sizes. There are several advantages of ICE over TEE: near-field imaging is better, particularly of the interatrial septum; esophageal trauma is not an issue; ICE does not require an additional echocardiographer, since the interventionalist typically performs the imaging; and ICE can be performed in the awake, unsedated patient. Its two major disadvantages are that the catheter is relatively large, such that experience in small children is limited (Patel et al., 2006) and only monoplane imaging is currently available (Kort, 2006; O'Leary, 2002). Undoubtedly, newer generation catheters and transducers will overcome these limitations as technology improves. Uses of ICE include guidance of transseptal puncture, percutaneous balloon valvuloplasty, cardiac biopsy, catheter placement, and radiofrequency ablation (Kort, 2006; O'Leary 2002). In pediatrics, ICE has primarily been used not only to guide device closure of ASD's, but also VSDs, fistulas, and valvuloplasty procedures (Cao et al., 2005; O'Leary, 2002; Rhodes et al., 2003; Patel et al., 2006).

Intravascular Ultrasound. Intravascular ultrasound (IVUS) is defined as ultrasonic navigation and imaging within small blood vessels (Kort, 2006). The scope of its utility is limited in pediatric cardiology, but IVUS appears to be useful in assessing blood vessel wall morphology following procedures or interventions. Investigators have now imaged branch pulmonary arterial wall morphology during balloon angioplasty

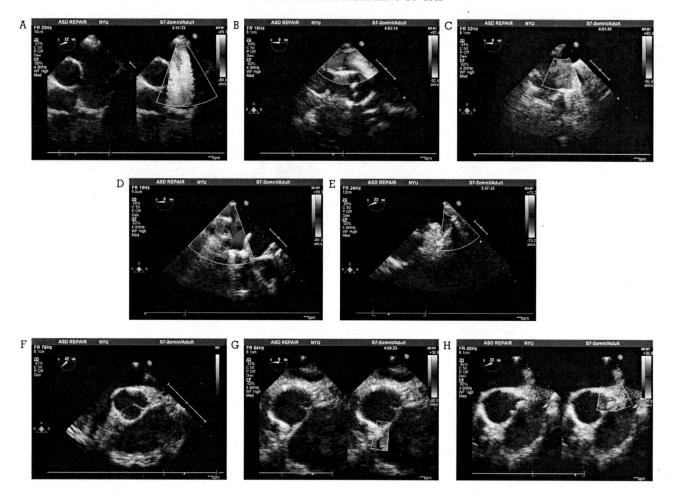

FIGURE 4–8. Representative images from a complete TEE examination. A: As one continues to position the TEE probe more superiorly, the pulmonary outflow tract can be seen. B: Rightward rotation brings the right pulmonary artery into view. C: Leftward rotation can in some cases bring the left pulmonary artery into view. D: Right pulmonary veins. E: Left pulmonary veins. F: With the TEE probe transducer at approximately a 30-degree rotation, the aortic valve is seen en face. G and H: Slight manipulations of the TEE probe during imaging of the aortic valve will yield the right coronary artery origin (G) and left coronary artery origin and course (H).

(Nakanishi et al., 1999), assessment of coronary wall morphology following arterial switch operation for transposition of the great arteries (Pedra et al., 2005), and assessment of transplant coronary arteriopathy (Nicolas et al., 2006). In all studies and similar to studies in adults, IVUS appears to be more sensitive to vessel wall alterations than angiography.

CARDIAC MAGNETIC RESONANCE IMAGING

Technological advances in MRI including advancements in computer hardware acquisition and post-processing times, have led to increased interest in cardiac imaging. The challenge in cardiac MRI is to cope with the cardiac motion and superimposed respiratory motion during the time needed for imaging sequences. In addition, high spatial and temporal resolutions are needed to obtain adequate information regarding cardiac structure, function, and flow. This is especially challenging in pediatric patients with CHD where the demands on spatial and temporal resolution are the greatest due to their small complex cardiac structures coupled with relatively rapid baseline heart rates. Developments of MRI systems, coil technology, and sequence techniques have led to considerably shortened acquisition times and improvements in overall image quality. High field imaging at 3T and multichannel coils result in improved spatial resolution, but may introduce other technical issues that need to be addressed. Acceleration techniques (e.g., parallel imaging) can further reduce scan acquisition time, but usually at the expense of spatial resolution. Hence, a combination of factors is often needed to optimize cardiac imaging protocols. With the progress in rapid MRI techniques, data acquisition is possible in just a

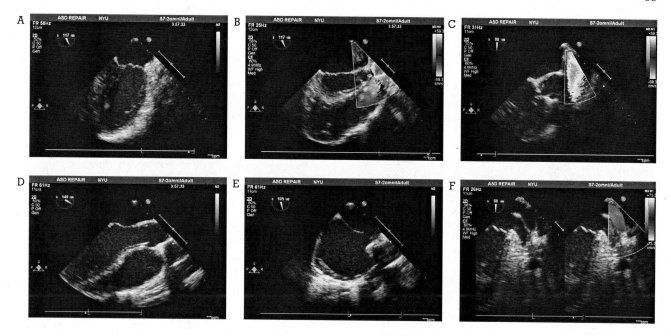

FIGURE 4–9. Representative images from a complete TEE examination, vertical or 90-degree plane of imaging. A: Far left rotation of the probe will demonstrate the left ventricle. B: As one rotates the probe rightward, the outflow tracts come into view. C: Main pulmonary artery. D: "Long axis" view of the aortic outflow tract and aortic valve. E: Interatrial septum. The SVC and IVC are not seen in this view, as they are slightly out of plane. F: Left upper pulmonary vein (red) adjacent to the left atrial appendage (blue) in the vertical/90-degree plane.

fraction of the heart cycle. However, synchronization with the heart cycle is still needed to obtain images without blurring throughout the cardiac cycle for both structural and functional analysis.

Basic Concepts

MRI is based on the concept that atoms act as tiny bar magnets when exposed to an external magnetic field. Over time, atoms align parallel to the external field with a net magnetization in the direction of the external field. Application of short radiofrequency (RF) pulses will cause some atoms to change their alignment and generate a signal as they relax back to their original alignment. Receiver coils are used to detect this signal. Differences in tissue contrast (T1, T2, proton-density, and T2*) are reflected by differences in the basic longitudinal and transverse relaxation times of the atoms that make up the tissues. Spatial localization within an imaging plane can be achieved by repetition with variation of frequency and phase encoding of the radiofrequency pulses. All the signals are collected in a data space referred to as k-space, which is then transformed into an image by a mathematical process called a Fourier transformation. Hydrogen is the most common atom in the body (occurring in water and fat) and provides one of the strongest magnetic signals, and thus the basis for clinical MRI. Magnetic field strengths of 1.5–3 T are currently used in clinical cardiac imaging.

Technical Considerations

Motion Compensation. Cardiac motion compensation usually relies on synchronization of image data to the ECG. Detected R-waves act as reference points for data acquisition, which can be performed in a prospective or retrospective manner (Figure 4–10). With prospective triggering, the detection of the R-wave triggers the execution of the next part of the imaging sequence. The search for the next trigger event is enabled after the completion of the sequence part. With retrospective gating, data acquisition occurs continuously with recording of the patient's ECG. Image data can then be referenced to the ECG and reconstructed with a user-definable temporal resolution. This type of gating is useful for studies of cardiac function, in which the complete heart cycle is covered during data acquisition. Additionally, arrhythmia rejection protocols can be employed to reject data acquired outside a user-definable heart cycle range.

Difficulties related to the magnetohydrodynamic effect of flowing blood can lead to an increase in the T-wave amplitude of the ECG, which may be misinterpreted as an R-wave and lead to mistriggering with consequent blurring of the image data. The development of vectorcardiography based triggering can classify cardiac events by comparing them with a previously calculated reference vector of the QRS complex of the heart cycle (Fischer et al., 1999). In this way, events with

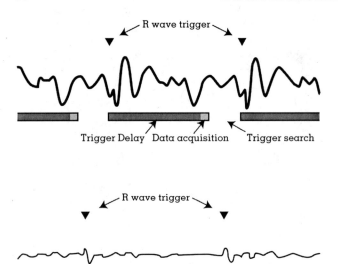

FIGURE 4–10. Demonstration of prospective data acquisition in MR imaging. A: Prospective; B: Retrospective.

the same magnitude but different phase as the R-wave are not misinterpreted as such. Alternatively peripheral pulse gating from pulse oximetry tracings can be used in a similar fashion to ECG gating. In addition, new methods such as self-gating techniques, which rely on previously acquired information regarding cardiac motion are in development to improve overall synchronization of image data acquisition to cardiac motion (Larson et al., 2004).

Cardiac MRI sequences are often acquired over multiple heart cycles and usually require a breath hold to avoid blurred images due to respiratory motion. With particularly long sequences and in patients unable to adequately hold their breaths, image acquisition can be applied multiple times and averaged to reduce overall respiratory motion artifact. In addition, navigator techniques, which track the movement of the diaphragm or cardiac border, have been used to acquire data during a particular phase of the respiratory cycle.

Another approach to motion compensation is the use of real-time sequences. The concept behind real-time sequences is to acquire MRI data fast enough to limit the amount of blurring seen with cardiac and respiratory motion. Recent technological advances in MRI have led to the development of real-time sequences capable of displaying images at 20–30 frames per second, but often at much reduced spatial resolution compared to the standard imaging sequences (Plein et al., 2001).

Acceleration Techniques. Although there has been a significant improvement in the speed of image acquisition that accompanies improvements in overall hardware performance, further improvements are often limited by patient related safety factors. There are several alternative approaches in shortening overall image acquisition time. Most involve omitting and/or sharing data acquired during image acquisition and applying correction factors to fill in the missing data. Common among these techniques are half-, and partial-Fourier transformations including parallel acquisition techniques (PAT) and shared k-space filling. In general, although image acquisition time is shortened, spatial and temporal resolution is often reduced with the potential for introducing imaging artifacts. Hence, the improvements in image acquisition speed need to be weighed against the reduced spatial and temporal resolution when applying these acceleration techniques.

Contrast Administration. Although the intrinsic T1, T2, and proton density differences of tissues can be used for generating image contrast between tissues, exogenous contrast agents are often administered to improve the detection and characterization of disease processes. Contrast agents that shorten T1 relaxation times are desirable since they lead to increased signal on T1-weighted images. Agents that demonstrate strong paramagnetic properties such as gadolinium or manganese based compounds have been used in cardiac imaging; however, gadolinium chelates are more frequently in clinical use due to their safety profile. Doses are often administered at 0.1–0.3 mmol/kg body weight with single dose referring to 0.1 mmol/kg and double dose referring to 0.2 mmol/kg. Large numbers of clinical safety studies have shown all agents to be safe and well tolerated with the total incidence of adverse events less than 5% (Lee et al., 2006).

Cardiac Acquisition Sequences

Tomographic Imaging. Most MR images can be characterized as either spin-echo or gradient-echo images; generally anatomic imaging is performed using either technique for evaluation of cardiac structure and morphology. Imaging features of spin-echo sequences include good tissue contrast, flowing blood appears dark, relative insensitivity to magnetic field inhomogeneities, generally longer acquisition time compared to gradient-echo techniques (Figure 4–11). The spin-echo sequences can be performed with T1 and T2 weighting, fat saturation, inversion recovery, and pre- and postcontrast administration to provide static high-resolution images with excellent contrast between the intracavitary blood flow and myocardium or other structures. (Winterer et al., 1999). Imaging features of gradient-echo techniques include flowing blood appears "bright," relative sensitivity to magnetic field

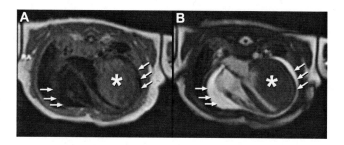

FIGURE 4–11. A: Dark blood spin echo and (B) corresponding bright blood gradient echo MR images from a patient with a large rhabdomyoma involving the lateral left ventricular wall (*). There is an associated pericardial effusion (arrows) that appears bright on the gradient echo image, but dark on the spin-echo images due to flow effects.

inhomogeneities, saturation effects that potentially reduce inherent tissue contrast, and shorter acquisition time compared to spin-echo techniques (Figure 4–11). The gradient-echo sequences provide a quick method for evaluating cardiac structure although tissue contrast is not as great as with spin-echo sequences. In general, gradient-echo sequences are widely used at present for assessment of functional characteristics of the heart.

Cine. Cine sequences used in cardiac MRI consist of a collection of images at the same spatial location covering one full period of the cardiac cycle. The imaging technique used is commonly a type of gradient-echo sequence since these can be acquired with relatively short acquisition times. The image acquisition utilizes cardiac gating in order to yield a multiphase sequence covering the cardiac cycle. As previously mentioned, data can be timed to the cardiac cycle in a prospective or retrospective manner. Data acquisition is often segmented over multiple cardiac cycles which are then pieced together to yield an image loop tracking the motion of tissues within the heart and/or vessels over the cardiac cycle (Figure 4–12).

The most commonly used cine sequence in clinical cardiac MRI is the steady-state free precession (SSFP), which is known by several proprietary names depending on the vendor including true fast imaging with steady precession (trueFISP), balanced fast field echo (FFE), and fast imaging employing steady state acquisition (FIESTA). Advantages of this imaging sequence include its short acquisition time (typically 4–10 seconds), sharp contrast between blood pool and myocardium in almost any imaging plane, and minimal motion-induced blurring. Its main disadvantage is its sensitivities to magnetic field inhomogeneities as may occur with implanted metallic devices such as surgical clips or stents. In addition, at higher field strengths, for example, 3T, artifacts related to magnetic field inhomogeneities become more problematic with SSFP imaging and as a consequence, cine imaging is often

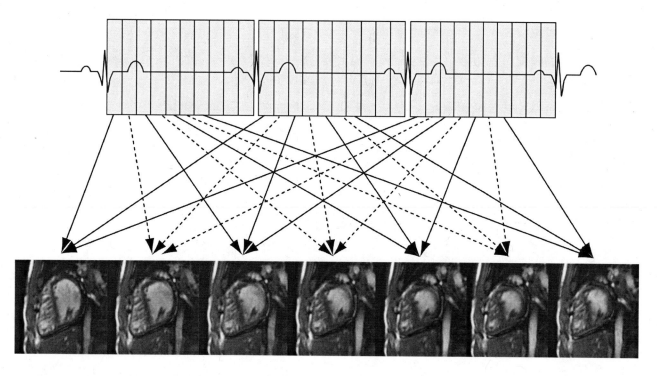

FIGURE 4–12. Schematic diagram demonstrating acquisition of gradient echo cine MR imaging at a mid short axis level of the heart in a patient with pulmonary hypertension.

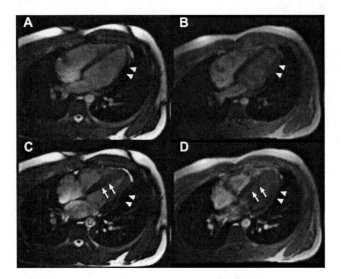

FIGURE 4–13. Four-chamber view of the heart in diastolic (A,B) and systolic (C,D) phases using steady state free precession (SSFP) imaging (A,C) and spoiled gradient-echo (SGE) (B,D) imaging. On the SSFP images, there is good endocardial border definition at both systolic and diastolic phases (small arrows) but a persistent artifact (arrowheads) noted along the lateral wall of the left ventricle. On SGE, which is less susceptible to inhomogeneities in the magnetic field, the artifact is no longer present. However, although good endocardial border definition is noted in the diastolic phase, this border becomes blurred during systolic phases (arrows).

performed using spoiled gradient echo (SGE) imaging fast low-angle shot (FLASH) imaging. In comparison to SSFP, spoiled gradient-echo cine imaging has longer acquisition time (8–16 seconds), slightly diminished contrast between blood pool and myocardium, especially in long axis planes, and less sensitivity to magnetic field inhomogeneities (Figure 4–13). Similar to SSFP, SGE sequences are referred to by proprietary names depending on vendor including FLASH, spoiled GRASS (SPGR), and FFE.

Tissue Tagging. Magnetic tissue tagging is a process in which landmarks on an MRI plane are introduced noninvasively prior to cine imaging (Figure 4–14). Presaturation pulses are used to create linear dark stripes or grid pattern over the myocardium. As systole proceeds, the pattern distorts in the direction corresponding with myocardial movement. This technique can be very useful in the analysis of the heart wall motion because it can provide temporal correspondence of material points within the heart wall, which can be assessed reproducibly and quantitatively.

Velocity Encoding Phase Contrast. Phase contrast MRI methods rely on the principle that spins from blood (or tissue) flowing through a magnetic field acquire a predictable phase shift. Using appropriate velocity encoding gradients, the motion-dependent phase effect can be used to directly determine the velocity of the flowing blood. Multiphase images are

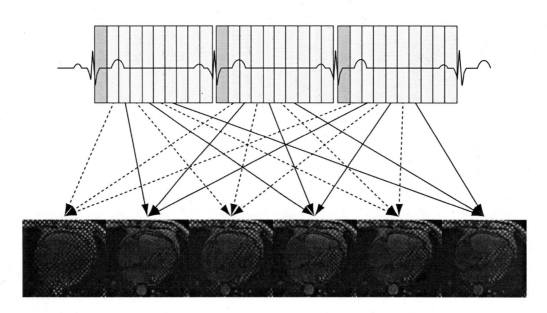

FIGURE 4–14. Schematic diagram demonstrating acquisition of tagged gradient echo cine MR imaging at a mid short axis level of the heart. The tagging sequence (gray) is applied just prior to cine imaging.

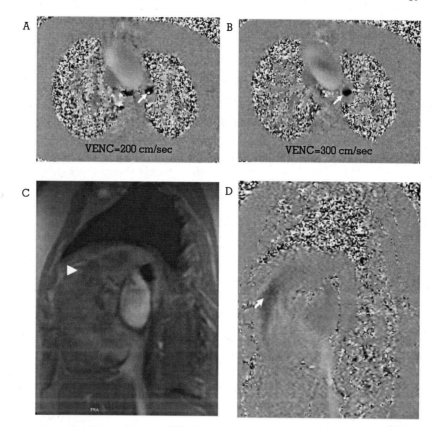

FIGURE 4–15. Through-plane velocity phase encoding (A,B) at a level of narrowing from aortic coarctation demonstrating aliasing of signal (A) from setting too low of VENC. With adjustment of the VENC, there is no longer aliasing of signal. Magnitude (C) and in-plane velocity phase encoding (D) of the right ventricular outflow tract demonstrating flail pulmonic valve leaflet (arrowhead) with associated pulmonary valve regurgitation (arrow).

constructed throughout the cardiac cycle and mapped where pixel color (black vs. white) represents velocity direction, and pixel brightness is proportional to spatial velocity (Figure 4–15). Phase change is measured on a circular scale, and is designed so that different flow velocities are displayed along the 360 degrees of phase shift depending on the velocity-encoding factor or VENC. For best results, the VENC is chosen to be slightly more than the maximum expected flow velocity in a region. However, if a higher velocity is encountered than that set for the VENC, it will be represented as a darker (or brighter depending on direction) pixel, otherwise known as velocity aliasing (Figure 4–15) Phase-encoded images are generally displayed as corresponding magnitude and phase display usually in encompassing an entire cardiac cycle (cine display). For the phase display, the flow information on flow direction (bright vs. black) and flow velocity (signal intensity) can be visually interpreted. Sequence acquisition can be performed through-plane or in-plane, and three orthogonal directions are needed to obtain a complete map of flow regardless of direction.

First Pass Perfusion. Dynamic first pass perfusion allow for the collection of multiple images during a single cardiac cycle and can be used to follow the flow of contrast into imaging planes during the first pass

of the contrast agent. A saturation recovery technique in combination with a gradient-echo-based sequence is used to maximize the T1 contrast in the imaging plane of interest. The contrast between the different perfused tissues is based on the very-short T1 generated by the contrast agent uptake into the tissues (Figure 4–16).

Contrast Enhanced MR Angiography. Depiction of blood vessels can be illustrated based on inherent differences between their T1 values, which are often lower, than the fat surrounding the blood vessels, which should have a higher T1 value. Additionally, T1-shortening agents such as gadolinium-based contrast can further reduce the T1 value of the blood to below 50 ms. As such, vessels of interest become much brighter than background fat and visualization of in-plane blood vessels is improved. This sequence is commonly performed as a T1-weighted 3-D spoiled gradient-echo pulse sequence with zero interpolation in the slice-selected direction and short TR and TE values. Contrast injection is timed with respect to the *k*-space acquisition such that peak enhancement coincides with optimal contrast imaging (Figure 4–17). This can be achieved with educated guess, bolus timing, or bolus tracking techniques as discussed previously. Alternatively, with improvements in acquisition time, time-resolved MR angiography can be performed

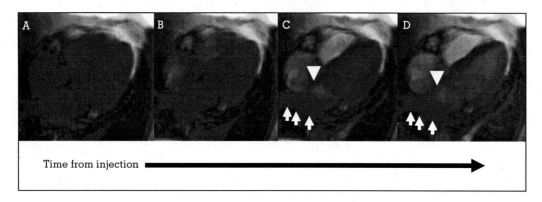

FIGURE 4–16. Dynamic first pass perfusion imaging demonstrating the passage of a compact bolus of contrast through the cardiac chambers. A: On initial images, the cardiac chambers still appear dark. B: Early imaging just after contrast injection demonstrates contrast opacification of the right heart chambers. Early opacification of the left atrium is noted via an atrial septal defect (arrowheads C and D) before contrast has reached the pulmonary veins (arrows C and D).

allowing acquisition and identification of specific phases of vascular opacification (e.g., pulmonary, arterial, venous phases).

Coronary MR Angiography.

Coronary artery imaging is one of the most technically challenging areas of MRI. In addition to the spatial requirements necessary to visualize the small coronary arteries, respiratory and cardiac motion provide further impediments to optimizing image quality. There have been numerous MRI sequences in use for imaging the coronary arteries with estimated in-plane spatial resolution of 0.6–1.0 mm depending on acquisition parameters. Variations on gradient-echo (bright blood) and spin-echo (dark blood) sequences have each been proposed. Furthermore, conventional gadolinium contrast agents and newer intravascular agents have also been utilized to improve image contrast. Both 2-D and 3-D sequences are available, each with their own pros and cons. The most widely available sequence in clinical use is a 2-D segmented *k*-space gradient-echo acquisition in which multiple thick slices are acquired through the vessel of interest. Variability in breath-holding and thick slices can limit the registration of images from slice to slice. 3D imaging methods including whole-heart volumetric sequences utilizing bright-blood techniques with fat suppression and free breathing are available, but suffer from relatively long acquisition times, which may result in image degradation due to shifts in diaphragmatic position during image acquisition despite navigator tracking techniques. These sequences can be performed with or without gadolinium-based contrast agents (Lee et al., 2006) (Figure 4–18).

Inversion Recovery (e.g., Delayed Enhancement Imaging).

The inversion recovery (IR) technique is often used in cardiac MRI to characterize tissue after the administration of contrast media. Normally perfused myocardium is often suppressed in order to better visualize areas with increased contrast uptake that

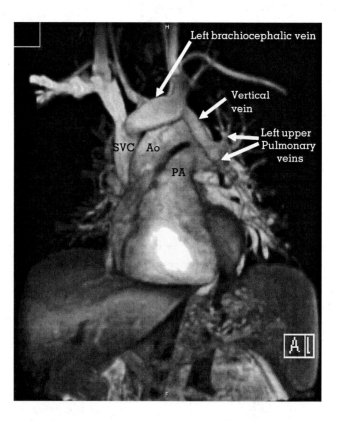

FIGURE 4–17. Volume-rendered MR image from contrast enhanced 3D gradient echo acquisition (MR angiography) viewed from a predominantly anterior projection demonstrating partial anomalous pulmonary venous return. The left upper lobe veins are noted to converge and ascend superiorly in a vertical vein to drain into the left brachiocephalic vein. *Abbreviations*: SVC, superior vena cava; Ao, aorta; PA, pulmonary artery.

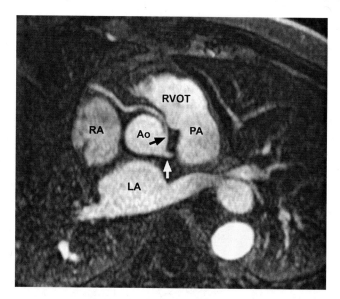

FIGURE 4–18. Multiplanar reformatted MR image from contrast enhanced thin slab 3D gradient echo acquisition demonstrating anomalous origin of the right coronary artery (black arrow) from the left sinus adjacent to the origin of the left coronary artery (white arrow). Additionally, the right coronary artery is noted to course between the pulmonary artery/right ventricular outflow tract and the aorta. *Abbreviations*: Ao, aorta; PA, pulmonary artery; RVOT, right ventricular outflow tract; RA, right atrium; LA, left atrium.

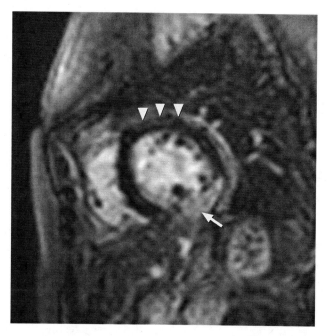

FIGURE 4–19. Delayed enhancement imaging using the inversion recovery technique to suppress the signal in normal myocardium (arrowheads) and as a consequence improve the visualization of areas of with increased contrast uptake (arrow) indicating some degree of myocardial inflammation and/or fibrosis in this patient with prior surgical repair for tetralogy of Fallot.

appear hyperintense (Figure 4–19). In conjunction with TSE imaging, the IR technique can be used to suppress fat in order to identify fatty infiltration seen in arrhythmogenic right ventricular dysplasia or to visual edema and tissue damage seen in acute myocardial infarctions.

A 180 degree RF inversion pulse is applied before data acquisition. As the longitudinal magnetization relaxes, the magnetization of different tissue types (fat, normal or hyper-intense, scarred myocardium) reaches zero at different times. Appropriate selection of inversion time (TI) can suppress the signal of relevant tissue and improve contrast between different tissue types with different T1 relaxation times. The challenge is in the choice of TI, which depends on the amount and time of contrast administration and continually changes during the examination.

Imaging Considerations and Postprocessing

Image Acquisition. MRI protocols vary depending on the structure of interest and the information desired. An overview of cardiovascular anatomy can be obtained using both spin-echo tomographic imaging and gradient-echo cine techniques. The vascular system can be further evaluated using 3-D MR angiography. An assessment of blood flow can be made using phase contrast velocity encoded mapping both for quantification of stenotic and regurgitant jets, calculation of shunt fraction, and calculation of differential blood flow (e.g., pulmonary artery system). Volumetric acquisition using cine MRI sequences can be used for quantification of chamber size and function, which is often important in the management and follow-up of patients with CHD.

Given the complexity of the cardiac anatomy and the individual variations unique to each patient, especially in the CHD, cardiac structures are often best understood using imaging planes defined with respect to the orientation of the heart. Hence, the most useful imaging planes are those that are parallel and perpendicular to the cardiac axes, which are based on internal cardiac landmarks. The most common standard views of the heart are demonstrated in Figure 4–20.

The two-chamber and four-chamber long-axis views along with the short-axis views are often used for visualization of the cardiac chambers and for evaluation of cardiac anatomy and function. The three-chamber view allows for visualization of the aortic root and provides the basis to demonstrate aortic valve and aortic root anatomy as well as for obtaining additional images of the ascending aorta. Depending on

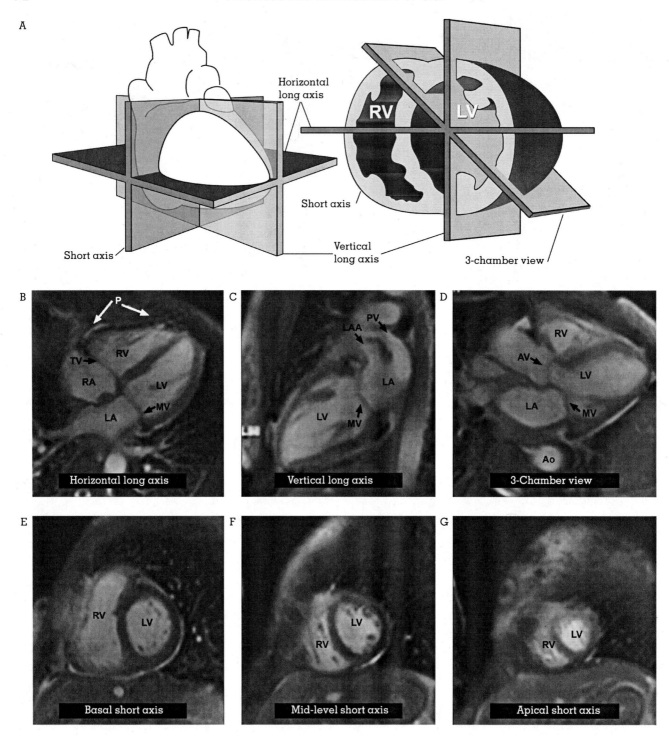

FIGURE 4–20. Standard imaging planes of the heart with corresponding 2D MR images. *Abbreviations*: RV, right ventricle; LV, left ventricle; RA, right atrium; LA, left atrium; LAA, left atrial appendage; MV, mitral valve; TV, tricuspid valve; AV, aortic valve; Ao, aorta; P, pericardium. (Reprinted with permission from Lee VS. *Cardiovascular MRI: Physical Principles to Practical Protocols*. Philadelphia, PA: Lippincott Williams & Wilkins; 2006.)

the structure of interest, additional imaging planes directed to best depict the anatomic relationships may be important for diagnosis (Figure 4–21). The use of volumetric data acquisition simplifies overall image acquisition. However, since in-plane spatial resolution is often better than through-plane spatial resolution, acquisition along the plane of interest often improves overall image quality.

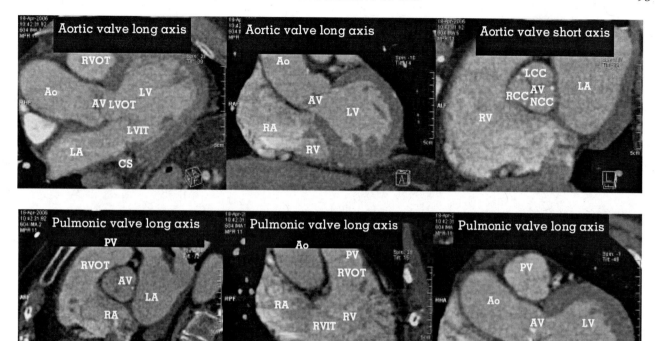

FIGURE 4-21. Additional imaging planes to demonstrate right ventricular, aortic valvular and pulmonary valvular anatomy shown using multiplanar reconstructed projections from CT volumetric image acquisition. *Abbreviations*: RV, right ventricle; RVOT, right ventricular outflow tract; RVIT, right ventricular inflow tract; RVA, right ventricular apex; LV, left ventricle; LVOT, left ventricular outflow tract; LVIT, left ventricular inflow tract; LVA, left ventricular apex; RA, right atrium; LA, left atrium; MV, mitral valve; AV, aortic valve; PV, pulmonary valve; Ao, aorta; NCC, noncoronary cusp; RCC, right coronary cusp; LCC, left coronary cusp; CS, coronary sinus.

Ventricular Analysis. Ventricular analysis requires acquisition of a volumetric cine imaging data set usually acquired in the true short-axis plane from the base of the heart to the apex (Figure 4–22), although long-axis orientations have also been used (Clay et al., 2006). Next, a selection of representative end-diastole (ED) and end-systole (ES) cardiac-phase images are chosen as phases with the largest and smallest ventricular volumes or the phase images obtained immediately before mitral valve closure (ED) and opening (ES). Once the selected phase images are chosen, the right and left ventricles are traced along the endocardial margin on each section obtained in the selected ED and ES phases from the cardiac apex to the section just prior to the one that depicts the mitral and tricuspid valve annuli. By convention, the tracings should exclude trabeculations. Papillary muscles are also commonly excluded, but may be included inside the endocardial margin, as long as there is consistency followed for both ED and ES phases (Figure 4–22). Typical calculations are demonstrated in Table 4–8.

Myocardial mass can be calculated by inclusion of the right ventricular and left ventricular epicardial borders during the ED phase. The interventricular septum is included with the left ventricle and excluded from the right ventricle tracing for myocardial mass calculation. The volumes of all sections are added, and the corresponding EDV is subtracted from the endocardial EDV to yield the myocardial volume. This result is then multiplied by the specific gravity of myocardium (i.e., 1.05 g/mL) to calculate the mass. Although this measure is useful for the assessment and follow-up of hypertrophic states, clinicians commonly also rely on the 1-D ED thickness measurement at specific segments throughout the left ventricle. Normal cardiac chamber dimensions in pediatric and adult patients are shown in Table 4–9.

Diastolic function of the ventricles can be measured by several different methods (Paelinck et al., 2002). Phase-contrast velocity mapping at the transtricuspid or transmitral level for calculation of time–velocity curves is a method similar to that used in Doppler echocardiography. Tagged MRI can also be used to measure global and regional diastolic function by calculation of diastolic strain rate (Edvardsen et al., 2006). However, the calculation of right and left ventricular time–volume curves is generally the most reliable method used in practice (Wintersperger and

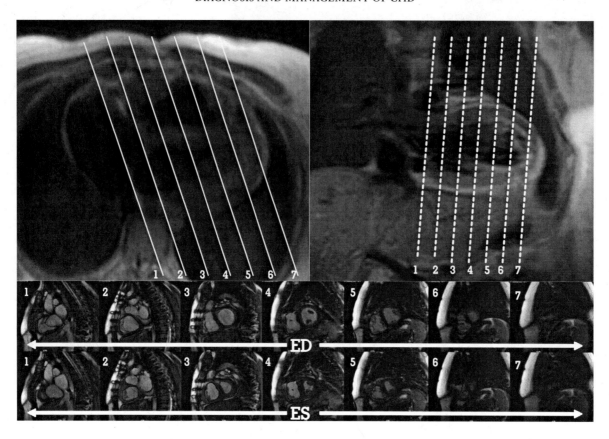

FIGURE 4–22. Volumetric acquisition of cine MR slices for calculation of ventricular volumes. Endocardial contours are drawn on all slices covering the ventricles at both end-diastole and end-systole for calculation of ventricular volumes, stroke volume, and ejection fraction.

Nikolaou, 2005). Diastolic function can be evaluated by several parameters related to both early and atrial filling. The early rapid filling phase can be characterized by parameters such as peak filling rate, time-to-peak filling rate, acceleration and deceleration slope of the early filling peak, deceleration time, and duration of the rapid filling period (Nishimura et al., 1989). The atrial filling peak is often quantified by peak filling rate. The ratio of early and atrial peak filling rate (E/A ratio) is another parameter that is commonly used.

Flow Analysis. Quantitative assessment of blood flow through the cardiac chambers, valves, and blood vessels is important in the management of cardiac patients. Phase contrast velocity measurements allow the assessment of the volume flow through a CSA of a vessel according to a simple relationship: $Q = VA$ where Q = blood flow in mL/s, V = velocity in cm/s, and A = lumen area in cm². Phase contrast velocity measurements have been validated and are currently used to quantify flow and other physiologic parameters such as stroke volume, valvular stenosis and regurgitation, and cardiac output, with an overall error in flow

measurement below 10% (Lotz et al., 2002). It should be noted that peak velocities might be underestimated with this method due to factors such as angle effects in the case of eccentric jets or low temporal resolution. Hence, imaging planes should be positioned orthogonal (through-plane) to the direction of the flow, and at least 16 phases of the cardiac cycle should be sampled with the VENC set well above the actual peak velocity in the region of interest in order to avoid aliasing (Wintersperger and Nikolaou, 2005).

Assessment of Intracardiac Shunts. Accurate assessment of the ratio of pulmonary (Qp) to systemic (Qs) flow is important in the management of patients with intracardiac left-to-right shunts. The Qp/Qs ratio is usually derived directly from heart catheterization oximetry, but noninvasive methods for calculation of this ratio can be made using Doppler echocardiography, radionuclide angiography and MRI. With phase-contrast velocity mapping MRI, flow quantification in both great arteries can be used to quantify Qp/Qs and has been shown to have good agreement with other methods for calculation of shunt size (Brenner et al., 1992; Hundley et al., 1995).

TABLE 4–8. *Common Quantitative Analyses*

Parameter	Calculation
LV EDV	ΣLV area(endocardial)$_{ED}$ × slice thickness
LV ESV	ΣLV area(endocardial)$_{ES}$ × slice thickness
RV EDV	ΣRV area(endocardial)$_{ED}$ × slice thickness
RV ESV	ΣRV area(endocardial)$_{ES}$ × slice thickness
SV	EDV – ESV
EF	SV/EDV × 100
CO	SV × HR
CI	(SV × HR)/BSA
LV MM	(ΣLV area(epicardial)$_{ED}$ × slice thickness – LV EDV) × 1.05 g/mL
RV MM	(ΣRV area(epicardial)$_{ED}$ × slice thickness – LV EDV) × 1.05 g/mL
MV RV	LV SV – aortic forward volume (from aortic flow quantification)
MV RF	MV RV/LV SV
TV RV	RV SV – MPA forward volume (from MPA flow quantification)
TV RF	TV RV/RV SV
AV RF	Aortic reverse volume/aortic forward volume (from aortic flow quantification)
PV RF	MPA reverse volume/MPA forward volume (from MPA flow quantification)

Abbreviations: AV RF, aortic valve regurgitant fraction; BSA, body surface area; CI, cardiac index; CO, cardiac output; EDV, end diastolic volume; EF, ejection fraction; ESV, end systolic volume; HR, heart rate; LV area(endocardial)$_{ED}$, left ventricular area enclosed by endocardial tracing at end-diastole; LV area(endocardial)$_{ES}$, left ventricular area enclosed by endocardial tracing at end-systole; LV area(epicardial)$_{ED}$, left ventricular area enclosed by epicardial tracing at end-diastole; LV, left ventricle; MM, myocardial mass; MPA, main pulmonary artery; MV RF, mitral valve regurgitant fraction; MV RV, mitral valve regurgitant volume; PV RF, pulmonic valve regurgitant fraction; RV area(endocardial)$_{ED}$, right ventricular area enclosed by endocardial tracing at end-diastole; RV area(endocardial)$_{ES}$, right ventricular area enclosed by endocardial tracing at end-systole; RV area(epicardial)$_{ED}$, right ventricular area enclosed by epicardial tracing at end-systole; RV, right ventricle; SV, stroke volume; TV RF, tricuspid valve regurgitant fraction; TV RV, tricuspid valve regurgitant volume.

3-D Reconstruction. Volumetric data sets acquired during MRI (e.g., MR angiography) can be evaluated in multiple planes "off-line" using a dedicated 3-D workstation. Image reconstructions can be visualized using multiplanar reformations, thick or thin maximum intensity projections, or using various shaded surface or volume rendering displays. These different projections are useful for evaluating abnormal vascular anatomy, especially when demonstrating abnormal connections (Figures 4–17 and 4–18).

Common Indications

Although echocardiography and cardiac catheterization are the primary cardiac imaging modalities in the assessment of patients with CHD, each have their own limitations. Echocardiography, though noninvasive with no radiation, is limited by a small field of view, acoustic windows, and operator dependence.

Conventional angiography is limited by the 2-D view with overlapping of adjacent vascular structures, catheter-related complications, and relatively high-exposure rates to ionizing radiation and iodinated contrast material.

No specific guidelines are in place regarding whether all patients with CHD should undergo further evaluation with MRI or CT . However, recently published guidelines suggest that MRI and CT imaging in complex CHD and for evaluation of anomalous coronary arteries are considered appropriate use of technology (Hendel et al., 2006). However, the decision to proceed with further imaging is largely patient and institution specific, since cardiovascular MRI and CT evaluation may not be widely available.

Patients are often referred for MRI as an adjunct to other imaging evaluation including echocardiography, cardiac catheterization, CT, and nuclear scintigraphy. MRI evaluation is particularly helpful in patients in whom diagnostic evaluation is incomplete, as an alternative to diagnostic cardiac catheterization, and for MRI specific evaluation such as tissue characterization. In particular, assessment of vascular anatomy including pulmonary arterial, pulmonary venous, systemic venous, and aortic anatomy is often best evaluated using MRI with its unrestricted imaging planes and unrestricted wide field of view. Right ventricular size and function is also a common evaluation better assessed with MRI than with echocardiography. Coronary artery anomalies are also better assessed with MRI than with echocardiography, although CT evaluation may eventually prove to be a better alternative. The reader is referred to other sources for MRI of specific lesions (see Fogel, 2006).

Patient Considerations

Patient-specific issues often dictate whether MRI examination is the optimal type of imaging test. MRI examination offers a large array of information for patients with CHD, and thus far, no known deleterious biologic effects related to MRI have been reported for clinical scanners in use today (Wolff et al., 1985). However, patients and accompanying individuals should be carefully screened for metallic objects or medical devices prior to entering the MRI suite. In addition to potential malfunction, implanted medical devices containing significant amount of ferromagnetic material are at risk for considerable torquing movements in an external magnetic field. Another potential hazard is heating of the devices due to deposited energy from the rapidly switching magnetic field gradients and RF pulses. Fortunately, most implants in patients with heart disease, including mechanical valves, sternal wires, stents, and occluding coils, are not considered a

TABLE 4–9. *Normal Measurements in Adult and Pediatric Patients*

Parameter	Normalized to BSA (m²)		Normalized to Height (cm)		Normalized to Weight (kg)	
	All (*n* = 75)	Pediatric (*n* = 8)	All (*n* = 75)	Pediatric (*n* = 8)	All (*n* = 75)	Pediatric (*n* = 8)
LVEDV (mL)	66±12 (44–89)	67±9 (49–85)	0.7±0.1 (0.4–1.0)	0.6±0.1 (0.4–0.9)	1.8±0.3 (1.2–2.4)	2.1±0.2 (1.7–2.5)
RVEDV (mL)	75±13 (49–101)	70±11 (49–91)	0.8±0.2 (0.4–1.1)	0.6±0.1 (0.4–0.9)	2.0±0.3 (1.4–2.6)	2.2±0.3 (1.6–2.8)
LVTM (g)	87±12 (64–109)	81±13 (56–106)	0.9±0.1 (0.8–1.0)	0.7±0.2 (0.4–1.1)	2.4±0.3 (1.8–2.9)	2.5±0.3 (1.9–3.1)
LVFWM (g)	57±8 (40–73)	53±8 (38–68)	0.6±0.0 (0.6–0.6)	0.5±0.1 (0.3–0.7)	1.6±0.2 (1.2–1.9)	1.6±0.2 (1.3–2.0)
IVSM (g)	30±4 (21–38)	28±5 (18–38)	0.3±0.1 (0.2–0.4)	0.3±0.1 (0.1–0.4)	0.8±0.1 (0.6–1.1)	0.9±0.1 (0.6–1.1)
RVFWM (g)	26±5 (17–34)	26±3 (20–32)	0.3±0.1 (0.2–0.4)	0.2±0.0 (0.2–0.3)	0.7±0.1 (0.5–1.0)	0.8±0.1 (0.7–0.9)
LVSV (mL)	45±8 (29–61)	44±7 (31–57)	0.5±0.1 (0.3–0.7)	0.4±0.1 (0.2–0.6)	1.2±0.2 (0.8–1.6)	1.4±0.2 (1.0–1.7)
RVSV (mL)	46±8 (30–62)	43±7 (28–58)	0.5±0.1 (0.3–0.7)	0.4±0.1 (0.2–0.6)	1.2±0.2 (0.8–1.7)	1.3±0.2 (0.9–1.8)
CO (L/min)	2.9±0.6 (1.74–4.03)	3.2±0.5 (2.17–4.28)				
LVEF	67±5% (57%–78%)					
RVEF	61±7% (47%–76%)					

Abbreviations: BSA, body surface area, 95% confidence intervals in parentheses (Lorenz, 2000); IVSM, interventricular septal mass; LVEDV; left ventricular end-diastolic volume; LVEF, left ventricular ejection fraction; LVTM, left ventricular total mass; LVFWM, left ventricular free wall mass; LVSV, left ventricular stroke volume; RVEDV, right ventricular end-diastolic volume; RVEF, right ventricular ejection fraction; RVFWM, right ventricular free wall mass; RVSV, right ventricular stroke volume.

contraindication to MRI (Ahmed and Shellock, 2001; Shellock and Crues, 2002). Pacemakers and implanted defibrillators are considered contraindication to MRI examination, though recent data suggest that in certain situations they may be acceptable (Nazarian et al., 2006). Information regarding the safety of individual devices is available either by consulting a published source on MRI safety (e.g., www.mrisafety.com) or by contacting the manufacturer. In addition to the safety concerns regarding particular devices, certain devices may produce imaging artifacts as a result of proximity to regions of interest, and depending on the imaging sequence used, these artifacts may be quite large, prohibiting accurate assessment of the structures of interest.

Preexamination planning is important in MRI of the CHD in order to optimize data acquisition. A thorough review of the patient's cardiovascular anatomy, including prior surgical or interventional procedures, is important in procedural planning. A supervising physician should also be present in order to optimize examination protocols in case of unexpected findings that may require adjustments in imaging planes, acquisition sequences and/or imaging parameters. Given the wide array of acquisition techniques available, it is also important to decide what type of information

is needed in order to optimize and limit overall examination times, especially given the possibility of truncated examination in an unstable patient due to their underlying disease process as well as concomitant use of sedatives, etc.

In order to obtain diagnostic-quality MR images, examination usually requires a patient to lie still for about an hour. Although this is usually not a problem for adolescents or adults, patients younger than 7 years of age and those older but with developmental delay usually require sedation or anesthesia in order to complete the examination. Additionally, patients who are even mildly claustrophobic will often require a sedative in order to complete the examination. Sedation can be administered via oral, rectal, or intravenous routes and is often specific to institutional policies. Particular care should be taken in monitoring the sedated child or infant with significant cardiac disease since the airway is now unprotected, and judicious use of cardiac anesthesia team is often helpful. An alternative is the use of general anesthesia in these patients, which has the added benefit of being able to suspend respiration during image acquisition. Again, particular sedation or anesthesia protocols for MRI examination in these patients is institution- and practitioner-specific.

Physician and Laboratory Standards

Medical specialists trained in cardiovascular medicine, radiology, and nuclear medicine are all involved in the cardiac imaging, and each provides differing perspectives. Clinical statements have been issued by the major medical societies regarding requirements for personnel involved in cardiac MRI examinations (Budoff et al., 2005; Weinreb et al., 2005). In particular, a familiarity with basic knowledge of MRI physics, scanner principles, safe contrast use, image postprocessing, and appropriate indications is needed. In general, the recommended cumulative time spent in the field of cardiac MRI is about 3 months (approximately 150 examinations) for physicians to perform and interpret cardiac MRI (Level 2 training) and at least 12 months (approximately 300 examinations) for physicians to serve as a director of a cardiac MRI laboratory (Level 3 training). Since the CHD requires a more special set of skills in order to evaluate complex lesions, postsurgical appearance, and postsurgical complications, it is recommended that practitioners wishing to specialize in CHD interpretation also include CHD cases as part of their training with a case load of 25 cases for Level 2 and 50 cases for Level 3 training with an additional 20 cases annually to maintain competence (Budoff et al., 2005). Training requirements as recommended by the American College of Radiology are slightly less rigorous owing to the fact that radiologists have background experience and residency training in cardiac anatomy and physics. Board certified radiologists are recommended to have supervised and interpreted 75 cardiac MRI cases within 36 months (Weinreb et al., 2005).

It is recommended that cardiac MRI studies be performed on scanners with field strength of 1.0 T or higher and a slew rate of at least 70 mT/m/s. Also, localized multichannel radiofrequency surface coils and electrocardiographic gating should be used. Technologists should be certified by the American Registry of Radiologic Technologists and/or have an unrestricted state license with documented training and experience in cardiac imaging procedures. In addition, documentation of advanced certification in MRI should also be provided. A continuous quality control program should be established with the assistance of a medical physicist and a Level 3-trained physician including periodic equipment calibration and a safety program. Patient safety should be assured through well-documented screening and evaluation for implanted devices.

COMPUTED TOMOGRAPHY

The advent of multidetector CT scanners in 1998 has led to increased interest and application of CT techniques for evaluation of cardiac structure and function. In addition, further advances in scanner technology have led to significant improvements in spatial resolution up to 0.4 × 0.4 × 0.4 mm and temporal resolution in the range of 85–210 ms depending on the scanner used.

Basic Concepts

CT uses rapidly rotating x-ray sources and detectors to create an image. The rotating unit is known as a gantry. The radiation that is not absorbed by the tissue passes into multiple detectors to yield a cross-sectional image. Images are acquired in an axial (transverse) plane in thin sections to yield isotropic voxels, matching that of in-plane spatial resolution. CT angiography (CTA) of the cardiovascular system refers to CT scanning that is performed during the injection of nonionic iodinated contrast agent. Although much information can be obtained from noncontrast CT, optimal evaluation of cardiac structures including vascular anatomy usually requires CTA.

Technical Considerations

Gantry Design. The gantry geometry of all MDCT generations is basically identical with only minor variations. However, detector geometry and postprocessing algorithms have become system-specific and somewhat dependent on the number of detectors used in gantry design and slices generated, currently anywhere from 4–256 slices (Flohr et al., 2004; Wintersperger and Nikolaou, 2005). Thin-slice collimations (0.5–0.625 mm) with reconstructed slice thickness of 0.4–0.7 mm allow for near isotropic voxels, which are important in postprocessing of coronary angiography studies. Gantry speed rotations of 330–420 ms/360 degree allow for high temporal resolution in the range of 165–190 ms, and new dual source technology (two sets of x-ray sources and detectors) allow for further improvement in temporal resolution down to 83 ms, which is important for functional assessment of the heart as well as in improving image quality for patients with fast heart rates.

Radiation dose exposure is largely dependent on the imaging protocol used. Typical effective radiation doses for coronary CT angiography are 5–12 mSv, although doses as high as 22 mSv have been reported with some protocols. In comparison, a typical radiation dose for chest CT is 5–7 mSv and that of a chest x-ray is <0.1 mSv. Fast table speeds (with fast heart rates) and ECG dose modulation schemes, in which tube current is lowered during acquisition of nondesired phases, can reduce the radiation dose received.

Motion Compensation. The rapid, constant motion of the heart is a source of significant motion artifact on conventional CT imaging. Although this is not usually a problem when visualizing larger vascular anatomy, optimal imaging of small cardiac structures requires some form of motion compensation. Hence, similar to MRI, synchronization of data acquisition to the cardiac cycle based on the ECG signal allows for combination of data acquired from consecutive gantry rotations in volumetric datasets with minimal blurring artifact related to cardiac motion. Again, data acquisition and reconstruction can be performed in a prospective or retrospective manner. In contrast to other CT spiral acquisitions, cardiac algorithms usually require very slow table movement through the gantry in order to allow image reconstruction at any time point of the cardiac cycle. As a result, increased radiation exposure can be expected compared with other conventional CT studies.

Temporal Resolution. Temporal resolution is the amount of time needed to acquire necessary scan data in order to reconstruct an image (Flohr and Ohnesorge, 2001). Temporal resolution in cardiac CT is primarily dependent on the rotation speed of the gantry. Data from only half a rotation (180 degree) can be used to create an image. As a result, temporal resolutions corresponding to half of a full 360° rotation, or 165 ms with a 330 ms/360 degree rotation speed are seen. Further improvements in temporal resolution can be achieved with multisector reconstruction algorithms, which are based on merging data of adjacent cardiac cycles (2–4 heartbeats) in order to fill a data segment more rapidly. Since dual source CT scanners have two sets of sources and detectors aligned 90 degree from one another, simultaneous scanning from the two sets of sources and detectors, can further reduce the temporal resolution down to 83 ms.

Given the limited temporal resolution offered by current CT technologies, image quality can also be improved by optimizing the patient's heart rate. Beta-blockers have been used to both lower the heart rate and promote regularity of the heart rhythm or decrease arrhythmias. Depending on the optimal diastolic time interval desired, oral or intravenous beta-blockers have been shown to be safe when administered to patients prior to CT scanning (Boudoulas, Lewis et al., 1979; Boudoulas, Rittgers et al., 1979; Shim et al., 2005). In patients unable to tolerate beta-blockers (e.g., severe asthmatics), calcium-channel blockers can often provide a similar benefit. The use of these medications in optimizing CT studies is institution and patient specific depending on the goal of imaging.

Spatial Resolution. Spatial resolution is mainly dependent on detector width, slice collimations and data sampling. The spatial resolution of four-detector CT scanners is 0.6 × 0.6 × 1.0 mm. With helical CT volume acquisition and reconstruction of overlapping sections, there is an improvement in the z-axis (through-plane) resolution, leading to near isotropic voxels. The resolution of 16 detector CT is 0.5 × 0.5 × 0.6 mm, and 64 slice systems is up to 0.4 × 0.4 × 0.4 mm (Nikolaou et al., 2004). These advances have greatly enhanced visualization of small structures such as the coronary arteries, but still remain inferior to conventional coronary angiography, which has a spatial resolution of 0.2 × 0.2 mm (Pannu et al., 2003).

Contrast Administration. Several considerations are important to be aware of with contrast use in cardiac imaging. First, since image quality is greatly affected by irregularity of the heart rhythm, nonionic contrast is used to prevent perturbations in the heart rate during image acquisition (Hill, 1993). Second, patients with cardiac disease may have low cardiac outputs, and as such, the timing of contrast arrival into the regions of interest can be variable. Hence, it becomes important to accurately track contrast-arrival times individually for each patient. Finally, the physiological impact of receiving contrast media must be taken into consideration as this can also affect the timing of contrast arrival.

Two types of contrast timing methods are employed in current CT scanning systems. The first involves determining the circulation time by giving a small volume test bolus (10–20 cc) of contrast and observing the time of its arrival in the heart, also known as a timing run. The second involves imaging a specific region of interest (e.g., ascending aorta) and once the contrast density attenuation reaches a prespecified point, the scanner turns on and starts imaging, also known as bolus tracking. Again, exact values are dependent on scanner type, contrast type, amount and delivery method, scan delay time, and individual preference.

Imaging Considerations and Postprocessing

CT imaging is a volumetric acquisition with high in-plane and through-plane spatial resolution. Due to the near-isotropic volumetric nature of the CT data, oblique multiplanar, and thin maximum intensity projection reconstructions, including curved reformations are used, in addition to standard axial 2-D evaluation of CT images in order to better understand cardiac structures. These oblique reconstructions are especially important for visualization of cardiac structures along imaging planes useful for understanding cardiac anatomy (see Figures 4–20 and 4–21) and great vessel and coronary artery anatomy throughout their course in both a longitudinal and axial plane to the vessel of interest. In addition to 2-D evaluations, volume and shaded surface rendered 3-D reconstructions with advanced visualization algorithms allow for the extraction of specific overlying structures such as bones, lung tissue and vessels, and soft tissue structures to focus on

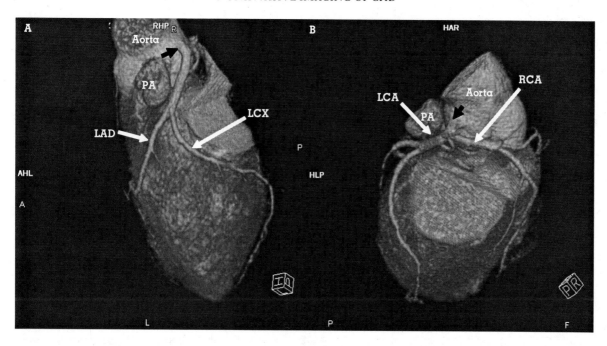

FIGURE 4-23. 3D Volume rendered CT images from a patient with history of Fontan repair for tricuspid atresia who was found to have a single coronary (black arrow) arising from the left cusp of the aorta and giving rise to the left and right coronary arterial systems. The left atrium has been removed from the image in order to better appreciate the proximal coronary arterial course. The small blind pouch of the proximal pulmonary artery is also seen. *Abbreviations*: PA, pulmonary artery; LAD, left anterior descending artery; LCX, left circumflex artery; LCA, left coronary artery; RCA, right coronary artery.

cardiac anatomy. These volume rendered 3-D images (Figure 4–23) are invaluable for understanding complex cardiac anatomy (e.g., anomalous coronary arteries) and in surgical planning. Shaded surface displays are commonly used for visualization of internal structures from a specified point simulating an endoscopic or angioscopic view and can provide the important information on the internal relationship of structures which may be important for guiding procedures (e.g., pulmonary vein isolation).

CT imaging protocol depends mainly on the structure of interest. As previously mentioned, evaluation of large vascular anatomy, including aortic and pulmonary arteries, usually does not require the use of cardiac gating. However, evaluation of cardiac function and coronary artery anatomy demands its use with resultant increase in radiation dose to the patient. In addition, depending on the type of scanner use, further optimization of image quality is achieved by the use of beta-blockers and nitrates. Evaluation of pericardial and mediastinal structures often does not require the use of contrast, but evaluation of vascular anatomy and internal cardiac structures demands it.

For patients with abnormalities in the vascular system, image acquisition is usually started a few centimeters above the aortic arch and continued to the diaphragm and even into abdominal structures depending on the anatomy. Since the CHD lesions often involves abnormalities in both the right and left heart chambers, the timing of data acquisition is set such that there is optimal contrast enhancement seen in both sides of the heart. In cases with intracardiac shunting, imaging can be performed early (within 5 seconds of contrast administration) and late (approximately 30 seconds after contrast administration) in order to determine the degree and direction of shunting (Funabashi et al., 2005).

Since CT data is volumetric and is often acquired with cardiac gating, slices in any arbitrary plane in 3-D space can be created during multiple phases of the cardiac cycle, similar to 3-D echocardiography. Although currently temporal resolution is still limited (83 ms at best), qualitative evaluation of wall motion and valve function can be made. Additionally, precise quantitative calculation of ventricular volumes and ejection fraction can be obtained from the data sets (Dirksen et al., 2002; Gilard et al., 2006; Mahnken et al., 2003; Juergens et al., 2004).

Common Indications

Similar to MRI, cardiovascular CT imaging is considered appropriate for the evaluation of complex CHD and evaluation of anomalous coronary arteries

(Hendel et al., 2006). Patients are often referred for CT evaluation to aid in assessment of patients with CHD, often when current evaluation is incomplete or as an alternative to invasive diagnostic cardiac catheterization. Alternatively, patients may often be referred for CT evaluation for noncardiac reasons and then incidentally are found to have congenital vascular or heart conditions. In particular, cardiovascular CT imaging is most helpful in the evaluation of vascular anomalies including anomalous coronary anomalies and in the evaluation of surgical graft patency. Although limited functional and flow information is obtainable, the benefit of CT evaluation lies mainly in its ability to provide high-resolution volumetric data on vascular anatomy in a matter of seconds.

Patient Considerations

Although CT imaging is in widespread use today, certain considerations need to be kept in mind when evaluating a patient with CHD. Since CT utilizes ionizing radiation in order to create images, optimization of image acquisition protocols is necessary in order to provide the information needed at as low a radiation dose as possible. In addition, risks of iodinated-contrast exposure also need to be weighed with regard to the lowest amount needed in order to provide adequate diagnostic information. Although important in any age group, these risks are particularly germane to the pediatric CHD population who are likely to undergo for future evaluations and resultant exposures.

Similar to MRI, preexamination planning is important in CT imaging of CHD. This is particularly important with regard to planning volumetric data acquisition and timing of contrast administration in order to capture the essential information needed. As such, CT protocols for CHD should be reviewed by an experienced physician familiar with the patient's cardiac disease and CT imaging protocols in order to ensure that data acquisition is optimal.

CT data acquisition time is short compared to corresponding MRI examinations. As such, patients often do not need to be sedated for examination. Patients do need to lie still for the examination, but given the short acquisition time (<15 seconds), this is usually not a problem, even with young kids. In addition, claustrophobia is usually not an issue given the short examination time and shorter length of the CT gantry compared to MRI. Unlike MRI, implanted medical devices do not pose a problem from a safety standpoint. However, depending on location, these devices may cause imaging artifacts on the resultant images. Fortunately, these artifacts are usually not as severe as with MRI and often do not preclude assessment of underlying or adjacent cardiovascular structures.

Physician and Laboratory Standards

Clinical statements have been issued by the major medical societies regarding requirements for personnel involved in cardiac CT examinations (Budoff et al., 2005; Weinreb et al., 2005). In particular, a familiarity with basic knowledge of CT physics, scanner principles, safe contrast use, image postprocessing, and appropriate indications is needed. In general, the recommended cumulative time spent in the field of cardiac CT is about 2 months (approximately 150 examinations) for physicians to perform and interpret cardiac CT (Level 2 training) and at least 6 months (approximately 300 examinations) for physicians to serve as a director of a cardiac CT laboratory (Level 3 training). Since the CHD needs a more special set of skills in order to evaluate complex lesions, postsurgical appearance and postsurgical complications, it is recommended that practitioners wishing to specialize in CHD interpretation also include CHD cases as part of their training with a case load of 25 cases for Level 2 and 50 cases for Level 3 training with an additional 20 cases annually to maintain competence (Budoff et al., 2005). Similar to MRI, training requirements as recommended by the American College of Radiology are less rigorous for radiologists recommending supervision and interpretation of at least 75 cardiac cases in 36 months (Weinreb et al., 2005).

Laboratory requirements and recommendations continue to change with the development of newer technologies. However, the availability of a multidetector CT or an electron-beam CT scanner is a requirement for cardiac imaging, especially for coronary artery imaging. In general, scanners used in cardiac CT should be at least 16 detectors and capable of temporal resolution of 500 ms or less with in-plane spatial resolution approaching 0.5 mm^3. For coronary imaging, thin-image sections <1 mm coupled with ECG gating is required. A powered contrast injector with programmable flow rates and volumes are a must. CT technologists specializing in cardiac CT should have advanced certification in CT in addition to regular certification by the American Registry of Radiologic Technologists and/or an unrestricted state license. A continuous quality control program should be established with the assistance of a medical physicist and a Level 3-trained physician.

REFERENCES

Echocardiography

Aldousany AW, DiSessa TG, Dubois R, Alpert BS, Willey ES, Birnbaum SE. Doppler estimation of pressure gradient in pulmonary stenosis: maximal instantaneous vs peak-to-peak, vs mean catheter gradient. *Pediatr Cardiol.* 1989;10:145–149.

American Academy of Pediatrics (AAP). Section on cardiology and cardiac surgery. Guidelines for pediatric cardiovascular centers. *Pediatrics.* 2002;109:544–549.

Amundsen BH, Helle-Valle T, Edvardsen T, et al. Noninvasive myocardial strain measurement by speckle tracking echocardiography: validation against sonomicrometry and tagged magnetic resonance imaging. *J Am Coll Cardiol.* 2006;47:789–793.

Ayres NA, Miller-Hance W, Fyfe DA, et al. Indications and guidelines for performance of transesophageal echocardiography in the patient with pediatric acquired or congenital heart disease. *J Am Soc Echocardiogr.* 2005;18:91–98.

Azhar AS, Habib HS. Accuracy of the initial evaluation of heart murmurs in neonates: do we need an echocardiogram? *Pediatr Cardiol.* 2006;27:234–237.

Banerjee A, Brook MM, Klautz RJ, Teitel DF. Nonlinearity of the left ventricular end-systolic wall stress-velocity of fiber shortening relation in young pigs: a potential pitfall in its use as a single-beat index of contractility. *J Am Coll Cardiol.* 1994;23:514–524.

Baumgartner H, Stefenelli T, Niederberger J, Schima H, Maurer G. "Overestimation" of catheter gradients by Doppler ultrasound in patients with aortic stenosis: a predictable manifestation of pressure recovery. *J Am Coll Cardiol.* 1999;33:1655–1661.

Bekeredjian R, Grayburn PA. Valvular heart disease. Aortic regurgitation. *Circulation.* 2005;112:125–134.

Bengur AR, Snider AR, Serwer GA, Peters J, Rosenthal A. Usefulness of the Doppler mean gradient in evaluation of children with aortic valve stenosis and comparison to gradient at catheterization. *Am J Cardiol.* 1989;64:756–761.

Bernstein HS, Brook MM, Silverman NH, Bristow J. Development of pulmonary arteriovenous fistulae in children after cavopulmonary shunt. *Circulation.* 1995;92(suppl 9):II309–314.

Bess RL, Khan S, Rosman HS, Cohen GI, Allebban Z, Gardin JM. Technical aspects of diastology: why mitral inflow and tissue Doppler imaging are the preferred parameters? *Echocardiography.* 2006;23:332–339.

Bezold LI, Ayres NA. Sedation and monitoring during diagnostic procedures. In: Garson A, Bricker JT, Fisher DJ, Neish SR, eds. *The Science and Practice of Pediatric Cardiology.* Philadelphia: Lippincott Williams & Wilkins; 1998:1065–1082.

Bleeker GB, Steendijk P, Holman ER, et al. Assessing right ventricular function: the role of echocardiography and complementary technologies. *Heart.* 2006;92 (suppl I):i19–i26.

Border WL, Michelfelder EC, Glascock BJ, et al. Color M-mode and Doppler tissue evaluation of diastolic function in children: simultaneous correlation with invasive indices. *J Am Soc Echocardiogr.* 2003;16:988–994.

Bossone E, Dino Bodini BD, Mazza A, Allegra L. Pulmonary arterial hypertension: the ket role of echocardiography. *Chest.* 2005;127:1836–1843.

Boucek RJ Jr, Martinez R. Echocardiographic determination of right ventricular function. *Cardiol Young.* 2005;15(suppl 1):48–50.

Brun P, Tribouilloy C, Duval AM, et al. Left ventricular flow propagation during early filling is related to wall relaxation: a color M-mode Doppler analysis. *J Am Coll Cardiol.* 1997;20:420–432.

Cao QL, Zabal C, Koenig P, Sandhu S, Hijazi ZM. Initial clinical experience with intracardiac echocardiography in guiding transcatheter closure of perimembranous ventricular septal defects: feasibility and comparison with transesophageal echocardiography. *Catheter Cardiovasc Interv.* 2005;66:258–267.

Carstensen EL, Duck FA, Meltzer RS, Schwarz KQ, Keller B. Bioeffects in echocardiography. *Echocardiography.* 1992;9:605–623.

Chan KL, Currie PJ, Seward JB, Hagler DJ, Mair DD, Tajik AJ. Comparison of three Doppler ultrasound methods in the prediction of pulmonary artery pressure. *J Am Coll Cardiol.* 1987;9:549–554.

Chang RK, Alejos JC, Atkinson D, et al. Bubble contrast echocardiography in detecting pulmonary arteriovenous shunting in children with univentricular heart after cavopulmonary anastomosis. *J Am Coll Cardiol.* 1999;33:2052–2058.

Cheitlin MD, Alpert JS, Armstrong WF, et al. ACC/AHA guidelines for the clinical application of echocardiography. A report of the American College of Cardiology/American Heart Association Task Force on Practice Guidelines (Committee on Clinical Application of Echocardiography). Developed in collaboration with the American Society of Echocardiography. *Circulation.* 1997;95:1686–744.

Cheitlin MD, Armstrong WF, Aurigemma GP, et al. American College of Cardiology; American Heart Association; American Society of Echocardiography. ACC/AHA/ASE 2003 guideline update for the clinical application of echocardiography: summary article: a report of the American College of Cardiology/American Heart Association Task Force on Practice Guidelines (ACC/AHA/ASE Committee to Update the 1997 Guidelines for the Clinical Application of Echocardiography). *Circulation.* 2003;108:1146–1162.

Cloutier A, Finley J. Telepediatric cardiology practice in Canada. *Telemed J E Health.* 2004;10:33–37.

Colan SD, Borow KM, Neumann A. Left ventricular end-systolic wall stress-velocity of fiber shortening relation: a load-independent index of myocardial contractility. *J Am Coll Cardiol.* 1984;4:715–724.

Colan SD, Parness IA, Spevak PJ, Sanders SP. Developmental modulation of myocardial mechanics: age- and growth-related alterations in afterload and contractility. *J Am Coll Cardiol.* 1992;19:619–629.

Danford DA, Murphy DJ Jr. Basic foundations of echocardiography and Doppler ultrasound. In: Garson A, Bricker JT, Fisher DJ, Neish SR, eds. *The Science and Practice of Pediatric Cardiology.* Philadelphia: Lippincott Williams & Wilkins; 1998:539–558.

Danford DA, Martin AB, Fletcher SE, Gumbiner CH. Echocardiographic yield in children when innocent murmur seems likely but doubts linger. *Pediatr Cardiol.* 2002;23:410–414.

Danford DA, Martin AB, Fletcher SE. Children with heart murmurs: can ventricular septal defect be diagnosed reliably without an echocardiogram? *J Am Coll Cardiol.* 1997;30:243–246.

Daniel WG, Mugge A. Transesophageal echocardiography. *N Engl J Med.* 1995;332:1268–1279.

Daubeney PE, Blackstone EH, Weintraub RG, Slavik Z, Scanlon J, Webber SA. Relationship of the dimension of cardiac structures to body size: an echocardiographic study in normal infants and children. *Cardiol Young.* 1999;9:402–410.

De Boeck BW, Oh JK, Vandervoort PM, Vierendeels JA, van der Aa RP, Cramer MJ. Colour M-mode velocity propagation: a glance at intra-ventricular pressure gradients and early diastolic ventricular performance. *Eur J Heart Fail.* 2005;7:19–28.

De Castro S, Caselli S, Papetti F, et al. Feasibility and clinical impact of live three-dimensional echocardiography in the management of congenital heart disease. *Echocardiography.* 2006;23:553–561.

DeGroff CG. Doppler echocardiography. *Pediatr Cardiol.* 2002;23:307–333.

Du ZD, Roguin N, Barak M. Clinical and echocardiographic evaluation of neonates with heart murmurs. *Acta Paediatr.* 1997;86:752–756.

Edler I, Hertz CH. Use of ultrasonic reflectoscope for the continuous recording of movements of heart walls. *Kungl Fyiogr Sallsk Lund Forl.* 1954;24:5.

Eidem BW, McMahon CJ, Cohen RR, et al. Impact of cardiac growth on Doppler tissue imaging velocities: a study in healthy children. *J Am Soc Echocardiogr.* 2004;17:212–221.

Feigenbaum H. Evolution of echocardiography. *Circulation*. 1996;93:1321–1327.

Frank DU, Minich LL, Shaddy RE, Tani LY. Is Doppler an accurate predictor of catheterization gradients for postoperative branch pulmonary stenosis? *J Am Soc Echocardiogr*. 2002;15:1140–1144.

Friedberg MK, Rosenthal DN. New developments in echocardiographic methods to assess right ventricular function in congenital heart disease. *Curr Opin Cardiol*. 2005;20:84–88.

Friedberg MK, Feinstein JA, Rosenthal DN. A novel echocardiographic Doppler method for estimation of pulmonary arterial pressures. *J Am Soc Echocardiogr*. 2006;19:559–562.

Frigiola A, Redington AN, Cullen S, Vogel M. Pulmonary regurgitation is an important determinant of right ventricular contractile dysfunction in patient with surgically repaired Tetralogy of Fallot. *Circulation*. 2004;110:153–157.

Frommelt PC, Whitstone EN, Frommelt MA. Experience with a DICOM-compatible digital pediatric echocardiography laboratory. *Pediatr Cardiol*. 2002;23:53–57.

Frommelt PC. Echocardiographic measures of diastolic function in pediatric heart disease. *Curr Opin Cardiol*. 2006;21:194–199.

Garcia MJ, Smedira NG, Greenberg NL, Main M, Firstenberg MS, Obadashian J, Thomas JD. Color M-mode Doppler flow propagation velocity is a preload insensitive index of left ventricular relaxation: animal and human validation. *J Am Coll Cardiol*. 2000;35:201–208.

Garg N, Agarwal BL, Modi N, Radhakrishnan S, Sinha N. Dextrocardia: an analysis of cardiac structures in 125 patients. *Int J Cardiol*. 2003;143–155.

Gerlis LM, Ho SY, Anderson RH, Branfoot AC. The anatomy of a collection. *Cardiovasc Pathol*. 1999;8:103–107.

Geva T. Echocardiography and Doppler ultrasound. In: Garson A, Bricker JT, Fisher DJ, Neish SR, eds. *The Science and Practice of Pediatric Cardiology*. Philadelphia: Lippincott Williams & Wilkins; 1998:789–843.

Geva T, van der Velde ME. Imaging techniques: echocardiography, magnetic resonance imaging, and computerized tomography. In: Keane JF, Lock JE, Fyler DC, eds. *Nadas' Pediatric Cardiology*. Philadelphia: Saunders Elsevier; 2006:183–212.

Ghaffar S, Haverland C, Ramaciotti C, Scott WA, Lemler MS. Sedation for pediatric echocardiography: evaluation of preprocedure fasting guidelines. *J Am Soc Echocardiogr*. 2002;15:980–983.

Giglio V, Pasceri V, Messano L, et al. Ultrasound tissue characterization detects preclinical myocardial structural changes in children affected by Duchenne muscular dystrophy. *J Am Coll Cardiol*. 2003;42:309–316.

Goens MB, Karr SS, Martin GR. Cyclic variation of integrated ultrasound backscatter: normal and abnormal myocardial patterns in children. *J Am Soc Echocardiogr*. 1996;9:616–621.

Gomez CA, Ludomirsky A, Ensing GJ, Rocchini AP. Effect of acute changes in load on left ventricular diastolic function during device closure of atrial septal defects. *Am J Cardiol*. 2005;95:686–688.

Goo HW, Park IS, Ko JK, Kim YH, Seo DM, Park JJ. Computed tomography for the diagnosis of congenital heart disease in pediatric and adult patients. *Int J Cardiovasc Imaging*. 2005;21:347–365.

Gowda RM, Khan IA, Vasavada BC, Sacchi TJ, Patel R. History of the evolution of echocardiography. *Int J Cardiol*. 2004;97:1–6.

Grech V. The evolution of diagnostic trends in congenital heart disease: a population-based study. *J Paediatr Child Health*. 1999;35:387–391.

Groundstroem KWE, Iivainen TE, Tavensaari T, Lahtela JT. Late postoperative follow-up of ostium secundum defect. *Eur Heart J*. 1999;20:904–999.

Gutgesell HP, Huhta JC, Latson LA, Huffines D, McNamara DG. Accuracy of two-dimensional echocardiography in the diagnosis of congenital heart disease. *Am J Cardiol*. 1985;55:514–518.

Gutgesell HP, Lindsey JH. Major advances in pediatric cardiology in the 20th century: I. Diagnostics. *J Pediatr*. 2000;137:431–433.

Hansen WH, Gilman G, Finnesgard SJ, et al. The transition from an analog to a digital echocardiography laboratory: the Mayo experience. *J Am Soc Echocardiogr*. 2004;17:1214–1224.

Harada K, Suzuki T, Shimada K, Takada G. Role of left ventricular mass/volume ratio on transmitral flow velocity patterns from infancy to childhood. *Int J Cardiol*. 1998;63:9–14.

Heistein LC, Ramaciotti C, Scott WA, Coursey M, Sheeran PW, Lemler MS. Chloral hydrate sedation for pediatric echocardiography: physiologic responses, adverse events, and risk factors. *Pediatrics*. 2006;117:e434–441.

Hlavacek AM, Crawford FA, Chessa KS, Shirali GS. Real-time three-dimensional echocardiography is useful in the evaluation of patients with atrioventricular septal defects. *Echocardiography*. 2006;23:225.

Hopkins WE, Waggoner AD, Gussak H. Quantitative ultrasonic tissue characterization of myocardium in cyanotic adults with an unrepaired congenital heart defect. *Am J Cardiol*. 1994;74:930–934.

Hurwitz RA, Caldwell RL. Should pediatric echocardiography be performed in adult laboratories? *Pediatrics*. 1998;102:e15. http://www.pediatrics.org/cgi/content/full/102/2/e15.

Irvine T, Li XK, Sahn DJ, Kenny A. Assessment of mitral regurgitation. *Heart*. 2002;88 (suppl IV):iv11–iv19.

Ishii M, Eto G, Tei C, et al. Quantitation of the global right ventricular function in children with normal heart and congenital heart disease: a right ventricular myocardial performance index. *Pediatr Cardiol*. 2000;21:416–421.

Ishii M, Himeno W, Sawa M, et al. Assessment of the ability of myocardial contrast echocardiography with harmonic power Doppler imaging to identify perfusion abnormalities in patients with Kawasaki disease at rest and during dipyridamole stress. *Pediatr Cardiol*. 2002;23:192–199.

Katz AM. *Physiology of the Heart*. 3rd ed. Philadelphia: Lippincott Williams & Wilkins; 2001.

Kavanaugh-McHugh A, Tobias JD, Doyle T, Heitmiller ES, Meagher C. Transesophageal echocardiography in pediatric congenital heart disease. *Cardiol Rev*. 2000;8:288–306.

Khanna D, Miller AP, Nanda NC, Ahmed S, Lloyd SG. Transthoracic and transesophageal echocardiographic assessment of mitral regurgitation severity: usefulness of qualitative and semiquantitative techniques. *Echocardiography*. 2005;22:748–769.

Khouri SJ, Maly GT, Suh DD, Walsh TE. A practical approach to the echocardiographic evaluation of diastolic function. *J Am Soc Echocardiogr*. 2004;17:290–297.

Kort S. Intracardiac echocardiography: evolution, recent advances, and current applications. *J Am Soc Echocardiogr*. 2006;19:1192–1201.

Krauss B, Green SM. Procedural sedation and analgesia in children. *Lancet*. 2006;367:766–780.

Lai WW, Geva T, Shirali G, et al. Guidelines and standards for performance of a pediatric echocardiogram: a report from the Task Force of the Pediatric Council of the American Society of Echocardiography. *J Am Soc Echocardiogr*. 2006;19:1413–1430.

Lang RM, Bierig M, Devereux RB, et al. American Society of Echocardiography's Nomenclature and Standards Committee; Task Force on Chamber Quantification; American College of Cardiology Echocardiography Committee; American Heart Association; European Association of Echocardiography, European Society of Cardiology. Recommendations for chamber quantification. *Eur J Echocardiogr*. 2006;7:79–108.

Lanzarini L, Fontana A, Lucca E, Campana C, Klersy C. Noninvasive estimation of both systolic and diastolic pulmonary artery pressure from Doppler analysis of tricuspid regurgitant velocity spectrum in patients with chronic heart failure. *Am Heart J.* 2002;144:1087–1094.

Larsson ES, Solymar L, Eriksson BO, de Wahl Granelli A, Mellander M. Bubble contrast echocardiography in detecting pulmonary arteriovenous malformations after modified Fontan operations. *Cardiol Young.* 2001;11:505–511.

Lemler MS, Valdes-Cruz LM, Shandas RS, Cape EG. Insights into catheter/Doppler discrepancies in congenital aortic stenosis. *Am J Cardiol.* 1999;83:1447–1450.

Lepper W, Belcik T, Wei K, Lindner JR, Sklenar J, Kaul S. Myocardial contrast echocardiography. *Circulation.* 2004;109:3132–3135.

Levine RA, Jimoh A, Cape EG, McMillan S, Yoganathan AP, Weyman AE. Pressure recovery distal to a stenosis: potential cause of gradient "overestimation" by Doppler echocardiography. *J Am Coll Cardiol.* 1989;13:706–715.

Li X, Mack GK, Rusk RA, et al. Will a handheld ultrasound scanner be applicable for screening for heart abnormalities in newborns and children? *J Am Soc Echocardiogr.* 2003;16:1007–1014.

Lipshultz SE, Easley KA, Orav EJ, et al. Cardiac dysfunction and mortality in HIV-infected children: The Prospective P2C2 HIV Multicenter Study. Pediatric Pulmonary and Cardiac Complications of Vertically Transmitted HIV Infection (P2C2 HIV) Study Group. *Circulation.* 2000;102:1542–1548.

Lopes LM, Damiano AP, Moreira GN, et al. The role of echocardiography as an isolated method for indicating surgery in patients with congenital heart disease. (Portuguese) *Arq Bras Cardiol.* 2005;84:381–386.

Mahle WT, Parks WJ, Fyfe DA, Sallee D. Tricuspid regurgitation in patients with repaired Tetralogy of Fallot and its relation to right ventricular dilatation. *Am J Cardiol.* 2003;92: 643–645.

Malviya S, Voepel-Lewis T, Ludomirsky A, Marshall J, Tait AR. Can we improve the assessment of discharge readiness? A comparative study of observational and objective measures of depth of sedation in children. *Anesthesiology.* 2004;100:218–224.

Marcus B, Steward DJ, Khan NR, et al. Outpatient transesophageal echocardiography with intravenous propofol anesthesia in children and adolescents. *J Am Soc Echocardiogr.* 1993;6:205–209.

Marek J, Skovranek J, Hucin B, et al. Seven-year experience of noninvasive preoperative diagnostics in children with congenital heart defects: comprehensive analysis of 2,788 consecutive patients. *Cardiology.* 1995;86:488–495.

Marx GR, Sherwood MC. Three-dimensional echocardiography in congenital heart disease: a continuum of unfulfilled promises? No. A presently clinically applicable technology with an important future? Yes. *Pediatr Cardiol.* 2002;23:266–285.

Mathewson JW, Perry JC, Maginot KR. Pediatric digital echocardiography: a study of analog-to-digital transition. *J Am Soc Echocardiogr.* 2000;13:561–569.

Mathewson JW, Dyar D, Jones FD, et al. Conversion to digital technology improves efficiency in the pediatric echocardiography laboratory. *J Am Soc Echocardiogr.* 2002;15:1515–1522.

Maurer G. Aortic regurgitation. *Heart.* 2006;92:994–1000.

McElhinney DB, Brook MM, Silverman NH. Echocardiography. In: Moller JH, Hoffman JIE, eds. *Pediatric Cardiovascular Medicine.* Churchill Livingstone, 2000:156–185.

McKendrick R, Owada CY. Real-time 3D echocardiography-guided transcatheter device closure of atrial septal defects. *Catheter Cardiovasc Interven.* 2005;65:442–446.

McMahon CJ, Ayres NA, Bezold LI, et al. Safety and efficacy of intravenous contrast imaging in pediatric echocardiography. *Pediatr Cardiol.* 2005;26:413–417.

McMahon CJ, Fraley JK, Kovalchin JP. Use of tissue harmonic imaging in pediatric echocardiography. *Cardiol Young.* 2001;11:562–564.

Mehta AR, Wakefield DS, Kienzle MG, Scholz TD. Pediatric tele-echocardiography: evaluation of transmission modalities. *Telemed J E Health.* 2001;7:17–25.

Meyer, RA. Echocardiography. In: Emmanouilides GC, Allen HD, Riemenschneider TA, Gutgesell HP eds. *Moss and Adams Heart Disease in Infants, Children, and Adolescents Including the Fetus and Young Adults.*

Milazzo AS Jr, Herlong JR, Li JS, Sanders SP, Barrington M, Bengur AR. Real-time transmission of pediatric echocardiograms using a single ISDN line. *Comput Biol Med.* 2002;32:379–388.

Minich LL, Tani LY, Pagotto LT, Shaddy RE, Veasy LG. Doppler echocardiography distinguishes between physiologic and pathologic "silent" mitral regurgitation in patients with rheumatic fever. *Clin Cardiol.* 1997;20:924–926.

Mondillo S, Giannotti G, Innelli P, Ballo PC, Galderisi M. Handheld echocardiography: its use and usefulness. *Int J Cardiol.* 2006;111:1–5.

Nakanishi T, Tobita K, Sasaki M, et al. Intravascular ultrasound imaging before and after balloon angioplasty for pulmonary artery stenosis. *Catheter Cardiovasc Interv.* 1999;46:68–78.

Nanda NC, Kisslo J, Lang R, et al. Examination protocol for three-dimensional echocardiography. *Echocardiography.* 2004;21:763–768.

Napoli KL, Ingall CG, Martin GR. Safety and efficacy of chloral hydrate sedation in children undergoing echocardiography. *J Pediatr.* 1996;129:287–291.

Nicolas RT, Kort HW, Balzer DT, et al. Surveillance for transplant coronary artery disease in infant, child and adolescent heart transplant recipients: an intravascular ultrasound study. *J Heart Lung Transplant.* 2006;25:921–927.

Nidorf SM, Picard MH, Triulzi MO, et al. New perspectives in the assessment of cardiac chamber dimensions during development and adulthood. *J Am Coll Cardiol.* 1992;19:983–988.

Noonan JA. A history of pediatric subspecialties: the development of pediatric cardiology. *Pediatr Res.* 2004;56:298–206.

Nyborg WL. Biological effects of ultrasound: development of safety guidelines. Part II: general review. *Ultrasound Med Biol.* 2001;27:301–333.

O'Leary PW. Intracardiac echocardiography in congenital heart disease: are we ready to begin the fantastic voyage? *Pediatr Cardiol.* 2002;23:286–291.

O'Leary PW, Durongpisitkul K, Cordes TM, et al. Diastolic ventricular function in children: a Doppler echocardiographic study establishing normal values and predictors of increased ventricular end-diastolic pressure. *Mayo Clin Proc.* 1998;73:616–628.

Okutan V, Lenk MK, Sarici SU, Dundaroz R, Akin R, Gokcay E. Efficacy and safety of rectal thiopental sedation in outpatient echocardiographic examination of children. *Acta Paediatr.* 2000;89:1340–1343.

Pasquini L, Sanders SP, Parness I, et al. Echocardiographic and anatomic findings in atrioventricular discordance with ventriculoarterial concordance. *Am J Cardiol.* 1988;62:1265–1262.

Patel A, Cao QL, Koenig PR, Hijazi ZM. Intracardiac echocardiography to guide closure of atrial septal defects in children less than 15 kilograms. *Catheter Cardiovasc Interv.* 2006;68:287–291.

Pedra SR, Pedra CA, Abizaid AA, et al. Intracoronary ultrasound assessment late after the arterial switch operation for transposition of the great arteries. *J Am Coll Cardiol.* 2005;45:2061–2068.

Pellett AA, Kerut EK. The Doppler equation. *Echocardiography.* 2004;21:197–198.

Pfammatter JP, Berdat P, Hammerli M, Carrel T. Pediatric cardiac surgery after exclusively echocardiography-based diagnostic work-up. *Int J Cardiol.* 2000;74:185–190.

Phoon CKL. Must doctors still examine patients? *Perspect Biol Med.* 2000;43:548–561.

Phoon CKL. Estimation of pressure gradients by auscultation: an innovative and accurate physical examination technique. *Am Heart J.* 2001;141:500–506.

Phoon CK, Bhardwaj N. Airway obstruction caused by transesophageal echocardiography in a patient with double aortic arch and truncus arteriosus. *J Am Soc Echocardiogr.* 1999;12:540–540.

Phoon CKL, Rutkowski M. Transesophageal imaging of the mid to distal left pulmonary artery in congenital heart disease. *J Am Soc Echocardiogr.* 1999;12:663–668.

Phoon CKL, Divekar A, Rutkowski M. Pediatric echocardiography: applications and limitations. *Curr Probl Pediatr.* 1999;29:157–192.

Pignatelli RH, McMahon CJ, Chung T, Vick GW 3rd. Role of echocardiography versus MRI for the diagnosis of congenital heart disease. *Curr Opin Cardiol.* 2003;18:357–365.

Pirat B, McCulloch ML, Zoghbi WA. Evaluation of global and regional right ventricular systolic function in patients with pulmonary hypertension using a novel speckle tracking method. *Am J Cardiol.* 2006;98:699–704.

Quiñones MA, Otto CM, Stoddard M, Waggoner A, Zoghbi WA. Recommendations for quantification of Doppler echocardiography: a report from the Doppler Quantification Task Force of the Nomenclature and Standards Committee of the American Society of Echocardiography. *J Am Soc Echocardiogr.* 2002;15:167–184.

Rhodes JF Jr, Qureshi AM, Preminger TJ, et al. Intracardiac echocardiography during transcatheter interventions for congenital heart disease. *Am J Cardiol.* 2003;92:1482–1484.

Roman MJ, Devereux RB. Kramer-Fox R, O'Loughlin. Two-dimensional echocardiographic aortic root dimensions in normal children and adults. *Am J Cardiol.* 1989;64:507–512.

Russell J, Justino H, Dipchand A, Yoo SJ, Kim YM, Freedom RM. Noninvasive imaging in congenital heart disease. *Curr Opin Cardiol.* 2000;15:224–237.

Sable C. Digital echocardiography and telemedicine applications in pediatric cardiology. *Pediatr Cardiol.* 2002;23:358–369.

Sable CA, Cummings SD, Pearson GD, et al. Impact of telemedicine on the practice of pediatric cardiology in community hospitals. *Pediatrics.* 2002 Jan;109:E3. http://www.pediatrics.org/cgi/content/full/109/1/e3.

Sanders SP, Colan SD, Cordes TM, et al. American Society of Echocardiography; Society of Pediatric Echocardiography; American College of Cardiology Foundation; American Heart Association; American College of Physicians Task Force on Clinical Competence (ACC/AHA/AAP Writing Committee to Develop Training Recommendations for Pediatric Cardiology). ACCF/AHA/AAP recommendations for training in pediatric cardiology. Task force 2: pediatric training guidelines for noninvasive cardiac imaging endorsed by the American Society of Echocardiography and the Society of Pediatric Echocardiography. *J Am Coll Cardiol.* 2005;46:1384–1388.

Schmitz L, Xanthopoulos A, Koch H, Lange PE. Doppler flow parameters of the left ventricular filling in infants: how long does it take for the maturation of the diastolic function in a normal left ventricle to occur? *Pediatr Cardiol.* 2004;25: 482–491.

Seifert BL, DesRochers K, Ta M, et al. Accuracy of Doppler methods for estimating peak-to-peak and peak instantaneous gradients across coarctation of the aorta: an in vitro study. *J Am Soc Echocardiogr.* 1999;12:744–753.

Seliem MA, Fedec A, Cohen MS, et al. Real-time 3-dimensional echocardiographic imaging of congenital heart disease using matrix-array technology: freehand real-time scanning adds instant morphologic details not well delineated by con-ventional 2-dimensional imaging. *J Am Soc Echocardiogr.* 2006;19:121–129.

Seward JB, Douglas PS, Erbel R, et al. Hand-carried cardiac ultrasound (HCU) device: recommendations regarding new technology. a report from the Echocardiography Task Force on New Technology of the Nomenclature and Standards Committee of the American Society of Echocardiography. *J Am Soc Echocardiogr.* 2002;15:369–373.

Shandas RS. Physics and instrumentation of ultrasound and Doppler imaging. In: Valdes-Cruz LM, Cayre RO, eds. *Echocardiographic Diagnosis of Congenital Heart Disease.* Philadelphia: Lippincott Williams & Wilkins, 1999:29–40.

Shanewise JS, Cheung AT, Aronson S, et al. ASE/SCA guidelines for performing intraoperative multiplane transesophageal echocardiography examination: recommendations of the American Society of Echocardiography Council for Intraoperative Echocardiography and the Society of Cardiovascular Anesthesiologists task force for certification in perioperative transesophageal echocardiography. *J Am Soc Echocardiogr.* 1999;12:884–900.

Sheil ML, Cartmill TB, Nunn GR, Sholler GF, Raitakari OT, Celermajer DS. Contrast echocardiography: potential for the in-vivo study of pediatric myocardial preservation. *Ann Thorac Surg.* 2003;75:1542–1548.

Silverman NH. *Pediatric Echocardiography.* Baltimore: Williams & Wilkins; 1993.

Silverman NH. Pediatric cardiac imaging—an historical perspective and future challenges. *Isr J Med Sci.* 1996;32:892–903.

Silvilairat S, Cabalka AK, Cetta F, Hagler DJ, O'Leary PW. Echocardiographic assessment of isolated pulmonary valve stenosis: which outpatient Doppler gradient has the most clinical validity? *J Am Soc Echocardiogr.* 2005;18:1137–1142.

Skorton DJ, Collins SM, Greenleaf JF, Meltzer RS, O'Brien WD Jr, Schnittger I, von Ramm OT. Ultrasound bioeffects and regulatory issues: an introduction for the echocardiographer. *J Am Soc Echocardiogr.* 1988;1:240–251.

Snider AR, Serwer GA, Ritter SB. *Echocardiography in Pediatric Heart Disease.* 2nd ed. Mosby-Year Book, Inc. 1997.

Spurney CF, Sable CA, Berger JT, Martin GR. Use of a hand-carried ultrasound device by critical care physicians for the diagnosis of pericardial effusions, decreased cardiac function, and left ventricular enlargement in pediatric patients. *J Am Soc Echocardiogr.* 2005;18:313–319.

Stanger P, Silverman NH, Foster E. Diagnostic accuracy of pediatric echocardiograms performed in adult laboratories. *Am J Cardiol.* 1999;83:908–914.

Stevenson JG. Comparison of several noninvasive methods for estimation of pulmonary artery pressure. *J Am Soc Echocardiogr.* 1989;2:157–171.

Stevenson JG, French JW, Tenckhoff L, Maeda H, Wright S, Zamberlin K. Video viewing as an alternative to sedation for young subjects who have cardiac ultrasound examinations. *J Am Soc Echocardiogr.* 1990;3:488–490.

Stugaard M, Brodahl U, Torp H, Ihlen H. Abnormalities of left ventricular filling in patients with coronary artery disease: assessment by color M-mode Doppler technique. *Eur Heart J.* 1994;15:318–327.

Stugaard M, Smiseth OA, Risoe C, Ihlen H. Intraventricular early diastolic filling during acute myocardial ischemia: assessment by multigated color M-mode Doppler. *Circulation.* 1993;88:2705–2713.

Sutherland GR, Di Salvo G, Claus P, D'hooge J, Bijnens B. Strain and strain rate imaging: a new clinical approach to quantifying regional myocardial function. *J Am Soc Echocardiogr.* 2004;17:788–802.

Tacy TA, Whitehead KK, Cape EG. In vitro Doppler assessment of pressure gradients across modified Blalock-Taussig shunts. *Am J Cardiol* 1998;81:1219–1223.

Takeuchi M, Nakai H, Kokumai M, Nishikage T, Otani S, Lang RM. Age-related changes in left ventricular twist assessed by two-dimensional speckle-tracking imaging. *J Am Soc Echocardiogr*. 2006;19:1077–1084.

Tani LY, Minich LL, Day RW, Orsmond GS, Shaddy RE. Doppler evaluation of aortic regurgitation in children. *Am J Cardiol*. 1997;80:927–931.

Taussig HB. *Congenital Malformations of the Heart*. New York: The Commonwealth Fund; 1947.

Thomas JD. Doppler echocardiographic assessment of valvar regurgitation. *Heart*. 2002;88:651–657.

Turner SP, Monaghan MJ. Tissue harmonic imaging for standard left ventricular measurements: Fundamentally flawed? *Eur J Echocardiogr*. 2006;7:9–15.

Tworetzky W, McElhinney DB, Brook MM, Reddy VM, Hanley FL, Silverman NH. Echocardiographic diagnosis alone for the complete repair of major congenital heart defects. *J Am Coll Cardiol*. 1999;33:228–233.

van den Bosch AE, Robbers-Visser D, Krenning BJ, et al. Real-time three-dimensional echocardiographic assessment of left ventricular volume and ejection fraction in congenital heart disease. *J Am Soc Echocardiogr*. 2006a;19:1–6.

van den Bosch AE, Harkel D-JT, McGhie JS, et al. Characterization of atrial septal defect assessed by real-time 3-dimensional echocardiography. *J Am Soc Echocardiogr*. 2006b;19:815–821.

Van Hare GF, Silverman NH. Contrast two-dimensional echocardiography in congenital heart disease: techniques, indications and clinical utility. *J Am Coll Cardiol*. 1989;13:673–686.

Villavicencio RE, Forbes TJ, Thomas RL, Humes RA. Pressure recovery in pediatric aortic valve stenosis. *Pediatr Cardiol*. 2003;24:457–462.

Ward CJB, Purdie J. Diagnostic accuracy of paediatric echocardiograms interpreted by individuals other than paediatric cardiologists. *J Paediatr Child Health*. 2001;37:331–336.

Weidemann F, Eyskens B, Sutherland GR. New ultrasound methods to quantify regional myocardial function in children with heart disease. *Pediatr Cardiol*. 2002;23:292–306.

Weyman AE, Scherrer-Crosbie M. Aortic stenosis: physics and physiology—what do the numbers really mean? *Rev Cardiovasc Med*. 2005;6:23–32.

Wheeler DS, Jensen RA, Poss WB. A randomized, blinded comparison of chloral hydrate and midazolam sedation in children undergoing echocardiography. *Clin Pediatr (Phila)*. 2001;40:381–387.

Widmer S, Ghisla R, Ramelli GP, et al. Tele-echocardiography in paediatrics. *Eur J Pediatr*. 2003;162:271–275.

Williams RV, Minich LL, Shaddy RE, Pagotto LT, Tani LY. Comparison of Doppler echocardiography with angiography for determining the severity of pulmonary regurgitation. *Am J Cardiol*. 2002;89:1438–1441.

Woodson KE, Sable CA, Cross RR, Pearson GD, Martin GR. Forward and store telemedicine using Motion Pictures Expert Group: a novel approach to pediatric tele-echocardiography. *J Am Soc Echocardiogr*. 2004;17:1197–1200.

Wright SB, Wienecke MM, Meyer KB, McKay CA, Wiles HB. Correlation of pediatric echocardiographic Doppler and catheter-derived valvar aortic stenosis gradients and the influence of aortic regurgitation. *Am J Cardiol*. 1996;77:663–665.

Yoganathan AP, Cape EG, Sung HW, Williams FP, Jimoh A. Review of hydrodynamic principles for the cardiologist: applications to the study of blood flow and jets by imaging techniques. *J Am Coll Cardiol*. 1988;12:1344–1353.

Zilberman MV, Witt SA, Kimball TR. Is there a role for intravenous transpulmonary contrast imaging in pediatric stress echocardiography? *J Am Soc Echocardiogr*. 2003;16:9–14.

Zoghbi WA, Enriquez-Sarano M, Foster E, et al. American Society of Echocardiography. Recommendations for evaluation of the severity of native valvular regurgitation with two-dimensional and Doppler echocardiography. *J Am Soc Echocardiogr*. 2003;16:777–802.

Cardiac MRI and Computed Tomography

Ahmed S, Shellock FG. Magnetic resonance imaging safety: implications for cardiovascular patients. *J Cardiovasc Magn Reson*. 2001;3(3):171–182.

Boudoulas H, Lewis RP, Rittgers SE, Leier CV, Vasko JS. Increased diastolic time: a possible important factor in the beneficial effect of propranolol in patients with coronary artery disease. *J Cardiovasc Pharmacol*. 1979;1(5):503–513.

Boudoulas H, Rittgers SE, Lewis RP, Leier CV, Weissler AM. Changes in diastolic time with various pharmacologic agents: implication for myocardial perfusion. *Circulation*. 1979;60(1):164–169.

Brenner LD, Caputo GR, Mostbeck G, et al. Quantification of left to right atrial shunts with velocity-encoded cine nuclear magnetic resonance imaging. *J Am Coll Cardiol*. 1992;20(5):1246–1250.

Budoff MJ, Cohen MC, Garcia MJ, et al. ACCF/AHA clinical competence statement on cardiac imaging with computed tomography and magnetic resonance: a report of the American College of Cardiology Foundation/American Heart Association/American College of Physicians Task Force on Clinical Competence and Training. *J Am Coll Cardiol*. 2005;46(2):383–402.

Clay S, Alfakih K, Radjenovic A, Jones T, Ridgway JP, Sinvananthan MU. Normal range of human left ventricular volumes and mass using steady state free precession MRI in the radial long axis orientation. *Magma*. 2006;19(1):1–5.

Dirksen MS, Bax JJ, de Roos A, et al. Usefulness of dynamic multislice computed tomography of left ventricular function in unstable angina pectoris and comparison with echocardiography. *Am J Cardiol*. 2002;90(10):1157–1160.

Edvardsen T, Rosen BD, Pan L, et al. Regional diastolic dysfunction in individuals with left ventricular hypertrophy measured by tagged magnetic resonance imaging—the Multi-Ethnic Study of Atherosclerosis (MESA). *Am Heart J*. 2006;151(1):109–114.

Fischer SE, Wickline SA, Pan L, et al. Novel real-time R-wave detection algorithm based on the vectorcardiogram for accurate gated magnetic resonance acquisitions. *Magn Reson Med*. 1999;42(2):361–370.

Flohr T, Ohnesorge B. Heart rate adaptive optimization of spatial and temporal resolution for electrocardiogram-gated multislice spiral CT of the heart. *J Comput Assist Tomogr*. 2001;25(6):907–923.

Flohr T, Stierstorfer K, Raupach R, Ulzheimer S, Bruder H. Performance evaluation of a 64-slice CT system with z-flying focal spot. *Rofo*. 2004;176(12):1803–1810.

Fogel MA, Guest Editor. Special Issue on CMR applications in congenital heart disease. *J Cardiovasc Magnet Reson*. 2006;8(4):567–670.

Funabashi N, Asano M, Sekine T, Nakayama T, Komuro I. Direction, location, and size of shunt flow in congenital heart disease evaluated by ECG-gated multislice computed tomography. *Int J Cardiol*. 2005;112(3):399–404.

Gilard M, Pennec PY, Cornily JC, et al. Multi-slice computer tomography of left ventricular function with automated analysis software in comparison with conventional ventriculography. *Eur J Radiol*. 2006;59(2):270–275.

Hendel RC, Patel MR, Kramer CM, et al. ACCF/ACR/SCCT/ SCMR/ASNC/NASCI/SCAI/SIR 2006 appropriateness criteria for cardiac computed tomography and cardiac magnetic resonance imaging: a report of the American College of Cardiology Foundation Quality Strategic Directions Committee Appropriateness Criteria Working Group, American College of Radiology, Society of Cardiovascular Computed Tomography, Society for Cardiovascular Magnetic Resonance, American Society of Nuclear Cardiology, North American Society for Cardiac Imaging, Society for Cardiovascular Angiography and Interventions, and Society of Interventional Radiology. *J Am Coll Cardiol.* 2006;48(7):1475–1497.

Hill JA. Nonionic contrast use in cardiac angiography. *Invest Radiol.* 1993;28 (suppl 5):S48–53;discussion S54.

Hundley WG., Li HF, Lange RA, et al. Assessment of left-to-right intracardiac shunting by velocity-encoded, phase-difference magnetic resonance imaging. A comparison with oximetric and indicator dilution techniques. *Circulation.* 1995;91(12):2955–2960.

Juergens KU, Grude M, Maintz D, et al. Multi-detector row CT of left ventricular function with dedicated analysis software versus MR imaging: initial experience. *Radiology.* 2004;230(2):403–410.

Larson AC, White RD, Laub G, McVeigh ER, Li D, Simonetti OP. Self-gated cardiac cine MRI. *Magn Reson Med.* 2004;51(1):93–102

Lee VS. *Cardiovascular MRI: Physical Principles to Practical Protocols.* Philadelphia, PA: Lippincott Williams & Wilkins; 2006.

Lorenz CH. The range of normal values of cardiovascular structures in infants, children, and adolescents measured by magnetic resonance imaging. *Pediatr Cardiol.* 2000;21(1):37–46.

Lotz J, Meier C, Leppert A, Galanski M. Cardiovascular flow measurement with phase-contrast MR imaging: basic facts and implementation. *Radiographics.* 2002;22(3):651–671.

Mahnken AH., Spuentrup E, Niethammer M, et al. Quantitative and qualitative assessment of left ventricular volume with ECG-gated multislice spiral CT: value of different image reconstruction algorithms in comparison to MRI. *Acta Radiol.* 2003;44(6):604–611.

Nazarian S, Roguin A, et al. Clinical utility and safety of a protocol for noncardiac and cardiac magnetic resonance imaging of patients with permanent pacemakers and implantable-cardioverter defibrillators at 1.5 tesla. *Circulation.* 2006;114(12):1277–1284.

Nikolaou K., Flohr T, Knez A, et al. Advances in cardiac CT imaging: 64-slice scanner. *Int J Cardiovasc Imaging.* 2004;20(6):535–540.

Nishimura RA, Abel MD, Hatle LK, Tajik AJ. Assessment of diastolic function of the heart: background and current applications of Doppler echocardiography. Part II. Clinical studies. *Mayo Clin Proc.* 1989;64(2):181–204.

Paelinck BP, Lamb HJ, Bax JJ, Van der Wall EE, de Roos A. Assessment of diastolic function by cardiovascular magnetic resonance. *Am Heart J.* 2002;144(2):198–205.

Pannu HK, Flohr TG, Corl FM, Fishman EK. Current concepts in multi-detector row CT evaluation of the coronary arteries: principles, techniques, and anatomy. *Radiographics.* 2003;23 Spec No:S111–S125.

Plein S, Smith WH, Ridgway JP, et al. Measurements of left ventricular dimensions using real-time acquisition in cardiac magnetic resonance imaging: comparison with conventional gradient echo imaging. *Magma.* 2001;13(2):101–108.

Shellock FG, Crues JV 3rd. MR Safety and the American College of Radiology White Paper. *AJR Am J Roentgenol.* 2002;178(6):1349–1352.

Shim SS., Kim Y, Lim SM. Improvement of image quality with beta-blocker premedication on ECG-gated 16-MDCT coronary angiography. *AJR Am J Roentgenol.* 2005;184(2):649–654.

Weinreb JC, Larson PA, Woodard PK, et al. American College of Radiology clinical statement on noninvasive cardiac imaging. *Radiology.* 2005;235(3):723–727

Winterer JT, Lehnhardt S, Schneider B, et al. MRI of heart morphology. Comparison of nongradient echo sequences with single- and multislice acquisition. *Invest Radiol.* 1999;34(8):516–522.

Wintersperger BJ, Nikolaou K. Basics of cardiac MDCT: techniques and contrast application. *Eur Radiol.* 2005;15(suppl 2):B2–9.

Wolff S, James TL, Young GB, et al. Magnetic resonance imaging: absence of in vitro cytogenetic damage. *Radiology.* 1985;155(1):163–165.

5

Novel Methods to Screen for Heart Disease in Infants

ROBERT I. KOPPEL

WILLIAM T. MAHLE

Congenital heart disease (CHD) occurs in 8 per 1000 live births. Approximately one-third of these children will have critical congenital heart disease (cyanotic congenital heart disease [CCHD]), which by definition requires surgery or catheter intervention in the first year of life (Botto et al., 2001). Currently, children with CCHD are diagnosed by a variety of methods. Newborns with CHD may be diagnosed in the newborn nursery based on the physical examination findings such as a heart murmur, tachypnea, or overt cyanosis. However, these findings are not always available, especially in the setting of hospital discharge at less than 48 hours of life. A study by Ainsworth et al. (1999) suggested that over 50% of children with CCHD did not have a clinically significant heart murmur by 48 hours of life. In addition, the ability to identify a pathologic heart murmur is dependent upon the skill of the practitioner. One study found that general pediatricians correctly identified a pathologic heart murmur 40% of the time (Danford et al., 2000). Approximately 20% of the newborns with CCHD may also present with tachypnea (Ramaciotti et al., 1993). In a detailed analysis of the diagnostic methods for CCHD in the United Kingdom, it has been determined that the routine physical examination of the newborns failed to detect CCHD in 69% of the cases. Interestingly, in a small but significant number of infants with CCHD, the disease was not diagnosed even during the routine physical examination of the infants at 6 weeks of age. Another important consideration is that a clinical examination that is suspicious for congenital heart defects does not always mean that a definitive evaluation for confirmation

of suspected diagnosis—an echocardiogram—will be performed on time. In a report from the United Kingdom, a small number of deaths were attributed to subjects with "suspected CCHD" who died before a definitive diagnosis could be obtained—either from echocardiography or examination by a pediatric cardiologist.

A common feature of many forms of CHD is hypoxemia, which results from mixing of the systemic and venous circulations or parallel circulations as one might see in transposition of the great arteries (TGA). Hypoxemia may result in obvious cyanosis. However, generally 4 g of deoxygenated hemoglobin is needed to produce visible cyanosis. For the typical newborn with a hemoglobin concentration of 20 g/dL, visible cyanosis will only be noted when arterial oxygen saturation is <80%. Children with mild hypoxemia, having an arterial oxygen saturation of 80%–95%, will not have visible cyanosis. Moreover, the identification of cyanosis is particularly difficult in African-American and Hispanic neonates due to skin pigmentation (Richmond and Wren, 2001).

Identification of hypoxemia in children with CCHD is of crucial importance as a majority of critical defects present with some degree of hypoxemia in the newborn period. Table 5–1 demonstrates the frequency of the most common forms of CCHD and the likelihood of having some degree of hypoxemia in the newborn period based on data obtained from the Metropolitan Atlanta Birth Defects Surveillance Program (Ainsworth et al., 1999). These data suggest that between 15 and 37 per 10,000 live births are likely to demonstrate hypoxemia that could be detected by pulse oximetry.

TABLE 5-1. *Critical CHD Lesions and Associated Clinical Characteristics*

Lesion	Rate	Hypoxemia	Ductal Dependent
Heterotaxias	1.4	All	Some
Corrected (L) transposition	0.7	Rare	No
Tetralogy of Fallot	6.1	Most	Rare
D-transposition of the great arteries	4.0	All	All
Double outlet right ventricle	1.7	Some	Some
Truncus arteriosus	1.0	All	None
TAPVC	1.2	All	None
Ebstein anomaly	0.6	Some	Some
Right obstructive defects			
Tricuspid atresia	0.5	All	Most
Pulmonary atresia, intact septum	0.8	All	All
Pulmonic stenosis, atresia	6.3	Some	Most
Hypoplastic left heart	3.3	All	All
Coarctation of the aorta	4.7	Rare	Most
Aortic arch atresia or hypoplasia	1.0	Rare	All
Aortic valve stenosis	1.6	Rare	Some
Other major heart defects	10.3	Some	Some

In addition, it is important to realize that newborns with CCHD are susceptible to profound, sudden worsening in clinical status with closure of the ductus arteriosus. In the normal newborns, closure of the ductus arteriosus, which typically occurs between 24 and 72 hours of life, does not result in significant changes in hemodynamics. Conversely, in neonates with CCHD, the ductus arteriosus is often essential for maintaining either the pulmonary or the systemic blood flow. These CCHD defects are considered "ductal-dependent lesions." Given that closure of the ductus arteriosus often occurs within the first several days of life, oximetry screening needs to be carried out in the setting of the newborn nursery rather than at subsequent well-child evaluations. Table 5–1 lists the CCHD lesions that are ductal-dependent. The timing of constriction or closure of the ductus arteriosus also explains why children with CCHD may be particularly vulnerable to cardiovascular collapse within several days of discharge from the newborn nursery. This is especially true in the current health care climate where newborns may be discharged to home at less than 48 hours of life.

Since the late 1980s, prenatal ultrasound scanning has been used to screen for congenital anomalies. An anatomical (or level II) ultrasound is typically performed between 18 and 20 weeks of gestation. During the procedure, many—but not all—cases of CCHD can be identified by a methodical scan. When CCHD is identified through this scan, the patient is often referred to a pediatric cardiologist for confirmatory imaging and counseling. With knowledge that the fetus

has CCHD, the newborn can be delivered in a hospital capable of providing intensive care, such as mechanical ventilation. The newborn can be stabilized and transferred to a congenital heart center. Theoretically, this prenatal ultrasound scanning should be able to identify most forms of CCHD. However, in the United States, it is estimated that only 20%–40% of cases of CCHD have a prenatal diagnosis (Montana et al., 1996). The reasons for this discrepancy are varied. An anatomical ultrasound scan is not performed on all pregnant women. The availability of anatomical ultrasound scanning may be limited in certain racial or low socioeconomic settings. The quality of anatomical ultrasound scans varies considerably (Queisser-Luft et al., 1998). A number of medical professionals including radiologists, perinatologists, and general obstetricians, with varying degrees of training, perform the ultrasound scanning procedure. The poor quality of obstetric ultrasound imaging was documented in a study in 1992 in which investigators reported that in 141 second-trimester sonograms—the sonogram that is most crucial for detecting defects in fetal structures—the heart, brain, spine, and kidneys were most often poorly or inadequately imaged. Of general obstetricians enrolling for a certification program for fetal ultrasound scanning, only 36% qualified for certification. Thus, even if all women were to undergo routine anatomical ultrasound scan, a significant proportion of CCHD cases are likely to be missed because of poor imaging.

Data regarding the prenatal detection rate for CHD in the United States are limited. A study from the CDC's Metropolitan Atlanta Congenital Defects Program (MACDP) reported that the prenatal detection rate for all congenital heart defects was only 12.7% in the mid-1990s (Montana et al., 1996). Detection rates for certain CHD such as hypoplastic left heart syndrome (HLHS) appear to be higher. Several single institution series from the United States have reported prenatal detection rates as high as 50% for HLHS; however, this number may be higher for a larger referral center than for the population at large. Detection rates for certain CCHD lesions such as TGA are less than 30% even in a number of contemporary series from U.S. centers. Other than the CDC study reported by Montana et al., there are no population-based series from the United States to provide an accurate assessment of the prenatal detection rates of CCHD. It is likely that detection rates will vary significantly among various regions in the United States for a variety of reasons including health care access, skill and experience of sonographer, and obstetric practices as outlined above. In the United Kingdom, prenatal detection rates for CCHD have been reported to be somewhat higher than in the United States. Hunter and colleagues reported that an intensive training program of sonographers achieved a detection rate of 36% for all forms of CHD (Hunter et al., 2000). However, the United Kingdom has a far more centralized obstetric imaging system with fetal sonography limited to a few regional centers. Such centralization and oversight are lacking in the United States. As such, a more comprehensive understanding of the patterns and sociodemographic factors associated with prenatal detection are of considerable importance in developing a strategy for improved early diagnosis of CCHD.

MORBIDITY DUE TO DELAYED DIAGNOSIS

Delayed diagnosis of CCHD may result in profound hypoxemia, hypoperfusion, and shock. A number of investigators have demonstrated severe end-organ damage or injury in this setting (Bonnet et al., 1999; Kumar et al., 1999; Mahle et al., 2001; Tworetzky et al., 2001). Tworetzky and colleagues (2001) reported that delayed diagnosis in the HLHS was significantly associated with ventricular dysfunction, tricuspid insufficiency, and a greater need for inotropic support preoperatively. Bonnet et al. (1999) examined the outcomes for children with TGA presenting to their center, and found that delayed diagnosis resulted in more severe metabolic acidosis and greater need for mechanical ventilation. Similarly, Kumar and colleagues (1999) examined both the TGA and HLHS populations. These investigators reported that delayed diagnosis was associated with impaired renal and liver functions, and that through supportive care, it may be possible to effectively treat such end-organ injury. However, in rare cases, damage may be so severe, as with hepatic dysfunction, to result in fulminant coagulopathy. Moreover, the ability to "reverse" injury to the brain may be limited as will be reported in some of our preliminary data.

DEATH DUE TO DELAYED DIAGNOSIS

While the delayed diagnosis of CCHD can result in impaired end-organ function, it is possible in many cases—as mentioned above—to support the infants medically until the organs can recover. Regrettably, however, there are a number of children who are so severely compromised at presentation that they die before surgical intervention. In a study from the Baltimore–Washington metro area in the 1980s, Kuehl and colleagues reported that of 4360 children with any form of CHD studied 76 (1.7%) died before the identification of the heart disease (Kuehl et al., 1999). Stated alternatively, 1.4 per 10,000 live births resulted in death, with CCHD being identified only on autopsy.

With the increased use of prenatal ultrasound scanning in the last decade, there is undoubtedly a reduction in the risk of death before diagnosis; however, the number of such deaths is still likely to be significant. A recent European study reported that children with TGA were at significant risk of death before diagnosis or adequate stabilization. In the analysis of infants with TGA, Bonnet and colleagues reported that 6% of the neonates with TGA died before surgical intervention could be made (Bonnet et al., 1999).

Failure to diagnose CCHD can result in death at home or during attempted stabilization. In addition, some authors have suggested that the impairment in cardiovascular function that occurs from delayed diagnosis can adversely impact survival for those who undergo neonatal cardiovascular surgery. Tworetzky and colleagues reported that patients diagnosed postnatally underwent surgery at a later age than those diagnosed prenatally—8.2 versus 5.9 days ($P = 0.02$) and that those diagnosed postnatally had an increased risk of postoperative mortality ($P = 0.04$). The benefit of early diagnosis in HLHS is not surprising given that numerous studies have shown that older age is associated with increased risk of death following the Norwood procedure (Forbess et al., 1995; Iannettoni et al., 1994; Mahle et al., 2000). In patients with TGA, it has also been suggested that early diagnosis with minimal preoperative organ injury is associated with improved postoperative survival. Examining outcomes after the arterial switch procedure for TGA, Bonnet and colleagues reported that the postoperative mortality was significantly less for those diagnosed prenatally than those diagnosed postnatally: 0% versus 10% ($P < 0.01$). This improved survival was attributed to lesser preoperative morbidity in the prenatally diagnosed group.

CLINICAL STUDIES OF OXIMETRY SCREENING

Pulse oximetry has gained wide acceptance as a noninvasive method to determine oxygen saturation (SpO_2). The method does not require calibration and is able to provide instantaneous data that correlates well with blood gas measurements. O'Brien et al. have defined reference data for oxygen saturation in healthy fullterm infants during their first 24 hours of life (O'Brien et al., 2000). The median value at 20–24 hours of life (97.8%) is similar to the results for healthy full-term infants between 2 and 7 days of age (97.6%) (Poets, 1999). Beginning in the 1990s, investigators began to explore the possible role of neonatal oximetry in identifying CCHD. Hoke and colleagues (2002) evaluated 32 newborns with CCHD to determine what percentage of the disease could be identified by oximetry.

Using a cutoff of 95% in lower extremity saturation, their data suggested that 26 of the 32 subjects (81%) with CCHD could be identified using oximetry. In addition, Hoke and colleagues studied oximetry in 2876 newborns admitted to a well-baby nursery. Using a cutoff of 92%, they found that 2% of infants had a leg saturation of <92%. Of these, 4 of the 57 had CCHD. Importantly, the investigators performed oximetry testing at less than 24 hours of life in many of the newborns evaluated, which might explain the relatively high number of false-positive results in this study. In the United Kingdom, Richmond and colleagues (2002) performed a similar study examining 6166 newborns with oximetry. These investigators performed oximetry measurements at two time periods: at 2 hours and before hospital discharge. They found that 1% of newborns had saturations of <95% before the planned discharge. The study discovered 4 subjects with CCHD and saturations of <95%, who had no other clinical findings suggestive of heart disease. Interestingly, the investigators also reported finding other clinically significant conditions such as persistent fetal circulation (PFC) or parenchymal lung disease based on oximetry screening alone, suggesting that oximetry screening may have benefits beyond the early identification of CCHD. In a study from Switzerland, Arlettaz and colleagues (2006) performed postductal oximetry measurements on 3262 newborns. They identified 17 cases of CHD, of which only one was a false-positive result. A group of investigators in Italy screened 5292 newborns and found two true-positives (.04%), one false-positive (.02%), and one false-negative (.02%) results, employing a single oximetry measurement at >24 h of age with a prespecified cutoff at <96% (Rosati et al., 2005). Bakr and Habib (2005) reported that oximetric screening increased the sensitivity of CCHD detection by clinical examination by 31%. Kawalec et al. (2006) reported the experience with oximetric screening in the Podkarpacie province of Poland. Obstetric ultrasound was performed on 99.3% of the pregnancies and fetal echocardiography on 9.2%. In this population of 27,200 screened newborns, the investigators found 7 cases of CCHD in asymptomatic newborns, with 13 false-positive and 1 false-negative (coarctation) results for a sensitivity of 87% and a specificity of 99.9%. Moreover, this study included an assessment of parental attitudes toward oximetric screening that revealed a 99.8% parental approval rating.

One of the concerns raised with oximetry screening is that it may not be well suited to detect lesions with isolated aortic arch obstructions. Some investigators have suggested that measurement of both the upper and the lower extremity saturations (preductally and postductally, respectively) may aid in identifying these patients. De-Wahl and colleagues recently reported the oximetry saturations of 66 newborns with CCHD and 200 healthy newborns at a median age of 2 days (de-Wahl et al., 2005). The authors reported that using lower extremity saturations of <95%, the test achieved a sensitivity of 89%. Importantly, all of the false-negative subjects had aortic arch obstruction. A sensitivity of 98.5% can be achieved when the difference between the saturation of the upper and lower extremities is higher than 3%. However, it is not clear as to how such a strategy is likely to perform in the setting of universal screening.

Several of the studies have reported incidental findings of PFC. In some reports, these cases have been reported as false-negative findings. In other studies, the investigators have emphasized the benefits of identifying these patients. Arlettaz and colleagues (2006) reported that 5 of the 3262 subjects who underwent screening had PFC, which was not otherwise been suspected clinically. From the other published reports, the number of subjects with PFC was somewhat less. Nonetheless, the finding of PFC in otherwise healthy newborns may be of benefit to medical care (Walton et al., 1991).

RELIABILITY OF ROUTINE OXIMETRY TO DETECT CCHD

As noted above, several institutions have reported that oximetry can be used to detect CCHD in the asymptomatic newborn population. However, questions have been raised regarding the quality of oximetry data when larger populations are examined, especially outside the setting of a clinical trial. Reich and colleagues (2005) retrospectively analyzed the quality of oximetric data obtained as part of a study of screening for CHD. In the initial portion of the study, the nurses or nursing technician were asked to acquire a single lower extremity oximetry measurement on all newborns. In the latter portion of the study, the nurses and nursing technicians were given more intensive instruction on the techniques to optimize data acquisition such as repositioning the probe. This study suggested that a failure to implement quality control measures resulted in a lower percentage (38%) high-quality oximetry measurements. However, with a quality improvement program, the reliability of the data acquisition can be considerably improved. This study points out the potential for human error in a universal screening program for CCHD.

Alternative Screening Strategies

Other screening strategies have been proposed for identification of CCHD (Li et al., 2003; Samson et al.,

2004). Some investigators have suggested that universal echocardiography would be sensitive as a screening tool for CCHD. However, the cost of an echocardiography screening program is likely to be exorbitantly high. A recent dossier from the Health Technology Assessment Program in the United Kingdom estimated that the cost to identify a single case of CCHD would be approximately U.S. $152,000 (Knowles et al., 2005). Given the risk that a case of delayed diagnosis of CCHD might result in death, the cost per life-year saved would be quite high. Moreover, the use of echocardiography in a universal screening setting is likely to yield a significant number of incidental cardiac findings that might produce unintended concern and anxiety for the parents. To date, genetic defects have been associated with numerous CCHD lesions. However, genetic testing does not appear to be a feasible screening strategy for CCHD in the near term.

Limitations of Oximetric Screening

Oximetric screening is, as the name implies, a screening test. As such, its performance characteristics are not on par with the gold standard diagnostic test of echocardiography. However, at this time, no other screening strategy has been shown to be effective and practical. Ideally, every atrial septal defect (ASD), ventricular septal defect (VSD), and patent ductus arteriosus (PDA) would be detected in the newborn nursery prior to discharge. However, these malformations will not be immediately life-threatening. Regrettably, oximetric screening is only useful for the detection of the malformations that can reasonably be expected to result in hypoxemia. The inability to detect critical lesions such as the aortic stenosis and the coarctation represent two very important limitations of this screening method. However, in these two instances, physical findings are often present that may raise clinical suspicion of an abnormality. Clearly, there is a need to develop a technology that can improve the ability of clinicians to detect these lesions as well.

Dissemination of Oximetric Screening

From early experiences reported in abstracts in the mid-1990s, there are now many published reports of relatively small, local, or regional experiences using oximetric screening. However, none are population-based with a sample size to provide adequate power for professional societies to endorse the method of oximetric screening. Unfortunately, despite the relative simplicity of the screening method, each of the published reports has unique aspects that make meta-analysis of the data difficult. Nevertheless, while data has been

accumulating, oximetric screening has been making gradual inroads into many parts of the world.

Screening for Long QT

In addition to efforts to improve early detection of CCHD, there has been interest in identifying neonates and infants at risk for sudden death due to cardiac arrhythmias. The most common arrhythmias leading to sudden death in this age population is long QT syndrome (LQTS). Congenital LQTS (prevalence about 1 in 5000) is a primarily familial disease with an autosomal dominant mode of disease transmission (Hoffman, 2001). Sudden death may be the first manifestation of the disease and, importantly, it may happen in infancy in up to 4% of the cases (Guntheroth et al., 2005; Wedekind et al., 2006). The duration of QT interval prolongation (>600 ms) as well as the presence of 2:1 atrioventricular (AV) block have been associated with increased risk of sudden death in infants (Schulze-Bahr et al., 2004).

A number of investigators have suggested that LQTS may be linked to a subset of sudden infant death syndrome (SIDS) (Hodgman and Siassi, 1999; Schwartz et al., 1998). SIDS has an incidence of 5 per 10,000 live births. The incidence of SIDS has decreased over the last 20 years. Factors associated with this decreased incidence include public health interventions such as recommendations for sleep position, decreased rates of parental smoking, and increased rates of breastfeeding (Kiechl-Kohlendorfer et al., 2001; Blair et al., 2006). In the majority of cases, an etiology for SIDS is not identified. However, primary cardiac arrhythmias have always been considered to be one of the possible causes (Skinner, 2000). Historically, authors have considered that arrhythmias such as LQTS might account for 2%–3% of SIDS cases (Maron et al., 2005). Data from Italy, however, suggested that QT prolongation may play a more important role in SIDS. Schwartz and colleagues reviewed electrocardiograms (ECGs) of over 30,000 infants. The ECG was performed on the third or fourth day of life. Of this initial birth cohort, there were 24 SIDS events. These investigators found that the infants who died of SIDS had a longer corrected QT interval (QTc) than did the survivors (mean [±standard deviation (SD)], 435 ± 45 vs. 400 ± 20 ms, $P < 0.01$). In addition, this study reported that 50% of the SIDS cases were found to have QT interval of >440 ms, which would be considered 2 SDs above the mean for that age. The authors concluded that prolongation of the QT interval in early neonatal period can be an important marker for SIDS. However, it is known that the ECG pattern undergoes transitional changes in early infancy, indicating that many infants with abnormal QTc intervals in the first week of life normalize in the subsequent weeks (Schwartz et al., 2002). Nonetheless, the findings did suggest that there may be a role for ECG screening. A number of criticisms of the aforementioned study have been published (Lucey, 1999; Maron et al., 2005; Phoon, 2000).

The last few years have witnessed a dramatic progress in our understanding of the molecular bases of congenital LQTS. Keating and colleagues (1991) reported the discovery of two genes causing LQTS. Subsequently, more genes have been identified. These genes, which encode ion channels subunits that are involved in the generation of the cardiac action potential, are responsible for maintaining electrical balance in the heart. One needs only to inherit one variant of these gene defects to have LQTS. However, about 40% of the families with LQTS have not yet been linked to any of the known genes (Priori and Cerrone, 2005). This means there are more genes yet to be identified. LQTS is a genetically heterogeneous ion channel disorder in which mutations either in cardiac potassium channel genes or in the cardiac sodium channel gene SCN5A (LQT3) cause the disease (Ackerman, 1998; Hoffman et al., 2001). The LQTS types are labeled LQT1 to LQT8. The LQT7 and LQT8 types have been discovered recently. In support of the potential link of LQTS and SIDS are reports that identify the presence of LQT gene mutations in cases of SIDS or near-miss SIDS (Ackerman et al., 2001; Eastman, 2003; SoRelle, 2000). In an analysis of 93 SIDS cases by Ackermann and colleagues, SCN5A mutation was identified in 2 subjects (2%). Other investigators have failed to identify mutations in postmortem analysis of SIDS cases (Bajanowski et al., 2001; Wedekind et al., 2006).

Much of the interest in early identification of LQTS in infants is based on the finding that pharmacologic interventions can significantly reduce the risk of sudden death because of this disorder. β-Blockers are the treatment of choice for most LQTS patients, potentially even in asymptomatic children. β-Blockers have been shown to reduce the risk of sudden death in LQT1 and LQT4 subtypes by 90% (Villain et al., 2004). β-Blockers are less efficacious for LQT2, whereas sodium channel blockers have specifically been proposed for treatment of the LQT3 subtype. In addition, some patients with malignant forms of LQTS may benefit from implantable cardiodefibrillators.

Given the potential benefits of early diagnosis of LQTS, there has been an interest in creating a newborn or infant screening program to identify long QT using electrocardiography (Wang et al., 2007; Weese-Mayer et al., 2007). As has been mentioned, the ECG undergoes a number of transitional changes in the first 2 weeks of life (Schwartz et al., 2002). Therefore, it would seem that an ECG-based screening strategy could improve sensitivity by waiting until 2 or more

weeks of age to perform the test. If one were to defer the ECG until much later in infancy, one could miss the opportunity to prevent SIDS deaths. In Italy, a prospective trial of ECG screening in neonates is underway. In this study, ECGs are recorded between the 15th and 25th day of life in 16 Italian centers and then transmitted to the coordinating center for analysis. The study plans to enroll 50,000 neonates. In 2004, the investigators of this study presented an interim analysis of 31,000 screened infants (Goulene et al., 2005). Of those screened, 0.9% had borderline prolonged QT intervals (440 ms) and 0.08% subjects had significantly prolonged QT intervals (>470 ms). Genotyping was carried out in these subjects with QT intervals >470 ms and 18% were found to have ion channel mutations. Importantly, the investigators described a number of collateral benefits to newborn ECG screening. In almost half the cases of marked QT prolongation (470 ms), the investigators were able to identify other family members with LQTS. This finding might ultimately result in preventive therapy that reduces risk of sudden death in other children and adults. In addition, the investigators reported that in 4 subjects, congenital defects that were otherwise not detected clinically were also identified. These defects included coarctation of the aorta ($n = 3$) and anomalous coronary artery from the pulmonary artery ($n = 1$). In addition, other recent data suggeststhat almost 10% of SIDS cases carry genetic variants in long QT genes (Arnestad et al., 2007). Such findings provide additional support for the important role of ECG screening in preventing SIDS.

One of the concerns of a universal screening strategy is the potential for misinterpretation of the ECG. One study in the United States found that the computer-generated interpretation of QT intervals had significant limitations. Miller and colleagues (2001) found that the computer-generated calculations were incorrect in 6 of the 23 subjects with genetically confirmed LQTS. These investigators emphasized the importance of having a physician familiar with LQTS interpret the ECG. The Italian study has been utilizing a central data interpretation to ensure uniformity. Others have been concerned that universal ECG screening in neonates is likely to generate a number of false-positive results, especially with respect to the voltage criteria (Lucey, 1999; Phoon, 2000). An understanding of the number of false-positives will be particularly important as public policy experts consider the cost-effectiveness of such a screening program.

To date, there have been several publications that have addressed the cost-effectiveness of neonatal or infant screening with ECG (Quaglini et al., 2006; Zupancic et al., 2000). Zupancic (2000) reported the incremental cost-effectiveness of neonatal ECG, assuming that a screening threshold of 440 ms would identify 50% of the cases. The base scenario calculated an incremental cost-effectiveness ratio of $18,465 per life-year saved. These calculations were based on the initial report by Schwartz et al., who performed screening at 3 days of age. More recently, Quaglini et al. (2006) have used data from the ongoing trial in Italy to determine the cost-effectiveness of neonatal ECG screening. This study assumed that the true positive rate for identifying LQTS is 80% and that ECG screening can be expected to identify rare cases of CHD that are otherwise asymptomatic (Quaglini et al., 2006). This model also assumes an overall false-positive rate of 1% for the initial screening ECG. Using a Markov model, the investigators reported a cost-effectiveness of €11,470 (U.S. $9176) per life-year saved. This would fall well within the range of acceptable cost-effectiveness (<$50,000 per life-year saved).

How a newborn or infant ECG screening strategy might be carried out in the United States requires further thought. The American Academy of Pediatrics (AAP) has recommended that newborns be evaluated by a physician or other knowledgeable and experienced health care professional at 2–3 weeks of age. This visit would provide an opportunity to perform the ECG. However, routine newborn care is provided in a number of settings in the United States including single physician or nurse-practitioner settings. Installing an ECG recording device and training allied health personnel to perform the study represents a barrier to implementing this screening strategy. Moreover, a central repository for review of ECG studies would be required. Timely review by a cardiologist is necessary to achieve early identification of ECG abnormalities.

OXIMETRY SCREENING AND ECG SCREENING COMPARED TO OTHER EXISTING NEWBORN SCREENING PROGRAMS

Newborn screening is typically thought of as a program that identifies newborns with conditions that are difficult to recognize but require immediate medical care. Most conditions for which newborn screening is performed depend upon the presence of marker analyte in a dried blood spot specimen. Universal newborn hearing screening was the first public health–sponsored newborn screening program that was not based on dried blood spot collection. These audiological tests performed in the newborn nursery have a high probability of identifying newborns with hearing defects that otherwise might not become evident until much later in life. The same tenets applied to traditional newborn screening were used by the AAP to justify universal [hearing] screening. Oximetric and ECG screening for heart disease may be evaluated in the same manner.

With any screening strategy, the frequency of the disorder, the effectiveness of the screening test, and the cost of a large-scale screening strategy need to be considered. While CCHD occurs in 2–3 per 1000 live births, the majority of cases are identified by prenatal ultrasound scanning or symptoms prompting a detailed investigation in the newborn nursery. Moreover, of those cases not diagnosed until after discharge from the hospital, a minority will have still have undiagnosed severe complications or may even die (sudden death). Nonetheless, it seems likely that the incidence of CCHD that results in death from delayed diagnosis may justify such a screening program. Similarly, LQTS is not always fatal. Nonetheless, it is a relatively common disorder occurring in 1 per 5000 live births. Even if only 3% of those with LQTS would die as a result of delayed diagnosis, this intervention would prevent 1 death for every 166,667 live births. For comparison, four disorders commonly included in blood spot screening that often result in death if not treated early (maple syrup urine disease [MSUD], homocystinuria, galactosemia, and biotinidase deficiency) occur in less than 1 per 100,000 live births—and these disorders are not uniformly fatal if diagnosis is delayed. Therefore, if only 1 in 100 newborns with CCHD dies from delayed diagnosis, universal newborn oximetry screening could save as many lives as several currently mandated screening tests. In addition to preventing death, early diagnosis has the potential to reduce morbidity and shorten length of stay in the hospital. Screening for MSUD and biotinidase deficiency cost approximately $2 each per newborn screened. The costs of oximetry screening may be less than or equal to $2 per newborn. The relative cost of newborn screening for a number of diseases commonly included in statewide screening panels is shown below for comparison (Table 5–2).

The effectiveness of oximetric or ECG screening has not been demonstrated in a randomized trial. However, there is an exception to the insistence on evidence from randomized trials for the poor prognosis of

TABLE 5–2. *Comparison of Cost and Prevalence of Newborn Screening for Various Diseases*

Disease	Cases/ 100,000 Births	Cost Test/ Specimen ($)	Cost Test Case Found, if 1 Specimen per Child ($)
Phenylketonuria	6.6	3.43	52,000
Maple syrup urine disease	0.6	2.49	415,000
Homocystinuria	0.4	0.84	210,000
Galactosemia	1.5	3.79	250,000
Biotinidase deficiency	1.1	1.83	170,000
Congenital hypothyroidism	39.6	4.59	12,000

the target disorder with delayed detection, for example phenylketonuria (PKU) and hypothyroidism. Under these circumstances, *any* intervention that improves prognosis is efficacious. As is the case with PKU and hypothyroidism, effective treatment exists for most forms of CCHD and for LQTS. The data regarding the frequency of delayed diagnosis leading to morbidity and mortality clearly demonstrate that there currently exists a burden of suffering that warrants screening.

REFERENCES

Ackerman MJ, Siu BL, Sturner WQ, et al. Postmortem molecular analysis of SCN5A defects in sudden infant death syndrome. *JAMA.* 2001;286(18):2264–2269.

Ackerman MJ. The long QT syndrome. *Pediatr Rev.* 1998;19(7):232–238.

Ainsworth S, Wyllie JP, Wren C. Prevalence and clinical significance of cardiac murmurs in neonates. *Arch Dis Child Fetal Neonatal Ed.* 1999;80(1):F43–F45.

Arlettaz R, Bauschatz AS, Monkhoff M, Essers B, Bauersfeld U. The contribution of pulse oximetry to the early detection of congenital heart disease in newborns. *Eur J Pediatr.* 2006;165(2):94–98.

Arnestad M, Crotti L, Rognum TO, et al. Prevalence of long-QT syndrome gene variants in sudden infant death syndrome. *Circulation.* 2007;115(3):361–367.

Bajanowski T, Rossi L, Biondo B, et al. Prolonged QT interval and sudden infant death—report of two cases. *Forensic Sci Int.* 2001;115(1–2):147–153.

Bakr AF, Habib HS. Combining pulse oximetry and clinical examination in screening for congenital heart disease. *Pediatr Cardiol.* 2005;26(6):832–835.

Blair PS, Sidebotham P, Berry PJ, Evans M, Fleming PJ. Major epidemiological changes in sudden infant death syndrome: a 20-year population-based study in the UK. *Lancet.* 2006;28;367(9507):314–319.

Bonnet D, Coltri A, Butera G, et al. Detection of transposition of the great arteries in fetuses reduces neonatal morbidity and mortality. *Circulation.* 1999;99(7):916–918.

Botto LD, Correa A, Erickson JD. Racial and temporal variations in the prevalence of heart defects. *Pediatrics.* 2001;107(3):E32.

Danford DA. Clinical and basic laboratory assessment of children for possible congenital heart disease. *Curr Opin Pediatr.* 2000;12(5):487–491.

de-Wahl GA, Mellander M, Sunnegardh J, Sandberg K, Ostman-Smith I. Screening for duct-dependant congenital heart disease with pulse oximetry: a critical evaluation of strategies to maximize sensitivity. *Acta Paediatr.* 2005;94(11):1590–1596.

Eastman Q. Genetics. Crib death exoneration could usher in new gene tests. *Science.* 2003;300(5627):1858.

Forbess JM, Cook N, Roth SJ, Serraf A, Mayer JE, Jr., Jonas RA. Ten-year institutional experience with palliative surgery for hypoplastic left heart syndrome. Risk factors related to stage I mortality. *Circulation.* 1995;92(9 suppl):II262–II266.

Goulene K, Stramba-Badiale M, Crotti L, et al. Neonatal Electrocardiographic screening of genetic arrhythmogenic disorders and congenital cardiovascular diseases: prospective data from 31,000 infants. *Eur Heart J.* 2005;26:214.

Guntheroth W, Spiers P. Long QT syndrome and sudden infant death syndrome. *Am J Cardiol.* 2005;96(7):1034.

Hodgman JE, Siassi B. Prolonged QTc as a risk factor for SIDS. *Pediatrics.* 1999;103(4 Pt 1):814–815.

Hoffman JI. The prolonged QT syndrome. *Adv Pediatr.* 2001;48:115–156.

Hoke TR, Donohue PK, Bawa PK, Mitchell RD, Pathak A, Rowe PC, Byrne BJ. Oxygen saturation as a screening test for critical congenital heart disease: a preliminary study. *Pediatr Cardiol.* 2002;23(4):403–409.

Hunter S, Heads A, Wyllie J, Robson S. Prenatal diagnosis of congenital heart disease in the northern region of England: benefits of a training programme for obstetric ultrasonographers. *Heart.* 2000;84(3):294–298.

Iannettoni MD, Bove EL, Mosca RS, et al. Improving results with first-stage palliation for hypoplastic left heart syndrome. *J Thorac Cardiovasc Surg.* 1994;107(3):934–940.

Kawalec M, Blaz W, Turska-Kmiec A, Zuk M, Helwich E, Tobota Z. Pulse oximetry as a population screening test in detection of critical congenital heart defects in presymptomatic newborns—Polish multicentre study. *Cardiol Young.* 2006;16[Suppl 2]:25–26.

Keating M, Atkinson D, Dunn C, Timothy K, Vincent GM, Leppert M. Linkage of a cardiac arrhythmia, the long QT syndrome, and the Harvey ras-1 gene. *Science.* 1991;252(5006):704–706.

Kiechl-Kohlendorfer U, Peglow UP, Kiechl S, Oberaigner W, Sperl W. Epidemiology of sudden infant death syndrome (SIDS) in the Tyrol before and after an intervention campaign. *Wien Klin Wochenschr.* 2001;113(1–2):27–32.

Knowles R, Griebsch I, Dezateux C, Brown J, Bull C, Wren C. Newborn screening for congenital heart defects: a systematic review and cost-effectiveness analysis. *Health Technol Assess.* 2005;9(44):1–168.

Kuehl KS, Loffredo CA, Ferencz C. Failure to diagnose congenital heart disease in infancy. *Pediatrics.* 1999;103(4 Pt 1):743–747.

Kumar RK, Newburger JW, Gauvreau K, Kamenir SA, Hornberger LK. Comparison of outcome when hypoplastic left heart syndrome and transposition of the great arteries are diagnosed prenatally versus when diagnosis of these two conditions is made only postnatally. *Am J Cardiol.* 1999;83(12):1649–1653.

Li X, Mack GK, Rusk RA, et al. Will a handheld ultrasound scanner be applicable for screening for heart abnormalities in newborns and children? *J Am Soc Echocardiogr.* 2003;16(10):1007–1014.

Lucey JF. Comments on a sudden infant death article in another journal. *Pediatrics.* 1999;103(4 Pt 1):812.

Mahle WT, Clancy RR, McGaurn SP, Goin JE, Clark BJ. Impact of prenatal diagnosis on survival and early neurologic morbidity in neonates with the hypoplastic left heart syndrome. *Pediatrics.* 2001;107(6):1277–1282.

Mahle WT, Spray TL, Wernovsky G, Gaynor JW, Clark BJ, III. Survival after reconstructive surgery for hypoplastic left heart syndrome: A 15-year experience from a single institution. *Circulation.* 2000;102(19 suppl 3):III136–III141.

Maron BJ. LQTS and SIDS linkage: clarifying the record. *Am J Cardiol.* 2005;96(2):323.

Miller MD, Porter C, Ackerman MJ. Diagnostic accuracy of screening electrocardiograms in long QT syndrome I. *Pediatrics.* 2001;108(1):8–12.

Montana E, Khoury MJ, Cragan JD, Sharma S, Dhar P, Fyfe D. Trends and outcomes after prenatal diagnosis of congenital cardiac malformations by fetal echocardiography in a well defined birth population, Atlanta, Georgia, 1990–1994. *J Am Coll Cardiol.* 1996;28(7):1805–1809.

O'brien LM, Stebbens VA, Poets CF, Heycock EG, Southall DP. Oxygen saturation during the first 24 hours of life. *Arch Dis Child Fetal Neonatal Ed.* 2000;83(1):F35–F38.

Phoon CK. Prolongation of the QT interval and SIDS. *N Engl J Med.* 2000;343(25):1896–1897.

Poets CF. Assessing oxygenation in healthy infants. *J Pediatr.* 1999;135(5):541–543.

Priori SG, Cerrone M.Molecular genetics: is it making an impact in the management of inherited arrhythmogenic syndromes? *Hellenic J Cardiol.* 2005;46(2):83–87.

Quaglini S, Rognoni C, Spazzolini C, Priori SG, Mannarino S, Schwartz PJ. Cost-effectiveness of neonatal ECG screening for the long QT syndrome. *Eur Heart J.* 2006;27(15):1824–1832.

Queisser-Luft A, Stopfkuchen H, Stolz G, Schlaefer K, Merz E. Prenatal diagnosis of major malformations: quality control of routine ultrasound examinations based on a five-year study of 20,248 newborn fetuses and infants. *Prenat Diagn.* 1998;18(6):567–576.

Ramaciotti C, Chin AJ. Noninvasive evaluation of newborns with congenital heart disease. *J Intensive Care Med.* 1993;8(3):130–143.

Reich JD, Connolly B, Bradley G, Littman S, Lewyscky P. The Reliability of Routine Pulse Oximetry to Detect Otherwise Undetectable Congenital Heart Disease in a Clinical Setting. Southeast Pediatric Cardiology Society 2005 Annual Meeting 2005;1, 17.

Richmond S, Reay G, Abu HM. Routine pulse oximetry in the asymptomatic newborn. *Arch Dis Child Fetal Neonatal Ed.* 2002;87(2):F83–F88.

Richmond S, Wren C. Early diagnosis of congenital heart disease. *Semin Neonatol.* 2001;6(1):27–35.

Rosati E, Chitano G, Dipaola L, De Felice C, Latini G. Indications and limitations for a neonatal pulse oximetry screening of critical congenital heart disease. *J Perinat Med.* 2005;33(5):455–457.

Samson GR, Kumar SR. A study of congenital cardiac disease in a neonatal population—the validity of echocardiography undertaken by a neonatologist. *Cardiol Young.* 2004;14(6):585–893.

Schulze-Bahr E, Fenge H, Etzrodt D, et al. Long QT syndrome and life threatening arrhythmia in a newborn: molecular diagnosis and treatment response. *Heart.* 2004;90(1):13–16.

Schwartz PJ, Garson A, Jr., Paul T, Stramba-Badiale M, Vetter VL, Wren C. Guidelines for the interpretation of the neonatal electrocardiogram. A task force of the European Society of Cardiology. *Eur Heart J.* 2002;23(17):1329–1344.

Schwartz PJ, Garson A, Jr., Paul T, Stramba-Badiale M, Vetter VL, Wren C. Guidelines for the interpretation of the neonatal electrocardiogram. A task force of the European Society of Cardiology. *Eur Heart J.* 2002;23(17):1329–14344.

Schwartz PJ, Stramba-Badiale M, Segantini A, et al. Prolongation of the QT interval and the sudden infant death syndrome. *N Engl J Med.* 1998;338(24):1709–1714.

Skinner J. Prolongation of the QT interval and SIDS. *N Engl J Med.* 2000;343(25):1896.

SoRelle R. Molecular link between Sudden Infant Death Syndrome and long-QT syndrome is "proof of concept". *Circulation.* 2000;102(8):E9014–E9015.

Tworetzky W, McElhinney DB, Reddy VM, Brook MM, Hanley FL, Silverman NH. Improved surgical outcome after fetal diagnosis of hypoplastic left heart syndrome. *Circulation.* 2001;103(9):1269–1273.

Villain E, Denjoy I, Lupoglazoff JM, et al. Low incidence of cardiac events with beta-blocking therapy in children with long QT syndrome. *Eur Heart J.* 2004;25(16):1405–1411.

Walton JP, Hendricks-Munoz K. Profile and stability of sensorineural hearing loss in persistent pulmonary hypertension of the newborn. *J Speech Hear Res.* 1991;34(6):1362–1370.

Wang DW, Desai RR, Crotti L, et al. Cardiac sodium channel dysfunction in sudden infant death syndrome. *Circulation.* 2007;115(3):368–376.

Wedekind H, Bajanowski T, Friederich P, et al. Sudden infant death syndrome and long QT syndrome: an epidemiological and genetic study. *Int J Legal Med.* 2006;120(3):129–137.

Weese-Mayer DE, Ackerman MJ, Marazita ML, Berry-Kravis EM. Sudden Infant Death Syndrome: review of implicated genetic factors. *Am J Med Genet A.* 2007;143(8):771–788.

Zupancic JA, Triedman JK, Alexander M, Walsh EP, Richardson DK, Berul CI. Cost-effectiveness and implications of newborn screening for prolongation of QT interval for the prevention of sudden infant death syndrome. *J Pediatr.* 2000;136(4):481–489.

6

Cardiac Catheterization

PHILLIP MOORE

The role of cardiac catheterization has evolved dramatically over the last 20 years from being the primary diagnostic tool for complex congenital heart disease to an adjunct diagnostic tool and the primary treatment tool for the most common forms of congenital heart disease including ASD, PDA, valvar PS, and valvar AS. Although displaced by echo, CT, and MRI as the primary tool for diagnosing complex disease, it remains the gold standard for evaluating physiology in complex disease, including assessment of cardiac flows, intracardiac shunting, and measurement of vascular resistances. As such, an understanding of the technique and the limitations of cardiac catheterization is crucial to the optimal management of children and adults with congenital heart disease.

PROCEDURAL CONSIDERATIONS

Diagnostic catheterization directly measures data including pressures, saturations, and thermodilution outputs, calculates data including cardiac flows, intracardiac shunts, and vascular resistances, and demonstrates anatomy with angiography. Direct measurements are made through a fluid-filled long thin plastic tube or catheter that is manipulated through the great vessels and cardiac chambers under fluoroscopic guidance. The catheter is inserted through a sheath with a valve, which prevents bleeding, placed percutaneously using the Seldinger technique (needle accesses the vessel, wire is placed through the needle into the vessel and the sheath is inserted over the wire). This sheath remains in the vessel throughout the procedure, allowing a variety of catheters to be inserted and removed for completion of the procedure. Depending on the patient's intracardiac anatomy and the information needed, antegrade

venous access is used to evaluate the right heart, while the left heart is evaluated either with antegrade venous access through a septal defect or with retrograde arterial access. The vessels most commonly used are the femoral vein and artery although the internal jugular veins, subclavian veins, and axillary arteries are also used. In very small patients, the carotid arteries are used by direct surgical cut down with surgical repair post catheterization. Patients with complex cardiac disease often require multiple catheterizations, which can result in limited central access due to obstruction of vessels. These patients are catheterized through direct percutaneous puncture of the hepatic veins, a technique known as transhepatic catheterization (Ebeid, 2007; Shim et al., 1995).

Cardiac catheterization can be effectively and safely performed in most children including premature infants and immediate postoperative patients, even those on ventricular assist support. A variety of catheter types and sizes are available to successfully reach all vascular and intracardiac areas of interest. At times, special wires are placed through the catheters to guide the tip into the desired position. New areas of research and development are under way to improve catheter manipulation including the use of echo and MRI imaging as well as magnetic directional guidance. Although many of these techniques look promising, none of them are presently in clinical use and fluoroscopic guidance thus remains the standard. Complications associated with cardiac catheterization are infrequent but can be quite severe and include infection requiring antibiotics, bleeding requiring transfusion, arrhythmia requiring medication, cardioversion or pacing, cardiac perforation with tamponade, vascular rupture or occlusion, and thrombotic or air embolus causing stroke or myocardial infarction.

Serious complications noted above occur in less than 1% of diagnostic catheterizations with risk factors of weight <2.5 kg, pulmonary hypertension > systemic, and decreased ventricular function (Vitiello et al., 1998). While I agree with the statement, I am not sure the reference supports the entire sentence. Consider the alternative—Serious complications noted above occur in less than 1% of diagnostic catheterizations (Vitiello et al., 1998). Risks are increased with weight <2.5 kg, pulmonary hypertension > systemic, and decreased ventricular function.

PRESSURE DATA

Direct pressure recordings are usually obtained sequentially throughout the cardiac chambers and vessels as the catheter is moved through the heart. As there is significant variability in cardiac pressures based on the heart rate, respiratory effort, level of sedation, mechanical ventilation, level of hydration, as well as the underlying cardiac pathology, it is important for the patient to be in a steady consistent state and for pressures to be measured in a timely fashion. If small differences are critical to detect, it is often necessary to measure multiple pressures simultaneously using multiple catheters. Accuracy of the pressure measurements must be insured by placing the transducer at the level of the heart, clearing the fluid-filled system of any air and re-zeroing the transducer regularly.

The volume of blood in a chamber or vessel, the size of the chamber or vessel, and the compliance of the walls will determine the pressure inside. This is a dynamic process because cardiac chambers contract and expand during the cardiac cycle. Abnormalities in cardiac pressures can be used to diagnose congenital cardiac disease; therefore an understanding of normal physiology is key to recognizing abnormalities. Table 6–1 lists normal cardiac and great vessel pressures as well as commonly detected abnormalities.

ATRIAL PRESSURES

Atrial pressures are reported as an "a" wave, "v" wave, and mean pressure. Although there is a "c" wave and an X and Y descent, they are rarely used to detect clinical abnormalities. The "a" wave is an increase in pressure that occurs at the end of ventricular diastole generated by contraction of the atrium so it starts with the "p" wave of the EKG. The "a" wave peaks as the atrium completes contraction and then the pressure decreases as the *atrioventricular* (AV) valves close

with ventricular systole (Figure 6–1A). Atrial pressure continues to decrease during early ventricular systole, the X descent, then increases in late ventricular systole creating the "v" wave as forward flow fills the atrium against closed AV valves. As the AV valves open at the start of ventricular diastole the atrial pressure falls, Y descent, resulting in early rapid filling of the ventricles in diastole.

Elevated atrial pressures signify increased intravascular volume, decreased compliance or hypoplasia of the atrium or decreased compliance of the downstream ventricle. Low atrial pressures typically indicate hypovolemia. Elevated "a" and "v" wave pressures indicate obstruction to emptying of the atria during diastole, either tricuspid or mitral stenosis or decreased ventricular compliance, a "stiff" ventricle" takes more pressure to fill (Figure 6–1B). Mitral or tricuspid insufficiency will increase the "v" wave and shift the peak earlier in the cardiac cycle, sometimes termed a "regurgitant wave." All of these relationships are dependent on normal sinus rhythm. If there is AV block, then this pattern will be disturbed and the ventricle will at times contract with an open AV valve resulting in a cannon "a" wave (Figure 6–1C).

VENTRICULAR PRESSURES

Ventricular pressures are reported as end diastolic and systolic, and no mean pressure is reported. In addition, the minimal ventricular pressure and the contour of the pressure tracing can be useful in detecting cardiac abnormalities. Normal ventricular pressure ranges are shown in Table 6–1. End diastolic pressure occurs just before systole begins and should be similar to the peak "a" wave atrial pressure. If the "a" wave is greater, this indicates AV valve stenosis. Elevation of the end diastolic pressure indicates decreased compliance of the ventricle commonly due to muscular hypertrophy or diastolic dysfunction. It also occurs if there is restriction or constriction as with pericardial tamponade. The normal ventricular systolic pressure trace has a square shape. Elevation of ventricular systolic pressure with a late peaked shape indicates dynamic ventricular outflow tract obstruction (sub AS or sub PS) (Figures 6–2A and 6–2B). Although not typically reported, the minimal pressure the ventricle reaches during the end of iso-volumetric relaxation should be below 4 mmHg (Udelson et al., 1990). The ventricle actively relaxes against closed AV and VA valves generating negative pressure until the AV valve opens and the ventricle begins to fill. Elevated minimal ventricular pressures and a rapid rise to end diastolic pressures (square root sign) indicate an abnormality with relaxation either

TABLE 6-1. *Common Pressure Abnormalities*

Measured Data

Site	Saturation (%)	Syst or A wave	Diast or V wave	Mean
RA	72–78	2–8	2–7	1–5
LA	96–100	3–12	5–13	2–10
RV	72–78	15–30	1–7	
LV	96–100	90–110	4–10	
PA	72–78	15–30	3–12	12–18
AAO	96–100	90–110	50–70	75–95
DAO	96–100	95–120	45–70	75–95

Calculated Data

Pulmonary Flow Qp (L/min/m^2)	3–4.5	
Systemic Flow Qs (L/min/m^2)	3–4.5	
Syst Vasc Resistance Rs (Woods u)	10–20	

		Mild	Moderate	Severe
Pulm Vasc Resistance Rp (Woods u)	<4	4–8	8–12	>12
Aortic Valve Area (cm^2/m^2)	>1.3	1.3–1.1	1–0.6	<0.6
Mitral Valve area (cm^2/m^2)	>2.3	2–1.5	1.5–0.6	<0.6

Common Pressure Abnormalities

RA			
↑ a and v waves	Tricuspid stenosis	RV dysfunction	
↑ v wave	Tricuspid regurgitation		
LA			
↑ a and v waves	Mitral stenosis	LV dysfunction	
↑ v wave	Mitral regurgitation		
RV			
↑ RVED	RV dysfunction	Pericardial constriction/ restriction	
↑ RV systolic	Sub or valvar PS	Branch PS	↑ PVR
LV			
↑ LVED	LV dysfunction	Peicardial constriction/ restriction	
↑ LV systolic	Sub or valvar AS	Coarctation	↑ SVR
PA			
↑ PA systolic, nl diastolic	Segmental PA stenoses		
↑ PA systolic and diastolic	↑ PVR	Pulm vein stenosis	LV dysfunction
↓ PA diastolic	Pulm insufficiency	Pulm AVM	
AAO			
↑ Systolic and Diastolic	Coarctation	↑ SVR	
↓ Diastolic	Aortic insufficiency	PDA	Cerebral AVM
DAO			
↓ Systolic	Coarctation		

due to diastolic dysfunction such as myocardial restriction or external limitation such as pericardial constriction (Figure 6–2C).

ARTERIAL PRESSURES

Normal pulmonary artery and aortic systolic, diastolic, and mean pressures are reported in Table 6–1. At peak systole, the pressure in the ventricle proximal to the artery should be identical to the artery. Elevation of the ventricular pressure suggests aortic or pulmonary valve stenosis (Figure 6–3A). Elevation of the arterial systolic pressure suggests downstream obstruction, either large vessel stenosis such as coarctation (Figures 6–3B and 6–3C) or pulmonary artery stenosis or small vessel vascular resistance elevation (pulmonary or systemic hypertension). Elevated arterial diastolic pressure suggests limited distal runoff due to elevated vascular resistance. Low diastolic pressures on the other hand suggest brisk distal runoff from low vascular resistance or some abnormal runoff such as aortic insufficiency, PDA, aortic window, or systemic arteriovenous malformation (AVM) in the systemic circulation or pulmonary insufficiency or pulmonary AVMs in the pulmonary circulation.

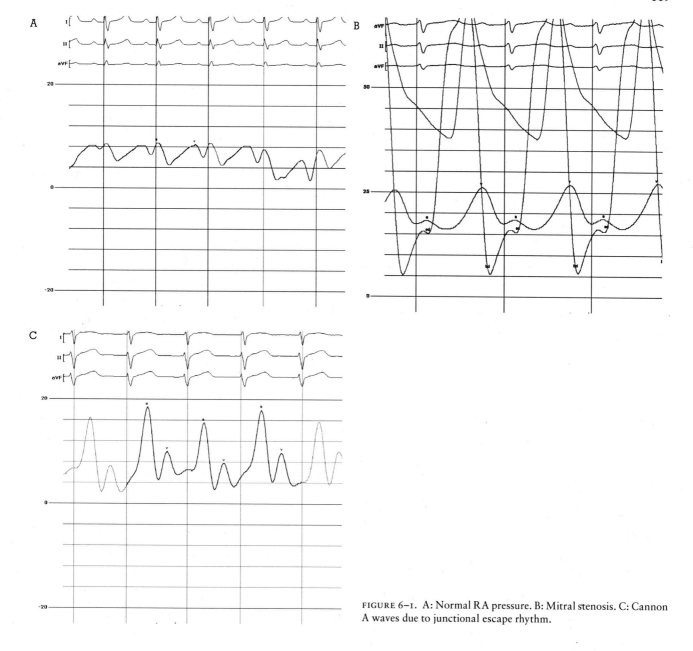

FIGURE 6–1. A: Normal RA pressure. B: Mitral stenosis. C: Cannon A waves due to junctional escape rhythm.

Flow Data

Saturations

Using the Fick method, saturations are obtained through out the cardiac chambers and vessels to determine degree and location of intracardiac and intrapulmonary shunting and the systemic and pulmonary flows (Fagard and Conway, 1990). Saturations are currently measured using spectrophotometric techniques based on the difference between the maximal wave length absorption of Hgb bound to O_2 (600 nm) versus deoxygenated Hgb (506.5 nm). Normal cardiac saturation data is shown in Table 6–1. Oxygen saturation in venous blood equals the arterial saturation of blood entering a tissue bed minus the amount of oxygen extracted by those tissues. Different tissue beds extract different amounts of oxygen, the heart and exercising skeletal muscle extracts a greater amount, whereas the kidneys and resting skeletal muscle extract a little amount. Therefore systemic venous saturations vary widely by location. A true measure of a mixed systemic venous saturation is best obtained from the pulmonary artery in the normal circulation. In complex congenital heart disease where intracardiac shunting occurs, this

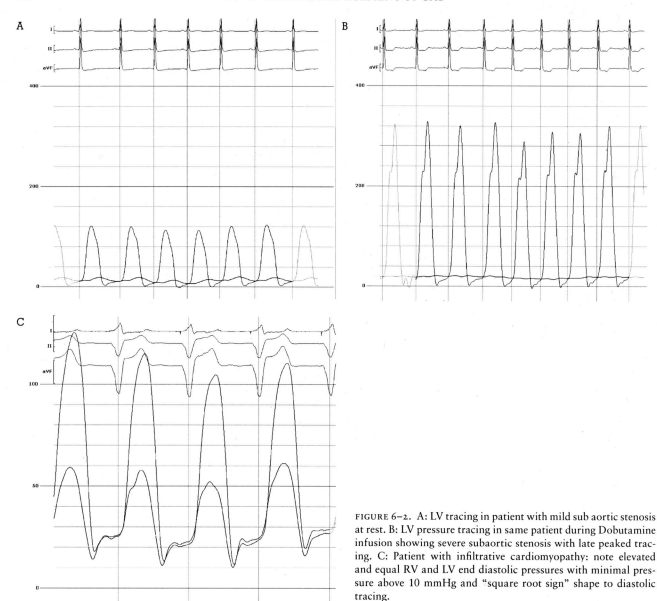

FIGURE 6–2. A: LV tracing in patient with mild sub aortic stenosis at rest. B: LV pressure tracing in same patient during Dobutamine infusion showing severe subaortic stenosis with late peaked tracing. C: Patient with infiltrative cardiomyopathy: note elevated and equal RV and LV end diastolic pressures with minimal pressure above 10 mmHg and "square root sign" shape to diastolic tracing.

measure is not true so mixed systemic venous saturation is estimated by the superior vena cava saturation. Although not perfect because the higher *inferior vena cava* (IVC) and much lower coronary sinus saturations are not accounted for, it remains the best estimate possible.

Normally saturations should vary little through the right heart, <4%, so any increase in saturation of >4%–6% indicates a significant left to right shunt (French et al., 1983). Theoretically, pulmonary venous saturations should be 100% since all the hemoglobin should bind O_2 as it passes through the pulmonary capillary bed. However, small areas of atelectasis can result in nonventilated but perfused lung, allowing for hemoglobin to pass through the lung without binding

to O_2. In addition, there is a small obligatory shunt from right to left in the form of bronchial flow to the lung tissue that supplies O_2 to the lung parenchyma with the deoxygenated venous blood entering directly into the pulmonary veins. Therefore pulmonary venous saturations, as low as 96%, are still considered normal. Lower saturations in the pulmonary veins indicate either parenchymal lung disease or pulmonary AVMs. Saturations should remain unchanged through the left heart. Any decrease in saturations of >4% suggests a right to left intracardiac shunt. As the location of a sample may vary within a cardiac chamber due to the position of the catheter tip, care must be exercised in determining the level of shunt from the saturations. Most often, the level of the shunt will occur in the

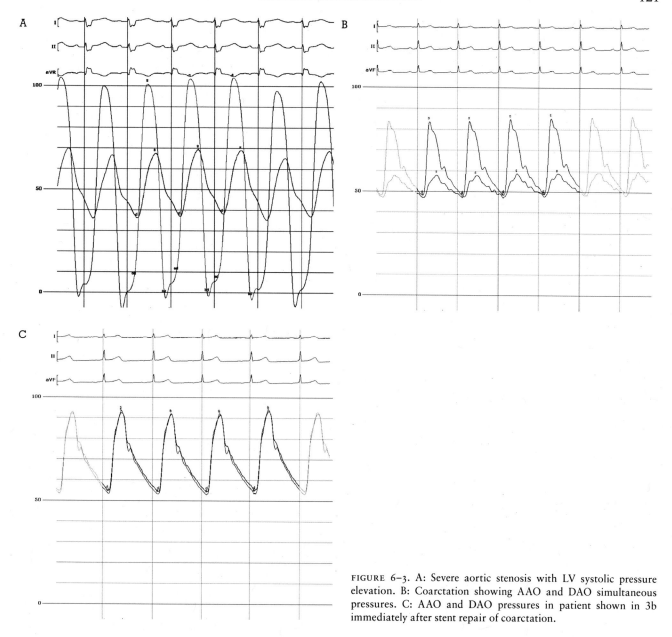

FIGURE 6–3. A: Severe aortic stenosis with LV systolic pressure elevation. B: Coarctation showing AAO and DAO simultaneous pressures. C: AAO and DAO pressures in patient shown in 3b immediately after stent repair of coarctation.

chamber where the saturation increase or decrease is noted, however it can occur just proximal to the sampling chamber or if there is valve insufficiency, distal to the sampling chamber.

Saturations are used to determine relative systemic and pulmonary flows and calculate the total right to left or left to right shunts. The formula to calculate Qp:Qs ratio when the patient is breathing room air is

$$Qp : Qs = \frac{Aortic\ sat - SVC\ sat}{Pulm\ Vein\ sat - Pulm\ art\ sat}$$

Fick Flow Calculations

Using the Fick principle and saturation data, specific pulmonary (Qp) and systemic (Qs) flows as well as the exact left to right and right to left shunts can be calculated. Fick showed that an indicator placed into a flowing liquid will disperse completely and the concentration of the indicator in the liquid will depend on the amount of indicator added and the flow. Therefore, if the amount of indicator added to blood and the concentration of the indicator in blood is known, blood flow can be calculated accurately. During catheterization, two indicators are commonly used. Temperature, the first commonly used indicator, is used with the thermodilution technique but is only applicable if there is no significant cardiac shunting and no more than moderate tricuspid or pulmonary insufficiency (Balik et al., 2002; Freed and Keane, 1978). Oxygen is the other commonly used indicator as it is easily measured by the saturation of a blood sample or, if needed, by blood gas measurement of PaO_2 for the dissolved content of blood. Since dissolved oxygen in blood makes up <3% of total oxygen in blood when breathing room air (compared to approximately 7% when breathing 100% O_2), dissolved O_2 is not typically included in the calculations unless patients are breathing high concentrations of supplemental oxygen. The amount of oxygen the body uses or takes in per minute is called the oxygen consumption (VO_2) and can be measured directly by comparing all the exhaled O_2 to the inhaled O_2 of a spontaneously breathing patient over 5 minutes. VO_2 is generally indexed to BSA and recorded as milliliter of O_2/minute/m^2 so that different sized patients can be compared. There are several commercially available machines appropriate for sedated supine patients undergoing catheterization (Lister et al., 1974). Although VO_2 varies by metabolic rate, temperature, respiratory rate, and heart rate, if direct measurement is not possible, it can be estimated from empiric data tables based on patient age and heart rate (LaFarge et al., 1970). For children <3 years VO_2, can be estimated at = 8.8 mL O_2/min/kg or 150 mL O_2/min time BSA. Due to individual variability, it is always best to measure VO_2 directly when possible.

The formulas for calculating flow from these measurements are

$$\text{Systemic flow Qs} = \frac{VO_2}{(Ao\,sat - SVC\,sat)13.6(Hgb)}$$

$$\text{Pulmonary flow Qp} = \frac{VO_2}{(PV\,sat - PA\,sat)13.6(Hgb)}$$

Flows are reported in liters/minute.

One additional flow is needed, effective flow, to accurately calculate shunts in patients with complex heart disease who have bidirectional shunting. Effective flow measures the amount of deoxygenated blood going to the lungs or the amount of oxygenated blood going to the body.

$$\text{Effective flow Qeff} = \frac{VO_2}{(PV\,sat - SVC\,sat)13.6(Hgb)}$$

Left to right shunt Q (L to R) = Qp − Qeff
Right to left shunt Q(R to L) = Qs − Qeff

Resistance Calculations

Vascular resistance reflects the state of the arterioles and capillary vessels of a vascular bed. It is calculated from the mean pressure difference across a vascular bed divided by the flow through the bed, $R = (\Delta P)/Q$ In congenital heart disease the focus is often on pulmonary vascular resistance: $PVR = (PAp - PVp)/Qp$ although systemic vascular resistance is also evaluated: $SVR = (AOp - Rap)/Qs$. Units of resistance are typically reported in mmHg/liters/minute also known as a Wood unit. This measurement is generally indexed to body surface area in congenital heart disease so different sized patients can be compared. In physiology studies and many adult cardiac catheterization laboratories, resistance is reported in metric units of dyne. second/cm^5 which = 80 × Wood unit.

The normal range for pulmonary vascular resistance (PVR) is shown in Table 6–1. Elevated PVR indicates either acute pulmonary vasoconstriction or reduced cross-sectional area of the pulmonary capillary bed. Vasoconstriction is reversible and typically due to either an acute insult such as hypoxia, hypecarbia, acidosis, or parenchymal lung injury, or to downstream obstruction such as pulmonary vein or mitral valve stenosis, or left ventricular failure. Reduction in the cross-sectional area of the pulmonary capillary bed is not reversible and is most often due to progressive vessel loss from shunt-associated pulmonary hypertension (Eisenmenger syndrome), chronic thrombo-embolic disease, or pulmonary hypoplasia. It is important to distinguish between reversible and nonreversible elevated PVR, particularly in the setting of repairable congenital heart disease to determine surgical risk and plan an optimal treatment strategy that may require pulmonary vasodilators. To determine reversibility, repeat hemodynamic assessment with calculation of flows and resistance is performed while the patient is given a pulmonary vasodilator. Current practice is 20–40 parts per million inhaled nitric oxide with 100% FiO_2 given by nasal cannula if the patient is spontaneously breathing or in the circuit if ventilated. Since there is significant variability in PVR measurements, a change of >25% would be considered significantly reactive.

Valve Area Calculations

The cross-sectional area of a valve or vessel most accurately reflects the degree of obstruction. Although pressure gradient is commonly used as a measure of obstruction, it is determined by the cross-sectional area of the obstruction and the blood flow through the obstruction. In patients with valvar aortic or mitral stenosis, the effective valve area can be calculated from cardiac flow and pressure measurements to help access the degree of obstruction more accurately. Gorlin and Gorlin in 1951 described a formula for calculating valve area that continues to be in use today (Gorlin and Gorlin, 1951, 1990). Flow through a valve only occurs during a portion of the cardiac cycle, during systole for the aortic valve and during diastole for the mitral valve, so this must be considered when calculating valve areas. Systolic ejection time is measured from simultaneous left ventricle (LV) and aortic pressure tracings by determining the duration in seconds the LV trace crosses the aortic trace in systole. Similarly, the diastolic filling time is measured from simultaneous LA (or pulmonary capillary wedge) and LV pressure tracings by determining the duration in seconds of the LV trace crossing the LA trace in diastole. The formula for valve areas are listed below:

$$\text{Aortic Valve Area}\left(\text{cm}^2\right)=\frac{\text{systolic flow}}{44.5\times\sqrt{\text{mean systolic gradient}}}$$

$$\text{Systolic flow}=\frac{\text{cardiac output}\times\text{R-R interval(secs)}}{60\times\text{systolic ejection time(secs)}}$$

$$\text{Mitral Valve Area}\left(\text{cm}^2\right)=\frac{\textit{diastolic flow}}{37.8\times\sqrt{\text{mean diastolic gradient}}}$$

$$\text{Diastolic flow}=\frac{\text{cardiac output}\times\text{R-R interval}}{60\times\text{diastolic ejection time}}$$

The mean gradient across a valve is most accurately determined by the area between the pressure tracings during ejection of blood through the valve. For the aortic valve, this would be the area between the LV and AO pressure tracings during systole and for the mitral the area between the LA and LV tracing during diastole. Current catheterization laboratory hemodynamic systems calculate these values easily, accurately, and automatically (Figure 6–4). Normal aortic and mitral valve areas are given in Table 6–1.

VASOACTIVE TESTING

There are two situations that are frequently encountered in the congenital catheterization laboratory where repeat measurement of pressures and flows during administration of a vasoactive drug can add important information for management. The first is in patients with pulmonary hypertension who are tested with 100% oxygen together with inhaled nitric oxide. The second is in patients with mild to moderate obstruction, such as aortic valve stenosis, coarctation, LVOT or RVOT subvalvar obstruction who are tested with Dobutamine infusion to increase contractility to simulate exercise.

Nitric Oxide with Oxygen

Inhaled nitric oxide at 40 ppm together with maximal O_2 (usually >90%) is given by nasal cannula in

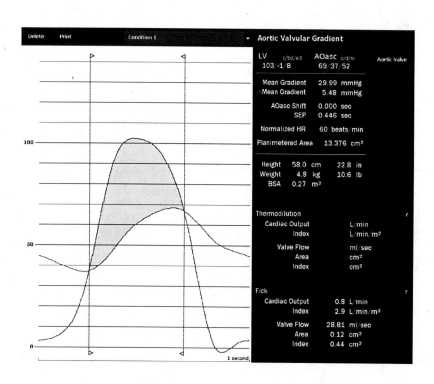

FIGURE 6–4. Aortic valve area calculation performed automatically by the hemodynamic monitoring system from simultaneous LV and AAO pressure tracings in a child with severe aortic stenosis.

spontaneously breathing patients and through the ventilator circuit in intubated patients. Repeat hemodynamic evaluation including SVC, PA, LA, and AO pressures and saturation are obtained so cardiac blood flows and resistances, particularly minimal PVR can be calculated. This information is often used to determine suitability for surgical repair, heart transplant, or outpatient pulmonary vasodilator therapy.

Dobutamine

Repeat measurements of pressures and flows during increased contractility and heart rate can be useful in patients with mild valvar, subvalvar, or aortic obstruction who have symptoms or hypertrophy out of proportion to their resting gradients. Dobutamine is given IV at 7.5 mcg/kg/min increasing the dose by 2.5 mcg/kg/min every 4 minutes to a maximum of 20 mcg/kg/min or a 15% increase in heart rate or pressures of interest from baseline. Once the end point is reached, repeat pressures and saturations are obtained. A dramatic worsening of the degree of obstruction during simulated activity may indicate the need for intervention sooner whereas minimal change in mild obstruction may allow for conservative observation (Figures 6–2A and 6–2B).

ANGIOGRAPHY

General Principles

Angiography is used to augment imaging data from echo, CT, and MRI. It remains particularly advantageous for evaluating vessel abnormalities in the pulmonary arteries (segmental stenosis or AVMs), systemic or pulmonary veins, and the aortic arch. In addition, it can often be helpful in evaluating complex LVOT obstruction and to subjectively determine relative size of left to right shunts in patients with more than one level of shunting (ASD + VSD + PDA) or in patients with multiple ventricular defects, particularly apical muscular.

Most congenital catheterization laboratories use biplane fluoroscopy so that complex anatomy can be viewed from two planes simultaneously reducing the contrast required. The fluoroscopic units can be rotated left and right oblique as well as cranial and caudal to focus on specific anatomical areas with the patient remaining supine on the table. New fluoroscopic systems still in development allow rapid rotational angiography that acquires image data from multiple angles during a single injection to allow reconstruction of 3-D images. In general, a fluoroscopy plane is angled perpendicular to the anatomic plane of interest for optimal visualization. Contrast is injected through catheters with multiple holes to allow large rapid bolus infusion that immediately opacifies the area of interest. A mechanical injector, which can inject contrast at a pressure of up to 1000 PSI at rates of 40 cc per second, is used. The amount of contrast given is increased with increasing size of the patient, larger site of injection, and larger blood flow through the area of interest, i.e., RV angiogram if a VSD with left to right shunting is present. A starting point is 1 cc contrast/kg body weight (maximum of 35 cc) over 1 second for injections in major vessels (aorta or main pulmonary artery) or chambers (atria or ventricles). Contrast agents are iodine-based low-osmolar nonionic to minimize complications such as allergic reaction and renal impairment.

Angiography poses a small risk to patients due to the use of iodine-based contrast and increased radiation exposure. The amount of radiation from a typical congenital diagnostic catheterization is 6 mSv, approximately twice the background exposure over 1 year in the United States and half of the exposure from a contrast CT scan (Bacher et al., 2005; Einstein et al., 2007). Lifetime mortality risk associated with radiation exposure-related cancers is highest in children under 1 year at 0.1% increased risk over a lifetime (Bacher et al., 2005).

Specific Views

A detailed description of angiography is beyond the scope of this chapter but general principles for specific areas or lesions of the heart are listed below. The goal of camera positioning is to have the plane of the x-ray beam perpendicular to the plane of the area of interest. If the plane of interest cannot be anticipated such as with complex single ventricle anatomy, the initial angiogram should be performed in straight AP and lateral projections so that general special relationships can be evaluated more easily. Table 6–2 shows a summary of recommended camera angles for common congenital lesions.

Atrial Septal Defects/Patent Foramen Ovale. To visualize the atrial septum, the cameras are positioned 20 degrees RAO/25 degrees cranial and 70 degrees LAO and 10 degrees cranial. The injection is performed in the mouth of the right upper pulmonary vein with 1 cc/kg (max 30 cc) contrast. This optimizes visualization of the septum and any left to right atrial shunting (Figures 6–5A and 6–5B). If right to left shunting is of concern as with a PFO, camera angles are the same but the catheter is placed in the low right atrium held rightward and posterior with a similar injection volume. A side hole catheter, such as a Berman or Gensini, can

TABLE 6–2. *Angiographic Camera Angles*

Lesion/Site of Interest	AP or A plane		LAT or B plane	
	RAO	Cran/Caud	LAO	Cran/Caud
ASD/PFO	20	25 Cran	70	10 Cran
AV canal/AV valves	40	25 Caud	40	35 Cran
VSD inlet	30	15 Caud	40	25 Cran
Peri-membranous or?	30	15 Caud	45	25 Cran
Muscular	30	15 Caud	60	25 Cran
Outlet	10	15 Caud	80	25 Cran
RV	0	0	0	0
RVOT/PV/MPA	0	15 Cran	0	0
Branch PAs	20	15 Caud	65	15 Cran
Selective RPA	25	20 Caud	65	25 Caud
Selective LPA	10	15 Caud	80	15 Cran
LV/LVOT/Ao valve	15	15 Caud	60	25 Cran
Aortic arch/coarctation	10 LAO	10 Caud	85	0
PDA	20	15 Caud	90	0
Glenn anastamosis	20	15 Caud	25	0
Fontan/single ventricle	0	0	90	0
Coronaries (Ao injection)	25	0	70	20 Caud
Selective left	20	20 Caud	70	20 Caud
Selective right	25	0	70	20 Cran
Coronaries (D-transposition)	30	0	60	30 Caud

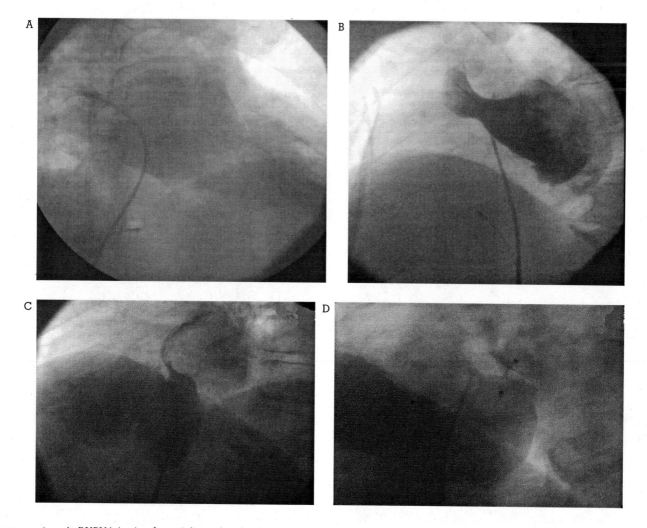

FIGURE 6–5. A: RUPV injection for atrial septal evaluation RAO/Cranial. B: RUPV injection evaluating the atrial septum LAO and Cranial. C: PFO injection in tunnel pre closure, 70 degrees LAO and 10 degrees cranial. D: RA injection post PFO device closure, 70 degrees LAO and 10 degrees cranial.

also be positioned straddling the PFO (Figures 6–5C and 6–5D).

AV Canal/AV Valve Regurgitation.

To evaluate the AV valves and posterior inlet ventricular septum, the catheter is placed in the RV apex, for the tricuspid valve, or LV apex for the mitral valve or inlet ventricular septum. Cameras are angled in the steep hepatoclavicular view with 40 degree RAO/20 degree caudal and 40 degree LAO/35 degree cranial.

Ventricular Septal Defects.

The ventricular septum is a curvilinear structure so a single camera angle will not adequately assess all types of ventricular septal defects. VSDs are seen best in the lateral plane and in general inlet VSDs, as noted above, are best seen with shallow LAO angulation of 40 degrees and 25 degrees of cranial, peri-membranous defects with 45 degrees LAO, muscular defects with 60 degrees LAO, and anterior muscular defects with very steep 80 degrees of LAO. If the location of the VSD is not known, then 45 degrees LAO/25 degrees cranial is best (Figure 6–6). The PA camera is typically angled orthogonal at 25 degrees caudal/45 degrees RAO. Injection is in the LV apex and the amount of contrast generous at 1.5 cc/kg if a significant shunt is present.

RV/RVOT Obstruction/Pulmonary Valve/MPA.

To visualize the RV, straight PA and lateral angulation is the best choice. To visualize the outflow tract and pulmonary valve, a straight PA with 15 degrees cranial angulation together with a straight lateral view is the best choice (Figures 6–7A and 6–7B). Contrast volume

of 1 cc/kg is adequate unless a VSD or significant PI is present, then the volume should be increased to 1.5 cc/kg (maximum 35 cc).

Branch Pulmonary Arteries.

Evaluating branch pulmonary arteries completely can require more than a single angiogram due to the complex nature of the vessels and the numerous planes involved when considering proximal and segmental arteries. In general, cameras angled 20 degrees RAO/15 degrees caudal

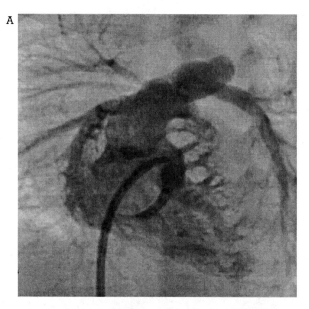

A

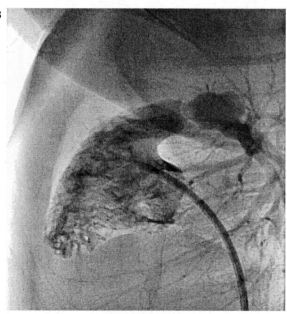

B

FIGURE 6–7. A: RV angiogram in patient with valvar pulmonic stenosis in A: 0 degrees/15 degrees cranial angulation. B: Straight lateral view at 90 degrees with 0 cranial.

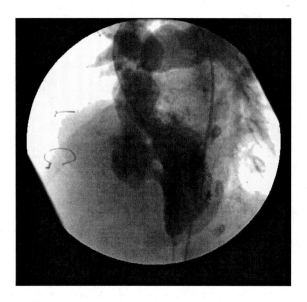

FIGURE 6–6. LV angiogram in 45 degrees LAO/25 degrees cranial.

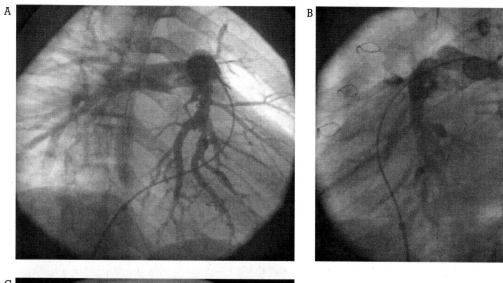

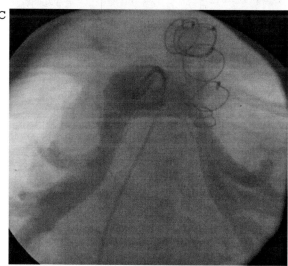

FIGURE 6-8. Angled MPA angiograms in patients with pulmonary artery stenoses. A: RAO caudal to evaluate the proximal RPA and distal LPA. B: LAO with cranial shows proximal LPA and distal RPA. C: RAO with steep caudal shows both proximal right and left PAs well ("pant leg view").

and 65 degrees LAO/15 degrees cranial will allow evaluation of both the right and left pulmonary arteries in both planes, visualizing both the branch origins as well as all segments (Figures 6–8A and 6–8B). The catheter is placed in the MPA or origin of one of the branches with 1 cc/kg of contrast adequate, more if a significant left to right shunt is present. Another approach is to perform two selective angiograms with injections in the proximal right and proximal left pulmonary arteries. To optimize visualization of a selective right pulmonary arteriogram, the cameras are angled 20 degrees RAO/20 degrees caudal and 65 degrees LAO/25 degrees caudal. It should be remembered that the volume of contrast should be reduced to 0.75 cc/kg for a selective PA injection. Cameras should be angled 10 degrees RAO/15 degrees caudal and 80 degrees LAO/15 degrees cranial for a selective LPA angiogram. To see the origins of both the right and left pulmonary artery, especially in patients with abnormal branch anatomy as with tetralogy of Fallot, shallow RAO with steep caudal angulation (+35 degrees) is the best choice (Figure 6–8C. Pant leg view).

LVOT/AO Valve Abnormalities. To evaluate the LVOT and aortic valve, cameras should be angled at 15 degrees RAO/15 caudal and 60 degrees LAO/25 degrees cranial. Injection is performed in the LV apex at 1 cc/kg, increased to 1.5 cc/kg if significant aortic insufficiency or LV dilation is present (Figure 6–9). In patients with transposition of the great arteries, straight AP and lateral angulation better demonstrates the outflow tract and aortic valve.

Aortic Arch/Coarctation. Camera position for evaluation of the aortic arch with coarctation is dependent on the location of coarctation. General assessment of

A

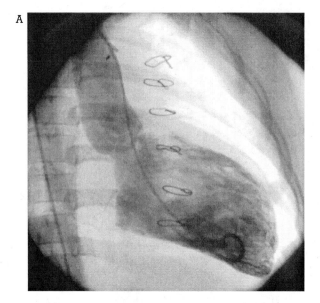

B

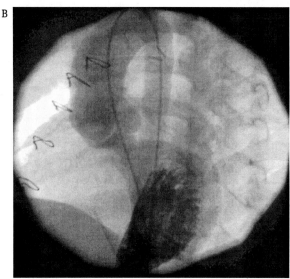

FIGURE 6–9. LV angiogram evaluating the outflow tract in a patient with subvalvar aortic stenosis, A: RAO/caudal angulation. B: LAO cranial.

A

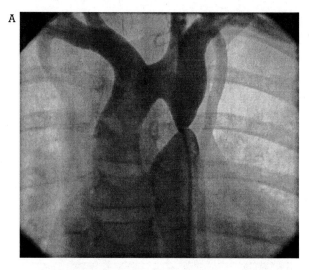

B

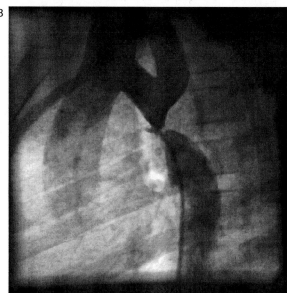

FIGURE 6–10. DAO angiogram of coarctation in A: LAO 10/15 caudal and B: straight lateral projections.

the arch can be performed in the straight PA and lateral projections. For a typical native coarctation located in the proximal descending aorta, the best camera positions are 10 degrees LAO/10 degrees caudal and 85 degrees LAO/0 degrees (Figures 6–10A and 6–10B).

Patent Ductus Arteriosus. Although ductal anatomy can vary typically the angiogram camera angles are 20 degrees RAO/15 degrees caudal and straight lateral. The side holes of the angiographic catheter should be positioned at or just inferior to the PDA in the proximal descending thoracic aorta (retrograde flow will fill the PDA with limited transverse arch filing minimizing

overlap). At least 1 cc/kg, up to 1.5 cc/kg if the duct is large, should be injected over 1 second (Figures 6–11A and 6–11B).

Glenn Anastamosis. Optimal camera angles for an SVC angiogram to evaluate a Glenn circulation are challenging due to overlap of important structures. Optimally the cameras should be positioned at 20 degrees RAO/15 degrees caudal and 25 degrees LAO/0 degrees. The catheter can be placed either in the SVC or in the left inominate vein injecting 1 cc/kg of contrast over a second. For evaluation of venous or arterial collaterals, straight PA and Lat projection is the best choice.

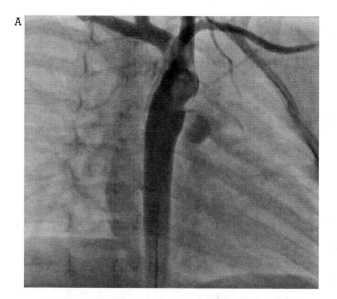

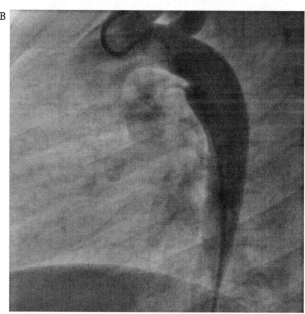

FIGURE 6–11. AAO angiogram for PDA. A: RAO with caudal angulation. B: straight lateral.

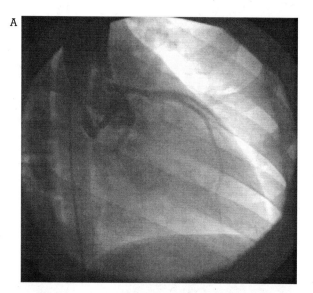

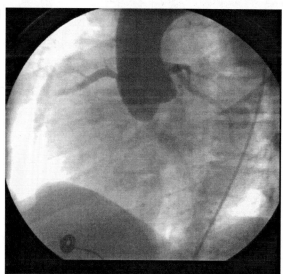

FIGURE 6–12. Aortic root angiogram in A: RAO projection showing the left main, LAD, distal circumflex nd mid and distal RCA, B: LAO projection showing the proximal and mid RCA, and circumflex arteries.

Fontan Repair/Complex Single Ventricle. Because of the variable anatomy found in surgical Fontan repairs and with single ventricles, initial angiograms are best performed in straight AP and lateral projections. Contrast should be given at 1 cc/kg over 1.5 seconds, due to the nonpulsatile nature of the circulation, at the IVC–Fontan junction. Make sure the frame rate or length of angiogram is adequate to include the levophase as flow through this circulation can be quite slow.

Coronary Arteries. Multiple angled views are required to evaluate all of the coronary arteries including the distal segments. However, most of congenital heart disease is concerned with the coronary origins and their proximal course since most of the patients are children or young adults in whom atherosclerotic coronary disease is uncommon. An aortic root injection at 1 cc/kg contrast given over 1 second with cameras angled at RAO 25 degrees/0 and LAO 70 degrees/20 degrees caudal will demonstrate both the right, left main, LAD, and circumflex in most patients (Figures 6–12A and 6–12B). Selective injections will give more information and are required if the aortic root injection is inadequate or if there is significant aortic insufficiency. For best visualization of the left coronary arteries, 20 degrees RAO/20 degrees caudal and 70 degrees LAO/20 degrees caudal is a good starting point. For the right coronary artery, 25 degrees RAO/0 and 70 degrees LAO/20 cranial will show all the artery including the origin in most patients. If the patient has transposition, the coronaries will arise from the posterior sinuses of the aorta, as the noncoronary sinus is anterior. Camera angles for visualization are 30 degree RAO/0 and 60 degrees LAO/30 degrees caudal, the latter view will give an en fas view of the aortic valve.

REFERENCES

Bacher K, Bogaert E, Lapere R, De Wolf D, Thierens H. Patient-specific dose and radiation risk estimation in pediatric cardiac catheterization. *Circulation.* 2005;111(1):83–89.

Balik M, Pachl J, Hendl J. Effect of the degree of tricuspid regurgitation on cardiac output measurements by thermodilution. *Intensive Care Med.* 2002;28(8):1117–1121.

Ebeid MR. Transhepatic vascular access for diagnostic and interventional procedures: techniques, outcome, and complications. *Catheter Cardiovasc Interv.* 2007;69(4):594–606.

Einstein AJ, Moser KW, Thompson RC, Cerqueira MD, Henzlova MJ. Radiation dose to patients from cardiac diagnostic imaging. *Circulation.* 2007;116(11):1290–1305.

Fagard R, Conway J. Measurement of cardiac output: Fick principle using catheterization. *Eur Heart J.* 1990;11 (suppl I):1–5.

Freed MD, Keane JF. Cardiac output measured by thermodilution in infants and children. *J Pediatr.* 1978;92(1):39–42.

French WJ, Chang P, Forsythe S, Criley JM. Estimation of mixed venous oxygen saturation. *Cathet Cardiovasc Diagn.* 1983;9(1):25–31.

Gorlin R, Gorlin SG. Hydraulic formula for calculation of the area of the stenotic mitral valve, other cardiac valves, and central circulatory shunts. I. *Am Heart J.* 1951;41(1):1–29.

Gorlin WB, Gorlin R. A generalized formulation of the Gorlin formula for calculating the area of the stenotic mitral valve and other stenotic cardiac valves. *J Am Coll Cardiol.* 1990;15(1):246–247.

LaFarge CG, Miettinen OS. The estimation of oxygen consumption. *Cardiovasc Res.* 1970;4(1):23–30.

Lister G, Hoffman JI, Rudolph AM. Oxygen uptake in infants and children: a simple method for measurement. *Pediatrics.* 1974;53(5):656–662.

Shim D, Lloyd TR, Cho KJ, Moorehead CP, Beekman RH, 3rd. Transhepatic cardiac catheterization in children. Evaluation of efficacy and safety. *Circulation.* 1995;92(6):1526–1530.

Udelson JE, Bacharach SL, Cannon RO III, Bonow RO. Minimum left ventricular pressure during beta-adrenergic stimulation in human subjects. Evidence for elastic recoil and diastolic "suction" in the normal heart. *Circulation.* 1990;82(4):1174–1182.

Vitiello R, McCrindle BW, Nykanen D, Freedom RM, Benson LN. Complications associated with pediatric cardiac catheterization. *J Am Coll Cardiol.* 1998;32(5):1433–1440.

7

Heritable Cardiac Channelopathies

MICHAEL J. ACKERMAN

The discipline of cardiac channelopathies or heritable arrhythmia syndromes unofficially commenced in 1995 with the discovery of mutations in genes encoding critical ion channels of the heart as the pathogenic basis for congenital long QT syndrome (LQTS) (Curran et al., 1995; Wang et al., 1995). Besides classical autosomal dominant (Romano-Ward) LQTS and autosomal recessive (Jervell and Lange-Nielsen) LQTS, the cardiac channelopathies now comprise Andersen-Tawil syndrome (ATS), Timothy syndrome (TS), drug-induced *torsades de pointes* (DI-TdP), short QT syndrome (SQTS), catecholaminergic polymorphic ventricular tachycardia (CPVT), Brugada syndrome (BrS), idiopathic ventricular fibrillation, inferolateral early repolarization syndrome, progressive cardiac conduction disease (PCCD) or familial atrioventricular conduction block (FAVCB) or Lev-Lenegre disease, and familial atrial fibrillation (FAF). Even primary cardiomyopathies like dilated cardiomyopathy (DCM) may stem from genetically mediated perturbations in ion channels, specifically the *SCN5A*-encoded cardiac sodium channel (Olson et al., 2005).

Cardiac channelopathies affect an estimated 1 in 2000 persons, may lie dormant for decades or present with sudden death during infancy, may or may not manifest signature electrocardiographic features, and in general represent very treatable conditions when properly recognized and diagnosed. The clinical presentation in general consists of abrupt onset of syncope, seizures, or sudden death. Sudden cardiac arrest (SCA) is uncommonly the sentinel event. It is estimated that nearly half of SCAs stemming from a cardiac channelopathy may have exhibited prior warning signs that went unrecognized (i.e., exertional syncope, positive family history of premature sudden death, etc.) An estimated 10% of sudden infant death syndrome (SIDS) and up to one-third of autopsy negative sudden unexplained deaths in the young (<40 years) may be precipitated by an underlying cardiac channelopathy (Ackerman et al., 2001; Arnestad et al., 2007; Tester and Ackerman, 2007).

In this chapter, the pathogenic basis, clinical evaluation and diagnosis, and therapeutic management of the QT syndromes, CPVT, and BrS will be examined.

QT-OPATHIES

Autosomal Dominant (Romano-Ward) Long QT Syndrome

Congenital LQTS is the prototypic cardiac channelopathy affecting an estimated 1 in 2500 persons. Clinically, LQTS is characterized by abnormal cardiac repolarization resulting in QT interval prolongation (Figure 7–1A), which predisposes patients to its trademark dysrhythmia of *torsade de pointes* (TdP, Figure 7–1B). If and when TdP occurs, the affected individual either exhibits the abrupt onset of syncope, seizures, or sudden death. The most common form of LQTS is autosomal dominant LQTS, previously known as Romano-Ward syndrome (Romano and Pongiglione, 1963; Ward, 1964). Autosomal recessive LQTS first described by Drs. Jervell and Lange-Nielsen (1957) affects about 1 in 1 million persons and is characterized by a severe cardiac phenotype as well as sensorineural hearing loss. Approximately 5%–10% of the time, LQTS originates as sporadic/spontaneous germline mutations.

With respect to its pathogenic mechanisms, hundreds of mutations in 12 distinct LQTS-susceptibility genes have been identified so far and they generally involve

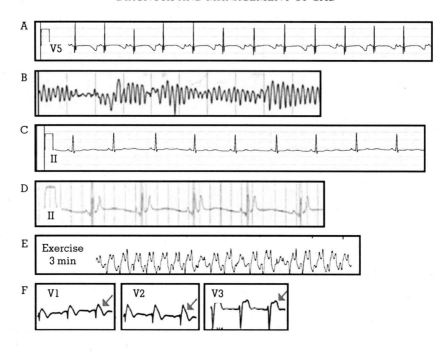

FIGURE 7–1. Signature electrocardiographic features of various channelopathies A: QT prolongation—an example of a patient with extreme QT prolongation (QTc > 650 ms). Note, the ST segment, T wave morphology would predict LQT3 but patient is among the 25% who are genotype negative. Also, the computer calculated QTc was 362 ms underscoring the mandate to independently compute the QTc. B: *Torsade de pointes* ("twisting of the points")—hallmark dysrhythmia of LQTS. C: Abnormal U wave in ATS—Although subtle, this lead II recording is quite abnormal characterized by normal QT interval, long isoelectric segment between the end of the T wave on the start of the U wave, and long duration U wave in this female with an ATS-associated mutation in *KCNJ2*. D: Short QT interval—QTc of approximately 250 ms. E: Exercise induced bi-directional VT seen in CPVT. F: Coved ST segment elevation in BrS (type I ECG pattern) in precordial leads V1 and V2 and a saddle back profile (type II ECG pattern) in V3.

either loss-of-function potassium channel mutations or gain-of-function sodium channel mutations (Table 7–1). Except for four rare subtypes that stem from perturbations in key cardiac channel interacting proteins (ChIPs) or structural membrane scaffolding proteins [ankyrin B-, caveolin 3-, yotiao-, and syntrophin alpha-LQTS] (Mohler et al., 2003; Vatta et al., 2006; Chen et al., 2007; Ueda et al., 2008), LQTS is a pure "channelopathy" stemming from mutations in cardiac channel alpha and beta subunits. The vast majority of LQTS is due to mutations in either the *KCNQ1*-encoded I_{Ks} potassium channel (LQT1, 30%–35%), or the *KCNH2*-encoded I_{Kr} potassium channel (LQT2, 25%–30%), or the *SCN5A*-encoded I_{Na} sodium channel (LQT3, 5%–10%) (Splawski et al., 2000; Tester et al., 2005).

The past decade of LQTS research has provided numerous genotype–phenotype relationships. Genotype–ECG relationships include broad based T waves in LQT1, low amplitude or notched T waves in LQT2, long ST isoelectric segment and normal T wave morphology in LQT3 (Moss et al., 1995; Zhang et al., 2000). Relatively gene-specific arrhythmogenic triggers have been observed including exertion, particularly swimming and LQT1, auditory triggers and the post-partum period in LQT2, and events during sleep in LQT3 (Ackerman et al., 1999; Khositseth et al., 2004; Moss et al., 1999; Schwartz et al., 2001; Wilde et al., 1999). Importantly, the response to standard LQTS pharmacotherapy (beta blockers) is strongly influenced by the underlying genotype (Moss et al., 2000). Beta blockers are extremely protective in LQT1, moderately protective in LQT2, and of no demonstrable protective benefit in LQT3. In 2004, LQTS genetic testing became a commercially available clinical diagnostic test involving a comprehensive open reading frame analysis of the translated exons for the genes associated with LQT1, LQT2, LQT3, LQT5, and LQT6. In the presence of a clinically robust presentation, the yield of LQTS genetic testing is about 75% (Tester et al., 2006). Indications for LQTS genetic testing are summarized in Table 7–2.

Electrocardiographically, individuals with LQTS may or may not display the hallmark repolarization abnormality of QT interval prolongation (Figure 7–1A). In fact, approximately 40%–50% of patients with genotype positive LQTS have a normal resting QTc (Priori

TABLE 7–1. *Molecular Basis of Cardiac Channelopathies*

Gene	Locus	Protein	Frequency in Patients (%)
Long QT Syndrome			
AKAP9	7q21–q22	Yotiao	Rare
ANKB	4q25–q27	Ankyrin B	Rare
CACNA1C	12p13.3	CaV1.2	Rare
CAV3	3p25	Caveolin-3	Rare
KCNE1	21q22.1	MinK	Rare
KCNE2	21q22.1	MiRP1	Rare
KCNH2 (LQT2)	7q35–36	Kv11.1	25–30
KCNJ2	17q23	Kir2.1	Rare
KCNQ1 (LQT1)	11p15.5	Kv7.1	30–35
SCN4B	11q23.3	NaV1.5 beta 4 subunit	Rare
SCN5A (LQT3)	3p21–p24	NaV1.5	5–10
SNTA1	20q11.2	Syntrophin-alpha 1	Rare
Catecholaminergic Polymorphic Ventricular Tachycardia			
CASQ2	1p13.3	Calsequestrin 2	Rare
RYR2 (CPVT1)	1q42.1–q43	Ryanodine Receptor 2/ calcium release channel	50–60
Brugada Syndrome			
CACNA1C	2p13.3	CaV1.2	5–10?
CACNB2	10p12	CaV1.2 beta 2 subunit	Rare
GPD1L	3p22.3	Glycerol-3-phosphate dehydrogenase 1-like	Rare
KCNE3	11q13.4	MiRP2	Rare
SCN1B	19	NaV1.5 beta 1 subunit	Rare
SCN5A (BrS1)	3p21–p24	NaV1.5	20–30
Short QT Syndrome			
KCNH2	7q35–36	Kv11.1	Rare
KCNJ2	17q23	Kir2.1	Rare
KCNQ1	11p15.5	Kv7.1	Rare

et al., 1999). This observation reinforces the critical role of genetic testing as the screening ECG has an unacceptable misclassification rate once the diagnosis of LQTS is established. In general, a heart rate–corrected QT interval (QTc) >480 ms in *postpubertal* females or >470 ms in *postpubertal* males should prompt a thorough investigation for LQTS as these values represent the 99th percentile in the distribution of QTc values. Previously, a QTc >440 ms (males) or >450 ms has been called borderline QT prolongation. While 50% of patients with genetically proven LQTS indeed exhibit a QTc < 460 ms, these cut-off values would result in an unacceptably high rate of false-positives if used as part of a screening program. By the aforementioned cut-off values, an estimated 15%–20% of the entire population has "borderline QT prolongation" (Figure 7–2). These QTc-based assessments presume an accurate determination of the QTc (Viskin et al., 2005). Here, it is absolutely critical to independently determine the QTc manually as reliance on the instrument derived QTc is unacceptable. Calculation of an average QTc from either lead II or V5 is recommended. Simply taking the beat yielding the maximum QTc will yield too many false-positives. Further, these QT distributions

do not apply to a 24-hour ambulatory ECG. In particular, recording of a maximum QTc at say 3 AM, that happens to exceed 500 ms is not sufficient evidence for a diagnosis of LQTS.

In an attempt to improve on the clinical diagnostic accuracy in the evaluation of LQTS, a composite clinical diagnostic scorecard has been developed ("Moss, Compton, and Schwartz LQTS score") and is detailed in Table 7–3 (Schwartz et al., 1993). This score includes ECG parameters (QT prolongation, *torsade de pointes*, T-wave alternans, notched T-wave, low heart rate for age), clinical history (syncope with or without stress, congenital deafness), and the family history (long QT, sudden death). A score >4 indicates high clinical probability for LQTS and is associated with a 75% likelihood of a positive LQTS genetic test result. While this diagnostic scorecard helps with the evaluation of the index case, it will miss many affected family members due to incomplete penetrance and variable expressivity.

Efforts to unmask individuals with concealed LQTS (genotype positive/resting ECG negative) include exercise stress testing and epinephrine QT stress testing (Ackerman et al., 2002; Shimizu et al., 2003; Vincent et al., 1991). With exercise stress testing, failure to

TABLE 7-2. *Indications for LQTS Genetic Testing*

1. Persons with unequivocal and unexplained QT prolongation (i.e., QTc >500 ms)
2. Persons with clinically suspected LQTS regardless of (i) baseline QTc or (ii) history of prior negative genetic testing in research laboratories or with commercially available targeted exon testing. (Rationale: Mutation detection methods over the past decade have changed significantly and false-negatives have been demonstrated. With respect to previous so-called targeted LQTS scans that comprises only 18 of the 60 translated exons in *KCNQ1*, *KCNH2*, *SCN5A*, *KCNE1*, and *KCNE2*, 35% of the LQTS-associated mutations detected in Mayo Clinic's Sudden Death Genomics Laboratory would have been missed.)
3. All first degree relatives of a genotype positive index case (genetic testing extended to other degrees of relatedness by "following the genetic trail" down the appropriate path of concentric first degree relatives). For example, confirmatory genetic testing demonstrates the index case's LQT1-associated mutation in the father. Accordingly, the father's parents and siblings (second degree relatives to the index case) should be offered testing. Next, if say the paternal aunt (to the index case) tests positive, now all of her children (cousins or 3rd degree relatives to the index case) should be tested and so forth.
4. Postmortem genetic testing for autopsy negative sudden unexplained death (debatable considering estimated 20% yield)
5. Persons with drug-induced TdP (debatable considering estimated 10% yield)
6. Postmortem genetic testing for sudden infant death syndrome (debatable considering estimated 5%–10% yield)

TABLE 7-3. *Moss, Compton, and Schwartz Score for the Clinical Diagnosis of LQTS*

Variable	Points
Electrocardiogram	
QTc (at rest, NOT during Holter or exercise stress testing)	
>480 ms	3
460–470 ms	2
450 ms (males)	1
Torsade de pontes	2
T-wave alternans	1
Notched T wave in 3 leads	1
Low heart rate for age	0.5
Clinical History	
Syncope	
With stress	2
Without stress	1
Congenital deafness	0.5
Family History	
Family member with long QT syndrome	1
Sudden death in a family member < 30 years of age	0.5
With no other identifiable cause	

Cumulative point score for risk of having congential LQTS:
≤1 low risk
2–3 intermediate
≥4 high risk (*)

*Note the yield of LQTS genetic testing is 75% for patients scoring >4.

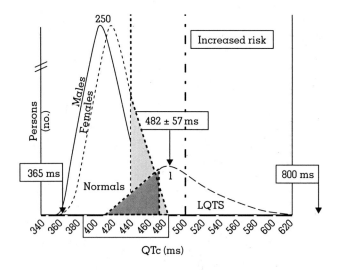

FIGURE 7-2. Distribution of QTc in health and LQTS. Shown are the normal distribution of QTc values among healthy postpubertal males (solid line) postpubertal females (dotted line), and patients with genotype positive LQTS from Mayo Clinic (dashed line). The triangles indicate the proportion of population with so-called *borderline* QT prolongation (> 440 ms, the vertical dashed line) and the proportion of patients with LQTS having QTc values that overlap with normals. The 3 annotated QTc values indicate the minimum, average, and maximum QTc values recorded in Mayo Clinic's Long QT Syndrome Clinic. The vertical line at 500 ms is an indicator of increased torsadogenic potential for both congenital LQTS and DI-TdP.

shorten the QT interval appropriately has been used to suggest LQTS. However, this failure to shorten the QT interval during exercise is principally a LQT1 specific response. So, the presence of normal QT interval shortening during exercise does NOT rule out LQTS. Similarly, during infusion of low-dose epinephrine (<0.1 mcg/kg/min), the presence of paradoxical lengthening (>30 ms) of the absolute QT interval is suggestive (75% positive predictive value) of concealed LQT1 (Vyas et al., 2006).

Overall, the annual mortality associated with LQTS is probably around 1% per year with the highest risk subset around 5%–8% per year, similar to hypertrophic cardiomyopathy. Indicators of increased risk include QTc >500 ms, history of LQTS-related symptoms, LQT2 or LQT3 genotype, and female gender after puberty (Hobbs et al., 2006; Priori et al., 2003). Both symptomatic and asymptomatic patients with LQTS must avoid concomitant exposure to medications that can aggravate the QT interval as an unwanted effect of the medication. In addition, patients should be alerted to maintain adequate hydration/electrolyte replenishment in the setting of vomiting and diarrheal illnesses that could precipitate hypokalemia. Asymptomatic patients >40 years of age probably do not require active intervention but this must be individualized.

In general, all symptomatic patients and all asymptomatic patients < 40 years of age at diagnosis should receive medical, surgical, and/or device-related therapy. Beta-blockers, preferably nadolol or propranolol, should be considered standard therapy in all patients with either LQT1 or LQT2 (Moss et al., 2000; Villain et al., 2004). In contrast, beta-blockers are not protective and may be theoretically proarrhythmic in LQT3. Genotype-targeted therapy with late sodium current blockers such as mexiletine, flecainide, or ranolazine should be considered in LQT3 instead (Moss et al., 2005; Schwartz et al., 1995). Indications for an internal cardioverter defibrillator (ICD) include (1) aborted cardiac arrest (regardless of genotype) as secondary prevention, (2) breakthrough cardiac event despite adequate medical therapy, (3) intolerance of primary pharmacotherapy, (4) symptoms plus QTc >550 ms (particularly in LQT2 women), and (5) LQT3 genotype (debatable).

In general, a single lead ICD system is preferred unless pacing is required. Conversely, there is probably very little role for a pacemaker as an only device therapy. In most instances, if a pacemaker is contemplated for therapy, then a dual chamber PM/ICD should be utilized instead. A left cardiac sympathetic denervation (LCSD) involving the surgical ablation of the lower half of the left stellate ganglion along with the left-sided thoracic ganglia T2 to T4 is indicated in patients receiving recurrent ventricular fibrillation (VF)-terminating ICD therapies (Moss and McDonald, 1971). LCSD could also be considered for the patients with a pharmacotherapeutic breakthrough event or as a "bridge to ICD" for those patients, such as infants and children, deemed at high risk for the disease but also at high risk for ICD-related complications. According to the 2005 Bethesda Conference #36 guidelines, competitive sports are restricted (except class IA activities of golf, cricket, bowling, billiards, and riflery) in all patients with symptomatic LQTS (except possibly LQT3) (Zipes et al., 2005). This competitive sports restriction may be loosened for patients with concealed LQTS (genotype positive but asymptomatic with QTc < 480 ms females/470 ms males).

Autosomal Recessive (Jervell and Lange-Nielsen) LQTS

In contrast to Romano-Ward LQTS, autosomal recessive LQTS (Jervell and Lange-Nielsen syndrome, JLNS) is extremely rare affecting 1 per million. The cardiac phenotype is generally more severe and in fact, primary prevention beta blocker plus ICD therapy or beta blocker plus LCSD therapy is clinically indicated for JLNS. Pathogenetically, JLNS involves homozygous or compound heterozygous ("double hits") mutations in

the I_{Ks} potassium channel (Table 7–1). Type 1 JLNS (JLN1) arises from such double mutations in KCNQ1 (i.e., LQT1) whereas type 2 JLNS (JLN2) stems from double mutations in KCNE1 (LQT5). These genes encode respectively the alpha subunit and the beta subunit of the critical phase 3 repolarizing potassium current, I_{Ks}. By definition, both parents of a child with JLNS are obligate-affected individuals with either LQT1 or LQT5. That is, the cardiac phenotype in JLNS is a dominant trait although the parents generally have an asymptomatic course and minimal, if any, manifest QT prolongation. In contrast, the deafness is a recessive trait. This same I_{Ks} potassium channel is critical for potassium homeostasis of the endolymph in inner ear.

Multisystem or Complex LQTS

Andersen-Tawil syndrome (ATS) is a multisystem disorder that includes skeletal and facial features, periodic paralysis, and abnormal cardiac repolarization. Loss-of-function mutations involving the KCNJ2-encoded inwardly rectifying potassium channel (Kir2.1) is implicated in the pathogenesis of at least 50% of ATS (Table 7–1) (Plaster et al., 2001). Unlike the classical forms of LQTS, however, the abnormal repolarization in ATS1 is better characterized as normal QT interval, prolonged QU intervals, with long duration U waves (Figure 7–1C) (Zhang et al., 2005). The incidence of sudden death is reportedly less in ATS then the major subtypes of LQTS.

Timothy syndrome (TS) is a rare multisystem disorder that includes abnormal cardiac repolarization, syncope, and sudden death, as well as syndactyly and significant learning disability. Mutations in the alpha subunit of the L-type calcium channel ($Ca_V1.2$) encoded by CACNA1C, particularly a specific missense mutation G406R, have been identified (Splawski et al., 2004). The mutation results in near complete loss of voltage-dependent channel inactivation of $Ca_V1.2$, producing QT prolongation secondary to increased calcium influx (i.e., gain-of-function phenotype). Although extremely rare, TS is associated with a very severe phenotype and primary prevention ICD therapy is probably indicated. Genetic testing for both ATS and TS remain largely confined to research laboratories.

Acquired LQTS

Besides mutant cardiac channels or cardiac ChIPs, abnormal cardiac repolarization, QT prolongation, and even TdP can result from numerous medical conditions (pheochromocytoma, anorexia, diabetes, hypertrophic cardiomyopathy to name just a few), electrolyte derangements particularly hypokalemia, and by over

TABLE 7-4. *Common Medications (Listed Alphabetically) Known to Prolong the QT Interval and Potentially Cause Torsades de Pointes (For a complete list see: [www.torsades.org or www.qtdrugs.org])*

Antiarrhythmias
Amiodarone (QT prolongation common, TdP extremely rare)
Dofetilide
Procainamide
Quinidine (QT prolongation common, 5%–10% prevalence of drug-induced TdP)
Sotalol

Antihistamines
Astemizole (withdrawn)
Terfenadine (withdrawn)

Antimicrobials
Azithromycin
Erythromycin
Gatifloxacin
Levofloxacin
Moxifloxacin

Psychotropics
Haloperidol
Phenothiazine
Thioridazine
Tricyclic antidepressants

Motility Agents
Cisapride (withdrawn)
Domperidone

Narcotics
Methadone

50 FDA-approved medications that can affect the QT interval (Roden, 2000). In fact, QT liability and drug-induced TdP (DI-TdP)/sudden death have been one of the most common reasons for drug withdrawal over the past 15 years (terfenadine, astemizole, propulcid, grepafloxacin, for example) (Fitzgerald and Ackerman, 2005). An Internet resource with an updated list of drugs exhibiting potential "QT liability" is maintained at the University of Arizona (www.torsades.org or www.qtdrugs.org). A list of common medications that can precipitate QT prolongation and possibly drug-induced TdP is provided in Table 7–4. The most potent QT-prolonging medications are the antiarrhythmic agents, particularly amiodarone, dofetilide, quinidine, and sotalol. While QT prolongation is extremely common with amiodarone, drug-induced TdP rarely occurs. In contrast, the drug with the most torsadogenic potential is probably quinidine.

The mechanism for the vast majority of potential QT-prolonging medications is pharmacological inhibition of the *KCNH2*-encoded HERG potassium channel. Thus, DI-TdP and LQT2 are partially phenocopies stemming from either pharmacologically or

genetically mediated perturbations in the I_{Kr} potassium channel. In fact, an estimated 10% of patients with DI-TdP actually possess quiescent LQTS-susceptibility mutations (Yang et al., 2002). An adverse drug reaction could be the sentinel event disclosing the presence of genetic LQTS. Presently, it is debatable whether clinical LQTS molecular genetic testing is indicated for all DI-TdP. At minimum, a careful personal and family history should be obtained as well as consideration for ECG screening of first degree relatives. In DI-TdP, management includes discontinuation of the offending medication, intravenous magnesium sulfate, temporary transvenous overdrive pacing, and isoproterenol infusion. These strategies are aimed to prevent the pause-dependent or bradycardia-associated triggering mechanism for DI-TdP.

Short QT Syndrome

In contrast to LQTS clinically described nearly 50 years ago, short QT syndrome (SQTS) is a relative newcomer with clinical descriptions first published in 2000 (Gussak et al., 2000). To date, there are three genetic subtypes of SQTS, each representing the antithesis of loss-of-function, potassium channel–mediated LQTS and ATS (Bellocq et al., 2004; Brugada et al., 2004; Priori et al., 2005). Instead, the 3 SQTS subtypes stem from gain-of-function mutations in *KCNH2*, *KCNQ1*, and *KCNJ2* (Table 7–1). These mutant potassium channels accelerate cardiac repolarization.

Electrocardiographically, the characteristic ECG finding is a short QT interval (QTc < 320 ms), with tall, symmetrical, peaked T-waves (Figure 7–1D). Clinically, these patients present with sudden death, syncope, palpitations, and sometimes paroxysmal atrial fibrillation. The age at which sudden death occurs varies greatly from 3 months to 70 years. Most patients have a family history of sudden death, with probable autosomal-dominant inheritance. The degree of incomplete penetrance, variable expressivity, and overall prevalence of SQTS are poorly understood. However, SQTS is felt to be much less common than LQTS and examples of family members who are genotype positive for a SQTS-associated mutation but a normal resting QT interval have been reported.

Most of these patients have easily inducible ventricular fibrillation during electrophysiological studies with revealed short atrial and ventricular refractory periods. The therapy of choice is implantation of an ICD. However, these patients are at increased risk of inappropriate therapies from T wave oversensing. ICD detection algorithms may decrease the risk of inappropriate shocks. Adjunctive pharmacotherapy with propafenone or quinidine may help prolong the QT interval and decrease the potential for VF.

Catecholaminergic Polymorphic Ventricular Tachycardia

Catecholaminergic polymorphic ventricular tachycardia (CPVT) is characterized by exercise-/stress-induced syncope and/or sudden death in the setting of a structurally normal heart with a normal QT interval (Leenhardt et al., 1995). CPVT clinically mimics concealed type 1 LQTS but is far more malignant than concealed (normal QT interval) LQTS. In fact, 3%–4% of patients referred for LQTS genetic testing actually hosted CPVT-associated mutations (Tester et al., 2005). Initially, CPVT was described in children, but more recent studies suggest that the age at presentation can vary from infancy to 40 years. In one-third of patients with CPVT, there is a family history positive for juvenile sudden death (Priori et al., 2002). The hallmark electrocardiographic feature of CPVT is exercise-/isoproterenol-induced ventriculary arrhythmias, particularly bidirectional VT (Figure 7–1E). However, bidirectional VT during exercise has been reported in ATS and LQTS. Nevertheless, a patient with a history of exertional syncope, normal QT interval at rest, and exercise-induced ventricular ectopy is far more likely to have CPVT than LQTS.

In contrast to the QT-opathies, the pathogenic substrates for CPVT involve key components of intracellular calcium-induced calcium release from the sarcoplasmic reticulum (Table 7–1). Type 1 CPVT (CPVT1) stems from mutations in the RYR2-encoded cardiac ryanodine receptor or calcium release channel and account for an estimated 50%–60% of CPVT (Laitinen et al., 2001; Prioriet al., 2001). Mutations in RYR2 confer a gain-of-function phenotype to the calcium release channel, resulting in increased calcium leak during sympathetic stimulation, particularly in diastole. In contrast to the autosomal dominant/sporadic CPVT1, CPVT2 is autosomal recessive, very rare, and is due to mutations in CASQ2-encoded calsequestrin (Lahat et al., 2001; Postma et al., 2002). Mutations in KCNJ2, the same gene for both ATS and SQTS, may also contribute to CPVT (Tester et al., 2006). Together, LQTS/CPVT-producing mutations provided a potential explanation for approximately 10% of sudden infant death syndrome and one-third of autopsy-negative sudden death after the first year of life (Ackerman et al., 2001; Arnestad et al., 2007; Tester and Ackerman, 2007; Tester et al., 2007). In 2008, CPVT genetic testing became a clinically available diagnostic test in North America with a targeted examination of < 40% of RYR2's 105 translated exons that host the vast majority of CPVT-associated mutations in RYR2. This genetic test would be expected to be positive in over half of the clinically robust cases of CPVT. Patients with symptomatic CPVT should be considered for either an ICD or LCSD as pharmacotherapy with either beta blockers or calcium channel blockers appears less protective in CPVT compared to LQT1 (Priori et al., 2002).

Brugada Syndrome

The BrS is characterized by typical ECG findings of coved-type ST elevation (type 1 BrS ECG, Figure 7–1F) in the right precordial leads (V1–3) in the presence or absence of incomplete or complete right bundle branch block morphology, and an increased risk of sudden death (Brugada and Brugada, 1992). The prevalence of a spontaneous Brugada ECG pattern in the general population is estimated to range from 0.05% to 0.6%. The characterization of a coved type ST elevation (type I ECG) or saddle back ST segment elevation (type II ECG) reflects distinct differences in the risk of sudden death. Overall, the saddle back type of ST elevation is more common in the general population and less specific for BrS.

In contrast, in patients that present with symptomatic Brugada syndrome, both in Europe and Japan, the majority have a coved type ST elevation (Antzelevitch et al., 2005). This type I ECG pattern may be present at rest or when unmasked with class I sodium channel blockers including ajmaline, flecainide, or procainamide. Provocative testing with class I antiarrhythmic agents is used strictly for diagnosis and is of no prognostic value. Superior performance with ajmaline during provocative testing has been demonstrated but this medication is not available in the United States. Increased sensitivity with the resting ECG is achieved by placing the right precordial leads of V1 thru V3 in the second intercostal space.

Patients are more often male, and often present symptomatically with sudden cardiac death due to ventricular fibrillation or with syncope due to polymorphic ventricular tachycardia. The age of diagnosis is variable, ranging from 2 months to 77 years, with a mean of approximately 40 years. In patients diagnosed with idiopathic ventricular fibrillation (IVF) initially, up to 20% have BrS. An estimated 10%–20% of patients with BrS also have atrial fibrillation.

In contrast to LQT3, which is due to gain-of-function mutations involving the SCN5A-encoded cardiac sodium channel $Na_V 1.5$, 20%–30% of BrS is due to loss-of-function mutations in SCN5A (BrS1, Table 7–1) (Chen et al., 1998; Vatta et al., 2002). To date, nearly 100 BrS1-causing mutations have been identified in SCN5A. Over the past two years, five novel BrS-susceptibility genes, GPD1L, CACNA1C, CACNB2, SCN1B, and KCNE3, have been identified (Table 7–1) (Antzelevitch et al., 2007; Delpon et al., 2008; Hiroshi et al., 2008; London et al., 2007). GPD1L-, SCN1B-, and *KCNE3*-BrS appear to be extremely uncommon (<1% frequency for each) and thus no meaningful genotype–phenotype relationships exist at this point. BrS secondary to dysregulation of the L-type calcium channel complex is more common (~10%). For the most part, there is no apparent difference in clinical outcome in patients with BrS1 versus the majority with *SCN5A*-negative BrS. Patients with BrS1 tend to have longer HV intervals. Genetic testing is available commercially for BrS bearing in mind the a priori yield of approximately 20% and its principal role in identifying asymptomatic carriers since there is less of a role in prognosis or treatment decisions.

The outcome of patients with BrS depends strongly on the presence/absence of symptoms and the spontaneous presence of a type I BrS ECG pattern. In patients who present with aborted sudden death, nearly two-thirds had documented ventricular fibrillation or sudden death in a 4.5-year follow-up period. In comparison, only 19% of patients who presented with syncope had ventricular fibrillation or sudden death. This percentage further decreased to 8% in asymptomatic patients. Therefore, all symptomatic patients (either ACA or syncope) with Brugada syndrome should be recommended an ICD (Antzelevitch et al., 2005).

The role of programmed electrical stimulation (PES) during an EPS in the risk stratification of asymptomatic individuals remains sharply debated (Brugada et al., 2003; Eckardt et al., 2005; Priori et al., 2002). Proponents of PES-EPS would advise ICD therapy as primary prevention in the asymptomatic patient with inducible VF whereas opponents suggest that there is no role for an EPS in the evaluation of BrS. Besides ICD therapy as secondary prevention, there may be a role for quinidine in the patient experiencing recurrent VF-terminating ICD therapies (Belhassen et al., 2004). Aggressive management of febrile illnesses is warranted as fever appears to be an arrhythmic trigger for patients with BrS (Antzelevitch and Brugada, 2002; Saura et al., 2002).

Summary of Class I/II Indications for ICD in Cardiac Channelopathies

Secondary Prevention
- History of aborted cardiac arrest (regardless of channelopathy)
- History of syncope in SQTS, CPVT, and BrS

Primary Prevention
- Failed pharmacotherapy in LQTS or CPVT (includes breakthrough syncopal episode or beta blocker intolerance)
- Jervell and Lange-Nielsen syndrome
- Asymptomatic LQTS with QTc >550 ms (regardless of genotype)

Controversial/Debatable Indications
- LQT2 with QTc >500 ms (particularly females)
- LQT3
- Asymptomatic/Genotype positive CPVT
- Asymptomatic BrS with inducible VF during PES-EPS

REFERENCES

Ackerman MJ, Khositseth A, Tester DJ, Hejlik J, Shen WK, Porter CJ. Epinephrine-induced QT interval prolongation: a gene-specific paradoxical response in congenital long QT syndrome. *Mayo Clin Proc.* 2002;77:413–421.

Ackerman MJ, Siu BL, Sturner WQ, et al. Postmortem molecular analysis of SCN5A defects in sudden infant death syndrome. *JAMA.* 2001;286(18):2264–2269.

Ackerman MJ, Tester DJ, Porter CJ. Swimming, a gene-specific arrhythmogenic trigger for inherited long QT syndrome. *Mayo Clin Proc.* 1999;74(11):1088–1094.

Antzelevitch C, Brugada R. Fever and Brugada syndrome. *Pacing Clin Electrophysiol.* 2002;25(11):1537–1539.

Antzelevitch C, Brugada P, Borggrefe M, et al.. Brugada syndrome: report of the second consensus conference. *Heart Rhythm.* 2005;2(4):429–440.

Antzelevitch C, Pollevick GD, Cordeiro JM, et al. Loss-of-function mutations in the cardiac calcium channel underlie a new clinical entity characterized by ST-segment elevation, short QT intervals, and sudden cardiac death. *Circulation.* 2007;115(4):442–449.

Arnestad M, Crotti L, Rognum TO, et al. Prevalence of long-QT syndrome gene variants in sudden infant death syndrome. *Circulation.* 2007;115(3):361–367.

Belhassen B, Glick A, Viskin S. efficacy of quinidine in high-risk patients with Brugada Syndrome 10.1161/01.CIR.0000143159.30585.90. *Circulation.* 2004;110(13):1731–1737.

Bellocq C, van Ginneken AC, Bezzina CR, et al. Mutation in the KCNQ1 gene leading to the short QT-interval syndrome. *Circulation.* 2004;109(20):2394–2397.

Brugada J, Brugada R, Brugada P. Determinants of sudden cardiac death in individuals with the electrocardiographic pattern of Brugada Syndrome and no previous cardiac arrest 10.1161/01.CIR.0000104568.13957.4F. *Circulation.* 2003;108(25):3092–3096.

Brugada R, Hong K, Dumaine R, et al. Sudden death associated with short-QT syndrome linked mutations in HERG. *Circulation.* 2004;109:30–35.

Chen L, Marquardt ML, Tester DJ, Sampson KJ, Ackerman MJ, Kass RS. Mutation of an A-kinase-anchoring protein causes long-QT syndrome. *Proc Natl Acad Sci.* 2007;104(52):20990–20995.

Chen Q, Kirsch GE, Zhang D, et al. Genetic basis and molecular mechanism for idiopathic ventricular fibrillation. *Nature.* 1998;392(6673):293–296.

Curran ME, Splawski I, Timothy KW, Vincent GM, Green ED, Keating MT. A molecular basis for cardiac arrhythmia: HERG mutations cause long QT syndrome. *Cell.* 1995;80(5):795–803.

Delpon E, Cordeiro JM, Nunez L, et al. functional effects of KCNE3 mutation and its role in the development of Brugada Syndrome 10.1161/CIRCEP.107.748103. *Circ Arrhythmia Electrophysiol.* 2008:CIRCEP.107.748103.

Eckardt L, Probst V, Smits JPP, et al. Long-term prognosis of individuals with right precordial st-segment-elevation Brugada Syndrome 10.1161/01.CIR.0000153267.21278.8D. *Circulation.* 2005;111(3):257–263.

Fitzgerald PT, Ackerman MJ. Drug-induced torsades de pointes: the evolving role of pharmacogenetics. *Heart Rhythm.* 2005;2:S30–S37.

Gussak I, Brugada P, Brugada J, et al. Idiopathic short qt interval: a new clinical syndrome? *Cardiology.* 2000;94(2):99–102.

Hiroshi Watanabe TTK, Solena Le Scouarnec, Tao Yang, et al. Sodium channel ß1 subunit mutations associated with Brugada syndrome and cardiac conduction disease in humans. *J Clin Invest.* 2008;118:2260–2268.

Hobbs JB, Peterson DR, Moss AJ, et al. Risk of aborted cardiac arrest or sudden cardiac death during adolescence in the long-QT syndrome. *JAMA.* 2006;296(10):1249–1254.

Jervell A, Lange-Nielsen F. Congenital deaf-mutism, functional heart disease with prolongation of the QT interval, and sudden death. *Am Heart J.* 1957;54:59–68.

Khositseth A, Tester DJ, Will ML, Bell CM, Ackerman MJ. Identification of a common genetic substrate underlying postpartum cardiac events in congenital long QT syndrome. *Heart Rhythm.* 2004;1:60–64.

Lahat H, Eldar M, Levy-Nissenbaum E, et al. Autosomal recessive catecholamine- or exercise-induced polymorphic ventricular tachycardia: clinical features and assignment of the disease gene to chromosome 1p13–21. *Circulation.* 2001;103:2822–2827.

Laitinen PJ, Brown KM, Piippo K, et al. Mutations of the cardiac ryanodine receptor (RyR2) gene in familial polymorphic ventricular tachycardia. *Circulation.* 2001;103(4):485–490.

Leenhardt A, Lucet V, Denjoy I, et al. Catecholaminergic polymorphic ventricular tachycardia in children: a 7-year follow-up of 21 patients. *Circulation.* 1995;91:1512–1519.

London B, Michalec M, Mehdi H, et al. Mutation in Glycerol-3-Phosphate Dehydrogenase 1 like gene (gpd1-l) decreases cardiac na+ current and causes inherited arrhythmias. *Circulation.* 2007;116(20):2260–2268.

Mohler PJ, Schott J-J, Gramolini AO, et al. Ankyrin-B mutation causes type 4 long-QT cardiac arrhythmia and sudden cardiac death. *Nature.* 2003;421:634–639.

Moss AJ, McDonald J. Unilateral cervicothoracic sympathetic ganglionectomy for the treatment of long QT interval syndrome. *N Engl J Med.* 1971;285(16):903–904.

Moss AJ, Robinson JL, Gessman L, et al. Comparison of clinical and genetic variables of cardiac events associated with loud noise versus swimming among subjects with the long QT syndrome. *Am J Cardiol.* 1999;84(8):876–879.

Moss AJ, Windle JR, Hall WJ, et al. Safety and efficacy of flecainide in subjects with Long QT-3 syndrome (DeltaKPQ mutation): a randomized, double-blind, placebo-controlled clinical trial. *Ann Noninvasive Electrocardiol.* 2005;10(suppl 4):59–66.

Moss AJ, Zareba W, Benhorin J, et al. ECG T-wave patterns in genetically distinct forms of the hereditary long QT syndrome. *Circulation.* 1995;92(10):2929–2934.

Moss AJ, Zareba W, Hall WJ, et al. Effectiveness and limitations of beta-blocker therapy in congenital long-QT syndrome. *Circulation.* 2000;101(6):616–623.

Olson TM, Michels VV, Ballew JD, et al. Sodium channel mutations and susceptibility to heart failure and atrial fibrillation. *JAMA.* 2005;293:447–454.

Plaster NM, Tawil R, Tristani-Firouzi M, et al. Mutations in Kir2.1 cause the developmental and episodic electrical phenotypes of Andersen's syndrome. *Cell.* 2001;105(4):511–519.

Postma AV, Denjoy I, Hoorntje TM, et al. Absence of calsequestrin 2 causes severe forms of catecholaminergic polymorphic ventricular tachycardia. *Circ Res.* 2002;91(8):e21–26.

Priori SG, Napolitano C, Gasparini M, et al. Natural history of Brugada syndrome: insights for risk stratification and management. *Circulation.* 2002;105:1342–1347.

Priori SG, Napolitano C, Memmi M, et al. Clinical and molecular characterization of patients with catecholaminergic polymorphic ventricular tachycardia. [see comment]. *Circulation.* 2002;106(1):69–74.

Priori SG, Napolitano C, Schwartz PJ. Low penetrance in the long-QT syndrome: clinical impact. *Circulation.* 1999;99(4): 529–533.

Priori SG, Napolitano C, Tiso N, et al. Mutations in the cardiac ryanodine receptor gene (hRyR2) underlie catecholaminergic polymorphic ventricular tachycardia. *Circulation.* 2001;103(2):196–200.

Priori SG, Pandit SV, Rivolta I, et al. A novel form of short QT syndrome (SQT3) is caused by a mutation in the KCNJ2 gene. *Circ Res.* 2005;96(7):800–807.

Priori SG, Schwartz PJ, Napolitano C, et al. Risk stratification in the long-QT syndrome. *N Engl J Med.* 2003;348:1866–1874.

Roden DM. Acquired long QT syndromes and the risk of proarrhythmia. *J Cardiovasc Electrophysiol.* 2000;11(8):938–940.

Romano C, Gemme G, Pongiglione R. Aritmie cardiache rare dell'eta'pediatrica. II. Accessi sincopali per fibrillazione ventricolare parossistica. *Clin Peditr (Bologna).* 1963;45:656–683.

Saura D, Garcia-Alberola A, Carrillo P, Pascual D, Martinez-Sanchez J, Valdes M. Brugada-like electrocardiographic pattern induced by fever. *Pacing Clin Electrophysiol.* 2002;25(5):856–859.

Schwartz PJ, Moss AJ, Vincent GM, Crampton RS. Diagnostic criteria for the long QT syndrome. An update. *Circulation.* 1993;88(2):782–784.

Schwartz PJ, Priori SG, Cerrone M, et al. Left cardiac sympathetic denervation in the management of high-risk patients affected by the long-QT syndrome. *Circulation.* 2004;109(15):1826–1833.

Schwartz PJ, Priori SG, Locati EH, et al. Long QT syndrome patients with mutations of the SCN5A and HERG genes have differential responses to Na+ channel blockade and to increases in heart rate. Implications for gene-specific therapy. *Circulation.* 1995;92(12):3381–3386.

Schwartz PJ, Priori SG, Spazzolini C, et al. Genotype-phenotype correlation in the long-QT syndrome: gene-specific triggers for life-threatening arrhythmias. *Circulation.* 2001;103:89–95.

Shimizu W, Noda T, Takaki H, et al. Epinephrine unmasks latent mutation carriers with LQT1 form of congenital long-QT syndrome. *J Am Coll Cardiol.* 2003;41:633–642.

Splawski I, Shen J, Timothy KW, et al. Spectrum of mutations in long-QT syndrome genes. KVLQT1, HERG, SCN5A, KCNE1, and KCNE2. *Circulation.* 2000;102(10):1178–1185.

Splawski I, Timothy KW, Sharpe LM, et al. Cav1.2 calcium channel dysfunction causes a multisystem disorder including arrhythmia and autism. *Cell.* 2004;119:19–31.

Tester DJ, Ackerman MJ. Postmortem long QT syndrome genetic testing for sudden unexplained death in the young. *J Am Coll Cardiol.* 2007;49(2):240–246.

Tester DJ, Arya P, Will M, et al. Genotypic heterogeneity and phenotypic mimicry among unrelated patients referred for catecholaminergic polymorphic ventricular tachycardia genetic testing. *Heart Rhythm.* 3(7):800–5, 2006.

Tester DJ, Dura M, Carturan E, et al. A mechanism for sudden infant death syndrome (SIDS): stress-induced leak via ryanodine receptors. *Heart Rhythm.* 2007;4(6):733–739.

Tester DJ, Kopplin LJ, Will ML, Ackerman MJ. Spectrum and prevalence of cardiac ryanodine receptor (RyR2) mutations in a cohort of unrelated patients referred explicitly for long QT syndrome genetic testing. *Heart Rhythm.* 2005;2(10):1099–1105.

Tester DJ, Will ML, Haglund CM, Ackerman MJ. Compendium of cardiac channel mutations in 541 consecutive unrelated patients referred for long QT syndrome genetic testing. *Heart Rhythm.* 2005;2(5):507–517.

Tester DJ, Will ML, Haglund CM, Ackerman MJ. Effect of clinical phenotype on yield of long QT syndrome genetic testing. *J Am Coll Cardiol.* 2006;47(4):764–768.

Ueda K, Valdivia C, Medeiros-Domingo A, et al. Syntrophin mutation associated with long QT syndrome through activation of the nNOS-SCN5A macromolecular complex. *Proc Natl Acad Sci.* 2008;105:9355–9360.

Vatta M, Ackerman MJ, Ye B, et al. Mutant caveolin-3 induces persistent late sodium current and is associated with long-QT syndrome. *Circulation.* 2006;114(20):2104–2112.

Vatta M, Dumaine R, Varghese G, et al. Genetic and biophysical basis of sudden unexplained nocturnal death syndrome (SUNDS), a disease allelic to Brugada syndrome. *Hum Mol Genet.* 2002;11:337–345.

Villain E, Denjoy I, Lupoglazoff JM, et al. Low incidence of cardiac events with B-blocking therapy in children with long QT syndrome. *Eur Heart J.* 2004;25:1405–1411.

Vincent GM, Jaiswal D, Timothy KW. Effects of exercise on heart rate, QT, QTc and QT/QS2 in the Romano-Ward inherited long QT syndrome. *Am J Cardiol.* 1991;68(5):498–503.

Viskin S, Rosovski U, Sands AJ, et al. Inaccurate electrocardiographic interpretation of long QT: the majority of physicians cannot recognize a long QT when they see one. *Heart Rhythm.* 2005;2(6):569–574.

Vyas H, Hejlik J, Ackerman MJ. Epinephrine QT stress testing in the evaluation of congenital long-QT syndrome: diagnostic accuracy of the paradoxical QT response. *Circulation.* 2006;113(11):1385–1392.

Wang Q, Shen J, Splawski I, et al. SCN5A mutations associated with an inherited cardiac arrhythmia, long QT syndrome. *Cell.* 1995;80(5):805–811.

Ward OC. A new familial cardiac syndrome in children. *J Irish Med Assoc.* 1964;54:103–106.

Wilde AA, Jongbloed RJ, Doevendans PA, et al. Auditory stimuli as a trigger for arrhythmic events differentiate HERG- related (LQTS2) patients from KVLQT1-related patients (LQTS1). *J Am Coll Cardiol.* 1999;33(2):327–332.

Yang P, Kanki H, Drolet B, et al. Allelic variants in long-QT disease genes in patients with drug-associated torsades de pointes. *Circulation.* 2002;105(16):1943–1948.

Zhang L, Benson W, Tristani-Firouzi M, et al. Electrocardiographic features in Andersen-Tawil syndrome patients with KCNJ2 mutations: characteristic T-U-wave patterns predict the KCNJ2 genotype. *Circulation.* 2005;111:2720–2726.

Zhang L, Timothy KW, Vincent GM, et al. Spectrum of ST-T-wave patterns and repolarization parameters in congenital long-QT syndrome: ECG findings identify genotypes. *Circulation.* 2000;102(23):2849–2855.

Zipes DP, Ackerman MJ, Estes NAr, Grant AO, Myerburg RJ, Van Hare G. Task Force 7: arrhythmias. *J Am Coll Cardiol.* 2005;45:1354–1363.

8

The Practice of Perinatal Cardiology

LISA K. HORNBERGER
STEPHEN G. MILLER

INTRODUCTION

Fetal and perinatal cardiology is an evolving practice with growing experience in the detection, natural intrauterine history, perinatal management, and outcome of structural, functional, and rhythm-related fetal heart disease. While the initial description of imaging of the fetal heart by B mode was published in 1972 (Winsberg, 1972), the foundation of two-dimensional (2-D) fetal echocardiography was established a decade later with documentation of normal fetal cardiac anatomy and growth, and initial descriptions of fetal cardiovascular pathology (Allan et al., 1980; Huhta et al., 1984; Kleinman et al., 1982, 1983; Lange et al., 1980; Sahn et al., 1980). Significant improvements in technology that have occurred over the past two decades, implementation of the four-chamber view in routine obstetrical ultrasound resulting in improved prenatal detection rates, further clinical experience, and recognition of the critical importance of collaboration between the subspecialties involved in the management of pregnant women have resulted in an ability to fine-tune the diagnosis of structural, functional, and rhythm-related fetal cardiovascular disorders and importantly improve the outcome of affected pregnancies.

Currently, introduction into fetal and perinatal cardiology is typically through fetal echocardiography which excludes or documents primary or secondary fetal cardiovascular pathology. When no fetal cardiac pathology is detected, reassurance is provided to the pregnant woman with or without plans for future assessments. When fetal cardiovascular pathology is identified, the pregnant woman or the couple is counseled regarding potential outcomes and pregnancy options; need for further testing, such as amniocentesis and comprehensive fetal ultrasound examination, is considered; and decisions are made regarding need for prenatal intervention, and the most appropriate perinatal and neonatal management.

Pregnant women are referred for fetal echocardiography when the fetus is at risk for structural or functional fetal heart disease or where a fetal dysrhythmia is suspected. Reasons for referral can be divided into three groups: maternal, fetal, and familial indications. Maternal indications include maternal metabolic disease such as type I or II diabetes and phenylketonuria, maternal congenital heart disease, and teratogen exposure (e.g., vitamin A derivatives, lithium and valproate). Fetal indications include the finding of fetal cardiac pathology at routine or level II fetal ultrasound, findings of extracardiac pathology, and chromosomal abnormalities in the fetus that are likely to be associated with prenatally detectable cardiac pathology including increased nuchal translucency in the late first trimester (Hyett et al., 1999; McAuliffe et al., 1486; Pandya et al., 1994), fetal dysrhythmia, and nonimmune hydrops. Finally familial indications include the history of a previously affected child or fetus, paternal heart disease, and genetic syndromes including tuberous sclerosis, Noonan, Ellis van Creveld, and DiGeorge syndromes.

While a large number of referrals for fetal echocardiography in most cardiology practices are assessed as a result of maternal and familial indications, in fact 85%–95% of pregnancies that are found to have fetal heart disease are referred as a result of a fetal indication, largely where a cardiac defect is suspected from a routine obstetrical ultrasound screening most often in low-risk pregnancies or where an extracardiac defect is identified (Sharland et al., 1991). As such the routine midtrimester fetal ultrasound screening, which is currently performed in most areas in North America and internationally in the majority of women, plays a critical role in the prenatal detection of cardiac defects. In general, fetal echocardiography, used as a screening method for at risk pregnancies, is often performed at 17–22 weeks of pregnancy. As the routine ultrasound screenings are typically performed in the same time period, referral for fetal echo where a fetal heart problem is suspected is often within the same period or within a few weeks of the initial ultrasound that suggests an abnormality. Unfortunately, though, many fetal heart defects are not identified until the late second or third trimester usually as a result of missed pathology at an earlier screening and rarely as a result of significant progression in the cardiac pathology from the time of an earlier screening. Finally in a few centers, fetal echocardiography may be provided prior to 17 weeks of pregnancy with the use of both transabdominal and transvaginal ultrasound approaches (Achiron et al., 1994; Bronshtein et al., 2002; Huggon et al., 2002; Mcauliffe et al., 2005).

BASIC FETAL ECHOCARDIOGRAM

Performing a fetal echocardiogram (ECG) requires consideration of the normal cardiac anatomy and function and unique aspects of the fetal circulation. Given the diminutive size of the fetal cardiovascular structures, a high frequency transducer (>5 MHz) is necessary in most cases. Lower frequencies may be helpful in certain instances to optimize Doppler interrogation. Image resolution can be optimized by maintaining high frame rates using the depth control, decreasing the sector width, positioning the focal zone, and choosing high-definition zoom features. Frame averaging options or persistence should be off or on low, in contrast to what is commonly used in general fetal anatomical surveys. A compress setting allowing for a narrow dynamic range (gray scale) has better sensitivity and defines the blood–tissue interfaces. Harmonic imaging can reduce image artifacts, haze and clutter, as well as increase contrast resolution and improve border delineation. Use of harmonic imaging can be very useful in the more challenging patients.

Guidelines for the performance of a fetal ECG have been established within the past 5 years through the American Society of Echocardiography (Rychik et al., 2004). Table 8–1 provides a list of the details of assessment in a thorough fetal ECG investigation. Determining fetal position, including the right–left, anterior–posterior, and superior–inferior orientation, is a critical first step in a fetal ECG. Once the fetal orientation is clear, evaluation of the fetal heart requires a somewhat creative approach as the standard postnatal

TABLE 8–1. *Fetal Echocardiographic Assessment—The Screen*

2-D Images
Visceral Situs
  Liver largely to the fetal right
  Stomach to the fetal left with spleen behind
  Sweep to the heart demonstrating levocardia
Cross-sectional/Axial Images
  IVC anterior and right of descending Ao and connecting to the RA
  Descending Ao anterior and to the left of the spine
  Four chamber view
    Cardiac axis 40 degrees
    Cardiac size- 1/3 the size of the thorax
    Cardiac position—levocardia but with RA to the right of the midline (no shift in cardiac position that could suggest extracardiac/ intrathoracic pathology)
  Pulmonary veins at least one right and one left connecting to the LA
  Foramen ovale with normal leftward billowing of septum primum towards the LA
  Tricuspid and mitral valves with offset, tricuspid valve with septal attachments and opening of the mitral valve towards the LV free wall
  RV and LV morphology, symmetry* and systolic function
  Intact ventricular septum (preferably perpendicular to the plane of the septum)
  Sweeps to the outflow tracts
    Thin normal appearing aortic and pulmonary valves
    LV to aorta and RV to pulmonary artery
    Crossing of the great arteries
    Symmetry
    3 vessel view demonstrating the main PA, aorta and SVC
  Cross-sectional image of the ductus arteriosus and aortic arches with normal relationship
  Both branch PAs

Sagital Images
  IVC and SVC connections to the right atrium
  Sweep towards the ventricular apex demonstrating the atria, atrial septum, AV valves, ventricles and outlets
  Long axis of the aortic and ductal arches
  LV and RV shortening fraction (if ruling out dysfunction)

Doppler Assessment
Color Doppler Ventricular Inlows, Outflows and Arches
Pulsed Doppler
  Mitral valve
  Pulmonary outflow
  IVC or hepatic vein
  Umbilical artery
  Tricuspid valve
  Ductus arteriosus
  Ductus venosus
  Aortic outflow
  1–2 pulmonary veins
  Umbilical vein

* Early in gestation the left and right heart structures are symmetric. later in gestation, however, mild asymmetry with dominant right heart structures is the norm.

views are not always feasible, and acoustic windows may be limited.

Doppler assessment is often performed throughout the study, however, as is true in many cases after birth, anatomical details may be missed if one is too eager to use either color or pulsed Doppler. Pulsed and color Doppler confirm the patency of the ventricular inflows and outflows as well as the arches. Color Doppler assists in the identification of abnormal flows such as valve regurgitation, obstruction, and abnormal direction of flows. Occasionally it may also assist in confirming normal anatomy, especially at earlier gestational ages when the image resolution is suboptimal. Pulsed Doppler should be routinely used to exclude evidence of ventricular diastolic function and elevated central venous pressures, which is poorly tolerated by the more passive umbilical venous return and fetal–placental circulation (Fontes-Pedra et al., 2002). Routine assessment of ventricular inflows, inferior vena caval flow, ductus venosus, and umbilical venous flow patterns in the normal fetuses facilitates the recognition of abnormal flow patterns suggestive of increased central venous pressures which occurs when there is abnormal function of the fetal heart and/or external compression of the heart that may alter ventricular filling and upstream pressures (Figure 8–1). While the majority of fetuses with cardiac pathology have normal placental function, the presence of placental insufficiency can significantly compromise an affected pregnancy. The finding of altered umbilical arterial flow suggestive of placental insufficiency in fetal heart disease should prompt closer observation, including serial fetal ECGs as well as obstetrical testing of fetal well-being, and may necessitate earlier delivery.

Finally pulsed Doppler and M-mode are very useful in the evaluation of the fetal heart rate and rhythm. These modalities, however, are only an indirect means of assessment through ventricular inflow and outflow tracings, or simultaneous superior vena cava and aortic tracings (Doppler), or mechanical contraction of the atria and ventricles (M-mode) (Figure 8–2). Tissue Doppler imaging techniques have recently been found to readily assist in the definition of the mechanisms of fetal dysrhythmias (Rein et al., 2002) and may ultimately contribute to the assessment of ventricular dysfunction.

FETAL CARDIOVASCULAR PATHOLOGY

Structural Heart Defects

The majority of major and most minor structural heart defects can be detected by fetal echocardiography. The pathologies identified prenatally tend to represent a more severe spectrum of heart disease than when encountered postnatally, and also tend to be more often associated with an abnormal four-chamber view such as hypoplastic left heart syndrome (HLHS) and single-ventricle type of lesions (Allan et al., 1985). In general the approach to the evaluation and diagnosis of structural heart defects in utero is similar to the approach after birth in defining as many of the details of the pathology as is possible, particularly those that

have the potential to impact perinatal and postnatal outcome. However, there are many unique aspects to the assessment of structural heart defects in utero. The fetal size and gestational age, orientation of the fetus, maternal habitus, and amniotic fluid levels all contribute to potential limitations in image resolution. One must rely entirely on the fetal echocardiographic assessment to define the pathology and pathophysiology. The fetal circulation with the presence of the foramen ovale and ductus arteriosus, which permit a redistribution of flow, and the presence of similar ventricular systolic pressures make the detection of certain conditions somewhat difficult. Retrograde ductal or aortic arch flows or foramen ovale flows, which are consistent with more critical obstruction (Berning et al., 1996), are not always present particularly at earlier gestational ages. In their absence, one must rely on indirect findings such as discrepancy in ventricular and great artery size, absolute size of structures relative to normal values, and subtle changes in Doppler flow signals. Finally, this information must be immediately presented to the pregnant woman/couple who must make a decision regarding the pregnancy based on the available data.

As with the normal examination, confirmation of fetal position including left–right orientation is critical and may be necessary several times through the examination, as the fetus changes position. Obtaining axial and sagittal images, as well as short-axis and long-axis images of the heart is often necessary. Documentation of the segmental anatomy including visceral and atrial situs, the atrioventricular (AV) connections, and ventricular looping as well as the great artery relationship and ventricular arterial connections should be performed in all cases. With a basic diagnosis, one can begin more detailed assessment of the anatomy that will be critical for perinatal management and outcome. Systemic and pulmonary venous connections, anatomy of the AV and semilunar valves, ventricular outlets, ventricular septal defect size and location, arches, and branch pulmonary arteries should be carefully evaluated. Subtle differences in atrial, ventricular, and great artery size may suggest the presence of an obstruction to filling or flow that cannot be fully appreciated due to the limitations in image resolution, but may become more obvious with a shift in fetal position, later in gestation or even after birth (Figure 8–3). Assumptions, including reliance on what is a more likely finding, may result in inaccurate information being provided at counseling.

Most of the diagnoses can be made through detailed 2-D imaging alone. Much of what is gleaned by spectral and pulsed Doppler can almost always be predicted based on the observations of the anatomy. For instance, with a significantly smaller main pulmonary artery, one can predict many times that there will

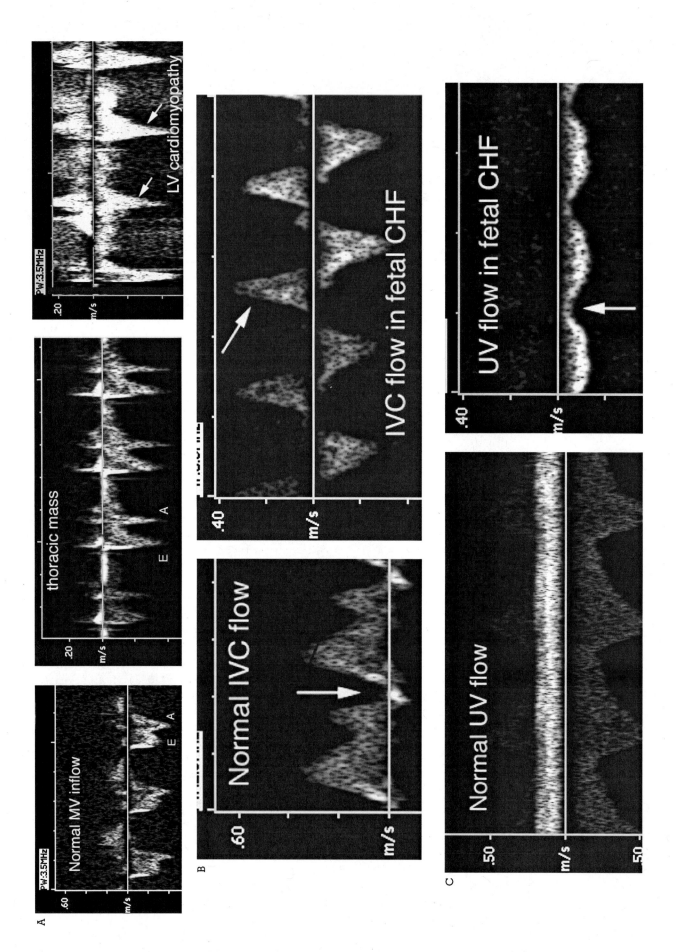

A

Normal MV inflow

thoracic mass

E A

E A

LV cardiomyopathy

B

Normal IVC flow

IVC flow in fetal CHF

C

Normal UV flow

UV flow in fetal CHF

be retrograde ductus arteriosus flow, suggesting more critical pulmonary outflow obstruction. Conversely, when left heart obstruction exists, billowing of the atrial septum toward the right atrium suggests left to right atrial flow. A dilated atrium suggests the presence of either significant AV valve regurgitation or abnormal right heart filling (Hornberger et al., 1994), both of which, for instance, may coexist in pulmonary outflow obstruction with an intact ventricular septum. Confirmation of these abnormal flows solidifies the diagnosis and severity of the condition.

Spectral Doppler assessment is also important for the assessment of function, with documentation of ventricular outputs, ventricular filling abnormalities, and changes in systemic venous and umbilical venous flow patterns that could be predictive of progressive cardiovascular compromise. Continuous-wave Doppler assists in documenting changes in ventricular pressures as well as gradients.

Evaluation of aspects of the cardiovascular pathology and pathophysiology that may compromise the fetus before or immediately after birth is critical for planning of prenatal management and delivery, and for counseling regarding the ultimate outcome of an affected fetus. For instance, identifying a severely restrictive atrial septal defect with evidence of left atrial hypertension as can be documented through pulmonary venous flow patterns will assist in planning the delivery and management of a fetus with HLHS (Figure 8–4) (Taketazu et al., 2004). It is also critical for counseling regarding the grim prognosis, particularly when the diagnosis is made in the second trimester. Documenting the evidence of foramen ovale restriction or ductus arteriosus constriction in the third trimester is important for planning immediate neonatal management in D-transposition of the great arteries (Maeno et al., 1999; Jouannic et al., 2004). Recognition of evolving abnormalities of left heart function using the Tei index, or the presence of progressive pulmonary insufficiency in fetal Ebstein's is important if the goal is to deliver the infant at a viable age before a sudden loss or the evolution of heart failure (Inamura et al., 2004).

There are certain lesions that may be more difficult to detect or exclude given the presence of the fetal circulation and limitations in image resolution. Such lesions include small to moderate-sized ventricular and atrial septal defects, apical muscular ventricular septal defects, minor valve pathology, partial anomalous venous drainage, lesions that may only evolve after birth such as a subaortic membrane, and coronary artery anomalies. There are also lesions that are unique to fetal/perinatal cardiology and such lesions are either never or rarely encountered after birth. These include echogenic focus of the papillary muscles, which are usually benign, ventricular aneurysms, prenatally lethal conditions, and conditions associated with the fetal shunts including agenesis of the ductus venosus, restriction of the foramen ovale, and constriction of even closure of the ductus arteriosus.

Potential for Progression. Most structural fetal heart defects have the potential to progress or evolve in some fashion before birth (Trines et al., 2004). Usually the progression occurs toward more severe structural pathology, often beginning with a simpler lesion that develops secondary cardiac pathology, which results in a worse overall prognosis of an affected fetus. Table 8–2 lists the potential mechanisms of progression of fetal heart disease. The best examples of this are critical aortic and pulmonary outflow obstruction (Hornberger et al., 1995, 1997; Simpson et al., 1997). When very severe outflow obstruction occurs in the midtrimester, in the absence of severe AV valve regurgitation, there is progressive hypertrophy followed by ventricular dilation as the ventricle is no longer able to maintain a normal output through the obstruction. With increasing ventricular filling and thus atrial pressures on the side of the obstruction, there is a redistribution of flow through the foramen ovale. As long as one of the ventricles is able to tolerate the added ventricular preload and is able to compensate for the other ventricle ejecting the equivalent of a biventricular output, the fetus continues to thrive. However, presumably, the lack of ventricular filling on the side of the obstruction leads to progressive hypoplasia of that

---

FIGURE 8-1. Doppler flow patterns in the absence and presence of cardiovascular compromise. A: Mitral valve inflow in utero is normally biphasic with a dominant A wave during atrial systole and a smaller E wave (left), however, when there is compression (middle) as was the case for this fetus with a large cystic adenomatous malformation, the E wave velocity increases and may even be dominant. When there is primary myocardial disease the mitral valve inflow may only consist of a single A wave (arrow) with little or no filling during early ventricular diastole (right). B: These spectra demonstrate the normal triphasic flow pattern in the inferior vena cava and hepatic veins with biphasic antegrade flow and only a brief, low velocity reversal of flow (arrow) during atrial systole (left). In contrast, when there is elevated ventricular filling pressures as observed in this a fetus with myocardial dysfunction, there is loss of forward flow in early ventricular diastole and an increased duration and velocity of flow in atrial systole (arrow) (right). Finally, C: demonstrates the normal laminar, minimally phasic flow in the umbilical vein of a healthy fetus (left). In contrast, when there is high central venous pressure due to myocardial dysfunction or significant cardiac compression, the umbilical venous flow becomes very phasic with so-called "pulsations" (right). The cessation of flow occurs during atrial systole.

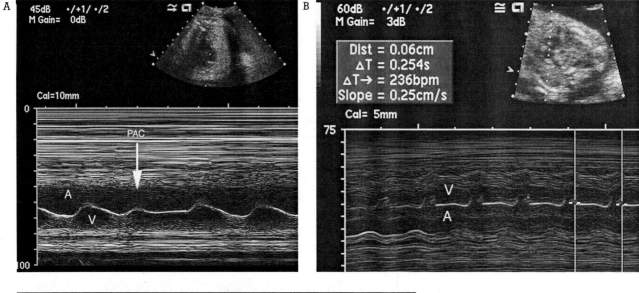

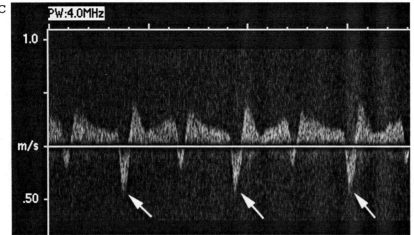

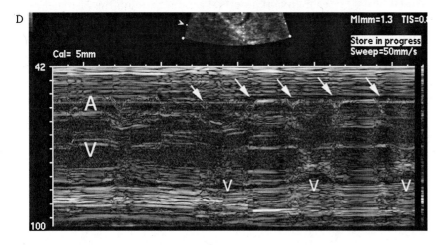

FIGURE 8–2. A: M mode tracing that demonstrates an atrial premature beat which is not conducted to the ventricle. A, right atrium; V, right ventricle; PAC, premature atrial beat. B: This m mode tracing was obtained in a 26 week hydropic fetus with incessant supraventricular tachycardia with 1:1 V-A conduction. (V-right ventricle, A-right atrium),With initiation of maternal antiarrhythmia medication, the rate of the tachycardia decreased from 240–190 bpm which resulted in resolution of the hydrops, permitting a delivery near term. C: This image demonstrates the Doppler specta obtained in the inferior vena cava of a fetus with 2:1 A-V block. One can see that every other a wave has a higher velocity (arrows) as the atria contract against a closed AV valve. D: This m mode tracing was obtained in a hydropic fetus with left atrial isomerism and complete A-V block. The atrial (A) rate was approximately 110 bpm and the ventricular (V) rate 45–50 bpm.

ventricle, the AV valve, and eventually the great artery beyond the obstruction. In critical aortic outflow tract obstruction, documentation of left to right atrial flow through the foramen ovale and retrograde aortic arch flow, irrespective of the size of the left ventricle, predicts that the left heart will become progressively more hypoplastic. Conversely retrograde ductus arteriosus flow in severe pulmonary outflow obstruction without

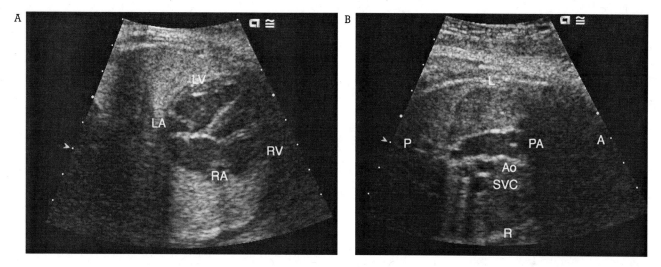

FIGURE 8–3. Follow up fetal echocardiogram performed in a 30 week gestational age fetus with persistant left-right. A: ventricular and B: great artery size discrepancy from 15 weeks, with significant ascending aortic and distal arch hypoplasia. The four chamber view showed a mildly smaller left ventricle (LV) compared to the right (RV). LA-left atrium, RA-right atrium. B: The three vessel view was particularly abnormal with the ascending aorta (Ao) having a similar diameter to the superior vena cava (SVC) and significantly smaller than the main pulmonary artery (PA). Coarctation of the aorta was considered the most likely diagnosis, although a posterior shelf was never observed in the distal arch. Postnatally, within the first month of life, while not a ductus arteriosus dependent lesion, the infant developed progressive valvar and supravalvar aortic stenosis and mild coarctation of the aorta, necessitating intervention. A, anterior; P, posterior; R, right; L, left.

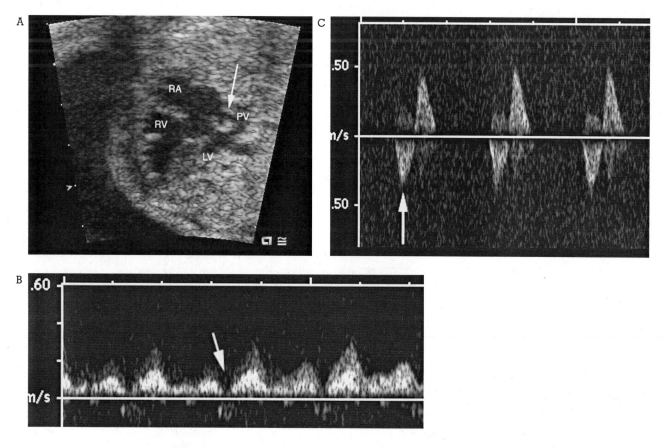

FIGURE 8–4. A: Fetal echocardiogram performed in a 28 week gestational age fetus with hypoplastic left heart syndrome, mitral and aortic atresia in whom the atrial septum was thickened and redundant (arrow), the pulmonary veins (PV) were dilated and the left atrial cavity diminutive. RA, right atrium; RV, right ventricle; LV-left ventricle. B: Normal spectral Doppler flow pattern in the pulmonary veins of a fetus without left atrial hypertension. There is mostly continuous forward flow with a brief reduction in the velocity during atrial systole (arrow). C: In contrast, pulsed Doppler interrogation of the pulmonary veins in the fetus with the thickened atrial septum revealed to and fro flow without forward flow in early ventricular diastole and with large reversal of flow during atrial systole. This was suggestive of severe left atrial hypertension. At birth the infant was severely cyanotic, requiring and emergent atrial septoplasty within hours of delivery.

TABLE 8–2. *Mechanisms of Antenatal Progression in Fetal Heart Disease*

1. Development or progression in the degree of AV valve, ventricular and great artery hypoplasia (e.g., left and right heart obstructive lesions)
2. Development or progression in the degree of branch pulmonary artery hypoplasia (e.g., tetralogy of Fallot, critical pulmonary outflow tract obstruction, restrictive foramen ovale in hypoplastic left heart syndrome)
3. Development or progression in degree of distal arch hypoplasia (coarctation of the aorta in isolation or associated with more complex intracardiac pathology with aortic outflow obstruction)
4. Development or progressive ventricular or great artery dilation (in the presence of AV or semilunar valve regurgitation, ductus arteriosus constriction, ventricular dysfunction, high output state)
5. Development or progressive AV valve stenosis or regurgitation (e.g., tricuspid valve dysplasia, AV septal defects)
6. Development or progressive semilunar valve stenosis or regurgitation (e.g., pulmonary stenosis, aortic stenosis, truncus arteriosus, tetralogy of Fallot absent pulmonary valve syndrome)
7. Development of foramen ovale restriction resulting in right (right heart obstruction) or left (left heart obstruction) atrial hypertension (also seen in D-transposition of the great arteries)
8. Development of ductus arteriosus constriction or aneurysm formation (the former in isolation, in response to maternal cyclo-oxygenase inhibitor therapy, or in D-transposition of the great arteries; the latter typically later in gestation)
9. Diminution in size or closure of ventricular septal defect
10. Development or progression in dysrhythmia (e.g., maternal autoantibody induced AV block, left atrial isomerism and AV block, tricuspid valve dysplasias and tumors for atrial ectopy and supraventricular tachyarrhythmias)
11. Development of myocardial dysfunction and heart failure (see section on myocardial dysfunction/heart failure)

significant tricuspid insufficiency is predictive of progressive right heart hypoplasia. Where there is aortic outflow obstruction or coarctation of the aorta, progressive arch hypoplasia may be observed (Hornberger et al., 1994). If there is myocardial dysfunction involving only one of the ventricles and the other is able to sustain the equivalent of a biventricular output in utero, there may be progressive hypoplasia of the abnormal ventricle as it fails to fill and progressive hypoplasia of even the great artery arising from the ventricle (Trines et al., 2004). Later in gestation and after birth, such fetuses may be indistinguishable from other fetuses with hypoplastic left and right heart complexes, which have evolved through other pathophysiological mechanisms. These observations provide new insight into the evolution of the spectrum of diseases observed postnatally and may alter our approach to counseling for recurrence risks and associated extracardiac pathology. There may be diminution in size or closure of a ventricular septal defect before birth. There may be restriction and even closure of the foramen ovale (Chobot et al., 1990). The ductus arteriosus may constrict in utero or even close completely (Leal et al., 1997; Tulzer

et al., 1991) and late in gestation may become aneurysmal (Dyamenahalli et al., 2000). There may be development or evolution in severity of dysrhythmias and myocardial dysfunction. Finally there may be development of fetal heart failure. Knowledge of the potential for progression is necessary for determining the need for serial assessment, and its timing and frequency. It is also critical for accurate prenatal counseling.

Prenatal Counseling. Counseling for fetal heart disease can be one of the most challenging aspects of prenatal management. Our role is to be the most "realistic" cardiologist, presenting to the families what is known and not known about the outcomes of affected fetuses and infants, often providing a spectrum of possible outcomes gleaned from our experience and knowledge and critical assessment of the literature. An outline of an approach to counseling is provided in Table 8–3. One must provide all of the information available to us based on our interpretation of the fetal ECG through presentation of the basic fetal cardiac anatomy. One must, however, be very cognizant of the potential pitfalls with fetal diagnosis, considering what can and cannot be diagnosed or excluded that would impact the outcome. Presentation of potential postnatal management algorithms may be necessary when the severity of the lesion after birth is not entirely certain such as one might consider for pulmonary outflow obstruction in a fetus with tricuspid atresia or for aortic coarctation, where prenatal diagnosis does not necessarily identify a ductus arteriosus-dependent lesion. Knowledge of the institution's most recent mortality and morbidity figures and treatment strategies is a necessary part of appropriate counseling. If the local institution does not manage such infants, it is critical that either the fetal/perinatal cardiologist provides outcomes of infants managed at other nearby regional programs or provides an opportunity for the affected family to have counseling from someone more familiar with outcomes of the lesion. Potential for progression of a lesion should also be explained and considered in the prenatal or postnatal algorithm of management as well as in the overall prognosis. The potential for extracardiac defects and chromosomal abnormalities and single-gene disorders should be considered. Fetal heart disease is associated with chromosomal abnormalitiesin 15%–25% of cases and extracardiac defects in 20%–40% (Allan et al., 1994; Copel et al., 1986; Fesslova et al., 1999; Paladini et al., 1993; Song et al., 2001), which are higher incidences than found in neonatal heart disease. Such additional abnormalities, which may or may not be identified before birth, in fact can have a greater overall impact on prognosis than the cardiac defect (Song et al., 2001). Finally, discussion regarding pregnancy options should be included. The

TABLE 8–3. *Counseling for Fetal Heart Disease: Considerations*

Description of Basic Cardiac Pathology
    Definitiveness of diagnosis (what can and cannot be determined among factors that influence prognosis)
    Potential for progression in structure and function (including risk of fetal heart failure and fetal demise)
Extracardiac pathology
    What can and cannot be prenatally diagnosed
    Impact of extracardiac pathology on overall outcome
Chromosomal abnormalities
    Timing of diagnosis and pregnancy options
Prenatal management
    Need for other investigations
    Chorionic villous sampling
    Amniocentesis
    Cordocentesis
    General fetal ultrasound
    Serial fetal echocardiography
    Options for prenatal intervention
Delivery Planning
    Gestational age at delivery
    Location of delivery
    Tertiary care center vs local hospital
    Mode of delivery (spontaneous vaginal, induced vaginal, caesarian delivery)
Neonatal Course
    Likely clinical status of baby at delivery
    Need for neonatal intensive care management versus discharge with mother
    Algorithms of cardiac management (particularly when severity and need for early intervention not definitive)
    Short-term outcome
    Morbidity/Mortality of planned surgery/intervention
    Length of stay in hospital
    Potential complications
    Home medications
Long term outcome/quality of life
Long term survival and need for re-operation
Learning disabilities/intelligence
Exercise tolerance/participation
Social work planning/family support
In-hospital services
Local/National support groups
Additional information (reputable internet sites, etc.)
Genetic counseling
Referral to appropriate genetics counselor
Risk for future pregnancies for mother

fetal cardiologist should be familiar with local regulations and availability with respect to absolute cutoffs for pregnancy terminations. Also, where possible, compassionate care and even delivery closer to home may be considered appropriate and be provided as an option for the pregnant woman.

Perinatal and Neonatal Management. In general, when a diagnosis of structural cardiac pathology is made in a fetus, exclusion of extracardiac disease should be sought, particularly if this would impact the decisions of the woman/couple regarding pregnancy options. Amniocentesis with additional FISH testing for *22q11.2* or chorionic villous sampling for earlier gestational ages should be offered at least for fetal heart

defects associated with chromosomal abnormalities including *22q11.2* deletion. Families can be informed that the risk of amniocentesis (1% fetal loss) is far lower in the setting of structural heart disease than the known associated risk of a chromosomal abnormality, which, if identified, may influence their decision regarding further management of the pregnancy. However, there are very few structural cardiac lesions, in which the risk of a chromosomal abnormality is lower than the risk of the amniocentesis including simple D-transposition of the great arteries and heterotaxy syndrome (Song et al., 2009), and in such cases, amniocentesis may be avoided. For cardiac defects associated with *22q11.2* deletion, the thymus, which is positioned anterior to the great arteries in the superior and anterior mediastinum, can be identified by fetal echocardiography (Barrea et al., 2003) (Figure 8–5). Absence of the thymus is consistent with *22q11.2* deletion and provides such information in a more timely manner. Detailed assessment and even serial assessment of the fetal anatomy should be performed given the increased risk of structural abnormalities, the incidence of which varies with the different cardiac lesions. Prenatal counseling regarding the potential for syndromes and the impact of extracardiac pathology on prognosis is important.

Most critical along every aspect of fetal cardiac diagnosis is the collaborative efforts and communication between obstetrical/perinatal, genetic, neonatal, fetal cardiology, and other pediatric and surgical subspecialty staff. When an affected pregnancy is continued, the timing, location, and mode of delivery must be considered. As the majority of fetal cardiac lesions detected before birth are severe pathologies that may require neonatal intervention, delivery of most affected pregnancies is carried out as close to term as possible in a tertiary-care center where the pediatric cardiology and cardiovascular surgical team are available to assist in the resuscitation and care. For most, normal vaginal delivery is sufficient with Caesarean section reserved largely for obstetrical/maternal indications, the most hydropic or compromised fetuses and those in whom fetal heart rate monitoring is difficult. An induced labor at 37–38 weeks may be elected, particularly for a mother who lives too far from the tertiary-care center or for the multiparous mother who could have a very short labor, not providing sufficient time to make it safely to the tertiary unit. Rarely, when less severe lesions are identified that are not likely to impact management in the first few weeks of life, one might consider a delivery at a local institution if pediatricians and family physicians are comfortable with the management of the infant. The infant can then be assessed within days to weeks by a nearby pediatric cardiologist. Isolated ventricular septal defects, atrial septal defects, AV septal defects, and minor valve abnormalities are

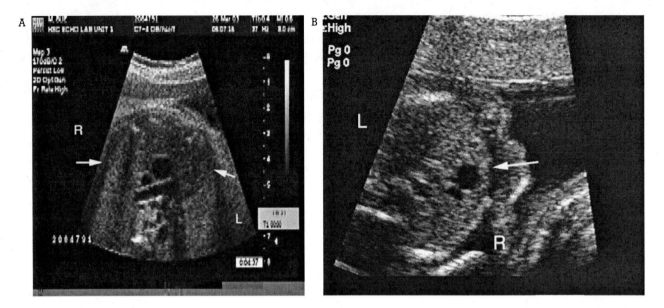

FIGURE 8–5. **A:** Echocardiogram obtained in a 32 week fetus with tetralogy of Fallot in whom an obvious thymus can be seen directly anterior to the three great vessels in the superior mediastinum, the superior vena cava, aorta and main pulmonary artery. The lung-thymus interface can be clearly seen and the thymus (arrows). This fetus had a normal karyotype and had a negative FISH for 22q11.2 deletion. **B:** In contrast, the ascending aorta is positioned closer to the anterior chest wall with little tissue in the separating space (arrow) and there is no obvious lung-thymus interface in this 28 week fetus with tetralogy of Fallot and pulmonary atresia. This latter fetus had confirmed 22q11.2 deletion.

examples of the types of lesions for which a term delivery close to home might be considered acceptable.

Functional Heart Defects

As is true after birth, myocardial dysfunction in the fetus can occur as a result of primary myocardial disease or secondary to other cardiac or extracardiac pathology. Primary myocardial abnormalities are often suspected following the exclusion of potentially treatable etiologies of myocardial dysfunction (Rychik et al., 2004). Primary myocardial disease may be due to intrinsic causes, such as single-gene disorders, mitochondrial disease, and chromosomal anomalies, or extrinsic causes, such as maternal autoantibodies with or without clinical autoimmune disease in the mother, maternal/fetal infection, and maternal diabetes. The cardiomyopathy observed in the recipient with twin–twin transfusion syndrome, which includes biventricular hypertrophy with early diastolic dysfunction and ultimately evolution of systolic dysfunction, may be considered a primary or secondary myocardial process (Barrea et al., 2004). Similar to the hypertrophic cardiomyopathy observed in infants of a diabetic mother, the cardiac pathology in fact resolves within several months after delivery as presumably the infant is no longer exposed to circulating intrauterine factors that lead to its evolution.

Certainly part of the pathology evolves secondary to increased systemic afterload and thus may also be considered a "secondary" lesion. Primary myocardial diseases from intrinsic causes, in general, have a uniformly poor prognosis with the majority succumbing either in utero or within the neonatal period (Rychik et al., 2004). By contrast, for certain lesions such as acute myocarditis, there may be improvement in function and for others, potential antenatal interventions may improve outcome.

Myocardial dysfunction may also occur in the presence of structural cardiac lesions including those associated with acute unilateral outflow tract obstruction, more chronic biventricular outflow obstruction, significant AV or semilunar valve regurgitation, and rhythm disturbances (Allan et al., 1986; Kleinman et al., 1982; Tsang et al., 2002). It may evolve secondary to fetal tachyarrhythmias and bradyarrhythmias. Myocardial dysfunction may evolve secondary to high output states including fetal anemia, acute fetal–fetal transfusion, arteriovenous malformations, agenesis of the ductus venosus, and acardiac twins (Brassard et al., 1999; Jaeggi et al., 2002). It may also evolve as a result of increased afterload as occurs in severe placental insufficiency (Makikallio et al., 2002) or reduced preload as may occur in the presence of an intrathoracic mass, diaphragmatic hernia, or ectopia cordis (Mahle et al., 2000). Recognition of the true etiology is critical for appropriate evaluation as well as prenatal, perinatal, and neonatal management.

Fetal Heart Failure. The discussion of myocardial dysfunction in utero would not be complete without a mention of fetal heart failure. In general, true fetal heart failure occurs when there is an increase in central venous pressures, usually due to abnormal ventricular filling that leads to changes in systemic venous, ductus venosus, and umbilical venous flow patterns. Ultimately this is manifested in its most severe form as fetal hydrops with placental edema, pleural and pericardial effusions, ascites, and skin edema. As mentioned above, umbilical venous flow is laminar and of low velocity with phases only during episodes of fetal breathing. Thus it is really a more passive circulation relying on the presence of very low downstream pressures. As a result of the fetal shunts, particularly the foramen ovale, redistribution of flow permits significant changes in function of one ventricle as long as there is no significant change in the function of the unaffected ventricle. The fetal circulation requires at least one patent ventricular inflow with a competent AV valve, one well-filling and ejecting ventricle, and one patent and competent semilunar valve. More chronically evolving ventricular outflow tract obstruction likely permits a gradual redistribution of the combined ventricular preload toward the "unaffected" ventricle. If the unaffected ventricle is able to accommodate the increased preload and eject the equivalent of the combined ventricular output, the fetus will thrive. In rare cases, though, the "unaffected" ventricle does not tolerate the additional preload or workload, which results in increasing atrial and thus central venous pressures, ultimately leading to hydrops (Figure 8–6). Acute univentricular outflow tract obstruction or ductus arteriosus constriction may in fact acutely impact the function of the "unaffected" ventricle as suggested recently from fetal lamb studies (Sonesson et al., 2004). The pathogenic mechanisms responsible are not entirely clear. In the context of severe AV valve regurgitation as occurs in Ebstein anomaly, the volume load of one ventricle influences the filling of the other and thus can impact both atrial pressures as well as the fetal output from the "unaffected" ventricle (Inamura et al., 2004) (Figure 8–7). Recognition of the pathogenic mechanism and the pathophysiology ultimately should result in improved management and identification of novel therapeutic strategies will ultimately improve outcome in such fetuses.

Dysrhythmias

The one area in which fetal and perinatal cardiology has made significant strides in defining mechanisms and improving associated fetal outcomes is in the case of fetal dysrhythmias. Dysrhythmias, which have thus far been documented in utero, include sinus bradycardia and tachycardia, premature atrial and ventricular beats, long and short V-A supraventricular tachycardia, ventricular tachycardia, long QT syndrome, and AV block (Chang et al., 2002; Ferrero et al., 2004; Fouron, 2004; Jaeggi, 2002; Jaeggi et al., 1998; Kleinman, 1986; Krapp et al., 2003; Lopez et al., 1996; Naheed et al., 1996; Ohkuchi et al., 1999; Simpson and Sharland, 1998; Van Engelen et al., 1994; Yamada et al., 1998). Among the supraventricular dysrhythmias, supraventricular tachycardia due to an accessory retrograde pathway is the most common diagnosis. The ability to more precisely define the temporal relationships between atrial and ventricular contraction through Doppler has resulted in our recognition of permanent junctional reciprocating tachycardia, junctional ectopic tachycardia, and ectopic atrial tachycardia before birth (Fouron, 2004). Atrial flutter is diagnosed in up to 30% of fetal supraventricular tachyarrhythmias (Jaeggi et al., 1998; Krapp et al., 2003). Recognition of the mechanism of tachyarrhythmia is critical for the most appropriate prenatal and perinatal management strategy.

Treatment algorithms for fetal supraventricular tachycardia have evolved primarily to prevent or ameliorate fetal heart failure, which may occur in up to 30%–40% of the cases with prenatally diagnosed fetal supraventricular tachyarrhythmia (Kleinman et al., 1986; Fouron, 2004). Fetuses at highest risk for the development of heart failure include those with more incessant supraventricular tachycardia (considered when present >50% of the assessment), when the presentation is at less than 32 weeks, and there is presence of structural heart disease (Naheed et al., 1996). The actual mechanism of supraventricular tachycardia and even the ventricular rate has as yet not been clearly identified as a risk factor. A fetus with rare and intermittent runs of supraventricular tachycardia, particularly in the third trimester, may only be serially assessed without intervention. If instead, the mother presents with intermittent fetal supraventricular tachycardia at less than 32 weeks or if the fetus has another risk factor for heart failure, maternal/transplacental therapy should be considered. Many fetal cardiologists recommend use of digoxin as first line of therapy, but for therapeutic levels of digoxin (1–2 mcg/dL), the mother may need up to 1000 mcg/day as an initial dose. This is as a result of such maternal factors as delayed gastric emptying and increased renal excretion (Ferrero et al., 2004). Furthermore, when the placenta is hydropic, transplacental passage of the drug may not be as effective. Long V-A tachyarrhythmias are also somewhat less responsive to digoxin, which should be considered

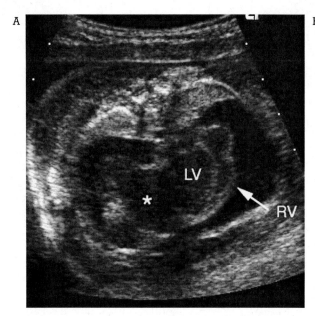

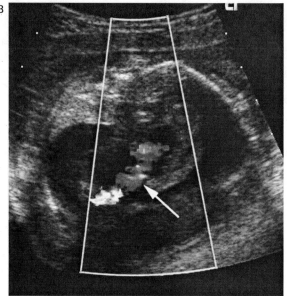

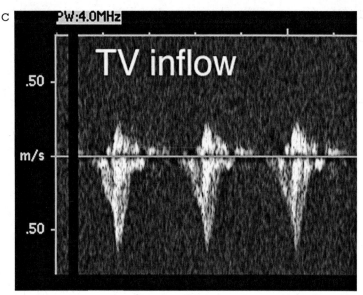

FIGURE 8–6. A: Massive left ventricular (LV) free wall aneurysm (*) in a 20 week gestational age fetus with a large pericardial effusion and progressive fetal hydrops. Right ventricular (RV) filling was clearly compromised by the very distended, poorly functioning left ventricle. B: Color flow mapping suggested that blood flow returned from the aneurysm to the left ventricle during diastole (arrow) which resulted in further dilatation of the left ventricle and compression of the right. C: Doppler flow through the tricuspid valve revealed reduced filling during early ventricular diastole with a more dominant A wave than usual for gestational age. Despite placement of an amnio-pericardial shunt with successful drainage of the pericardial effusion, progressive hydrops ensued and there was a fetal demise at 24 weeks.

in the management strategy of an affected pregnancy (Krapp et al., 2003). One must always be cautious with use of other agents in conjunction with digoxin such as amiodorone, which could increase the digoxin levels to more toxic limits. In addition, caution with use of digoxin should be exercised in the third trimester given the presence of substances that can interfere with the radioimmunoassay (Ferrero et al., 2004). A measured level that is within a therapeutic range in the third trimester could underestimate the true plasma level which may in fact be in a toxic range.

In more recent years, some fetal and perinatal cardiologists have chosen to be more aggressive in the prenatal treatment of fetal supraventricular tachycardia, not only when a fetus has heart failure, but even when the fetus is at least at a significant risk, or has a long V-A tachyarrhythmia. Use of a more potent antiarrhythmic agents such as sotalol, flecainide, or procainamide may be considered in the initial treatment to achieve more rapid conversion. This should be considered especially when the fetus is already hydropic as death may be imminent. If one of these potentially proarrhythmic drugs is to be used, the mother should be fully evaluated from a cardiovascular standpoint, preferably by an adult cardiologist who can exclude important underlying maternal heart disease that might contraindicate the use of the medication. In addition, when initiating such medications, as one would do for an

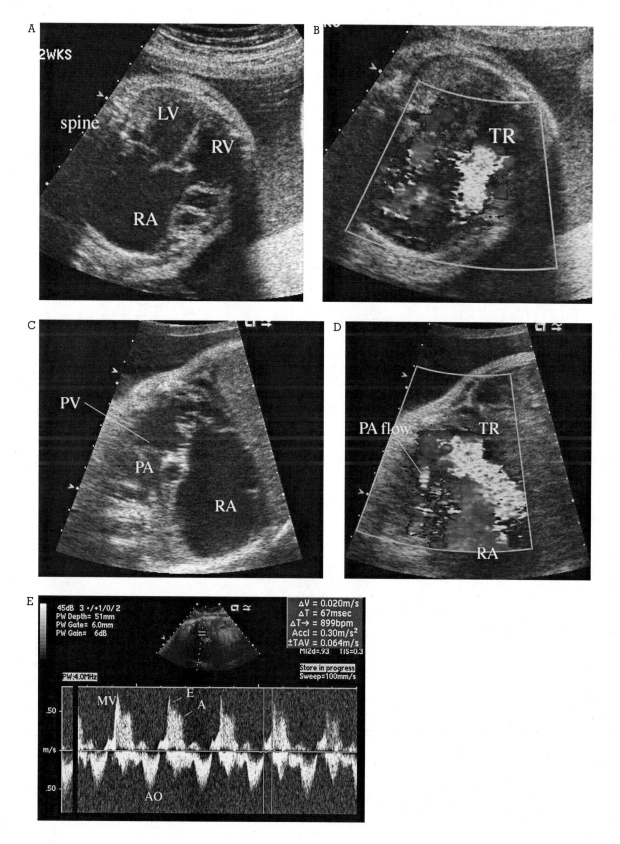

FIGURE 8–7. A thirty-two week fetus with Ebstein's anomaly of the tricuspid valve. A: The four chamber view demonstrated significant cardiomegaly with severe dilation of the right atrium (RA) and ventricle (RV). LV—left ventricle. B: Color Doppler confirmed the presence of severe tricuspid regurgitation (TR) that originated mid-way in the right ventricle. C: From short-axis images, the pulmonary valve (PV) was demonstrated in a fixed-closed position in systole, (PA-pulmonary artery) but D: by color flow mapping retrograde pulmonary arterial (PA) flow and even pulmonary valve regurgitation could be demonstrated suggesting the presence of a patent pulmonary valve. In this situation, although the pulmonary valve was patent it was surmised that the right ventricle was unable to generate a sufficient pressure to eject as a consequence of the severe tricuspid regurgitation. E: With the severely dilated right heart, very abnormal left ventricular filling was demonstrated including a dominant E (early ventricular filling) versus A (flow during atrial contraction), the reverse of normal, and a prolonged isovolumic relaxation time (measured) of 67 ms) (normal <42 ms.) AO, aortic flow; MV, mitral valve flow. The impact of severe tricuspid insufficiency on left ventricular filling placed the fetus at risk for both sudden demise as well as hydrops fetalis.

affected infant or child, the mother and fetus should be monitored in the hospital until a therapeutic dose is achieved without evidence of any important side effects in the mother. Even after discharge, the mother should continue to be frequently assessed for potential side effects, including use of serial ECG, and should have frequent fetal ECG for reassessment of the fetal rhythm and cardiovascular function. Frequent biophysical profiles and nonstress tests (the latter when the fetus is in a sinus rhythm) should also be considered by the physician to be absolutely certain of the fetal well-being. With effective therapy and close monitoring, the delivery near term is often possible. As observed after birth, no one antiarrhythmia medication is effective in every fetus, and occasionally more than one medication may be necessary to achieve conversion to sinus rhythm or at least ventricular rate control (Van Engelen et al., 1994). Often where the fetal dysrhythmia is difficult to treat, it is also difficult to treat after birth. As such, accepting rate control with no evolution of or actual resolution of hydrops, for instance, may be a better option than an early delivery.

Atrioventricular block is another dysrhythmia that may be encountered before birth. Differentiation of true AV block from atrial bigeminy with AV block is a critical first step as the latter is both much more common and certainly more benign. Nearly half of the cases of fetal AV block are associated with structural heart disease, most commonly left atrial isomerism or polysplenia and L-transposition of the great arteries (Jaeggi et al., 2005; Schmidt et al., 1991). The perinatal mortality risk, particularly for the former is very high, which may be due to the very low ventricular escape rates, and associated structural and functional cardiovascular pathology.

Among cases of isolated fetal AV block, more than 95% are associated with maternal autoantibodies: anti-Ro and anti-La (Jaeggi et al., 2002). The AV block in this condition is "acquired" in the midtrimester at the time in which the transplacental passage of maternal IgG occurs. While these autoantibodies are often found in women with systemic lupus erythematosus and Sjogren syndrome, 70%–80% of the mothers of affected fetuses and infants with autoimmune mediated AV block have clinically asymptomatic mothers (Jaeggi et al., 2002). For most cases, the diagnosis of autoantibodies is only made after the detection of AV block in the fetus or infant. While we have recently found up to 2.8% of pregnant women to have these autoantibodies (Spence et al., 2003) it is still unclear who among these mothers is truly at risk for having a fetus develop AV block in the midtrimester. Further delineation of the at-risk population perhaps through identification of a unique repertoire of associated autoantibodies, and elucidation of the pathogenic mechanism of this disease may ultimately lead to therapeutic strategies aimed at preventing the development of the condition perhaps even in the late first, early second trimester. In the meantime, we are left with using maternally administered corticosteroids to reduce inflammation where the antibodies have been deposited. Use of maternal dexamethasone at 4–8 mg/day has been shown, in rare cases, to resolve fetal heart failure and even reduce the degree of AV block (Bierman et al., 1988; Saleeb et al., 1999). More recently, it has been shown that routine use of dexamethasone, as well as beta- sympathomimetic agents such as terbutaline along with frequent surveillance and aggressive perinatal and neonatal management significantly improves the outcome of affected pregnancies (Jaeggi et al., 2004). An improvement in survival from 43%–87% in more recent years has also been shown with this management strategy. With a new diagnosis of isolated AV block of any degree at least in the midtrimester, the mother should have serology testing, particularly for anti-Ro and anti-La antibodies. Even prior to receiving the result, one might consider initiating at least low-dose dexamethasone in the mother. Weekly to biweekly monitoring by fetal echocardiography should be provided to be certain that the fetal heart function remains normal to hyperdynamic without evidence of evolving compromise. For fetal heart rates of less than 55 bpm or where there is evolving heart failure beta-sympathomimetic therapy might be considered to improve the fetal ventricular rate and/or myocardial function (Groves et al., 1995; Jaeggi et al., 2004). Worsening fetal heart function, slowing of the ventricular rate, or ventricular ectopy may prompt an early delivery at a viable gestational age. Such fetuses frequently require pacemaker insertion in the neonatal period, even within hours of life. Serial general ultrasound assessment should also be performed to document sufficient growth of the fetus and to watch for oligohydramnios which is a side effect of maternal corticosteroid use. Development of oligohydramnios may prompt a tapering of the dexamethasone dose with eventual discontinuation.

IMPACT OF FETAL AND PERINATAL CARDIOLOGY

Prenatal diagnosis of structural, functional, and rhythm-related fetal cardiovascular pathology has significantly impacted the field of pediatric cardiology and perinatology and will likely continue to do so even more in the future. Observations of the natural evolution of fetal heart diseases before birth have provided insight into the spectrum of pathology that we encounter after birth. Many initial studies evaluating impact of prenatal diagnosis on postnatal morbidity and mortality failed to show a benefit for patients diagnosed prenatally. Factors involving study size and era, and methods of data collection may have contributed to this initial failure. Significant perinatal morbidity and mortality in undiagnosed infants is underrepresented when these patients are not transferred to regional centers where data is surveyed. Similarly, patients with poor prognoses due to abnormal karyotypes and extracardiac abnormalities, more likely to be referred for prenatal echocardiography, are often overrepresented in prenatally diagnosed populations. Still more recent studies have documented a significant reduction in the preoperative morbidity and perioperative mortality of critical neonatal congenital heart disease when prenatally diagnosed compared to infants in whom the diagnosis is made only after birth (Bonnet et al., 1999; Eapen et al., 1998; Franklin et al., 2002; Kumar et al., 1999; Mahle et al., 2001; Satomi et al., 1999; Tworetzsky et al., 2001; Verheijen et al., 2001; Yates, 2004). In infants with HLHS, for instance, a significant reduction in metabolic acidosis, right ventricular dysfunction, tricuspid insufficiency, and need for inotropic support and bicarbonate, and improved postoperative survival have been documented where a prenatal diagnosis has been made (Eapen et al., 1998; Kumar et al., 1999; Tworetzsky et al., 2001). Delayed neurological morbidity has also been shown in infants with a prenatal diagnosis of HLHS (Mahle et al., 2001). Bonnet and colleagues have also demonstrated both improved preoperative condition and improved pre- and postoperative survival in infants with a prenatal diagnosis of transposition of the great arteries as compared to infants diagnosed only after birth (Bonnet et al., 1999). A significant reduction in mortality and overall hospital expense has also been demonstrated for infants with complex biventricular heart defects requiring surgical intervention in the neonatal period (Copel et al., 1997). As discussed above, prenatal diagnosis of fetal rhythm disturbances with appropriate therapeutic intervention has also significantly impacted the outcome of affected pregnancies. While not clearly demonstrated as yet, for many conditions, reduced morbidity and mortality is likely to be ultimately shown for other cardiovascular conditions in which there may be hemodynamic compromise in utero or spontaneous fetal loss. The growing interest in antenatal intervention for cardiovascular disorders will no doubt ultimately have an even more critical impact on the overall survival and morbidity rates through reduction of development of such secondary pathology as hypoplastic ventricles or fetal heart failure (see Chapter 11).

Timely prenatal detection with appropriate prenatal counseling not only prepares the family for having an affected infant, but also provides an opportunity for the couple to consider the option of termination of pregnancy. For certain more severe congenital heart defects, and for those associated with important extracardiac pathology and chromosomal abnormalities, termination rates are quite high. Prenatal detection of congenital heart disease has already begun to alter the spectrum of diseases encountered among live births. Allan and colleagues initially documented this in the early 1990s for HLHS (Allan et al., 1991). This has also been shown for pulmonary atresia with intact ventricular septum (Daubeney et al., 1998). These changes in the spectrum of cardiac pathology encountered after birth will no doubt increase in the future as the prenatal detection rates increase.

FUTURE DIRECTIONS IN FETAL AND PERINATAL CARDIOLOGY

Technological Advances

The future of fetal and perinatal cardiology at least in part will involve an expansion in technology and interventional techniques that have existed over the past decade. Three-dimensional fetal echocardiography, initially introduced in the mid 1990s, has continued to be of growing interest to fetal sonographers and as technology improves, its clinical utility is better defined. Three-dimensional imaging has the potential to improve both prenatal detection and definition of congenital heart defects (Figure 8–8). With acquisition of volumetric data from a single acoustic window, it has the potential to reduce scanning time, operator dependence, and even window dependence (Sklansky, 2004). The data could be electronically transmitted from a more remote site to a regional center of experts for interpretation. Three-dimensional echo has already been shown to provide accurate volumetric data in the evaluation of the normal fetal heart (Prakash et al., 2004). It also has the potential to significantly facilitate knowledge acquisition of individuals in the field, who can manipulate the volumetric data set to obtain various planes of imaging that will aid the comprehension of the relationship of cardiovascular structures from 2-D images.

Early diagnosis of fetal heart disease, even in the first trimester, has also continued to be of interest over the past decade, particularly with the development, and implementation of transvaginal ultrasound. Since the initial description of a 12-week fetus with left atrial isomerism (Gembruch et al., 1990), numerous reports have been published documenting late first and early second trimester fetal cardiovascular diagnoses (Achiron et al., 1994; Bronshtein et al., 2002; Fong et al., 2004; Huggon et al., 2002; Mcauliffe et al., 2005). Early assessment provides more time for

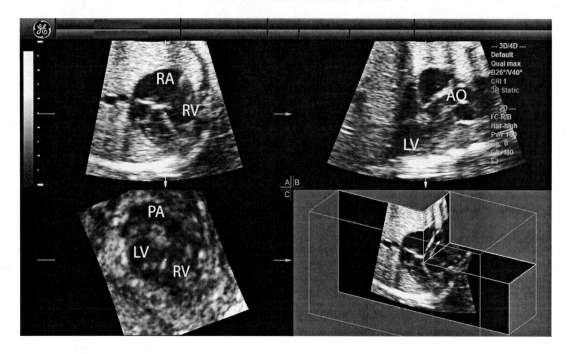

FIGURE 8–8. Three-dimensional images obtained in normal fetal heart at 28 weeks. The upper left image demonstrates a four chamber equivalent on a B scan plane, the right upper image represents a short-axis image through the ventricles and the left lower demonstrates a long-axis image obtained through the left ventricular outflow tract. The orthogonal planes from which these images were obtained are shown in the right lower image. (These images were kindly contributed by Dr. Aarti Bhat, University of California, Davis.)

additional tests such as fetal karyotyping when an abnormality is identified, permits earlier termination of pregnancy (which is both safer and emotionally easier for the pregnant woman), and provides reassurance of a normalcy of the pregnancy in case of pregnancies at risk for fetal heart disease. However, imaging of the fetal heart at very early gestational ages pushes the spatial resolution of ultrasound, and as such the detailed assessment that is possible at 20 weeks in the majority of pregnancies is not possible in most at 10–14 weeks. Limited planes of imaging and range of motion reduces the efficacy of transvaginal imaging at the earlier gestational ages even further. Furthermore, the potential for significant progression during this period of very rapid fetal growth must be taken into consideration. As a result of these limitations, early fetal echocardiography before 16 weeks of pregnancy is typically only reserved for the pregnancies at increased risk of fetal heart disease and should still be followed by reassessment at 17–20 weeks. Recognition of the association between increased nuchal translucency in the 10–14-week gestational fetus and aneuploidy, and cardiovascular disorders even in the absence of aneuploidy, has resulted in an increased need for earlier assessment of a larger population of pregnancies (Hyett et al., 1999; McAuliffe et al., 1486; Pandya et al., 1994). Finally earlier fetal echocardiographic assessment may ultimately provide insight into hemodynamic etiologies of pregnancy loss in the first trimester.

Fetal Cardiovascular Intervention

An area of fetal and perinatal cardiology of tremendous potential is that of fetal cardiovascular intervention. The knowledge of the potential for progression with development of secondary structural pathology and heart failure has led to a focus on invasive strategies to improve the outcome of various fetal heart defects. This has been particularly true for critical semilunar valve obstruction and for restrictive atrial septum in critical left heart obstruction, primarily HLHS (Arzt et al., 2003; Kohl et al., 2000; Marshall et al., 2004; Presbitero et al., 1996; Tworetzky et al., 2004). While the first reports of balloon dilation of the aortic valve in utero in late second and third trimester fetuses were largely unsuccessful (Kohl et al., 2000), a renewed interest in fetal cardiovascular intervention has recently developed. With experience and development of the tools to effectively dilate the aortic valve, there is clearly potential to alter the growth of left heart structures in some affected fetuses (Tworetzky et al., 2004) (Figure 8–9). The fetal group, in whom the intervention will be effective, with normalization of left heart systolic and diastolic function and with

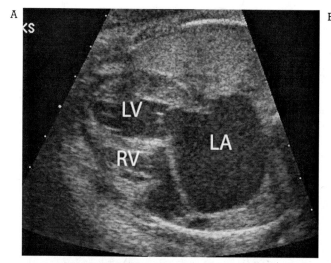

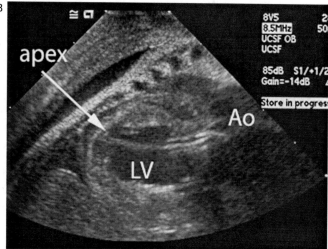

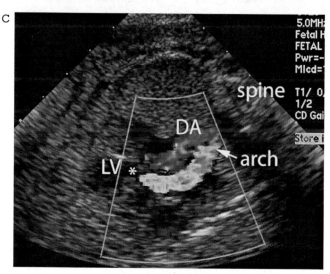

FIGURE 8–9. A: Four chamber view obtained in a 27 week gestational age with critical aortic valve stenosis, left ventricular (LV) hypertrophy and severely reduced left ventricular systolic function. There was left (LA) to right atrial flow and retrograde aortic arch flow consistent with severe left heart obstruction. No forward flow was demonstrated through the valve. B: Within days of the fetal diagnosis, balloon valvuloplasty of the fetal aortic valve was performed at the University of California, San Francisco Fetal Treatment Center. Under ultrasound guidance the catheter was introduced through the uterus, fetal thorax, and apex of the left ventricle and then advanced to the aortic valve as shown in this image. (Ao-ascending aorta). C: Follow up color Doppler demonstrated antegrade flow through the valve (*) and aortic arch in systole. (DA-ductus arteriosus)

growth of the left ventricle, aortic valve, and aorta, is still to be fully defined. Similarly there is much work to be done in delineating the efficacy of procedures for relief of atrial level restriction in left heart lesions, in altering hemodynamics, and in changing postnatal outcomes in this population. Distinction between the primary versus secondary lesion is of critical importance if the invasive interventional strategies are to be adequately applied and for their efficacy. For instance, a primary left ventricular endocardial fibroelastosis may result in abnormal filling and thus abnormal growth of the left ventricle with secondary aortic valve pathology (Sharland et al., 1991). Ten percent of recipient twins in twin–twin transfusion syndrome demonstrate development of structural right ventricular outflow obstruction, from mild pulmonary stenosis to pulmonary atresia and intact ventricular septum, which is thought to be secondary to right ventricular diastolic and/or systolic dysfunction

(Lougheed et al., 2001). Right ventricular outflow obstruction may also develop secondary to severe tricuspid valve disease with tricuspid insufficiency (Hornberger et al., 1991). Finally a more timely diagnosis of the primary simple valve pathology, particularly earlier in their course will significantly improve the impact of this field.

An area of fetal intervention that has already begun to impact outcome of affected pregnancies is in disruption of vascular pathologies that lead to cardiovascular compromise including arteriovenous malformations (e.g., sacrococcygeal teratoma), acardiac twins and twin–twin transfusion syndrome (Alkazaleh et al., 2002; Gallot et al., 2003; Paek et al., 2001; Quintero, 2003). In such pathologies, fetal echocardiography can assist in determining the need for, timing of, and subsequent efficacy of the intervention.

Administration of maternal/transplacental and intraumbilical medications and agents will likely play a more important role in the future as we better understand the basic etiologies of fetal myocardial dysfunction. For instance, transplacental or intraumbilical corticosteroids and gamma globulin may be effective in reducing inflammation and improving myocardial function in certain primary myocardial pathologies such as myocarditis and maternal autoantibody-mediated endocardial fibroelastosis (Fontes-Pedra et al., 2002). While there have been isolated reports on the use of digoxin and lasix in fetal heart failure, the results have been variable (Chavkin et al., 1996; Hsieh et al., 1998; Koike et al., 1997).

Fetal gene therapy may be another potential direction in the field of fetal and perinatal cardiology. The first description of vascular gene therapy in utero has recently been published by Mason and colleagues (Mason, 1999). In this study, gene therapy was used to alter formation of intimal cushions in the ductus arteriosus in third-trimester fetal lambs to prevent ductal constriction after birth. These investigators used a decoy of a translational protein critical for upregulation of fibronectin that allows migration of vascular smooth muscle cells that ultimately contribute to ductus arteriosus constriction. The design of this study was ultimately to develop a means of maintaining ductal patency in fetuses with a ductus arteriosus-dependent systemic or pulmonary circulation prior to postnatal intervention whether that be complete repair, surgical palliation, or cardiac transplantation. While we are still years away from its clinical application, Mason and her colleagues paved the way for further research in this area. Gene therapy to promote growth of fetal cardiovascular structures or improve myocardial function may be possible in the future. We have shown that fetal cardiac myocyte proliferation in response to mitogens is dramatically enhanced in response to pulsatile mechanical stretch, which may mimic the mechanical force of ventricular filling (Hornberger et al., 1999). Furthermore, ventricular filling may play a role in organization and function of the myocardium. Knowledge of the cellular and molecular mechanisms that are responsible for the conversion of the mechanical stimulus to growth promoting signals, for instance, may lead ultimately to novel strategies of promoting growth of a hypoplastic ventricle.

Improvements in Detection Rates

Finally, there is no doubt that one of the ongoing critical directions of our field is in education of our colleagues who perform routine obstetrical ultrasounds. While more than 90% of major congenital heart defects can be diagnosed before birth, our current detection rates are less than 55% (Grembruch, 1997; Hafner et al., 1998; Hofbeck et al., 1999; Jaeggi et al., 2001;

Rustico et al., 1995). Most of the pathology encountered in fetal cardiology programs are identified not in the high-risk pregnancies but rather low-risk pregnancies in which pathology is found during routine fetal ultrasound. While many academic institutions and larger regional hospitals often achieve excellent prenatal detection rates, the majority of low-risk pregnancies are screened in smaller community practices, which may or may not adhere to nationally recognized standards of obstetrical ultrasound performance. As such most fetal pathology continues to be missed, and the impact of fetal cardiology remains limited. More regulation of ultrasound screening practices, personnel, and technology either through national organizations such as the American Institute of Ultrasound in Medicine, American College of Obstetrics and Gynecology, and the American College of Radiology, or through legislation would lead to the greater improvements in prenatal detection. Furthermore, routine use of not only four-chamber screening but also imaging of the outlets and great arteries will contribute to improvements in prenatal detection of fetal heart disease.

It is both an exciting and challenging time to participate in the field of fetal and perinatal cardiology. Certainly, as the genetic and environmental factors responsible for the development of structural and functional congenital heart disease are discovered, there will be an even greater need for fetal echocardiography in the future including a need for earlier diagnoses. Continued collaboration with other colleagues in fetal and perinatal cardiology, perinatology, neonatology, and fetal surgery is critical for the development of timely and effective interventional strategies, and for improvements in the perinatal and neonatal management and outcome of affected fetuses. Our greatest challenge, however, is in the area of obstetrical ultrasound screening, as without improvements in this area, which will include ongoing education of those responsible, our field will never reach its full potential.

REFERENCES

Achiron R, Rotstein Z, Lipitz S, Mashiach S, Hegesh J. First-trimester diagnosis of fetal congenital heart disease by transvaginal ultrasonography. *Obstet Gynecol.* 1994;84:69–72.

Alkazaleh F, Barrea C, Hornberger LK, Seaward G, Greg R. Outcome and acute changes of the cardiovascular manifestations in the recipient twin after laser therapy for severe twin-to-twin transfusion syndrome (TTTS). *J Soc Gynecol Invest.* 2002;9:70A.

Allan LD, Cook A, Sullivan I, Sharland GK. Hypoplastic left heart syndrome: effects of fetal echocardiography on birth prevalence. *Lancet.* 1991;337(8747):959–961.

Allan LD, Crawford DC, Anderson RH, et al. Spectrum of congenital heart disease detected echocardiographically in prenatal life. *Obstet Gynecol.* 1985;54:523–526.

Allan LD, Crawford DC, Sheridan R, Chapman MG. Aetiology of non-immune hydrops: the value of echocardiography. *Br J Obstet Gynaecol.* 1986;93;223–225.

Allan LD, Sharland GK, Milburn A, et al. Prospective diagnosis of 1,006 consecutive cases of congenital heart disease in the fetus. *J Am Coll Cardiol.* 1994;23:1452–1458.

Allan, LD, Tynan MJ, Campbell S, et al. Echocardiographic and anatomical correlates in thefetus. *Obstet Gynecol.* 1980;44:444–447.

Arzt W, Tulzer G, Aigner M, Mair R, Hafner E. Invasive intra-uterine treatment of pulmonary atresia/intact ventricular septum with heart failure. *Ultrasound Obstet Gynecol.* 2003 Feb;21(2):186–188.

Barrea C, Alkazaleh F, Ryan G, McCrindle BW, Roberts A, Bigras J-L, Barrett J, Seaward G, Smallhorn J, Hornberger LK. Prenatal cardiovascular manifestations in twin-to-twin transfusion syndrome (TTTS) and the impact of therapeutic amnioreduction. *Am J Obstet Gynecol.* 2005;192(3):892–902.

Barrea C, Yoo S-J, Chitayat D, et al. Assessment of the thymus at echocardiography in fetuses at risk for 22q11.2 deletion. *Prenat Diagn.* 2003:23(1):9–15.

Berning RA, Silverman NH, Villegas M, Sahn DJ, Martin GR, Rice MJ. Reversed shunting across the ductus arteriosus or atrial septum in utero heralds severe congenital heart disease. *J Am Coll Cardiol.* 1996 Feb;27(2):481–486.

Bierman FZ, Baxi L, Jaffe E, Driscoll J. Fetal hydrops and congenital complete heart block: response to maternal steroid therapy. *J Pediatr.* 1988;112:646–648.

Bonnet D, Coltri A, Butera G, et al. Prenatal diagnosis of transposition of the great vessels reduces neonatal morbidity and mortality. *Arch Mal Coeur Vaiss* .1999;92:637–640.

Brassard M, Fouron JC, Leduc L, Grignon A, Proulx F. Prognostic markers in twin pregnancies with an acardiac fetus. *Obstet Gynecol.* 1999 Sep;94(3):409–414.

Bronshtein M, Zimmer EJ. The sonographic approach to the detection of fetal cardiac anomalies in early pregnancy. *Ultrasound Obstet Gynecol.* 2002;19:360–365.

Chang IK, Shyu MK, Lee CN, Kau ML, Ko YH, Chow SN, Hsieh FJ. Prenatal diagnosis and treatment of fetal long QT syndrome: a case report. *Prenat Diagn.* 2002;22:1209–1212.

Chavkin Y, Kupfersztain C, Ergaz Z, Guedj P, Finkel AR, Stark M. Successful outcome of idiopathic nonimmune hydrops treated by maternal digoxin. *Gynecol Obstetr Invest.* 1996;42:137–139.

Chobot V, Hornberger LK, Hagen-Ansert S, Sahn DJ. Prenatal detection of restrictive foramen ovale. *J Am Soc Echocardiogr.* 1990;3 (1):15–19.

Copel JA, Pilu G, Kleinman CS. Congenital heart disease and extracardiac anomalies: associations and indications for fetal echocardiography. *Am J Obstet Gynecol.* 1986;154:1121–1124.

Copel JA, Tan AS, Kleinman CS. Does a prenatal diagnosis of congenital heart disease alter short-term outcome? *Ultrasound Obstet Gynecol.* 1997 Oct;10(4):237–241.

Daubeney PE, Sharland GK, Cook AC, Keeton BR, Anderson RH, Webber SA. Pulmonary atresia with intact ventricular septum:impact of fetal echocardiography on incidence at birth and postnatal outcome. UK and Eire Collaborative Study of Pulmonary Atresia with Intact Ventricular Septum. *Circulation.* 1998;98:562.

Dyamenahalli U, Smallhorn JF, Geva T, et al. Isolated ductus arteriosus aneurysm in the fetus and infant: A multi-institutional experience. *J Am Coll Cardiol.* 2000;36:262–269.

Eapen RS, Rowland DG, Franklin WH. Effect of prenatal diagnosis of critical left heart obstruction on perinatal morbidity and mortality. *Am J Perinatol.* 1998;15:237–242.

Ferrero S, Colombo BM, Ragni N. Maternal arrhythmias during pregnancy. *Arch Gynecol Obstetr.* 2004;269:244–253.

Fesslova V, Nava S, Villa I. Fetal cardiology study group of the Italian society of pediatric cardiology. Evolution and long term outcome in cases with fetal diagnosis of congenital heart disease: Italian multicentre study. *Heart.* 1999;82:594–599.

Fong KW, Toi A, Hornberger LK, Keating SJ, Johnson J. Detection of fetal structural abnormalities with US during early pregnancy. *Radiographics.* 2004 Jan–Feb;24(1):157–174.

Fontes-Pedra SRF, Smallhorn J, Ryan G, et al. Fetal cardiomyopathies: etiologies, hemodynamic findings and clinical outcome. *Circulation.* 2002;106:585–591.

Fouron JC. Fetal arrhythmias: the Sainte-Justine hospital experience. *Prenat Diagn.* 2004;24:1068–1080.

Franklin O, Burch M, Manning N, et al. Prenatal diagnosis of coarctation of the aorta improves survival and reduces morbidity. *Heart.* 2002;87:67–69.

Gallot D, Laurichesse H, Lemery D. Selective feticide in monochorionic twin pregnancies by ultrasound-guided umbilical cord occlusion.*Ultrasound Obstet Gynecol.* 2003 Oct;22(4):409–419.

Gembruch U, Knopfle G, Chatterjee M, Bald R, Hansmann M. First-trimester diagnosis of fetal congenital heart disease by transvaginal two-dimensional and Doppler echocardiography. *Obstet Gynecol.* 1990 75:496–498

Grembruch U. Prenatal diagnosis of congenital heart disease. *Prenat Diagn.* 1997 Dec;(13):1283–298.

Groves AMM, Allan LD, Rosenthal E. Therapeutic trial of sympathomimetics in three cases of complete heart block in the fetus. *Circulation.* 1995;92:3394–3396.

Hafner E, Scholler J, Schuchter K, Sterniste W, Philipp K. Detection of fetal congenital heart disease in a low-risk population. *Prenat Diagn.* 1998;18:808–815.

Hofbeck M, Rauch R, Beinder E, Buheitel G, Leipold G, Rauch A, Singer H. Rate of prenatal detection of congenital heart defects. *Z geburtshilfe Neonatol.* 1999;Sep–Oct;203(5):207–212.

Hornberger L, Sanders SP, Rein AJJT, et al. Left heart obstructive lesions and left ventricular growth in the midtrimester fetus. A longitudinal study. *Circulation.* 1995;92:1531–1538.

Hornberger LK, Benacerraf BR, Bromley BS, Spevak PJ, Sanders SP. Prenatal detection of severe right ventricular outflow tract obstruction: valvar pulmonary stenosis and pulmonary atresia with intact ventricular septum. *J Ultrasound Med.* 1994;13:743–750.

Hornberger LK, Need L, Benacerraf BR. Development of significant left and right ventricular hypoplasia in the second and third trimester fetus. *J Ultrasound Med.* 1996;15:60–65.

Hornberger LK, Sahn DJ, Kleinman C, Copel J, Silverman N. Antenatal diagnosis of coarctation of the aorta: a multicenter experience. *J Am Coll Cardiol.* 1994:23:417–423.

Hornberger LK, Sahn DJ, Kleinman CS, Copel JA, Reed Kl. Tricuspid valve disease with significant tricuspid insufficiency in the fetus: diagnosis and outcome. *J Am Coll Cardiol.* 1991;17:167–173.

Hornberger LK, Singhroy S, Cavalle-Garrido T, Rabinovitch M. Pulsatile mechanical stretch used to simulate preload dramatically enhances fetal ventricular myocyte proliferative response to mitogens. *Circulation.* 1999:100:1–41.

Hsieh YY, Lee CC, Chang CC, Tsai HD, Yeh LS, Tsai CH. Successful prenatal digoxin therapy for Ebstein's anomaly with hydrops fetalis. A case report. *J Reprod Med.* 1998 Aug;43(8): 710–712.

Huggon IC, Ghi T, Cook AC, Zosmer N, Allan LD, Nicolaides KH. Fetal cardiac abnormalities identified prior to 14 weeks' gestation. *Ultrasound Obstet Gynecol.* 2002 Jul;20(1):22–29.

Huhta JC, Hagler DJ, Hill LM. Two-dimensional echocardiographic assessment of normal fetal cardiac anatomy. *J Reprod Med.* 1984;29:162–165.

Hyett J, Perdu M, Sharland G, Snijders R, Nicolaides KH. Using fetal nuchal translucency to screen for major congenital cardiac defects at 10–14 weeks of gestation: population based cohort study. *Br Med J.* 1999;318:81–85.

Inamura N, Taketasu M, Smallhorn JF, Hornberger LK. Left ventricular myocardial performance in the fetus with severe tricuspid valve disease and tricuspid insufficiency. *Am J Perinatol.* 2005;22(2):91–97.

Jaeggi E, Fouron JC, Drblik SP. Fetal atrial flutter: diagnosis, clinical features, treatment, and outcome. *J Pediatr.* 1998;132:335–339.

Jaeggi ET, Fouron J-C, Hornberger LK, Proulx F, Iberhaensli-Weiss I, Fermont L. Agenesis of the ductus venosus associated with extrahepatic umbilical vein drainage: clinical presentation, echocardiographic features and fetal outcome. *Am J Obstet Gynecol.* 2002;187:1031–1037.

Jaeggi ET, Fouron JC, Silverman ED, Ryan G, Smallhorn J, Hornberger LK. Transplacental fetal treatment improves the outcome of prenatally diagnosed complete atrioventricular block without structural heart disease. *Circulation.* 2004;110:1542–1548.

Jaeggi ET, Hamilton RM, Silverman ED, Zamora SA, Hornberger LK. Outcome of children with fetal, neonatal or childhood diagnosis of isolated congenital atrioventricular block. A single institution's experience of 30 years. *J Am Coll Cardiol.* 2002;39:130–137.

Jaeggi ET, Hornberger LK, Smallhorn JF, Fouron J-C. Prenatal diagnosis of compete atrio-ventricular block associated with structural heart disease since 1990: combined experience of 2 tertiary care centers and review of the literature. *Ultrasound Obstet Gynecol.* 2005 Jul;26(1):16–21.

Jaeggi ET, Sholler GF, Jones OD, Cooper SG. Comparative analysis of pattern, management and outcome of pre- versus postnatally diagnosed major congenital heart disease: a population-based study. *Ultrasound Obstet Gynecol.* 2001;17:380–385.

Jouannic JM, Gavard L, Fermont L, et al. Sensitivity and specificity of prenatal features of physiological shunts to predict neonatal clinical status in transposition of the great arteries. *Circulation.* 2004 Sep 28;110(13):1743–1746.

Kleinman CS, Connerstein RL, DeVore GR, et al. Fetal Echocardiography for evaluation of in utero congestive heart failure: a technique for study of nonimmune fetal hydrops. *N Eng J Med.* 1982;306:568–75.

Kleinman CS, Donnerstein RL, DeVore GR, et al. Fetal echocardiography for the evaluation of in utero congestive heart failure. *N Engl J Med.* 1982;306:568–571.

Kleinman CS, Donnerstein RL, Jaffe CC, et al. Fetal echocardiography: a tool for evaluation of in utero cardiac arrhythmias and monitoring of in utero therapy:Analyisi of 71 patients. *Am J Cardiol.* 1983;51:237–242.

Kleinman CS. Prenatal diagnosis and management of intrauterine arrhythmias. *Fetal Ther.* 1986;1:92–95.

Kohl T, Sharland G, Allan LD, et al. World experience of percutaneous ultrasound-guided balloon valvuloplasty in human fetuses with severe aortic valve obstruction. *Am J Cardiol.* 2000 May 15;85(10):1230–1233.

Koike T, Minakami H, Shiraishi H, Ogawa S, Matsubara S, Honma Y, Sato I. Digitalization of the mother in treating hydrops fetalis in monochorionic twin with Ebstein's anomaly. Case report. *J Perinat Med.* 1997;25:295–297.

Krapp M, Kohl T, Simpson JM, Sharland GK, Katalinic A, Gembruch U. Review of diagnosis, treatment, and outcome of fetal atrial flutter compared with supraventricular tachycardia. *Heart.* 2003 Aug;89(8):913–917.

Kumar K, Newburger JW, Gauvreau K, Kamenir SA, Hornberger LK. Comparison of the outcome when hypoplastic left heart syndrome and transposition of the great arteries are diagnosed prenatally versus when diagnosis of these two conditions is made only postnatally. *Am J Cardiol.* 1999;83:1649–1653.

Lange IW, Sahn DJ, Allen HD, et al. Qualitative real-time cross-sectional echocardiographic imaging of the human fetus during the second half of pregnancy. *Circulation.* 1980;62:799–805.

Leal SD, Cavalle-Garrido T, Ryan G, Farine D, Heilbut M, Smallhorn JF. Isolated ductal closure in utero diagnosed by fetal echocardiography. *Am J Perinatol.* 1997 Apr;14(4):205–210.

Lopez LM, Cha SC, Scanavacca MI, Tuma-Cali VM, Zugaib M. Fetal idiopathic ventricular tachycardia with nonimmune hydrops: benign course. *Pediatr Cardiol.* 1996;17:192–193.

Lougheed J, Sinclair BG, Fung KFK, et al. Acquired right ventricular outflow tract obstruction in the recipient twin in twin-twin transfusion syndrome. *J Am Coll Cardiol.* 2001;38:1533–1538.

Maeno Y, Kamenir SA, Sinclair B, Smallhorn JF, Vandervelde M, Hornberger LK. Prenatal features of ductus arteriosus constriction and foramen ovale restriction in D-transposition of the great arteries. *Circulation.* 1999;99:1209–1214.

Mahle WT, Clancy RR, McGaurn SP, et al. Impact of prenatal diagnosis on survival and early neurologic morbidity in neonates with the hypoplastic left heart sydrome. *Pediatrics.* 2001;107:1277–1282.

Mahle WT, Rychik J, Tian ZY, et al. Echocardiographic evaluation of the fetus with congenital cystic adenomatoid malformation. *Ultrasound Obstet Gynecol.* 2000;16:620–624.

Makikallio K, Vuolteenaho O, Jouppila P, Rasanen J. Ultrasonographic and biochemical markers of human fetal cardiac dysfunction in placental insufficiency. *Circulation.* 2002 Apr 30;105(17):2058–2063.

Marshall AC, van der Velde ME, Tworetzky W, et al. Creation of an atrial septal defect in utero for fetuses with hypoplastic left heart syndrome and intact or highly restrictive atrial septum. *Circulation.* 2004 Jul 20;110(3):253–258.

Mason CA, Bigras JL, O'Blenes SB, et al. Gene transfer in utero biologically engineers a patent ductus arteriosus in lambs by arresting fibronectin-dependent neointimal formation. *Nat Med.* 1999 Feb;5(2):176–182.

McAuliffe FM, Hornberger LK, Winsor S, Chitayat D, Chong K, Johnson J. Fetal cardiac defects and increased nuchal translucency thickness, a prospective study. *Am J Obstet Gynecol.* 2004 Oct;191(4):1486–1490.

Mcauliffe FM, Trines T, Nield LE, Chitayat D, Jaeggi E, Hornberger LK. Early fetal echocardiography—a reliable prenatal diagnosis tool. *Am J Ob Gyn.* 2005:193:1253–1259.

Naheed ZJ, Strasburger JF, Deal BJ, Benson DW Jr, Gidding SS. Fetal tachycardia: mechanisms and predictors of hydrops fetalis. *J Am Coll Cardiol.* 1996;27:1736–1740.

Ohkuchi A, Shiraishi H, Minakami H, Eguchi Y, Izumi A, Sato I. Fetus with long QT syndrome manifested by tachyarrhythmia: a case report. *Prenat Diagn.* 1999;19:990–992.

Paek BW, Jennings RW, Harrison MR, et al. Radiofrequency ablation of human fetal sacrococcygeal teratoma. *Am J Obstetr Gynecol.* 2001;184:503–507.

Paladini D, Calabro R, Palmieri S, D'Andrea T. Prenatal diagnosis of congenital heart disease and fetal karyotyping. *Obstet Gynecol.* 1993;81(5 Pt 1):679–682.

Pandya PP, Brizot ML, Khun P, Snijders RJ, Nicolaides KH. First-trimester fetal nuchal translucency thickness and risk for trisomies. *Obstet Gynecol.* 1994;84:420–423.

Prakash K, Li X, Hejmadi A, Hashimoto I, Sahn DJ. Determination of asymmetric cavity volumes using real-time three-dimensional echocardiography: an in vitro balloon model study. *Echocardiography.* 2004 Apr;21(3):257–263.

Presbitero P, Prever SB, Brusca A. Interventional cardiology in pregnancy. *Eur Heart J.* 1996 Feb;17(2):182–188.

Quintero RA. Twin-twin transfusion syndrome. *Clin perinatol.* 2003;30:591–600.

Rein AJJT, O'Donnell CO, Geva T, et al. Use of tissue velocity imaging in the diagnosis of fetal cardiac arrhythmias. *Circulation.* 2002;106:1827–1833.

Rustico MA, Benettoni A, D'Ottavio G, et al. Fetal heart screening in low-risk pregnancies. *Ultra Obstet Gynecol.* 1995 Nov;50:331–339.

Rychik J, Ayres N, Cuneo B, et al. American Society of Echocardiography guidelines and standards for performance of the fetal echocardiogram. *J Am Soc Echocardio.* 2004;17:803–810.

Sahn DJ, Lange LW, Allen HD, et al. Quantitative real-time cross-sectional echocardiography in the developing normal human fetus and newborn. *Circulation.* 1980;62:588–603.

Saleeb S, Copel J, Friedman D, Buyon JP. Comparison of treatment with fluorinated glucocorticoids to the natural history of auto-antibody.associated congenital heart block. *Arthritis Rheum.* 1999;42:2335–2345.

Satomi G, Yasukochi S, Shimizu T, et al. Has fetal echocardiography improved the prognosis of congenital heart disease? Comparison of patients with hypoplasti left heart syndrome with and without a prenatal diagnosis. *Pediatr Int.* 1999;41:728–732.

Schmidt KG, Ulmer HE, Silverman NH, Kleinman CS, Copel JA. Perinatal outcome of fetal complete atrioventricular block: a multicenter experience. *J Am Coll Cardiol.* 1991;17:1360–1366.

Sharland GK, Chita SK, Fagg NL, et al. Left ventricular dysfunction in the fetus: relation to aortic valve anomalies and endocardial fibroelastosis. *Br Heart J.* 1991;66:419–424.

Sharland GK, Lockhart SM, Chita SK, Allan LD. Factors influencing the outcome of congenital heart disease detected prenatally. *Arch Dis Child.* 1991;66:284–287.

Simpson JM, Sharland GK. Fetal tachycardias: management and outcome of 127 consecutive cases. *Heart.* 1998;79:576–581.

Simpson JM, Sharland GK. Natural history and outcome of aortic stenosis diagnosed prenatally. *Heart.* 1997;77:205–210.

Sklansky M. Advances in fetal cardiac imaging. *Pediatr Cardiol.* 2004 May–Jun;25(3):307–321.

Sonesson SE, Fouron JC, Teyssier G, Skoll A, Chartrand C. Immediate and short-term effects of pulmonary artery banding on left ventricular performance in foetal sheep. *Acta Paediatr.* 2004 Apr;93(4):540–544.

Song MS, Dyamenahalli U, Chitayat D, et al. Extracardiac defects and chromosomal abnormalities associated with major fetal heart defects: a comparison of intrauterine, postnatal and postmortem diagnoses. *Ultrasound Obstet Gynecol.* 2009;33:552–559.

Spence D, Ng L, Hornberger L, Windrim R, Wyatt P, Silverman E. Results of a prenatal screening program for anti-Ro &/or anti-La antibodies. *Am J Rheumatol.* 2006;33:167–170.

Taketazu M, Barrea C, Smallhorn J, Hornberger LK. Pulmonary vein flow in fetal hypoplastic left heart syndrome. *J Am Coll Cardiol.* 2004;43:1902–1907.

Trines J, Hornberger LK. Evolution of heart disease in utero. *Pediatr Cardiol.* 2004 May–Jun;25(3):287–298.

Tsang W, van der Velde Mary, Windrim R, Smallhorn JF, Hornberger LK. Hydrops Fetalis: Primary Cardiovascular Etiologies and Clinical Outcome in 98 Affected Pregnancies. American College of Cardiology Scientific Session, Atlanta, GA. *J Am Coll Cardiol.* 39(suppl A),415A; March 2002. AV malformations.

Tulzer G, Gudmundsson S, Sharkey AM, Wood DC, Cohen AW, Huhta JC. Doppler echocardiography of fetal ductus arteriosus constriction versus increased right ventricular output. *J Am Coll Cardiol.* 1991;18:532–536.

Tworetzky W, McElhinney DB, Reddy VM, Brook MM, Hanley FL, Silverman NH. Improved surgical outcome after fetal diagnosis of hypoplastic left heart syndrome. *Circulation.* 2001;103:1269–1273.

Tworetzky W, Wilkins-Haug L, Jennings RW, et al. Balloon dilation of severe aortic stenosis in the fetus: potential for prevention of hypoplastic left heart syndrome: candidate selection, technique, and results of successful intervention. *Circulation.* 2004 Oct 12;110(15):2125–2131.

Van Engelen AD, Weijtens O, Brenner JI, et al. Management, outcome and follow-up of fetal tachycardia. *J Am Coll Cardiol.* 1994;24:1371–1375.

Verheijen PM, Lisowski LA, Stoutenbeek P, et al. Prenatal diagnosis of congenital heart disease affects preoperative acidosis in the newborn patient. *J Thoraci Cardiovasc Surg.* 2001;121:798–803.

Winsberg F. Echocardiography of the fetal newborn heart. *Invest Radiol.* 1972;7:152–158.

Yamada M, Nakazawa M, Momma K. Fetal ventricular tachycardia in long QT syndrome. *Cardiol Young.* 1998;8:119–122.

Yates RS. The influence of prenatal diagnosis on postnatal outcome in patients with structural congenital heart disease. *Prenat Diagn.* 2004;24:1143–1149.

9

Intracardiac Left to Right Shunt Lesions

CRAIG A. SABLE

ATRIAL SEPTAL DEFECTS

Morphology

The anatomy of the atrial septum is shown in Figure 9–1. The fossa ovalis is located where septum primum fuses to septum secundum. Up to 25% of the adult population has persistence of the foramen ovale (Hagen et al., 1984), which is a normal communication in fetal life. There are three major types of atrial septal defects: secundum, sinus venosus, and primum atrial septal defects. Secundum defects, the most common type, usually represent a defect or defects in septum primum but can also be a stretched foramen ovale without deficiency in septum primum. The location, size, shape, and number of secundum atrial septal defects are highly variable (Webb and Gatzoulis, 2006). The anatomy can impact the ability to close these defects percutaneously with transcatheter devices. Eccentric defects with deficient retroaortic rims, very large defects, and multiple defects may be more difficult to close with catheter-based devices.

Primum defects fall within the spectrum of atrioventricular septal defects and will be discussed in the section on atrioventricular septal defects. Sinus venosus defects are most commonly located in the posterior aspect of the junction of the right atrium and superior vena cava but can also occur in the right atrial/inferior vena cava junction. Sinus venosus defects are commonly associated with partial anomalous venous drainage of the right pulmonary veins to the superior vena cava or right atrium. Coronary sinus defects, which are much less common than the other three types of atrial septal defects, are considered the fourth type of atrial septal defect as they do represent a left to right atrial shunt.

Embryology

Septation begins at day 31 of gestation and is complete by day 49. During looping of the heart, the main veins that feed the sinus venosus (right anterior and posterior cardinal veins as well as the left anterior cardinal vein) become incorporated into the posterior wall of the right atrium (Abdulla et al., 2004; Anderson et al., 2003; Moore and Persaud, 2003; Sadler 2004). This process includes formation of left and right sinus venosus valves. The anterior portion of these valves fuses to form septum primum, which is connected to the anterior portion of the atrioventricular canal. Two atria are initially formed and ostium primum is normally closed as septum primum fuses with the cushion like rims of the atrioventricular septum. During normal growth of septum primum, a fenestration forms, known as ostium secundum. The secondary septum (septum secundum) forms from a fold in the roof of the right atrium and grows to cover the ostium secundum and fuse with septum primum to form the foramen ovale (Figure 9–2). A secundum atrial septal defect may result if this fusion is not complete (from deficient septum secundum, deficient septum primum, or additional fenestrations in septum primum). Completion of atrial septation occurs at gestation day 39–42. However, permanent fusion and closure of the foramen ovale does not normally occur until several weeks after birth and persists in a significant minority of adults.

Hemodynamics

The direction and magnitude of shunting through an atrial septal defect is determined primarily by the relative compliances of the two ventricles and size of the

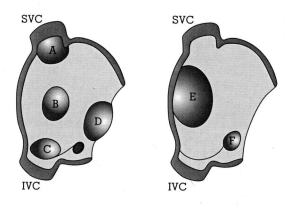

FIGURE 9–1. Types of atrial septal defects as seen from the right atrium—A: superior sinus venosus septal defect; B: secundum atrial septal defect; C: inferior sinus venosus septal defect, D: ostium primum atrial septal defect; E: secundum atrial septal defect with deficient posterior rim; F: coronary sinus atrial septal defect. *Abbreviations*: IVC, inferior vena cava; SVC, superior vena cava.

actual defect. The right ventricle becomes more compliant as the pulmonary vascular resistance undergoes its normal decline in the first few weeks of life. Thus, flow will transition from a normal right to left shunt in fetal life to predominantly left to right shunting within 1 month of life. In patients with moderate or large defects, left to right shunting will lead to volume overload of the right side of the heart, secondary dilation of the right atrium and ventricle, and significant increase in pulmonary blood flow. However, most patients in the first two decades of life have normal or only mildly elevated pulmonary artery pressure and normal pulmonary vascular resistance. Pulmonary hypertension is more common in patients with moderate or large defects, which is present in adulthood, but significant elevation of pulmonary vascular resistance is still uncommon (Vogel et al., 1999). Development of systemic hypertension and left ventricular diastolic dysfunction in older patients may significantly increase the amount of left to right shunting in someone with an unrepaired defect as they age.

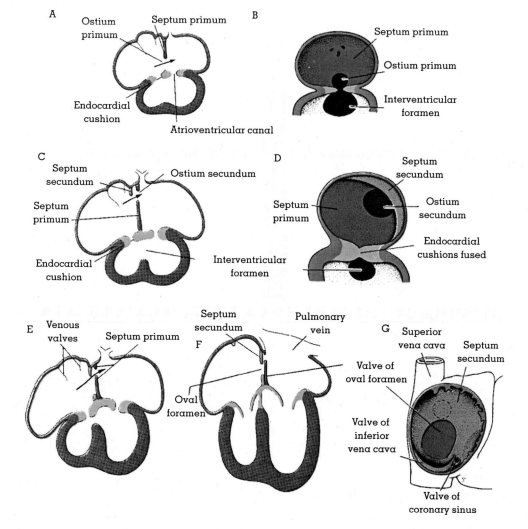

FIGURE 9–2. Embryology of atrial septum from frontal view (A, C, E, and F) and right atrial view (B, D, and G).

Atrial shunting also occurs secondary to other cardiac and noncardiac diseases. Cyanosis, secondary to right to left shunting, is very uncommon in isolated atrial septal defects, but can occur if an atrial septal defect is present in combination with other conditions such as right ventricular outflow obstruction, primary pulmonary hypertension, and significant pulmonary disease. Patients with left-sided disease including mitral stenosis, left ventricular dysfunction, and left-sided outflow obstruction may develop significant left to right shunting.

Clinical Features

Many patients with atrial septal defects are asymptomatic. Children and adults with large left to right shunts may complain of some degree of exercise intolerance with exertional dyspnea. Occasionally, moderate to large defects may be associated with poor growth and more frequent respiratory infections. Adults with unrepaired defects may develop atrial flutter or fibrillation, but rarely before age 40 (Gatzoulis et al., 1999; Webb and Gatzoulis, 2006). Embolic cerebral vascular accident or transient ischemic attack can be the first presentation of an atrial septal defect or patent foramen ovale.

Most children diagnosed with atrial septal defects are referred for a heart murmur. Increasingly, small atrial defects are being diagnosed as incidental findings in the first few months of life as echocardiography has become universally available. Examination findings in patients with moderate to large defects are secondary to right ventricular volume overload and increased tricuspid and pulmonary blood flow. In older children with a large defect, a precordial bulge and hyperdynamic right ventricular impulse may be present. A fixed split second heart sound due to delay in the pulmonary component of the second heart sound is often heard at the left upper sternal border. However, this finding may be difficult to assess in infants with high heart rates. A systolic ejection murmur grade 2–3 is usually heard at the left upper sternal border and radiates to the axilla and back, secondary to increased pulmonary blood flow. Increased tricuspid flow may result in a soft mid-diastolic murmur at the left sternal border. Patients with primum atrial septal defects may also have a holosystolic regurgitant murmur at the apex secondary to mitral regurgitation. In adults with unrepaired defects and pulmonary hypertension, the split second heart sound is absent and a loud pulmonary component of the second heart sound may be present. Cyanosis is rarely found in isolated atrial septal defects but may be present if right ventricular outflow obstruction, anomalous pulmonary venous drainage, or pulmonary hypertension is present.

Patients with small atrial septal defects often have normal electrocardiograms. In patients with moderate or large defects, right axis deviation and right atrial enlargement is frequently present. An rSR' pattern (right ventricular conduction delay or incomplete right bundle branch block), indicative of right ventricular volume overload, is often present in lead V1. Sinus rhythm is usually present; older patients may have first degree atrioventricular block. An abnormal P wave axis with P wave inversion in the inferior precordial leads may be indicative of a sinus venosus defect. Leftward or superior axis is often found with primum atrial septal defects. Chest radiography is nonspecific and not usually part of the initial diagnostic workup. Cardiomegaly secondary to right heart enlargement may be present. A prominent main pulmonary artery shadow may be seen and increased pulmonary vascularity may be appreciated.

Transthoracic echocardiography is the mainstay of diagnosis of atrial septal defects. The presence of a patent foramen ovale or small atrial septal defect is almost universal in the newborn period and independent of other findings. An aneurysm of septum primum may also be present in the newborn period as a normal variant. The presence of right ventricular volume overload is often apparent on initial parasternal long axis images, which reveal a large right ventricle even before the actual septal defect is seen. Parasternal short axis imaging shows an enlarged right ventricle with diastolic interventricular septal flattening. The differential diagnosis of this finding includes atrial septal defects, anomalous pulmonary venous return, tricuspid regurgitation, and pulmonary insufficiency.

Although atrial septal defects may be seen from parasternal and apical windows, false positive and negative findings may occur because the thin septum is parallel to the beam of sound. Subcostal windows provide the most specific diagnostic information about morphology, size, shape, location, and number of atrial septal defects because the transducer beam angle is perpendicular to the atrial septum. Multiplane (coronal, sagittal, and oblique) imaging can put together a detailed three-dimensional assessment of the atrial septum as well as location of systemic and pulmonary veins. Secundum defects can be round or elliptical, central, or eccentric, and single or multiple (including one or more fenestrations in septum primum). Color flow Doppler is very helpful to determine the direction and amount of shunting as well as venous abnormalities. Newer real-time transthoracic 3-D echocardiography transducers can provide additional information with biplane, surface rendered, and "en-face" views to aid in better delineating the borders of defects relative to surrounding structures (Figure 9–3). This information can be very important in determining the

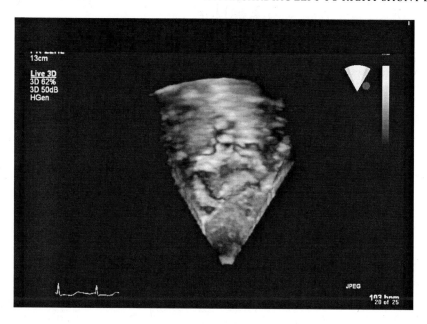

FIGURE 9–3. Three-dimensional echocardiographic subcostal sagittal plane image as seen from right atrium demonstrating superior sinus venosus septal defect and partial anomalous pulmonary venous return. Right upper pulmonary veins (arrows) and septal defect (asterisk) are shown. *Abbreviations*: IVC, inferior vena cava; SVC, superior vena cava.

suitability for transcather closure, especially in patients with large defects and concern for deficiency of the retroaortic rim.

Subcostal windows provide exquisite imaging in infants, but may be more challenging in older children. In all patients, even infants, using lower frequency transducers to improve penetration and imaging from the right of center and lower down to optimize the positive acoustic properties of transhepatic imaging will maximize image quality. In older patients, asking the patient to inspire will significantly improve subcostal image quality. High right parasternal imaging with the transducer in near straight sagittal orientation and patient lying on his or her right side can also provide detailed assessment of the atrial septum, including the relationship of the defect to right pulmonary veins in sinus venosus defects.

Hemodynamic information can also be provided by echocardiography. The ratio of pulmonary to systemic blood flow can be estimated from spectral Doppler and 2-D assessment of the left and right ventricular outflow tracks. However, this estimation has some degree of error and should be interpreted in combination with other findings on echocardiography. In patients with a history of embolic stroke and suspected right to left atrial shunting, color flow Doppler may not detect any shunting. Saline contrast injection through a peripheral vein may be helpful to detect a small right to left shunt but needs to be performed with enough volume and speed to completely opacify the right atrium. Mixing a small amount of blood or air with saline, "agitating" the saline with two syringes and a stopcock, and having the patient valsalva during the injection can increase the sensitivity of the test.

Transesophageal echocardiography is an excellent modality to image the atrial septum, but is rarely needed to make a primary diagnosis in children. In adults with poor transthoracic windows, it may be needed to define the anatomy of the atrial septum. Transesophageal echocardiography is more sensitive to rule out small defects and right to left shunts in patients with suspected cerebral embolic events. Transesophageal and intracardiac echocardiography are both used to help guide transcatheter device closure of atrial septal defects.

Cardiac magnetic resonance imaging (MRI) and computed tomography scanning technology has dramatically improved and can provide useful information about atrial septal defects. Information about ventricular size and shunting as well as the anatomic location of the defects can be obtained. The most useful clinical scenario for cardiac MRI is in patients with abnormal pulmonary venous return. Cardiac catheterization has little role for diagnosis in children with atrial septal defects other than those with complex pulmonary vein abnormalities. Catheterization may be important in older adults with suspected pulmonary hypertension and for preoperative evaluation of coronary arteries in patients over age 50 (Webb and Gatzoulis, 2006).

Management

Anticongestive therapy is rarely indicated as most patients are asymptomatic. However, older children and adults, in third world countries, with large defects and shunts who do not have access to treatment may benefit from digoxin and diuretics. The two main management questions for secundum atrial septal defects are whether or not to close the defect and to make a choice between catheter device and surgical closure (Du et al., 2002). Consideration of the natural history of atrial septal defects is an important principle in guiding management. Almost all defects under 3 mm, and the majority of defects under 8 mm, diagnosed in infancy undergo spontaneous closure by 2–4 years of life (Brassard et al., 1999; Radzik et al., 1993). However, a study following atrial septal defects diagnosed that at a mean age of 4 years of life, the defects enlarged in 65% of cases, including some defects that became too large for catheter device closure (McMahon et al., 2002). Unrepaired moderate to large defects have increased long term morbidity and mortality. Sinus venosus and primum atrial septal defects almost never undergo spontaneous closure and are not amenable to current catheter device techniques for closure.

The ideal timing for closure of a secundum atrial septal defect is based on the size and consideration of data presented above (Kharouf et al., 2008). Moderate and large defects that do not show any signs of decrease in size by 2–3 years of life are referred for closure. Rarely closure may be indicated in the first year of life for infants with large defects and congestive heart failure (Mainwaring et al., 1996). The utility of closing small (<6 mm) defects is less clear, but any defect large enough to cause any degree of right-sided volume overload or an estimated Qp:Qs of 1.5:1 are also referred for closure. The ideal timing for closure of sinus venosus and primum defects is similar to secundum defects, although some centers refer primum defects in the first year to optimize long-term atrioventricular valve function. In patients with significant right ventricular hypertension, significantly impaired right ventricular compliance, or severe left atrial hypertension (i.e., mitral stenosis), atrial septal defect closure may be contraindicated as the defect may be functioning as a critical "pop off" for the right or left ventricle.

Surgical closure via cardiopulmonary bypass has been practiced since the 1950s with excellent outcome and safety results in the modern era. The approach can be through a traditional sternotomy or limited lower sternotomy. Surgical series of secundum defects report 100% survival, no significant residual defects, and no neurological defects. Long-term outcomes of patients repaired under age 25 are not different than the general population (Murphy et al., 1990). However, adults repaired after age 40 have lower actuarial survival than the general population, with pulmonary hypertension being the most significant risk factor (Webb and Gatzoulis, 2006). Median length of hospital stay for limited sternotomy is under 3 days. The only significant complication was postpericardiotomy syndrome.

Adults with atrial septal defects repaired after age 25 have worse long-term outcomes. Smaller secundum defects can be closed primarily, large defects require patch closure.

Repair of sinus venosus defects often requires baffling of some or all of the right pulmonary veins to the left atrium as part of the patch closure of the defect (Jost et al., 2005). If the right upper pulmonary veins enter the superior vena cava superiorly, baffling may not be possible. In these situations, the superior vena cava is transected above the pulmonary veins and reattached to the right atrial appendage while the inferior portion of the superior vena cava and right upper pulmonary veins are directed to the left atrium (Warden Procedure) (Shahriari et al., 2006).

Catheter closure of secundum atrial septal defects has been available for several years; initial reports date back to the 1970s. Since 2008 catheter closure has become the more common route of closure for defects that meet acceptable criteria and is guided by transesophageal or intracardiac echocardiography. Several different devices exist; most of the experiences are with the Amplatzer and CardioSEAL/STARFlex devices (Figures 9–4 and 9–5). Patients are treated with low-dose aspirin for 3–6 months after device closure. The advantages of catheter closure include no surgical wound, minimal pain, and shorter hospital stay and recovery. Five- to 10-year follow-up studies show complete closure at 3 years with no deaths or significant complications (Masura et al., 2005). However, there have been rare reports of device embolization and erosion (0.1%), most but not all occurring in the first 72 hours post procedure (Amin et al., 2004; Delaney et al., 2007). Thrombus formation has been reported in up to 1% of patients, but not in the Amplatzer device. Correct patient selection, device sizing, and operator experience are the most critical factors in preventing these complications.

Relative contraindications to device closure are very large defects (balloon stretch diameter is more than 36 mm in adults, upper limit will be lower in children) (Varma et al., 2004), inadequate septal rims, and very close proximity to vena cava, coronary sinus, and right pulmonary veins. Patients with multiple defects are more challenging to address with transcatheter devices, but can be closed with a single or multiple devices. The risk/benefit ratio of catheter closure versus surgery for each patient should be presented to parents (and older patients) in helping to decide which modality is most appropriate for each patient.

There have been several reports of transcatheter closure of patent foramen ovale in patient with cryptogenic stroke (Slottow et al., 2007). However, this issue remains controversial. Although catheter closure of patent foramen ovale has the potential to decrease the

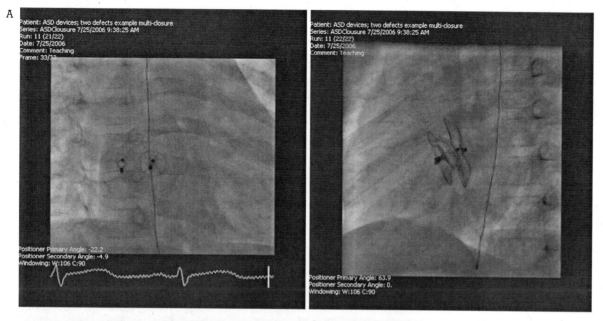

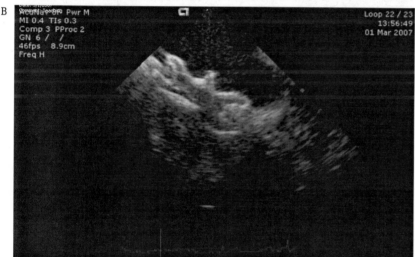

FIGURE 9–4. Angiographic (A) and intracardiac echocardiographic (B) images of an Amplatzer atrial septal defect device.

risk of recurrent stroke, there have been no randomized trials to prove the efficacy of this strategy.

VENTRICULAR SEPTAL DEFECTS

Morphology

The morphologic classification of ventricular septal defects is based on the four components of the ventricular septum (Figure 9–6) as viewed from the right ventricle (Anderson and Wilcox, 1992; Hagler et al., 1985; Soto et al., 1980). The inlet septum separates the tricuspid and mitral valves. The muscular septum is bordered by tricuspid valve chordal attachments, right ventricular apex, and crista supraventricularis. The outlet or infundibular septum is bordered inferiorly by the crista supraventricularis and superiorly by the pulmonary valve. The membranous septum, the smallest portion of the septum, is bordered by the other three parts of the septum.

Inlet ventricular septal defects, which make up 5%–8% of ventricular septal defects, are often part of the spectrum of the atrioventricular septal defects and can include abnormalities of the mitral and tricuspid valve. Muscular defects can be located in the apical, anterior, mid or posterior muscular septum, can be multiple, and make up 5%–20% of ventricular septal defects (Roguin et al., 1995). The term "Swiss cheese heart" is used for patients with multiple muscular

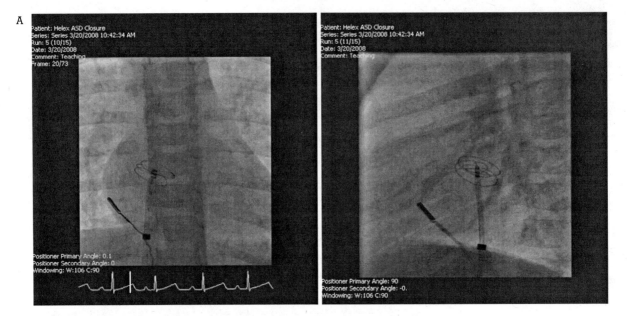

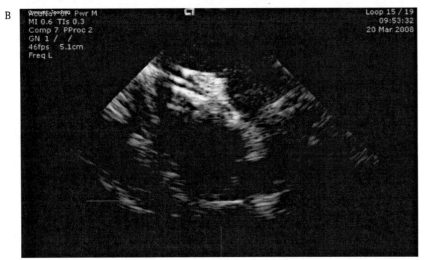

FIGURE 9–5. Helix atrial septal defect device as seen from anterior posterior (A left) and lateral (A right) angiographic and intracardiac echocardiographic (B) images. Solid arrow shows device just prior to release. *Abbreviations:* LA, left atrium: RA, right atrium.

ventricular septal defects. Several terms have been used for defects in the outlet septum including supracristal, subpulmonary, conal, conalseptal hypoplasia, infundibular, and doubly committed subarterial. Many of these terms are confusing and some have significant overlap with other cardiac defects (e.g., subpulmonary used for patients with double outlet right ventricle). Supracristal defects make up 5%–7% of ventricular septal defects but are significantly more common in the Far Eastern countries. The right, and less commonly left, aortic valve cusps frequently prolapse into supracristal defects and can be associated with aortic insufficiency (Eroglu et al., 2003; Lun et al., 2001).

Defects in the membranous septum often extend into the inlet, muscular, or outlet septum and are often referred to as perimembranous defects. These defects, which make up 75%–80% of ventricular septal defects, are often in direct continuity with the tricuspid and aortic valves. The septal leaflet of the tricuspid valve often forms a pouch or aneurysm in a perimembranous defect, which can partially or completely close the defect. Prolapse of the right cusp of the aortic valve may also be seen (Eroglu et al., 2003). Small perimembranous defects can be associated with development of a prominent midcavity obstruction or double-chambered right ventricle. Malalignment of the outlet and anterior muscular septum as seen in tetralogy of Fallot and double outlet right ventricle (anterior malalignment) and interrupted aortic arch (posterior malalignment) may be classified as a subset of perimembranous defects. However, these defects have significantly different anatomy, physiology, and natural history and

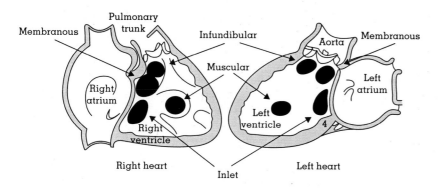

FIGURE 9–6. Morphology of ventricular septum showing four major types of defects from right and left ventricle.

are probably more appropriately classified as a fifth type of defect—conoventricular septal defects.

Embryology

Ventricular septation, which occurs during weeks 5 and 6 of gestation, is a complex process that involves several structures positioned at different planes (Figure 9–7)

(Abdulla et al., 2004; Anderson et al., 2003; Moore and Persaud, 2003; Mooreman et al., 2003; Sadler, 2004). It can be divided into inlet, muscular, and outflow septation. The three different regions grow toward one another and coalesce to form the membranous septum. The muscular portion of the ventricular septum is formed from a primary muscular fold that arises from the apex of the primitive ventricle and grows toward

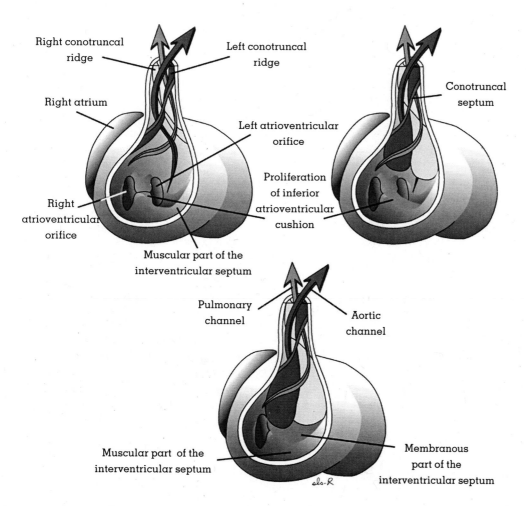

FIGURE 9–7. Embryology of ventricular septum.

the atrioventricular valves. The inlet septum, which forms at the same time in a slightly different plane, grows toward the muscular septum. Positioning of the tricuspid orifice over the right ventricle and the mitral orifice over the left ventricle results from the secondary formation and outgrowth of the inflow portion of the right ventricle. Abnormalities in this process can lead to malposition of the tricuspid valve partially (straddling or overriding) or completely (double inlet left ventricle) over the left ventricle and underdevelopment of the right ventricular inflow tract (tricuspid atresia) (Gittenberger-DeGroot et al., 2005).

Physiology

The assessment of ventricular septal defect physiology includes evaluation of pressure drop and flow across the defect. The primary factors impacting volume of flow through a ventricular septal defect are size of the defect and relative pulmonary and systemic vascular resistance. The size of the defect is best compared to that of the aortic annulus. Small defects are less than one-third the diameter of the left ventricular outflow and large defects approach or are greater than the diameter of the left ventricular outflow.

Shunting across ventricular septal defects without right ventricular outflow obstruction or advanced pulmonary vascular disease is primarily left to right and occurs during systole defects with significant flow going across them, resulting in volume overload of the left atrium and left ventricle. The right ventricle serves as a conduit for increased pulmonary flow in systole but does not undergo volume overload. Small defects do not allow a significant amount of blood flow through the septum and will create a significant pressure drop across the defect. Moderate size defects will also create a pressure drop across the defect but can allow significant flow across the defect if the pulmonary vascular resistance is significantly lower than the systemic vascular resistance. Large defects equalize pressure across the defect; flow across the defect is entirely determined by the relative resistances across the pulmonary and systemic vascular beds.

Pulmonary vascular resistance normally falls over the first 1–4 weeks of life. During fetal life and in the first week of life, there will be little flow across any size defect. As resistance falls, patients with moderate and large ventricular septal defects develop increased flow across the defect. The high pulmonary pressure, high pulmonary flow, low pulmonary vascular resistance state is first seen between 2 and 6 weeks of life and results in symptoms of congestive heart failure. Compensatory mechanisms in these infants include increased endogenous catecholamine release and ventricular hypertrophy. If the defect is repaired in a timely manner (first 3–6 months of life) pulmonary artery pressure will be normal or near normal in the postoperative period (Rabinovitch et al., 1984). Over time (several years), if the defect is not repaired, damage to the pulmonary vascular bed occurs, pulmonary resistance rises, the left to right shunt decreases and ultimately, right to left shunting occurs. This phenomenon is known as Eisenmenger syndrome (Minette and Sahn, 2006).

A subset of patients with large ventricular septal defects do not undergo the normal fall in pulmonary resistance. These patients will develop as much increased left to right shunting despite having a moderate or large hole. This phenomenon is observed more frequently in children with trisomy 21. Paradoxically, these children may be less symptomatic and experience more normal growth. However, they may be at higher risk for pulmonary hypertension postoperatively.

Patients with moderate size defects that are pressure restrictive may allow enough shunting to allow for slow growth and symptoms of congestive heart failure, but are unlikely to pose a significant risk for development of pulmonary vascular obstructive disease in the first two decades of life. Shunting across small ventricular septal defects is not impacted by pulmonary vascular resistance; the size of the hole limits blood flow.

Clinical Features

The clinical features of ventricular septal defects are directly related to defect size and physiology (van den Heuvel et al., 1995). Symptoms in children with small defects do not occur. Children with moderate and large defects may have a "honeymoon" period in the first few weeks of life. However, as pulmonary vascular resistance falls and pulmonary blood flow increases, symptoms of congestive heart failure including slow growth, tachypnea, slow feeding and diaphoresis with feeding, and increased respiratory infections are seen (Artman and Graham, 1982). The rapidity and severity is dependent on how large the hole is and the normal fall in pulmonary resistance. Patients with moderate size defects may have only mild growth delay and tachypnea, which may resolve if the defect decreases in size.

Physical examination findings in a ventricular septal defect are related to the pressure drop across the defect and the amount of pulmonary blood flow. Precordial activity is normal in small defects. A thrill may be present. As the pulmonary vascular resistance falls, a harsh systolic regurgitant murmur will be heard throughout the precordium and is related directly to the pressure difference across the defect. The murmur most often starts in early systole and obscures the first heart sound. In small muscular defects, ventricular contraction may limit blood flow in late systole, resulting in shorter duration of the murmur. The patient with a large ventricular septal defect is likely to have an increased left ventricular impulse. The pulmonic component of the second heart sound will be increased. The murmur is primarily related to excess pulmonary blood flow. A prominent systolic ejection murmur is heard at the left upper sternal border and radiates to the lung fields. A mid-diastolic rumble may also be heard at the apex from increased pulmonary venous return and mitral flow. Patients with moderate size defects have examination findings of both small and large defects. The precordial activity is increased, the systolic murmur is usually a holosystolic and regurgitant and a diastolic rumble may be present. Development of a double-chambered right ventricle will cause a harsh systolic ejection murmur; however, the murmur may only be subtly different and can be difficult to recognize clinically unless there is a high suspicion. The presence of a diastolic decrescendo murmur at the left sternal border likely indicates aortic valve insufficiency secondary to prolapse of the aortic valve. Patients with large defects and pulmonary vascular obstructive disease will appear cyanotic and may have evidence of digital clubbing. The right ventricular impulse will be increased and a lift may be present. Shunting through the defect, which is bidirectional or right to left, does not produce a murmur; however, a holosystolic regurgitant murmur of tricuspid regurgitation may be present.

The electrocardiogram is usually normal in patients with small ventricular septal defects. Left ventricular hypertrophy is seen with moderate and large defects. A significant number of patients may also have right or biventricular hypertrophy. Attention should be paid to the voltage standard to avoid underestimating the degree of hypertrophy. Left axis deviation is frequently seen in inlet ventricular septal defects. Right ventricular hypertrophy may be seen in double-chambered right ventricle in patients with obstructive pulmonary vascular disease. Chest radiography will show increased pulmonary vascular markings and cardiomegaly in moderate to large defects. The lateral film will show left atrial enlargement, which may also be inferred from the posterior-anterior film from elevation of the left mainstem bronchus.

Echocardiography is the mainstay of diagnosis of ventricular septal defects (Cheatham et al., 1981; Pieroni et al., 1993). Anatomy and physiology can be ascertained. Black and white and color Doppler imaging from parasternal, apical, and subxyphoid windows is used to define the location, size, and number of defects as well as associated findings such as tricuspid valve aneurysm tissue, aortic valve prolapse, and double-chamber right ventricle (Hagler et al., 1985). The relative anterior/posterior position of each defect as well as its relation to all heart valves is very important, especially in patients who are referred for surgical repair. The morphology of multiple muscular defects may not be readily apparent until all views are assessed and a three-dimensional understanding of the defects is possible.

The distinction between perimembranous and supracristal defects is made by assessing the relation of the defect to the aortic, tricuspid, and pulmonary valves. On parasternal long axis and apical four-chamber views, a perimembranous defect will be next to the tricuspid and aortic valves while a supracristal defect will be closer to the pulmonary valve. On short axis imaging, a perimembranous defect is seen just inferior to the right aortic valve cusp near the tricuspid valve and right/non aortic valve commissure (9–10 o'clock relative to the aortic valve from parasternal short axis, Figure 9–8). Tricuspid valve aneurysm tissue partially closing the defect is often present. A supracristal defect is found adjacent to the pulmonary valve and right/left aortic valve commissure (12–1 o'clock relative to the aortic valve from parasternal short axis, Figure 9–9). There is often deficiency or absence of conal septum in supracristal defects, giving the appearance that the two valves are touching (instead of the normal appearance of them being separated by conal septum).

Color Doppler can be used to determine the direction of shunting, although a small amount of right to left shunting during isovolumic relaxation occurs in almost all defects. Spectral Doppler of flow across the ventricular septal defect using the modified, Bernoulli equation, can be used to estimate the pressure drop across the defect when combined with a concurrent measure of systolic systemic blood pressure (Houston et al., 1988). Tricuspid regurgitation velocity Doppler can also be used to estimate right ventricular systolic pressure. Patients with high-velocity flow across the defect (more than 4 m/s) almost always have normal right ventricular and pulmonary artery systolic pressure.

There are pitfalls that need to be recognized while using spectral Doppler to estimate right ventricular and pulmonary pressure. The angle of flow should be parallel to flow or the gradient may be underestimated. The amount of flow across a very small defect may not be adequate to obtain a clean envelope. Patients with large defects and low velocity flow are likely to have near systemic or systemic pulmonary artery systolic pressure. However, the pulmonary artery diastolic and mean pressure may be subsystemic. Spectral Doppler represents the peak instantaneous pressure gradient across the defect. Left ventricular pressure rises earlier in systole then the right ventricular pressure; the peak instantaneous gradient may overestimate the true gradient and thus underestimate the right ventricular

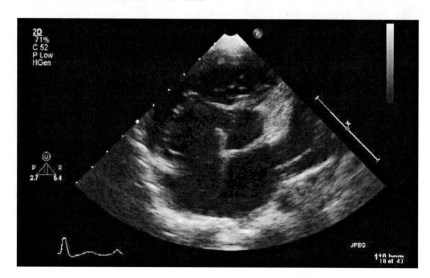

FIGURE 9–8. Parasternal short axis transthoracic echocardiographic of a large membranous ventricular septal defect.

pressure. In patients with double-chambered right ventricle, a high-velocity signal may be interpreted as evidence of normal right ventricular pressure but may actually represent midcavity obstruction with normal pressure in the right ventricular outflow but elevated pressure in the proximal right ventricle. Careful subxyphoid imaging of the right ventricular outflow, especially from the sagittal short axis plane and correlation with tricuspid valve regurgitation velocity, is important to exclude a double-chambered right ventricle. Assessment of right ventricular pressure in postoperative patients and those with inlet ventricular septal defects may be complicated by the presence of a left ventricle to right atrial shunt. This may be interpreted as an elevated right ventricular pressure when actually it is a measure of left ventricular pressure.

Echocardiography cannot directly measure pulmonary vascular resistance. However, combining assessment of pulmonary artery pressure and degree of left to right shunting based on left atrial and ventricular enlargement can provide an estimation of whether a patient with a moderate or large defect has significant elevation of pulmonary resistance. Spectral Doppler and two-dimensional diameters of the left and right ventricular outflow tracks can also be used to estimate the ratio of pulmonary to systemic blood flow.

Cardiac catheterization can provide important anatomic and hemodynamic information. Pulmonary artery pressure, pulmonary vascular resistance, and pulmonary to systemic flow ratio can be directly measured and calculated. Response to pulmonary vasodilators can be assessed. Angiography can provide

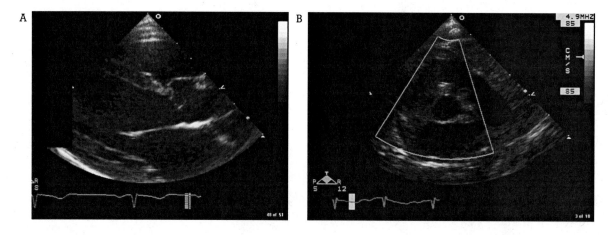

FIGURE 9–9. Parasternral long (A) and short axis (B) images of supracristal ventricular septal defect partially closed by prolapse of right aortic valve cusp. *Abbreviations*: AoV, aortic valve; LA, left atrium; LV, left ventricle; RA, right atrium, RV, right ventricle; VSD, ventricular septal defect.

morphologic details of location and number of defects and associated anatomic defects. Most infants with ventricular septal defects who are referred for surgery do not undergo cardiac catheterization prior to surgery. Catheterization is more commonly performed in older patients with borderline shunts or with concern for significant pulmonary vascular resistance elevation and in patients with residual defects after surgical repair.

Management

Infants with moderate or large defects who develop signs and symptoms of congestive heart failure may benefit from anticongestive therapy. The first line therapy is often furosemide or other diuretic with or without digoxin. Although there is a large experience with digoxin and improvement in symptoms is observed in some patients, the efficacy has not been completely proven (Kimball et al., 1991). Afterload reduction, most commonly angiotensin-converting enzyme inhibitors, has been shown to decrease pulmonary flow (Montigny et al., 1989). Other supportive medical therapy in infancy includes nutritional supplementation with high calorie formula and prophylaxis against respiratory syncytial virus. Infants with moderate size pressure restrictive defects may only have mild symptoms and only require frequent outpatient assessment. A significant number of membranous and muscular defects that initially have significant shunts will decrease in size to the point that symptoms completely abate or the defects close all together. Patients with small membranous defects do not require any medical intervention but do need to be followed-up for development of aortic valve prolapse or double-chambered right ventricle. A majority of small muscular defects diagnosed in infancy will undergo spontaneous closure. The most recent guidelines from the American Heart Association advise that antibiotic prophylaxis for endocarditis is not indicated for ventricular septal defects, except for patients with postoperative peripatch leaks (Wilson et al., 2007).

Indications for surgical closure of ventricular septal defects include large shunt with congestive heart failure, moderate size shunt with some growth delay and/or risk for long-term development of pulmonary vascular disease, associated double-chamber right ventricle, aortic valve prolapse with aortic insufficiency (Yacoub et al., 1997), and recurrent bacterial endocarditis. Although medical therapy for moderate to large defects in infancy may have some efficacy, surgical therapy is the definitive treatment and has a very low risk, even in the first 2 months of life. In patients with anatomic substrate for spontaneous closure such as a membranous defect with tricuspid valve aneurysm tissue partially

closing the defect, some period of delay may be warranted (Krovetz, 1998; Moe and Guntheroth, 1987). In general, defects that have not undergone spontaneous closure or significant reduction in size by the age 2 are unlikely to close further.

Inlet and perimembranous defects are usually approached through the atrium and supracristal defects are most commonly approached through the pulmonary valve. Muscular defects may be able to be approached through the tricuspid valve; more apical defects may require a ventriculotomy. The short- and long-term results of ventricular septal defects repair are excellent (Kidd et al., 1993; Roos-Hesselin et al., 2004). The risk of perioperative heart block is less than 5% in modern series.

Catheter device closure of ventricular septal defects is not as established as for atrial septal defects but there is extensive experience with muscular defects (Figure 9–10) (Arora et al., 2004; Bacha et al., 2005; Butera et al., 2007). Long-term closure rates of over 90% have been reported, but significant complications including heart block have been reported in over 25% of patients. Weight less than 10 kg was a significant risk for complications. A hybrid approach, placing the device through the right ventricle in the operating room, may be more appropriate in smaller children with defects that are more difficult to access surgically. A membranous ventricular septal defect device is also undergoing clinical trials (Fu et al., 2006). A phase 1 clinical trial showed a 96% closure rate by 6 months with a complication rate of 9%. There is also successful experience with transcatheter closure of postoperative residual ventricular septal defects (Knauth et al., 2004).

ATRIOVENTRICULAR SEPTAL DEFECTS

Morphology

In a normal heart, the small area of septum between the right atrium and left ventricle (above the septal tricuspid valve leaflet and below the septal mitral valve leaflet) is the atrioventricular septum. Atrioventricular septal defects (also called atrioventricular canal defects or endocardial cushion defects) are a defect in the atrioventricular septum. There is a wide anatomic and physiological spectrum but the most consistent feature is a common atrioventricular connection, the right- and left-sided components of the atrioventricular valves inserted at the same level (Anderson et al., 1998; Fugelstad et al., 1988). Atrioventricular septal defects are subdivided into partial (separate atrioventricular orifices) and complete (common atrioventricular orifice) defects (Figure 9–11). A partial atrioventricular

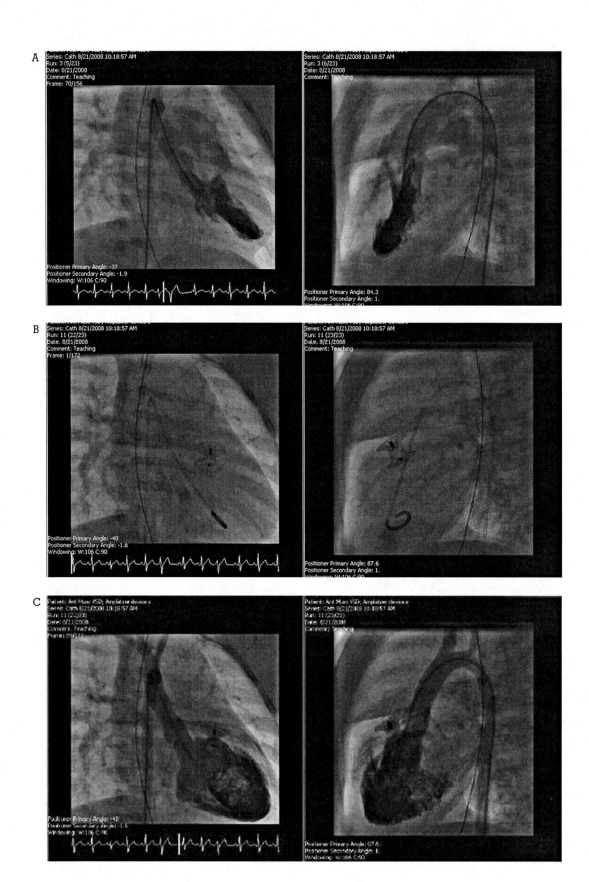

FIGURE 9–10. Angiographic images of mid muscular ventricular septal defect showing defect (A), Amplatzer device in place (B), and lack of residual defect (C).

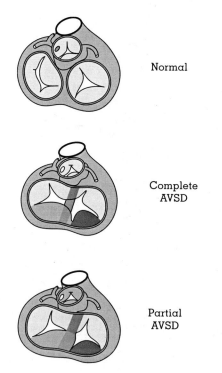

Normal

Complete
AVSD

Partial
AVSD

FIGURE 9–11. Morphology of atrioventricular valve in normal and partial and complete atrioventricular septal defects as seen from cross sectional image at crux of heart. *Abbreviation:* AVSD, atrioventricular septal defect.

septal defect consists of a primum atrial septal defect and cleft in the anterior mitral valve leaflet. A secundum atrial septal defect may also be present.

A complete atrioventricular septal defect contains a common atrioventricular valve, most often with five leaflets, an inlet ventricular septal defect, and primum atrioventricular septal defect. The Rastelli classification is used to describe the morphology of the common anterior atrioventricular valve leaflet. In type "A" atrioventricular septal defects, the anterior bridging leaflet is divided and has chordal attachments to the crest of the interventricular septum. These attachments can limit or completely occlude the ventricular septal defect component of the atrioventricular septal defect. Type "B" atrioventricular septal defects are the least common. The anterior leaflet is not divided but does have attachments to the right ventricle septal or moderator band and these attachments straddle the interventricular septum. In type "C" defects, the anterior bridging leaflet is described as free floating; the leaflet is not divided and has no chordal attachments to the crest of the septum. As a result, there is a large ventricular septal defect.

Transitional atrioventricular septal defects have features of both type "A" defects and partial defects. Chordal attachments partially close the ventricular

septal defect, resulting in a small ventricular component. In some cases, the ventricular component can be completely closed by septal attachments, giving the appearance of two separate orifices. The nomenclature can get confusing, and it is important to have an accurate description of the valve morphology.

Atrioventricular septal defects can be associated with other cardiac and noncardiac defects. There is a strong association with trisomy 21 (Marino et al., 1990); almost one half of whom have a congenital heart defect and one half of these are atrioventricular septal defects. Type "A" complete atrioventricular septal defects are the most common type seen in trisomy 21, although Type "C" defects are also frequently seen. Type "C" defects can be associated with tetralogy of Fallot (Uretzky et al., 1984) and this combination is commonly seen in trisomy 21. The association of type "C" atrioventricular septal defect with double outlet right ventricle and pulmonary venous anomalies is seen in patients with heterotaxy, most often asplenia. Atrioventricular septal defects can be balanced or associated with hypoplastic left or right ventricles.

Embryology

Cardiac looping results in a primitive atrioventricular canal, primitive right ventricle, and primitive left ventricle. Endocardial cushion tissue initially forms bulges at the atrioventricular groove. Superior and inferior endocardial cushions grow toward one another, fusing to divide the atrioventricular canal into left and right orifices (Figure 9–12), (Abdulla et al., 2004; Anderson et al., 2003; Moore and Persaud, 2003; Sadler, 2004). When this process does not occur normally, the result is an atrioventricular septal defect (also known as endocardial cushion defect or atrioventricular canal defect). This disease spectrum ranges from a primum atrial septal defect to a complete atrioventricular septal defect. This process also results in the initial formation of the inlet ventricular septum (Van Mierop, 1976). As the atria and inlet portion of the ventricles enlarge, a flap of tissue attached to the endocardial cushions is formed and ultimately becomes the atrioventricular valves. At the same time a portion of the ventricular inlet is undermined and forms the valve chordal apparatus.

Physiology

The physiology of an atrioventricular septal defect depends on the size of the atrial and ventricular septal defects. Patients with partial atrioventricular septal defects have physiology similar to patients with atrial septal defects. Those with transitional atrioventricular septal defects have physiology similar to patients with small ventricular septal defects and those with complete atrioventricular septal defects have physiology of large ventricular septal defects (Haworth, 1986). The presence of significant atrioventricular valve regurgitation may cause additional volume load on the left ventricle. In many cases, left-sided atrioventricular valve regurgitation is directed into the right atrium causing significant right atrial enlargement.

Patients with trisomy 21 and complete atrioventricular septal defects may have higher pulmonary vascular resistance than patients with similar heart defects without trisomy 21 (Hals et al., 1993). This may be secondary to the presence of airway obstruction, central hypoventilation, and more frequent respiratory infections in patients with trisomy 21.

Clinical Findings

Historical findings in patients with partial atrioventricular septal defects mimic those found in patients with moderate size atrial septal defects. If significant mitral regurgitation is present, symptoms of congestive heart failure might develop in infancy with complaints of rapid breathing and slow weight gain. In the absence of significant atrioventricular valve regurgitation, mild symptoms may be present in early childhood, but in other patients, they may present later in childhood or adulthood. The examination of a patient with a partial atrioventricular septal defect depends on the presence or absence of significant atrioventricular valve regurgitation. When present, a loud holosystolic regurgitant murmur will be heard at the apex or left lower sternal border and the patient may have tachypnea, retractions, and hepatomegaly. The examination is more typical of a large atrial septal defect when there is no significant atrioventricular valve regurgitation.

The history and physical examination findings in a complete atrioventricular septal defect depend on the size of the ventricular septal defect and presence of atrioventricular valve regurgitation. An infant with a transitional defect and very small ventricular shunt may have minimal or no symptoms on the examination of a small restrictive ventricular septal defect. Conversely, patients with large ventricular septal defects present with signs and symptoms of early congestive heart failure with a loud pulmonic component of the second heart sound, systolic pulmonary flow murmur, and possible mitral rumble.

The electrocardiogram is often very helpful in the diagnosis of atrioventricular septal defects. The bundle of His is inferiorly displaced and atrioventricular node is posteriorly deviated near the coronary sinus (Feldt et al., 1970). This results in a leftward or superior frontal plane QRS axis (figure) usually between −30° and −120° (Figure 9–13). There is qR pattern seen in leads I and AVL and absence of the normal qR pattern in leads II, III, and AVF. Additional findings will depend on degree shunting and valvar regurgitation.

Echocardiography is the primary mode of diagnosis for all types of atrioventricular septal defects (Minich et al., 1992; Silverman et al., 1986; Smallhorn, 2001). The presence and size of atrial and ventricular septal defects, atrioventricular valve morphology and function, relative sizes (Cohen et al., 1996) of the left and right atrium, ventricles, and atrioventricular valve components, and associated defects are clearly delineated by a combination of parasternal, apical, and subxyphoid windows. Apical four chamber windows provide excellent details about the presence of defects and balance (Figure 9–14). It is important to sweep from posterior to anterior to gauge the extent of the ventricular septal defect. Color flow Doppler helps define and quantify the degree of atrioventricular valve regurgitation. Spectral Doppler of tricuspid regurgitation may be used to estimate right ventricular pressure, but many patients have left ventricular to right atrial shunts, which will cause falsely elevated estimation of right ventricular pressure.

Subxyphoid coronal imaging at the plane of the atrioventricular valve provides a cross-sectional view of the valve leaflets and gives the best anatomic information about the valve morphology and relative distribution over each ventricle (Figure 9–15). The anterior leaflet can be assessed for being free floating or divided

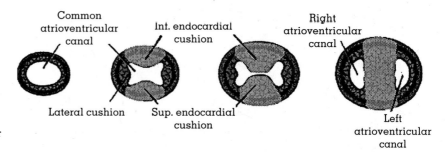

FIGURE 9–12. Embryology of atrioventricular junction/canal.

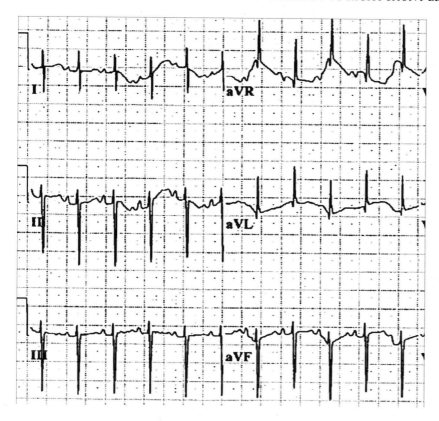

FIGURE 9-13. Electrocardiogram showing limb leads in patient with atrioventricular septal defect. There is left axis deviation with a frontal plane QRS axis of −45 degree (lead I is has a positive QRS deflection and lead aVF has a negative QRS deflection).

as well as for the presence or absence of attachments to the crest of the ventricular septum (figures). Apical sweeping from this view can provide information about the number and spacing of left ventricular papillary muscles.

Echocardiography is very important in the intraoperative and postoperative setting to assess for residual defects including left ventricle to right atrial shunts, presence of left and right sided atrioventricular valve regurgitation and subaortic obstruction. The presence

of accessory atrioventricular valve tissue as well as superior displacement of the aorta can result in subaortic stenosis in a small but significant number of patients after repair. In assessing residual left-sided atrioventricular valve regurgitation, it is important to try to assess if the leak is from a residual cleft or secondary to poor coaptation and leak through a commissure.

Cardiac catheterization is not commonly performed as a diagnostic test for atrioventricular septal defects. However, in unrepaired patients with a concern for

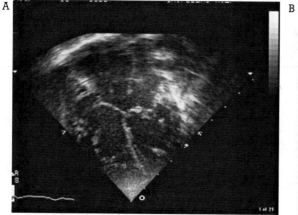
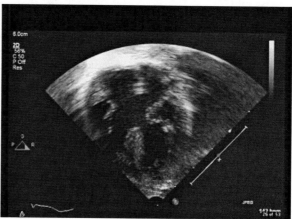

FIGURE 9-14. Apical four-chamber transthoracic echocardiographic images of partial (A) and complete (B) atrioventricular septal defects (arrows). *Abbreviations*: LA, left atrium; LV, left ventricle; RA, right atrium; RV, right ventricle.

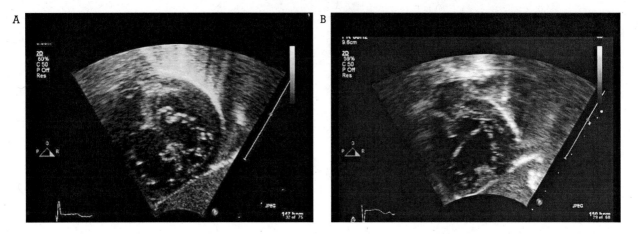

FIGURE 9–15. Subcostal coronal plane transthoracic echocardiographic images of complete Rastelli type A atrioventricular septal defect with divided anterior bridging leaflet (A) and complete Rastelli type C atrioventricular septal defect with undivided anterior bridging leaflet (B). Solid and thatched arrows show anterior and posterior atrioventricular valve leaflets respectively.

pulmonary vascular disease over 1 year of life, hemodynamic assessment of pulmonary vascular resistance may be warranted. The left ventriculogram reveals the "gooseneck deformity" of the superiorly displaced left ventricular outflow track.

Management

The natural history of atrioventricular septal defects is much less ambiguous than that of atrial and ventricular septal defects (Craig, 2006). Atrioventricular septal defects do not undergo spontaneous closure. Additionally, the underlying valve abnormalities can lead to progressive valve leak and annular dilation. Medical management with anticongestive therapy may be helpful in ameliorating some congestive heart failure symptoms in patients with large ventricular shunts but the primary treatment is surgical.

The timing of repair for complete defects with significant ventricular level shunting is usually in the first 2–4 months of life (Hanley et al., 1993). Despite the concern of increased pulmonary vascular resistance in trisomy 21, outcomes in this population are not different (Al-Hay et al., 2003; Rizzoli et al., 1992; Vet and Ottenkamp, 1989). The timing of repair for partial or transitional atrioventricular septal defects in patients without symptoms is more debatable. Repair in the neonatal period is not needed; however, repair later in the first year of life may decrease the risk of significant postoperative atrioventricular valve regurgitation (El-Najdawi et al., 2000). Adults with partial atrioventricular septal defects can undergo successful repair (Bergin et al., 1995).

Different surgical approaches to repair of complete atrioventricular septal defect include single patch (Nicholsan et al., 1999), double patch, and Australian repair (common atrioventricular leaflets are sutured directly to crest of ventricular septum). All techniques include creation of functional tricuspid and mitral valves with some degree of mitral valve cleft closure. Results of complete atrioventricular septal defect repair are quite good with mortality well under 5% (Najm et al., 1997). However, there is a significant (up to 10%) risk of need for subsequent mitral valve repair (Rhodes et al., 1997). Risk factors for this include older age at surgery, significant residual valve leak post operatively, and failure to close the cleft. The risk of recurrent mitral regurgitation requiring surgery is not decreased in primum atrial septal defects.

REFERENCES

Abdulla R, Blew GA, Holterman MJ. Cardiovascular embryology. *Pediatr Cardiol.* 2004;25:191–200.

Al-Hay AA, MacNeil SJ, Yacoub M, Shore DF, Shinebourne EA. Complete atrioventricular septal defect, Down syndrome, and surgical outcome: risk factors. *Ann Thorac Surg.* 2003;75(2):412–421.

Amin Z, Hijazi ZM, Bass JL, Cheatham JP, Hellenbrand WE, Kleinman CS. Erosion of Amplatzer septal occluder device after closure of secundum atrial septal defects: review of registry of complications and recommendations to minimize future risk. *Catheter Cardiovasc Interv.* 2004;63:496–502.

Anderson R, Webb S, Brown N, et al. Development of the heart: (2) Septation of the atrial and ventricles. *Heart.* 2003;89:949–958.

Anderson RH, Ho SY, Falcao S, Daliento L, Rigby ML. The diagnostic features of atrioventricular septal defect with common atrioventricular junction. *Cardiol Young.* 1998;8(1):33–49.

Anderson RH, Wilcox BR. The surgical anatomy of ventricular septal defect. *J Cardiac Surg.* 1992;7:17–34.

Arora R, Trehan V, Thakur AK, Mehta V, Sengupta PP, Nigam M. Transcatheter closure of congenital muscular ventricular septal defect. *J Interv Cardiol.* 2004;17:109–115.

Artman M, Graham TP Jr. Congestive heart failure in infancy: recognition and management. *Am Heart J.* 1982;103:1040–1055.

Attenhofer Jost CH, Connolly HM, Danielson GK, et al. Sinus venosus atrial septal defect: long-term postoperative outcome for 115 patients. *Circulation.* 2005;112:1953–1958.

Bacha EA, Cao QL, Galantowicz ME, et al. Multicenter experience with perventricular device closure of muscular ventricular septal defects. *Pediatr Cardiol.* 2005;26:169–175.

Bergin ML, Warnes CA, Tajik AJ, Danielson GK. Partial atrioventricular canal defect: long-term follow-up after initial repair in patients > or = 40 years old. *J Am Coll Cardiol.* 1995;25:1189–1194.

Brassard M, Fouron JC, van Doesburg NH, et al. Outcome of children with atrial septal defect considered too small for surgical closure. *Am J Cardiol.* 1999;83:1552–1555.

Butera G, Chessa M, Carminati M. Percutaneous closure of ventricular septal defects. *Cardiol Young.* 2007;17(3):243–253.

Cheatham JP, Latson LA, Gutgesell HP. Ventricular septal defect in infancy detection with two-dimensional echocardiography. *Am J Cardiol.* 1981;47:85–89.

Cohen M, Jacobs ML, Weinberg PM, Rychik J. Morphometric analysis of unbalanced common atrioventricular canal using two-dimensional echocardiography. *J Am Coll Cardiol.* 1996; 28:1017–1023.

Craig B. Atrioventricular septal defect: from fetus to adult. *Heart.* 2006;92:1879–1885.

Delaney JW, Li JS, Rhodes JF. Major complications associated with transcatheter atrial septal occluder implantation: a review of the medical literature and the manufacturer and user facility device experience (MAUDE) database. *Congenit Heart Dis.* 2007;2(4):256–264.

Du ZD, Hijazi ZM, Kleinman CS, Silverman NH, Larntz K. Comparison between transcatheter and surgical closure of secundum atrial septal defect in children and adults: results of a multicenter nonrandomized trial. *J Am Coll Cardiol.* 2002;39:1836–1844.

El-Najdawi E, Driscoll D, Puga F, et al. Operation for partial atrioventricular septal defect: a 40-year review. *J Thorac Cardiovasc Surg.* 2000;119:880–889.

Eroglu AG, Öztunç F, Saltik L Dedeoǧlu S, Bakari S, Ahunbay G. Aortic valve prolapse and aortic regurgitation in patients with ventricular septal defect. *Pediatr Cardiol.* 2003;24:36–39.

Feldt RH, DuShane JW, Titus JL. The atrioventricular conduction system in persistent common atrioventricular canal defect: correlations with electrocardiogram. *Circulation.* 1970;42:437–444.

Fu Y-C, Bass J, Amin Z, Radtke W, et al. Transcatheter closure of perimembranous ventricular septal defects using the new Amplatzer membranous VSD occluder: result of the U.S. Phase I trial. *J Am Coll Cardiol.* 2006;47:319–325.

Fugelstad SJ, Danielson GH, Puga FJ, Edwards WD. Surgical pathology of the common atrioventricular valve: a study of 11 cases. *Am J Cardiovasc Pathol.* 1988;2:49–55.

Hagen PT, Scholz DG, Edward WD. Incidence and size of patent foramen ovale during the first 10 decades of life: An autopsy study of 965 normal hearts. *Mayo Clin Proc.* 1984;59:17–20.

Hagler DJ, Edwards WD, Seward JB, Tajik AJ. Standardized nomenclature of the ventricular septum and ventricular septal defects, with applications for two-dimensional echocardiography. *Mayo Clin Proc.* 1985;60:741–752.

Hals J, Hagemo PS, Thaulow E, Sørland SJ. Pulmonary vascular resistance in complete atrioventricular septal defect: a comparison between children with and without Down syndrome. *Acta Paediatr.* 1993;82:595–598.

Hanley FL, Fenton KN, Jonas RA, et al. Surgical repair of complete atrioventricular canal defects in infancy. Twenty-year trends. *J Thorac Cardiovasc Surg.* 1993;106:387–394.

Haworth SG. Pulmonary vascular bed in children with complete atrioventricular septal defect: relation between structural and hemodynamic abnormalities. *Am J Cardiol.* 1986;57:833–839.

Houston AB, Lim MK, Doig WB, Reid JM, Coleman EN. Doppler assessment of the interventricular pressure drop in patients with ventricular septal defects. *Br Heart J.* 1988;60:50–56.

Gatzoulis MA, Freeman MA, Siu SC, Webb GD, Harris L. Atrial arrhythmia after surgical closure of atrial septal defects in adults. *N Engl J Med.* 1999;340:839–846.

Gittenberger-DeGroot AC, Bartelings MM, Deruiter MC, Poelmann RE. Basics of cardiac development for understanding of congenital heart malformations. *Pediatr Res.* 2005;57:169–176.

Kharouf R, Luxenberg DM, Khalid O, Abdulla R. Atrial septal defect: spectrum of care. *Pediatr Cardiol.* 2008;29(2): 271–280.

Kidd L, Driscoll DJ, Gersony WM, et al. Second natural history study of congenital heart defects: results of treatment of patients with ventricular septal defects. *Circulation.* 1993;87(suppl I):I38–I51.

Kimball TR, Daniels SR, Meyer RA, Hannon DW, Tian J, Shukla R, Schwartz DC. Effect of digoxin on contractility and symptoms in infants with a large ventricular septal defect. *Am J Cardiol.* 1991;68:1377–1382.

Knauth AL, Lock JE, Perry SB, et al. Transcatheter device closure of congenital and postoperative residual ventricular septal defects. *Circulation.* 2004;110:501–507.

Krovetz JL. Spontaneous closure of ventricular septal defect. *Am J Cardiol.* 1998;81:100–101.

Lun K, Li H, Leung MP, et al. Analysis of indications for surgical closure of subarterial ventricular septal defect without associated aortic cusp prolapse and aortic regurgitation. *Am J Cardiol.* 2001;87:1266–1270.

Mainwaring RD, Mirali-Akbar H, Lamberti JJ, Moore JW. Secundum-type atrial septal defects with failure to thrive in the first year of life. *J Cardiol Surg.* 1996;11:116–120.

Marino B, Vairo U, Corno A, et al. Atrioventricular canal in Down syndrome. Prevalence of associated cardiac malformations compared with patients without Down syndrome. *Am J Dis Child.* 1990;144:1120–1122.

Masura J, Gavora P, Podnar T. Long-term outcome of transcatheter secundum-type atrial septal defect closure using Amplatzer septal occluders. *J Am Coll Cardiol.* 2005;45:505–507.

McMahon CJ, Feltes TF, Fraley JK, et al. Natural history of growth of secundum atrial septal defects and implications for transcatheter closure. *Heart.* 2002;87:256–259.

Minette MS, Sahn DJ. Ventricular septal defects. *Circulation.* 2006;114(20):2190–2197.

Minich LA, Snider AR, Bove EL, Lupinetti FM, Vermilion RP. Echocardiographic evaluation of atrioventricular orifice anatomy in children with atrioventricular septal defect. *J Am Coll Cardiol.* 1992;19:149–153.

Moe DG, Guntheroth WG. Spontaneous closure of uncomplicated ventricular septal defect. *Am J Cardiol.* 1987;60:674–678.

Moore K, Persaud T. *The Developing Human.* 7th ed. Philadelphia: W.B. Saunders Company; 2003.

Moorman A, Webb S, Brown N, Lamers W, Anderson RH. Development of the heart: (1) Formation of the cardiac chambers and arterial trunks. *Heart.* 2003;89:806–814.

Montigny M, Davignon A, Fouron JC, Biron P, Fournier A, Elie R. Captopril in infants for congestive heart failure secondary to a large ventricular left-to-right shunt. *Am J Cardiol.* 1989; 63:631–633.

Murphy JG, Gersh BJ, McGoon MD, et al. Long-term outcome after surgical repair of isolated atrial septal defect: follow-up at 27 to 32 years. *N Engl J Med.* 1990;323:1645–1650.

Najm HK, Coles JG, Endo M, et al. Complete atrioventricular septal defects: results of repair, risk factors, and freedom from reoperation. *Circulation.* 1997;96:311–315.

Nicholson IA, Nunn GR, Sholler GF, et al. Simplified single patch technique for the repair of atrioventricular septal defect. *J Thorac Cardiovasc Surg.* 1999;118:642–646.

Pieroni DR, Nishimura RA, Bierman FZ, et al. Second natural study of congenital heart defects: ventricular septal defect; echocardiography. *Circulation.* 1993;87(suppl I):I80–I88.

Rabinovitch M, Keane JF, Norwood WI, Castaneda AR, Reid L. Vascular structure in lung tissue obtained at biopsy correlated with pulmonary hemodynamic findings after repair of congenital heart defects. *Circulation.* 1984;69:655–667.

Radzik D, Davignon A, Van Doesburg N, Fournier A, Marchand T, Ducharme G. Predictive factors for spontaneous closure of atrial septal defects diagnosed in the first 3 months of life. *J Am Coll Cardiol.* 1993;22:851–853.

Rhodes J, Warner KG, Fulton DR, Romero BA, Schmid CH, Marx GR. Fate of mitral regurgitation following repair of atrioventricular septal defect. *Am J Cardiol.* 1997;80:1194–1197.

Rizzoli G, Mazzucco A, Maizza F, Daliento L, Rubino M, Tursi V, Scalia D. Does Down syndrome affect prognosis of surgically managed atrioventricular canal defects? *J Thorac Cardiovasc Surg.* 1992;104:945–953.

Roguin N, Du Z-D, Barak M, Nasser N, Hershkowitz S, Milgram E. High prevalence of muscular ventricular septal defect in neonates. *J Am Coll Cardiol.* 1995;26:1545–1548.

Roos-Hesselin JW, Meijboom FJ, Spitaels SE, et al. Outcome of patients after surgical closure of ventricular septal defect at young age: longitudinal follow-up of 22–34 years. *Eur Heart J.* 2004;25:1057–1062.

Sadler T. *Langman's Medical Embryology.* 10th ed. Philadelphia: Lippincott, Williams and Wilkins; 2004.

Shahriari A, Rodefeld MD, Turrentine MW, Brown JW. Caval division technique for sinus venosus atrial septal defect with partial anomalous pulmonary venous connection. *Ann Thorac Surg.* 2006;81:224–229.

Silverman NJ, Zuberbuhler JR, Anderson RH. Atrioventricular septal defects: cross-sectional echocardiographic and morphologic comparisons. *Int J Cardiol.* 1986;13:309–331.

Slottow TL, Steinberg DH, Waksman R. Overview of the 2007 Food and Drug Administration Circulatory System Devices Panel meeting on patent foramen ovale closure devices. *Circulation.* 2007;116(6):677–682.

Smallhorn JF. Cross-sectional echocardiographic assessment of atrioventricular septal defect: basic morphology and preoperative risk factors. *Echocardiography.* 2001;18:415–432.

Soto B, Becker AE, Moulaert AJ, Lie JT, Anderson RH. Classification of ventricular septal defects. *Br Heart J.* 1980;43:332–343.

Uretzky G, Puga FJ, Danielson GK, et al. Complete atrioventricular canal associated with tetralogy of Fallot: morphologic and surgical considerations. *J Thorac Cardiovasc Surg.* 1984;87:756–766.

van den Heuvel F, Timmers T, Hess J. Morphological, haemodynamic, and clinical variables as predictors for management of isolated ventricular septal defect. *Br Heart J.* 1995;73:49–52.

Van Mierop LHS. Embryology of the atrioventricular canal region and pathogenesis of endocardial cushion defects. In: Feldt RH, McGoon DC, Ongley PA, et al., eds. *Atrioventricular Canal Defects.* Philadelphia: W.B. Saunders, 1976:1–129.

Varma C, Benson LN, Silversides C, et al. Outcomes and alternative techniques for device closure of the large secundum atrial septal defect. *Catheter Cardiovasc Interv.* 2004;61:131–139.

Vet TW, Ottenkamp J. Correction of atrioventricular septal defect: results influenced by Down syndrome? *Am J Dis Child.* 1989;143:1361–1365.

Vogel M, Berger F, Kramer A, Alexi-Meshkishvili V, Lange PE. Incidence of secondary pulmonary hypertension in adults with atrial septal or sinus venosus defects. *Heart.* 1999;82:30–33.

Webb G and Gatzoulis M. Atrial septal defect in adults: recent progress and overview. *Circ* 2006;114:1645–53.

Wilson W, Taubert K, Gewitz M, et al. Prevention of endocarditis: guidelines from the American Heart Association. *Circulation.* 2007;116:1736–1754.

Yacoub MH, Khan H, Stavri G, et al. Anatomic correction of the syndrome of prolapsing right coronary aortic cusp, dilation of the sinus of Valsalva, and ventricular septal defect. *J Thorac Cardiovasc Surg.* 1997;113:253–261.

10

Anomalous Pulmonary Venous Connections

WELTON M. GERSONY

TOTAL ANOMALOUS PULMONARY VENOUS CONNECTIONS

Total anomalous pulmonary venous connections (TAPVC) is a rare congenital anomaly in which the pulmonary veins do not connect to the left atrium, and thus completely drain via embryonic connections into the systemic venous circulation or directly into the right atrium through the coronary sinus. The type of connection and the degree of obstruction of pulmonary venous blood flow determine the natural history and clinical course of infants with this anomaly (Cooper and Gersony, 2006; Freedom et al., 1992; Garson et al., 1998; Moss et al., 1997).

TAPVC is classified as one of these four types:

- *Supracardiac* is the most common type, accounting for slightly over half of all cases. Pulmonary venous blood flows from a common pulmonary vein to a persistent left superior vena cava (vertical vein) to the innominate vein to the superior vena cava and right atrium (Figure 10–1). Less commonly, the common pulmonary vein connects directly to the right superior vena cava.
- In the *intracardiac* type, the common pulmonary vein blood flows through the left superior vena cava directly to the coronary sinus and right atrium.
- In the *infracardiac* type, pulmonary venous blood flows inferiorly through the embryonic cardinal veins to the portal system and the liver, entering the right atrium through the inferior vena cava.
- The *mixed* type is quite rare; pulmonary venous blood enters the right atrium directly through two or more connections.

Genetics

Isolated TAPVC had not been reported in association with a specific genetic loci. However, a number of individual reports and family series have identified various genetic abnormalities (Bleyl et al., 1994; Harris et al., 2004). These include the report of a large family in which TAPVC occurred as an autosominal dominant trait with a disease locus in the region of chromosome 4 (Bleyl et al., 1994). TAPVC as a component of specific genetic syndromes such as cat eye syndrome and Holt-Oram syndrome have been reported (Bleyl et al., 1994). Anomalies of pulmonary venous return occurs in virtually all cases of asplenia syndrome (bilateral right sidedness) (Cooper and Gersony, 2006; Freedom et al., 1992; Garson et al., 1998; Moss et al., 1997). However, in most instances, TAPVC occurs sporadically with no family history or association with congenital heart disease in siblings. Undoubtedly, genetic markers for this congenital heart defect will continue to be identified.

Natural History

The natural history of TAPVC is essentially determined by the degree of obstruction to pulmonary venous return (Cooper and Gersony, 2006). With severe obstruction, most commonly occurring in the infracardiac subdiaphragmatic type, the infant presents with cyanosis and severe respiratory distress in the first few day of life, and if untreated will succumb with pulmonary edema and low cardiac output. With lesser degrees of obstruction, heart failure will appear later and infants may live several months or somewhat longer. In patients who have virtually no pulmonary venous obstruction,

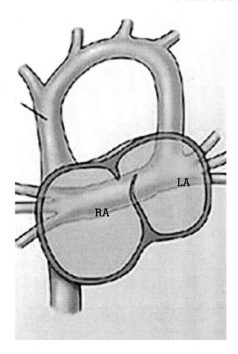

FIGURE 10–1. Schematic of supracardiac TAPVC. Common pulmonary vein is posterior to the left atrium and drains superiorly via a left superior vena cava (vertical vein) to the right superior vena cava and right atrium. The left atrium is filled via the foramen ovale.

the natural history is similar to individuals with large atrial septal defects; such patients will often survive through late childhood into adult life.

Pathophysiology

In patients with TAPVC, the entire pulmonary venous return reaches the right atrium. Systemic cardiac output is maintained by blood reaching the left heart through a dilated foramen ovale or an atrial septal defect to the left atrium, left ventricle, and aorta. Severe obstruction to pulmonary venous return results from narrowing of the common venous channel at some level between the common pulmonary vein and right atrium. Obstruction is virtually universal in TAPVC of the subdiaphragmatic type, and also occurs often with direct connection to the right superior vena cava, and occasionally with the more common superior type to the innominate vein. The natural opening of the foramen ovale rarely results in obstruction between the right and left atrium.

If obstruction is mild, there will be increased pulmonary blood flow leading to hyperkinetic pulmonary hypertension and heart failure, usually during early infancy. When there is no obstruction, cardiac failure does not occur because despite the large left to right shunt, pulmonary pressure remains relatively normal and the increased pulmonary blood flow is well tolerated.

CLINICAL FEATURES

Severe Obstruction

Neonates with severe pulmonary venous obstruction present with signs and symptoms of marked pulmonary hypertension and low pulmonary blood flow. The findings are similar to the clinical picture of severe mitral stenosis with pulmonary edema secondary to severe obstruction. A baby with obstructed TAPVC will become markedly symptomatic within the first few days of life. In the absence of a diagnostic fetal or neonatal echocardiogram, the infant may be considered to have severe lung disease, since a cardiac murmur or other signs leading to the diagnosis of heart disease are most often not apparent. The patient presents with cyanosis, marked tachypnea, tachycardia, and signs of low cardiac output. The great majority of these babies will have subdiaphragmatic venous connections, but rare infants with direct communications to the right superior vena cava or right atrium will have similar presentations.

The electrocardiogram shows right ventricular hypertrophy, at times beyond the usual newborn pattern, with ST-T wave changes, indicating a strain pattern over the right precordium. The chest x-ray shows a small cardiac silhouette with a diffuse pulmonary edema pattern, often characterized as a ground glass appearance (Figure 10–2). This may create confusion with primary pulmonary diseases of the newborn, such as respiratory distress syndrome. Arterial oxygen saturation may be as low as 60%–80%, and there is a high umbilical venous saturation (90%–100%). The infant with mild to moderate pulmonary venous obstruction, usually of the supracardiac or cardiac type will present with markedly increased pulmonary blood flow and pulmonary hypertension. The findings are that of congestive heart failure; tachycardia, tachypnea, and hepatomegaly are prominent.

The patient will be only mildly cyanotic. In contrast to the markedly obstructed form of TAPVC, the chest x-ray shows a large cardiac silhouette with markedly increased pulmonary vascular markings, but the pulmonary edema pattern characteristic of the obstructive type is not noted. The ECG will show right ventricular hypertrophy; the arterial saturation is usually in the 85%–95% range.

Some patients with TAPVC do not have pulmonary venous obstruction, and this rather uncommon presentation is most often seen with TAPVC to the coronary sinus. Pulmonary blood flow is markedly increased, but

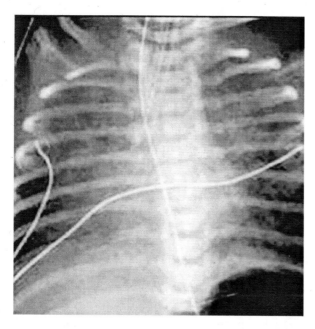

FIGURE 10-2. Chest x-ray of newborn with obstructed TAPVC. Note "ground glass" appearance of pulmonary vascularity. The heart size is normal.

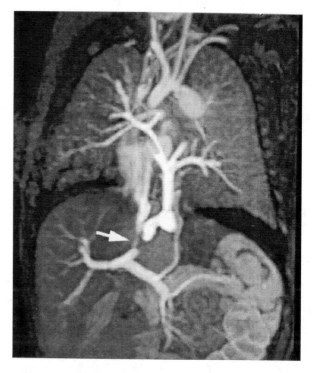

FIGURE 10-3. MRI of infant with TAPVC below the diaphragm. Pulmonary venous return enters inferior segment of a persistent venous structure, courses below the diaphragm, and enters the liver, where an obstruction is noted (arrow). Flow then continues into the inferior vena cava and right atrium.

pulmonary artery pressure is in the normal range. The large left to right shunt is well tolerated in the absence of pulmonary hypertension, and most patients will be asymptomatic through early childhood and may not be recognized until later in life. The electrocardiogram will display right ventricular enlargement, often with an RSR prime pattern in the right precordial leads. The chest x-ray will show a large cardiac silhouette with increased pulmonary blood flow.

ECHOCARDIOGRAPHY

Modern echocardiography should diagnose all types of TAPVC by demonstrating pulmonary venous confluence draining to the supra- or infracardiac veins, or directly to the heart via the coronary sinus. An MRI or CT scan will be used to confirm the diagnosis when echocardiographic studies are not definitive (Figure 10-3).

CARDIAC CATHETERIZATION

In most cases, advances in 2-D echocardiogram and Doppler color technology have eliminated the need for cardiac catheterization; potential preoperative morbidity is thus avoided. Occasionally, hemodynamic studies are required in order to evaluate associated cardiac or pulmonary disease, as well as possible postsurgical

residual anatomic abnormalities. Angiographic studies readily identify the abnormal pulmonary venous drainage (Freedom et al., 1997). Balloon septostomy of the atrial septum is rarely required for this anomaly because obstruction is unusual with right to left shunting at the atrial level. Therefore, in most cases, definitive surgical intervention is carried out without preoperative balloon septostomy.

MANAGEMENT

Medical management of symptomatic patients is transient until surgery can be accomplished (Cooper and Gersony, 2006; Freedom et al., 1992; Garson et al., 1998; Moss et al., 1997). In rare instances, prostaglandin E1 may be utilized to maintain patency of the ductus arteriosis. The use of diuretics and inotropes on a temporary basis may be useful.

Total anomalous pulmonary venous connections always require surgical repair (Cooper and Gersony, 2006; Stark and Deleval, 1983). In the vast majority of cases, operative intervention should be carried out at the time of diagnosis. There are no reasons for delay, since progressive cardiac failure is inevitable in neonates and infants with this congenital abnormality.

The rare older patient who is asymptomatic with no obstruction may be scheduled for elective repair.

Surgical correction consists of redirection of pulmonary venous return to the left atrium and closure of the atrial septal defect or foramen ovale. A large anastamosis between the common pulmonary vein and left atrium is established. To achieve this result, enlargement of the left atrium by moving the atrial septal rightward may be required. The vertical vein is ligated.

TAPVC into the coronary sinus requires a different type of operation. The coronary sinus is opened within the left atrium through a right atriotomy. The atrial septal defect is closed, resulting in all of the coronary sinus blood flowing into the left atrium. This allows all of the pulmonary venous return to enter the left atrium, along with coronary venous blood. There will be mild systemic arterial oxygen desaturation due to blood from the coronary sinus entering the systemic circulation, but this is not clinically significant.

In the modern era, mortality for surgical correction of TAPVC is extremely low, even among severely ill newborns. If TAPVC is associated with other complicated defects, such as single ventricle, polysplenia syndrome, or transposition of the great arteries, mortality, and morbidity can be expected to be more significant.

Aside from postoperative complications that might occur after any cardiac surgical procedure in an infant, the most common issue is possible residual obstruction of pulmonary venous drainage due to an insufficiently large anastamosis. However, there are also a few patients who have stenoses of individual pulmonary veins as they enter the common pulmonary vein site. In extremely rare instances, pulmonary veinule disease may result in intractable obstruction, leading to a fatal outcome.

A fully corrected patient with total anomalous pulmonary venous return has an excellent prognosis, and late reoperation is virtually never required. Although cardiac arrhythmia might be expected to be more frequent due to the surgical incisions in the atria, in practice, late supraventricular abnormalities or sick sinus syndrome are extremely rare events.

PARTIAL ANOMALOUS PULMONARY VENOUS CONNECTIONS

The hemodynamics of partial anomalous pulmonary venous connection (PAPVC) is similar to a large atrial septal defect in that there is right ventricular volume overload as a result of the left to right shunt (Freedom et al., 1992; Garson et al., 1998; Moss et al., 1997). The anomalous pulmonary venous connections may arise from either the right or left lung and may drain into the right atrium, vena cava, innominate vein, or coronary sinus. The most common type of pulmonary venous connection is from the right upper middle lobe into the right atrium or proximal SVC, and this abnormality is frequently associated with a sinus venosus type atrial septal defect. Left pulmonary vein drainage into the innominate vein and a right pulmonary vein connected to the IVC also occur with some frequency. When pulmonary venous drainage connects directly from the right lung into the IVC, the anomaly is often referred to as "scimitar syndrome," based on the x-ray images. There may be associated hypoplasia of the right lung and pulmonary artery and/or sequestration of a lobe of the right lung.

Although a single anomalous pulmonary vein would theoretically drain only one-fourth to one-third of the pulmonary arterial blood flow to the lungs, the left to right shunt will be greater because decreased resistance to venous return into the lower pressure right atrium rather than the left atrium will result in increased blood flow through the affected lung segment.

When surgical repair for PAPVC is carried out in a patient with an associated sinus venosus atrial septal defect, an ASD patch must redirect blood from the anomalous pulmonary vein into the left atrium (Gatzoulis et al., 1999; King et al., 1986). This operation often requires augmentation of the superior vena cava with a pericardial patch, in order to prevent SVC syndrome. The decision as to whether to carry out surgical tunneling of a right sided pulmonary venous connection to the left atrium is determined both by the size of the left to right shunt, and the requirements for correction of the pulmonary abnormalities. Redirection of a small anomalous right pulmonary vein that requires channeling to the left atrium, results in a low pressure blood flow channel, which may be subject to thrombosis. In such cases, small veins with minimal shunting may be left untouched, without the expectation of late cardiac manifestations.

REFERENCES

Bleyl S, Ruttenberg HD, Carey JC, Ward K. Familial total anomalous pulmonary venous return: A large utah-idaho family. *Am J Med Gen.* 1994;52:462–466.

Cooper RS, Gersony WM. Anomalous pulmonary venous connections. In: Alpert JS, ed. *The AHA Clinical Cardiac Consult.* 2nd ed. Lippincott Williams & Wilkins, Baltimore, New York, London, Buenos Aires, Hong Kong, Sydney, Tokyo; 2001:22–23, 2nd ed. 2006.

Freedom RM, Benson LN, Smalhorn JF. *Neonatal Heart Disease.* New York: Springer-Verlag; 1992.

Freedom RM, Mawson JB, Yoo S, et al. *Congenital Heart Disease—Text Book of Angiocardiology.* New York: Futura; 1997.

Garson A Jr, Bricker JT, Fisher DJ, Neish SR. *The Science and Practice of Pediatric Cardiology.* 2nd ed. Baltimore: Lippincott Williams & Wilkins; 1998.

Gatzoulis MA, Hechter S, Webb GD, Williams WG. Surgery for partial atrioventricular septal defect in the adult. *Ann Thorac Surg.* 1999;67(2):504.

Harris DL, Sui BL, Hummel M, et al. Mosaic ring 12p and total anomalous pulmonary venous return. *Am J Med Gen.* 2004;131A:91.

King RM, Puga FJ, Danielson GK, et al. Prognostic factors and surgical treatment of partial atrioventricular canal. *Circulation.* 1986;74:142.

Moss AJ, Adams FH, Emmanouilides GC. *Heart Disease in Infants Children and Adolescents.* 2nd ed. Baltimore: Williams & Wilkins; 1997.

Stark J, Deleval M. *Surgery for Congenital Heart Defects.* New York: Grune & Stratton; 1983.

11

Left Ventricular Outflow Tract Obstruction

SHARON E. O'BRIEN

VALVULAR AORTIC STENOSIS

The most common form of left ventricular outflow tract obstruction in the pediatric population is valvular aortic stenosis (AS) which accounts for 70%–86% of the cases (Kitchiner et al., 1994). In the pediatric population, the most frequent etiology of valvular AS is bicuspid (or bicommissural) aortic valve (BAV). Generally, it is accepted that the incidence of BAV is 1%–2% (Lewis and Grant et al., 1923). The true prevalence is underestimated because AS often only becomes apparent in the adult years and at that point a congenitally BAV may be indistinguishable from one with acquired stenosis (Emmanouilides, 1995). Valvular AS occurs in 3%–6% of patients with congenital heart disease (CHD). It occurs in males more than in females at a ratio of ~4:1. Associated cardiac defects, including most commonly patent ductus arteriosus, PDA and coarctation of the aorta, are found in up to 20% of cases (Braunwald et al., 1963). Conversely, a BAV occurs in 20%–85% of cases of coarctation of the aorta (Presbitero et al., 1987; Stewart, 1993; Tawes, 1969). One study also showed BAV present in 27% of cases of interrupted aortic arch, implicating a common developmental pathogenesis for abnormalities of the aortic valve and arch (Roberts et al., 1962). Ventricular septal defects and isolated pulmonary stenosis have also been reported with valvular AS but less frequently.

Pathology

The underlying abnormality of valvular AS is most commonly restricted leaflet motion, resulting in obstruction to left ventricular outflow. This may be due to thickening of the leaflet tissue, causing rigidity and/or varying degrees of fusion of one or more of the commissures. A hypoplastic valve annulus is often present with more severe degrees of AS. Most commonly, the valve will be bicuspid with unequal cusp sizes, have a central raphe, and eccentric orifice. Fusion of the intercoronary commissure is more common than fusion of the right-non commissure. Fusion of the left-non commissure is very rare (Fernandes et al., 2004). Less commonly, the valve may be unicuspid. Calcification of the valve is increasingly prominent from the fourth decade of life on. The left ventricle (LV) responds to chronic pressure overload and a hemodynamically significant obstruction will lead to the development of concentric left ventricular hypertrophy (LVH). As the afterload on the LV increases, the wall stress increases as well. The LV will develop concentric hypertrophy, which will reduce the wall stress. Poststenotic dilation of the ascending aorta may also develop with chronic pressure overload. Aortic sclerosis refers to leaflet thickening and calcification with adequate leaflet motion and normal Doppler velocity.

Severely restricted left ventricular outflow due to valvular AS may result in hypoplastic left heart syndrome in utero with endocardial fibroelastosis and small left-sided structures (see Chapter 17).

Natural History

Congenital valvular AS is frequently a progressive disorder. Worsening of obstruction is a result of increased cardiac output that occurs with growth. A decrease in the area of the effective valve orifice may also be noted and contribute to worsening of the obstruction. Patients with gradients of <25 mmHg can be followed-up medically. However, they are at risk for progression of the disease and 20% will end up requiring intervention. With gradients beyond 50 mmHg, there is a risk of arrhythmias and possibly sudden death. Complications of BAV are common and include AS, regurgitation,

TABLE 11–1. *Assessing Severity of Aortic Stenosis*

Degree of AS	Peak to Peak Systolic Gradient at Catheterization (mmHg)	Mean Echo Doppler Gradient (CW) (mmHg)	Peak Instantaneous Echo Doppler Gradient (CW) (mmHg)
Mild	<30	<25	<40
Moderate	30–50	25–40	40–70
Severe	>50	>40	>70

infective endocarditis, and aortic dissection. With the decline in the incidence of rheumatic fever in North America, rheumatic AS now represents <10% of cases of acquired AS (Schoen, 2005).

From the Natural History Study, which reports on a group of patients studied between the late 1950s and the late 1970s, the 25-year survival rate was 85% overall. This was slightly higher at 92% for those patients with initial gradients of 50 mmHg or less. The survival was slightly lower, 80%, in patients with initial gradient of greater than 50 mmHg. Sudden death was a rare event occurring in 5% of the patients. The majority of the deaths (75%) occurred in postoperative patients and in the remaining 25%, death occurred as a result of endocarditis (Wagner et al., 1977).

Physiology

The AS affects the valve, the LV, and the systemic vasculature. The degree of AS is best described as the pressure drop across the aortic valve during systole. Because the flow across a stenotic valve is turbulent, the relationship between the transvalvar gradient and transvalvar flow is not linear but instead is directly proportional to the square of the flow across the valve. Therefore, any alteration in the patient's physiologic state requiring an increased cardiac output will result in a proportionally greater increase in the gradient across the aortic valve (Gorlin, 1951). The transvalvar gradient is also affected by the contractile state of the LV and the systemic vascular resistance even without a change in the cardiac output. Heart rate will also affect the transvalvar gradient. With increasing heart rates, diastole is shortened relatively more than systole, which allows more time for the flow across the valve at any given cardiac output. Therefore the gradient alone cannot always be used as an accurate determination of the severity of AS.

Measurement of the aortic valve orifice is another method for assessing the severity of AS. The effective systolic orifice area of the valve can be calculated by using the Gorlin formula: area (cm^2) = cardiac output (mL/min)/[heart rate (beats/min) × systolic ejection period (s)√ mean gradient (mmHg)] × 44.3 (Gorlin and Gorlin, 1951). The normal orifice area is ~2.0 cm^2/m^2; areas of 0.5–0.8 cm^2/m^2 signify moderate obstruction while areas of > 0.8 cm^2/m^2 signify mild obstruction.

Table 11–1 summarizes the definitions of mild, moderate, and severe AS put forth by the task force on CHD and competitive sports at the 36th Bethesda conference (Graham et al., 2005).

In most pediatric patients with AS, the resting cardiac output remains normal and increases along with the transvalvar systolic gradient during the exercise due to the increased left ventricular pressure and total cardiac workload. LVH develops in response to chronic pressure overload and this increased wall thickness results in a normal or lower than normal wall stress despite the elevated LV pressure. Studies have also revealed a higher than normal ejection fraction and mean velocity of fiber shortening in patients with AS (Donner et al., 1983; Grahm et al., 1970).

A mismatch between myocardial oxygen demand and delivery is a significant concern in this group of patients. In the setting of elevated LV pressures, flow to the subendocardium may occur only in diastole, which is shortened in AS due to the prolonged systolic ejection time of a stenotic valve. With increased heart rates, diastole is shortened even further, which decreases the perfusion time. Additionally, coronary artery perfusion pressure is reduced if the LV end-diastolic pressure is elevated, as will occur with LV failure; or if aortic diastolic pressure is low, as will occur with aortic regurgitation (Lewis et al., 1974). The above may result in chronic ischemia and infarction.

LVH, while it helps to maintain normal wall stress in the AS patient, also contributes to impaired early diastolic filling. Adult studies have indicated that abnormal diastolic function precedes impaired myocardial contractility (Villari et al., 1992). When the LV failure occurs, cardiac output decreases; the left ventricular end-diastolic pressure, left atrial pressure, and the pulmonary artery pressure increase.

Clinical Features

Most children with AS are asymptomatic and the defect is uncovered during evaluation of a murmur. Patients who are symptomatic may complain of dyspnea with exertion or fatigability, both usually are indicators of at least moderate AS. Exertional syncope is an ominous sign, indicating the inability to maintain adequate cardiac output and cerebral perfusion during exercise and is associated with severe stenosis. Complaints of exertional chest pains are less common.

On physical examination, there may be a systolic thrill in the supraclavicular notch. More severe stenosis may present with a thrill at the right sternal border. An ejection click is typically heard best at the apex in mild or moderate stenosis followed by a harsh crescendo-decrescendo murmur best heard in the right second intercostal space. This murmur will typically transmit to the neck. The click may be absent if the valve cusps are sufficiently rigid (Shaver and Salerni, 1994; Sutton et al., 1996). S2 may be narrowed by prolonged aortic ejection time and delay of the aortic valve closure. Occasionally the aortic valve will close after the pulmonary valve, causing reversed splitting of S2. A high-pitched early diastolic murmur of aortic regurgitation may also be heard. The pulse pressure of AS is typically smaller than normal, a finding known as pulsus parvus.

Critical AS is generally well tolerated in the fetus because the right ventricle (RV) supports the majority of the combined cardiac output and due to the presence of the ductus arteriosus, which supports systemic circulation. However, cases of depressed LV function, hydrops fetalis, and endocardial fibroelastosis have been reported (McCaffrey et al., 1997; Strasburger et al., 1984). Severe AS in utero may lead to underdevelopment of left-sided structures and possibly hypoplastic left heart syndrome. Fetal echocardiography is key to detecting patients at risk and identifying those patients who may potentially benefit from in utero intervention (Makikallio, 2006).

Postnatally, signs and symptoms of heart failure may develop as the ductus arteriosus closes and adequate cardiac output cannot be maintained. Infarction of the papillary muscles may lead to significant mitral regurgitation, which worsens the heart failure. The infant may present with increased work of breathing, irritability, and poor feeding. The patient may be cyanotic on examination—from intrapulmonary shunting, tachypneic, tachycardic, and hypotensive. On physical examination, the precordium may be hyperactive with preserved ventricular function or quiet in the setting of severe ventricular dysfunction. Generally, a click is not appreciated. The systolic murmur of AS may be soft or absent due to decreased transvalvar flow. The murmur may increase with medical intervention if cardiac output increases and it may be best heard at the lower left sternal border. The murmur of mitral regurgitation may be heard at the apex. Hepatomegaly may be present and peripheral pulses will be poor. This clinical situation requires immediate intervention.

The infant with severe AS presents in infancy with signs and symptoms of heart failure. Patients typically demonstrate tachypnea, poor feeding, and irritability.

A hyperdynamic precordium is usually present and a thrill may be present. Typically, a click is not heard with severe stenosis. The systolic ejection murmur of severe AS is atypical and heard along the left sternal border radiating to the neck. Pulses are diminished.

ECG. There is a wide range of findings on the electrocardiogram (ECG) of a patient with AS depending on the degree of obstruction. With mild gradients, the ECG may be normal. With more severe obstruction, the ECG may reveal increased left ventricular voltage, decreased right ventricular forces, and ST–T wave changes consistent with strain.

CXR. The chest X-ray (CXR) may be normal in patients with mild disease. In infants with congestive heart failure, there will be cardiomegaly and increased pulmonary vascular markings. Poststenotic dilation of the ascending aorta may be visible in the CXR. If there is an associated coarctation, rib notching indicative of collateral vessels may be observed.

ECHO. 2-D echocardiography is an excellent method of evaluating the morphology of the aortic valve. The number of commissures, whether or not these commissures are partially or completely fused, the size of the leaflets, and thickening of the leaflets are all examined from the parasternal short-axis views. The dimension of the aortic valve annulus and leaflet mobility is best demonstrated from the parasternal long-axis views. Color Doppler will reveal flow turbulence at the level of the valve annulus and is best demonstrated from the apical or parasternal long-axis views. Color Doppler will also reveal the presence of aortic regurgitation that is frequently associated with AS. The apical and parasternal views are best to measure the vena contracta, which is a parameter for assessing severity of AR. Color Doppler in the parasternal short-axis view will indicate the origin of the regurgitant jet. 3-D echocardiography is useful for determining the exact mechanism of the regurgitation.

In the infant with severe or critical AS, markedly diminished mobility of the aortic valve in association with poststenotic dilation of the ascending aorta will be observed and LVH and RV dilation will be seen. Left-to-right shunting at high velocity at the atrial level is observed with left atrial hypertension. Full examination of the cardiac anatomy should be performed to assess for additional cardiovascular malformations. In particular, examination of the mitral valve annulus size and left ventricular volumes should be undertaken to assess for hypoplastic left heart. The supramitral valve area and the subaortic valve region should be evaluated because obstruction at these levels may occur in the Shone syndrome. Careful assessment of the aortic arch should be made to assess for arch obstruction because coexisting coarctation of the aorta occurs in 6% of cases with BAV (Roberts, 1970).

With recent advances in echocardiography, Doppler routinely measures aortic valve pressure gradients. Although Doppler measures the maximum instantaneous pressure gradient as opposed to the peak-to-peak pressure gradient obtained in the catheterization laboratory, it is a useful technique for serial studies given its noninvasive nature. It is not useful, however, as a sole marker of disease severity. The maximum instantaneous gradient obtained by Doppler tends to routinely overestimate the peak-to-peak gradient obtained in the catheterization laboratory. In adults, the Doppler mean gradient has been shown to be a more reliable estimation of the peak-to-peak gradient (Currie et al., 1986).

Cardiac Catheterization. Cardiac catheterization is useful for therapeutic as well as diagnostic measures. However, given the advances in noninvasive imaging, it is increasingly rare to take an AS patient to the catheterization laboratory for hemodynamic reasons alone. Indications for cardiac catheterization and possible balloon dilation include the following:

1. Episodes of fainting
2. Chest pain thought to be cardiac in origin
3. ST or T wave changes on ECG at rest or with exercise
4. A maximum instantaneous gradient MIG of 60 mmHg or more by echocardiography
5. Ventricular ectopy

The peak-to-peak pressure gradient across the aortic valve is measured and the balloon dilation performed if the gradient is more than 50 mmHg and aortic regurgitation is no more than mild.

Angiography can provide valuable anatomical information. A contrast injection in the ascending aorta will reveal the degree of aortic regurgitation, outline the aortic valve, and in particular delineate the fused commissure of a bicommissural valve (Keane et al., 2006).

Exercise Stress Testing. Exercise stress testing (EST) is useful in asymptomatic patients with normal or borderline findings. The development of ST or T wave changes with exercise could indicate significant obstruction. An EST is particularly useful in those patients wanting to participate in competitive sports.

Management

Differentiation between mild, moderate, and severe AS is based on the physical examination, ECG, echocardiography, and if required cardiac catheterization. Symptomatic patients including those with lightheadedness, dizziness, syncope, chest pain, or pallor with exercise warrant a complete evaluation possibly including cardiac catheterization and EST. Indications for cardiac catheterization are mentioned above.

For asymptomatic patients with a peak-to-peak gradient at catheterization of <25 mmHg, and normal ECG and EST, careful monitoring during annual evaluations with no restrictions on activity is reasonable. For asymptomatic patients with a gradient of 25–49 mmHg, and normal ECG and EST, no intervention is warranted, but strenuous activity should be avoided. Careful monitoring of this group on an annual basis is required. For patients with a gradient greater than 50 mmHg and no more than mild aortic regurgitation, balloon dilation is warranted (Keane, 1993). In general, balloon valvuloplasty is successful in dilating or tearing the aortic valve leaflets with a decrease in the transvalvar gradient by at least 50% being the rule. Aortic regurgitation is a common complication and although generally mild, it can at times be significant. Long-term survival is excellent although the incidence of repeat intervention at 8 years is 50% (Moore et al., 1996).

Severe or critical AS in the infant requires immediate intervention. Supportive medical management including the use of prostaglandins to maintain the patency of the ductus arteriosus is used as an adjunct to balloon dilation. One study of 113 infants undergoing balloon valvuloplasty demonstrated that there was a reduction in the gradient by 50% with 15% of patients developing significant aortic regurgitation. Approximately 50% of patients required reintervention by 5 years. Early mortality was significantly lower for those undergoing intervention between 1994 and 2002 as compared to 1985 and 1993 (4% vs. 22%) (McElhinney et al., 2005).

In the fetus with severe AS, balloon valvuloplasty has the ability to increase forward flow across the LV and left ventricular outflow tract LVOT, potential reversing the development of critical AS with small left-sided structures, endocardial fibroelastosis, or even frank hypoplastic left heart syndrome (Latson, 2005; Marshall et al., 2005).

Balloon dilation is generally ineffective in adults because of calcification of the valves. Aortic valve replacement is the preferred treatment option in this group of patients especially if more than mild aortic regurgitation is present (Rosenfeld, 1994).

Patients with moderate to severe aortic regurgitation are not candidates for balloon valvotomy. Patients with aortic regurgitation and stable, moderately dilated LVs may be medically managed with the afterload reducing agents. Patients who develop syncope, chest pain, ventricular arrhythmias, or signs or symptoms of congestive heart failure should undergo surgical intervention. When possible, a valvuloplasty will be performed. Other options include aortic valve replacement with a prosthesis and long-term anticoagulation. The Ross operation with replacing the aortic valve with the pulmonary valve has met with success at some centers.

At the 36th Bethesda Conference, Task Force 2 on CHD outlined the following recommendations for patients with untreated aortic valve disease participating in competitive sports:

Asymptomatic athletes with mild AS can participate in all competitive sports if they have a normal ECG, EST, and no tachyarrhythmias associated with symptoms.

Asymptomatic athletes with moderate AS can participate in low-static/low-to-moderate-dynamic and moderate-static/low-to-moderate dynamic (classes IA, IB, and IIA) competitive sports if: they have mild or no LVH by echocardiography and no LV strain pattern by ECG, they have a normal EST without evidence of myocardial ischemia or tachyarrhythmias and with normal EST duration and BP response. Althetes with supraventricular tachycardia (SVT) or multiple or complex ventricular tachyarrhythmias at rest or with exercise can participate only in low-intensity competitive sports (classes IA and IB).

Athletes with severe AS should not participate in competitive sports (Graham et al., 2005).

In 2007, the American Heart Association revised the guidelines regarding antiobiotic prophylaxis to prevent bacterial endocarditis. Patients with valvular AS no longer require prophylaxis. However, if there is a prosthetic valve, a history of endocarditis, a history of repair requiring prosthetic material, prophylaxis would be required for 6 months following the procedure; or if there were history of a repair with a residual defect adjacent to prosthetic material in which case prophylaxis is continued indefinitely (Walter, 2007).

SUBAORTIC STENOSIS

Subaortic stenosis, also referred to as subvalvar AS, encompasses a group of lesions that create obstruction to left ventricular outflow at a level beneath the aortic valve. It accounts for approximately 10%–14% of AS cases (Kitchiner et al., 1994; Liu et al., 1997) and is the second most common cause of AS. Subaortic stenosis may be fixed or dynamic. The latter is usually related to hypertrophic cardiomyopathy and will not be reviewed in this section. Subaortic stenosis is a condition seldom present in infancy although it is associated with other CHD in 50%–65% of cases (Choi ans Sullivan, 1991; Leichter, 1989). Associated CHD

lesions can include coarctation of the aorta, interrupted aortic arch, patent ductus arteriosus, mitral stenosis, and ventricular septal defects. Progression of subaortic stenosis during childhood is well recognized. Often there is a deformation of the aortic valve caused by the high-velocity jet of blood across the subaortic stenosis. This constant injury/damage to the aortic valve may lead to aortic regurgitation. The etiology of subaortic stenosis remains unclear. The rarity of this condition in infancy and the natural history for progression with time has caused many to consider this an acquired lesion as opposed to congenital (Firpo et al., 1990). In 1992, Gelwillig and colleagues proposed the theory that abnormal flow patterns are present in patients with subaortic stenosis and that chronic flow disturbances stimulate the endothelium to undergo transformation, creating thickening and fibrosis, which leads to the stenosis and its recurrence (Gewillig et al., 1992). However, there is good evidence for a genetic predisposition. This includes the description of familial subaortic stenosis in Newfoundland dogs (Pyle et al., 1976) and humans (Urbach et al., 1985). Additionally it has been demonstrated that among children who undergo repair of VSD, coarctation of the aorta, or both and subsequently develop subaortic stenosis, there is a LVOT abnormality characterized by a wider mitral–aortic separation, an exaggerated aortic override, and a steeper aortoseptal angle (Kleinert and Geva, 1993).

Pathology

There are four types of subaortic stenosis, the most common of them being the discrete membrane located at a variable distance from the aortic valve. The term "membrane" is somewhat misleading in as much as the tissue is often thickened. At times, this membrane is located so close to the aortic valve that the surgeon has to peel it away from the valve tissue. Commonly the membrane is circumferential.

The tunnel type of subaortic stenosis is less common and involves a greater length of obstruction beneath the aortic valve. Frequently hypoplasia of the aortic annulus is present as well as LVH. This type also tends to involve the anterior leaflet of the mitral valve (Maron et al., 1976).

Hypertrophy of the ventricular septum produces a dynamic obstruction to left ventricular outflow.

Occasionally, accessory tissue presumed to be derived from the endocardial cushions can billow in to the outflow region during systole and create obstruction. Additionally, there can be abnormal attachments from the anterior leaflet of the mitral valve to the ventricular septum, which creates stenosis.

Natural History

Subaortic stenosis is generally thought of as a progressive disease. It is very rarely severe in infancy but can progress rapidly during childhood. However, the rate of progression of mild subaortic stenosis is variable and some patients may remain stable for years (De Vries et al., 1992; Leichter et al., 1989). Not unexpectedly, patients diagnosed in adulthood as having subaortic stenosis have a slower rate of progression of their disease. Oliver et al. showed a progression of only 2.25 ± 4.7 mmHg per year of follow-up (Oliver et al., 2001). Aortic regurgitation may develop or progress as the systolic gradient worsens, if the patient undergoes a procedure or if the patient were to develop endocarditis. Risk factors for increased aortic regurgitation appear to be a Doppler gradient >50 mmHg, history of endocarditis, or a history of intervention (Aboulhosn and Child, 2006). Congestive heart failure secondary to subaortic stenosis alone is virtually nonexistent. Early studies looking at recurrence of subaortic stenosis after surgical intervention reported a recurrence rate of approximately 20% or more. In more recent years, circumferential enucleation of the fibrous membrane occasionally with myomectomy appears to provide more satisfactory results; however the problem of recurrence still exists (Gersony, 2001). Subacute bacterial endocarditis is a known complication of subaortic stenosis. One study reported a 12% rate of occurrence of subacute bacterial endocarditis in cases of subaortic stenosis (Wright et al., 1983).

Physiology

It is theorized that subaortic stenosis results from an abnormal geometry of the LVOT, which promotes abnormal flow patterns in this region and over time leads to progressive thickening, fibrosis, and the development of subaortic stenosis. The severity of subaortic stenosis may be masked by other lesions such as obstructive lesions distal to the subaortic region, (e.g., coarctation of the aorta), large VSDs, or a right-to-left shunting ductus arteriosus that supplies the distal systemic circulation.

Aortic regurgitation may be present and is thought to result from chronic insult to the aortic valve from the high-pressure jet of the subaortic stenosis; however, direct extension of the fibrous material into the aortic valve has been cited as an etiology as well (Feigl et al., 1984). Prevention of aortic valve injury is often presented as an indication for early surgery. This is controversial and it has been reported that aortic regurgitation is more prominent in patients after surgical repair than in unoperated patients (Oliver et al., 2001). In 2004,

McMahon et al. showed that a peak gradient of ≥50 mmHg was a significant predictor of at least moderate aortic regurgitation (McMahon et al., 2004).

Clinical Features

Isolated subaortic stenosis is rare in the infant population (Leichter et al., 1989) and mild subaortic stenosis typically leaves a patient asymptomatic. Therefore, isolated subaortic stenosis typically presents in childhood or later following progression of the stenosis. The recognition of subaortic stenosis may occur earlier in patients being evaluated for associated heart defects. It may develop in the unoperated patient or may progress following surgical correction of the associated defect. The murmur of subaortic stenosis is a systolic-ejection murmur at the mid-left sternal border. This is similar to the murmur of valvular AS, however, only rarely there is a systolic click. One study reports that the majority of affected patients have a murmur during the first year of life, which becomes more typical of subaortic stenosis as the child gets older (Newfeld et al., 1976). A thrill may be palpable. If aortic regurgitation is present, an early, high-pitched, diastolic blowing murmur may be heard as well. The murmur of a fixed obstruction like subaortic stenosis will be accentuated by squatting and diminished by standing or a Valsalva maneuver. This is in contrast to the murmur of a dynamic LVOT obstruction such as hypertrophic cardiomyopathy in which the murmur is accentuated by standing or Valsalva maneuver and diminished by squatting.

ECG. The ECG usually reveals LVH in proportion to the degree of obstruction.

CXR. The CXR in isolated subaortic stenosis is rarely revealing. Typically there is no cardiomegaly or dilation of the aortic root. If associated cardiac lesions are present, abnormalities may be seen in the chest x-ray.

ECHO. 2-D echocardiography is the gold standard for confirming the diagnosis of a subaortic stenosis and delineating any associated cardiac anomalies. A fibrous membrane is typically seen arising from the septal surface just proximal to junction of the septum with the aortic root. Occasionally, the membrane may arise from a thickened muscular ridge located more proximally in the left ventricular outflow tract. An attachment of the fibrous membrane to the anterior leaflet of the mitral valve can frequently be seen. 3-D echocardiography can usually demonstrate the circumferential nature of the membrane. A measurement of the distance between the subaortic obstruction and the aortic valve annulus should be made. The aortic valve leaflets can be assessed for thickening. Pulse- and continuous-wave Dopplers are used to estimate the degree of subaortic obstruction. The maximum instantaneous gradient obtained by Doppler often overestimates, by as much as 37%, the peak-to-peak gradient obtained in the cardiac catheterization laboratory (Currie et al., 1986). It is therefore recommended by many that the mean gradient obtained by Doppler be used for the purpose of making management decisions given that this number correlates much more closely with the peak-to-peak gradient in the cardiac catheterization laboratory (Bengur et al., 1989; Rosenfeld et al., 1994). Color and pulse Doppler will identify any aortic regurgitation. LVH is usually in proportion to the degree of obstruction in isolated subaortic stenosis.

Cardiac Catheterization. Cardiac catheterization can provide both hemodynamic and anatomical data including the gradient across the LVOT, cardiac output, the degree of aortic regurgitation, and any associated heart defects. Catheterization is particularly useful in complex cases with associated defects and multiple levels of obstruction but is not generally performed on isolated subaortic membranes.

Management

Balloon dilation is ineffective for the relief of subaortic stenosis. Therefore, definitive repair includes surgical resection of the fibrous material and potentially a myomectomy in cases of tunnel like obstruction. These include the Konno procedure with septal incision and patch augmentation of the LVOT.

The timing of the surgery in this lesion has been controversial given the high rate of recurrence balanced against the long-term effects including the potential for rapid progression and the development of aortic regurgitation. More recently, it has been recognized that the progression of mild subaortic stenosis is very variable and can remain stable for years.

Often the presence of aortic regurgitation is identified as a reason for early surgery. However, this has become more controversial with the recognition that aortic regurgitation rarely progresses to a moderate degree in the unoperated patient whereas there have been higher levels of regurgitation documented in the postoperative patient.

Many agree on the following management strategies:

1. During early childhood, patients with a maximum instantaneous gradient of <30 mmHg and no significant LVH should be followed closely, especially during the first several years of life when progression may be rapid. Patients can be seen regularly at 6-month intervals if stable or sooner if there is a change in the examination, if they develop symptoms referable to the cardiovascular system, or if there is an indication of progression of the disease. Echocardiography is performed for any change in examination or symptoms. The limitations of echocardiography must be recognized and cardiac catheterization pursued if it is unclear as to whether the gradient is significant or not.

   Some advocate for surgical intervention for a gradient >30 mmHg in this age group (Gersony, 2001) while others would not proceed with surgery for a maximum instantaneous gradient of <60 mmHg without LVH in the first decade of life (Brown and Keane, 2006).
2. Older children with gradients of <30 mmHg can be followed-up with at less frequent intervals until there is evidence by echocardiography or cardiac catheterization of significant progression of the subaortic obstruction.
3. Adult patients with a gradient of <50 mmHg and no significant LVH should be followed at regular intervals since they too may develop progressive subaortic obstruction and eventually require intervention.
4. The desire to prevent aortic regurgitation is not an indication for surgery. Un-operated patients rarely develop hemodynamically significant aortic regurgitation. However, the progression of aortic regurgitation in this lesion has been used as an indication for intervention (Gersony, 2001).

In 2007, the American Heart Association revised the guidelines regarding antibiotic prophylaxis to prevent bacterial endocarditis. Patients with isolated subaortic stenosis no longer require prophylaxis unless there is a history of endocarditis, a history of repair requiring prosthetic material in which case prophylaxis would be required for 6 months following the procedure, or if there were history of a repair with a residual defect adjacent to prosthetic material in which case prophylaxis is continued indefinitely (Walter, 2007).

SUPRAVALVAR AORTIC STENOSIS

The defining feature of congenital supravalvar aortic stenosis (SVAS) is narrowing at the level of the sinotubular junction although narrowing of the entire ascending aorta and arch vessels has been recognized as well. This lesion is the rarest of the left ventricular obstructive lesions accounting for 8%–14% of cases of congenital AS (Kitchiner et al., 1994; Liu et al., 1997). The underlying cause of this lesion, which can be sporadic or inherited, has been identified as a mutation of the elastin gene on chromosome *7q11.23*. This mutation results in an obstructive arteriopathy, which can involve the systemic and pulmonary arteries but which is most prominent at the aortic sinotubular junction. This localization can impact the functioning of the aortic valve and the coronary arteries. Two anatomic variants have been recognized, discrete and diffuse, the former being more common. There is relatively little clinical experience with SVAS and general treatment guidelines have not been established. Various modifications of surgical treatments have been proposed but it is unclear if these will have true long-term benefits over traditional surgical approaches.

Pathology

SVAS is caused by a loss-of-function mutation on chromosome *7q11.23*. A single gene on this chromosome encodes for tropoelastin, which is the soluble precursor to elastin. Tropoelastin is formed in concentric rings alternating with layers of smooth muscle cells. Affected individuals produce less tropoelastin during development, resulting in an overall reduction of elastin content in the large arteries with disorganized arrangement of the elastin lamellae. Large arteries have the majority of elastin fibers in the media to absorb the energy in systole and disperse energy during diastole. The loss of elasticity in affected individuals may lead to increased shear stress on the arterial wall, triggering hypertrophy of smooth muscle cells and increased deposition of collagen, resulting in marked thickening of the media (Li, Brooke et al., 1998; Li, Faury et al., 1998). The predominant histologic findings are of the media and include an increased number of hypertrophied smooth muscle cells, increased amounts of collagen, and abnormal elastic tissue with coarse and stumpy or scant and slender disorganized elastin fibers. Marked intimal thickening has been reported as well (Vaideeswar et al., 2001).

Clinically, SVAS is recognized in four different forms: an inherited, autosomal dominant familial form; an isolated, sporadic form; in patients with familial hypercholesterolemia (FH); and in association with William's syndrome, an entity that also includes mental retardation, hypercalcemia, distinctive facial features, and peripheral pulmonary artery stenosis. In addition to the disruption of the elastin gene, patients with Williams syndrome also have a disruption of neighboring genes, which account for the other features observed (Eronen et al., 2002). In one study, the sporadic form accounted for the majority (52%) of SVAS cases (Flaker et al., 1983).

Currently there are two recognized anatomic forms of SVAS. The discrete form is the most common, accounts for 60%–75% of cases and exhibits the classic hourglass deformity creating a discrete narrowing at the level of the sinotubular junction (Flaker et al.,

1983; Morrow et al., 1959). The diffuse form is seen in 25%–40% of cases and exhibits a diffuse narrowing for a variable distance along the ascending aorta. Involvement of the pulmonary, arch, renal, common iliac, and coronary arteries can also occur.

Abnormal coronary blood flow has been reported frequently in SVAS. The coronary artery ostia can be obstructed by a thickened aortic or sinus wall. Additionally, the coronary artery blood flow can be restricted by adhesion of the leaflet edge to the sinotubular junction. The left coronary sinus of Valsalva seems to be involved most frequently. The coronary arteries can become dilated and tortuous secondary to the high, prestenotic pressures and premature atherosclerosis may develop (Kim et al., 1999; Stamm et al., 1997). The development of LVH, increased myocardial mass, and elevated intramyocardial pressures can result in significant mismatch of myocardial demand and perfusion, which in turn can lead to subendocardial ischemia. Chronic ischemic changes including myocyte necrosis and subendocardial fibrosis have been described (Van Son et al., 1994).

Abnormalities of the aortic valve leaflets have been described in up to 50% of surgical SVAS patients (Stamm et al., 2001). These abnormalities include severely thickened leaflets that are adherent to the narrowed sinotubular junction. In normal hearts, the aortic root and sinotubular junction expand during systole, allowing the leaflet edges to straighten, thus maintaining a constant strain and minimizing fatigue stress (Brewer et al., 1976). A stiff, fixed sinotubular junction and redundant aortic leaflets do not permit the leaflet edges to straighten, which results in premature degeneration of the valve leaflets. Aortic regurgitation is common being present in ~41% of cases.

Natural History

Narrowing of the aortic lumen results in progressive left ventricular hypertension and hypertrophy. Thickening of the aortic leaflets and aortic regurgitation may develop due to the rigid sinotubular junction and redundant aortic valve leaflets. Impaired coronary artery blood flow can occur and lead to a perfusion mismatch, resulting in chronic ischemia and its associated findings. Associated vascular obstructions including coarctation of the aorta can also be progressive.

Physiology

The physiology is similar to that of valvular AS with the development of a hypertensive, hypertrophied LV. This is complicated by the coronary artery abnormalities described above with impaired coronary artery perfusion.

Clinical Features

Up to 30% of patients with SVAS have Williams syndrome and its associated clinical findings such as elfin facies, short stature, mental retardation, hypercalcemia, and defects in visuospatial cognition. In the absence of Williams syndrome, the clinical features of SVAS are mainly due to the LVOT obstruction, but may also include findings due to the coronary artery abnormalities with possible ischemia and the findings associated with other obstructive lesions such as coarctation of the aorta or renal artery stenosis.

The blood pressure may be higher in the right arm as compared to the left arm due to the Coanda effect. This phenomenon is due to the systolic jet of SVAS that transfers the kinetic energy to the innominate artery by hugging the aortic wall. Hypertension may be present if coarctation of the aorta or renal artery stenosis is present.

SVAS patients typically have a loud systolic ejection murmur heard best at the first right intercostal space and the suprasternal notch with a thrill often present at the latter. There is the notable absence of a systolic click, which is typically heard in valvular AS. The diastolic murmur of mild aortic regurgitation may be present. Murmurs of peripheral pulmonary stenosis may be heard over the axillae and back. The murmur of renal artery stenosis may be heard over the abdomen.

ECG. LVH with or without a strain pattern will be evident if LVOT obstruction is significant. Findings of coronary artery ischemia may be present if there is significant perfusion mismatch.

CXR. The heart may be enlarge but otherwise the CXR is typically unremarkable.

ECHO. The diagnosis is made with echocardiography. The supravalvar narrowing is best seen from parasternal long-axis views. Careful examination of the aortic valve leaflets, sinuses of Valsalva, coronary arteries, sinotubular junction, and ascending, transverse, and descending aorta must be made. Imaging of the arch vessels should be performed. Color and spectral Doppler should be used to estimate the gradient across the supravalvar narrowing. Evaluation of left ventricular mass and function should be made. Branch pulmonary arteries should be evaluated for stenosis and right ventricular systolic pressure estimated.

MRI. Magnetic resonance imaging (MRI) can provide excellent anatomical detail and is useful when echocardiographic imaging is limited or when associated obstructive lesions are suspected. Otherwise echocardiography alone is adequate.

Cardiac Catheterization. In the straightforward patient with SVAS, cardiac catheterization is unnecessary. In cases of distal branch pulmonary stenosis, however cardiac catheterization is useful to relieve these obstructions, which otherwise might be inaccessible to the surgeon.

Management

The 2007 American Heart Association guidelines on the prevention of bacterial endocarditis do not recommend prophylaxis for patients with SVAS. The exceptions are patients with a history of endocarditis, history of prosthetic material in which case prohylaxis is recommended for the first 6 months following surgery, or in patients with prosthetic material and a residual defect in which case prophylaxis is continued indefinitely.

The definitive treatment of SVAS is surgical with the main goal of surgery being the relief of the left ventricular pressure overload.

Indications for surgery are debatable because experience is limited. Since surgery can be curative for the discrete form of SVAS, it is recommended for symptomatic disease and for instantaneous gradients exceeding 30 mmHg at cardiac catheterization (Castaneda et al., 1994).

Surgical techniques vary and include simple patch enlargement of the sinotubular junction above the noncoronary sinus, bifurcated patch augmentation of the right coronary sinus, and noncoronary sinus, and separate patches of all three sinuses after transaction of the aorta. It is controversial whether three-sinus reconstructions are superior to simple patch augmentation of the noncoronary sinus (Stamm et al., 2001).Treatment of the diffuse form of SVAS is more complicated and options include extensive endarterectomy and patch aortoplasty, resection of stenotic segment with end-to-end anastomosis, and adjunct therapy with transcatheter stent placement (Brown et al., 2002).

Surgical outcomes depend upon the form of SVAS and associated lesions. Operative mortality ranges from 1%–9%, 20 year survival ranges from 77%–97%, and freedom from reoperation ranges from 81%–85%. Diffuse stenosis and associated aortic valve disease were the predictors of worse outcome (Brown et al., 2002).

COARCTATION OF THE AORTA

Coarctation of the aorta was first described by Morgagni in 1760 from an autopsy case (Aboulhosn and Child, 2006). It is a common defect accounting for approximately 7% of CHD with a male predominance of 2:1. Coarctation usually presents as a discrete narrowing just opposite the insertion of the ductus arteriosus, the "juxta-ductal" coarctation. A prominent posterior shelf due to an infolding of the posterior wall is usually present. Pathological specimens reveal intimal hyperplasia and medial thickening that may create the posterolateral ridge that narrows the aortic lumen. However, a wide range of anatomical and physiological variations of coarctation can be found. It can present as a lesion proximal or distal to the left subclavian or even in the abdominal aorta (Refenstein et al., 1947). It can be a complicated lesion with involvement of the more proximal arch, tortuosity of the arch, or a long segment of narrowing. BAV is seen in 22%–42% of the cases. Additional cardiac lesions can include ventricular septal defects, patent ductus arteriosus, mitral stenosis, and AS either at the subvalvar, valvar, or supravalvar levels. Intracranial aneurysms are the most important noncardiac associated malformation and affect up to 10% of the patients (Connolly et al., 2003). Previously, familial recurrence was thought to be rare. However, recent studies have shown evidence of an increased familial risk for left ventricular outflow tract obstructive lesions including coarctation of the aorta (McBride et al., 2005; Wessels et al., 2005). Patients with Turner's syndrome also have an increased incidence of BAV, which is seen in approximately 30% of the patients and coarctation of the aorta seen in approximately 10% of the patients (Jones and Kenneth, 1997).

Pathology

Coarctation of the aorta may be a congenital or acquired lesion. In the normal fetus, the aortic arch develops during the sixth to eighth week of gestation. The left fourth aortic arch persists to form the thoracic aortic arch and the isthmus distally. The distal part of the left sixth aortic arch forms the ductus arteriosus. Therefore, the typical coarctation of the aorta most likely involves an abnormality of the fourth or sixth aortic arches. The exact underlying mechanism that gives rise to the development of coarctation of the aorta is not completely understood but is thought to be due to either reduced antegrade aortic arch blood flow during fetal life, which leads to an underdevelopment of the aortic arch or as a result of constriction of ductal tissue that extends into the aorta itself (Rudolph, 2001; Rudolph et al., 1972; Talner et al., 1975). In fetal life, the aortic isthmus receives only 10% of combined cardiac output accounting for its relatively smaller size compared to the ascending aorta. Abnormalities, which restrict the amount of flow across the ascending aorta, could contribute to underdevelopment of the aortic isthmus and coarctation of the aorta (Rudolph et al., 1972; Shinebourne and Elseed, 1974).

Acquired coarctation of the aorta can be associated with inflammatory diseases such as Takayasu arteritis where the midthoracic or abdominal aorta is often the site of involvement (Pagni et al., 1996).

Natural History

Unoperated adult patients invariably present with systemic hypertension in the upper extremities. Measurements of the upper and lower extremity blood pressures will make the diagnosis of coarctation of the aorta. In the normal patient, the lower extremity blood pressure should be higher by 5–10 mmHg. When the upper extremity measurement is >10 mmHg higher than the lower extremity measurement coarctation of the aorta must be ruled out. Coarctation is a progressive disease with increased collateral circulation as the arch obstruction worsens. Patients who do not undergo intervention for their coarctation have an average life span of 35 years with a 76% mortality rate by age 46 (Cambell, 1970). Death may result from congestive heart failure, rupture of the aorta, endocarditis, or intracranial hemorrhage.

Physiology

In utero, only 10% of the cardiac output crosses the aortic isthmus with 90% of the cardiac output crossing the patent ductus arteriosus into the descending aorta. After birth, systemic vascular resistance increases dramatically as the umbilical cord is cut and the infant is separated from the low-resistance circuit of the placenta. Pulmonary vascular resistance drops as the infant takes the first breath and inflates the lungs. An increased PaO_2 and dropping PGE level promote closure of the DA and 100% of the cardiac output must now cross the aortic arch. The arch obstruction itself primarily accounts for the hypertension in the upper extremities. However, hypoperfusion of the kidneys leads to increased renin production, volume expansion, and hypertension as well. Left ventricular pressure is elevated by the obstruction across the arch. Various mechanisms help compensate for the increased obstruction to flow including LVH. This helps to maintain normal left ventricular function and to normalize wall stress. Other mechanisms include activation of the sympathetic pathway to increase heart rate and contractility, and an increase in LV end-diastolic volume to maintain normal stroke volume.

In the neonate with rapidly developing coarctation due to ductal closure, there is inadequate time to develop LVH and wall stress therefore increases markedly. If cardiac output is compromised, there can be a significant mismatch in myocardial oxygen demand and delivery that can contribute to the cascade of LV systolic dysfunction, elevated end-diastolic pressure, elevated left atrial pressures, and pulmonary congestion. The neonatal myocardium is relatively resistant to sympathetic activation and relatively noncompliant, and therefore less able to maintain stroke volume using the Frank–Starling mechanism.

Clinical Findings

The clinical findings associated with a coarctation will vary depending on the age of the patient, the location, and the severity of the obstruction as well as any associated lesions.

The newborn with a coarctation of the aorta may remain asymptomatic if the ductus arteriosus is patent or if the obstruction is mild. Femoral pulses may be delayed when compared to brachial pulses but the amplitude of the pulse may appear normal. A bicuspid valve will be present in 22%–42% of the cases and a systolic ejection click may be appreciated as a result of this. A murmur may be heard over the precordium if there is an associated lesion like AS, PDA, or a ventricular septal defect VSD. The murmur associated with the coarctation itself is typically heard at the left parascapular region.

The newborn with severe obstruction and a closing or closed ductus arteriosus usually presents critically ill with congestive heart failure or shock that can develop suddenly. Frequently, these are complicated cases with associated intracardiac defects. Multisystem organ failure can develop quickly unless definitive intervention is undertaken immediately. There is often a history of recent feeding intolerance or irritability. They will appear pale, tachypneic, and diaphoretic. Femoral pulses will typically be absent, but pulses may be diminished or absent in all four extremities due to poor cardiac output.

As in adults, the major clinical manisfestation of coarctation of the aorta in children is systemic hypertension in the upper extremities with a higher systolic blood pressure in the upper extremities compared to the lower extremities. The diastolic blood pressures are typically similar (Brickner et al., 2000). Any patient with systemic hypertension should have the blood pressures measured in both arms and at least one leg. The pulses in both arms and legs should be palpated to compare the amplitude and upstroke of the impulse. The classic finding in coarctation is diminished and/or delayed femoral pulses as compared to the brachial. In most cases, the left subclavian artery is proximal to the coarctation and therefore the blood pressure is elevated in both arms. Occasionally, the left subclavian origin is distal to the coarctation, resulting in the left arm blood pressure being equal to that of the legs and the left arm pulse being diminished when compared to

the right arm. Rarely, in ~3% of cases, both the right and left subclavian arteries arise distal to the area of coarctation, resulting in diminished blood pressures and pulses in all the four extremities. In these cases, an active precordium with dynamic carotid pulses can be a clue to the presence of coarctation.

ECG. The ECG will vary depending on the age of the patient and the severity of the coarctation. Infants with severe obstruction will typically exhibit findings of right ventricular hypertrophy (RVH), LVH is most often absent as the LV has not had time to hypertrophy in reponse to the increased pressure load. Older children may exhibit findings of LVH and ST or T-wave changes on their ECGs. A normal ECG does not rule out coarctation of the aorta.

CXR. The CXR will vary with age of the patient and severity of coarctation. Infants with severe obstruction will most typically exhibit signs of congestive heart failure with cardiomegaly and increased pulmonary vascular markings consistent with pulmonary edema. In older children, one may be able to discern notching of the posterior ribs due to erosion from large collateral vessels that can develop. The classic "3-sign" is seen on the A-P projection and is created by the indentation of the coarctation contrasted with the pre- and post-stenotic dilation of the aorta.

ECHO. 2-D echocardiography is typically excellent for delineating the site of coarctation, the anatomy of the arch and head vessels, and any associated cardiac defects such as BAV. 2-D imaging may reveal narrowing of the aorta in the region of the ductus arteriosus or one may visualize the characteristic finding of a posterior shelf off the posterior–lateral aspect of the aorta even in the presence of a patent ductus arteriosus. The severity of the obstruction can be estimated by pulsed- and continuous-wave Doppler. Continuos-wave Doppler may reveal the classic double envelop Doppler pattern with the low-velocity flow representing precoarctation flow and the high-velocity flow representing flow through the area of coarctation and distal to it. Doppler of the abdominal aorta may reveal a blunted upstroke of the aortic Doppler pattern in association with delayed deceleration and continuous antegrade diastolic flow.

In the infant with a persistently patent ductus arteriosus, the classic 2-D and Doppler findings of coarctation may not be present. Therefore, it is important to realize that coarctation of the aorta cannot be completely excluded in the setting of a patent ductus arteriosus.

MRI. MRI is useful in delineating the site and severity of coarctation of the aorta particularly if the tarnsthoracic echocardiographic images are not clear. MRI will also detect the extent of aortopulmonary collateral formation and any associated cardiac defects. Additionally, MRI is useful for assessment for aneurysm formation or restenosis in the postintervention period.

Cardiac Catheterization.

Given the excellent imaging available by echocardiography and MRI, routine diagnostic cardiac catheteriziation is not warranted in the patient with uncomplicated coarctation of the aorta.

Management

The current therapy for coarctation of the aorta is either surgical or transcatheter based. Intervention is indicated in the patient with uncomplicated coarctation of the aorta if there is a gradient of 20 mmHg or more across the area of obstruction. Intervention should be undertaken as soon as possible after the diagnosis is made since delayed correction may result in residual hypertension despite successful relief of the obstruction (Bhat et al., 2001; O'Sullivan et al., 2002).

The preferred method of surgical repair is resection of the area of coarctation and end-to-end anastomosis. The use of prosthetic overlay grafts and subclavian patch aortoplasty is infrequent because of potential aneurysm formation. Tube grafts or conduits are rarely used.

Transcatheter balloon angioplasty with or without stent placement has been used in the treatment of certain coarctations. However, the risk of aneurysm formation or restenosis is higher in this group. Transcatheter intervention is most suitable for the discrete stenosis in the older child or in patients with recoarctation. Stenting the area of coarctation has reduced the risk of aneurysm formation (Aboulhosn and Child, 2006).

In 2007, the American Heart Association revised the guidelines regarding antibiotic prophylaxis to prevent bacterial endocarditis. Patients with isolated coarctation of the aorta no longer require prophylaxis unless there is a history of endocarditis, a history of repair requiring prosthetic material in which case prophylaxis would be required for 6 months following the procedure, or if there were history of a repair with a residual defect adjacent to prosthetic material in which case prophylaxis is continued indefinitely (Bhat et al., 2001).

REFERENCES

Aboulhosn J, Child JS. Left ventricular outflow obstruction: subaortic stenosis, bicuspid aortic valve, supravalvar aortic stenosis, and coarctation of the aorta. *Circulation.* 2006;114:2412–2422.

Bengur AR, Snider AR, Serwer GA, et al. Usefulness of the Doppler mean gradient in evaluation of children with aortic valve stenosis and comparison to gradient at catheterization. *Am J Cardiol.* 1989;64:756.

Bhat MA, Neelakandhan KS, Unnikrishnan M, et al. Fate of hypertension after repair of coarctation of the aorta in adults. *British J Surg.* 2001;88(4):536.

Braunwald E, Goldblatt A, Aygen MM, et al. Congenital aortic stenosis. I: clinical and hemodynamic findings in 100 patients. *Circulation.* 1963;27:426–462.

Brewer RJ, Deck D, Capati B, Nolan SP. The dynamic aortic root. Its role in aortic valve function. *J Thorac Cardiovasc Surg.* 1976;72:413.

Brickner ME, Hillis LD, Lange RA. Congenital heart disease in adults. First of two parts. *N Engl J Med.* 2000;342:256.

Brown D, Keane JF. Subvalvar aortic stenosis (subaortic stenosis). *UpToDate.* April 2006.

Brown JW, Ruzmetov M, Vijay P, Turretine MW. Surgical repair of congenital supravalvar aortic stenosis in children. *Eur J Cardiothorac Surg.* 2002;21:50.

Cambell M. Natural history of coarctation of the aorta. *Br Heart J.* 1970;32:633–640.

Choi JY, Sullivan ID. Fixed subaortic stenosis: anatomical spectrum and nature of progression. *Br Heart J.* 1991;65:280.

Connolly HM, Husto J III, Brown RD Jr, Warnes CA, Ammash NM, Tajik AJ. Intracranial aneurysms in patients with coarctation of the aorta: a prospective magnetic resonance angiography study of 100 patients. *Mayo Clin Proc.* 2003;78:1491.

Currie PJ, Hagler DJ, Seward JB, et al. Instantaneous pressure gradient: a simultaneous Doppler and dual catheter correlative study. *J Am Coll Cardiol.* 1986;7:800.

De Vries AG, Hess J, Witsenburg M, et al. Management of fixed subaortic stenosis: a retrospective study of 57 cases. *J Am Coll Cardiol.* 1992;19:1013–1017.

Donner R, Carabello BA, Black I, Spann JF. Left ventricular wall stress in compensated aortic stenosis in children. *Am J Cardiol.* 1983;51:946.

Emmanouilides GC, ed. Heart disease in infants, children, and adolescents. Baltimore: Williams and Wilkins, 1995:1087.

Eronen M, Peippo M, Hiippala A, Raatikka M. Cardiovascular manisfestations in 75 patients with Williams syndrome. *J Med Genet.* 2002;39:554.

Feigl A, Feigl D, Lucas RV Jr, Edwards JE. Involvement of the aortic valve cusps in discrete subaortic stenosis. *Pediatr Cardiol.* 1984;5:185.

Fernandes SM, Sanders S, Khairy P, et al. Morphology of bicuspid aortic valve in children and adolescents. *J Am Coll Cardiol.* 2004;44:16.

Firpo C, Azcarate MJ, Quero-Jiminez M, Saravalli O. Discrete subaortic stenosis (DSS) in childhood: a congenital or acquired disease? Follow-up in 65 patients. *Eu Heart J.* 1990;11:1033–1040.

Flaker G, Teske D, Kilman J, Hosier D, Wooley C. Supravalvar aortic stenosis. A 20-year clinical perspective with patch aortoplasty. *Am J Cardiol.* 1983;51:256.

Flaker G, Teske D, Kilman J, Hosier D, Wooley C. Supravalvar aortic stenosis. A 20-year clinical perspective with patch aortoplasty. *Am J Cardiol.* 1983;51:256.

Gersony WM. Natural history of discrete subvalvar aortic stenosis: management implications. *J Am Coll Cardiol.* 2001;38;843.

Gewillig M, Daenen W, Dumoulin M, Van der Harwert L. Rheologic genesis of discrete subvalvular aortic stenosis: A Doppler echocardiographic study. *J Am Coll Cardiol.* 1992;19:818.

Gorlin R, Gorlin SG. Hydraulic formula for calculation of area of stenotic mitral valve and other cardiac valves, and central circulation shunts. *Am Heart J.* 1951;41:1–29.

Graham TP, Driscoll DJ, Gersony WM. Newburger JW, Rocchini A, Towbin JA. 36th Bethesda Conference: congenital heart disease. *J Am Coll Cardiol.* 2005;45(8):1326–1333.

Grahm, TP, Louis, BJ, Jarmakani, JM, Canent, RV, Copp, MP. Left heart volume and mass quantification in children with left ventricular pressure overload. *Circulation.* 1970;41:201.

Jones, KL. *Smith's Recognizable Patterns of Human Malformation.* 5th ed. Philadelphia: W.B. Saunders Company; 1997.

Keane JF, Driscoll DJ, Gersony WM, et al. Second natural history study of congenital heart defects: results of treatment of patients with aortic valvar stenosis. *Circulation.* 1993;87:116.

Keane JF, Fyler DC. Aortic outflow abnormalities. In: Keane JF, Fyler DC, eds. *Nadas' Pediatric Cardiology.* Philadelphia: Elsevier; 2006:585.

Kim YM, Yoo SJ, Choi JY, Kim SH, Bae EJ, Lee YT. Natural course of supravalvar aortic stenosis and peripheral pulmonary stenosis in Williams syndrome. *Cardiol Young.* 1999;9:37.

Kitchiner D, Jackson M, Malaiya N, et al. Incidence and prognosis of obstruction of the left ventricular outflow tract in Liverpool (1960–91): a study of 313 patients. *Br Heart J.* 1994;71:588.

Kleinert S, Geva T. Echocardiographic morphometry and geometry of the left ventricular outflow tract in fixed subaortic stenosis. *J Am Coll Cardiol.* 1993;22;1501.

Latson LA. Aortic valvuloplasty in the fetus: technically possible but is it ready for prime time? *J Pediatr.* 2005;147:424.

Leichter DA, Sullivan I, Gersony WM. "Acquired"discrete subalvar aortic stenosis: natural history and hemodynamics. *J Am Coll Cardiol.* 1989;14:1539.

Lewis AL, Heymann MA, Stanger P, Hoffman JIE, Rudolph AM. Evaluation of subendocardial ischemia in valvar aortic stenosis in children. *Circulation.* 1974;49:978.

Lewis T, Grant RT. Observations relating to sub-acute infective endocarditis. *Heart.* 1923;10:21–99.

Li DY, Brooke B, Davis EC, et al. Elastin is an essential determinant of arterial morphogenesis. *Nature.* 1998;393:276.

Li DY, Faury G, Taylor DG, et al. Novel arterial pathology in mice and humans hemizygous for elastin. *J Clin Invest.* 1998;102:1783.

Liu CW, Hwang B, Lee BC, Lu JH. Aortic stenosis in children: 19-year experience. *Zhonghua Yi Xue Za Zhi (Taipei).* 1997;59:107.

Makikallio K, McElhinney DB, Levine JL, et al. Fetal aortic valve stenosis and the evolution of hypoplastic left heart syndrome: patient selection for fetal intervention. *Circulation.* 2006;113:1401.

Maron GJ, Redwood DR, Roberts WC, et al. Tunnel subaortic stenosis: left ventricular outflow tract obstruction produced by fibromuscular tubular narrowing. *Circulation.* 1976;54:404.

Marshall AC, Tworetzky W, Bergersen L, et al. Aortic valvuloplasty in the fetus: technical characteristics of successful balloon dilation. *J Pediatr.* 2005;147:535.

McBride KL, Pignatelli R, Lewin M, et al. Inheritance analysis of congenital left ventricular outflow tract obstruction malformations: segregation, multiplex relative risk, and heritability. *Am J Med Genet A.* 2005;134:180.

McCaffrey FM, Sherman FS. Prenatal diagnosis of severe aortic stenosis. *Pediatr Cardiol.* 1997;18:276.

McElhinney DB, Lock JE, Keane JF, et al. Left heart growth, function and re-intervention after balloon aortic valvuloplasty for neonatal aortic stenosis. *Circulation.* 2005;111:451.

McMahon CJ, Gauvreau K, Edwards JC, Geva T. Risk factors for aortic valve dysfunction in children with discrete subvalvar aortic stenosis. *Am J Cardiol.* 2004;94:459.

Moore P, Egito E, Mowrey H, Perry SB. Midterm results of balloon dilation of congenital aortic stenosis: predictors of success. *J Am Coll Cardiol.* 1996;27:1257.

Morrow AG, Waldhausen JA, Peters RL, Bloodwell RD, Braunwald E. Supravalvar aortic stenosis. Clinical, hemodynamic and pathologic observations. *Circulation.* 1959;20:1003.

Newfeld EA, Muster AJ, Paul MH, et al. Discrete subvalvular aortic stenosis in childhood. Study of 51 patients. *Am J Cardiol.* 1976;38:53.

O'Sullivan JJ, Derrick G, Dranell R. Prevalence of hypertension in children after early repair of coarctation of the aorta: a cohort study using casual and 24 hour blood pressure measurement. *Heart.* 2002;88(2):163–166.

Obstruction of the left ventricular outflow tract. In: Castaneda AR, Jonas RA, Mayer JE, Hanley FL, eds. *Cardiac Surgery of the Neonate and Infant.* Philadelphia: WB Saunders; 1994:315.

Oliver JM, Gonzalez A, Gallego P, Sanchez-Recalde FB, Mesa JM. Discrete subaortic stenosis in adults:increased prevalence and slow rate of progression of the obstructionand aortic regurgitation. *J Am Coll Card.* 2001;38:835–842.

Pagni S, Denatale RW, Boltax RS. Takayasu's arteritis: the middle aortic syndrome. *Am Surg.* 1996;62:409.

Presbitero P, Demarie D, Villani M, et al. Long term results (15–30 years) of surgical repair of aortic coarctation. *Br Heart J.* 1987;57:162 167.

Pyle RL, Patterson DF, Chacko S. The genetics and pathology of discrete subaortic stenosis in the Newfoundland dog. *Am Heart J.* 1976;92:324.

Refenstein GH, Levine SA, Gross RE. Coarctation of the aorta: a review of 104 autopsied cases of the "adult type", 2 years of age or older. *Am Heart J.* 1947;33:146.

Roberts WC, Morrow AG, Braunwald E. Complete interruption of the aortic arch. *Circulation.* 1962;26:39–59.

Roberts, WC. The congenitally bicuspid aortic valve. A study of 85 autopsy cases. *Am J Cardiol.* 1970;26:72.

Rosenfeld HM, Landzberg MJ, Perry SB, et al. Balloon aortic valvuloplasty in the young adult with congenital heart disease. *Am J Cardiol.* 73:112, 1994.

Rudolph A. Aortic arch obstruction. In: Rudolph A, ed. *Congenital Diseases of the Heart.* New York: Futura Publishing; 2001:367.

Rudolph AM, Heymann MA, Spitznas U. Hemodynamic considerations in the development of narrowing of the aorta. *Am J Cardiol.* 1972;30:514.

Schoen FJ. Cardiac valves and valvular pathology update on function, disease, repair, and replacement *Cardiovasc Pathol.* 2005;14(4):189–194.

Shaver JA, Salerni R. Auscultatation of the heart. In: Schlant RC, Alexander RW, eds. *The Heart.* New York: McGraw-Hill, 1994:261.

Shinebourne EA, Elseed AM. Relation between fetal flow patterns, coarctation of the aorta, and pulmonary blood flow. *Br Heart J.* 1974;36:492.

Stamm C, Friehs I, Yen Ho S, Moran AM, Jonas RA, del Nido PJ. Congenital supravalvar aortic stenosis: a simple lesion? *Eur J Cardiothorac Surg.* 2001;19(2):195.

Stamm C, Li J, Ho SY, Redington AN, Anderson RH. The aortic root in supravalvar aortic stenosis: the potential surgical relevance of morphologic findings. *J Thorac Cardiovasc Surg.* 1997;114:16.

Stewart AB, Ahmed R, Travill CM, et al. Coarctation of the aorta, life and health 20–44 years after surgical repair. *Br Heart J.* 1993: 69:65–70.

Strasburger JF, Kugler JD, Cheatham JP, McManus BM. Nonimmunologic hydrops fetalis associated with congenital aortic valvular stenosis. *Am Heart J.* 1984;108:1380.

Sutton GC. Examination of the cardiovascular system. In: Julian, DG, Camm AJ, Fox KM, et al. eds. *Diseases of the Heart.* 2nd ed. Philadelphia: W.B. Saunders; 1996:140.

Talner NS, Berman MA. Postnatal development of coarctaion of obstruction in coarctation of the aorta: role of the ductus arteriosus. *Pediatrics*. 1975;56:562.

Tawes RL Jr, Berry CL, Aberdeen E. Congenital bicuspid aortic valve associated with coarctation of the aorta in children. *Br Heart J*. 1969;31:127–128.

Urbach J, Glaser J, Balkin J, et al. Familial membranous subaortic stenosis. *Cardiology*. 1985;72:214.

Vaideeswar P, Shankar V, Deshpande JR, Sivaraman A, Jain N. Pathology of the diffuse variant of supravalvar aortic stenosis. *Cardiovascular Path*. 2001;10(1):33.

Van Son JAM, Edwards WD, Danielson GK. Pathology of coronary arteries, myocardium, and great arteries in supravalvar aortic stenosis. *J Thorac Cardiovasc Surg*. 1994;108:21.

Villari B, Hess OM, Kaufmann P, Krogmann ON, Grimm J, Krayenbuehl HP. Effect of aortic valve stenosis (pressure overload) and aortic regurgitation (volume overload) on left ventricular systolic and diastolic function. *Am J Cardiol*. 1992;69:927.

Wagner HR, Ellison RC, Keane JF, et al. Clinical course in aortic stenosis. Report form the Joint Study of the Natural History of Congenital Heart Defects. *Circulation*. 1977;(suppl 1):56.

Wilson W, Taubert KA, Gewitz M, et al.; for the American Heart Association Rheumatic Fever, Endocarditis, and Kawasaki Disease Committee, Council on Cardiovascular Disease in the Young, and the Council on Clinical Cardiology, Council on Cardiovascular Surgery and Anesthesia, and the Quality of Care and Outcomes Research Interdisciplinary Working Group. Prevention of infective endocarditis. *Circulation*. 2007;115.

Wessels MW, Berger RM, Frohn-Mulder IM, et al. Autosomal dominant inheritance of left ventricular outflow tract obstruction. *Am J Med Genet A*. 2005;134:171.

Wright GB, Keane JF, Nadas AS, et al. Fixed subaortic stenosis in the young: medical and surgical course in 83 patients. *Am J Cardiol*. 1983;52:830.

12

Right Ventricular Outflow Tract Obstruction

MARK D. PARRISH

ANITA J. MOON-GRADY

JEFFERY MEADOWS

PULMONARY ATRESIA WITH INTACT VENTRICULAR SEPTUM

Introduction

Pulmonary atresia with intact ventricular septum is a structural heart defect that usually consists of situs solitus, with normal systemic and pulmonary venous connections. With rare exceptions, atrioventricular and ventriculo-arterial relationships are concordant. The primary feature of the defect is the absence of continuity between the right ventricle and the pulmonary artery. Despite this simple description, the defect includes a large degree of heterogeneity in tricuspid valve, right ventricular, and coronary artery anatomy. Variations in anatomy are the principal determinants of treatment options for patients with this heart defect.

Morphology

The tricuspid valve anatomy is usually abnormal in patients with pulmonary atresia and intact ventricular septum (Choi et al., 1998; Daubeney et al., 2002; Freedom et al., 1978). Valve leaflets are frequently thick, with restricted valve apparatus and short chordae tendineae. The valve annulus is often hypoplastic. However, approximately 10% of patients have Ebstein malformations of the tricuspid valve, with redundant, dysplastic, sail-like anterior leaflets, and downward displacement of the septal and/or posterior tricuspid leaflet. In rare cases, there may be virtually no effective valve tissue at all, leaving an "unguarded" tricuspid orifice (Anderson et al., 1990).

The atrial situs and structure is usually normal; however, the right atrium is mildly to massively enlarged, depending upon the anatomy of the tricuspid valve. A giant right atrium occurs in cases with severe tricuspid regurgitation due to an Ebstein malformation, or an "unguarded" tricuspid valve. There is either an atrial septal defect or a patent foramen ovale. Rarely, significant structural abnormalities occur in the atria, including persistence of the right venous valve, coronary sinus to left atrial fenestration, or aneurysm of the septum primum, with herniation through the mitral valve.

Right ventricular morphology may be quite variable (Bharati et al., 1977; Browlin et al., 1982; Santos and Azevedo, 2004). The ventricular wall may be extremely thin in children with severe tricuspid valve regurgitation due to Ebstein anomaly. In others, muscular obliteration of the apical trabecular cavity and/or the infundibulum or outlet portion results in a small "bipartite" right ventricle in approximately one-third of cases, and a "unipartite" chamber in an additional 7% (Figures 12–1A and 12–1B). Nearly 60% of children have a "tripartite" right ventricle. Anatomy of the right ventricle–pulmonary artery obstruction correlates to some degree with ventricular size and development. The atretic segment of the right ventricular outflow tract may be a long muscular segment or it may consist of a short segment with an imperforate valve or membrane. Tripartite hearts usually have a valvar or membranous atresia, whereas unipartite hearts have a muscular atresia. Bipartite hearts may have either membranous or muscular atresia. Overall, atresia is membranous in approximately 75% of cases, and muscular in the remaining 25%. In patients with a well-formed right ventricle, the membranous atretic "valve" may be quite thin, consisting of complete fusion between commissures of three semilunar cusps (Figure 12–1C). Other cases have a more primitive membranous structure, with a thick, plate-like obstruction.

Coronary artery abnormalities occur in slightly less than half of the patients with pulmonary atresia and intact ventricular septum (Gittenberger-de Groot et al., 1988; Oosthoek et al., 1995; Selamet et al., 2004). These abnormalities include right ventricular to coronary fistulas, arterial stenoses, and interruptions and ectasias of the coronary arteries. For those cases with communication between the right ventricular cavity and coronary system, there may be portions of the myocardium dependent upon perfusion from the right ventricle (Figure 12–2) and this occurs in approximately 9% of the cases. Alternatively, there may be a "steal" phenomenon, with excessive coronary diastolic flow into the right ventricular cavity. These patients may also have reversal of flow during systole, with coronary "run-off" into the ascending aorta. At the capillary level, there may be extensive regions of the myocardium with low capillary density. These areas of low capillary density correlate with the areas of fibrosis, low myocyte density, and myocardial disarray. Low capillary density occurs most commonly in hearts with significant right ventricular hypoplasia.

Children with pulmonary atresia and intact ventricular septum often have well-developed pulmonary arteries. However, rare cases occur with very small but confluent pulmonary arteries or discontinuous pulmonary arteries (Albanese et al., 2002; Milanesi et al., 1990). For the more common case, with normal-sized proximal vessels, the small, distal pulmonary vessels may be abnormal (Tanaka et al., 1996). There is a tendency toward thinning of the media in these small resistance vessels. This medial thinning may worsen with prolonged prostaglandin E1 treatment. One speculation is that the medial thinning may promote permanent injury to the intima in the distal vessels. If true, this mechanism could explain the development of early pulmonary vascular disease in some patients with pulmonary atresia and intact ventricular septum.

The anatomy of the ductus arteriosus is frequently different between patients with pulmonary atresia and intact ventricular septum, compared to those with pulmonary atresia with a ventricular septal defect (Santos et al., 1980). In those with an intact septum, the ductus is usually left sided and the inferior angle of the ductus arteriosus at the aortic junction is obtuse; whereas in cases with a ventricular septal defect, the angle is commonly acute ("reverse-oriented ductus"). It has been speculated that the more "normal" ductal and pulmonary artery anatomy in patients with pulmonary

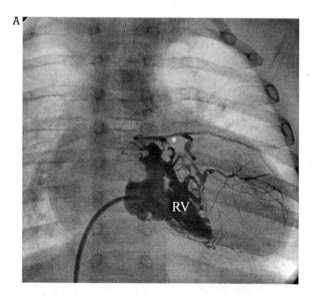
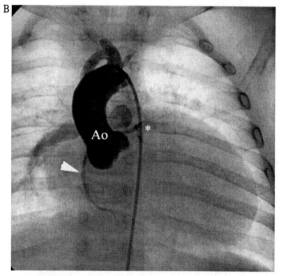

FIGURE 12–1. Range of morphologies observed in pulmonary atresia with intact ventricular septum. A: Frontal projection right ventricular angiogram from an older child with pulmonary atresia with intact ventricular septum who has undergone a superior cavopulmonary anastamosis. There is a small inlet portion (I) and significant fistulae (*). The trabecular and outlet portions are absent, making the ventricle "unipartite." B: Right ventricular angiogram in frontal projection. The ventricle is somewhat small but there are distinct inlet (I), trabecular (T) and outlet (O) portions, so-called "tripartite." C: Lateral projection angiogram with simultaneous injections in the right ventricular outflow tract (antegrade venous catheter) and main pulmonary artery (retrograde with a catheter passing from the aorta through a patent ductus arteriosus to the pulmonary artery) during transcatheter valve perforation and balloon pulmonary valvuloplasty in an attempt to establish a two-ventricle circulation. The tricuspid valve is clearly visible, as are the well-formed semilunar cusps and main pulmonary artery (MPA) separated from the right ventricular outflow by an imperforate valve (arrow).

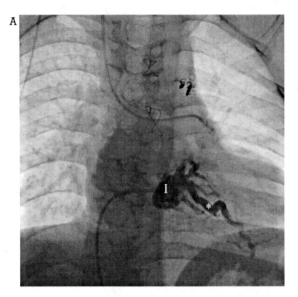

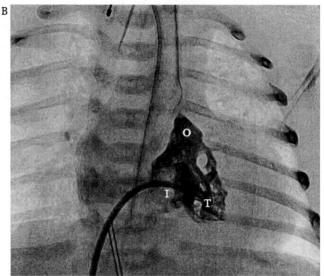

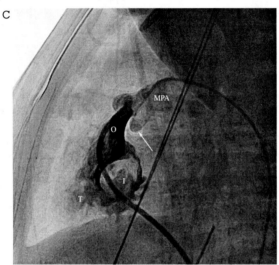

FIGURE 12–2. Coronary artery abnormalities in pulmonary atresia with intact ventricular septum. A: shows a frontal projection right ventricular angiogram demonstrating filling of the right ventricle (RV) with opacification of a majority of the left coronary system via fistulous connections with the RV cavity. The left main coronary is seen on this injection (*). B: shows a frontal projection aortic root (AO) angiogram in the same patient. Note that as opposed to figure A, the right coronary artery is seen in this injection (arrowhead). The left main opacifies (*) but little is seen of the remainder of the left system. An argument may be made that the left coronary system is dependent on the right ventricle for perfusion in this patient despite clear evidence of coronary artery stenoses.

atresia and intact ventricular septum, reflects the fact that this defect occurs late in the development of the cardiovascular system, after the cardiac septation is complete (Kutsche and Van Mierop, 1983).

Occasionally, left heart abnormalities occur in patients with pulmonary atresia and intact ventricular septum (Kobayashi et al., 2005; Razzouk et al., 1992; Zuberbuhler et al., 1979). Although obstruction of both the right and left ventricular outflow tracts is very uncommon in live-born infants, aortic valve stenosis has been described a number of times in patients with pulmonary atresia and intact ventricular septum. A convexity of the left-sided outlet portion of the interventricular septum also occurs in patients with small and hypertensive right ventricles. Due to this bulge in the septum, severe left ventricular outflow obstruction can occur following a Fontan operation.

Etiology

The estimated incidence of pulmonary atresia with intact ventricular septum is 132 per million live births (Hoffman and Kaplan, 2002). This comprises approximately 9.5% of infants born with cyanotic heart disease and 1% of infants born with all forms of congenital heart disease, including trivial conditions. However, the incidence of pulmonary atresia with intact ventricular septum in live births is likely to change with aggressive fetal diagnosis and pregnancy termination programs. In the United Kingdom, one group found a pregnancy termination rate of 61% in fetuses with a diagnosis of pulmonary atresia with intact ventricular septum (Daubeney et al., 1998).

The cause of this defect is unknown. Extracardiac malformations are rare. There are sporadic reports of familial occurrence or specific chromosomal anomalies (Frober et al., 2001; Grossfeld et al., 1997; Gucer et al., 2005; Li et al., 2003). One group speculated that the defect might be due to an inflammatory process during fetal gestation, but there is currently no specific pathologic evidence to support this hypothesis (Kutsche and Van Mierop, 1983).

Hemodynamics

The dynamics of returning systemic venous blood depends upon the tricuspid valve and coronary artery anatomy. In the absence of a dilated right ventricle with severe tricuspid valve regurgitation, the majority of systemic venous blood returns to the right atrium and traverses the atrial septum to mix with the pulmonary venous return in the left atrium. Some of the systemic venous blood in the right atrium may enter the right ventricle, and perfuse the coronary system through ventricular–coronary fistulas.

Structural coronary anomalies, such as fistulous communications with the right ventricle, coronary stenoses, or atresia of a major coronary artery, may all affect hemodynamics and ventricular function. In the presence of large right ventricle to coronary fistulas and suprasystemic right ventricular pressures, there may be a high volume systolic "run-off" between the right ventricle and aortic root. In diastole, blood flow may reverse, creating the potential of a "coronary steal" as coronary artery blood flows into the right ventricle. Coronary stenoses may further aggravate the risk for myocardial ischemia.

The presence of an Ebstein malformation, with a giant right atrium and severe tricuspid valve regurgitation, may importantly affect hemodynamics. The loss of kinetic energy as systemic venous blood returns to a cavernous right atrium and right ventricle can lead to decreased left ventricular filling and thus decreased left heart stroke volumes. The decreased stroke volume from the left heart adversely affects both the systemic and pulmonary blood flow and increases the risks for circulatory collapse and death.

The right atrial mean pressure is equal to or slightly greater than the left atrial mean pressure when the interatrial communication is nonrestrictive. With restriction of the interatrial communication, the pressure difference between the two atria will increase. Occasionally, a restrictive interatrial communication produces clinically important right atrial hypertension, requiring intervention to create a larger septal opening. A significantly restrictive atrial communication may be a cause for in utero fetal demise.

The left atrium and left ventricle receive both systemic and pulmonary venous return. Left ventricular end-diastolic pressure and left atrial pressure may be slightly increased, related to the increase in left ventricular filling. However, large increases in left heart filling pressures suggest abnormal diastolic compliance of the left ventricle due to myocardial injury or ventricular–ventricular interaction, or both.

At birth, patients with pulmonary atresia and intact ventricular septum are entirely dependent upon flow from the aorta to the pulmonary artery to supply blood to the lungs for oxygenation. Usually this occurs through a patent ductus arteriosus, since significant accessory collateral vessels from aorta to pulmonary artery are rare. Ductal and pulmonary arterial sizes are, therefore, very important determinants of the quantity of blood available to the lungs for oxygenation. However, additional physiological factors may contribute to determining the quantity of pulmonary blood flow, including pulmonary vascular resistance, systemic vascular resistance, intrathoracic pressure, left heart filling pressure, left ventricular stroke volume, and systemic cardiac output.

The arterial oxygen saturation is largely dependent upon the quantity of high-saturation pulmonary venous return mixing with low-saturation systemic venous return, in the left atrium. Low mixed venous saturations, as a result of low systemic cardiac output, may further lower systemic arterial saturations, as the systemic output consists of both the systemic and pulmonary venous blood. Assuming relatively normal oxygenation of blood traversing the lungs and relatively normal systemic cardiac output, the systemic arterial blood saturation serves as a rough measure of the quantity of pulmonary blood flow. Thus, with normal ventilation and normal lungs, a very low arterial saturation may be seen when pulmonary blood flow is low and a high saturation when pulmonary blood flow is high. When arterial oxygen saturations are above 90%, this reflects excessive pulmonary blood flow, leading to a pulmonary "overperfusion" syndrome. This syndrome consists of left heart volume overload and pulmonary edema due to the large quantity of pulmonary blood flow.

Hemodynamics outside the neonatal period depends to some degree upon the treatment strategy chosen for a particular patient. However, there are two long-term issues to consider in virtually all children undergoing surgical palliation for pulmonary atresia with intact ventricular septum: ventricular function and the coronary circulation.

Left ventricular end-systolic elastance and ventriculo-arterial coupling were assessed from cardiac catheterization data in a cohort of children with pulmonary atresia and intact ventricular septum and were compared to children with tricuspid valve atresia (Tanoue et al., 2004). Both groups were studied before bidirectional Glenn procedure, before Fontan procedure, and approximately 1 year following Fontan procedure.

Although the groups did not differ before a bidirectional Glenn procedure, thereafter the pulmonary atresia group showed a significant worsening of left ventricular contractility and efficiency.

Right ventricular performance may also deteriorate over time. In one study, progressive dilatation of the right ventricle was noted in children undergoing a two-ventricle repair of pulmonary atresia (Mishima et al., 2000). This finding was linked to the development of postoperative arrhythmias.

Other studies provide insight into the possible etiology of ventricular dysfunction. One group (Akiba and Becker, 1994) examined eight hearts with pulmonary atresia and intact ventricular septum. They found high values of interfiber collagen, suggesting chronic ischemia. Other investigators (Fyfe et al., 1986) examined 17 hearts and found that myocardial ischemia was common and did not consistently relate to observed coronary abnormalities or the type of operation. In contrast, another group found a greater severity of coronary arterial abnormalities significantly associated with left ventricular dysfunction (Dyamenahalli et al., 2004).

Therefore, long-term hemodynamic concerns in children with pulmonary atresia and intact ventricular septum should include consideration of myocardial ischemia and left ventricular dysfunction. Although children with severely hypoplastic right ventricles and recognized coronary abnormalities may be at increased risk for this problem, the issues are not limited entirely to this subgroup.

Clinical Features

Newborns with pulmonary atresia and intact ventricular septum typically present with cyanosis. Hypoxemia worsens coincident with ductal constriction. Since the ductus usually begins to constrict shortly after birth, most infants with this defect become cyanotic within the first 24 hours of birth. Presentation is delayed if ductal constriction occurs late or the infant is anemic (making the visual signs of hypoxemia less obvious).

Other findings of the physical examination are often normal or quite subtle. The baby may be mildly tachypneic, but the work of breathing is not usually increased. There may be a regurgitant systolic murmur at the left lower sternal border due to tricuspid valve regurgitation. With a severe Ebstein malformation of the tricuspid valve, the physical examination findings may include a gallop rhythm and a mid-diastolic rumble due to increased inflow through the tricuspid orifice. Hepatic engorgement suggests the possibility of a restrictive interatrial communication.

Signs of congestive heart failure or shock are not typical presenting features for pulmonary atresia with intact ventricular septum. The exceptions to this caveat include infants with restriction of the interatrial communication, those with severe tricuspid regurgitation with a large thin-walled right ventricle, those with left ventricular dysfunction due to ischemia, or patients with delayed diagnosis, severe hypoxemia, and acidosis.

Differential Diagnosis

Simple ancillary studies can help confirm the presence of a cyanotic heart disease but are not adequate to arrive at a specific anatomic diagnosis. The arterial blood gas shows hypoxemia that is not responsive to oxygen, and mild hypocarbia due to tachypnea. Both of these features suggest that the cyanosis is caused by congenital heart disease rather than lung disease. The chest x-ray shows a normal to mildly enlarged cardiac silhouette, unless there is a significant tricuspid regurgitation. In the presence of Ebstein malformation with severe tricuspid valve regurgitation, there is massive enlargement of the cardiac silhouette. The vascularity observable in the lung fields on the chest x-ray may appear oligemic, normal, or hyperemic, depending upon the quantity of blood flow through the ductus arteriosus. The electrocardiogram shows normal sinus rhythm and a mean QRS axis in the frontal plane of +30 degrees to +90 degrees. Right ventricular forces are decreased with right atrial enlargement, and there is left ventricular dominance or hypertrophy.

Developing an understanding of the anatomic details of an individual patient's defect begins with echocardiography. Two-dimensional echocardiography begins with precise identification of the systemic and pulmonary venous connections, which are usually normal. Next, atrial anatomy including presence and size of interatrial communications is assessed. Atrioventricular valve morphology including tricuspid valve size and presence or absence of Ebstein malformation; left and right ventricular size, morphology, and function; and outflow tract size and morphology are evaluated. Measurements of the tricuspid valve annulus size from the apical four-chamber window may be especially helpful in designing surgical strategy (Hanley et al., 1993), though right ventricular volume or end-diastolic area measurement in comparison with left ventricle has also been used (Schmidt et al., 1992) to predict success of two-ventricle repair. Assessment of right ventricular hypertrophy and cavity size (including inlet, trabecular body, and infundibulum or outlet) is best done using orthogonal planes utilizing the subcostal approach. The pulmonary valve annulus diameter should be measured, generally from the parasternal short axis window, and the right ventricular outflow tract and infundibular region evaluated as a potential additional source of obstruction if surgical valvotomy or balloon valvuloplasty for reestablisment of patency of the valve are being contemplated. The branch pulmonary arteries should be evaluated for confluency and size, as well as for potential for acquired stenosis of the left pulmonary artery at the time of ductal closure (Moon-Grady et al., 2006). The aortic valve is usually normal unless genetic abnormalities are present, though bicuspid aortic valve may be seen. Aortic arch anatomy should be assessed but is usually normal. The ductus arteriosus is often abnormal even on 2-D imaging with a "vertical" proximal takeoff from the aorta and a tortuous course before inserting at the main-left pulmonary artery region.

Doppler echocardiography is quite helpful in evaluation of the physiology as well as anatomy of these patients. Doppler interrogation of the interatrial septum should be performed to evaluate for restriction. Tricuspid regurgitation should be evaluated by color Doppler and continuous wave Doppler to assess the severity and to determine the right ventricular pressure, which may be very low (particularly in the presence of the Ebstein anomaly) or suprasystemic (in which case one should have a high index of suspicion for the presence of coronary artery sinusoids). Particular attention should be paid to color Doppler assessment of the pulmonary valve and main pulmonary artery, as some patients with lower right ventricular pressure and a large left-to-right ductal shunt may exhibit "functional" rather than true anatomic pulmonary valve atresia; trace of pulmonary valve insufficiency may be the only clue to outflow tract patency in these patients. The mitral and aortic valves should be evaluated, the latter in particular for presence of subaortic obstruction due to hypertrophy of the interventricular septum, which may cause dynamic and progressive obstruction. Ductal patency can be confirmed by color Doppler but stenosis of the arterial duct may be difficult to appreciate; therefore, unexplained moderate to severe desaturation in a patient with an apparently patent duct should prompt evaluation by cardiac catheterization. Color Doppler can be used at lower Nyquist limits to evaluate regions of the right ventricular myocardium to identify coronary artery fistulae with the right ventricular cavity (Sanders et al., 1989), though precise anatomic definition and evaluation for coronary artery stenosis or interruption is not yet feasible using this technique. Some have used pulsed-wave Doppler within the main coronary artery systems to assess for forward and reversed flow due to fistulous connections (Garcia et al., 1998; Satou et al., 2000), but angiography remains the mainstay of coronary evaluations in these patients.

Because the right ventricle may be hypoplastic beginning fairly early in gestation, especially in moderate to severe forms of pulmonary atresia with intact ventricular septum, it is possible to detect the defect on routine prenatal screening. Fetal echocardiographic evaluation for confirmation of the diagnosis will also include evaluation for the presence and velocity of tricuspid regurgitation, right ventricular size, and presence of coronary artery sinusoids, as the prognosis and counseling differ significantly when these findings are present. Less severe right ventricular hypoplasia associated with plate-like valvar atresia is less likely to be detected prenatally; only when the right ventricular outflow tract is interrogated with Doppler or when reverse ductal Doppler flow is noted is the diagnosis clear. Serial evaluation in such cases, especially when discovered in the early second trimester, is indicated as pulmonary annulus and right ventricular hypoplasia clearly may be progressive in utero (Hornberger et al., 1994; Maeno et al., 1999; Sharland, 2000), with dramatic implications for surgical management (single-ventricle palliation vs. two-ventricle repair) at birth.

Cardiac catheterization may augment the information obtained from echocardiography, although the role of this diagnostic modality varies depending upon institutional philosophy. One approach is to base the timing of diagnostic catheterization upon the initial echocardiographic findings. If the echocardiogram demonstrates that the patient is unsuitable for a two-ventricle repair, catheterization is deferred until the infant is ready to undergo evaluation for a bidirectional cavopulmonary shunt. However, if the echocardiogram suggests that the patient is a potential candidate for a two-ventricle repair, then a newborn diagnostic catheterization is performed to augment the evaluation of right ventricular size, tricuspid valve size and physiology, and coronary artery anatomy and physiology. Some centers believe that a clear understanding of coronary anatomy and physiology is important in all infants, regardless of the surgical treatment plan. Angiography in both the right ventricle and aortic root is deemed necessary to develop a complete understanding of the coronary anatomy. Occasionally, selective coronary injections are necessary to clarify this anatomy.

Management

Initial treatment of the infant with pulmonary atresia and intact ventricular septum focuses on stabilization of the pulmonary blood flow. A continuous infusion of prostaglandin E1 at a dose of 0.05–0.1 µg/kg/min can dilate the ductus and stabilize the pulmonary blood flow. In cyanotic neonates for whom there is a high suspicion of congenital heart disease, prostaglandin therapy is often initiated prior to transfer to a tertiary care facility, even before the exact anatomic diagnosis is known. As prostaglandin may cause apnea, close attention to ventilation is needed, especially during transport. After stability of the infant is assured, prostaglandin dosage can be reduced to 0.02–0.03 μg/kg/min, in order to minimize side effects. Treatment strategy thereafter depends upon results of the diagnostic evaluation.

Treatment strategy at many institutions falls into one of the two categories: (1) create continuity between the right ventricle and pulmonary artery, and stabilize the pulmonary blood flow or (2) just provide a stable source of pulmonary blood flow. Choice between these two strategies depends upon the specific anatomy in each patient. When the treating team believes that the patient is a candidate for two-ventricular physiology, right ventricular to pulmonary artery continuity should be created in the newborn. If the treating team considers two-ventricular physiology to be impossible, newborn treatment usually consists of stabilization of the pulmonary blood flow only.

Several anatomic details are predictive of failure for a two-ventricle physiology. These predictive features include right ventricular dependent coronary circulation, a unipartite right ventricle, and severe tricuspid regurgitation with a dilated, thin-walled right ventricle (Ashburn et al., 2004; Minich et al., 2000; Odim et al., 2006; Yoshimura et al., 2003). A tricuspid annulus Z score of less than −3, or a tricuspid/mitral annulus ratio of less than 0.5 are sometimes used as surrogate indicators of severe right ventricular hypoplasia and also predict failure of a two-ventricle strategy. In the presence of any of these predictive features, many institutions choose to simplify the newborn treatment and just establish a stable communication between the aorta and pulmonary artery. However, if these features are not present, many institutions will attempt to create continuity between the right ventricle and the pulmonary artery in the newborn, encouraging antegrade flow and decreasing the right ventricular pressure. This is frequently termed the "two-ventricle" strategy.

When a two-ventricle repair seems inappropriate due to unsuitable anatomy or comorbid conditions, stable pulmonary blood flow can be established by placing a tube graft between the systemic circuit and the pulmonary artery (modified Blalock-Tausig shunt). Usually, the ductus arteriosus is ligated with this approach. Alternatively, some institutions have chosen to stabilize pulmonary blood flow by placing a stent in the ductus arteriosus, thus avoiding a sternotomy or thoracotomy (Schneider et al., 1998). Infants in this situation then undergo comprehensive reevaluation with echocardiography and cardiac catheterization between 3 and 6 months of age. If anatomy and physiology seem suitable at that age, a bidirectional cavopulmonary shunt is performed. For those patients with right-ventricle-dependent coronary circulation, there may be some

advantage to performing the cavopulmonary shunt as early as possible, since this intervention does increase oxygen saturation of the blood in the right ventricular cavity that supplies the coronary circulation by as much as 40% (Miyaji et al., 2005). If the patient does well following the cavopulmonary shunt, a comprehensive reevaluation is performed between 2 and 4 years of age before considering treatment with a modified Fontan procedure.

A number of treatment strategies have been attempted to alter the coronary physiology in patients with large right ventricle to coronary communications. These techniques include tricuspid valvectomy, thrombotic or coil occlusion of the right ventricle, an aortic to right ventricular conduit, or ligation of large fistulae (Sauer et al., 2006). Mortality remains quite high in patients undergoing these procedures, most likely due to the complexity of coronary physiology. Procedures that lower right ventricular pressures or obliterate the right ventricular cavity may lead to myocardial ischemia if a portion of ventricular muscle is dependent upon right ventricular perfusion. Alternatively, decompression of the right ventricle may worsen a coronary steal, leading to further myocardial ischemia. Angiography cannot always predict the effect of decompression or obliteration of the right ventricle on coronary physiology.

For the newborn who is a candidate for a two-ventricle repair, the initial intervention consists of creating continuity between the right ventricle and the pulmonary artery. When this continuity is established surgically, the procedure usually consists of resection of all obstructive valvar and infundibular tissue, with a transannular right-ventricular outflow tract patch to enlarge both the outflow tract and pulmonary valve annulus. If continuity is established in the catheterization laboratory, several methodologies are available to perforate the obstructing membrane (Siblini et al., 1997). After creating a perforation, balloon dilation is performed in an effort to eliminate as much obstruction as possible. When continuity is established between the right ventricle and the pulmonary artery, the ventricle may grow very well, sometimes achieving normal dimensions (Schmidt et al., 1992). However, occasionally a hypoplastic ventricle does not grow, even with continuity to the pulmonary artery, and the patient becomes a candidate for a bidirectional cavopulmonary shunt and eventually modified Fontan palliation.

The choice between surgery to create right ventricle to pulmonary artery continuity, versus the catheter technique, is often dictated by the anatomy of the right ventricular infundibulum and the length of the atretic segment (see Figure 12–1). If the outflow from the right ventricle is diffusely hypoplastic, with severe annular hypoplasia, creation of unobstructed flow into the pulmonary artery may not be possible in the catheterization laboratory. In general, catheter perforation and balloon dilation leaves a significantly greater risk that the patient will require early reintervention compared to surgical right ventricular outflow reconstruction. However, the catheter technique significantly decreases the risk of postprocedural low cardiac output state (Mi et al., 2005).

Frequently, after the right ventricular–pulmonary artery continuity is established, the pulmonary blood flow remains inadequate due to abnormal right ventricular compliance. Although compliance usually improves with time, the newborn may need a supplementary source of pulmonary blood flow. Pulmonary flow can be stabilized by maintaining patency of the ductus arteriosus for some period, or surgically creating a systemic-to-pulmonary artery shunt. Eventually, if right ventricular compliance improves and antegrade flow from the right ventricle to pulmonary artery becomes sufficient, the systemic-to-pulmonary artery shunt can be occluded in the catheterization laboratory. At the same time, any persistent atrial septal defect can be evaluated for device closure.

Long-term outcomes for children with pulmonary atresia and intact ventricular septum are difficult to ascertain due to variations between institutions and a paucity of population-based data. One recent population-based study from the United Kingdom and Ireland reported outcomes for a cohort of 183 children with pulmonary atresia and intact ventricular septum (Daubeney et al., 2005). With 9 years of follow-up, they found an overall mortality of 41%. Twenty-nine percent of patients achieved a biventricular repair, 10.5% a univentricular repair, and 3% had right ventricular outflow tract reconstruction but then received a bidirectional cavopulmonary shunt (one and one-half ventricle repair). The remaining children died or had not yet achieved a surgical end point. Low birth weight, unipartite right ventricular morphology, and a dilated right ventricle were independent risk factors for death. Another population-based study from Sweden evaluated outcomes for children born between 1980 and 1999 (Ekman et al., 2001). Eighty-four children with pulmonary atresia and intact ventricular septum were born during this period, with a median follow-up of 6 years. Mortality for this group was 38%. Incremental risk factors for death included low birth weight, male sex, muscular pulmonary atresia, and having a systemic-to-pulmonary shunt as the sole initial intervention.

Surprisingly, published studies have failed to show any significant long-term functional difference between patients undergoing a univentricular repair compared to those with a biventricular repair. One group compared exercise performance of 19 patients undergoing biventricular repair compared to 10 with univentricular repair (Sanghavi et al., 2006). Most patients in each group had subnormal peak oxygen consumption. There was a trend toward impaired performance with increasing age regardless of type of repair. Another group evaluated quality of life in children with pulmonary atresia and intact ventricular septum (Ekman-Joelsson et al., 2004). They found no significant difference between those with biventricular repair, univentricular repair, and a normal reference group.

VALVAR PULMONIC STENOSIS

Introduction

Valvar pulmonic stenosis is one of the most prevalent structural heart defects. Although a structurally abnormal pulmonary valve can be seen in association with numerous other cardiac abnormalities, pulmonary valve stenosis is most commonly seen as an isolated structural anomaly, with otherwise normal systemic and pulmonary venous drainage, normal atrial situs, atrioventricular concordance, and ventriculo-arterial concordance. The clinical spectrum of pulmonary valve stenosis is broad, primarily due to variations in the severity of valvar obstruction.

Morphology

The anatomy of the abnormal pulmonary valve can be divided into two categories. The first and most common category is the dome-shaped valve. Pulmonary valves in this category have mild thickening of valve leaflets, with fusion or adhesions between leaflets (Altrichter et al., 1989; Gikonyo et al., 1987; Stamm et al., 1998). The adhesions cause variable degrees of restriction to valve motion, leading to a dome-shaped valve during ventricular systole (Figure 12–3). In approximately 20% of children with a dome-shaped valve, there are only two valve cusps, as opposed to the usual three cusps. In older children and adults, these doming valves occasionally develop small verrucous vegetations or calcifications around the valve edges. The second anatomic category, accounting for approximately 10%–15% of abnormal pulmonary valves, is the dysplastic valve. In this group, the valve leaflets are markedly thickened due to increased myxomatous tissue within the leaflet. The valve leaflets are relatively immobile, creating obstruction to flow due to this lack of mobility (Koretzky et al., 1969; Rodriguez-Fernandez et al., 1972).

Additional morphological changes may be seen, which are usually due to the pulmonary valve abnormality. The first of these is the dilation of the main pulmonary artery. This dilation may be prominent and is believed to be secondary to the systolic jet of blood

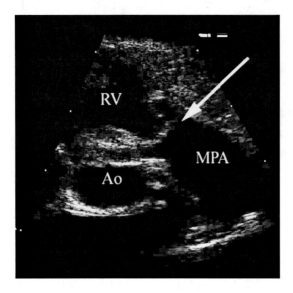

FIGURE 12-3. Valvar pulmonary stenosis. Parasternal short-axis echocardiographic image demonstrates the characteristic systolic "doming" of the pulmonary valve (arrow) as well as dilation of the main pulmonary artery (MPA). *Abbreviations*: AO, aortic valve; RV, right ventricular outflow.

through the abnormal doming valve, striking the main pulmonary artery wall. The degree of dilation does not appear to correlate with the severity of stenosis. The abnormally dilated pulmonary artery is only seen with the doming type of pulmonary valve and does not occur with a dysplastic valve.

Right ventricular hypertrophy may also occur in patients with valvar pulmonic stenosis. The degree of hypertrophy correlates with the severity of the valvar obstruction. Sometimes this muscular hypertrophy is particularly prominent in the right ventricular outflow tract, creating the potential for an additional level of obstruction proximal to the valve. Occasionally, the tricuspid valve is thickened, leading to moderate or severe tricuspid valve insufficiency and secondary right atrial dilation.

Abnormalities of the coronary circulation do occasionally occur in patients with severe pulmonary valve stenosis and illustrate the similarity of this disease with pulmonary valve atresia. Right ventricle to coronary artery sinusoidal connections have been described in cases of severe pulmonary valve stenosis (Bonnet et al., 1998).

Etiology

The estimated incidence of isolated pulmonary valve stenosis is 729 per 1 million live births (Hoffman and Kaplan, 2002). This comprises approximately 5.4% of infants born with all forms of congenital heart disease, including trivial conditions. The incidence of congenital heart disease in siblings of patients with valvar pulmonic stenosis is reported to be between 1.1% and 2.1% (Campbell, 1962; Driscoll et al., 1993).

For the majority of children born with pulmonary valve stenosis, the cause of the defect is unknown. However, a number of genetic syndromes associated with pulmonary valve stenosis have been described (Andiran et al., 2002; Digillo et al., 2006; Grech et al., 2000; Ishizawa et al., 1996; Kula et al., 2004; Lin et al., 2002; Wieczorek et al., 1997). These include Noonan syndrome, Leopard syndrome (also referred to as multiple lentigines syndrome), cardio-facio-cutaneous syndrome, Costello syndrome, Mayer-Rokitansky-Kuster-Hauser syndrome, congenital cutis laxa, and congenital nephritic syndrome.

Pulmonary valve stenosis has also been associated with a number of "nonsyndromic" conditions, including hemophilia A (Ackerman et al., 1986), Takayasu's disease (Rangel et al., 1996), and following twin–twin transfusion (Murakoshi et al., 2000). In addition, a viral etiology has been suggested, supported by the finding in valve tissue of viral antigens to adenovirus, coxsackie B virus, and parvovirus B19 (Oyer et al., 2000).

Hemodynamics

Hemodynamics in the infant with valvar pulmonic stenosis is determined by the severity of obstruction. Myocardial muscle hypertrophy and/or hyperplasia occur as a secondary phenomenon, proportional to the severity of obstruction. A pressure gradient between right ventricle and pulmonary artery of greater than 10 mmHg, in the quietly resting patient, is considered abnormal. If the right ventricular pressure is less than 50% of the left ventricular pressure, the patient is considered to have mild stenosis. Moderate pulmonary stenosis is defined as a right ventricular systolic pressure between 50% and 75% of the left ventricular pressure. Severe stenosis is defined as a right ventricular pressure greater than 75% of left ventricular pressure.

With mild pulmonary valve stenosis, the right atrial, right ventricular end-diastolic, and pulmonary artery pressures are normal. However, with moderate or severe obstruction, the right ventricular end-diastolic pressure may be increased, due to thickening of the right ventricular wall. In the presence of severe obstruction, the right ventricle may fail, leading to a drop in cardiac output, with a marked elevation of the right ventricular end-diastolic pressure. In this situation, the atrial mean pressure and "a" wave may increase in response to the abnormal right ventricular filling characteristics. With severe obstruction, the pulmonary artery pressure will decrease, with a dampened pulse amplitude. This effect may be more pronounced in the area immediately distal to the valve than in the peripheral pulmonary arteries due to the Bernoulli effect. Pressure in the right pulmonary artery is sometimes lower than left pulmonary artery, even without any evidence of branch pulmonary artery stenosis (Muster et al., 1982). This phenomenon may be due to the different orientation of the branch pulmonary arteries relative to the high-velocity systolic jet coming through the pulmonary valve.

The infant with severe pulmonary stenosis may present with a hemodynamic profile very much like the baby with pulmonary valve atresia. The tricuspid valve may develop mild or moderate regurgitation. Shunting of blood from right-to-left across the atrial septum may lead to varying degrees of systemic desaturation. Antegrade pulmonary blood flow is sometimes severely diminished and the infant may depend upon the ductus arteriosus to maintain adequate oxygenation.

In the older child with moderate or severe pulmonary stenosis, abnormal hemodynamics are particularly notable during exercise. Abnormal right ventricular compliance may lead to a fall in stroke volume as the patient becomes tachycardic, producing an abnormal blood pressure response to exercise (Krabill et al., 1985). With milder degrees of obstruction, both right and left ventricular performance during exercise is usually normal (Louie et al., 1995; Oosterhof et al., 2006).

Clinical Features

As noted earlier, the infant with severe pulmonary valve stenosis may present very much like the baby with pulmonary valve atresia. The patient may become desaturated and may depend upon ductal flow to maintain adequate pulmonary blood flow. Severe pulmonary stenosis can also present as shock, with severe right ventricular dysfunction due to the obstruction. However, after infancy, the majority of children with pulmonary stenosis present for evaluation of a murmur, and symptomatic right heart failure is rare. Growth and development are usually normal.

Palpation of the precordium may reveal abnormal findings in the presence of severe pulmonary valve stenosis. The right ventricle may be hypertrophied and hyperdynamic, leading to a prominent parasternal lift or heave. There may also be a palpable vibration or thrill at the left upper sternal border and suprasternal notch, corresponding to the systolic murmur.

Auscultatory findings in the most common form of valvar pulmonic stenosis consist of an early systolic ejection click followed by a crescendo-decrescendo murmur, which is best heard at the left upper sternal border, radiating to the back. The ejection click is thought to be due to a mobile but doming and stenotic valve snapping open. The click increases in intensity during expiration, and decreases during inspiration, probably because of partial opening of the pulmonary valve during late diastole with the increased right heart filling associated with inspiration. The click is not heard in children with a dysplastic valve. With increasing severity of pulmonary valve stenosis, the murmur increases in intensity, unless the child develops a low cardiac output due to right ventricular failure. Additional auscultatory findings with worsening stenosis include a movement of the ejection click to earlier in systole until it merges with the first sound, as well as a softening of the pulmonary component of the second heart sound until this becomes inaudible. With severe stenosis, the murmur becomes longer and may obscure the sound of aortic valve closure as well. The second heart sound is often widely split in the presence of pulmonary valve stenosis, but this may not be helpful from a diagnostic standpoint, since the pulmonary component of this sound can be difficult to hear.

Electrocardiographic abnormalities correlate in a general way with the severity of pulmonary valve obstruction. Patients with mild obstruction often have a normal electrocardiogram. Increases in right ventricular pressure may manifest early by "inversion" of the normal downgoing T-wave in the right and mid-precordial leads. However, with worsening degrees of stenosis, the electrocardiogram tends to show more signs of right ventricular hypertrophy. There may be right axis deviation, and with more severe obstruction, evidence of atrial enlargement may appear. Some patients with a dysplastic pulmonary valve have a superior axis.

The chest x-ray may be entirely normal, even in the presence of moderate or severe stenosis. However, in the presence of a doming pulmonary valve, the main pulmonary artery segment can be quite dilated and easily seen in the anterior–posterior view. The presence of the finding, though, does not correlate with the severity of stenosis. In the patient with a failing right ventricle, cardiomegaly would be expected on the chest x-ray.

Echo. Echocardiography complements physical examination and electrocardiographic findings and allows for establishment of the diagnosis, exclusion of other significant abnormalities (most commonly atrial and ventricular septal defects), and allows for noninvasive longitudinal assessment of the degree of obstruction. Two-dimensional echocardiographic evaluation allows for visualization of right ventricular hypertrophy, dilation, and function. Especially in infants and young children, exquisite detail of the precise anatomy of the abnormal pulmonary valve is possible. Pulmonary annulus size measurement (from the parasternal short-axis view) and assessment of the infundibulum as a potential source for obstruction should be performed if intervention is being entertained. The interatrial septum should be evaluated for the presence of interatrial communication, and if found, Doppler interrogation to assess the degree and direction of shunting may be useful, especially in patients with cyanosis. Doppler evaluation of the degree and velocity of tricuspid regurgitation is helpful and may in fact provide a better estimate of the degree of outflow tract obstruction than Doppler gradients obtained in the outflow tract, especially if there are multiple levels of obstruction present. Both mean and peak systolic gradients are often reported. Though in a large natural history study reported in 1993 (Nishimura et al., 1993), the mean gradient was used in stratification of patients for severity of obstruction, the authors acknowledged that there may be better agreement between Doppler-derived peak instantaneous gradient and catheter-derived peak-to-peak gradient (Currie et al., 1986; Lima et al., 1983) and the peak instantaneous pressure gradient observed at cardiac catheterization has been shown to correlate well with the highest peak Doppler gradient (Frantz and Silverman, 1988) when multiple sonographic transducer positions are used to obtain the maximal Doppler gradient.

Prenatal diagnosis of valvar pulmonary stenosis is unusual but if seen should be followed up with serial examination by fetal echocardiography as the lesion may progress significantly in utero and may in fact present at birth as pulmonary atresia (see preceding section) (Allan et al., 1994, Todros et al., 1988). Cardiac catheterization is now seldom necessary unless undertaken for the purpose of balloon valvuloplasty or if the distal pulmonary arterial anatomy is in question.

Differential Diagnosis

Frequent physical examination alone can produce a high level of confidence in the diagnosis of pulmonary valvar stenosis. However, mild stenosis is sometimes confused with an atrial septal defect. The midsystolic click found in mitral valve prolapse may lead to the inclusion of this defect in the differential diagnosis. With findings that suggest moderate or severe stenosis, ventricular septal defects and tetralogy of Fallot may need inclusion in the differential diagnosis. Supravalvar or infundibular pulmonic stenosis is sometimes confused with valvar obstruction on physical examination. Echocardiography is usually sufficient to clarify the diagnosis and rule out any unsuspected associated defects.

Management

For infants, management decisions require some insight into the natural history of this disease. In the first year of life, the natural history of both mild and moderate stenosis is quite variable. Often, stenosis that is thought to be mild in infancy will rapidly worsen, becoming moderate or severe over the course of weeks or months (Anand and Mehta, 1997; Rowland et al., 1997). However, this clinical course cannot be reliably predicted, since moderate obstruction in the first year of life may also improve spontaneously over the course of time (Kirk et al., 1988; Lueker et al., 1970; Tomita et al., 1995). Due to the variable natural history in the first year of life, infants with valvar pulmonic stenosis who do not meet criteria for immediate treatment should be followed closely over time to detect any significant worsening of obstruction that might occur.

The infant with severe or critical obstruction of the pulmonary valve needs urgent treatment. The options for this treatment are similar to those in patients with complete pulmonary atresia and depend upon specific anatomic considerations. However, most often the right ventricle is reasonably well developed, and treatment consists of an intervention to decrease the severity of obstruction. This intervention can be either catheter-based (angioplasty), or surgical, depending upon the anatomy and institutional preferences.

Many investigators have reported that beyond the first year of life, mild pulmonary valve stenosis (right ventricular pressure less than 50% of left ventricular pressure) remains mild or shows spontaneous improvement (Lange et al., 1985; Mody, 1975). In rare cases, mild stenosis may become moderate (right ventricular pressure 50%–75% of left ventricular pressure). Older patients with mild stenosis require periodic cardiac evaluations, but otherwise need no treatment or restriction of activities. No significant adverse outcomes have been seen in the long-term follow-up studies (Hayes et al., 1993; Nugent et al., 1977). The most recent guidelines of the American Heart Association and American Dental Association do not recommend antibiotic prophylaxis for dental or other procedures for patients with pulmonary stenosis (Wilson et al., 2007).

For patients older than 1 year of age, with moderate obstruction, natural history studies suggest that some will develop progressive right ventricular hypertrophy and outflow tract obstruction. In addition, older patients may develop systolic and diastolic dysfunction (Krabill et al., 1985). For these reasons, most centers recommend treatment of children older than 1 year of age with moderate or severe pulmonary valve stenosis.

Balloon valvuloplasty is accepted as the best initial therapy for patients with valvar pulmonic stenosis. In infants with critical pulmonary valve obstruction, balloon dilation may be the only required treatment in 85% of the cases. However, up to 15% of newborns may require surgery to relieve the obstruction (Fedderly et al., 1995; Tabatabaei et al., 1996). If the infant has right ventricular hypoplasia, near complete relief of obstruction is important, to give the ventricle a good opportunity to grow (Gournay et al., 1995). Following balloon pulmonary valvuloplasty, the right ventricular hypertrophy may cause residual infundibular obstruction. Often this will resolve over time, although some have used beta-adrenergic blockers to minimize obstruction as the hypertrophy regresses (Thapar and Rao, 1989).

Results of treatment depend upon patient characteristics and the treatment method. One long term follow-up study of 150 children suggests that 90% of treated infants and children remain free of re-intervention 1 year post treatment, whereas only 77% had not required additional treatment after 15 years (Garty et al., 2005). In this series, 57% of the children had moderate or severe pulmonary regurgitation, although other studies have found the incidence of moderate pulmonary regurgitation to be less than 5% (Masura et al., 1993; McCrindle et al., 1993). Pulmonary regurgitation that is initially mild may increase with longer term follow-up (Poon and Menahem, 2003). Suboptimal relief of obstruction has been shown to correlate with dysplasia of the pulmonary valve, smaller annulus size, and use of balloons—with a balloon:annulus ratio of less than 120%. However, use of larger balloons correlates with the development of pulmonary valve insufficiency. Important complications occur in less than 10% of patients, with overall mortality of 0.2% (Stanger et al., 1990). Complication risks increase in neonates and infants.

DOUBLE CHAMBER RIGHT VENTRICLE

Introduction

Double chamber right ventricle is a structural heart defect that consists of situs solitus, with normal systemic and pulmonary venous connections. Atrioventricular and ventriculo-arterial relationships are concordant. The primary feature of the defect is the presence of anomalous hypertrophied muscular bands that divide the right ventricle into a high-pressure inflow portion and an outlet portion with normal or low pressures.

Morphology

The anomalous muscle bundle originates from the ventricular septum, near the insertion of the septal leaflet of the tricuspid valve. The muscle may be bifid, with an anterior segment attaching to the free wall of the right ventricle, and a more posterior segment attaching to the base of the anterior papillary muscle. The obstruction created by this anomaly is proximal to the infundibulum. There is frequently an associated ventricular septal defect, which often communicates with the low-pressure portion of the right ventricle.

Etiology

The etiology of double chamber right ventricle is unknown but when associated with ventricular septal defect is thought to be due to progressive right ventricular hypertrophy.

Hemodynamics

This defect produces a variable degree of intracavitary obstruction in the right ventricle, depending upon size and slight variations in the position of the anomalous bundle. The obstruction may be dynamic, increasing with catecholamine stimulation. If there is an associated ventricular septal defect, it usually communicates with the low pressure portion of the right ventricle. This produces a left-to-right shunt, the severity of which depends primarily upon the size of the ventricular septal defect. Occasionally a ventricular defect communicates with the high-pressure portion of the right ventricular cavity, which can lead to a right-to-left shunt and systemic desaturation.

Clinical Features

If there is an associated ventricular septal defect, the clinical features of double chamber right ventricle may be dominated by this component of the anomaly. However, if the ventricular defect is small or not present, clinical features are similar to other forms of pulmonary outflow obstruction. There is usually a systolic crescendo-decrescendo murmur, which is best heard along the mid to upper left sternal border. The electrocardiogram may show signs of right ventricular hypertrophy, depending upon the severity of obstruction. The chest x-ray is often normal unless a significant ventricular left-to right-shunt is present. Unlike in patients with pulmonary valve stenosis, there is no ejection click and no dilation of the main pulmonary artery in patients with double chamber right ventricle.

Differential Diagnosis

Different forms of right ventricular outflow obstruction have similar clinical features. When pulmonary stenosis is suspected, echocardiography is the best tool to determine the specific anatomy and level of obstruction. Both two-dimensional and Doppler inter-rogation of the right ventricle, outflow tract, pulmonary valve, and supravalvar area are necessary, as multiple levels of obstruction may exist. Two-dimensional appearance, as opposed to valvar stenosis, will show a normal pulmonary valve with right ventricular hyper-trophy and characteristic anomalous muscle bundles in the infundibular region (Figure 12–4A). These muscle bundles can be assessed from the parasternal short axis position and as well as from the subcostal windows, but Doppler interrogation from the subcos-tal window will often be most helpful in determining the precise site and degree of obstruction due to poor angles of insonance obtained with the transducer in the parasternal position (Figure 12–4B). Tricuspid regurgitation, if present, can be extremely helpful in determining the true degree of obstruction as the application of the modified Bernoulli equation for determining pressure gradients through the complex tunnel-like outflow tract may be flawed. Identification by transesophageal echocardiography is also possible and should be actively sought out intraoperatively dur-ing ventricular septal defect closure as elimination of a left-to-right ventricular shunt may unmask obstruc-tion in this region.

Cardiac catheterization can add additional infor-mation about associated ventricular septal defects and further identify the anatomy and severity of the right ventricular outflow obstruction, but it usually is not needed.

Management

If treatment is needed, the right ventricular outflow obstruction must be corrected surgically. Visualization of the anomalous muscle bundle is usually best through the tricuspid valve and a ventriculotomy is seldom necessary.

PERIPHERAL PULMONARY ARTERY STENOSIS

Introduction

Peripheral pulmonary artery stenosis is a defect with several distinct anatomic variants and a wide spectrum of severity. It may occur as an isolated defect or in asso-ciation with other forms of congenital heart disease.

Morphology

Stenosis may occur in the main pulmonary artery, at either of the main pulmonary artery branches, or in the peripheral pulmonary arteries. Diffuse pulmonary artery hypoplasia also occurs, often in combination

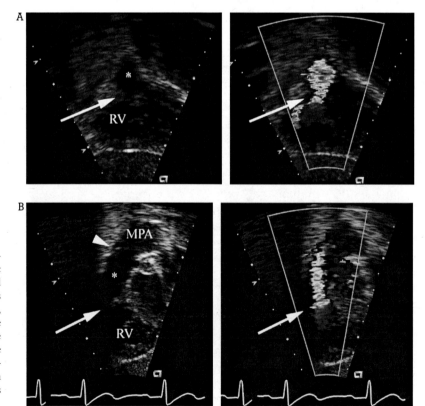

FIGURE 12–4. "Double-chambered" right ven-tricle. A: Subcostal coronal echocardiographic images, two-dimensional and with superimposed color Doppler. The abnormal muscle bundles (arrow) divide the ventricle into the trabecular, high-pressure portion (RV) and a low-pressure outlet (*) proximal to the pulmonary valve. The color aliasing clearly begins at the region of the muscle bundles. B: Subcostal sagital images dem-onstrating similar anatomy. The obstruction (arrow), by both 2D and color Doppler, begins well below the pulmonary valve (arrowhead).

with tetralogy of Fallot or other complex structural heart defects.

Etiology

Peripheral pulmonary artery stenosis occurs in association with a number of syndromes. Congenital rubella is associated with multiple stenoses of the distal pulmonary arteries. Williams syndrome is associated with supravalvar pulmonic stenosis, branch pulmonary artery stenosis, multiple peripheral pulmonary artery stenoses, and supravalvar aortic stenosis. Diffuse hypoplasia of the pulmonary arteries is seen in Alagille syndrome. Peripheral and branch pulmonary artery stenoses are seen in association with the Noonan syndrome, Ehlers-Danlos syndrome, Silver-Russell syndrome, congenital cutis laxa, and twin–twin transfusion syndrome. A murmur due to flow acceleration at the origin of the right and left branch pulmonary arteries ("physiological peripheral pulmonary stenosis") occurs as a normal anatomic variant in approximately 10% of newborns (Arlettaz et al., 1998). The mild stenosis that produces this murmur usually disappears by 6 months of age.

Hemodynamics

Stenosis of the main pulmonary artery, or bilateral stenosis of branch or peripheral pulmonary arteries, raises proximal systolic pressures to a degree consistent with the severity of stenosis. Proximal pulmonary artery diastolic pressures, though, are usually low and frequently equal right ventricular end-diastolic pressures. With unilateral stenosis, systolic pressures proximal to the obstruction are normal, although blood flow is proportionally increased to the unobstructed lung.

Clinical Features

Auscultatory findings vary depending upon the site and severity of the stenosis. Peripheral pulmonary artery stenosis produces a crescendo-decrescendo murmur that correlates with the severity of the stenosis when the obstruction is in the main pulmonary artery. Due to the potential redistribution of blood flow with branch pulmonary artery stenosis, the intensity of the murmur may not correlate with the severity of obstruction for this lesion. When the stenosis occurs in one of the branch pulmonary arteries, the murmur may radiate quite well into the axilla on the affected side. Distal branch pulmonary artery stenosis may produce a continuous murmur, indicating both a systolic and diastolic gradient across the obstruction. When branch pulmonary artery stenosis is bilateral and severe, pulmonary valve closure may be increased in intensity.

The electrocardiogram may be normal, even in the presence of severe branch stenosis. However, severe main pulmonary artery obstruction usually produces right ventricular hypertrophy, which can be identified by the electrocardiogram. If there is severe unilateral stenosis, the chest x-ray may reveal asymmetrical pulmonary vascularity.

Differential Diagnosis

The echocardiographic appearance of this spectrum of defects is dependent on site and severity of obstruction. In the majority of patients with peripheral stenosis, the echocardiogram is normal. There may be evidence of right ventricular hypertrophy depending on the severity of distal obstruction, and tricuspid regurgitant jet velocity may be elevated; however, these findings are nonspecific and may also be indicative of pulmonary hypertension. More proximal stenosis, at the proximal origin of the right or left pulmonary arteries, may be detected on two-dimensional and Doppler evaluation, best appreciated from the parasternal or suprasternal notch coronal views. Supravalvar narrowing and acceleration are easily appreciated on parasternal imaging and Doppler evaluation, though accurate assessment of gradients may be difficult.

Additional imaging studies are usually needed to evaluate the branch and distal pulmonary artery anatomy. Magnetic resonance imaging can produce excellent definition of the pulmonary artery anatomy. However, cardiac catheterization permits a detailed angiographic evaluation of pulmonary artery anatomy, an assessment of pulmonary artery pressures, and an opportunity for catheter-based treatment of some forms of obstruction.

Management

Criteria for treatment of peripheral pulmonary stenosis are not well established. Certainly, obstruction that produces a moderate or severe elevation of right ventricular pressure is worth considering for treatment for the same reasons that this level of stenosis is treated when the obstruction is valvar. However, since unilateral obstruction may severely alter distribution of the pulmonary blood flow without changing the right ventricular pressure, additional indications for treatment must be considered. In the presence of unilateral branch or segmental pulmonary artery stenosis, some institutions assess the distribution of pulmonary blood flow with radionuclide flow studies. When one lung or one segment shows a marked reduction in flow, treatment is considered. Additionally, many cardiologists feel that it is important to treat moderate to severe branch or segmental obstruction in the univentricular heart, where flow through the lung will be passive and nonpulsatile.

Techniques for treating peripheral pulmonary artery stenosis include both surgical and interventional catheterization methods. Selection of particular treatment strategies depends upon institutional expertise, patient age, associated conditions, and anatomy of the pulmonary artery obstruction. Frequently, children with complex forms of peripheral pulmonary artery stenosis will need multiple interventions using both interventional catheterization and surgical treatments. Surgical methods for excising, patching, and enlarging stenotic pulmonary arteries can produce excellent long-term results. However, various factors, including patient size, presence of multiple stenoses, and presence of distal obstructions, may make surgical intervention extremely difficult or impossible. The interventional cardiologist possesses a complementary set of techniques that may provide excellent palliation for certain forms of pulmonary artery obstruction. High-pressure balloons, inflated up to 25 atm, as well as cutting balloons can successfully increase luminal diameter for many patients with peripheral pulmonary artery stenosis. For unresponsive stenoses, the interventional cardiologist can often place a balloon expandable stent to increase the luminal diameter. The risk of balloon dilation and stent placement include pulmonary artery rupture, aneurysms, pulmonary edema, and thrombotic occlusion of ileofemoral veins. Some centers have attempted to control these risks and improve outcomes by taking a "hybrid" approach, and placing stents and balloon catheter with the chest open in the operating room. This carries the advantage of permitting the placement of larger stents, and potentially allows control of bleeding complications.

Infundibular Pulmonary Stenosis

Infundibular pulmonary stenosis with an intact ventricular septum is a rare defect. This defect can be caused by fibromuscular thickening of the right ventricular wall and septum. Treatment considerations are similar to those for patients with anomalous right ventricular muscle bundle.

REFERENCES

Ackerman Z, Koren G, Gotsman M, Eldor A. Pulmonary valve stenosis and hemophilia A. Report of three cases and discussion of a possible genetic linkage. *Arch Intern Med.* 1986;146:2233–2234.

Akiba T, Becker AE. Disease of the left ventricle in pulmonary atresia with intact ventricular septum. The limiting factor for long-lasting successful surgical intervention? *J Thorac Cardiovasc Surg.* 1994;108:1–8.

Albanese SB, Carotti A, Toscano A, Marino B, Di Donato RM. Pulmonary atresia with intact ventricular septum and systemic-pulmonary collateral arteries. *Ann Thorac Surg.* 2002;73:1322–1324.

Allan LD, Sharland GK, Milburn A, et al. Prospective diagnosis of 1,006 consecutive cases of congenital heart disease in the fetus. *J Am Coll Cardiol.* 1994;23:1452–1458.

Altrichter PM, Olson LJ, Edwards WD, Puga FJ, Danielson GK. Surgical pathology of the pulmonary valve: a study of 116 cases spanning 15 years. *Mayo Clin Proc.* 1989;64:1352–1360.

Anand R, Mehta AV. Natural history of asymptomatic valvar pulmonary stenosis diagnosed in infancy. *Clin Cardiol.* 1997;20:377–380.

Anderson RH, Silverman NH, Zuberbuhler JR. Congenitally unguarded tricuspid orifice: its differentiation from Ebstein's malformation in association with pulmonary atresia and intact ventricular septum. *Pediatr Cardiol.* 1990;11:86–90.

Andiran N, Sarikayalar F, Saraclar M, Caglar M. Autosomal recessive form of congenital cutis laxa: more than the clinical appearance. *Pediatr Dermatol.* 2002;19:412–414.

Arlettaz R, Archer N, Wilkinson AR. Natural history of innocent heart murmurs in newborn babies: controlled echocardiographic study. *Arch Dis Child Fetal Neonatal Ed.* 1998;78: F166–F170.

Ashburn DA, Blackstone EH, Wells WJ, et al. Determinants of mortality and type of repair in neonates with pulmonary atresia and intact ventricular septum. *J Thorac Cardiovasc Surg.* 2004;127:1000–1007.

Bharati S, McAllister HAJ, Chiemmongkaltip P, Lev M. Congenital pulmonary atresia with tricuspid insufficiency: morphologic study. *Am J Cardiol.* 1977;40:70–75.

Bonnet D, Gautier-Lhermitte I, Bonhoeffer P, Sidi D. Right ventricular myocardial sinusoidal-coronary artery connections in critical pulmonary valve stenosis. *Pediatr Cardiol.* 1998;19:269–271.

Braunlin EA, Formanek AG, Moller JH, Edwards JE. Angiopathologic appearances of pulmonary valve in pulmonary atresia with intact ventricular septum: interpretation of nature of right ventricle from pulmonary angiography. *Br Heart J.* 1982;47:281–289.

Campbell M. Factors in the etiology of pulmonary stenosis. *Br Heart J.* 1962;24:625–632.

Choi YH, Seo JW, Choi JY, Yun YS, Kim SH, Lee HJ. Morphology of tricuspid valve in pulmonary atresia with intact ventricular septum. *Pediatr Cardiol.* 1998;19:381–389.

Currie PJ, Hagler DJ, Seward JB et al. Instantaneous pressure gradient: a simultaneous Doppler and dual catheter correlative study. *J Am Coll Cardiol.* 1986;7(4):800–806.

Daubeney PE, Delany DJ, Anderson RH, et al. Pulmonary atresia with intact ventricular septum: range of morphology in a population-based study. *J Am Coll Cardiol.* 2002;39:1670–1670.

Daubeney PE, Wang D, Delany DJ, et al. Pulmonary atresia with intact ventricular septum: predictors of early and medium-term outcome in a population-based study. *J Thorac Cardiovasc Surg.* 2005;130:1071–1074.

Daubeney PE, Sharland GK, Cook AC, Keeton BR, Anderson RH, Webber SA. Pulmonary atresia with intact ventricular septum: impact of fetal echocardiography on incidence at birth and postnatal outcome. UK and Eire Collaborative Study of Pulmonary Atresia with Intact Ventricular Septum. *Circulation.* 1998;98:562–566.

Digillio MC, Sarkozy A, de Zorzi A, et al. LEOPARD syndrome: clinical diagnosis in the first year of life. *Am J Med Genet A.* 2006;140:740–746.

Driscoll DJ, Michels VV, Gersony WM, et al. Occurrence risk for congenital heart defects in relatives of patients with aortic stenosis, pulmonary stenosis or ventricular septal defect. *Circulation*. 1993;87(supp 3):I114–I120.

Dyamenahalli U, McCrindle BW, McDonald C, et al. Pulmonary atresia with intact ventricular septum: management of, and outcomes for, a cohort of 210 consecutive patients. *Cardiol Young*. 2004;14:299–308.

Ekman-Joelsson BM, Berntsson L, Sunnegardh J. Quality of life in children with pulmonary atresia and intact ventricular septum. *Cardiol Young*. 2004;14:615–621.

Ekman-Joelsson BM, Sunnegardh J, Hanseus K, et al. The outcome of children born with pulmonary atresia and intact ventricular septum in Sweden from 1980 to 1999. *Scand Cardiovasc J*. 2001;35:192–198.

Fedderly RT, Lloyd TR, Mendelsohn AM, Beekman RH. Determinants of successful balloon valvulotomy in infants with critical pulmonary stenosis or membranous pulmonary atresia with intact ventricular septum. *J Am Coll Cardiol*. 1995;25:460–465.

Frantz EG, Silverman NH. Doppler ultrasound evaluation of valvar pulmonary stenosis from multiple transducer positions in children requiring pulmonary valvuloplasty. *Am J Cardiol*. 1988;61:844–849.

Freedom RM, Dische MR, Rowe RD. The tricuspid valve in pulmonary atresia and intact ventricular septum: a morphological study of 60 cases. *Arch Pathol Lab Med*. 1978;102:28–31.

Frober R, Kohoutek T, Kahler C, et al. Pulmonary atresia with hypoplastic right ventricle. A clinical embryological study. *Fetal Diagn Ther*. 2001;16:274–279.

Fyfe DA, Edwards WD, Driscoll DJ. Myocardial ischemia in patients with pulmonary atresia and intact ventricular septum. *J Am Coll Cardiol*. 1986;8:402–406.

Garcia JA, Zellers TM, Weinstein EM, Mahony L. Usefulness of Doppler echocardiography in diagnosing right ventricular coronary arterial communications in patients with pulmonary atresia and intact ventricular septum and comparison with angiography. *Am J Cardiol*. 1998;81:103–104.

Garty Y, Veldtman G, Lee K, Benson L. Late outcomes after pulmonary valve balloon dilatation in neonates, infants and children. *J Invasive Cardiol*. 2005;17:318–322.

Gikonyo BM, Lucas RV, Edwards JE. Anatomic features of congenital pulmonary valvar stenosis. *Pediatr Cardiol*. 1987;8:109–116.

Gittenberger-de Groot AC, Sauer U, Bindl L, Babic R, Essed CE, Buhlmeyer K. Competition of coronary arteries and ventriculocoronary arterial communications in pulmonary atresia with intact ventricular septum. *Int J Cardiol*. 1988;18:243–258.

Gournay V, Piechaud JF, Delogu A, Sidi D, Kachaner J. Balloon valvulotomy for critical stenosis or atresia of pulmonary valve in newborns. *J Am Coll Cardiol*. 1995;26:1725–1731.

Grech V, Chan MK, Vella C, Attard-Montalto S, Rees P, Trompeter RS. Cardiac malformations associated with the congenital nephrotic syndrome. *Pediatr Nephrol*. 2000;14:1115–1117.

Grossfeld PD, Lucas VW, Sklansky MS, Kashani IA, Rothman A. Familial occurrence of pulmonary atresia with intact ventricular septum. *Am J Med Genet*. 1997;72:294–296.

Gucer S, Ince T, Kale G, et al. Noncardiac malformations in congenital heart disease: a retrospective analysis of 305 pediatric autopsies. *Turk J Pediatr*. 2005;47:159–166.

Hanley FL, Sade RM, Blackstone EH, Kirklin JW, Freedom RM, Nanda NC. Outcomes in neonatal pulmonary atresia with intact ventricular septum. A multiinstitutional study. *J Thorac Cardiovasc Surg*. 1993;105:406–427.

Hayes CJ, Gersony WM, Driscoll DJ, et al. Second natural history study of congenital heart defects. Results of treatment of patients with pulmonary valvar stenosis. *Circulation*. 1993;87(suppl 2):I28–I37.

Hoffman JIE, Kaplan S. The incidence of congenital heart disease. *J Am Coll Cardiol*. 2002;39:1890–1900.

Hornberger LK, Benacerraf BR, Bromley BS, Spevak PJ, Sanders SP. Prenatal detection of severe right ventricular outflow tract obstruction: pulmonary stenosis and pulmonary atresia. *J Ultrasound Med*. 1994;13:743–750.

Ishizawa A, Oho S, Dodo H, Katori T, Homma SI. Cardiovascular abnormalities in Noonan syndrome: the clinical findings and treatments. *Acta Paediatr Jpn*. 1996;38:84–90.

Kirk CR, Wilkinson JL, Qureshi SA. Regression of pulmonary valve stenosis due to a dysplastic valve presenting in the neonatal period. *Eur Heart J*. 1988;9:1027–1029.

Kobayashi T, Momoi N, Fukuda Y, Suzuki H. Percutaneous balloon valvuloplasty of both pulmonary and aortic valves in a neonate with pulmonary atresia and critical aortic stenosis. *Pediatr Cardiol*. 2005;26:839–842.

Koretzky ED, Muller JH, Korus ME, Schwartz CT, Edwards JE. Congenital pulmonary stenosis resulting from dysplasia of the valve. *Circulation*. 1969;40:43–53.

Krabill KA, Wang Y, Einzig S, Moller JH. Rest and exercise hemodynamics in pulmonary stenosis: comparison of children and adults. *Am J Cardiol*. 1985;56:360–365.

Kula S, Saygili A, Tunaoglu FS, Olgunturk R. Mayer-Rokitansky-Kuster-Hauser syndrome associated with pulmonary stenosis. *Acta Paediatr*. 2004;93:570–572.

Kutsche LM, Van Mierop LH. Pulmonary atresia with and without ventricular septal defect: a different etiology and pathogenesis for the atresia in the 2 types? *Am J Cardiol*. 1983;51:932–935.

Lange PE, Onnasch DG, Heintzen PH. Valvular pulmonary stenosis. Natural history and right ventricular function in infants and children. *Eur Heart J*. 1985;6:706–709.

Li C, Chudley AE, Soni R, Divekar A. Pulmonary atresia with intact ventricular septum and major aortopulmonary collaterals: association with deletion 22q11.2. *Pediatr Cardiol*. 2003;24:585–587.

Lima CO, Sahn DJ, Valdes-Cruz LM, et al. Noninvasive prediction of transvalvular pressure gradient in patients with pulmonary stenosis by quantitative two-dimensional echocardiographic Doppler studies *Circulation*. 1983;67(4):866–871.

Lin AE, Grossfeld PD, Hamilton RM, et al. Further delineation of cardiac abnormalities in Costello syndrome. *Am J Med Genet*. 2002;111:115–129.

Louie EK, Lin SS, Reynertson SI, Brundage BH, Levitsky S, Rich S. Pressure and volume loading of the right ventricle have opposite effects on left ventricular ejection fraction. *Circulation*. 1995;92:819–824.

Lueker RD, Vogel JH, Blount SG. Regression of valvular pulmonary stenosis. *Br Heart J*. 1970;32:779–782.

Maeno YV, Boutin C, Hornberger LK, et al. Prenatal diagnosis of right ventricular outflow tract obstruction with intact ventricular septum, and detection of ventriculocoronary connections. *Heart*. 1999;81:661–668.

Masura J, Burch M, Deanfield JE, Sullivan ID. Five-year follow-up after balloon pulmonary valvuloplasty. *J Am Coll Cardiol*. 1993;21:132–136.

McCrindle BW. Independent predictors of long-term results after balloon pulmonary valvuloplasty. *J Am Coll Cardiol*. 21:132–136.

Mi YP, Chau AK, Chiu CS, Yung TC, Lun KS, Cheung YF. Evolution of the management approach for pulmonary atresia with intact ventriculoar septum. *Heart*. 2005;91:657–663.

Milanesi O, Daliento L, Thiene G. Solitary aorta with bilateral ductal origin of non-confluent pulmonary arteries in pulmonary atresia with intact ventricular septum. *Int J Cardiol*. 1990;29:90–92.

Minich LL, Tani LY, Ritter S, Williams RV, Shaddy RE, Hawkins JA. Usefulness of the preoperative tricuspid/mitral valve ratio for predicting outcome in pulomonary atresia with intact ventricular septum. *Am J Cardiol.* 2000;85:1325–1328.

Mishima A, Asano M, Sasaki S, et al. Long-term outcome for right heart function after biventricular repair of pulmonary atresia and intact ventricular septum. *Jpn J Thorac Cardiovasc Surg.* 2000;48:145–152.

Miyaji K, Murakami A, Takasaki T, Ohara K, Takamoto S, Yoshimura H. Does a bidirectional Glenn shunt improve the oxygenation of right ventricle-dependent coronary circulation in pulmonary atresia with intact ventricular septum? *J Thorac Cardiovasc Surg.* 2005;130:1050–1053.

Mody MR. The natural history of uncomplicated valvular pulmonic stenosis. *Am Heart J.* 1975;90:317–321.

Moon-Grady AJ, Teitel DF, Hanley FL, Moore P. Ductus-associated proximal pulmonary artery stenosis in patients with right heart obstruction. *Int J Cardiol.* 2007;114:41–45.

Murakoshi T, Yamamori K, Tojo Y, et al. Pulmonary stenosis in recipient twins in twin-to-twin transfusion syndrome: report on 3 cases and review of literature. *Croat Med J.* 2000;41: 252–256.

Muster AJ, van Grondelle A, Paul MH. Unequal pressures in the central pulmonary arterial branches in patients with pulmonary stenosis. The influence of blood velocity and anatomy. *Pediatr Cardiol.* 1982;2:7–14.

Nishimura RA, Pieroni DR, Bierman FZ, et al. Second natural history study of congenital heart defects. Pulmonary stenosis: echocardiography. *Circulation.* 1993;87(suppl 2):I73–I79.

Nugent EW, Freedom RM, Nora JJ, Ellison RC, Rowe RD, Nadas AS. Clinical course in pulmonic stenosis. *Circulation.* 1977;56(suppl 1):15–28.

Odim J, Laks H, Plunkett MD, Tung TC. Successful management of patients with pulmonary atresia with intact ventricular septum using a three tier grading system for right ventricular hypoplasia. *Ann Thorac Surg.* 2006;81:678–684.

Oosterhof T, Tulevski II, Vliegen HW, Spijkerboer AM, Mulder BJ. Effects of volume and/or pressure overload secondary to congenital heart disease (tetralogy of fallot or pulmonary stenosis) on right ventricular function using cardiovascular magnetic resonance and B-type natriuretic peptide levels. *Am J Cardiol.* 2006;97:1051–1055.

Oosthoek PW, Moorman AF, Sauer U, Gittenberger-de Groot AC. Capillary distribution in the ventricles of hearts with pulmonary atresia and intact ventricular septum. *Circulation.* 1995;91:1790–1798.

Oyer CE, Ongcapin EH, Nhi J, Bowles NE, Towbin JA. Fatal intrauterine adenoviral endomyocarditis with aortic and pulmonary valve stenosis: diagnosis by polymerase chain reaction. *Hum Pathol.* 2000;31:1433–1435.

Poon LK, Menaham S. Pulmonary regurgitation after percutaneous balloon valvoplasty for isolated pulmonary valvar stenosis in childhood. *Cardiol Young.* 2003;13:444–450.

Rangel A, Badui E, Jara LJ, et al. Pulmonary valvular stenosis associated with Takayasu's Disease. Favorable response to corticosteroids. A case report. *Angiology.* 1996;47:717–724.

Razzouk A, Freedom RM, Cohen AJ, et al. The recognition, identification of morphological substrate, and treatment of subaortic stenosis after a Fontan operation: an analysis of 12 patients. *J Thorac Cardiovasc Surg.* 1992;104:938–944.

Rodriguez-Fernandez HC, Char F, Kelly DT, Rowe RD. The dysplastic pulmonary valve and the Noonan Syndrome. *Circulation.* 1972;98(suppl 2):45–46.

Rowland DG, Hammill WW, Allen HD, Gutgesell HP. Natural course of isolated pulmonary valve stenosis in infants and children utilizing Doppler echocardiography. *Am J Cardiol.* 1997;79:344–349.

Sanders SP, Parness IA, Colan SD. Recognition of abnormal connections of coronary arteries with the use of Doppler color flow mapping. *J Am Coll Cardiol.* 1989;13:922–926.

Sanghavi DM, Flanagan M, Powell AJ, Curran T, Picard S, Rhodes J. Determinants of exercise function following univentricular versus biventricular repair for pulmonary atresia/intact ventricular septum. *Am J Cardiol.* 2006;97:1638–1643.

Santos MA, Moll JN, Drumond C, Araujo WB, Romao N, Reis NB. Development of the ductus arteriosus in right ventricular outflow tract obstruction. *Circulation.* 1980;62:818–822.

Santos MA, Azevedo VM. Angiographic morphologic characteristics in pulmonary atrresia with intact ventricular septum. *Arq Bras Cardiol.* 2004;82:420–425.

Satou GM, Perry SB, Gauvreau K, Geva T. Echocardiographic predictors of coronary artery pathology in pulmonary atresia with intact ventricular septum. *Am J Cardiol.* 2000;85:1319–1324.

Sauer U, Gittenberger-de Groot AC, Heimisch W, Bindl L. Right ventricle to coronary artery connections (fistulae) in pulmonary atresia with intact ventricular septum: clinical and histopathological correlations. *Prog Pediatr Cardiol.* 2006;22: 187–204.

Schmidt KG, Cloez JL, Silverman NH. Changes of right ventricular size and function in neonates after valvotomy for pulmonary atresia or critical pulmonary stenosis and intact ventricular septum. *J Am Coll Cardiol.* 1992;19:1032–1037.

Schneider M, Zartner P, Sidiropoulos A, Konertz W, Hausdorf G. Stent implantation of the arterial duct in newborns with duct-dependent circulation. *Eur Heart J.* 1998;19:1401–1409.

Selamet SE, Hsu DT, Thaker HM, Gersony WM. Complete atresia of coronary ostia in pulmonary atresia and intact ventricular septum. *Pediatr Cardiol.* 2004;25:67–69.

Sharland G. Pulmonary valve abnormalities. In: Allan L, Hornberger LK, Sharlan G, eds. *Textbook of Fetal Cardiology.* London: Greenwich Medical Media; 2000:233–247.

Siblini G, Rao PS, Singh GK, Tinker K, Balfour IC. Transcatheter management of neonates with pulmonary atresia and intact ventricular septum. *Cathet Cardiovasc Diagn.* 1997;42: 395–402.

Stamm C, Anderson RH, Ho SY. Clinical anatomy of the normal pulmonary root compared with that in isolated pulmonary valvular stenosis. *J Am Coll Cardiol.* 1998;31:1420–1425.

Stanger P, Cassidy SC, Girod DA, Kan JS, Lababidi Z, Shapiro. Balloon pulmonary valvuloplasty: results of the valvuloplasty and angioplasty of congenital anomalies registry. *Am J Cardiol.* 1990;65:775–783.

Tabatabaei H, Bautin C, Nykanen DG, Freedom RM, Benson LN. Morphologic and hemodynamic consequences after percutaneous balloon valvotomy for neonatal pulmonary stenosis: medium-term follow-up. *J Am Coll Cardiol.* 1996;27:473–478.

Tanaka T, Yamaki S, Kakizawa H. Histologic study of the small pulmonary arteries in 38 patients with pulmonary atresia and intact ventricular septum. *Jpn Circ J.* 1996;60:293–299.

Tanoue Y, Kado H, Maeda T, Shiokawa Y, Fuswazaki N, Ishikawa S. Left ventricular performance of pulmonary atresia with intact ventricular septum after right heart bypass surgery. *J Thorac Cardiovasc Surg.* 2004;128:710–717.

Thapar MK, Rao PS. Significance of infundibular obstruction following balloon valvuloplasty for valvar pulmonic stenosis. *Am Heart J.* 1989;118:99–103.

Todros T, Presbitero P, Gaglioti P, Demarie D. Pulmonary stenosis with intact ventricular septum: documentation of development of the lesion echocardiographically during fetal life. *Int J Cardiol.* 1988;19:355–362.

Tomita H, Ikeda K, Iida K, Chiba S. Mild to moderate pulmonary valvular stenosis in infant sometimes improves to the condition unnecessary to do PTPV: Doppler echocardiographic observation. *Tohoku J Exp Med.* 1995;176:155–162.

Wieczorek D, Majewski F, Gillessen-Kaesbach G. Cardio-facio-cutaneous (CFC) syndrome—a distinct entity? Report of three patients demonstrating the diagnostic difficulties in delineation of CFC syndrome. *Clin Genet.* 1997;52:37–46.

Wilson W, Taubert KA, Gewitz M et al. Prevention of infective endocarditis: guidelines from the American Heart Association. *Circulation.* 2007;116:1736–1754.

Yoshimura N, Yamaguchi M, Ohashi, et al. Pulmonary atresia with intact ventricular septum: strategy based on right ventricular morphology. *J Thorac Cardiovasc Surg.* 2003;126:1417–1426.

Zuberbuhler JR, Anderson RH. Morphological variations in pulmonary atresia with intact ventricular septum. *Br Heart J.* 1979;41:281–288.

13

Nonsyndromic Conotruncal Anomalies

ELLEN DEES

H. SCOTT BALDWIN

THOMAS DOYLE

DAVID BICHELL

THOMAS P. GRAHAM

PRELIMINARY COMMENTS

This chapter details four specific conotruncal lesions under the heading "nonsyndromic" anomalies. We will focus on the clinical aspects of these defects, which are for the most part independent of the genetic etiology. However, it is important to point out that this group of anomalies is often associated with a genetic syndrome. In particular, the DiGeorge syndrome, associated most often with a large deletion within chromosome 22 (22q11) including the gene *Tbx1*, among others, often accompanies the conotruncal lesions described below. This has been shown in several large population studies (Botto et al., 2003; Goldmuntz et al., 1998; Marino et al., 2001). In a prospective study of 251 patients with conotruncal anomalies, Goldmuntz et al. reported the 22q11 deletion in 50% of patients with interrupted aortic arch (IAA), 34.5% with truncus arteriosus, and 16% with tetralogy of Fallot (TOF) (Goldmuntz et al., 1998). DiGeorge syndrome is associated with increased morbidity and mortality in patients undergoing repair of their congenital heart disease (Carotti et al., 2006), and this syndrome is described in detail in Chapter 31.

The conotruncus of the heart is embryologically complex, as reviewed in Part I of this book. This region of the heart is formed not only from the embryologic conotruncus of the primitive heart tube, but also has contributions from several other sources. These include: (1) a secondary heart field of anterior mesoderm, (2) migrating neural crest cells that arise from the branchial arches, (3) endocardial cushion cells, and (4) the developing vasculature of the heart. All of these cell populations must coordinate their arrival, proliferation, and differentiation to achieve four important tasks. First is septation of the entire conotruncus in a spiral fashion to create two great vessels, with pulmonary artery anterior and aorta posterior. Second is formation of the two semilunar valves of the heart, pulmonary and aortic. Third is to complete septation of the ventricles such that the anterior right ventricle (RV) egress is exclusively via the pulmonary artery and the posterior left ventricle is via the aorta. Finally, the main coronary arteries must "plug in" to their correct positions just superior to the aortic valve, thereby connecting the coronary circulation to its blood supply (Bernanke et al., 2002). Given the precision necessary for these functions, and the multiple cell populations involved, it follows that there are many varieties of conotruncal defects. We will discuss these major varieties below, including the current understanding of the embryologic cause, the resulting physiology and clinical presentation, the key features of diagnosis, and the medical and surgical management.

TETRALOGY OF FALLOT

Pathology

The original description of TOF dates to 1888 and consists of (1) ventricular septal defect (VSD), (2) pulmonic

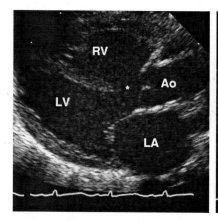 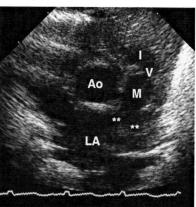

FIGURE 13-1. Echocardiogram in TOF. Left: long-axis view, showing the aorta (Ao) and chambers as labeled (LA, left atrium; LV, left ventricle; RV, hypertrophied right ventricle). The large VSD with aortic override is marked *. Right: short-axis view. The RVOT components are labeled: I, infundibulum; V, dysplastic pulmonary valve; M, main pulmonary artery; ** right and left pulmonary arteries.

stenosis (PS), (3) aortic override, and (4) right ventricular hypertrophy (RVH) (Fallot et al., 1963). The necessary details of the anatomy to merit the diagnosis have been debated since. The VSD is generally large and perimembranous, with anterior malalignment of the infundibular septum. This anterior deviation of the infundibular septum is associated with narrowing of the infundibulum of the RV, and contributes to hypoplasia of the pulmonic valve and pulmonary arteries, which can manifest with a wide range of severity. Both the overriding aorta and the RVH have been considered by some to be secondary to the VSD and PS. In fact, Van Praagh and colleagues (1970) have suggested that the entire entity of TOF stems from a single anomaly, namely, underdevelopment of the subpulmonary infundibulum. In this theory, the VSD results from failure of the crista supraventricularis to be moved posteriorly by the developing infundibulum, such that it cannot line up over the inferior portion of the ventricular septum. The aortic override is a consequence of its position to the right and anterior from normal, secondary to the underdeveloped subpulmonary infundibulum. Mitral–aortic continuity is retained, but with severe pulmonary infundibular hypoplasia. The aortic root may be rotated such that the mitral–aortic continuity may only involve the left coronary leaflet, rather than both the left and noncoronary leaflets as in the normal heart. Finally, the RVH is a postnatal physiologic consequence of the right ventricular outflow tract (RVOT) obstruction and large VSD (Van Praagh et al., 1970). This interesting way of describing TOF emphasizes that the disorder is a continuum from mild hypoplasia of the infundibulum (the so-called "pink tetralogy" patient with little RVOT obstruction) to severe ("pulmonary atresia, tetralogy type").

Tetralogy of Fallot is highly associated with several other cardiac and vascular abnormalities, not directly related to the hypoplasia of the subpulmonary infundibulum. Up to 85% of patients have an atrial septal defect. A right aortic arch is seen in 25% of patients,

sometimes with an aberrant left subclavian artery (3%) (McManus et al., 1982). There may also be an aberrant right subclavian artery from the descending aorta in patients with a left aortic arch (1%). A persistent left superior vena cava drains to the coronary sinus in 11% of patients. Increased incidence of well-developed aorticopulmonary (AP) collaterals is seen with TOF, even without pulmonary atresia, and the lungs and intrapulmonary arteries may also be generally underdeveloped (Rabinovitch et al., 1981). This has been used as an argument for early repair, to optimize chances for normalized growth of these structures (Kolcz and Pizarro, 2005). Coronary anomalies are seen in 3%–6% of patients and are important to define, as many involve a major branch crossing the RVOT and thus could be damaged at surgery (McManus et al., 1982). These include left anterior descending artery arising from the right coronary artery, single coronary origin, and large conal branches arising from the right coronary artery. The aortic valve and root are generally enlarged, and may further dilate over time. This has often been assumed to be secondary to hemodynamic stress, but several studies indicate a primary abnormality of the aorta with fragmentation of elastic fibers suggestive of primary pathology (Aru et al., 2006; Chong et al., 2006; Niwa, 2005; Tan et al., 2006).

Two variants of TOF that deserve special mention are tetralogy with absent pulmonary valve, and tetralogy in combination with complete atrioventricular septal defect (AVSD). In TOF with absent pulmonary valve, the annulus is usually severely hypoplastic with dysplastic leaflet tissue often contributing to the obstruction, while allowing pulmonary regurgitation. The main and proximal branch pulmonary arteries are dilated, sometimes massively, presumably from poststenotic dilation. The pulmonary arteries can cause significant airway obstruction that can be acutely life-threatening in the neonatal period and/or can be longstanding by causing bronchomalacia. Intubation in the delivery room with mechanical ventilation in the prone position can be lifesaving in these infants. These infants are often born without a ductus arteriosus, and if present, the ductus arteriosus may be supplying a discontinuous left pulmonary artery, a variant seen in up to 14% of cases (McCaughan et al., 1985). Tetralogy in combination with complete AV canal is not common, but occurs in 1%–2% of tetralogy patients. Here, there is also hypoplasia of the subpulmonary infundibulum, accompanied by fibrous continuity of the anterior bridging leaflet of the common AV valve with the aorta. Patients with Down syndrome more often have TOF with complete AV canal than TOF in isolation.

Physiology

The cardiac output of a patient with TOF will be normal to increased, depending on the net degree of shunt. This in turn depends on the balance between resistances to pulmonary and systemic vascular flow. Thus the physiology of TOF depends primarily on the severity of the pulmonary stenosis, and on the size of the VSD. Patients can range at presentation from ductal-dependent to asymptomatic. Pulmonary atresia or severe PS will cause ductal dependence. These infants will become profoundly cyanotic as the ductus arteriosus closes, and most of the RV output is across the VSD (right to left shunt) instead of the obstructed RVOT. The presence of AP collaterals can mitigate the cyanosis to some extent, and there is a continuum here between TOF and pulmonary atresia/VSD with multiple AP collateral arteries discussed in a following section. Restoring ductal patency with prostaglandins similarly provides an avenue of left to right shunt to maintain adequate pulmonary blood flow and oxygenation of blood. At the other end of the spectrum, a patient with a large VSD and mild pulmonary stenosis may be at first asymptomatic, with gradual development of congestive heart failure over a few weeks to months as the pulmonary vascular resistance falls and

left to right shunting predominates. Such patients are commonly referred to as "pink TOF," and are clinically similar to patients with an isolated large VSD.

It is important to carefully assess the level or levels and severity of pulmonary stenosis. RVOT obstruction is the most dynamic feature of the disease, both acutely and chronically. The pulmonary stenosis can be infundibular, valvar, supravalvar, and involving the branch pulmonary arteries. Many patients have obstruction at multiple levels, and the relative contribution of each often evolves over time. In particular, the infundibular stenosis tends to worsen as RVH progresses, but any of the components may progress. The newborn physiology of a "pink" TOF patient can thus evolve over a few months to a patient with significant RVOT obstruction and cyanosis. This progression is not due to lack of flow, as these patients have a significant left to right shunt, but rather it is likely to be an intrinsic feature of the abnormally developed infundibulum and pulmonary arteries themselves (Geva et al., 1995).

The pulmonary stenosis can also be acutely dynamic, a clinical feature that is very important to recognize. Stenoses of the pulmonic valve and of the pulmonary arteries create a static obstruction, that is, one that does not change on a minute-to-minute basis. The infundibulum, however, is a muscular structure, and thus can constitute a dynamic obstruction. This is the basis for the hypercyanotic or "Tet spells," a risk particularly for infants between 2 and 4 months of age. Part of the basis for these sudden paroxysms of cyanosis is thought to be catecholamine release in times of stress (crying, feeding) that causes spasm of the infundibulum (Kothari, 1992). The hallmark of these spells is agitation, tachypnea, and cyanosis with decreased intensity (or even absence) of the cardiac murmur. The treatment is to calm the infant and shift the balance toward higher systemic vascular resistance (knee–chest position, or in extreme cases pharmacologic alpha agonists such as Neo-Synephrine) and lower pulmonary

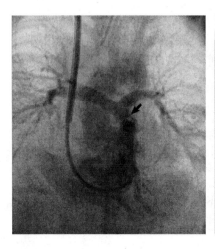 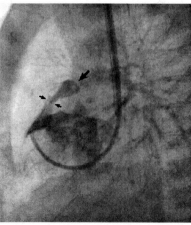

FIGURE 13-2. AP and lateral projections of a right ventriculogram in TOF, showing a thickened, doming pulmonic valve (large arrows). In the lateral projection, severe, dynamic infundibular narrowing is appreciated (opposing arrows). This patient had multiple medical problems precluding early surgical repair, and underwent successful pulmonary balloon valvuloplasty at this procedure. Note catheter pass is via the internal jugular vein because of thrombus in the inferior vena cava system.

vascular resistance (oxygen or morphine/sedatives). Increasing preload with intravascular volume administration may be very effective by acutely expanding the RV volume.

Clinical Diagnosis

Physical examination findings depend on the physiologic features reviewed above. Cyanosis may be profound or absent. Signs of cardiac output, including pulses, perfusion, and blood pressure should be normal. Precordial activity is most often normal, but an RV lift may be present as severe RVH develops. The first heart sound is normal. The second heart sound (S2) is most often single, as the pulmonary pressures are low—even subnormal—rendering the pulmonic component of S2 inaudible. The aortic component may be louder than normal because of the prominence and relatively anterior position of the aorta. If the second heart sound is normally split and is of relatively normal intensity, mild pulmonary stenosis is suggested. There is generally a systolic ejection murmur of pulmonary stenosis, which will vary in intensity and duration depending on severity. A pulmonic valve click is not usually present. Hepatomegaly is not prominent, except in cases where there is congestive heart failure from either left to right shunt in the "pink" TOF patients or advanced RV failure from severe obstruction.

The hallmark of chest x-ray is a concave pulmonary artery segment, creating an upturned appearance to the apex and a so-called boot-shaped heart. The heart is generally not significantly enlarged and pulmonary vascular markings are decreased or normal, depending on the degree of pulmonary stenosis. A right aortic arch may be detectable.

Electrocardiogram (EKG) findings reflect the degree of RVH. There is often concomitant right axis deviation.

The diagnosis may be most firmly established by echocardiography. The essential four features can be well-characterized: the VSD size and location; the degree of infundibular hypertrophy, pulmonary valve, supravalvar, and branch pulmonary artery stenosis; the degree of aortic override; and presence and severity of RVH. Assessment of alignment of the conal septum with the inferior septal rim, that is, the degree of anterior deviation of the conal septum, may help predict the potential for worsening infundibular stenosis. Mitral–aortic continuity should be present, although may be altered by rotation of the aorta rightward and anteriorly. Absence of mitral–aortic continuity and/or greater than 50% aortic override suggest a diagnosis of double-outlet RV with subaortic VSD and pulmonary stenosis, which can also be considered within a spectrum with TOF. There may be secondary VSDs in the muscular septum; these should be actively sought as their presence may complicate the surgical and postoperative management. The size of the branch pulmonary arteries should be quantitatively assessed, using the established McGoon and Nakata indices. The McGoon index is the sum of the branch pulmonary artery diameters divided by the diameter of the descending aorta measured at the diaphragm (McGoon et al., 1975; Piehler et al., 1980). In a series of 27 patients reported by this group, the average McGoon index prior to intervention was 0.65 ± 0.19, with a range of 0.3–1 (Piehler et al., 1980). The Nakata index similarly uses a ratio of the sum of the right and left branch pulmonary artery cross-sectional area to body surface area. Normal is 330 ± 30 mm^2/m^2, and severe hypoplasia is less than 150 mm^2/m^2. This index removes the variable of the descending aorta diameter, which may be smaller than normal in patients with tetralogy (Nakata et al., 1984). The aortic valve and root generally measure large and there may be aortic insufficiency, typically mild. There is usually an ASD, occasionally large with significant shunting. The aortic arch and coronary anatomy should be carefully assessed. Variants including TOF/ absent pulmonary valve or TOF/AVSD, and DORV with pulmonary stenosis should be considered.

Cardiac catheterization is not usually necessary for diagnosis in the current era, but may be indicated if there is question about the coronary anatomy, or complex anatomy of the RVOT and pulmonary arteries. Some centers advocate pulmonary balloon valvuloplasty in cases in which the infant is not a good neonatal surgery candidate, and if valvar pulmonary stenosis appears to be a significant contributor to RVOT obstruction. Wu et al. (2006) reported 22 infants in Taiwan who underwent pulmonary balloon valvuloplasty for either low oxygen saturation or repeated hypercyanotic spells. Weight at procedure ranged from 2 to 5 kg. There were no complications, almost all had improved oxygen saturations after the procedure, and 12 of the 22 were able to avoid systemic to pulmonary shunt placement (Wu et al., 2006). Stent placement in the RVOT as palliative treatment for premature neonates has been reported as a successful bridge to later complete repair (Laudito et al., 2006). Computer tomography (CT) angiography has been shown to be very accurate in delineating pulmonary artery and coronary anatomy (Dogan et al., 2007; Wang et al., 2007), as has cardiac magnetic resonance angiography (Bernardes et al., 2006; Dorfman and Geva, 2006). Each of these modalities can also be important in long-term management of TOF patients. Cardiac catheterization continues to play a definitive role in older patients following repair, for assessment and rehabilitation of stenotic branch pulmonary arteries and of residual outflow tract obstruction, and for assessment of RV volumes and function. Cardiac

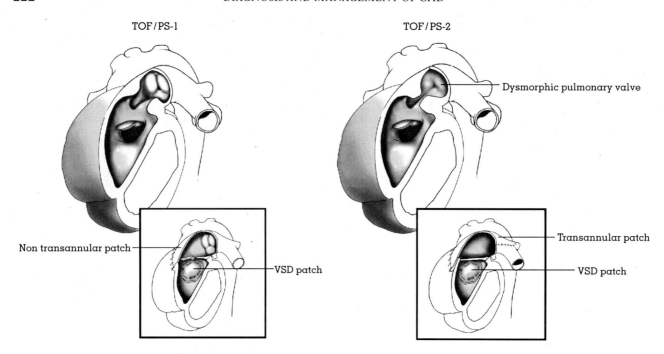

FIGURE 13–3. Anatomy and repair of tetralogy of Fallot (TOF). On the left is TOF with primarily infundibular pulmonary stenosis, managed with a valve-sparing repair depicted below. On the right, TOF with severe valvar pulmonary stenosis, repaired with a transannular patch depicted below.

magnetic resonance imaging (MRI) is also extremely helpful in assessing older patients following repair, particularly for RV volume and function assessment, and as a guide for timing of pulmonary valve replacement (see below).

Current Principles of Medical and Surgical Management

Timing of surgical correction depends on symptoms, primarily the degree of cyanosis caused by RVOT obstruction. The goals of repair are to close the VSD and completely relieve the RVOT obstruction, leaving a competent pulmonary valve if possible.

Operative mortality for TOF repair was reported as 20% in the 1950s to early 1960s (Murphy et al., 1993), 9.5% in the early 1970s (Chiariello et al., 1975), and 0%–0.8% in recent years (Giannopoulos et al., 2005; Karl et al., 1992; Lee et al., 2006). Early in the history of tetralogy repair, the optimal timing of corrective surgery was considered to be 6–10 years of age (Chiariello et al., 1975). In the current era, complete repair is performed in neonates with severe cyanosis at some centers (Derby and Pizarro, 2005; Kolcz and Pizarro, 2005), and is deferred until at least 6–12 months of age when there is milder cyanosis (Karl et al., 1992). The traditional TOF repair involves a right ventriculotomy, with patch augmentation of the infundibulum and pulmonary annulus (transannular patch), with extension

onto the pulmonary arteries as needed (Gott, 1990; Lillehei et al., 1986). This procedure was first done in 1954 at the University of Minnesota, using cross-circulation prior to the development of cardiopulmonary bypass. The transannular patch technique remains in common use. A potential improvement introduced in 1967 and still in use for some patients is the insertion of a monocusp valve in the RVOT to prevent laminar pulmonary insufficiency (Marchand, 1967). The monocusp valve can be fashioned from pericardium, cut from an aortic homograft leaving a single aortic valve leaflet in place, or are commercially available (Bigras et al., 1996). The monocusp valve has been thought to be beneficial in the short term for postoperative recovery of a stressed, volume-loaded RV. Favorable acute hemodynamics in the immediate postoperative period have been reported by some authors (Gundry et al., 1994; Revuelta et al., 1983; Anagnostopoulos et al., 2007) but not by others (Bigras et al., 1996; Sievers et al., 1983). Long-term benefits from monocusp valves have generally not been demonstrated because the monocusp valves rapidly lose competence (Bigras et al., 1996; Gundry et al., 1994; Sievers et al., 1983).

Another innovation in surgical repair of TOF is the valve-sparing repair (Karl et al., 1992; Stewart et al., 2005). This is generally done using a transatrial approach for closure of the VSD and resection of infundibular muscle bundles. Patch augmentation of the pulmonary arteries and a pulmonary valvotomy is

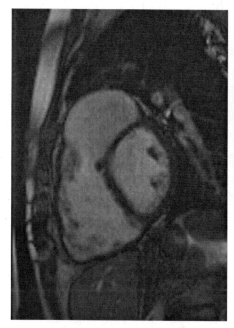
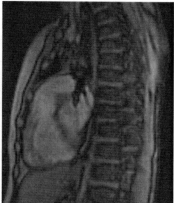
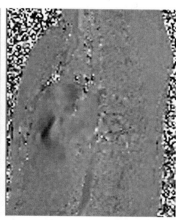

FIGURE 13–4. Cardiac MRI. Left, steady state free procession (SSFP) short-axis view shows severe RV dilation. Right two panels, velocity encoding gradient echo sequence in plane of the RVOT. The magnitude image (left, PC mag 39) shows the RVOT. The phase-image with in-plane velocity encoding (right, PC mag 40) demonstates pulmonary regurgitation (dark signal).

also often combined with this approach. Stewart et al. reviewed their results at Children's Memorial Hospital in Chicago using this approach in 2005. The authors reported 102 patients, 82 repaired as above and 20 with transannular patch. A pulmonary annulus Z-score of less than −4 indicated a need for transannular patch, with a "gray zone" Z score between −3 and −4. A postoperative RV pressure of more than 70% systemic was an indicator of eventual need for reoperation; only 6% of patients who had a valve-sparing repair compared to 10% of patients who had a transannular patch required reoperation (Stewart et al., 2005).

In patients with severe cyanosis, intervention must be performed soon after birth. This has traditionally been done by placing a palliative systemic to pulmonary artery shunt. There is evidence that this approach fosters pulmonary artery growth (Gale et al., 1979; Sabri et al., 1999). A retrospective study by Sabri et al. published in 1999 showed a 40% increase of the Nakata index when measured 6–120 days after shunting and a 60% increase when measured beyond this (Sabri et al., 1999). The authors considered the early changes to be related primarily to pulmonary artery distensibility, and the later to growth. However, there are also reports of pulmonary artery distortion and stenosis following systemic to pulmonary artery shunts that require later intervention (Gladman et al., 1997). An alternative approach favored in some centers is placement of an RV outflow patch as a palliative step to encourage branch pulmonary artery growth, without closing the VSD. Seipelt reported this approach in 15 infants with severe branch pulmonary stenosis. There was significant early morbidity from congestive

heart failure, although oxygen saturations increased significantly, and branch pulmonary artery growth was demonstrated angiographically. Subsequent complete repair was performed (Seipelt et al., 2002). This approach has the disadvantage of requiring cardiopulmonary bypass and hypothermic arrest for both the palliation and the subsequent repair.

Increasingly, centers are reporting good success performing the primary complete repair in early infancy. Kolcz and Pizarro reported 46 neonatal TOF repairs performed at a median age of 5 days between 1998 and 2004. These patients were compared to 20 nonneonatal patients ranging in age from 1 to 5 months. All repairs were done with cardiopulmonary bypass and deep hypothermic arrest using a right ventriculotomy, most (88%) with a transannular patch extending into the left pulmonary artery. There were three early deaths, and no late deaths; two of the three neonates who died had significant other congenital malformations. Improvement in the Nakata index was statistically significant at follow-up only for the neonatal group. There was no difference in the need for reintervention. The neonatal group had a higher incidence of left pulmonary artery stenosis; this was treated by balloon dilation in the cardiac catheterization laboratory. The authors conclude that elective neonatal repair has excellent results in the absence of other congenital anomalies (Kolcz and Pizarro, 2005). The long-term complication rates of this approach remain to be determined (Derby and Pizarro, 2005; Kolcz and Pizarro, 2005). Some centers continue to advocate systemic to pulmonary shunt in symptomatic neonates to avoid placement of a transannular patch (Stewart et al., 2005).

Long-Term Outcome

Most patients with TOF do very well in long-term follow-up analyses. Lillehei et al. (1986) from the University of Minnesota published 30-year follow-up results for patients repaired in or before 1960. There were 106 patients who underwent surgery between 4 months and 45 years of age and survived to hospital discharge. Actuarial survival in these patients was 77% over 30 years, and freedom from reoperation was 91%. Patients were described to have led full and productive lives, little encumbered by their cardiac surgery history (Lillehei et al., 1986). A similar study from Mayo Clinic was published in 1993, reporting 30-year follow-up data on 163 hospital survivors repaired between 1955 and 1960. Thirty-year actuarial survival overall was 86%; in a subgroup repaired at an age older than 12 years, survival was considerably lower at 76% (Murphy et al., 1993). More recent era follow-up data suggests 3–4-year survival of 97.5%–100% (Giannopoulos et al., 2005; Karl et al., 1992), with freedom from early reoperation of approximately 93% (Kirklin et al., 1989; Stewart et al., 2005).

In the future, freedom from long-term reoperation, however, will be significantly less than the Minnesota experience. This is as a result of numerous studies reporting the detrimental effects on RV function of long-standing pulmonary insufficiency and the resultant chronic volume overload (Chowdhury et al., 2006; del Nido, 2006; Giardini et al., 2006; Grothoff et al., 2006; Knauth et al., 2006; Laudito et al., 2006; Menteer et al., 2005; Oosterhof, 2006; Redington, 2006). Any residual RVOT obstruction will compound this by increasing the afterload faced by the RV, affecting both systolic and diastolic performance (Helbing et al., 1996; Redington, 2006). Cardiac MRI has proven to be an effective modality to demonstrate such changes in the RV, in particular using delayed enhancement techniques to demonstrate fibrosis (Babu-Narayan et al., 2006; Oosterhof et al., 2005, 2006). Diastolic dysfunction per se appears to predispose to arrythmias, as does significant RV dilation and evidence of fibrosis (Cheung et al., 2005; Grothoff et al., 2006; Karamlou et al., 2006; Redington, 2006). Because of these findings, patients with evidence of RV dilation and dysfunction and/or arrhythmias are now undergoing pulmonary valve replacement, most often in teenage years or early adulthood. Precise indications for this vary from study to study, but include progressive RV dilation with exercise intolerance and/or ventricular tachycardia (Bove et al., 1985; Kleinveld et al., 2006; Therrien et al., 2005; Yemets et al., 1997). Therrien et al. showed a decrease in RV end-diastolic volume in patients who underwent pulmonary valve replacement from a mean of 163 mL/m² preoperatively to 107 mL/m² postoperatively, as assessed by cardiac MRI. Importantly, patients with an RV end-diastolic volume in excess of 170 mL/m² failed to normalize RV volume postoperatively. It was recommended based on this finding that pulmonary valve replacement be performed prior to dilation of the RV to 170 mL/m², regardless of symptoms (Therrien et al., 2005). In addition, Davlouros et al. suggest in a 2004 review that pulmonary valve replacement also be performed in patients with documented symptoms of exercise intolerance, those undergoing surgery for other hemodynamically significant lesions (e.g., residual shunts), and patients who have significant arrythmias. In the latter case, cryoablation may be part of the procedure (Davlouros et al., 2004). There is good evidence that postvalve replacement patients demonstrate sustained improvement in RV volumes and function (Bove et al., 1985; Kleinveld et al., 2006; Therrien et al., 2005), in exercise tolerance (Bove et al., 1985; Kleinveld et al., 2006; Yemets et al., 1997), and may have less progressive QRS prolongation (Kleinveld et al., 2006).

PULMONARY ATRESIA WITH VENTRICULAR SEPTAL DEFECT

Pathology

In pulmonary atresia with VSD (PAVSD), there is no direct communication between the RV and the pulmonary circulation. All pulmonary blood flow is derived from the systemic circulation, via either a ductus arteriosus and/or AP collateral vessels. Such vessels develop from the bronchial arterial plexus (Norgaard et al., 2006) and other AP artery connections that normally remain underdeveloped. These arise most commonly from the descending thoracic aorta or subclavian arteries (Norgaard et al., 2006), or rarely from the abdominal aorta or even coronary arteries (Amin et al., 2000). If a ductus arteriosus is present, it is often to one lung or one lung segment, with the remaining segments supplied by collaterals. The main pulmonary arteries are almost always present, and may range in size from near normal to extremely hypoplastic (1 mm or less). The caliber of the central pulmonary arteries is directly related to blood flow, and inversely related to the number and size of alternate sources of pulmonary blood flow. In general, the more distally the collateral vessels insert into the pulmonary circulation, the more hypoplastic the central pulmonary arteries become. The atresia probably occurs very early in development, likely just after septation of the conotruncus and before ventricular septation. This is distinct from pulmonary atresia with intact septum, in which the pulmonary arteries are generally well developed, likely occurring much

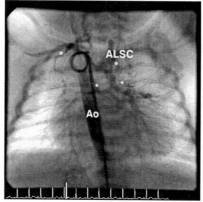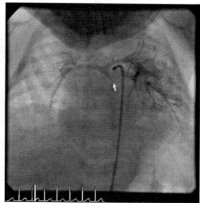

FIGURE 13-5. Aortogram (left) and selective descending aorta collateral injection (right) in two patients with PA/VSD and multiple AP collateral vessels. In the aortogram, the pigtail catheter is positioned in the transverse arch; note there is a right aortic arch. Contrast fills the aberrant left subclavian artery (ALSC), which gives rise to several collateral vessels (*) and to the true pulmonary arteries (not well seen in this frame). The selective descending aorta collateral injection reveals the patient's true main pulmonary artery (arrow) and branches.

later in gestation (Kutsche and Van Mierop, 1983). PAVSD was once considered to be a variant of truncus arteriosus (so called type IV truncus, or pseudotruncus), but this designation is not accurate embryologically (Bharati et al., 1975). The left ventricular outflow is a true aorta, not a common trunk, and the pulmonary arteries do not originate directly from the aorta, but from collateral arteries as described above. It is more accurate to consider pulmonary artresia with VSD to be at the extreme end of a spectrum of TOF. The VSD is in the perimembranous septum, and there is aortic override with dilation of the aorta. The RV is hypertrophied. The infundibulum ends blindly and may have a normal shape and length, or may be significantly shortened. Associated abnormalities are similar to those associated with TOF and include the right aortic arch (26%–50%) sometimes with an aberrant left subclavian artery, aberrant right subclavian artery with left arch, an atrial septal defect, a persistent left superior vena cava, and occasional coronary anomalies. Usually there is enlargement of the conal branch of the right coronary artery because of RVH, even when coronary anatomy is normal.

Physiology

Some patients can be identified prenatally by fetal echocardiography with high accuracy (90%) (Vesel et al., 2006). Most are not suspected prenatally and manifest soon after birth with severe cyanosis. A few patients have well enough developed collateral circulation to be minimally cyanotic for months after birth. Some of these infants are diagnosed because they begin to develop congestive heart failure, and others because of prominent continuous murmurs heard on routine examination. Eventually, virtually all patients will become cyanotic as they outgrow their relatively fixed pulmonary blood supply. Further, the natural history of AP collateral arteries is to acquire stenoses and to involute over time, particularly if there are many

collateral vessels to divide the blood volume. Likewise, a patent ductus arteriosus may close over time, leading to severe cyanosis. Infants with PAVSD have normal to increased systemic cardiac output, with normal pulses and blood pressure. There may be a wide pulse pressure in patients with large collateral arteries and high pulmonary blood flow, from the diastolic "run-off." Some patients who have sufficient pulmonary blood flow to survive unoperated for many years, although they tend to be very symptomatic by the second or third decade of their life. Belli et al. reported 27 patients undergoing late surgery for PAVSD, at a median age of 20 years (15–43 years). Eight of these were undergoing their very first surgery; the rest had had at least one palliative shunt (Belli et al., 2007).

Clinical Diagnosis

On physical examination, most infants will have cyanosis, an increased RV impulse, and continuous murmurs heard over the precordium and back. The murmurs may be subtle or absent in newborns, and become increasingly prominent as pulmonary vascular resistance falls. The second heart sound is single because there is no pulmonic closure. On chest x-ray, the heart is generally not enlarged and has the concave pulmonary artery segment and upturned apex, or boot-shaped heart, as seen in TOF. The pulmonary blood flow pattern is abnormal, with absence of the normal arborization of pulmonary arteries, and a more heterogeneous distribution. The EKG is similar to that in TOF, with right axis deviation and RVH. Echocardiography usually establishes the diagnosis accurately, particularly the intracardiac anatomy. The most common misdiagnoses come from confusion between PAVSD and truncus arteriosus, both prenatally (Volpe et al., 2003) and postnatally. In PAVSD, there will be some development of the RVOT, whereas this is absent in truncus arteriosus. The origin of the central pulmonary arteries from the ascending aorta should be identifiable in patients with truncus arteriosus, as may be the abnormalities of the truncal valve (Vargas Barron et al., 1983). Delineation of the entire pulmonary blood supply is not always possible by echocardiography. Acherman et al. reported echo findings in 42 consecutive patients diagnosed with PAVSD. In all patients, the presence or absence and site collateral vessel origin were correctly identified, and the correct number of collateral vessels was identified in two-thirds of patients. Careful color-flow mapping, with attention to retrograde flow in the pulmonary arteries signaling entry of a collateral vessel, was important in identifying these vessels. However, a small central pulmonary artery was missed in at least one patient (Acherman et al., 1996). For this reason, most infants diagnosed with this condition still undergo cardiac catheterization with an aortogram and selective injections into collateral arteries to determine their segmental distribution within the lung. It is also important to identify which segments of lung have a single blood supply, and which have dual or multiple sources. It is important to determine the distance between the RV infundibulum and the central pulmonary arteries, as this can vary from near continuity to separation of a centimeter or more and dictates the type of RVOT reconstruction. CT angiography (Greil et al., 2006; Murai et al., 2004) and cardiac MRI (Bernardes et al., 2006) are proving fully as accurate as cardiac catheterization and angiography in identifying pulmonary blood supply in patients with PAVSD. In an MRI study, Bernardes et al. found 25 collateral vessels in 15 patients with pulmonary atresia, whereas only 21 were identified angiographically (Bernardes et al., 2006).

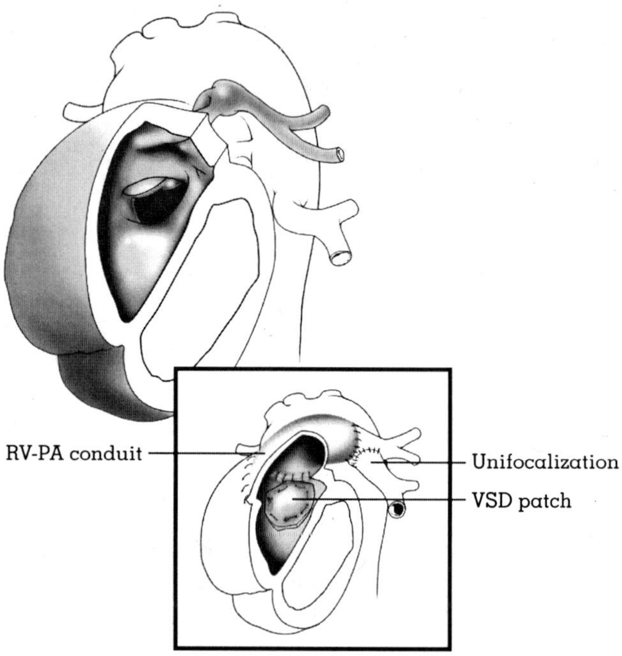

Current Principles of Medical and Surgical Management

In patients with good-sized central pulmonary arteries and minimal separation between the RV and central pulmonary arteries, neonatal surgical approaches and considerations are essential as discussed above for TOF. Decisions for primary neonatal repair versus AP shunting and delayed repair depend on whether the central pulmonary arteries are sufficient to support full pulmonary flow, on the presence of other complicating factors such as prematurity or extracardiac anomalies, and on surgeon/institution preferences (Pagani et al., 1995; Reddy et al., 1995; Yagihara et al., 1996). Unlike patients with TOF, patients with PAVSD and multiple collateral vessels as primary pulmonary blood flow often require a multistage surgical approach. The goals of this multistage approach are to (1) promote growth of the true pulmonary arteries, (2) incorporate as much as possible of the pulmonary blood flow into the true pulmonary arteries, or at least into a central arterial confluence, (3) establish continuity of the pulmonary

TOF/PA/MAPCAS

RV-PA conduit — Unifocalization — VSD patch

FIGURE 13–6. Pulmonary atresia/VSD and multiple AP collateral vessels. Anatomy depicted above, large perimembranous VSD with aortic override, main pulmonary artery arising from PDA, and large collateral artery from descending aorta. Repair depicted below, with VSD patch closure, conduit joining RV to central pulmonary artery, and unifocalization of the descending aorta collateral to the central pulmonary artery.

arteries with the RV, and (4) close the VSD with a RV pressure as low as possible (Metras et al., 2001).

Growth of the pulmonary arteries has often been promoted with systemic to pulmonary artery shunts, sometimes bilaterally (Sabri et al., 1999). This approach has been noted to have significant limitations in the degree of pulmonary artery growth actually achieved (Cotrufo et al., 1989). Further, it has been argued that establishing continuity between the RV and the central pulmonary artery by age 3 months is critical to long-term success. Antegrade pulmonary flow is thought to promote better growth of the central pulmonary arteries and their proximal branches, improve oxygenation, and provide access for cardiac catheter-based intervention in the branch pulmonary arteries. This can be accomplished by placing a conduit, or by direct aorta to pulmonary artery anastomosis. The latter is favored for pulmonary arteries less than 1.5 mm in diameter (Pagani et al., 1995).

The conventional approach to multiple collateral vessels is known as unifocalization, referring to a surgical anastomosis of two or more vessels into a confluence. Optimally, this confluence is the true pulmonary artery, but in patients with no true central pulmonary artery, a

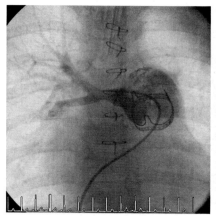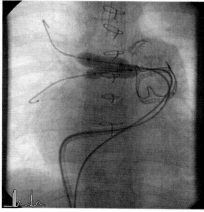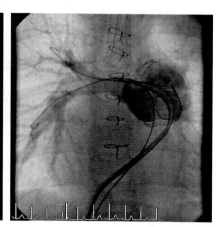

FIGURE 13-7. Right pulmonary artery rehabilitation in the cardiac catheterization lab. Note this patient has already had pulmonary valve replacement. Here, balloon angioplasty is used for a discrete right pulmonary artery stenosis occurring just proximal to a bifurcation of the vessel. Balloons placed into each branch are simultaneously inflated for even pressure, avoiding distortion of the branches.

central confluence may be created from xenograft material, such as pericardium or vein segments (Yagihara et al., 1996). The unifocalization can involve side-to-side or oblique end-to-side anastomosis between two collateral vessels, or between a collateral vessel and a pulmonary artery. Patch augmentation of stenotic segments is often required. Ligation of collaterals with dual connections to the aorta and pulmonary artery may also be indicated, such that the aortic connection is lost and continuity with the pulmonary artery is maintained (Yagihara et al., 1996). The goal is to achieve as normal pulmonary arborization as possible. As this requires working posteriorly in the chest, sometimes a significant distance peripheral to the hilum, unifocalization is often performed via a lateral thoracotomy (Pagani et al., 1995; Reddy et al., 1995; Yagihara et al., 1996). Often repeat procedures are required, on both sides, before all vessels are brought into continuity. However, some recent success with single-stage repair via a median sternotomy, including extensive unifocalization, has been reported in infants with severely hypoplastic branch pulmonary arteries (Lofland, 2000; Reddy et al., 1997; Tireli et al., 2002). Acute mortality ranged from 0% to 10%. Lofland noted the importance of normothermic bypass during the dissection portion of the procedure, both for ease of dissection and to prevent hypoxemia. Reddy and Tireli pointed out the difficulty in knowing when to close the VSD as part of the procedure, given the radical changes in hemodynamics resulting from the procedure. Leaving the VSD open was associated with severe congestive heart failure secondary to excessive pulmonary blood flow; closing it inappropriately was associated with hypertension and failure of the RV (Reddy et al., 1995; Tireli et al., 2002). In cases where the pulmonary arteries are borderline, an intraoperative pump flow study was advocated. This consisted of

measuring the mean pulmonary pressure during simulated full pulmonary flow, while venting the left atrium. A mean pulmonary pressure of less than 24 mmHg during flow of 2.5 mL/min/m^2 was found to be predictive of successful VSD closure (Carotti et al., 2006; Reddy et al., 1997).

Complications of unifocalization are bleeding, which may be difficult to control, phrenic nerve palsy, and bronchospasm (Reddy et al., 1995; Schulze-Neick et al., 2000; Tireli et al., 2002). An important and probably under recognized complication of unifocalization is necrosis of focal areas of the bronchi or trachea from compromised blood supply. Schulze-Neick et al. recently reported severe bronchospasm after unifocalization in 3 of 16 patients. Bronchoscopy revealed areas of focal necrosis in the airways. Autopsy in one of the three patients demonstrated a significant peribronchial blood supply arising from the unifocalized collateral; a separate autopsy series confirmed such connections in 7/14 patients with PAVSD (Schulze-Neick et al., 2000).

Cardiac catheterization is an essential part of an integrated approach to patients with PAVSD. In a large series from Birmingham, AL, DeGiovanni et al. reported an average of 2.3 catheterization procedures prior to complete repair in 164 patients (De Giovanni, 2004). Stenosis of the branch pulmonary arteries can be aggressively balloon dilated or stented (Carotti et al., 2003; Brown et al., 1998; El-Said et al., 2000), especially once RV to pulmonary artery continuity is established. Brown et al. (1998) reported this to be successful in 83% of vessels in which it was attempted, with infrequent complications including vasospasm and aneurism/dissection. In future procedures, the vessels can be dilated repeatedly, either with or without stenting (De Giovanni, 2004). Collaterals can also be coil occluded or device occluded when this is determined by angiography to be appropriate (Tissot et al., 2007). Given that many patients with PAVSD will require multiple operations, both for conduit replacements, and not for unifocalization procedures, the ability to rehabilitate pulmonary arteries in the cardiac catheterization laboratory is critical in the care of these patients. These are technically challenging procedures, but can allow incorporation of vessels too distal for surgical intervention. In this way, surgery and cardiac catheterization are complementary and allow for an aggressive, proactive approach to this difficult disease (De Giovanni, 2004).

The distance between the infundibulum of the RV and the pulmonary arteries in patients with PAVSD most often necessitates placement of a conduit to connect the two. This is an important distinction from TOF, in which a transannular patch type repair uses native tissue that will grow with the patient. All conduits must be periodically replaced, due to patient growth in childhood, and for acquired calcification and stenosis in adulthood. There is an extensive literature on advantages and disadvantages of various types of conduits over the past 30 years (Brown et al., 2006; Chiappini et al., 2007; Corno et al., 1988; Crupi et al., 1978; Lecompte et al., 1982; Molina, 1986; Perron et al., 1999; Shebani et al., 2006; Turrentine et al., 2002; Willems et al., 1996; Yankah et al., 1984). In the 1970s–1980s, tube grafts made of Dacron (Corno et al., 1988; Crupi et al., 1978) or Gore-Tex (Molina, 1986) were used to reconstruct the RVOT. These had the problem of pseudointimal formation and stenosis, and laminar insufficiency. The addition of a valve, either bioprosthetic (Corno et al., 1988), xenograft (Yankah et al., 1984), or homograft (Lofland, 2000; Perron et al., 1999; Willems et al., 1996), was the next step and improved hemodynamics were reported. By the mid-1980s, homografts were the preferred method in most institutions (Brown et al., 2006). Still, these have the problem of high expense and low availability, and acquired calcification and stenosis. In a review by Perron et al. of homograft containing conduits placed in infants less than 3 months of age, the median time to replacement was 3.1 years (Perron et al., 1999). This is as good or better than palliative procedures such as AP shunts; homograft survival is still significantly shorter in PAVSD patients than in pulmonary autograft patients (Brown et al., 2006; Willems et al., 1996). Finally, Willems et al. noted in their series that pulmonary homografts had superior structural durability than aortic, and that younger age of the homograft donor may adversely affect durability (Willems et al., 1996).

In the last few years, several reports have been published using "Contegra" conduits (Medtronic,

Minneapolis, MN) made from bovine jugular vein segments including a venous valve (Barbero-Marcial et al., 1995; Brown et al., 2006; Chiappini et al., 2007; Shebani et al., 2006). The advantages of this approach include lower cost and higher availability, wide range of sizes, and sufficient length proximal to the valve to allow flexibility in shaping of the infundibular anastomosis without additional materials. In 2006, Brown et al. reported using these in 62 patients ranging from 2 weeks to 18 years of age, in sizes of 12–22 mm. Only one had required complete revision; seven others had required intervention for acquired stenosis of the distal anastomosis (6 via balloon angioplasty and 1 surgical). Time of reintervention ranged from 3 to 27 months. These short-term results were judged to be as good or better than with homografts (Brown et al., 2006). Similarly, Shebani reported a series of 62 patients, ages less than 1 month to 20 years, with follow-up of 0–38 months (median 14 months). Four patients required explantation during the follow-up period, for endocarditis (one patient) or progressive dilation (three patient), and 16 patients required interventional catheterization, again mostly for stenosis at the distal anastomosis. Smaller conduits and high postoperative RV pressure were predictive of conduit failure. The conduits removed for dilation showed pathologic changes of neointimal proliferation, calcification, thrombus, and chronic inflammation (Shebani et al., 2006). Longer-term follow-up is needed to fully assess the use of these conduits in this challenging patient population (Barbero-Marcial et al., 1995; Brown et al., 2006; Shebani et al., 2006).

Long-Term Outcomes

Long-term outcomes in patients with PAVSD and diminutive pulmonary arteries are improving. In 1978, Crupi et al. referred to these patients as "hopeless" in their report of successful palliation with a Dacron conduit without VSD closure (Crupi et al., 1978). Dinarevic et al. published results from the Royal Brompton National Heart and Lung Hospital in London with 54 patients referred in the first year of life with PAVSD (56% with ductal supply to continuous pulmonary arteries and 44% with collaterals only) between 1972 and 1992. During the first decade, corrective surgery was attempted in less than 10% of patients with 42% mortality. During the second decade, corrective surgery was performed in 39% of patients with 26% mortality. Differences were attributed to increasing availability of prostaglandins, the use of selective angiography to delineate the pulmonary arteries, and advances in surgical approaches including unifocalization (Dinarevic et al., 1995). Reddy et al. published results from 1992 to 2000 at the University of California, San Francisco, with 85 patients. Fifty-six underwent single-stage complete repair, and the rest had staged repair. There were no early deaths but seven late deaths; 24 patients required reintervention on the neopulmonary arteries. The actuarial 3-year survival was 80% (Reddy et al., 2000). The authors point out room for improvement, especially given the natural history of survival of approximately 50% in unoperated patients at 2 years of age (Belli et al., 2007; Reddy et al., 1997). The unoperated survival is associated with significant morbidity, however, which is improved with intervention (Belli et al., 2007; Leonard et al., 2000).

TRUNCUS ARTERIOSUS COMMUNIS

Pathology

In truncus arteriosus, a single artery arises from the base of the heart and gives rise directly to the coronary circulation and to the pulmonary arteries. Embryologically this is due to failure of septation of the arterial trunk and of the conal septum. This leaves a single great artery with a single (truncal) valve overriding a VSD that is typically large. In a chick embryo model, ablation of the neural crest causes persistent truncus arteriosus (Besson et al., 1986; Leatherbury et al., 1991, 1993; Nishibatake et al., 1987), and there is a significant association with the DiGeorge 22q11 deletion in humans, as discussed in the introduction. More recently, several specific gene defects, many involved in neural crest signaling and cell survival, have been associated with this lesion. These include Alk5, a TGFβ type 1 receptor important in neural crest cell survival (Wang et al., 2006); Sox4, a transcription factor important for conotruncal septation and semilunar valve formation (Ya et al., 1998); Fgf8, a growth factor with dose-dependent effects in the developing conotruncus (Hutson et al., 2006); and retinaldehyhde dehydrogenase 2, an enzyme critical for retinoic acid synthesis in the developing heart (Niederreither et al., 2001; Vermot et al., 2003, 2006).

The Collett and Edwards classification system of truncus Arteriosus devised in 1949 (Collett and Edwards, 1949) remains the most widely used, and is based on the pulmonary artery configuration. In Collett and Edwards type I truncus, there is a short pulmonary truck arising from the aorta, which gives rise to both left and right pulmonary arteries. In type II, the branch pulmonary arteries arise separately from the truncus, but the origins are close together. There is a spectrum between types I and II such that it may be difficult to discern if there are one or two true origins. In type III truncus, the pulmonary arteries arise separately from opposite aspects of the common trunk. What was originally termed type IV truncus is actually

PAVSD with multiple collateral vessels, and should be described as such, rather than as "pseudotruncus." There are some rare variants that this system does not address. Van Praagh and Van Praagh proposed an alternate nomenclature, with Type A designating the presence of a VSD, and type B an intact ventricular septum (extremely rare). Further delineations included A or B type 1, common pulmonary trunk giving rise to left and right pulmonary arteries; type 2, separate pulmonary left and right artery origins; type 3, absence of one branch pulmonary artery with AP collateral supply to that lung; and type 4, truncus arteriosus associated with interruption, coarctation, or hypoplasia of the aortic arch (Van Praagh, and Van Praagh, 1965). Van Praagh type A3 truncus is also commonly called hemitruncus, and constituted 11% in a Mayo clinic series (Fyfe et al., 1985). Arch anomalies are most commonly right aortic arch (up to 35%) or IAA (11%–19%). The latter presents special surgical challenges, which are discussed below. The truncal valve also shows significant heterogeneity, which can likewise present surgical challenges. Most truncal valves are trileaflet, but they can be quadricuspid (22%) or bicuspid (9%) (Crupi et al., 1977). Dysplasia and size discrepancy of the valve cusps may be present and cause either stenosis, insufficiency, or both. The ductus arteriosus is absent in at least 50% of patients. There may be coronary artery anomalies (Chaudhari et al., 2006), including single coronary origin, both ostia arising from the same sinus, and high ostial origin. These coronary abnormalities may have the same implications as in TOF, because of the necessity of performing a right ventriculotomy to place a conduit from the RV to the pulmonary artery confluence.

Physiology

Infants with truncus arteriosus are usually diagnosed soon after birth. Symptoms depend on pulmonary flow, on competence of the truncal valve, and on associated anomalies. Pulmonary flow may be markedly increased once pulmonary vascular resistance falls, leading to early congestive heart failure. Alternately, if the pulmonary flow relatively balanced, either from pulmonary artery stenosis or persistent pulmonary hypertension, patients may be relatively asymptomatic. A competent truncal valve may result in normal systemic cardiac output, although the excess runoff to the pulmonary circulation may compromise systemic perfusion. This runoff may also impair diastolic coronary blood flow, resulting in ischemia and/or sudden death. Severe truncal stenosis results in low systemic cardiac output, which can lead to ventricular failure and shock. Severe truncal insufficiency also compromises systemic cardiac output, leading to severe ventricular dilation

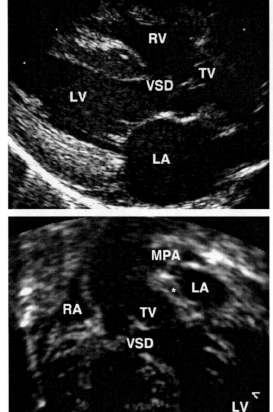

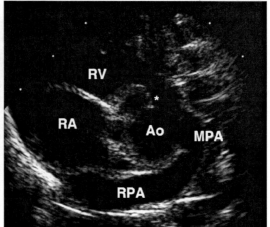

FIGURE 13–8. Echocardiographic views of truncus arteriosus. Top left, long-axis view of VSD with overriding truncal valve. Note chamber enlargement from congestive heart failure. Top right, short-axis view above the truncal valve. A truncal valve leaflet is just in the plane (*) and the pulmonary artery is seen arising from the proximal ascending aorta. The left pulmonary artery is out of plane. Below, subcostal coronal view in a different patient. The truncal valve overrides the VSD and the pulmonary artery arises from the aorta just above the origin of the left main coronary artery; the distal left coronary is labeled (*). LA, left atrium; LV, left ventricle; RA, right atrium; RV, right ventricle; VSD, ventricular septal defect; TV, truncal valve; Ao, aorta; MPA, main pulmonary artery; RPA, right pulmonary artery.

and failure, and is associated with sudden death prior to repair (McElhinney et al., 1998). Patients with truncus arteriosus and associated IAA are dependent on the ductus arteriosus for systemic output and will rapidly develop shock if the ductus closes. Such patients are prostaglandin-dependent until surgical repair. On the other hand, the ductus is often absent in patients with isolated truncus arteriosus, and prostaglandins may exacerbate congestive heart failure by causing pulmonary vasodilation. Patients with truncus arteriosus usually have only minimal cyanosis, as the pulmonary to systemic flow ratio (Q_p/Q_s) is sufficiently high that the arterial saturation is greater than 90%. Preferential streaming, of deoxygenated blood from the RV to the pulmonary arteries and of oxygenated blood from the left ventricle to the aorta, often occurs, improving systemic oxygen saturation as well.

Clinical Diagnosis

Physical examination findings in patients with truncus arteriosus also depends on the truncal valve morphology and competence, and on the pulmonary blood flow. S1 is normal, and S2 single. An ejection click is often heard with truncal valves, especially if they have abnormal cusp morphology or number. A systolic ejection murmur is usually heard as well, and more pronounced in the presence of truncal stenosis. A high pitched diastolic murmur along the left sternal border and bounding pulses are indicative of significant truncal insufficiency. Otherwise, pulses tend to be normal, reflecting normal systemic cardiac output. Severe cyanosis is a sign of significant pulmonary artery stenosis, and is not usually present; milder cyanosis may be present with net right to left shunting from persistent pulmonary hypertension. Patients with high pulmonary blood flow will have near-normal saturation and develop congestive heart failure. Signs of congestive heart failure, including tachypnea and hepatomegaly, occur after the pulmonary vascular resistance falls. EKG shows a normal to rightward axis, and evidence of left ventricular hypertrophy or often biventricular hypertrophy. Conduction times are generally normal, with sinus rhythm. Chest x-ray generally shows cardiomegaly with increased pulmonary vascular markings. If there is pulmonary artery stenosis, there may instead be decreased pulmonary markings. In hemitruncus, there will be asymmetry of pulmonary blood flow, markedly diminished on the side with the absent pulmonary artery. A right arch may be detected, as may the abnormally high takeoff of the left pulmonary artery. Echocardiography generally reveals all of the necessary details of the anatomy, and care must be taken to distinguish truncus arteriosus from PAVSD or severe TOF, and from AP window. The VSD of truncus arteriosus, PA/VSD, and tetralogy is of the same morphologic type; the distinguishing feature is the pulmonary artery origin (Vargas et al., 1983. This may be difficult to determine at first glance. A high short-axis view, well above the semilunar valve, is helpful in locating the pulmonary origin or origins, as are subcostal sweeps. Distinguishing these entities on the basis of the semilunar valve morphology can be misleading. The aortic annulus is dilated in TOF and PAVSD, and may be stenotic or insufficient in rare cases thus resembling a truncal valve. AP window can be distinguished from truncus arteriosus by the absence of a VSD (almost always) and by the presence of a normal pulmonary artery, with dropout of the AP septum superior to the pulmonic valve. Cardiac catheterization is not often necessary in patients with truncus arteriosus, unless there the anatomy is not clear from echocardiography, for example, in cases of hemitruncus where a branch pulmonary artery is absent and there is collateral flow to that lung.

Fetal echocardiography can be successful in correctly diagnosing truncus arteriosus (Duke et al., 2001; Volpe et al., 2003), and there is at least one case report that fetal MRI may yield better definition of the pulmonary artery anatomy (Muhler et al., 2004). In a multicenter series, Volpe et al. reported 23 of 24 diagnoses of truncus arteriosus to be correct; the patient misdiagnosed as truncus arteriosus had PAVS. Overall survival was 34.8% (Volpe et al., 2003). Duke et al. reported 14 of 16 firm diagnoses of truncus arteriosus to be correct. Truncal stenosis was reliably identified by Doppler velocities. There was a relatively high prenatal mortality, both spontaneous and elective abortions, with additional pre and postoperative deaths for an overall survival in prenatally diagnosed patients of only 29% (42% in patients with intent to treat) (Duke et al., 2001).

Current Principles of Medical and Surgical Management

The first successful surgical repair of truncus arteriosus was performed by McGoon and others in 1967, using an aortic homograft to connect the RV to the pulmonary artery. Repair consists of closure of the VSD such that the left ventricle ejects to the truncal valve, transection of the pulmonary arteries at their origin with patch closure of the ascending aorta, and establishment of continuity between the RV and the pulmonary arteries. Use of a homograft is generally still the method of choice for the latter, although xenografts and patch-augmented direct anastomosis have also been used. Danton et al. reported that direct anastomosis of the pulmonary artery confluence to the RV with anterior patch placement, either simple or with a monocusp valve, had similar short- and long-term outcomes to homografts, and improved freedom from reoperation over xenografts (Danton et al., 2001). As a novel alternative to extensive patching, an alternate technique recently reported is transaction of a ring of aorta containing the pulmonary artery origins. The aorta is then reconnected end-to-end, and the pulmonary artery–containing segment is used as the neo-main pulmonary artery (Kaczmarek et al., 2006). This is particularly useful for Collett and Edwards type III truncus, in which the pulmonary arteries arise from opposite sides of the aorta, but is reported by the authors to be useful in all subtypes (Kaczmarek et al., 2006). The truncal valve can present a significant surgical challenge, and may require commisurotomy, valve repair, or even replacement when severely insufficient (Bove et al., 1993; Elzein et al., 2005; McElhinney et al., 1998). Valve repair can be accomplished by stabilizing the valve leaflet with sutures, although Mavroudis and Backer report better results excising a prolapsing valve leaflet and performing annuloplasty to bring the remaining cusps together (Mavroudis and Backer, 2001). More than moderate insufficiency is associated with a high incidence of eventual replacement (McElhinney et al., 1998; Imamura et al., 1999). Truncal valve replacements in neonates are done either with homografts or mechanical valves (Bove et al., 1993; McElhinney et al., 1998), with poor survival (McElhinney et al., 1998).

Finally, truncus arteriosus with IAA is a particular challenge, as it combines several time-consuming and extensive repairs. The largest series of these patients is a Congenital Heart Surgeon's Society study reported by Konstantinov et al. This multi-institution study of 50 infants with truncus arteriosus and IAA repaired between 1987 and 1997 reported 47% mortality in 38 patients who underwent complete repair, and 86% mortality in staged repair (usually arch reconstruction with subsequent truncal repair and VSD closure). Most of the deaths were from low-output cardiac failure, related possibly to coronary insufficiency (Konstantinov et al., 2006). A trend toward improved results in more recent years, and toward better results in certain centers was noted. More recent but smaller

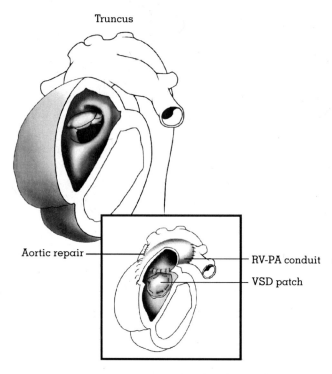

FIGURE 13–9. Truncus arterosus and repair. Above is the anatomy, with the main pulmonary artery arising from the ascending aorta and a perimembranous VSD. Below is the repair, with VSD patch and RV to PA conduit. The aorta is repaired where the pulmonary artery or arteries are detached.

single institution results reported by Tlaskal et al. and by Jahangiri et al. reported more favorable outcomes, with seven of eight (87%) and nine of nine (100%) survivors, respectively. Neither series reported reinterventions for the aortic arch, but there were numerous reinterventions for conduit revisions at less than 3 years (Jahangiri et al., 2000; Tlaskal et al., 2005). The Tlaskal series reported other reinterventions for branch pulmonary artery stenoses and truncal valve insufficiency. These patients thus remain a significant challenge. For selected patients with particularly unfavorable anatomy, cardiac transplantation has been pursued instead of repair (Akintuerk et al., 2006; Konstantinov et al., 2006).

Age of repair of truncus arteriosis has steadily declined since the first intervention attempts. An early approach was to perform a palliative procedure such as pulmonary artery banding in infancy, to protect from pulmonary vascular disease, deferring complete repair until older childhood (Bove et al., 1993). This approach was associated with high mortality (McElhinney et al., 1998). Later, elective primary repair in infancy timed similarly to elective VSD closure at 3–6 months of age was advocated (Bove et al., 1993; Hanley et al., 1993). Neonatal repair was first adopted in the late 1980s, and in the current era this has become the standard (Bove

et al., 1993; Danton et al., 2001; Hanley et al., 1993; Urban et al., 1998). Hanley et al. compared elective primary repair at 3 months of age to neonatal repair in 63 patients in a 1993 retrospective review from Boston Children's Hospital. The older patients had higher surgical mortality, and more problems with pulmonary hypertension postoperatively, both in terms of greater number of pulmonary hypertensive crises and higher mean pulmonary artery pressures, than the neonates. Other risk factors for poor outcome in this series were truncal valve insufficiency, IAA, and coronary artery anomalies. Neonates without any of these risk factors had 100% early survival (Hanley et al., 1993). In the same journal issue, Bove et al. (1993) reported their experience in 46 infants, 38 of whom were less than 1 month at repair. Hospital mortality was 11%, with three late deaths (all within 4 months of operation) for an overall mortality of 17%. Five patients required truncal valve replacement. Importantly, there was no association between mortality and age, weight, or associated cardiac anomalies; only one of nine patients with truncus arteriosus and IAA died (11%). The authors advocate repair of patients with truncus arteriosus before 1 month of age (Bove et al., 1993). Urban et al. reported a series of 46 patients in Germany with a 4% hospital mortality, with one additional late death for overall mortality of 6%. This series covered the years 1987–1997, with older age at repair (median 62 days). There were no truncal valve replacements, and the two hospital deaths were patients with severe truncal regurgitation and with IAAs (Urban et al., 1998). Thompson et al. reported 65 patients from University of California, San Francisco operated on at a median age of 10 days with 5% early mortality and 11% overall mortality. Weight less than 2.5 kg at operation and need for truncal valve replacements were negative predictors of survival. Thus, neonatal repair, deferred repair, and staged repair all have their proponents with data to support success with each. Clearly, results are improving with time in the neonatal repair approach. Truncal valve insufficiency, and associated IAA in some series, both remain surgical challenges in this repair.

Long-Term Outcomes

Follow-up studies in truncus arteriosus repair have shown good long-term results, with severe truncal insufficiency remaining a source of mortality and morbidity. Rajasinghe et al. reported a 20-year follow-up on the patients from the University of California, San Francisco. Data were available for 140 of 165 patients, operated on at a median age of 3.5 months followed for a median of 10.5 years (Rajasinghe et al., 1997; Reddy et al., 1998). Late mortality was 16%, with just under half of these deaths occurring at reoperation. Conduit replacement was required in 76% of patients at a median of 5.5 years after first operation. The other significant group of reoperations were truncal valve replacements, in 19% of patients, most of whom had significant truncal insufficiency prior to initial repair (Rajasinghe, et al., 1997; Reddy et al., 1998). Brown et al. reported a similar time to conduit replacement (59.1 months) in their series of 60 patients operated on at Riley Children's hospital in Indiana (Brown et al., 2001).

INTERRUPTED AORTIC ARCH

Pathology

Interruption of the aortic arch refers to loss of luminal continuity between the ascending and descending aorta (Tchervenkov et al., 2005). As a conotruncal lesion, this is a true anatomic separation, with the descending aorta in continuity with the ductus arteriosus. There are three anatomic subtypes, defined by the location of the interruption. Type A occurs distal to the left subclavian artery, such that none of the branches arise from the descending aorta. This is anatomically most similar to a coarctation of the aorta, and some authors have suggested a spectrum between Type A interruption and coarctation (Kreutzer et al., 2000). Type B occurs distal to the left carotid artery, such that only the left subclavian artery arises from the descending aorta. This type is most often associated with the DiGeorge syndrome and other chromosomal disorders, and has a female preponderance (Kreutzer et al., 2000). Type C occurs distal to the innominate artery, such that the left carotid and left subclavian arteries both arise from the descending aorta. It is very rare. IAA of all types

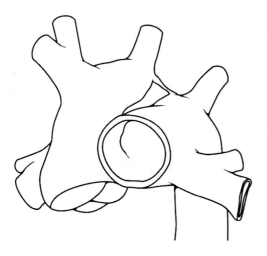

FIGURE 13–10. IAA, type B. Note the atretic aortic segment distal to the left carotid artery. The left subclavian artery and the descending aorta are supplied by the ductus arteriosus.

is usually associated with a large malalignment VSD (93%), as in other conotruncal anomalies. Here the malaligment is posterior, with consequent tendency for narrowing of the left ventricular outflow tract (LVOT) (Kreutzer and Van Praagh, 2000). The aortic valve may be bicuspid and is often small. Other associated lesions include AP window, aberrant right subclavian artery, truncus arteriosus (see section above), transposed great arteries, and complex intracardiac lesions such as double outlet RV and various forms of single ventricle (Brown et al., 2006; Kreutzer and Van Praagh, 2000; McCrindle et al., 2005; Oosterhof et al., 2004; Serraf et al., 1996; Tlaskal et al., 1998). The pathogenesis of arch interruption, especially type B, appears tied to neural crest cell migration into the conotruncal regions in the embryo (Kreutze and Van Praagh, 2000), causing abnormal branchial arch development (Bockman et al., 1987, 1989) and likely the malalignment of the conal septum as well. Coarctation, also associated with VSD and bicuspid aortic valves, may be within the spectrum of type A interruption, but there are important distinctions. A severe coarctation may result in a functionally IAA, but with anatomic continuity between the ascending and descending aorta. The associated VSD may be malaligned, but is more often perimembranous, and the tendency to develop LVOT obstruction is much less (Kreutzer and Van Praagh, 2000).

Physiology

Patients with IAA are entirely dependent on the ductus arteriosus for blood flow to the descending aorta, and to any head and neck vessels arising from the descending aorta. If the ductus begins to close prior to diagnosis, patients rapidly develop signs of shock from the low cardiac output, with acidosis, renal and hepatic insufficiency and high risk of necrotizing enterocolitis. If the ductus remains patent, patients will develop congestive heart failure from high pulmonary flow associated with large VSD, or with single ventricle physiology, especially in combination with LVOT obstruction. Hence, these patients are often quite ill by the time they present, unless diagnosed prenatally (Volpe, Marasiniet al., 2003; Volpe, Paladini et al., 2003) or very soon after birth and prostaglandins are initiated immediately. In a large series from Toronto, Oosterhoff et al. reported a median age of presentation of 3 days, with range from prenatal to 7 months, in a cohort of 119 patients. Clinical signs prompting the diagnosis were congestive heart failure (37%), murmur (31%), circulatory collapse (28%), cyanosis (24%), and tachypnea (12%). Only five patients were first detected because of weak femoral pulses (Oosterhof et al., 2004).

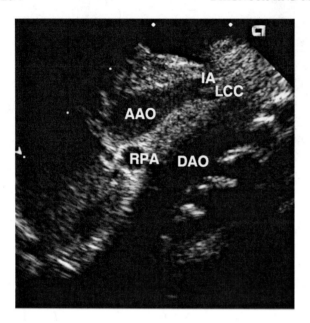

FIGURE 13–11. Type B IAA, suprasternal notch echocardiographic view. AAO, ascending aorta; DAO, descending aorta; IA, innominate artery; LCC, left common carotid artery; RPA, right pulmonary artery.

Diagnosis

Physical examination findings mirror the physiology as discussed above. Infants in heart failure will have hepatomegaly and a hyperdynamic precordium with a gallop and outflow murmur. A systolic click is common in those patients with a bicuspid aortic valve. Because there is obligatory right to left shunting at the ductus arteriosus, oxygen saturation in the lower extremities will be lower than in the right arm. Infants presenting in shock with poor pulses, poor perfusion, and depressed consciousness, require rapid institution of prostaglandins. The EKG shows RVH, given the persistent dependence of systemic output on the RV. The chest x-ray shows nonspecific cardiomegaly and pulmonary edema; the arch anomaly is not generally readily apparent. The echocardiogram is usually diagnostic, including delineation of the anatomic subtype (A, B, or C) as well as any associated anomalies. It can be difficult to image both the ascending and descending aorta in the same plane with standard suprasternal notch views. The ascending aorta may be in the usual position and appear to travel straight superiorly without branching, especially in type B or C. In type B interruption, the left carotid can be seen with slight rotation. It is important to confirm branching of the innominate artery, as an aberrant right subclavian artery may be present and will arise from the descending aorta. The size and flow through the ductus arteriosus, and Doppler patterns of the aorta at the diaphragm, are important to assess

systemic output to the descending aorta. Careful evaluation of the intracardiac anatomy for associated lesions, and of the ascending aorta and pulmonary arteries for AP window is important. In patients with an IAA without a VSD, AP windows are almost always present. The LVOT must be carefully assessed for stenosis, with measurements and pulsed Doppler interrogation. Tchervenkov et al. report a simple index their group uses to determine adequacy of the LVOT. If the diameter of the LVOT in millimeters is less than the infant's weight in kilograms, an AP anastomosis with RV to PA conduit or BT shunt (modified Norwood operation) is indicated. If the LVOT diameter is greater than the infant's weight plus 2, a two-ventricle approach is safe; measurements in between are equivocal and are to be determined case-by-case (Tchervenkov and Roy, 2000). Geva et al. (1993) found that the cross-sectional area of the LVOT in systole, measured in the short-axis view prior to surgical intervention, was predictive of subsequent outflow tract obstruction. Their "cutoff value" was less than or equal to $0.7 \text{ cm}^2/\text{m}^2$. Other imaging modalities useful in delineating anatomy in IAA and associated abnormalities include 64 slice CT (Wong et al., 2007) and CT angiogram with 3D reconstruction (Lee et al., 2006).

Current Medical and Surgical Management

Arch reconstruction generally must be done in the newborn period, as these infants tend to become increasingly unstable over time even with prostaglandins. The more traditional approach is staged, with arch reconstruction and pulmonary artery band followed by elective complete repair at a few months of age. Brown et al. (2006) recently reported their experience at Riley Children's hospital in Indiana with 65 patients repaired between 1982 and 2005. The majority (52 patients) had a staged repair, while 13 underwent complete neonatal repair. The approach for arch reconstruction most often used was trans-section of the left carotid artery and incorporation of the proximal segment into the arch repair. They had five early and ten late deaths for overall survival of 92% at 1 year, 81% at 5 years, and 76% at 15 years. Fifteen-year survival was better for less complex patients (interrupted arch with VSD, AP window, and/or LVOT obstruction; 81%) than for more complex patients (Taussig-Bing double outlet RV or truncus arteriosus with arch interruption; 54%). Importantly, they reported no seizures or neurologic deficits in their patients after sacrifice of the left common carotid artery (Brown et al., 2006). Others have reported similar success using primarily a single-stage repair. Serraf et al. reported 79 patients repaired in France between 1985 and 1995, 64 with single-stage repair and 15 multistage repairs (Serraf

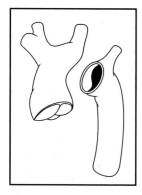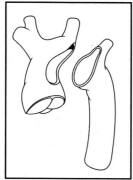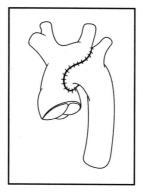

FIGURE 13–12. IAA repair. Three panels depict the sequence of arch reconstruction. First, the ductal insertion is excised from the proximal descending aorta, next, an incision is made in the transverse arch, and finally the two are anasthamosed together. Here the left carotid is spared; it can be incorporated into the proximal segment of the repair if needed, as can patch material.

et al., 1996). Median age at operation was just 9 days, but most patients were reported to have congestive heart failure. Twenty-four patients had complex intracardiac anatomy. Arch repair was primarily via direct anastomosis (59 patients), with patch augmentation in 8 and conduits in 12. LVOT obstruction was addressed by placing the VSD patch on the left side in 15 patients, myomectomy in 5, and conversion to single ventricle physiology with AP anastomosis and RV to PA conduit in 4. Overall postoperative mortality was 18.9 %, with improvement to 12% in the period from 1990 to 1995. Factors adversely affecting survival included preoperative intracranial hemorrhage, preoperative renal failure, earlier date of operation, and number of cardioplegia injections (Serraf et al., 1996). Kostelka et al. (2004) reported a series of 24 patients who underwent single-stage neonatal repair in Leipzig, Germany with no mortality. It is important to note that half of the patients had severe coarctation and not truly interrupted arch; 8 of the 12 true interrupted arches were type B. These authors report a technique of selective brain perfusion via the innominate artery and selective coronary perfusion via the aortic root during arch reconstruction in all patients. Several others have reported excellent success with regional perfusion of the innominate artery and aortic root, with a "nonworking, beating heart" (Lim et al., 2007). This can be performed during arch reconstruction to minimize the myocardial and cerebral ischemia associated with deep hypothermic circulatory arrest (Harrington et al., 2004; Korkola et al., 2002; Lim et al., 2007; Takeda et al., 2005).

SUMMARY

Conotruncal defects comprise a significant percentage of complex congenital heart defects. Maldevelopment of the outflow tracts, with associated malalignment of the outflow tracts with the conal septum, underlies the pathology and physiology of this group of lesions.

Improved diagnostic capabilities, including fetal echocardiography and other noninvasive imaging techniques such as CT and MRI, coupled with advanced medical and surgical options have led to overall earlier age of intervention, fewer palliative instead of reparative procedures, and generally improved survival. Long-term management of RV function and of RVOT and branch pulmonary arteries remain a challenge in patients with TOF and TOF variants, while continuing LVOT obstruction affects patients with interrupted arches. Patients with truncus arteriosus face bilateral outflow tract complications over time. Novel transcatheter techniques compliment surgical advances in the ongoing care of patients with each of these lesions.

ACKNOWLEDGMENTS

The authors would like to thank Dominic Doyle and David Parra for valuable assistance with illustrations and figures.

REFERENCES

Acherman RJ, Smallhorn JF, Freedom RM. Echocardiographic assessment of pulmonary blood supply in patients with pulmonary atresia and ventricular septal defect. *J Am Coll Cardiol.* 1996;28:1308–1313.

Akinturek H, Goerlach G, Valeske K, et al. Transplantation in truncus arteriosus combined with interrupted aortic arch. *Ann Thorac Surg.* 2006;82:1535–1537.

Amin Z, McElhinney DB, Reddy VM, Moore P, Hanley FL, Teitel DF. Coronary to pulmonary artery collaterals in patients with pulmonary atresia and ventricular septal defect. *Ann Thorac Surg.* 2000;70:119–123.

Anagnostopoulos P, Azakie A, Natarajan S, Alphonso N, Brook MM, Karl TR. Pulmonary valve cusp augmentation with autologous pericardium may improve early outcome for tetralogy of Fallot. *J Thorac Cardiovasc Surg.* 2007;133:640–647.

Aru GM, Juraszek A, Moskowitz I, Van Praagh R. Tetralogy of Fallot with congenital aortic valvar stenosis: the tetralogy-truncus interrelationship. *Pediatr Cardiol.* 2006;27:354–359.

Babu-Narayan SV, Kilner PJ, et al. Ventricular fibrosis suggested by cardiovascular magnetic resonance in adults with repaired tetralogy of fallot and its relationship to adverse markers of clinical outcome. *Circulation.* 2006;113:405–413.

Barbero-Marcial M, Baucia JA, Jatene A. Valved conduits of bovine pericardium for right ventricle to pulmonary artery connections. *Semin Thorac Cardiovasc Surg.* 1995;7:148–153.

Belli E, Mace L, Ly M, et al. Surgical management of pulmonary atresia with ventricular septal defect in late adolescence and adulthood. *Eur J Cardiothorac Surg.* 2007;31:236–241.

Bernanke DH, Velkey JM. Development of the coronary blood supply: changing concepts and current ideas. *Anat Rec.* 2002;269:198–208.

Bernardes RJ, Marchiori E, Bernardes PM, Monzo Gonzaga MB, Simoes LC. A comparison of magnetic resonance angiography with conventional angiography in the diagnosis of tetralogy of Fallot. *Cardiol Young.* 2006;16:281–288.

Besson WT III, Kirby ML, Van Mierop LH, Teabeaut JR, II. Effects of the size of lesions of the cardiac neural crest at various embryonic ages on incidence and type of cardiac defects. *Circulation.* 1986;73:360–364.

Bharati S, Paul MH, Idriss FS, Potkin RT, Lev M. The surgical anatomy of pulmonary atresia with ventricular septal defect: pseudotruncus. *J Thorac Cardiovasc Surg.* 1975;69:713–721.

Bigras JL, Boutin C, McCrindle BW, Rebeyka IM. Short-term effect of monocuspid valves on pulmonary insufficiency and clinical outcome after surgical repair of tetralogy of Fallot. *J Thorac Cardiovasc Surg.* 1996;112:33–37.

Bockman DE, Redmond ME, Kirby ML. Alteration of early vascular development after ablation of cranial neural crest. *Anat Rec.* 1989;225:209–217.

Bockman DE, Redmond ME, Waldo K, Davis H, Kirby ML. Effect of neural crest ablation on development of the heart and arch arteries in the chick. *Am J Anat.* 1987;180:332–341.

Botto LD, May K, Fernhoff PM, et al. A population-based study of the 22q11.2 deletion: phenotype, incidence, and contribution to major birth defects in the population. *Pediatrics.* 2003;112:101–107.

Bove EL, Lupinetti FM, Pridjian AK, et al. Results of a policy of primary repair of truncus arteriosus in the neonate. *J Thorac Cardiovasc Surg.* 1993;105:1057–1065; discussion 1065–1066.

Bove EL, Kavey RE, Byrum CJ, Sondheimer HM, Blackman MS, Thomas FD. Improved right ventricular function following late pulmonary valve replacement for residual pulmonary insufficiency or stenosis. *J Thorac Cardiovasc Surg.* 1985;90: 50–55.

Brown JW, Ruzmetov M, Okada Y, Vijay P, Rodefeld MD, Turrentine MW. Outcomes in patients with interrupted aortic arch and associated anomalies: a 20-year experience. *Eur J Cardiothorac Surg.* 2006;29:666–673; discussion 673–674.

Brown JW, Ruzmetov M, Okada Y, Vijay P, Turrentine MW. Truncus arteriosus repair: outcomes, risk factors, reoperation and management. *Eur J Cardiothorac Surg.* 2001;20:221–227.

Brown JW, Ruzmetov M, Rodefeld MD, Vijay P, Darragh RK. Valved bovine jugular vein conduits for right ventricular outflow tract reconstruction in children: an attractive alternative to pulmonary homograft. *Ann Thorac Surg.* 2006;82:909–916.

Brown SC, Eyskens B, Mertens L, Dumoulin M, Gewillig M. Percutaneous treatment of stenosed major aortopulmonary collaterals with balloon dilatation and stenting: what can be achieved? *Heart.* 1998;79:24–28.

Carotti A, Albanese SB, Di Donato RM. Unifocalization and repair of pulmonary atresia with ventricular septal defect and major aortopulmonary collateral arteries. *Acta Paediatr Suppl.* 2006;95:22–26.

Carotti A, Albanese SB, Minniti G, Guccione P, Di Donato RM. Increasing experience with integrated approach to pulmonary atresia with ventricular septal defect and major aortopulmonary collateral arteries. *Eur J Cardiothorac Surg.* 23:719–726; discussion 726–727.

Chaudhari M, Hamilton L, Hasan A. Correction of coronary arterial anomalies at surgical repair of common arterial trunk with ischaemic left ventricular dysfunction. *Cardiol Young.* 2006;16:179–181.

Cheung MM, Konstantinov IE, Redington AN. Late complications of repair of tetralogy of Fallot and indications for pulmonary valve replacement. *Semin Thorac Cardiovasc Surg.* 2005;17:155–159.

Chiappini B, Barrea C, Rubay J. Right ventricular outflow tract reconstruction with contegra monocuspid transannular patch in tetralogy of Fallot. *Ann Thorac Surg.* 2007;83:185–187.

Chiariello L, Meyer J, Wukasch DC, Hallman GL, Cooley DA. Intracardiac repair of tetralogy of Fallot. Five-year review of 403 patients. *J Thorac Cardiovasc Surg.* 1975;70:529–535.

Chong WY, Wong WH, Chiu CS, Cheung YF. Aortic root dilation and aortic elastic properties in children after repair of tetralogy of Fallot. *Am J Cardiol.* 2006;97:905–909.

Chowdhury UK, Pradeep KK, Patel CD, et al. Noninvasive assessment of repaired tetralogy of Fallot by magnetic resonance imaging and dynamic radionuclide studies. *Ann Thorac Surg.* 2006;81:1436–1442.

Collett R, Edwards J. Persistant truncus arteriosus: a classification according to anatomic subtypes. *Surg Clinic North Am.* 1949;1245–1270.

Corno A, Giamberti A, Giannico S, et al. Long-term results after extracardiac valved conduits implanted for complex congenital heart disease. *J Card Surg.* 1988;3:495–500.

Cotrufo M, Arciprete P, Caianiello G, et al. Right pulmonary artery development after modified Blalock-Taussig shunt (MBTS) in infants with pulmonary atresia, VSD and confluent pulmonary arteries. *Eur J Cardiothorac Surg.* 1989;3:12–15.

Crupi G, Locatelli G, Villani M, Tiraboschi R, Parenzan L. Open-heart palliative surgery for pulmonary atresia with ventricular septal defect and hypoplastic pulmonary arteries. *Thorax.* 1978;33:625–628.

Crupi G, Macartney FJ, Anderson RH. Persistent truncus arteriosus. A study of 66 autopsy cases with special reference to definition and morphogenesis. *Am J Cardiol.* 1977;40:569–578.

Danton MH, Barron DJ, Stumper O, et al. Repair of truncus arteriosus: a considered approach to right ventricular outflow tract reconstruction. *Eur J Cardiothorac Surg.* 2001;20:95–103 discussion 103–104.

Davlouros PA, Karatza AA, Gatzoulis MA, Shore DF. Timing and type of surgery for severe pulmonary regurgitation after repair of tetralogy of Fallot. *Int J Cardiol.* 2004;97 Suppl 1: 91–101.

De Giovanni JV. Timing, frequency, and results of catheter intervention following recruitment of major aortopulmonary collaterals in patients with pulmonary atresia and ventricular septal defect. *J Interv Cardiol.* 2004;17:47–52.

del Nido PJ. Surgical management of right ventricular dysfunction late after repair of tetralogy of fallot: right ventricular remodeling surgery. *Semin Thorac Cardiovasc Surg Pediatr Card Surg Annu.* 2006;29–34.

Derby CD, Pizarro C. Routine primary repair of tetralogy of Fallot in the neonate. *Expert Rev Cardiovasc Ther.* 2005;3:857–863.

Dinarevic S, Redington A, Rigby M, Shinebourne EA. Outcome of pulmonary atresia and ventricular septal defect during infancy. *Pediatr Cardiol.* 1995;16:276–282.

Dogan OF, Karcaaltincaba M, Yorgancioglu C, et al. Demonstration of coronary arteries and major cardiac vascular structures in congenital heart disease by cardiac multidetector computed tomography angiography. *Heart Surg Forum.* 2007;10:E90–E94.

Dorfman AL, Geva T. Magnetic resonance imaging evaluation of congenital heart disease: conotruncal anomalies. *J Cardiovasc Magn Reson.* 2006;8:645–659.

Duke C, Sharland GK, Jones AM, Simpson JM. Echocardiographic features and outcome of truncus arteriosus diagnosed during fetal life. *Am J Cardiol.* 2001;88:1379–1384.

El-Said HG, Clapp S, Fagan TE, Conwell J, Nihill MR. Stenting of stenosed aortopulmonary collaterals and shunts for palliation of pulmonary atresia/ventricular septal defect. *Catheter Cardiovasc Interv.* 2000;49:430–436.

Elzein C, Ilbawi M, Kumar S, Ruiz C. Severe truncal valve stenosis: diagnosis and management. *J Card Surg.* 2005;20:589–593.

Fallot A. [Contribution To The Pathological Anatomy Of Blue Disease (Cardiac Cyanosis).]. *Mars Med.* 1963;100:779–797.

Fyfe DA, Driscoll DJ, Di Donato RM, et al. Truncus arteriosus with single pulmonary artery: influence of pulmonary vascular obstructive disease on early and late operative results. *J Am Coll Cardiol.* 1985;5:1168–1172.

Gale AW, Arciniegas E, Green EW, Blackstone EH, Kirklin JW. Growth of the pulmonary anulus and pulmonary arteries after the Blalock-Taussig shunt. *J Thorac Cardiovasc Surg.* 1979;77:459–465.

Geva T, Ayres NA, Pac FA, Pignatelli R. Quantitative morphometric analysis of progressive infundibular obstruction in tetralogy of Fallot. A prospective longitudinal echocardiographic study. *Circulation.* 1995;92:886–892.

Geva T, Hornberger LK, Sanders SP, Jonas RA, Ott DA, Colan SD. Echocardiographic predictors of left ventricular outflow tract obstruction after repair of interrupted aortic arch. *J Am Coll Cardiol.* 1993;22:1953–1960.

Giannopoulos NM, Chatzis AC, Tsoutsinos AI, et al. Surgical results after total transatrial/transpulmonary correction of tetralogy of Fallot. *Hellenic J Cardiol.* 2005;46:273–282.

Giardini A, Specchia S, Coutsoumbas G, et al. Impact of pulmonary regurgitation and right ventricular dysfunction on oxygen uptake recovery kinetics in repaired tetralogy of Fallot. *Eur J Heart Fail.* 2006;8:736–743.

Gladman G, McCrindle BW, Williams WG, Freedom RM, Benson LN. The modified Blalock-Taussig shunt: clinical impact and morbidity in Fallot's tetralogy in the current era. *J Thorac Cardiovasc Surg.* 1997;114:25–30.

Goldmuntz E, Clark BJ, Mitchell LE, et al. Frequency of 22q11 deletions in patients with conotruncal defects. *J Am Coll Cardiol.* 1998;32:492–498.

Gott VL. C. Walton Lillehei and total correction of tetralogy of Fallot. *Ann Thorac Surg.* 1990;49:328–32.

Greil GF, Schoebinger M, Kuettner A, et al. Imaging of aortopulmonary collateral arteries with high-resolution multidetector CT. *Pediatr Radiol.* 2006;36:502–509.

Grothoff M, Spors B, Abdul-Khaliq H, et al. Pulmonary regurgitation is a powerful factor influencing QRS duration in patients after surgical repair of tetralogy of Fallot: a magnetic resonance imaging (MRI) study. *Clin Res Cardiol.* 2006;95:643–649.

Gundry SR, Razzouk AJ, Boskind JF, Bansal R, Bailey LL. Fate of the pericardial monocusp pulmonary valve for right ventricular outflow tract reconstruction. Early function, late failure without obstruction. *J Thorac Cardiovasc Surg.* 1994;107:908–912; discussion 912–913.

Hanley FL, Heinemann MK, Jonas RA, et al. Repair of truncus arteriosus in the neonate. *J Thorac Cardiovasc Surg.* 1993;105:1047–1056.

Harrington DK, Walker AS, Kaukuntla H, et al. Selective antegrade cerebral perfusion attenuates brain metabolic deficit in aortic arch surgery: a prospective randomized trial. *Circulation.* 2004;110: II231–236.

Helbing WA, Niezen RA, Le Cessie S, et al. Right ventricular diastolic function in children with pulmonary regurgitation after repair of tetralogy of Fallot: volumetric evaluation by magnetic resonance velocity mapping. *J Am Coll Cardiol.* 1996;28:1827–1835.

Hutson MR, Zhang P, Stadt HA, et al. Cardiac arterial pole alignment is sensitive to FGF8 signaling in the pharynx. *Dev Biol.* 2006;295:486–497.

Imamura M, Drummond-Webb JJ, Sarris GE, Mee RB. Improving early and intermediate results of truncus arteriosus repair: a new technique of truncal valve repair. *Ann Thorac Surg.* 1999;67:1142–1146.

Jahangiri M, Zurakowski D, Mayer JE, del Nido PJ, Jonas RA. Repair of the truncal valve and associated interrupted arch in neonates with truncus arteriosus. *J Thorac Cardiovasc Surg.* 2000;119:508–514.

Kaczmarek I, Schmauss D, Reichart B, Daebritz SH. Complete autologous reconstruction of the aorta and the pulmonary bifurcation in truncus arteriosus communis. *Eur J Cardiothorac Surg.* 2006;30:675–677.

Karamlou T, Silber I, Lao R, et al. Outcomes after late reoperation in patients with repaired tetralogy of Fallot: the impact of arrhythmia and arrhythmia surgery. *Ann Thorac Surg.* 2006;81:1786–1793; discussion 1793.

Karl TR, Sano S, Pornviliwan S, Mee RB. Tetralogy of Fallot: favorable outcome of nonneonatal transatrial, transpulmonary repair. *Ann Thorac Surg.* 1992;54:903–907.

Kirklin JK, Kirklin JW, Blackstone EH, Milano A, Pacifico AD. Effect of transannular patching on outcome after repair of tetralogy of Fallot. *Ann Thorac Surg.* 1989;48:783–791.

Kleinveld G, Joyner RW, Sallee D III, Kanter KR, Park, WJ. Hemodynamic and electrocardiographic effects of early pulmonary valve replacement in pediatric patients after transannular complete repair of tetralogy of Fallot. *Pediatr Cardiol.* 2006;27:329–335.

Knauth AL, Gauvreau K, Powell AJ, et al. Ventricular size and function assessed by cardiac MRI predict major adverse clinical outcomes late after tetralogy of Fallot repair. *Heart.* 2008;94:211–216.

Kolcz J, Pizarro C. Neonatal repair of tetralogy of Fallot results in improved pulmonary artery development without increased need for reintervention. *Eur J Cardiothorac Surg.* 2005;28: 394–399.

Konstantinov IE, Karamlou T, Blackstone EH, et al. Truncus arteriosus associated with interrupted aortic arch in 50 neonates: a Congenital Heart Surgeons Society study. *Ann Thorac Surg.* 2006;81:214–222.

Korkola SJ, Tchervenkov CI, Shum-Tim D. Aortic arch reconstruction without circulatory arrest: review of techniques, applications, and indications. *Semin Thorac Cardiovasc Surg Pediatr Card Surg Annu.* 2002;5:116–125.

Kostelka M, Walther T, Geerdts I, et al. Primary repair for aortic arch obstruction associated with ventricular septal defect. *Ann Thorac Surg.* 2004;78:1989–1993; discussion 1993.

Kothari SS. Mechanism of cyanotic spells in tetralogy of Fallot—the missing link? *Int J Cardiol.* 1992;37:1–5.

Kreutzer J, Van Praagh R. Comparison of left ventricular outflow tract obstruction in interruption of the aortic arch and in coarctation of the aorta, with diagnostic, developmental, and surgical implications. *Am J Cardiol.* 2000;86:856–862.

Kutsche LM, Van Mierop LH. Pulmonary atresia with and without ventricular septal defect: a different etiology and pathogenesis for the atresia in the 2 types? *Am J Cardiol.* 1983;51:932–935.

Laudito A, Bandisode VM, Lucas JF, Radtke WA, Adamson WT, Bradley SM. Right ventricular outflow tract stent as a bridge to surgery in a premature infant with tetralogy of Fallot. *Ann Thorac Surg.* 2006;81:744–746.

Laudito A, Graham EM, Stroud MR, et al. Complete repair of conotruncal defects with an interatrial communication: oxygenation, hemodynamic status, and early outcome. *Ann Thorac Surg.* 2006;82:1286–1291; discussion 1291.

Leatherbury L, Connuck DM, Gauldin HE, Kirby ML. Hemodynamic changes and compensatory mechanisms during early cardiogenesis after neural crest ablation in chick embryos. *Pediatr Res.* 30:509–12.

Leatherbury L, Connuck DM, Kirby ML. Neural crest ablation versus sham surgical effects in a chick embryo model of defective cardiovascular development. *Pediatr Res.* 1993;33:628–631.

Lecompte Y, Neveux JY, Leca F, et al. Reconstruction of the pulmonary outflow tract without prosthetic conduit. *J Thorac Cardiovasc Surg.* 1982;84:727–733.

Lee C, Lee CN, Kim SC, et al. Outcome after one-stage repair of tetralogy of Fallot. *J Cardiovasc Surg (Torino).* 2006;47: 65–70.

Lee HY, Lee W, Chung JW, Park JH, Yeon KM. Interrupted aortic arch with aberrant subclavian artery: a rare form of arch anomaly demonstrated with multidetector CT and 3D reconstruction. *Pediatr Radiol.* 2006;36:272–273.

Leonard H, Derrick G, O'Sullivan J, Wren C. Natural and unnatural history of pulmonary atresia. *Heart.* 2000;84:499–503.

Lillehei CW, Varco RL, Cohen M, et al. The first open heart corrections of tetralogy of Fallot. A 26–31 year follow-up of 106 patients. *Ann Surg.* 1986;204:490–502.

Lim HG, Kim WH, Jang WS, et al. One-stage total repair of aortic arch anomaly using regional perfusion. *Eur J Cardiothorac Surg.* 2007;31:242–248.

Lofland GK. The management of pulmonary atresia, ventricular septal defect, and multiple aorta pulmonary collateral arteries by definitive single stage repair in early infancy. *Eur J Cardiothorac Surg.* 2000;18:480–486.

Marchand P. The use of a cusp-bearing homograft patch to the outflow tract and pulmonary artery in Fallot's tetralogy and pulmonary valvular stenosis. *Thorax.* 1967;22:497–509.

Marino B, Digilio MC, Toscano A, et al. Anatomic patterns of conotruncal defects associated with deletion 22q11. *Genet Med.* 2001;3:45–48.

Mavroudis C, Backer CL. Surgical management of severe truncal insufficiency: experience with truncal valve remodeling techniques. *Ann Thorac Surg.* 2001;72:396–400.

McCaughan BC, Danielson GK, Driscoll DJ, McGoon DC. Tetralogy of Fallot with absent pulmonary valve. Early and late results of surgical treatment. *J Thorac Cardiovasc Surg.* 1985;89:280–287.

McCrindle BW, Tchervenkov CI, Konstantinov IE, et al. Risk factors associated with mortality and interventions in 472 neonates with interrupted aortic arch: a Congenital Heart Surgeons Society study. *J Thorac Cardiovasc Surg.* 2005;129:343–350.

McElhinney DB, Reddy VM, Rajasinghe HA, Mora BN, Silverman NH, Hanley FL. Trends in the management of truncal valve insufficiency. *Ann Thorac Surg.* 1998;65:517–524.

McGoon DC, Baird DK, Davis GD. Surgical management of large bronchial collateral arteries with pulmonary stenosis or atresia. *Circulation.* 1975;52:109–118.

McGoon DC, Rastelli GC, Ongley PA. An operation for the correction of truncus arteriosus. *JAMA.* 1968;205:69–73.

McManus BM, Waller BF, Jones M, Epstein SE, Roberts WC. The case for preoperative coronary angiography in patients with tetralogy of Fallot and other complex congenital heart diseases. *Am Heart J.* 1982;103:451–456.

Menteer J, Weinberg PM, Fogel MA. Quantifying regional right ventricular function in tetralogy of Fallot. *J Cardiovasc Magn Reson.* 2005;7:753–761.

Metras D, Chetaille P, Kreitmann B, Fraisse A, Ghez O, Riberi A. Pulmonary atresia with ventricular septal defect, extremely hypoplastic pulmonary arteries, major aorto-pulmonary collaterals. *Eur J Cardiothorac Surg.* 2001;20:590–596; discussion 596–597.

Molina JE. Preliminary experience with GORE-TEX grafting for right ventricle-pulmonary artery conduits. *Tex Heart Inst J.* 1986;13:137–142.

Muhler MR, Rake A, Schwabe M, et al. Truncus arteriosus communis in a midtrimester fetus: comparison of prenatal ultrasound and MRI with postmortem MRI and autopsy. *Eur Radiol.* 2004;14:2120–2124.

Murai S, Hamada S, Yamamoto S, et al. Evaluation of major aortopulmonary collateral arteries (MAPCAs) using three-dimensional CT angiography: two case reports. *Radiat Med.* 2004;22:186–189.

Murphy JG, Gersh BJ, Mair DD, et al. Long-term outcome in patients undergoing surgical repair of tetralogy of Fallot. *N Engl J Med.* 1993;329:593–599.

Nakata S, Imai Y, Takanashi Y, et al. A new method for the quantitative standardization of cross-sectional areas of the pulmonary arteries in congenital heart diseases with decreased pulmonary blood flow. *J Thorac Cardiovasc Surg.* 1984;88:610–619.

Niederreither K, Vermot J, Messaddeq N, Schuhbaur B, Chambon P, Dolle P. Embryonic retinoic acid synthesis is essential for heart morphogenesis in the mouse. *Development.* 2001;128:1019–1031.

Nishibatake M, Kirby ML, Van Mierop LH. Pathogenesis of persistent truncus arteriosus and dextroposed aorta in the chick embryo after neural crest ablation. *Circulation.* 1987;75:255–264.

Niwa K. Aortic root dilatation in tetralogy of Fallot long-term after repair—histology of the aorta in tetralogy of Fallot: evidence of intrinsic aortopathy. *Int J Cardiol.* 2005;103:117–119.

Norgaard, MA, Alphonso N, Cochrane AD, Menahem S, Brizard CP, d'Udekem Y. Major aorto-pulmonary collateral arteries of patients with pulmonary atresia and ventricular septal defect are dilated bronchial arteries. *Eur J Cardiothorac Surg.* 2006;29:653–658.

Oosterhof T, Azakie A, Freedom RM, Williams WG, McCrindle BW. Associated factors and trends in outcomes of interrupted aortic arch. *Ann Thorac Surg.* 2004;78:1696–1702.

Oosterhof T, Mulder BJ, Vliegen HW, de Roos A. Cardiovascular magnetic resonance in the follow-up of patients with corrected tetralogy of Fallot: a review. *Am Heart J.* 2006;151:265–722.

Oosterhof T, Mulder BJ, Vliegen HW, de Roos A. Corrected tetralogy of Fallot: delayed enhancement in right ventricular outflow tract. *Radiology.* 2005;237:868–871.

Oosterhof T, Tulevski II, Vliegen HW, Spijkerboer AM, Mulder BJ. Effects of volume and/or pressure overload secondary to congenital heart disease (tetralogy of fallot or pulmonary stenosis) on right ventricular function using cardiovascular magnetic resonance and B-type natriuretic peptide levels. *Am J Cardiol.* 2006;97:1051–1055.

Pagani FD, Cheatham JP, Beekman RH III, Lloyd TR, Mosca RS, Bove EL. The management of tetralogy of Fallot with pulmonary atresia and diminutive pulmonary arteries. *J Thorac Cardiovasc Surg.* 1995;110:1521–1532; discussion 1532–1533.

Perron J, Moran AM, Gauvreau K, del Nido PJ, Mayer JE Jr, Jonas RA. Valved homograft conduit repair of the right heart in early infancy. *Ann Thorac Surg.* 1999;68:542–548.

Piehler JM, Danielson GK, McGoon DC, Wallace RB, Fulton RE, Mair DD. Management of pulmonary atresia with ventricular septal defect and hypoplastic pulmonary arteries by right ventricular outflow construction. *J Thorac Cardiovasc Surg.* 1980;80:552–567.

Rabinovitch M, Herrera-deLeon V, Castaneda AR, Reid L. Growth and development of the pulmonary vascular bed in patients with tetralogy of Fallot with or without pulmonary atresia. *Circulation.* 1981;64:1234–1249.

Rajasinghe HA, McElhinney DB, Reddy VM, Mora BN, Hanley FL. Long-term follow-up of truncus arteriosus repaired in infancy: a twenty-year experience. *J Thorac Cardiovasc Surg.* 1997;113:869–878; discussion 878–879.

Reddy VM, Hanley F. Late results of repair of truncus arteriosus. *Semin Thorac Cardiovasc Surg Pediatr Card Surg Annu.* 1998;1:139–146.

Reddy VM, Liddicoat JR, Hanley FL. Midline one-stage complete unifocalization and repair of pulmonary atresia with ventricular septal defect and major aortopulmonary collaterals. *J Thorac Cardiovasc Surg.* 1995;109:832–844; discussion 844–5.

Reddy VM, McElhinney DB, Amin Z, et al. Early and intermediate outcomes after repair of pulmonary atresia with ventricular septal defect and major aortopulmonary collateral arteries: experience with 85 patients. *Circulation.* 2000;101:1826–1832.

Reddy VM, Petrossian E, McElhinney DB, Moore P, Teitel DF, Hanley FL. One-stage complete unifocalization in infants: when should the ventricular septal defect be closed? *J Thorac Cardiovasc Surg.* 1997;113:858–866; discussion 866–868.

Redington AN. Physiopathology of right ventricular failure. *Semin Thorac Cardiovasc Surg Pediatr Card Surg Annu.* 2006;3–10.

Revuelta JM, Ubago JL, Duran CM. Composite pericardial monocusp patch for the reconstruction of right ventricular outflow tract. Clinical application in 7 patients. *Thorac Cardiovasc Surg.* 1983;31:156–159.

Sabri MR, Sholler G, Hawker R, Nunn G. Branch pulmonary artery growth after blalock-taussig shunts in tetralogy of fallot and pulmonary atresia with ventricular septal defect: a retrospective, echocardiographic study. *Pediatr Cardiol.* 1999;20:358–363.

Schulze-Neick I, Ho SY, Bush A, et al. Severe airflow limitation after the unifocalization procedure: clinical and morphological correlates. *Circulation.* 2000;102:III142–147.

Seipelt RG, Vazquez-Jimenez JF, Sachweh JS, Seghaye MC, Messmer BJ. Antegrade palliation for diminutive pulmonary arteries in Tetralogy of Fallot. *Eur J Cardiothorac Surg.* 2002;21:721–724; discussion 724.

Serraf A, Lacour-Gayet F, Robotin M, et al. Repair of interrupted aortic arch: a ten-year experience. *J Thorac Cardiovasc Surg.* 1996;112:1150–1160.

Shebani SO, McGuirk S, Baghai M, et al. Right ventricular outflow tract reconstruction using Contegra valved conduit: natural history and conduit performance under pressure. *Eur J Cardiothorac Surg.* 2006;29:397–405.

Sievers HH, Lange PE, Regensburger D, et al. Short-term hemodynamic results after right ventricular outflow tract reconstruction using a cusp-bearing transannular patch. *J Thorac Cardiovasc Surg.* 1983;86:777–783.

Stewart RD, Backer CL, Young L, Mavroudis C. Tetralogy of Fallot: results of a pulmonary valve-sparing strategy. *Ann Thorac Surg.* 2005;80:1431–1438; discussion 1438–9.

Takeda Y, Asou T, Yamamoto N, Ohara K, Yoshimura H, Okamoto H. Arch reconstruction without circulatory arrest in neonates. *Asian Cardiovasc Thorac Ann.* 2005;13:337–340.

Tan JL, Gatzoulis MA, Ho SY. Aortic root disease in tetralogy of Fallot. *Curr Opin Cardiol.* 2006;21:569–572.

Tchervenkov CI, Jacobs JP, Sharma K, Ungerleider RM. Interrupted aortic arch: surgical decision making. *Semin Thorac Cardiovasc Surg Pediatr Card Surg Annu.* 2005;8:92.

Tchervenkov CI, Roy N. Congenital Heart Surgery Nomenclature and Database Project: pulmonary atresia—ventricular septal defect. *Ann Thorac Surg.* 2000;69: S97–105.

Therrien J, Provost Y, Merchant N, Williams W, Colman J, Webb G. Optimal timing for pulmonary valve replacement in adults after tetralogy of Fallot repair. *Am J Cardiol.* 2005;95:779–782.

Tireli E, Basaran M, Kafali E, Soyler I, Camci E, Dayioglu E. Single-stage unifocalization and correction with median sternotomy in complex pulmonary atresia. *Cardiovasc Surg.* 2002;10:600–604.

Tissot C, da Cruz E, Beghetti M, Aggoun Y. Successful use of a new Amplatzer Vascular plug for percutaneous closure of a large aortopulmonary collateral artery in a pulmonary atresia with ventricular septal defect prior to complete repair. *Int J Cardiol.* 2007;116: e39–41.

Tlaskal T, Hucin B, Hruda J, et al. Results of primary and two-stage repair of interrupted aortic arch. *Eur J Cardiothorac Surg.* 1998;14:235–242.

Tlaskal T, Hucin B, Kucera V, et al. Repair of persistent truncus arteriosus with interrupted aortic arch. *Eur J Cardiothorac Surg.* 2005;28:736–741.

Turrentine MW, McCarthy RP, Vijay P, McConnell KW, Brown JW. PTFE monocusp valve reconstruction of the right ventricular outflow tract. *Ann Thorac Surg.* 2002;73:871–879; discussion 879–80.

Urban AE, Sinzobahamvya N, Brecher AM, Wetter J, Malorny S. Truncus arteriosus: ten-year experience with homograft repair in neonates and infants. *Ann Thorac Surg.* 1998;66: S183–188.

Van Praagh R, Van Praagh S, Nebesar RA, Muster AJ, Sinha SN, Paul MH. Tetralogy of Fallot: underdevelopment of the pulmonary infundibulum and its sequelae. *Am J Cardiol.* 1970;26:25–33.

Van Praagh R, Van Praagh S. The anatomy of common aorticopulmonary trunk (truncus arteriosus communis) and its embryologic implications. A study of 57 necropsy cases. *Am J Cardiol.* 1965;16:406–425.

Vargas Barron J, Sahn DJ, Attie F, et al. Two-dimensional echocardiographic study of right ventricular outflow and great artery anatomy in pulmonary atresia with ventricular septal defects and in truncus arteriosus. *Am Heart J.* 1983;105:281–286.

Vermot J, Messaddeq N, Niederreither K, Dierich A, Dolle P. Rescue of morphogenetic defects and of retinoic acid signaling in retinaldehyde dehydrogenase 2 (Raldh2) mouse mutants by chimerism with wild-type cells. *Differentiation.* 2006;74:661–668.

Vermot J, Niederreither K, Garnier JM, Chambon P, Dolle P. Decreased embryonic retinoic acid synthesis results in a DiGeorge syndrome phenotype in newborn mice. *Proc Natl Acad Sci U S A.* 2003;100:1763–1768.

Vesel S, Rollings S, Jones A, Callaghan N, Simpson J, Sharland GK. Prenatally diagnosed pulmonary atresia with ventricular septal defect: echocardiography, genetics, associated anomalies and outcome. *Heart.* 2006;92:1501–1505.

Volpe P, Marasini M, Caruso G, et al. 22q11 deletions in fetuses with malformations of the outflow tracts or interruption of the aortic arch: impact of additional ultrasound signs. *Prenat Diagn.* 2003;23:752–757.

Volpe P, Paladini D, Marasini M, et al. Common arterial trunk in the fetus: characteristics, associations, and outcome in a multicentre series of 23 cases. *Heart.* 2003;89:1437–1441.

Wang J, Nagy A, Larsson J, Dudas M, Sucov HM, Kaartinen V. Defective ALK5 signaling in the neural crest leads to increased postmigratory neural crest cell apoptosis and severe outflow tract defects. *BMC Dev Biol.* 2006;6:51.

Wang XM, Wu LB, Sun C, et al. Clinical application of 64-slice spiral CT in the diagnosis of the Tetralogy of Fallot. *Eur J Radiol.* 2007;64:296–301.

Willems TP, Bogers AJ, Cromme-Dijkhuis AH, et al. Allograft reconstruction of the right ventricular outflow tract. *Eur J Cardiothorac Surg.* 1996;10:609–614; discussion 614–615.

Wong MN, Chan LG, Sim KH. Interrupted aortic arch and aortopulmonary window demonstrated on 64-slice multidetector computed tomography angiography. *Heart.* 2007;93:95.

Wu ET, Wang JK, Lee WL, Chang CC, Wu MH. Balloon valvuloplasty as an initial palliation in the treatment of newborns and young infants with severely symptomatic tetralogy of Fallot. *Cardiology.* 2006;105;52–56.

Ya J, Schilham MW, de Boer PA, Moorman AF, Clevers H, Lamers WH. Sox4-deficiency syndrome in mice is an animal model for common trunk. *Circ Res.* 1998;83:986–994.

Yagihara T, Yamamoto F, Nishigaki K, et al. Unifocalization for pulmonary atresia with ventricular septal defect and major aortopulmonary collateral arteries. *J Thorac Cardiovasc Surg.* 1996;112:392–402.

Yankah AC, Lange PE, Sievers HH, et al. Late results of valve xenograft conduits between the right ventricle and the pulmonary arteries in patients with pulmonary atresia and extreme tetralogy of Fallot. *Thorac Cardiovasc Surg.* 1984;32:250–252.

Yemets IM, Williams WG, Webb GD, et al. Pulmonary valve replacement late after repair of tetralogy of Fallot. *Ann Thorac Surg.* 1997;64:526–530.

14

Hypoplastic Left Ventricle

MATTHEW A. STUDER

HENRI JUSTINO

INTRODUCTION

Hypoplastic left heart syndrome is the extreme form of a spectrum of cardiac abnormalities involving atresia or severe stenosis of the aortic and mitral valves (Figure 14–1). First described in 1952 by Lev (1952), the term hypoplastic left heart syndrome was used to describe a series of hearts with aortic tract hypoplasia and an underdeveloped left ventricle that was unable to sustain the systemic circulation.

Before 1980, hypoplastic left heart syndrome was deemed inoperable, and was almost invariably fatal in infancy, with only extremely rare cases of survival into childhood or even adulthood (Moodie et al., 1972; Morris et al., 1990; Noonan and Nadas, 1958). In 1980, Norwood et al. (1980) and Doty et al. (1980) independently described the first successful palliation of this congenital heart defect. Enabled by the advent of prostaglandin therapy to maintain ductal patency in the 1970s (Hastreiter et al., 1982; Yabek and Mann, 1979) along with the success of the Fontan operation for palliating single-ventricle hearts, the Norwood procedure became the cornerstone of therapy for this devastating condition. In the last three decades, an astounding number of medical and surgical advances have been made in the management of these fragile infants. Whereas mortality was previously almost certain with this condition, nowadays, practitioners have witnessed a dramatic improvement in both the short-, medium-, and long-term survival (Gandhi et al., 2007; Goldberg et al., 2000; Mahle et al., 2000b).

EPIDEMIOLOGY

Hypoplastic left heart syndrome is a rare form of cyanotic congenital heart disease, yet it is the leading cause of death in infants, under the age of 1 year, with congenital heart disease (Gillum, 1994; Samanek et al., 1988). There is regional variability in the incidence of hypoplastic left heart syndrome (Ferencz et al., 1985; Pradat et al., 2003). In the United States, the New England Regional Infant Cardiac Program reported a prevalence of 0.164 per 1000 live births (Fyler, 1980), while the Baltimore–Washington Infant Study (Ferencz et al., 1985) and California Birth Defects Monitoring Program (Croen et al., 1991) reported a slightly higher prevalence of 0.267 and 0.210 per 1000, respectively. Internationally, the prevalence of hypoplastic left heart syndrome was found to be similar to that reported in the Baltimore–Washington Infant Study and California Birth Defects Monitoring Program, at 0.228 per 1000 in the Central–Eastern France Registry (Robert et al., 1988), and 0.199 per 1000 in the Swedish Child Cardiology Registry (Carlgren et al., 1987).

Hypoplastic left heart syndrome demonstrates both an ethnic variability and a male predominance with a male to female ratio of 1.74:1 (Pradat et al., 2003). Fixler et al. demonstrated that Caucasian and African-American infants are twice as likely to be born with hypoplastic left heart syndrome compared to Hispanic infants (Fixler et al., 1993), whereas Shapiro et al. documented Caucasian infants to have a 1.8 times greater incidence compared to African-American infants (Shapiro et al., 1958). The California Birth Defects

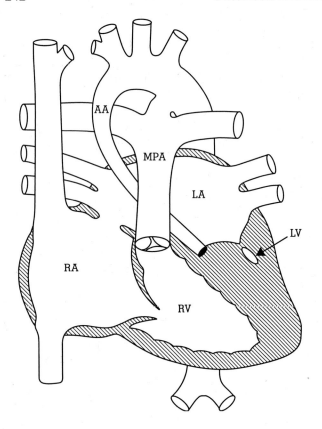

FIGURE 14–1. Hypoplastic left heart syndrome with aortic and mitral atresia. RA, right atrium; RV, right ventricle; LA, left atrium; LV, left ventricle; MPA, main pulmonary artery (MPA); AA, ascending aorta. (Adapted from Congenital Heart Disease: A Diagrammatic Atlas, by C.E. Mullins and D.C. Mayer, Copyright 1988 Alan R Liss. This material is reproduced with permission of Wiley-Liss, Inc., a subsidiary of John Wiley & Sons, Inc.)

Monitoring Program showed a slightly different ethnic distribution, but found that Caucasian infants remained the most common ethnic background associated with hypoplastic left heart syndrome. They reported a rate for Caucasians of 0.230, Asians 0.189, Hispanics 0.16, and African-Americans 0.146 per 1000 (Croen et al., 1991).

MORPHOLOGY

Over the past 55 years, a number of pathologic reports in the literature have elucidated the morphology of hypoplastic left heart syndrome (Bharati and Lev, 1984; Hastreiter et al., 1983; Kanjuh et al., 1965; Lev, 1952; Mahowald et al., 1982; Noonan and Nadas, 1958; Roberts, 1984). The general anatomic findings most commonly associated with hypoplastic left heart syndrome followed by variations in the fundamental anatomy will be discussed in this chapter.

Levocardia is the norm, with the cardiac apex formed by the right ventricle (Bharati and Lev, 1984; Hastreiter et al., 1983; Kanjuh et al., 1965; Lev, 1952; Mahowald et al., 1982; Noonan and Nadas, 1958; Roberts, 1984). The heart size, with few exceptions, is enlarged, with the preponderance of cardiac muscle composed of a dilated right atrium and right ventricle. Other than a few cases reported in the literature (Oppido et al., 2004; Raines and Armstrong, 1989) there is most often atrial and visceral situs solitus. The atrioventricular relationship is concordant (Bharati and Lev, 1984; Hastreiter et al., 1983; Kanjuh et al., 1965; Lev, 1952; Mahowald et al., 1982; Noonan and Nadas, 1958; Roberts, 1984) although histopathologically there may be an absence of any true left atrioventricular connection (Aiello et al., 1990). The ventriculoarterial relationship is also most often concordant with normally related, but markedly size-discrepant, great vessels.

In the presence of a hypoplastic left ventricle, the right ventricle exhibits compensatory enlargement (dilation and hypertrophy), due to the fact that it supports both the pulmonary and systemic circulations; these changes are seen both in utero and after birth. The right ventricle is apex forming and, despite its greater size, maintains its right ventricular morphologic characteristics (Bharati and Lev, 1984; Kanjuh et al., 1965; Mahowald et al., 1982). Given that the majority of the cardiac output (or the entirety, in the case of aortic atresia) during development is directed through the right ventricle, the main pulmonary artery and patent ductus arteriosus are also enlarged, providing prograde systemic blood flow to both the upper and lower body. The ductus arteriosus is typically short and very wide, distinctly different from the ductal morphology of pulmonary atresia, which is characteristically long and tortuous.

Hypoplasia of the ascending aorta is the hallmark of hypoplastic left heart syndrome, with little or no prograde blood flow across the atretic or severely stenotic aortic valve. As such, the carotid, subclavian, and coronary arterial circulation is dependent upon retrograde blood flow supplied by a patent ductus arteriosus. The transverse aortic arch may range in size from severely hypoplastic to normal size. The aortic arch is usually left-sided with a normal branching pattern of the head and neck vessels (Kanjuh et al., 1965). In the case of aortic atresia, the aortic valve may consist of a fibrous imperforate membrane, whereas in the case of aortic valve stenosis, the valve is small and thickened with partially fused leaflets that may be unicuspid, bicuspid, or tricuspid (Bharati and Lev, 1984; Kanjuh et al., 1965; Lev, 1952). The ascending aorta may measure less than 1 mm in diameter, but is always patent and serves as a functional common coronary artery

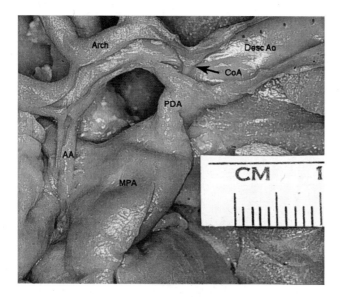

FIGURE 14–2. Severe hypoplasia of the ascending aorta (AA) with mild hypoplasia of the aortic arch (Arch); compare with the normal size of the descending aorta (Desc Ao). Note the patent ductus arteriosus (PDA) and dilated main pulmonary artery (MPA). There is a discrete juxtaductal coarctation (CoA) with evidence of a posterior shelf (arrow). (Courtesy of Debra L. Kearny, MD, Texas Children's Hospital.)

(Neufeld et al., 1962), supplying retrograde blood flow to both the right and left coronary arteries.

Of anatomic significance and particular clinical concern is the association of coarctation of the aorta with hypoplastic left heart syndrome (Elzenga and Gittenberger-de Groot, 1985) (Figure 14–2). Von Rueden determined that coarctation of the aorta was present in 75% of pathologic specimens with hypoplastic left heart syndrome (Von Rueden et al., 1975). Aiello noted a significant association between an ascending aorta size of less than 3 mm and the presence of coarctation (Aiello et al., 1990). The location of coarctation has been described as pre-, juxta-, or postductal in relation to the ductus arteriosus in pathological reports (Elzenga and Gittenberger-de Groot, 1985; Mahowald et al., 1982) with the proposed etiology being that of ductal tissue extending into the aortic wall (Von Rueden et al., 1975).

The mitral valve in hypoplastic left heart syndrome is markedly abnormal, preventing the normal egress of blood from the left atrium to the left ventricle. As is the case with the aortic valve, the mitral valve may demonstrate complete atresia or severe stenosis. In the case of mitral valve atresia, there may be a blind-dimple at the floor of the left atrium or membranous area where the valve would be expected, however, there may grossly and histopathologically be no discernable valvular

tissue (Bharati and Lev, 1984; Kanjuh et al., 1965). In the case of stenosis, the mitral valve leaflets are often severely dysplastic with thickened leaflets, and with short, thick chordae and papillary muscles (Bharati and Lev, 1984).

The aforementioned pathologic abnormalities involving the aortic and mitral valves culminate in a left ventricle that, as the term hypoplastic left heart syndrome would imply, is frequently diminutive and virtually noncontributory to the systemic circulation. However, the degree of left ventricular hypoplasia may vary from complete absence to normal dimensions for the body surface area of the patient (Bharati and Lev, 1984; Hastreiter et al., 1983; Kanjuh et al., 1965; Lev, 1952; Mahowald et al., 1982; Noonan and Nadas, 1958; Pellegrino and Thiene, 1976; Roberts, 1984). This sometimes makes the term hypoplastic left heart syndrome confusing, and care should be taken when using it interchangeably with aortic or mitral atresia, as 5%–7% of patients with aortic atresia will have a normal-sized left ventricle due to the presence of a large ventricular septal defect that allows egress of blood from the left ventricle (Pellegrino and Thiene, 1976; Thiene et al., 1979). The in utero development of the left ventricle is predominantly determined by the degree of mitral valve stenosis and/or the presence of a ventricular septal defect (Freedom et al., 1977; Kanjuh et al., 1965; Mahowald et al., 1982; Thiene et al., 1979). In the case of mitral and aortic atresia with an intact ventricular septum, the left ventricle may be nonexistent or simply a blind-ending cavity with a lumen that is often referred to as "slit-like" without inlet or outlet components. There may be a more discernable left ventricular cavity in the setting of mitral stenosis. The ventricular free wall is often hypertrophied relative to the lumen dimensions (Bharati and Lev, 1984; Kanjuh et al., 1965). A common association with a patent mitral valve is evidence of endomyocardial fibroelastosis within the left ventricle (Aiello et al., 1990; Bharati and Lev, 1984; Lev, 1952; Kanjuh et al., 1965; Mahowald et al., 1982). One may also see myocardial sinusoids that communicate with the left ventricular lumen, and on occasion, blood clots within the ventricular cavity (Bharati and Lev, 1984).

Pathologic series have noted the presence of a ventricular septal defect in 0.9%–14% of specimens (Aiello et al., 1990; Bharati and Lev, 1984; Kanjuh et al., 1965; Mahowald et al., 1982). Defects may occur at any location along the ventricular septum to include infundibular septal malalignment type, perimembranous, muscular, or inlet septal defects (Aiello et al., 1990; Bharati and Lev, 1984; Mahowald et al., 1982).

In the setting of atresia or severe stenosis of the mitral valve, pulmonary venous return to the left atrium must bridge an interatrial communication via either a patent foramen ovale or true atrial septal defect to reach the right atrium. Pathologic reports have demonstrated a variety of different atrial septal configurations with the most common being a patent foramen ovale (Kanjuh et al., 1965; Mahowald et al., 1982; Aiello et al., 1990). The septum primum may be seen herniating into the right atrium. Additional septal configurations that allow blood to communicate between the two atria include true secundum atrial septal defects, fenestration of the septum primum, ostium primum defects in the presence of an unbalanced atrioventricular canal defect, and finally, as described by Weinberg and colleagues, an anomalous leftward and malaligned attachment of the septum primum to the posterosuperior left atrial wall (Weinberg et al., 1986). Rarely, but of important clinical concern, an atrial septal communication may be either restrictive or completely absent. The incidence of an intact atrial septum with hypoplastic left heart syndrome ranges from 0% to 10% (Bharati and Lev, 1984; Mahowald et al., 1982; Weinberg et al., 1986). Some of these patients will have an alternate route for the egress of blood from the pulmonary veins in the way of anomalous pulmonary venous return, or a levoatrial cardinal vein. In others, no discernable route can be established, resulting in severe pulmonary venous congestion and a significant association with early neonatal mortality (Daebritz et al., 2000; Photiadis et al., 2005).

Early debate surrounding the anatomy of the atrial septum and its association with hypoplastic left heart syndrome resulted in the notion that restriction in the foramen ovale might alter the normal right-to-left flow across the atrial septum early in development, resulting in secondary underdevelopment of the left-sided structures (Lev, 1952; Noonan and Nadas, 1958). This is no longer the prevailing view, and it is currently believed that an underdevelopment of the aortic and/or mitral valve primarily results in hypoplasia of the left ventricle (Aiello et al., 1990; Anderson et al., 2004).

The tricuspid valve is often enlarged and may demonstrate a range of morphological abnormalities. Early pathologic case series reported near-normal trileaflet appearance of the tricuspid valve in hypoplastic left heart syndrome (Mahowald et al., 1982). However, following the success of the Norwood procedure, more attention has been focused on this anatomical structure, revealing a number of abnormalities. Stamm et al., in a series of 82 specimens with hypoplastic left heart syndrome, specifically evaluated the tricuspid valve and noted an increased incidence of structural anomalies, demonstrating that any of the tricuspid valve leaflets may be thickened and/or have redundant tissue (Stamm et al., 1997). Additional reports have demonstrated abnormal papillary muscle attachments, and rarely, a double orifice or Ebstein malformation

(Aiello et al., 1990; Bharati and Lev, 1984; Stamm et al., 1997). Occasionally some specimens may have clefts in the septal leaflet, often seen as part of a persistent, common atrioventricular canal defect with a hypoplastic left ventricle (a hypoplastic left heart syndrome variant) (Mahowald et al., 1982). There may be varying degrees of tricuspid valvular regurgitation postnatally, which may be the result of a morphologically dysplastic valve, but in most cases appears to depend on the degree of annular dilation (Barber et al., 1988).

Lloyd et al., in their evaluation of coronary blood flow in hypoplastic left heart syndrome, found areas of focal myocytolysis and large regions of necrosis involving the right ventricle in their pathologic series (Lloyd et al., 1986). The necrotic regions found in the right ventricle were subendocardial or transmural, and of varying age, suggesting abnormalities in coronary perfusion along with discrepancies between supply and demand of oxygen to the myocardium. They did not find an association between these right ventricular findings and the size of the ascending aorta or coronary arteries. They theorized that the degree of myocardial necrosis suggested an early insult possibly related to the altered hemodynamics of this cardiac lesion (Lloyd et al., 1986).

GENETICS

Like many forms of congenital heart disease, hypoplastic left heart syndrome involves a complex interplay between genetic abnormalities and phenotypic expression (Mu et al., 2005). While no single genetic defect has been identified as a causative factor, 12%–19% of first-degree relatives of children born with hypoplastic left heart syndrome have been reported to have some form of cardiovascular malformation primarily affecting the left side of the heart, with bicuspid aortic valve being the most common reported abnormality (Brenner et al., 1989; Loffredo et al., 2004). Hinton et al. recently studied 38 probands with hypoplastic left heart syndrome, demonstrating a recurrence risk of hypoplastic left heart syndrome in first-degree relatives of 3.5% and of other cardiovascular malformations of 18%, suggesting that heritability plays an important role in the occurrence of hypoplastic left heart syndrome (Hinton, Jr. et al., 2007).

A small but important subset of infants born with hypoplastic left heart syndrome has an identifiable chromosomal abnormality or an extracardiac anomaly. In a review of three large registries of congenital malformations, Harris et al. reported a 4.2% incidence of identifiable chromosomal anomalies in infants with hypoplastic left heart syndrome (Pradat et al., 2003).

Natowicz et al. found a higher percentage of identifiable chromosomal abnormalities or single-gene defects in their hypoplastic left heart syndrome population, reporting a 15% incidence (Natowicz et al., 1988). Of the chromosomal anomalies identified with hypoplastic left heart syndrome, Turner syndrome is the most common (Allen et al., 2005; Jacobs et al., 1998; Natowicz and Kelley, 1987). In contrast to children born with Turner syndrome without hypoplastic left heart syndrome, the combination of the two findings portends a poor prognosis with only 20% survival through the second-stage palliation (Reis et al., 1999). Other chromosomal disorders identified with hypoplastic left heart syndrome include trisomy 13 and 18 (Allen et al., 2005; Tennstedt et al., 1999), trisomy 21 (Allen et al., 2005), Noonan syndrome (Morris et al., 1990), Holt-Oram, Apert, Smith-Lemli-Opitz syndromes (Natowicz et al., 1988), and a variety of chromosomal deletions and translocations (Allen et al., 2005; Consevage et al., 1996; Jacobs et al., 1998; Morris et al., 1990).

Of equal importance is the presence of extracardiac malformations seen with hypoplastic left heart syndrome. Virtually any organ system may be affected, with a reported incidence of extracardiac anomalies of 13%–38% in these patients (Allen et al., 2005; Natowicz et al., 1988; Tennstedt et al., 1999). Extracardiac defects seen with hypoplastic left heart syndrome include facial clefts, diaphragmatic hernia, splenic malformations, and intestinal malrotation. Disorders of the central nervous system, however, are the most prevalent associated anomaly (Pradat et al., 2003). Glauser et al. demonstrated that among infants with hypoplastic left heart syndrome and central nervous system abnormalities, 27% had microcephaly and 21% had an immature cortical mantle (Glauser et al., 1990). The presence of any extracardiac malformation appears to adversely affect the long-term prognosis of these patients (Bove and Lloyd, 1996; Jacobs et al., 1998; Stasik et al., 2006).

CLINICAL PRESENTATION

Prior to the era of surgical palliation, hypoplastic left heart syndrome was a uniformly fatal disease (Roberts et al., 1976; Samanek et al., 1988). Only a few scattered case reports exist of children with hypoplastic left heart syndrome surviving beyond infancy (Noonan and Nadas, 1958; Moodie et al., 1972; Morris et al., 1990). Samanek et al. (1988), in their evaluation of the distribution of age at death in children with congenital heart disease, reported that all 102 infants born with hypoplastic left heart syndrome died by the age of 10 months with the majority (89%) dying before the first month of life. Noonan and Nadas (1958), in

their review of 101 pathologic cases of hypoplastic left heart syndrome, reported that 82% of infants died by 3 months of age.

The majority of infants with hypoplastic left heart syndrome are born at term with an appropriate weight for gestational age (Morris et al., 1990; Rosenthal et al., 1991). However, data from the Baltimore–Washington Infant Study found that infants born with hypoplastic left heart syndrome were more likely than infants born with other forms of congenital heart disease to be small for gestational age, reporting that 20% of infants with hypoplastic left heart syndrome had a birth weight less than the 10th percentile for gestational age (Rosenthal et al., 1991).

Except for those with intact or nearly-intact atrial septum, term infants born with hypoplastic left heart syndrome who do not have extracardiac defects are typically asymptomatic at the time of birth without evidence of respiratory distress or profound cyanosis (Noonan and Nadas, 1958). The onset of symptoms may occur in the first few hours of life, either due to ductal closure or due to the gradual drop in the pulmonary vascular resistance. Infants without a prenatal diagnosis of hypoplastic left heart syndrome may present within the first few hours or days of life, and on rare occasion may present a few weeks after birth (Watson and Rowe, 1962; Morris et al., 1990) with a spectrum of signs and symptoms that range from mild tachypnea to complete circulatory collapse and death. Hypoplastic left heart syndrome may be a challenging diagnosis to make in the immediate newborn period in infants who are initially asymptomatic. Infants typically have a normal respiratory rate and work of breathing, appear vigorous, and lack any obvious cyanosis early after birth (Watson and Rowe, 1962). Physical examination may reveal a prominent right ventricular impulse on palpation of the chest (Watson and Rowe, 1962). The infant should have a normal S1 and a single S2 (Watson and Rowe, 1962). Absence of a murmur is not uncommon, however, at times an infant may have a nonspecific, soft systolic ejection murmur heard best over the left sternal border (Roberts et al., 1976; Sinha et al., 1968; Watson and Rowe, 1962). As the pulmonary vascular resistance drops, the infant may develop signs of pulmonary overcirculation. The infant will at first appear comfortably tachypneic with eventual hepatomegaly, a gallop rhythm, and a diastolic rumble secondary to an increased volume of blood flow across the atrioventricular valve. With progressive impairment of the infant's cardiac output, lactic acidosis develops. Worsening tachypnea is often the first sign of a compensatory mechanism to correct the metabolic acidosis. Infants may have decreased or absent femoral pulses (Sinha et al., 1968; Watson and Rowe, 1962).

The role of the ductus arteriosus in this lesion is often misunderstood. It is important to understand that ductal constriction in the setting of hypoplastic left heart syndrome does not result in increased cyanosis. In lesions that are ductal-dependent for pulmonary blood flow (e.g., pulmonary atresia), ductal constriction reduces pulmonary blood flow, leading to a drop in the measured oxygen saturation and appearance of clinical cyanosis. The reverse scenario occurs in lesions that are ductal-dependant for systemic blood flow, such as hypoplastic left heart syndrome: ductal constriction reduces the amount of blood that crosses the duct from the main pulmonary artery into the systemic circulation, obliging more blood to enter the pulmonary circulation. The result is increased pulmonary blood flow at the expense of the systemic blood flow. Hence, ductal constriction in hypoplastic left heart syndrome results in an increase in the measured oxygen saturation. The clinical appearance of the infant may not reflect this increase in saturation, as the child may not necessarily look pinker, but rather pale, mottled, or even gray, as the systemic blood flow falls to critically low levels. If unrecognized, infants often rapidly progress from a compensated to a decompensated state of shock with profound respiratory distress, hypotension, and acidosis. Tachypnea, dyspnea, tachycardia, hypotension, pallor, and lethargy all precede impending cardiovascular collapse. Auscultation of the heart may reveal a harsh systolic ejection murmur of blood flow through a constricting ductus arteriosus (an uncommon occurrence), and/or a holosystolic murmur consistent with tricuspid valve regurgitation due to progressive right ventricular dilation and dysfunction. A prominent gallop is often appreciated over the apex of the heart, also indicating right ventricular dilation and dysfunction (Watson and Rowe, 1962). Without aggressive cardiopulmonary resuscitative measures, including the initiation of prostaglandin (Yabek and Mann, 1979), the infant will not survive.

Taken in context with the child's physical examination, any of the above findings should alert the practitioner to the potential presence of congenital heart disease. The differential diagnosis includes other forms of ductal-dependent left-sided obstructive lesions (e.g., critical coarctation, critical aortic stenosis). In addition, respiratory distress syndrome, neonatal sepsis, and metabolic disorders can present with symptoms of low cardiac output and acidosis and should be considered in the differential diagnosis during the initial assessment of the child.

DIAGNOSIS

There is no single electrocardiographic finding that is unique to hypoplastic left heart syndrome. A number of nonspecific electrocardiographic abnormalities, including right or northwest QRS axis deviation, right ventricular hypertrophy, right atrial enlargement, and nonspecific ST and T wave abnormalities may be present (Noonan and Nadas, 1958; Watson and Rowe, 1962). Roberts et al. found right ventricular hypertrophy in 46% of patients and diminished left ventricular forces in 36% of patients with hypoplastic left heart syndrome (Roberts et al., 1976).

Radiographic findings are also nonspecific in the presence of hypoplastic left heart syndrome. Patients may show relatively normal cardiac size and normal pulmonary vascularity initially and then progress to considerable cardiomegaly and pulmonary congestion (Sinha et al., 1968; Noonan and Nadas, 1958; Watson and Rowe, 1962). Roberts et al. (1976) demonstrated cardiomegaly in 73% of infants with hypoplastic left heart syndrome and increased pulmonary vascular markings in 68%.

Echocardiography

Echocardiography is the modality of choice for diagnosing hypoplastic left heart syndrome (Bass et al., 1980; Farooki et al., 1976; Suzuki et al., 1982), and typically provides sufficient information to proceed with the Norwood operation (Bash et al., 1986). The transthoracic echocardiogram should include a detailed assessment of the mitral and aortic valve morphology and patency (atresia vs. stenosis). This can be accomplished in the parasternal long axis and apical four-chamber views (Figures 14–3 and 14–4). In some cases of aortic and mitral atresia, the mitral valve, aortic valve, and left ventricle may be so small as to be unidentifiable by two-dimensional echocardiography. In the setting of mitral stenosis, an echo-bright appearance of the left ventricular endocardium is consistent with the presence of endomyocardial fibroelastosis.

The size of the ascending and transverse aorta and aortic isthmus should all be assessed from a high-parasternal and/or suprasternal view. The presence or absence of coarctation of the aorta must be assessed given its frequent association with hypoplastic left heart syndrome (Aiello et al., 1990; Lang et al., 1985; Mahowald et al., 1982). As there is inadequate or absent prograde flow through the aortic valve in hypoplastic left heart syndrome, blood supply to the carotid, subclavian, and coronary arteries must be supplied in a retrograde fashion via the ductus arteriosus. In fact, the presence of retrograde flow in the transverse aortic arch and ascending aorta is one of the hallmarks of aortic atresia and an essential component of the echocardiographic assessment. In the setting of aortic stenosis, the flow pattern in the ascending aorta may be normal rather than retrograde.

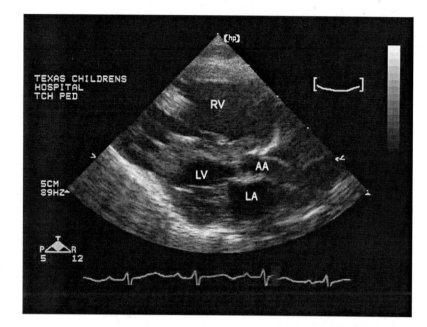

FIGURE 14–3. Two-dimensional echocardiogram, parasternal long axis view of hypoplastic left heart syndrome with aortic and mitral stenosis. Note the hypoplastic ascending aorta (AA) and hypoplastic, nonapex-forming left ventricle (LV). The right ventricle (RV) is severely dilated (LA, left atrium).

From the subcostal view, the adequacy of the interatrial communication should be thoroughly assessed to be certain there is no obstruction to blood flow from the left-to-right atrium. A widely patent interatrial communication with low-velocity flow across the atrial septum is satisfactory for the early postnatal period; however, a mildly restrictive atrial septal defect may be favorable, delaying the progression of pulmonary overcirculation in the infant before their first palliative procedure (Chin et al., 1990). In contrast, a severely restrictive interatrial communication, which prevents adequate egress of blood from the left atrium, is life-threatening and must be readily identified and emergently addressed (Vlahos et al., 2004; Atz et al., 1999). Rychik et al. (1999), in a review of echocardiograms of infants with restrictive atrial septal defects, noted three distinct morphologies described as types A, B, and C (Rychik et al., 1999). Type A included a thick septum secundum and thin septum primum adherent to each other coupled with a large left atrium, type B was a

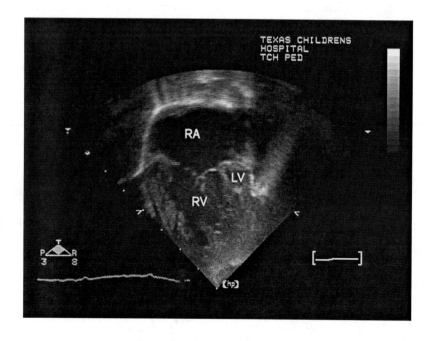

FIGURE 14–4. Two-dimensional echocardiogram, apical four-chamber view of hypoplastic left heart syndrome with severe mitral stenosis. A small remnant of the left ventricle (LV) can be identified. Note the echogenic endocardial layer of the left ventricle consistent with endomyocardial fibroelastosis. The right atrium (RA) and right ventricle (RV) exhibit compensatory enlargement.

thick "spongy" muscular atrial septum without clear distinction between the septum primum and septum secundum with a small muscular left atrium, and type C was a thin septum primum and septum secundum that bulged into the right atrium coupled with a giant left atrium and severe mitral regurgitation. In the presence of an intact or severely restrictive atrial septum, the left atrium should be immediately decompressed by means of a balloon or blade atrial septostomy, or a balloon atrial septoplasty with or without stent placement across the atrial septum (Gossett et al., 2006; Justino et al., 2001; Leonard et al., 2006; Vlahos et al., 2004).

From the apical four-chamber view, the competency of the tricuspid valve is easily evaluated. In one report, over half the patients with hypoplastic left heart syndrome had some degree of tricuspid valve regurgitation (Barber et al., 1988). Finally, not only the size of the ductus arteriosus, but also the pattern of blood flow across the ductus arteriosus must be assessed. The pulmonary vascular resistance will dictate the pattern of flow of blood across the ductus arteriosus which may either be exclusively right-to-left, indicating elevated pulmonary vascular resistance or bidirectional (right-to-left during systole, and left-to- right during diastole), indicating a relatively lower pulmonary vascular resistance. Diastolic flow reversal in the descending thoracic or abdominal aorta may be observed and also indicates a relatively low pulmonary vascular resistance.

Fetal echocardiography can accurately diagnose hypoplastic left heart syndrome, with a positive predictive value of 96%–100% at some centers (Chang et al., 1991; Stumpflen et al., 1996). There is debate surrounding the benefits of prenatal diagnosis of hypoplastic left heart syndrome, with some, but not all, studies demonstrating improved outcomes in infants with a prenatal diagnosis (Kumar et al., 1999; Mahle et al., 2001; Tworetzky et al., 2001). Issues pertaining to the fetal diagnosis of hypoplastic left heart syndrome, in particular the role of fetal intervention, will be discussed later in this chapter.

TREATMENT

Preoperative Management

Following the diagnosis of hypoplastic left heart syndrome, the goal of preoperative care is to maintain ductal patency and ensure adequate systemic end-organ perfusion by achieving a satisfactory balance between the pulmonary and systemic perfusion. The aim is to send the patient for surgical palliation in as optimal a hemodynamic state as can be achieved. This has historically been achieved with the use of intravenous prostaglandin therapy, diuretics, and inotropic support as needed. In the current era, more attention has been directed toward manipulation of the relative resistances of the parallel pulmonary and systemic circulations as a means to optimize cardiac output and limit pulmonary blood flow in the preoperative setting (Nelson et al., 2004). As we shall discuss, a variety of strategies exist to attempt to stabilize the fragile circulation of an infant with hypoplastic left heart syndrome, however, there is a paucity of robust data to favor one management practice over another (Johnson et al., 2008).

Initiation of prostaglandin therapy to maintain patency of the ductus arteriosus should begin shortly after birth, or immediately following diagnosis. In the case of an infant presenting in shock, aggressive resuscitative measures such as mechanical ventilation, fluid resuscitation, and inotropic support should be implemented to treat ventricular dysfunction, augment cardiac output, correct acidosis, and ultimately preserve vital end-organ function. The relentless drop in pulmonary vascular resistance leads to a severely unbalanced circulation that favors pulmonary blood flow at the expense of systemic perfusion. In order to correct this unbalanced circulation, the pulmonary vascular resistance must be increased while the systemic vascular resistance must be decreased. If these maneuvers are successful, the patient's systemic oxygen saturation should drop, ideally into the 80s. Oxygen saturations in the mid 90s may be indicative of excessive pulmonary blood flow, and may be a sign that the ideal balance between pulmonary and systemic vascular resistances has not been achieved. However, it is important to emphasize that the goal of therapy is to maintain adequate organ perfusion and cardiac output. As such, obtaining a given target oxygen saturation should not be regarded as the primary goal. The systemic oxygen saturation should be viewed as only one of many important variables that should be monitored closely, including mixed venous oxygen saturation, pH, lactic acid levels, urine output, etc. Accordingly, some neonates with hypoplastic left heart syndrome may exhibit systemic oxygen saturations in the 90s and yet maintain adequate organ perfusion.

One important caveat in assessing the systemic oxygen saturation in infants with hypoplastic left heart syndrome is the patient with aortic stenosis and a modest amount of prograde flow: such patients may eject enough blood into the ascending aorta to elevate the oxygen saturation measured in the right arm (in the case of a normal arch branching pattern) to close to 100%. In this setting, one will usually detect a significantly lower saturation if the pulse oximetry probe is placed in the left arm or on the foot. In patients such as these pulse oximetry measured in the right arm is misleading and should not be utilized to gauge the relative pulmonary and systemic blood flows.

Mechanisms by which the pulmonary vascular resistance can be raised include mechanical ventilation with administration of sedation and/or neuromuscular blockade, so as to rigidly control ventilation in a manner that allows for permissive hypercapnia via diminished tidal volumes and low ventilatory rates. Another way to raise the pCO_2 is to ventilate the patient with a gas mixture containing 3%–5% CO_2 (Jobes et al., 1992; Mora et al., 1994).

In addition to raising the pCO_2, another possible strategy to raise the pulmonary vascular resistance is to lower the FiO_2 (oxygen being a potent pulmonary vasodilator). Therefore infants with hypoplastic left heart syndrome with signs of pulmonary overcirculation should receive ambient air, and supplemental oxygen should be avoided. Furthermore, a hypoxic gas mixture may be considered to further increase the degree of pulmonary vasoconstriction. This can be achieved by addition of supplemental nitrogen into the inhaled gas mixture, so as to administer subambient oxygen levels (fractional concentration of oxygen of 17%–19%) (Shime et al., 2000). The use of inspired hypoxic (nitrogen) or hypercapnic (carbon dioxide) gas mixtures remains controversial and there are few data addressing their impact on outcomes. Ramamoorthy et al. (2002), in a trial comparing these two alternatives, prospectively demonstrated that although each gaseous mixture resulted in an increase in pulmonary vascular resistance, only 3% inspired carbon dioxide increased cerebral oxygen saturations and increased mean arterial pressure. The long-term effects of these hemodynamic changes have yet to be identified, but the authors suggest that a strategy of supplemental CO_2 confers a better hemodynamic state as compared to hypoxic gas mixture, with potentially improved neuroprotection.

In recent years, the preoperative management strategy has shifted toward manipulation of the systemic vascular resistance rather than the pulmonary vascular resistance. Accordingly, mechanical ventilation to rigidly control pCO_2 and alterations in the inhaled gas mixture are less commonly utilized. Instead, a decrease in the systemic vascular resistance is achieved with systemic arterial vasodilators. At Texas Children's Hospital, milrinone is frequently utilized as an adjunct to prostaglandin and diuretic therapy due to its dual role as both an inotrope and a systemic arterial vasodilator. Although there are abundant published data on the use of milrinone in the postoperative period in children with a variety of cardiac defects, there is scant literature on its use in the preoperative period. Other centers have successfully used sodium nitroprusside or phenoxybenzamine as an alternative means of lowering

systemic vascular resistance in the preoperative setting (Stieh et al., 2006).

Medical stabilization of the critically ill infant with hypoplastic left heart syndrome may be extremely difficult. Ultimately, surgical palliation is necessary and should take place as soon as the infant has been hemodynamically stabilized. Unnecessary delay in surgical therapy should be avoided. There is no consensus as to the ideal age for surgical palliation, however, a number of studies have indicated that older age at Norwood operation (beyond 2–4 weeks) is a risk factor for mortality (Ashburn et al., 2003; Bove, 1998; Mahle et al., 2000a).

Surgical Management

Most medical centers in developed countries currently advocate surgical palliation of hypoplastic left heart syndrome, while some institutions offer neonatal heart transplantation. There is ongoing debate as to which is the best practice (Bailey, 2004; Chrisant, 2004; Elliott, 2004; Jacobs, 2004; Wernovsky). We will predominantly discuss the Norwood procedure and its modifications, as this is the most commonly applied palliative approach.

The Norwood procedure is the first in a series of palliative surgical procedures for hypoplastic left heart syndrome. Following the Norwood procedure, patients typically undergo staged operations toward the Fontan operation. Most centers perform a bidirectional–cavopulmonary anastomosis around the ages of 4–6 months, and culminate with a Fontan operation between the ages of 18 months to 4 years. As the bidirectional–cavopulmonary anastomosis and Fontan procedures will be covered elsewhere in this textbook, we will focus this discussion on the issues unique to this first-stage palliation of hypoplastic left heart syndrome.

The Norwood procedure has undergone a series of technical modifications over the past three decades, although its fundamental principles have not changed. It involves a series of three modifications to the anatomy of the hypoplastic left heart with the goal of achieving balanced pulmonary and systemic circulations. Simply stated, the intent of the Norwood procedure is to accomplish the following: (1) create an unobstructed systemic circulation, (2) ensure a widely patent interatrial communication, and (3) regulate pulmonary blood flow (Figure 14–5).

In order to achieve the first of the three goals described above, namely an unobstructed systemic circulation, the Norwood procedure requires modifying the pulmonary artery in a way that allows the right ventricle to support the systemic circulation. In the presence of a hypoplastic ascending aorta, the surgeon

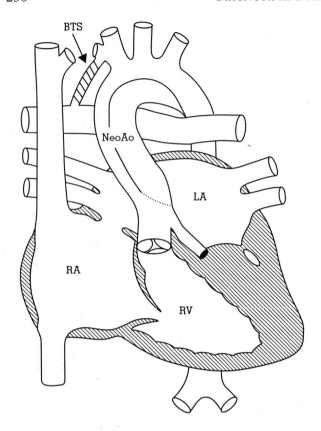

FIGURE 14–5. The Norwood procedure. The "neoaorta" (NeoAo) is an anastomosis of the proximal main pulmonary artery with the ascending and descending aorta, allowing the right ventricle (RV) to support the systemic circulation. The atrial septum has been widely resected, allowing unrestrictive blood flow from the left atrium (LA) to right atrium (RA). A Blalock-Taussig shunt (BTS) regulates pulmonary blood flow. (Adapted from Congenital Heart Disease: A Diagrammatic Atlas, by C.E. Mullins and D.C. Mayer, Copyright 1988 Alan R Liss. This material is reproduced with permission of Wiley-Liss, Inc., a subsidiary of John Wiley & Sons, Inc.)

must create a "neoaorta" by joining the proximal main pulmonary artery and ascending aorta to the descending aorta, allowing unobstructed blood flow from the right ventricle to the systemic circulation and coronary arteries.

Despite multiple modifications of this technique, stenosis of the reconstructed aortic arch remains a well-described complication (Bartram et al., 1997; Helton et al., 1986; Meliones et al., 1990), with an incidence of arch obstruction ranging from 13% to 33% (Bartram et al., 1997; Fraser, Jr. and Mee, 1995; Helton et al., 1986; Meliones et al., 1990; Tworetzky et al., 2000). The etiology of recoarctation may be caused by incomplete resection of the ductal tissue from the native aorta, excessive or redundant patch material, which may fold into the lumen of the neoaorta (Ishino et al., 1999), stenosis caused by suture lines, or stenosis of

the prosthetic portion of the distal end of the reconstructed arch (Bartram et al., 1997). Azakie et al. (2001) reported that the only significant independent factor associated with recoarctation of the neoaorta was an ascending aortic diameter of less than 3 mm. Any residual postoperative coarctation should be aggressively treated given that the increased afterload it places on the right ventricle is deleterious to ventricular function and is associated with increased risk of postoperative mortality (Bartram et al., 1997; Mahle et al., 2000b). Recoarctation may be treated either by transcatheter means (balloon angioplasty with or without stent implantation) or by surgical patch augmentation (Tworetzky et al., 2000).

Other potential complications arising from the reconstructed neoaorta include compression of the left pulmonary artery and left bronchus due to downward tension imposed on these structures by the arch reconstruction (Alboliras et al., 1989). Additionally, patency of both the native ascending aorta and coronary ostia is crucial to allow for unobstructed retrograde blood flow to the right and left coronary arteries. The surgeon must take great care to ensure the neoaortic reconstruction does not impinge upon or kink the native ascending aorta. Bartram et al. (1977) demonstrated that impaired coronary artery perfusion was the number one cause of death in an autopsy series of 122 patients undergoing the Norwood procedure.

The second goal of the Norwood procedure is to ensure creation of a widely patent interatrial communication whereby oxygenated blood returning to the left atrium can freely shunt across to the right atrium. Via a right atrial incision, the surgeon must widely resect the secundum and primum atrial septal tissue to allow for free communication between the atria.

The final goal of the Norwood procedure involves the regulation of pulmonary blood flow. Historically this has been accomplished with the placement of a modified Blalock-Taussig (BT) shunt from the right innominate or proximal right subclavian artery to the proximal right pulmonary artery. The ideal shunt size to allow for adequately balanced systemic and pulmonary blood flow in the Norwood procedure is subject to debate. The current surgical practice is to place polytetrafluoroethylene (PTFE) shunts in the range of 3–4 mm, thereby restricting pulmonary blood flow and reducing the volume load on the right ventricle. Most centers advocate for a weight-based approach for selection of shunt size (Krasemann et al., 2005; Pearl et al., 2002), although other factors such as patient age greater than 1 month (Bove, 1998), or the presence of preoperative risk factors for the development of elevated pulmonary vascular resistance (Pearl et al., 2002; Tweddell et al., 2000) may necessitate the use of a larger shunt size. In addition to shunt diameter, the length can also be modified to further control pulmonary blood flow. Survival after the Norwood procedure in the early to mid-1980s may have been adversely affected by the excessive pulmonary blood flow due to relatively oversized BT shunts compared to current standards (Bartram et al., 1997). Despite recent trends toward smaller BT shunts, data on the relationship between shunt size and survival remain elusive. Tweddell reported that a larger shunt size indexed to body surface area, by univariate analysis, was a risk factor against survival to second-stage palliation (Tweddell et al., 2002), however, other studies have not shown such an association (Azakie et al., 2001; Krasemann et al., 2005). Other complications universal to the BT shunt include, issues related to diminished pulmonary blood flow, such as kinking of the shunt or shunt thrombosis. A trade-off exists: smaller shunt size may avoid pulmonary overcirculation, but may lead to an increased risk of shunt thrombosis (Bartram et al., 1997).

The physiology of a BT shunt (with continuous pulmonary blood flow during both systole and diastole) leads to a series of physiologic consequences. First, continuous flow across the BT shunt throughout the cardiac cycle may result in excessive pulmonary blood flow, which imposes an excessive volume load on the single right ventricle. Second, diastolic flow across the shunt results in lower aortic diastolic pressures (and thus a wide pulse pressure), resulting in a "steal" of blood flow from the systemic circulation during diastole. The phenomenon of systemic steal may result in inadequate tissue perfusion to all systemic vascular beds, but most importantly, to the coronary circulation, which is predominantly perfused in diastole. In combination, these factors may be deleterious to the function of the systemic right ventricle: the volume-loaded ventricle has increased workload (and thus increased myocardial oxygen consumption) and yet may have impaired myocardial perfusion. The Sano modification was devised in order to provide a theoretically more stable circulation thus minimizing the potential for the complications associated with a BT shunt (Sano et al., 2003, 2004). Although this remains an institution-specific preference, the Sano modification has received increasing recognition as an important evolution in the Norwood procedure.

First described by Sano in 2003 (Sano et al., 2003), this most recent surgical modification to the Norwood procedure alters the source of pulmonary blood flow, while the other components of the Norwood procedure (aortic arch reconstruction and atrial septectomy) remain essentially unchanged. The fundamental difference is that the BT shunt is replaced by a 4–6 mm nonvalved right ventricle to pulmonary artery conduit. The procedure requires a small 5–10 mm ventriculotomy just below the pulmonary valve where the proximal end of the conduit is anastomosed. The distal end of the conduit is then placed anterior and leftward of the neoaorta and anastomosed to the distal main pulmonary artery or proximal left pulmonary artery. Pulmonary blood flow is maintained during systole only, thus eliminating diastolic runoff into the pulmonary artery.

Proponents of this modification report that the benefit of this change in the postoperative physiology relates directly to the creation of a more stable circulation through the avoidance of diastolic runoff into the pulmonary arteries, thereby preventing the phenomenon of systemic "steal." The resultant increase in diastolic blood pressure improves systemic circulation and coronary artery perfusion, and reduces the volume load on the right ventricle thus potentially improving ventricular function (Sano et al., 2003, 2004). Hughes et al. (2004), with the use of strain Doppler echocardiography, demonstrated that despite the need for a ventriculotomy, there was improved ventricular longitudinal systolic contractility in hypoplastic left heart syndrome patients palliated with a right ventricle to pulmonary artery conduit over those with a BT shunt. Some centers have reported improved hospital and interstage survival with the use of a right ventricle to pulmonary artery conduit over the use of a BT shunt, demonstrating a statistically significant rise in the postoperative diastolic blood pressures and lower Qp:Qs ratio at follow-up catheterization (Mair et al., 2003; Malec et al., 2003). One criticism of these data, however, is that they involve comparisons between patients palliated in different eras. The results of more contemporary studies have been at odds with these findings. Nonrandomized, single-center studies comparing simultaneous outcomes of Norwood patients with a BT shunt versus right ventricle to pulmonary artery conduit have shown equivalent survival results (Bradley et al., 2004; Ghanayem et al., 2006; Mahle et al., 2003; Tabbutt et al., 2005). Despite a significantly higher diastolic blood pressure in patients undergoing the Sano modification, there did not appear to be demonstrable postoperative differences in patient hemodynamic stability (Bradley et al., 2004; Ghanayem et al., 2006; Tabbutt et al., 2005), oxygen delivery (Bradley et al., 2004; Ghanayem et al., 2006; Tabbutt et al., 2005), or Qp:Qs (Ghanayem et al., 2006; Mahle et al., 2003). Cua et al. (2006), in their comparison of the two groups, did show that patients who had the Sano modification had a shorter time to sternal closure, fewer days of mechanical ventilation, shorter intensive care unit stay, and shorter time to establishment of feeding, indirect evidence suggesting that this modification may potentially lead to more favorable postoperative hemodynamics. However, they too failed to show a statistical difference in hospital or interstage mortality. In the face of these conflicting data on the postoperative condition of these patients, some centers will reserve the Sano modification for low-birth-weight infants. Sano et al. (2004) reported successful palliation with this surgical technique in 5 of 6 infants weighing less than 2 kg. Beyond the potential hemodynamic benefits, the Sano modification also carries certain unique risks, including aneurysm formation at the site of the ventriculotomy (Mahle et al., 2003), progressive and early cyanosis requiring earlier promotion to stage II palliation (Cua et al., 2006; Sano et al., 2004; Tabbutt et al., 2005), a higher incidence of reoperation due to the need for conduit revisions (Tabbutt et al., 2005), and impaired growth of the pulmonary arteries (Sano et al., 2004). At present, it remains unclear whether the standard Norwood or the Sano modification should be considered the preferred approach. The Single Ventricle Reconstruction Trial, a multicenter randomized clinical trial, is currently underway; until this and other large, prospective, randomized trials are performed, it is too early to determine if one approach is superior to the other.

Alternative Treatment Options

Two additional treatment options, though less widely utilized, are available to infants born with hypoplastic left heart syndrome. The first is a combined surgical and transcatheter approach to establish the first stage of a palliated circulation, sometimes referred to as a "hybrid" Norwood procedure. The second is neonatal cardiac transplantation.

The combination of surgical and transcatheter techniques to palliate infants with hypoplastic left heart syndrome was first reported by Gibbs et al. (1993) as an alternative to the traditional Norwood surgical palliation (Figure 14–6). This treatment approach, which we will refer to as the "hybrid" Norwood procedure, involves two main components (Akintuerk et al., 2002; Gibbs et al., 1993; Lim et al., 2006). The transcatheter component includes placement of a ductal stent to maintain its patency, and, if necessary, widening the interatrial communication via either a balloon, or blade atrial septostomy, or with placement of an intravascular stent across the atrial septum. The second step involves surgical banding of both pulmonary arteries to regulate pulmonary blood flow. Recently, Chan et al. (2006) reported successful use of a new experimental intravascular pulmonary artery band, allowing for the procedure to be performed without surgical intervention. Unlike the standard Norwood operation, the hybrid approach possesses the unique benefits of avoiding cardiopulmonary bypass and hypothermic circulatory arrest. Following a hybrid procedure, infants may

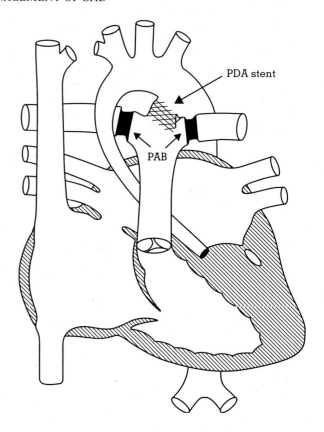

FIGURE 14–6. The "hybrid" Norwood procedure. Note the stent in the patent ductus arteriosus (PDA stent) to maintain its patency, and bilateral pulmonary artery banding (PAB) to regulate pulmonary blood flow. (Adapted from Congenital Heart Disease: A Diagrammatic Atlas, by C.E. Mullins and D.C. Mayer, Copyright 1988 Alan R Liss. This material is reproduced with permission of Wiley-Liss, Inc., a subsidiary of John Wiley & Sons, Inc.)

be promoted on a similar timetable as those treated with the standard Norwood procedure to a bidirectional cavopulmonary anastomosis around the age of 4–6 months. However, the benefits of avoiding cardiopulmonary bypass and hypothermic circulatory arrest at the initial palliation may be mitigated by the much greater complexity of the second stage of palliation, which requires not only the arch reconstruction of the Norwood procedure but also the excision of the ductal stent, followed by creation of the bidirectional cavopulmonary anastomosis. Currently, a relatively small number of patients have been treated with this hybrid strategy. Short-term data point to its successful application as the first-stage palliative procedure for both low- and high-risk infants with hypoplastic left heart syndrome (Akinturk et al., 2007; Lim et al., 2006). At present, there are insufficient data comparing outcomes between the hybrid and the Norwood procedures.

Pediatric cardiac transplantation is a remarkably successful, albeit limited, therapeutic option for infants born with hypoplastic left heart syndrome (Chiavarelli et al., 1993). Since his first report of a neonatal cardiac xenotransplantation (Bailey et al., 1985), Bailey has been a strong proponent of infant cardiac transplantation for this condition (Bailey, 2004). Unfortunately, cardiac transplantation as a primary means of therapy is limited by the paucity of available donors. Accordingly, a large proportion of deaths occur while infants wait for a suitable organ (Chiavarelli et al., 1993; Chrisant et al., 2005). Infants historically have been maintained on intravenous prostaglandin while awaiting heart transplantation, but the hybrid procedure has also been utilized as a bridge to cardiac transplantation, allowing the pulmonary vasculature to remain protected until an organ becomes available (Akinturk et al., 2007; Chan et al., 2006; Michel-Behnke et al., 2003; Mitchell et al., 2003). Cardiac transplantation is the only means of restoring a biventricular circulation in these infants; however, it is far from being considered a "cure" as recipients of heart transplantation face lifelong immunosuppression, vigilance for organ rejection, and the possibility of repeat organ transplantation due to graft failure.

POSTOPERATIVE MANAGEMENT

The postoperative management of infants following the Norwood procedure has evolved in parallel with surgical advances and should be credited with playing a significant role in improved outcomes. Without question, the first 24–48 hours of a Norwood patient's postoperative care is a uniquely challenging endeavor that requires extensive cardiovascular intensive care expertise, advanced monitoring, and a multidisciplinary team that understands the unique physiology of this surgical palliation. Similar to preoperative management strategies, recognition of the patient's parallel circulations and the interplay between pulmonary (Qp) and systemic (Qs) blood flow is paramount, with the goal of avoiding excessive pulmonary blood flow while maximizing cardiac function and systemic oxygen delivery (Barnea et al., 1994; De Oliveira et al., 2004; De Oliveira and Van Arsdell, 2004; Li et al., 2007; Pearl et al., 2002; Tweddell et al., 1999, 2000). Numerous postoperative issues require meticulous attention including selection of appropriate inotropic agents to improve the contractile performance of the single right ventricle, mechanical ventilation strategies, monitoring of end-organ function, and provision of adequate sedation and pain control. Importantly, the immediate postoperative care of the patient who has undergone a Norwood operation should focus on manipulation of the respective pulmonary and systemic vascular resistances. Lowering the Qp:Qs ratio

(i.e., preferentially limiting pulmonary blood flow while raising systemic blood flow) will improve cardiac output and the delivery of oxygen to end-organs. It would appear that this is more readily accomplished by decreasing the systemic vascular resistance through the use of intravenous afterload-reducing agents such as phenoxybenzamine, sodium nitroprusside, or milrinone, as opposed to raising the pulmonary vascular resistance via manipulations in mechanical ventilation (Hoffman et al., 2004; Pearl et al., 2002; Tweddell et al., 1999). Li et al. (2007) demonstrated, in a cohort of 14 postoperative patients who had undergone the Norwood operation, that despite dramatic changes in individual hemodynamics and oxygen transport during the first few postoperative days, the balance of Qp/Qs and therefore delivery of oxygen was best achieved by lowering systemic vascular resistance, lowering oxygen consumption rates, and ensuring higher hemoglobin levels. Interestingly, changes in the pulmonary vascular resistance had little effect on the balance between Qp and Qs. The authors expounded a postoperative management strategy that is followed in many surgical centers: optimize the systemic vascular resistance, limit pulmonary blood flow, ensure an appropriate hemoglobin level, and minimize factors that increase oxygen consumption.

Many of the finer details related to postoperative management of the Norwood operation remain institution specific, with each center espousing different strategies with regard to the timing of chest closure, medication selection, ventilator management, and feeding. Important areas of ongoing research pertaining to postoperative care include monitoring techniques such as continuous mixed venous oxygen sampling and near-infrared spectroscopy (NIRS), and clarification of the role of early mechanical support such as extracorporeal membrane oxygenation (ECMO) and ventricular assist devices.

OUTCOMES

The past three decades have demonstrated dramatic improvements in the short- and intermediate-term survival of patients born with hypoplastic left heart syndrome. The literature commonly refers to different eras of success in regard to outcomes following surgical palliation. In the early years of the Norwood procedure, reported survival to hospital discharge was poor, ranging between 21% and 56%, with the majority of deaths occurring during the first 24–48 hours postoperatively (Mahle et al., 2000b; Meliones et al., 1990). In the current era, however, institutions report a marked improvement in survival to hospital discharge, ranging between 64% and 90% (Ashburn et al., 2003; Stasik et al., 2006). Azakie reported data from Toronto's Hospital for Sick Children on overall survival for infants undergoing the Norwood procedure during the 1990s (Azakie et al., 2001). Although they reported an overall survival at 1 month of 59%, when stratified into different eras, the survival clearly improved during the latter years, from 43% between 1990 and 1993, to 80% between 1998 and 2000. Similar findings were reported by Tweddell from Wisconsin (Tweddell et al., 2002) who demonstrated a dramatic rise in survival to hospital discharge from 53% between 1992 and 1996, to 93% after 1996. Mahle from the Children's Hospital of Philadelphia (Mahle et al., 2000b) also reported an improvement in short-term survival during the 1990s, from 71% between 1995 and 1998, to 77% after 1998. An additional consistent finding in a number of studies is that the attrition rate is much lower once infants are transitioned to a cavopulmonary circulation (Ashburn et al., 2003; Forbess et al., 1997; Jonas, 1991). The majority of the mortality, regardless of era or institution, occurs primarily between the first and second stage of repair (Ashburn et al., 2003).

The greatly improved overall survival seen in this patient population has resulted in an increased interest in identifying which patient characteristics continue to portend a poor prognosis. The anatomic subtype of hypoplastic left heart syndrome had been considered an important predictor of outcome, with aortic atresia/mitral atresia reportedly having a worse prognosis than aortic stenosis/mitral stenosis (Jonas et al., 1994), although more recent reports have generally not supported this finding (Azakie et al., 2001; Mahle et al., 2000b; Murdison et al., 1990; Stasik et al., 2006). Other anatomic risk factors, such as a small ascending aorta (Poirier et al., 2000; Ashburn et al., 2003) and the presence of a restrictive or intact atrial septum (Daebritz et al., 2000; Photiadis et al., 2005; Rychik et al., 1999) have also been considered to herald a poorer prognosis. Moderate-to-severe tricuspid regurgitation may also negatively impact the outcomes of the infant following the Norwood procedure (Barber et al., 1988) and if severe, may require surgical repair (Ohye et al., 2004). As mentioned above, chromosomal defects (Glauser et al., 1990) or extracardiac congenital anomalies (Bove and Lloyd, 1996; Jacobs et al., 1998; Stasik et al., 2006) are associated with a worse prognosis. In addition, there is mounting evidence that premature infants (Elliott, 2004) and/or infants weighing less than 2.5 kg (Ashburn et al., 2003; Artrip et al., 2006; Jacobs et al., 1998; Krasemann et al., 2005; Mahle et al., 2000b; Stasik et al., 2006) have significantly higher mortality rates. Nonetheless, a birth weight of 2.5 kg or less, in isolation, should not be considered a contraindication to surgical palliation (Weinstein et al., 1999).

A number of single-institution studies have published conflicting data in regard to the significance of preoperative conditions such as age at time of surgery, need for mechanical ventilation or inotropic support, acidosis and organ dysfunction and the risk they pose for negative outcomes (Ashburn et al., 2003; Kern et al., 1997; Mahle et al., 2000b; Stasik et al., 2006; Tweddell et al., 2000). To date, no consensus has been reached on the relative importance of each of these factors. However, it appears reasonable to surmise that the outcomes from surgical palliation are likely to be superior if the patient's preoperative hemodynamic condition can be improved, and in particular, if cardiogenic shock can be avoided. Hence, one might hypothesize that a prompt diagnosis may mitigate the need for invasive preoperative support. Given that hypoplastic left heart syndrome frequently presents with cardiovascular collapse in the first week of life due to delayed postnatal diagnosis, one might postulate that prenatal diagnosis of hypoplastic left heart syndrome by means of fetal echocardiography could improve survival by allowing appropriate medical care to be provided to affected infants immediately after birth, thereby averting the relentless downward spiral that culminates in cardiogenic shock. In that regard, literature reports are conflicting, and a survival benefit to those patients prenatally diagnosed has not consistently been demonstrated (Kumar et al., 1999; Mahle et al., 2001; Stieh et al., 2006; Tworetzky et al., 2001; Vida et al., 2007).

Despite improvements in preoperative, intraoperative, and postoperative care, there is an important ongoing attrition among patients affected with hypoplastic left heart syndrome, and long-term survival rates are sobering. This is true for those recipients of all varieties of surgical palliations as well as for heart transplant recipients. The Pediatric Heart Transplantation Study Group reported a 5-year survival of 72% for infants born with hypoplastic left heart syndrome who underwent successful transplantation (Chrisant et al., 2005). Of great importance is the observation that in this same cohort of patients, 25% died while awaiting transplantation, such that the 5-year survival of the total number of infants with hypoplastic left heart syndrome listed for transplantation was 54%. In a multi-institutional study, Jacobs reported that the 3-year survival rate of infants who are designated for transplantation as compared to those treated with surgical palliation did not significantly differ, and approached 50% in both groups (Jacobs et al., 1998). Artrip showed similar short-term survival outcomes when comparing the two groups (Artrip et al., 2006). A clear distinction between the two treatment options, however, is that infants who are successfully transplanted under favorable conditions (i.e., within the first 30 days of life) and survive beyond the first month posttransplantation, have a remarkable 5-year survival rate that approaches 85% (Chiavarelli et al., 1993; Chrisant et al., 2005; Gandhi et al., 2007).

With improving short and intermediate term outcomes, attention has begun to shift toward long-term survival characteristics and neurodevelopmental outcomes of patients born with hypoplastic left heart syndrome (Goldberg et al., 2000; Mahle et al., 2000a; Rychik, 2005). A thorough discussion of this important topic will be covered in a separate chapter.

FUTURE DIRECTIONS

The next challenge in the continual quest to improve the survival and quality of life for patients with hypoplastic left heart syndrome is perhaps to prevent altogether the development of left ventricular hypoplasia sufficiently early in gestation. A subset of infants born with hypoplastic left heart syndrome have a normally developed left ventricle during the second and into the third trimester of fetal life before eventual regression in its size (Hornberger et al., 1995; McCaffrey and Sherman, 1997; Trines and Hornberger, 2004). This raises the hypothesis that at least a subset of patients do not develop early hypoplasia of the left ventricle as a result of failed embryogenesis, but rather evolve into left ventricular dysfunction and eventual hypoplasia due to the deleterious hemodynamic effects of preexisting aortic stenosis (Hornberger et al., 1995; McCaffrey and Sherman, 1997; Trines and Hornberger, 2004). A number of studies have evaluated fetal anatomic and hemodynamic features with the aim of predicting which fetuses will go on to develop a normal left ventricle and which will demonstrate left ventricular hypoplasia (Trines and Hornberger, 2004; Makikallio et al., 2006). Makikallio et al. (2006) demonstrated that following an initial fetal diagnosis of aortic stenosis with a normal left ventricle, physiologic observations such as retrograde blood flow in the transverse aortic arch, left-to-right flow across the foramen ovale, monophasic mitral inflow, and significant left ventricular dysfunction were all findings highly specific for progression to hypoplastic left heart syndrome. They found that anatomic features such as aortic valve and mitral valve size were not as useful in predicting the progression towards hypoplastic left heart syndrome.

The recent application of fetal cardiac interventional techniques to attempt to alter the pathologic evolution of aortic stenosis into hypoplastic left heart syndrome is a highly controversial subject (Kleinman, 2006). Fetal aortic balloon valvuloplasty may be applied to salvage fetuses with severely dilated and dysfunctional left ventricles with evidence of hydrops, as well as in fetuses without evidence of hydrops but in whom the aortic stenosis is of sufficient severity to presumably result in progression into hypoplastic left heart syndrome (Kohl et al., 2000; Tworetzky et al., 2004; Makikallio et al., 2006). The proportion of fetuses who receive a fetal aortic valvuloplasty that ultimately achieve a biventricular circulation remains unknown at this time. Although the procedural risk to the fetus and mother appears low, the procedure may not necessarily result in a biventricular circulation; hence those factors must be weighed against the improving outcomes of single-ventricle palliation. A separate chapter will elaborate on the current status of fetal interventions and their role in patient management in the current era.

End-of-Life Care

A final consideration should be discussed in regard to infants born with hypoplastic left heart syndrome. Despite improved treatment success, a significant number of pregnancies with affected fetuses end in elective termination following a fetal diagnosis, although rates vary widely in different countries (Elliott, 2004). Other families choose to deliver the affected infant but provide only end-of-life comfort care after birth (Vandvik and Forde, 2000), although it appears that the proportion of families who choose this option is steadily decreasing in the United States (Chang et al., 2002). Families with a fetus or infant diagnosed with hypoplastic left heart syndrome deserve honest, open dialogue and the support of their caregivers when they are grieving the news of this diagnosis while contending with the immensely complicated medical decisions regarding the variety of treatment options before them. In that regard, there are limited, but compelling data on the role of the caregiver in the decision-making process of affected families, suggesting that physicians do not consistently offer all management options to families affected with a child with hypoplastic left heart syndrome. This may occur for a variety of reasons, including the referral patterns and the availability of certain treatment strategies within the physicians' own institutions (Kon et al., 2004). Furthermore, the role of physicians in influencing the choice of treatment strategies by affected families appeared to be highly dependent on the specialty of the physician, with surgeons being most directive in their counseling of families (Kon, 2004). Sadly, few studies have addressed the anguish that parents face when having to make treatment decisions for their infant with hypoplastic left heart syndrome. In a published report, parents who chose to only provide end-of-life comfort care to their affected infant did so in effort to avoid what they perceived to be lifelong suffering for their child, while those who opted for surgical palliation did so because they perceived this to be the only acceptable option (Vandvik and Forde, 2000). The critical state of the infant coupled with the need to make a rapid decision within the first few hours or days of life place the parents in a harrowing emotional state. Caregivers should accordingly strive to provide abundant compassion and empathy, while counseling families as accurately as possible by portraying realistic expectations of outcomes.

CONCLUSION

Hypoplastic left heart syndrome represents a broad spectrum of anatomic abnormalities involving underdevelopment of the mitral valve, left ventricle, aortic valve, and aorta, with the salient feature being the inability of the left-sided heart structures to support the systemic circulation. In the last three decades, a remarkable evolution in medical and surgical management approaches has resulted in a dramatic improvement in the survival of those afflicted with this condition. Still, the survival rates are comparatively poor in relation to those conditions amenable to biventricular repair strategies, hence the need for ongoing research. Large-scale studies are needed to identify the role of a number of exciting innovations in the care of these children, such as the Sano modification, hybrid Norwood procedure, improved perioperative myocardial and cerebral protection strategies, and fetal interventional strategies.

REFERENCES

Aiello VD, Ho SY, Anderson RH, Thiene G. Morphologic features of the hypoplastic left heart syndrome—a reappraisal. *Pediatr Pathol.* 1990;10:931–943.

Akintuerk H, Michel-Behnke I, Valeske K, et al. Stenting of the arterial duct and banding of the pulmonary arteries: basis for combined Norwood stage I and II repair in hypoplastic left heart. *Circulation.* 2002;105:1099–1103.

Akinturk H, Michel-Behnke I, Valeske K, et al. Hybrid transcatheter-surgical palliation: basis for univentricular or biventricular repair: the Giessen experience. *Pediatr Cardiol.* 2007;28:79–87.

Alboliras ET, Chin AJ, Barber G, Helton JG, Pigott JD, Norwood WI. Pulmonary artery configuration after palliative operations for hypoplastic left heart syndrome. *J Thorac Cardiovasc Surg.* 1989;97:878–885.

Allen RH, Benson CB, Haug LW. Pregnancy outcome of fetuses with a diagnosis of hypoplastic left ventricle on prenatal sonography. *J Ultrasound Med.* 2005;24:1199–1203.

Anderson RH, Smith A, Cook AC. Hypoplasia of the left heart. *Cardiol Young.* 2004;14(suppl 1):13–21.

Artrip JH, Campbell DN, Ivy DD, et al. Birth weight and complexity are significant factors for the management of hypoplastic left heart syndrome. *Ann Thorac Surg.* 2006;82:1252–1257.

Ashburn DA, McCrindle BW, Tchervenkov CI, et al. Outcomes after the Norwood operation in neonates with critical aortic stenosis or aortic valve atresia. *J Thorac Cardiovasc Surg.* 2003;125:1070–1082.

Atz AM, Feinstein JA, Jonas RA, Perry SB, Wessel DL. Preoperative management of pulmonary venous hypertension in hypoplastic left heart syndrome with restrictive atrial septal defect. *Am J Cardiol.* 1999;83:1224–1228.

Azakie A, Merklinger SL, McCrindle BW, et al. Evolving strategies and improving outcomes of the modified Norwood procedure: a 10-year single-institution experience. *Ann Thorac Surg.* 2001;72:1349–1353.

Bailey LL. Transplantation is the best treatment for hypoplastic left heart syndrome. *Cardiol Young.* 2004;14 Suppl 1:109–111.

Bailey LL, Nehlsen-Cannarella SL, Concepcion W, Jolley WB. Baboon-to-human cardiac xenotransplantation in a neonate. *JAMA.* 1985;254:3321–3329.

Barber G, Helton JG, Aglira BA, et al. The significance of tricuspid regurgitation in hypoplastic left-heart syndrome. *Am Heart J.* 1988;116:1563–1567.

Barnea O, Austin EH, Richman B, Santamore WP. Balancing the circulation: theoretic optimization of pulmonary/systemic flow ratio in hypoplastic left heart syndrome. *J Am Coll Cardiol.* 1994;24:1376–1381.

Bartram U, Grunenfelder J, Van PR. Causes of death after the modified Norwood procedure: a study of 122 postmortem cases. *Ann Thorac Surg.* 1997;64:1795–1802.

Bash SE, Huhta JC, Vick GW, III, Gutgesell HP, Ott DA. Hypoplastic left heart syndrome: is echocardiography accurate enough to guide surgical palliation? *J Am Coll Cardiol.* 1986;7:610–616.

Bass JL, Ben-Shachar G, Edwards JE. Comparison of M mode echocardiography and pathologic findings in the hypoplastic left heart syndrome. *Am J Cardiol.* 1980;45:79–86.

Bharati S, Lev M. The surgical anatomy of hypoplasia of aortic tract complex. *J Thorac Cardiovasc Surg.* 1984;88:97–101.

Bove EL. Current status of staged reconstruction for hypoplastic left heart syndrome. *Pediatr Cardiol.* 1998;19:308–315.

Bove EL, Lloyd TR. Staged reconstruction for hypoplastic left heart syndrome. Contemporary results. *Ann Surg.* 1996;224:387–394.

Bradley SM, Simsic JM, McQuinn TC, Habib DM, Shirali GS, Atz AM. Hemodynamic status after the Norwood procedure: a comparison of right ventricle-to-pulmonary artery connection versus modified Blalock-Taussig shunt. *Ann Thorac Surg.* 2004;78:933–941.

Brenner JI, Berg KA, Schneider DS, Clark EB, Boughman JA. Cardiac malformations in relatives of infants with hypoplastic left-heart syndrome. *Am J Dis Child.* 1989;143:1492–1494.

Carlgren LE, Ericson A, Kallen B. Monitoring of congenital cardiac defects. *Pediatr Cardiol.* 1987;8:247–256.

Chan KC, Mashburn C, Boucek MM. Initial transcatheter palliation of hypoplastic left heart syndrome. *Catheter Cardiovasc Interv.* 2006;68:719–726.

Chang AC, Huhta JC, Yoon GY, et al. Diagnosis, transport, and outcome in fetuses with left ventricular outflow tract obstruction. *J Thorac Cardiovasc Surg.* 1991;102:841–848.

Chang RK, Chen AY, Klitzner TS. Clinical management of infants with hypoplastic left heart syndrome in the United States, 1988–1997. *Pediatrics.* 2002;110:292–298.

Chiavarelli M, Gundry SR, Razzouk AJ, Bailey LL. Cardiac transplantation for infants with hypoplastic left-heart syndrome. *JAMA.* 1993;270:2944–2947.

Chin AJ, Weinberg PM, Barber G. Subcostal two-dimensional echocardiographic identification of anomalous attachment of septum primum in patients with left atrioventricular valve underdevelopment. *J Am Coll Cardiol.* 1990;15:678–681.

Chrisant MR, Naftel DC, Drummond-Webb J, et al. Fate of infants with hypoplastic left heart syndrome listed for cardiac transplantation: a multicenter study. *J Heart Lung Transplant.* 2005;24:576–582.

Consevage MW, Seip JR, Belchis DA, Davis AT, Baylen BG, Rogan PK. Association of a mosaic chromosomal 22q11 deletion with hypoplastic left heart syndrome. *Am J Cardiol.* 1996;77:1023–1025.

Croen LA, Shaw GM, Jensvold NG, Harris JA. Birth defects monitoring in California: a resource for epidemiological research. *Paediatr Perinat Epidemiol.* 1991;5:423–427.

Cua CL, Thiagarajan RR, Gauvreau K, et al. Early postoperative outcomes in a series of infants with hypoplastic left heart syndrome undergoing stage I palliation operation with either modified Blalock-Taussig shunt or right ventricle to pulmonary artery conduit. *Pediatr Crit Care Med.* 2006;7:238–244.

Daebritz SH, Nollert GD, Zurakowski D, et al. Results of Norwood stage I operation: comparison of hypoplastic left heart syndrome with other malformations. *J Thorac Cardiovasc Surg.* 2000;119:358–367.

De Oliveira NC, Ashburn DA, Khalid F, et al. Prevention of early sudden circulatory collapse after the Norwood operation. *Circulation.* 2004;110:II133–II138.

De Oliveira NC, Van Arsdell GS. Practical use of alpha blockade strategy in the management of hypoplastic left heart syndrome following stage one palliation with a Blalock-Taussig shunt. *Semin Thorac Cardiovasc Surg Pediatr Card Surg Annu.* 2004;7:11–15.

Doty DB, Marvin WJ Jr, Schieken RM, Lauer RM. Hypoplastic left heart syndrome: successful palliation with a new operation. *J Thorac Cardiovasc Surg.* 1980;80:148–152.

Elliott MJ. A European perspective on the management of hypoplastic left heart syndrome. *Cardiol Young.* 2004;14(suppl 1):41–46.

Elzenga NJ, Gittenberger-de Groot AC. Coarctation and related aortic arch anomalies in hypoplastic left heart syndrome. *Int J Cardiol.* 1985;8:379–393.

Farooki ZQ, Henry JG, Green EW. Echocardiographic spectrum of the hypoplastic left heart syndrome: a clinicopathologic correlation in 19 newborns. *Am J Cardiol.* 1976;38:337–343.

Ferencz C, Rubin JD, McCarter RJ, et al. Congenital heart disease: prevalence at livebirth. The Baltimore-Washington Infant Study. *Am J Epidemiol.* 1985;121:31–36.

Fixler DE, Pastor P, Sigman E, Eifler CW. Ethnicity and socioeconomic status: impact on the diagnosis of congenital heart disease. *J Am Coll Cardiol.* 1993;21:1722–1726.

Forbess JM, Cook N, Serraf A, Burke RP, Mayer JE Jr, Jonas RA. An institutional experience with second- and third-stage palliative procedures for hypoplastic left heart syndrome: the impact of the bidirectional cavopulmonary shunt. *J Am Coll Cardiol.* 1997;29:665–670.

Fraser CD Jr, Mee RB. Modified Norwood procedure for hypoplastic left heart syndrome. *Ann Thorac Surg.* 1995;60:S546–S549.

Freedom RM, Culham JA, Rowe RD. Aortic atresia with normal left ventricle distinctive angiocardiographic findings. *Cathet Cardiovasc Diagn.* 1977;3:283–295.

Fyler DC. Report of the New England Regional Infant Cardiac Program. *Pediatrics.* 1980;65:375–461.

Gandhi SK, Canter CE, Kulikowska A, Huddleston CB. Infant heart transplantation ten years later—where are they now? *Ann Thorac Surg.* 2007;83:169–172.

Ghanayem NS, Jaquiss RD, Cava JR. Right ventricle-to-pulmonary artery conduit versus Blalock-Taussig shunt: a hemodynamic comparison. *Ann Thorac Surg.* 2006;82:1603–1609.

Gibbs JL, Wren C, Watterson KG, Hunter S, Hamilton JR. Stenting of the arterial duct combined with banding of the pulmonary arteries and atrial septectomy or septostomy: a new approach to palliation for the hypoplastic left heart syndrome. *Br Heart J.* 1993;69:551–555.

Gillum RF. Epidemiology of congenital heart disease in the United States. *Am Heart J.* 1994;127:919–927.

Glauser TA, Rorke LB, Weinberg PM, Clancy RR. Congenital brain anomalies associated with the hypoplastic left heart syndrome. *Pediatrics.* 1990;85:984–990.

Goldberg CS, Schwartz EM, Brunberg JA, et al. Neurodevelopmental outcome of patients after the fontan operation: a comparison between children with hypoplastic left heart syndrome and other functional single ventricle lesions. *J Pediatr.* 2000;137:646–652.

Gossett JG, Rocchini AP, Lloyd TR, Graziano JN. Catheter-based decompression of the left atrium in patients with hypoplastic left heart syndrome and restrictive atrial septum is safe and effective. *Catheter Cardiovasc Interv.* 2006;67:619–624.

Hastreiter AR, van der Horst RL, DuBrow IW, Eckner FO. Quantitative angiographic and morphologic aspects of aortic valve atresia. *Am J Cardiol.* 1983;51:1705–1708.

Hastreiter AR, van der Horst RL, Sepehri B, DuBrow IW, Fisher EA, Levitsky S. Prostaglandin E1 infusion in newborns with hypoplastic left ventricle and aortic atresia. *Pediatr Cardiol.* 1982;2:95–98.

Helton JG, Aglira BA, Chin AJ, Murphy JD, Pigott JD, Norwood WI. Analysis of potential anatomic or physiologic determinants of outcome of palliative surgery for hypoplastic left heart syndrome. *Circulation.* 1986;74:I70–I76.

Hinton RB Jr, Martin LJ, Tabangin ME, Mazwi ML, Cripe LH, Benson DW. Hypoplastic left heart syndrome is heritable. *J Am Coll Cardiol.* 2007;50:1590–1595.

Hoffman GM, Tweddell JS, Ghanayem NS, et al. Alteration of the critical arteriovenous oxygen saturation relationship by sustained afterload reduction after the Norwood procedure. *J Thorac Cardiovasc Surg.* 2004;127:738–745.

Hornberger LK, Sanders SP, Rein AJ, Spevak PJ, Parness IA, Colan SD. Left heart obstructive lesions and left ventricular growth in the midtrimester fetus. A longitudinal study. *Circulation.* 1995;92:1531–1538.

Hughes ML, Shekerdemian LS, Brizard CP, Penny DJ. Improved early ventricular performance with a right ventricle to pulmonary artery conduit in stage 1 palliation for hypoplastic left heart syndrome: evidence from strain Doppler echocardiography. *Heart.* 2004;90:191–194.

Ishino K, Stumper O, De Giovanni JJ, et al. The modified Norwood procedure for hypoplastic left heart syndrome: early to intermediate results of 120 patients with particular reference to aortic arch repair. *J Thorac Cardiovasc Surg.* 1999;117:920–930.

Jacobs ML. Staged reconstructive surgery—the most appropriate therapy for hypoplastic left heart syndrome. *Cardiol Young.* 2004;14(suppl 1):105–108.

Jacobs ML, Blackstone EH, Bailey LL. Intermediate survival in neonates with aortic atresia: a multi-institutional study. The Congenital Heart Surgeons Society. *J Thorac Cardiovasc Surg.* 1998;116:417–431.

Jobes DR, Nicolson SC, Steven JM, Miller M, Jacobs ML, Norwood WI Jr. Carbon dioxide prevents pulmonary overcirculation in hypoplastic left heart syndrome. *Ann Thorac Surg.* 1992;54:150–151.

Johnson BA, Mussatto K, Uhing MR, Zimmerman H, Tweddell J, Ghanayem N. Variability in the preoperative management of infants with hypoplastic left heart syndrome. *Pediatr Cardiol.* 2008;29:515–520.

Jonas RA. Intermediate procedures after first-stage Norwood operation facilitate subsequent repair. *Ann Thorac Surg.* 1991;52:696–700.

Jonas RA, Hansen DD, Cook N, Wessel D. Anatomic subtype and survival after reconstructive operation for hypoplastic left heart syndrome. *J Thorac Cardiovasc Surg.* 1994;107:1121–1127.

Justino H, Benson LN, Nykanen DG. Transcatheter creation of an atrial septal defect using radiofrequency perforation. *Catheter Cardiovasc Interv.* 2001;54:83–87.

Kanjuh V, Eliot RS, Edwards JE. Coexistent mitral and aortic valvular atresia: a pathologic study of 14 cases. *Am J Cardiol.* 1965;15:611–621.

Kern JH, Hayes CJ, Michler RE, Gersony WM, Quaegebeur JM. Survival and risk factor analysis for the Norwood procedure for hypoplastic left heart syndrome. *Am J Cardiol.* 1997;80:170–174.

Kleinman CS. Fetal cardiac intervention: innovative therapy or a technique in search of an indication? *Circulation.* 2006;113:1378–1381.

Kohl T, Sharland G, Allan LD, et al. World experience of percutaneous ultrasound-guided balloon valvuloplasty in human fetuses with severe aortic valve obstruction. *Am J Cardiol.* 2000;85:1230–1233.

Kon AA. Assessment of physician directiveness: using hypoplastic left heart syndrome as a model. *J Perinatol.* 2004;24:500–504.

Kon AA, Ackerson L, Lo B. How pediatricians counsel parents when no "best-choice" management exists: lessons to be learned from hypoplastic left heart syndrome. *Arch Pediatr Adolesc Med.* 2004;158:436–441.

Krasemann T, Fenge H, Kehl HG, et al. A decade of staged Norwood palliation in hypoplastic left heart syndrome in a midsized cardiosurgical center. *Pediatr Cardiol.* 2005;26:751–755.

Kumar RK, Newburger JW, Gauvreau K, Kamenir SA, Hornberger LK. Comparison of outcome when hypoplastic left heart syndrome and transposition of the great arteries are diagnosed prenatally versus when diagnosis of these two conditions is made only postnatally. *Am J Cardiol.* 1999;83:1649–1653.

Lang P, Jonas RA, Norwood WI, Mayer JE Jr, Castaneda AR. The surgical anatomy of hypoplasia of aortic tract complex. *J Thorac Cardiovasc Surg.* 1985;89:149–150.

Leonard GT, Justino H, Carlson KM, et al. Atrial Septal Stent Implant: Atrial Septal Defect Creation in the Management of Complex Congenital Heart Defects in Infants. *Congenital Heart Disease.* 2006;1:129–135.

Lev M. Pathologic anatomy and interrelationship of hypoplasia of the aortic tract complexes. *Lab Invest.* 1952;1:61–70.

Li J, Zhang G, McCrindle BW, et al. Profiles of hemodynamics and oxygen transport derived by using continuous measured oxygen consumption after the Norwood procedure. *J Thorac Cardiovasc Surg.* 2007;133:441–448.

Lim DS, Peeler BB, Matherne GP, Kron IL, Gutgesell HP. Risk-stratified approach to hybrid transcatheter-surgical palliation of hypoplastic left heart syndrome. *Pediatr Cardiol.* 2006;27:91–95.

Lloyd TR, Evans TC, Marvin WJ Jr. Morphologic determinants of coronary blood flow in the hypoplastic left heart syndrome. *Am Heart J.* 1986;112:666–671.

Loffredo CA, Chokkalingam A, Sill AM, et al. Prevalence of congenital cardiovascular malformations among relatives of infants with hypoplastic left heart, coarctation of the aorta, and d-transposition of the great arteries. *Am J Med Genet A.* 2004;124:225–230.

Mahle WT, Clancy RR, McGaurn SP, Goin JE, Clark BJ. Impact of prenatal diagnosis on survival and early neurologic morbidity in neonates with the hypoplastic left heart syndrome. *Pediatrics.* 2001;107:1277–1282.

Mahle WT, Clancy RR, Moss EM, Gerdes M, Jobes DR, Wernovsky G. Neurodevelopmental outcome and lifestyle assessment in school-aged and adolescent children with hypoplastic left heart syndrome. *Pediatrics.* 2000a;105:1082–1089.

Mahle WT, Cuadrado AR, Tam VK. Early experience with a modified Norwood procedure using right ventricle to pulmonary artery conduit. *Ann Thorac Surg.* 2003;76:1084–1088.

Mahle WT, Spray TL, Wernovsky G, Gaynor JW, Clark BJ, III. Survival after reconstructive surgery for hypoplastic left heart syndrome: a 15-year experience from a single institution. *Circulation.* 2000b;102:III136–III141.

Mahowald JM, Lucas RV Jr, Edwards JE. Aortic valvular atresia. Associated cardiovascular anomalies. *Pediatr Cardiol.* 1982;2:99–105.

Mair R, Tulzer G, Sames E, et al. Right ventricular to pulmonary artery conduit instead of modified Blalock-Taussig shunt improves postoperative hemodynamics in newborns after the Norwood operation. *J Thorac Cardiovasc Surg.* 2003;126:1378–1384.

Makikallio K, McElhinney DB, Levine JC, et al. Fetal aortic valve stenosis and the evolution of hypoplastic left heart syndrome: patient selection for fetal intervention. *Circulation.* 2006;113:1401–1405.

Malec E, Januszewska K, Kolcz J, Mroczek T. Right ventricle-to-pulmonary artery shunt versus modified Blalock-Taussig shunt in the Norwood procedure for hypoplastic left heart syndrome—influence on early and late haemodynamic status. *Eur J Cardiothorac Surg.* 2003;23:728–733.

McCaffrey FM, Sherman FS. Prenatal diagnosis of severe aortic stenosis. *Pediatr Cardiol.* 1997;18:276–281.

Meliones JN, Snider AR, Bove EL, Rosenthal A, Rosen DA. Longitudinal results after first-stage palliation for hypoplastic left heart syndrome. *Circulation.* 1990;82:IV151–IV156.

Michel-Behnke I, Akintuerk H, Marquardt I, et al. Stenting of the ductus arteriosus and banding of the pulmonary arteries: basis for various surgical strategies in newborns with multiple left heart obstructive lesions. *Heart.* 2003;89:645–650.

Mitchell MB, Campbell DN, Boucek MM, et al. Mechanical limitation of pulmonary blood flow facilitates heart transplantation in older infants with hypoplastic left heart syndrome. *Eur J Cardiothorac Surg.* 2003;23:735–742.

Moodie DS, Gallen WJ, Friedberg DZ. Congenital aortic atresia. Report of long survival and some speculations about surgical approaches. *J Thorac Cardiovasc Surg.* 1972;63:726–731.

Mora GA, Pizarro C, Jacobs ML, Norwood WI. Experimental model of single ventricle. Influence of carbon dioxide on pulmonary vascular dynamics. *Circulation.* 1994;90:II43–II46.

Morris CD, Outcalt J, Menashe VD. Hypoplastic left heart syndrome: natural history in a geographically defined population. *Pediatrics.* 1990;85:977–983.

Mu TS, McAdams RM, Bush DM. A case of hypoplastic left heart syndrome and bicuspid aortic valve in monochorionic twins. *Pediatr Cardiol.* 2005;26:884–885.

Mullins CE, Mayer DC. *Congenital Heart Disease: A Diagrammatic Atlas.* New York: Alan R. Liss, Inc; 1988.

Murdison KA, Baffa JM, Farrell PE Jr, et al. Hypoplastic left heart syndrome. Outcome after initial reconstruction and before modified Fontan procedure. *Circulation.* 1990;82:IV199–IV207.

Natowicz M, Chatten J, Clancy R, et al. Genetic disorders and major extracardiac anomalies associated with the hypoplastic left heart syndrome. *Pediatrics.* 1988;82:698–706.

Natowicz M, Kelley RI. Association of Turner syndrome with hypoplastic left-heart syndrome. *Am J Dis Child.* 1987;141:218–220.

Nelson DP, Schwartz SM, Chang AC. Neonatal physiology of the functionally univentricular heart. *Cardiol Young.* 2004;14(suppl 1):52–60.

Neufeld HN, Adams P Jr, Edwards JE, Lester RG. Diagnosis of aortic atresia by retrograde aortography. *Circulation.* 1962;25:278–280.

Noonan JA, Nadas AS. The hypoplastic left heart syndrome: an analysis of 101 cases. *Pediatr Clin North Am.* 1958;5:1029–1056.

Norwood WI, Kirklin JK, Sanders SP. Hypoplastic left heart syndrome: experience with palliative surgery. *Am J Cardiol.* 1980;45:87–91.

Ohye RG, Gomez CA, Goldberg CS, Graves HL, Devaney EJ, Bove EL. Tricuspid valve repair in hypoplastic left heart syndrome. *J Thorac Cardiovasc Surg.* 2004;127:465–472.

Oppido G, Napoleone CP, Martano S, Gargiulo G. Hypoplastic left heart syndrome in situs inversus totalis. *Eur J Cardiothorac Surg.* 2004;26:1052–1054.

Pearl JM, Nelson DP, Schwartz SM, Manning PB. First-stage palliation for hypoplastic left heart syndrome in the twenty-first century. *Ann Thorac Surg.* 2002;73:331–339.

Pellegrino PA, Thiene G. Aortic valve atresia with a normally developed left ventricle. *Chest.* 1976;69:121–122.

Photiadis J, Urban AE, Sinzobahamvya N, et al. Restrictive left atrial outflow adversely affects outcome after the modified Norwood procedure. *Eur J Cardiothorac Surg.* 2005;27:962–967.

Poirier NC, Drummond-Webb JJ, Hisamochi K, Imamura M, Harrison AM, Mee RB. Modified Norwood procedure with a high-flow cardiopulmonary bypass strategy results in low mortality without late arch obstruction. *J Thorac Cardiovasc Surg.* 2000;120:875–884.

Pradat P, Francannet C, Harris JA, Robert E. The epidemiology of cardiovascular defects, part i: a study based on data from three large registries of congenital malformations. *Pediatr Cardiol.* 2003;24:195–221.

Raines KH, Armstrong BE. Aortic atresia with visceral situs inversus with mirror-image dextrocardia. *Pediatr Cardiol.* 1989;10:232–235.

Ramamoorthy C, Tabbutt S, Kurth CD, et al. Effects of inspired hypoxic and hypercapnic gas mixtures on cerebral oxygen saturation in neonates with univentricular heart defects. *Anesthesiology.* 2002;96:283–288.

Reis PM, Punch MR, Bove EL, van DV. Outcome of infants with hypoplastic left heart and Turner syndromes. *Obstet Gynecol.* 1999;93:532–535.

Robert E, Francannet C, Robert JM. [Registries of malformations in the Rhone-Alps/Auvergne region. Value and limits of monitoring teratogenesis. 11 years' experience (1976–1986)]. *J Gynecol Obstet Biol Reprod* (Paris). 1988;17:601–607.

Roberts WC. The worst heart disease. *Am J Cardiol.* 1984;54:1169.

Roberts WC, Perry LW, Chandra RS, Myers GE, Shapiro SR, Scott LP. Aortic valve atresia: a new classification based on necropsy study of 73 cases. *Am J Cardiol.* 1976;37:753–756.

Rosenthal GL, Wilson PD, Permutt T, Boughman JA, Ferencz C. Birth weight and cardiovascular malformations: a population-based study. The Baltimore-Washington Infant Study. *Am J Epidemiol.* 1991;133:1273–1281.

Rychik J. Hypoplastic left heart syndrome: from in-utero diagnosis to school age. *Semin Fetal Neonatal Med.* 2005;10:553–566.

Rychik J, Rome JJ, Collins MH, DeCampli WM, Spray TL. The hypoplastic left heart syndrome with intact atrial septum: atrial morphology, pulmonary vascular histopathology and outcome. *J Am Coll Cardiol.* 1999;34:554–560.

Samanek M, Benesova D, Goetzova J, Hrycejova I. Distribution of age at death in children with congenital heart disease who died before the age of 15. *Br Heart J.* 1988;59:581–585.

Sano S, Ishino K, Kado H, et al. Outcome of right ventricle-to-pulmonary artery shunt in first-stage palliation of hypoplastic left heart syndrome: a multi-institutional study. *Ann Thorac Surg.* 2004;78:1951–1957.

Sano S, Ishino K, Kawada M, et al. Right ventricle-pulmonary artery shunt in first-stage palliation of hypoplastic left heart syndrome. *J Thorac Cardiovasc Surg.* 2003;126:504–509.

Shapiro RN, Eddy W, Fitzgibbon J, O'Brien G. The incidence of congenital anomalies discovered in the neonatal period. *Am J Surg.* 1958;96:396–400.

Shime N, Hashimoto S, Hiramatsu N, Oka T, Kageyama K, Tanaka Y. Hypoxic gas therapy using nitrogen in the preoperative management of neonates with hypoplastic left heart syndrome. *Pediatr Crit Care Med.* 2000;1:38–41.

Sinha SN, Rusnak SL, Sommers HM, Cole RB, Muster AJ, Paul MH. Hypoplastic left ventricle syndrome. Analysis of thirty autopsy cases in infants with surgical considerations. *Am J Cardiol.* 1968;21:166–173.

Stamm C, Anderson RH, Ho SY. The morphologically tricuspid valve in hypoplastic left heart syndrome. *Eur J Cardiothorac Surg.* 1997;12:587–592.

Stasik CN, Gelehrter S, Goldberg CS, Bove EL, Devaney EJ, Ohye RG. Current outcomes and risk factors for the Norwood procedure. *J Thorac Cardiovasc Surg.* 2006;131:412–417.

Stieh J, Fischer G, Scheewe J, et al. Impact of preoperative treatment strategies on the early perioperative outcome in neonates with hypoplastic left heart syndrome. *J Thorac Cardiovasc Surg.* 2006;131:1122–1129.

Stumpflen I, Stumpflen A, Wimmer M, Bernaschek G. Effect of detailed fetal echocardiography as part of routine prenatal ultrasonographic screening on detection of congenital heart disease. *Lancet.* 1996;348:854–857.

Suzuki K, Hirata K, Eto Y, et al. [Echocardiographic assessment of anatomical detail in patients with hypoplastic left heart syndrome]. *J Cardiogr.* 1982;12:991–1008.

Tabbutt S, Dominguez TE, Ravishankar C, et al. Outcomes after the stage I reconstruction comparing the right ventricular to pulmonary artery conduit with the modified blalock taussig shunt. *Ann Thorac Surg.* 2005;80:1582–1591.

Tennstedt C, Chaoui R, Korner H, Dietel M. Spectrum of congenital heart defects and extracardiac malformations associated with chromosomal abnormalities: results of a seven year necropsy study. *Heart.* 1999;82:34–39.

Thiene G, Gallucci V, Macartney FJ, Del TS, Pellegrino PA, Anderson RH. Anatomy of aortic atresia. Cases presenting with a ventricular septal defect. *Circulation.* 1979;59:173–178.

Trines J, Hornberger LK. Evolution of heart disease in utero. *Pediatr Cardiol.* 2004;25:287–298.

Tweddell JS, Hoffman GM, Fedderly RT, et al. Phenoxybenzamine improves systemic oxygen delivery after the Norwood procedure. *Ann Thorac Surg.* 1999;67:161–167.

Tweddell JS, Hoffman GM, Fedderly RT, et al. Patients at risk for low systemic oxygen delivery after the Norwood procedure. *Ann Thorac Surg.* 2000;69:1893–1899.

Tweddell JS, Hoffman GM, Mussatto KA, et al. Improved survival of patients undergoing palliation of hypoplastic left heart syndrome: lessons learned from 115 consecutive patients. *Circulation.* 2002;106:I82–I89.

Tworetzky W, McElhinney DB, Burch GH, Teitel DF, Moore P. Balloon arterioplasty of recurrent coarctation after the modified Norwood procedure in infants. *Catheter Cardiovasc Interv.* 2000;50:54–58.

Tworetzky W, McElhinney DB, Reddy VM, Brook MM, Hanley FL, Silverman NH. Improved surgical outcome after fetal diagnosis of hypoplastic left heart syndrome. *Circulation.* 2001;103:1269–1273.

Tworetzky W, Wilkins-Haug L, Jennings RW, et al. Balloon dilation of severe aortic stenosis in the fetus: potential for prevention of hypoplastic left heart syndrome: candidate selection, technique, and results of successful intervention. *Circulation.* 2004;110:2125–2131.

Vandvik IH, Forde R. Ethical issues in parental decision-making. An interview study of mothers of children with hypoplastic left heart syndrome. *Acta Paediatr.* 2000;89:1129–1133.

Vida VL, Bacha EA, Larrazabal A, et al. Hypoplastic left heart syndrome with intact or highly restrictive atrial septum: surgical experience from a single center. *Ann Thorac Surg.* 2007;84:581–585.

Vlahos AP, Lock JE, McElhinney DB, van DV. Hypoplastic left heart syndrome with intact or highly restrictive atrial septum: outcome after neonatal transcatheter atrial septostomy. *Circulation.* 2004;109:2326–2330.

Von Rueden TJ, Knight L, Moller JH, Ewards JE. Coarctation of the aorta associated with aortic valvular atresia. *Circulation.* 1975;52:951–954.

Watson DG, Rowe RD. Aortic-valve atresia. Report of 43 cases. *JAMA.* 1962;179:14–18.

Weinberg PM, Chin AJ, Murphy JD, Pigott JD, Norwood WI. Postmortem echocardiography and tomographic anatomy of hypoplastic left heart syndrome after palliative surgery. *Am J Cardiol.* 1986;58:1228–1232.

Weinstein S, Gaynor JW, Bridges ND, et al. Early survival of infants weighing 2.5 kilograms or less undergoing first-stage reconstruction for hypoplastic left heart syndrome. *Circulation.* 1999;100:II167–II170.

Wernovsky G, Chrisant MR. Long-term follow-up after staged reconstruction or transplantation for patients with functionally univentricular heart. *Cardiol Young.* 2004;14(suppl 1):115–126.

Yabek SM, Mann JS. Prostaglandin E1 infusion in the hypoplastic left heart syndrome. *Chest.* 1979;76:330–331.

15

Ebstein Anomaly: A Disorder Involving the Right Ventricle and the Tricuspid Valve

PATRICK W. O'LEARY

FRANK CETTA

JOSEPH A. DEARANI

DEFINITION OF THE LESION

Ebstein anomaly is often thought of as a disorder of the tricuspid valve. However, it is actually a manifestation of abnormal development of *both* the heart muscle (myocardium) and its valvar components. Ebstein anomaly primarily affects the right ventricle (RV) and tricuspid valve (TV). In this condition, the TV leaflets remain variably adherent to the underlying RV and septal myocardium. This "adherence" is secondary to incomplete separation (delamination) of leaflet tissue from the inner section of the RV myocardium (the endomyocardium) during fetal development. Such failure to delaminate results in the characteristic displacement of the tricuspid valve's annular attachments—away from their usual position at the junction of the right atrium (RA) and the RV (right atrioventricular groove/junction). The functional tricuspid valve is spirally displaced into the right ventricle's cavity toward the RV outflow tract. In the most severe cases, the functional leaflet tissue may be positioned within the outlet from the RV (the infundibulum). The adherent TV leaflets usually have reduced motion. This reduced motion impairs the function of the TV, invariably leading to backward flow of blood from the RV to the RA (regurgitation) or rarely to narrowing of the valve (stenosis).

In addition to the valvular malformation, the right ventricular myocardium is always abnormal in patients with Ebstein anomaly. The degree of right ventricular dysfunction in a specific patient is variable. In many,

but not all, cases, the degree of myocardial dysfunction mirrors the severity of the valvular deformity.

Ebstein anomaly almost exclusively affects the right heart, which normally supports the lung (pulmonary) circulation. However, in combined atrioventricular and ventriculoarterial discordance (congenitally corrected transposition), an Ebstein-like deformity can be seen involving the systemic atrioventricular (AV) valve. In these hearts, the systemic AV valve is morphologically a tricuspid valve and is associated with the body's (aortic) circulation. The nature of the annular displacement and the adherence of the septal and posterior leaflets to the myocardium are similar to what is seen in right-sided Ebstein anomaly, but the anterior leaflet tends to be smaller in these cases (Mann and Lie, 1979).

HISTORY

In 1864, a 19-year-old laborer was admitted to All Saints' Hospital in Breslau, Poland. He complained of shortness of breath and irregular heart rhythms (Mann and Lie, 1979). He had pronounced cyanosis (low oxygen level), marked pulsation of his neck veins, and was thought to have congenital heart disease. He died 1 week later and Wilhelm Ebstein performed a postmortem examination. Ebstein described three cardiac abnormalities: a severe malformation of the tricuspid valve, absence of a thebesian valve (a small structure within the right atrium), and a defect in the atrial septum (patent foramen ovale). He concluded

261

that the most important abnormality was that of the tricuspid valve. He published his case report (Ebstein, 1866) in *Archiv für Anatomie, Physiologie und Wissenschaftliche Medicin* in January 1866, emphasizing the circulatory disturbances caused by the abnormal tricuspid valve and explaining the genesis of the systolic and diastolic murmurs. In 1900, William G. MacCallum, an assistant professor of pathology at Johns Hopkins University, described a museum specimen that appeared to be identical to Ebstein case. This was the first case to appear in the English literature. In 1927, Alfred Arnstein published the 14th case report and concluded that this abnormality with the characteristic tricuspid valve deformity should be called *Ebsteinsche Krankheit* (Ebstein disease) (Anderson et al., 1978).

ANATOMY

Displacement of Tricuspid Valve Leaflets

The septal and posterior (inferior) leaflet annular attachments are displaced apically, away from the right atrioventricular groove and the crux of the heart. Echocardiography is the most common imaging method used to diagnose and serially evaluate patients with this malformation.

The commissure between the septal and inferior leaflets is the point of maximal displacement and lies at the posterior border of the ventricular septum. These two leaflets are dysplastic and of variable size. In most hearts with Ebstein anomaly, the leaflets are truly displaced, and in a smaller percentage, the leaflets are extensively adherent to the ventricular wall (resulting in displacement of the functional segment of the leaflet).

Anterior Leaflet

The annular attachment of the anterior leaflet is usually not displaced, but the leaflet itself is larger than normal. In classic cases, it has been described as "sail-like," due to its large, redundant belly. Any of the valve leaflets may be fenestrated, but fenestrations are found most often in the anterior leaflet and contribute to the regurgitation seen in these cases. In the most severe forms of Ebstein anomaly (Figure 15–2), even the anterior leaflet may fail to delaminate and be adherent to the endocardium of the right ventricle.

Atria and Atrioventricular Junction

The right atrium is dilated (often severely), and the right atrioventricular junction, or true annulus of the

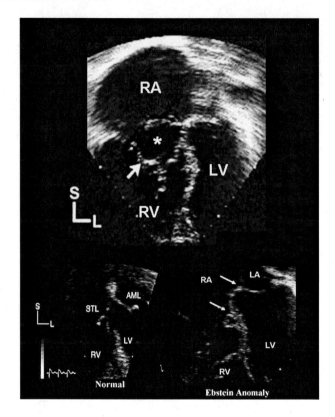

FIGURE 15–1. Series of echocardiographic images that point out the abnormalities seen in Ebstein anomaly. The upper panel is an apical four-chamber image. The image is displayed with the right heart chambers to the viewer left (as if looking at the patient face to face). The right atrium and ventricle (RA and RV) are severely enlarged. The TV leaflets are displaced into the RV (arrow). The area between the anatomic TV anulus and the coaptation point of the functional TV leaflets is referred to as the "atrialized" portion of the RV (*). The displacement of the septal tricuspid leaflet (STL) is easily seen in the lower panels of the figure. The left panel shows the normal relationship of the STL and the anterior mitral leaflet (AML) as they arise from the septum [the central cardiac wall that divides the RV from the left ventricle (LV)]. The arrows in the right panel highlight the displacement of the STL into the cavity of the RV and away from the insertion of the AML.

tricuspid valve, is enlarged circumferentially. The valve of the inferior vena cava (eustachian valve) is often very prominent.

Right Ventricle

The right ventricular myocardium is always abnormal in patients with Ebstein anomaly. In addition to cavity enlargement, the ventricular wall is thinner than normal and there is an absolute decrease in the number of myocardial fibers present. The displaced tricuspid valve divides the ventricle into two zones. The inlet portion (proximal to the valve) has walls composed of

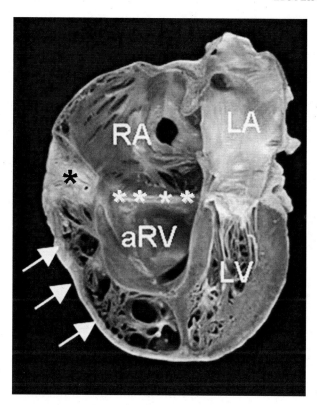

FIGURE 15–2. Four-chamber view of an anatomic specimen displaying an extremely severe form of Ebstein anomaly. There is no functional valve tissue present within anatomic the inflow tract, the entire anterior leaflet is adherent to the RV free wall (arrows). The mobile segments of the valve are displaced anteriorly and apically and are out of the plane of this image. The right heart is globally enlarged and the vestiges of the anterior TV leaflet are attached at multiple points to the RV walls by direct muscular connections (arrows). The area between the anatomic TV anulus and the coaptation point of the functional TV leaflets is referred to as the "atrialized" portion of the RV (aRV). The anatomic anulus is located adjacent to the right atrioventricular groove and is marked with an asterisk in the figure.

ventricular myocardium, but the pressures within the cavity are "atrial." This area has therefore been referred to as the "*atrialized* right ventricle" (Figure 15–2). The trabecular and outlet portions of the ventricle distal to the displaced coaptation point of the valve are referred to as the "functional right ventricle." The atrialized ventricle usually has a thinner wall than the functional right ventricle and may contain segments that are very thin and have no contractile elements. Uhl's anomaly of the right ventricle may closely resemble Ebstein anomaly, due to the right heart enlargement and thin ventricular myocardium. However, in Uhl's anomaly, there is no displacement of the tricuspid annular insertion and the tricuspid valve leaflets are completely delaminated from the underlying myocardium (Uhl, 1952).

Imperforate Ebstein Anomaly

Approximately 10% of hearts with Ebstein anomaly have an imperforate tricuspid valve. In this situation, the leading edge of the anterior leaflet is directly attached to the myocardium and totally separates the atrialized segment of the right ventricle from the functional portion. This has been called Ebstein anomaly with tricuspid atresia.

Coronary Arteries

In Ebstein anomaly, the coronary arteries are generally normal. The right coronary artery may be displaced superiorly and posteriorly (coursing in the atrioventricular sulcus) because of the dilated, atrialized portion of the right ventricle.

Conduction Tissue

Limited studies have been performed on the specialized conduction tissue in hearts with Ebstein anomaly (Anderson et al., 1979; Lev et al., 1955). The sinoatrial node appears to be normally positioned, as is the proximal part of the atrioventricular conduction tissue. However, various abnormalities of the right bundle branch have been reported. It may (a) be located superficially in the subendocardium of the atrialized ventricle, (b) fan out in a fashion similar to that of the normal left bundle branch, (c) give off small communications high to the right-side of the septum, and/or (d) be encased in dense fibroelastic tissue. In addition, accessory atrioventricular conduction pathways bridging the right atrioventricular sulcus and giving rise to the Wolff Parkinson White pattern on the electrocardiogram have been reported (Lev et al., 1955). These pathways play an important role in generating one of the rhythm disturbances (supraventricular tachycardia [SVT]) that many patients with Ebstein anomaly develop. Accessory pathways in Ebstein anomaly can be broad or multiple, making catheter ablation challenging in this group of patients.

Associated Anomalies

A patent foramen ovale or secundum atrial septal defect is found in approximately 90% of patients with Ebstein anomaly. Pulmonary stenosis occurs in a small percentage of patients and complete atresia of the pulmonary valve can also be seen. Ventricular septal defects are rare.

Left Ventricle

Even though Ebstein anomaly involves primarily the right heart, some patients manifest abnormalities of the left ventricle as well. Microscopic examination of left ventricular myocardium from patients with Ebstein anomaly has shown variable amounts of fibrosis, hypertrophy, and nonspecific dysplasia (Celermajer, 1992; Ng, 1979). Left ventricular dysfunction has been clinically attributed to abnormal bowing of the ventricular septum and mitral valve prolapse (Hurwitz, 1994). Recent echocardiographic reports have described left ventricular findings, resembling noncompaction syndrome in 18% of patients with Ebstein anomaly (Attenhofer, in press). Although uncommon, these left heart findings suggest that Ebstein anomaly may be better thought of as a cardiomyopathy that includes abnormal tricuspid valve development, rather than as a primary valvular disorder.

EPIDEMIOLOGY, ENVIRONMENTAL FACTORS, AND GENETICS

Ebstein anomaly is a rare congenital heart defect, found in 1 per 1000 autopsies of patients with congenital cardiac lesions (Abbott, 1936); the suggested incidence is 1 per 210,000 live births (Keith, 1958). This defect is believed to constitute less than 1% of all congenital heart defects (Keith, 1958). Of 2251 infants with cardiac disease who qualified for entry into the New England Regional Infant Cardiac Program, only 13 (0.5%) had Ebstein anomaly (Fyler and Bernhard, 1980). There were equal numbers of male and female patients with Ebstein disease (Bialostozky, 1972; Giuliani et al., 1979).

Based on retrospective case reporting, lithium therapy during the first trimester of pregnancy was once thought to be strongly associated with the occurrence of Ebstein anomaly in the fetus (Nora et al., 1974). However, more recent cohort and case–control epidemiologic studies have not confirmed these initial findings (Cohen et al., 1994). In contrast, these more rigorous studies found that while the frequency of all congenital malformations was increased with gestational lithium exposure, the relative risk for any malformation (not only cardiac) was only 2–3 times that of nontreated mothers. More importantly, although the frequency of all congenital cardiac malformations was greater in lithium-exposed pregnancies, there was no increase in the frequency of Ebstein anomaly relative to controls. Given the rarity of Ebstein anomaly, these studies do not have the power to completely exclude a connection between lithium and the development of Ebstein anomaly. However, they do conclusively demonstrate that the relative "risk" of lithium therapy during pregnancy is much less than was originally estimated from the retrospective case reports (Cohen et al., 1994).

The majority of cases of Ebstein anomaly are sporadic, but some familial cases have been reported. There continues to be a difference of opinion as to whether there is a major hereditary basis for transgenerational transmission in Ebstein anomaly (Emanuel et al., 1976; Rosenmann, 1976).

Pathophysiology

The findings and symptoms seen in patients with Ebstein anomaly are dependent on many factors and are influenced by the age at which the patient comes to clinical attention. In children and adults, cyanosis, heart murmur, cardiac enlargement on chest x-ray, tachycardia/palpitations, and reduced exercise tolerance are the most common presenting problems. The broad range of anatomic severity seen in Ebstein anomaly, combined with the variable myopathy, produce a wide spectrum of clinical and hemodynamic manifestations. The pathophysiologic changes in the patient with Ebstein anomaly are related to several factors: (a) functional status of the tricuspid valve (degree of regurgitation or more rarely, stenosis); (b) the presence (or absence) and size of the atrial septal communication; (c) degree of right ventricular dysfunction; and (d) amount of left ventricular dysfunction. To a lesser degree, the pathologic substrates predisposing to tachyarrhythmias produce an additional dimension contributing to the pathophysiology.

Atrial septal defects in a patient with Ebstein anomaly often allow desaturated (low oxygen content or "blue") blood to cross to the left heart circulation without passing through the lungs. This right to left shunt causes clinical cyanosis (a dusky blue color in the skin) when the amount of shunt is significant. Often the cyanosis increases with exertion/exercise because the inefficient right heart cannot increase its output as much as the left ventricle, elevating RA and systemic venous pressure and augmenting the flow across the atrial septum.

The dysfunctional nature of the right ventricular myocardium and the coexisting tricuspid valve abnormalities impair flow through the right heart and the pulmonary circulation. The interaction between the dilated right atrium and the atrialized segment of the right ventricle are perhaps just as important in the creation of ineffective flow patterns within the right heart. During ventricular systole, the atrialized right ventricular myocardium is contracting. However, no valve tissue separates this area from the true atrial chamber and the great veins. This results in increased venous pressure and effectively increases "resistance" to forward flow. This decreases the ability of the great veins to empty into the right atrium while its muscle fibers are "relaxed" (atrial mechanical diastole/relaxation occurs during ventricular systole/contraction). The increase in "resistance" to flow out of the atrium will also augment the amount of right to left shunt that crosses any coexisting atrial septal communication.

Later in the cardiac cycle, the atrialized portion of the right ventricle relaxes; it will expand and can even "balloon outwards" during atrial contraction (which occurs during ventricular diastole). This creates a reservoir for venous blood and decreases the amount of effective forward flow that crosses the abnormal tricuspid valve to reach the functional right ventricular zone and the pulmonary arteries. This to and fro flow pattern (between the right atrium and the atrialized right ventricle) not only decreases effective right heart output, but also provides an ongoing stimulus for atrial dilation and atrial arrhythmias—even when there is little "trans-valvular" regurgitation. The degree of functional impairment experienced by patients with Ebstein anomaly has been directly related to these anatomic and physiologic abnormalities. Shiina and colleagues (1984) found that (a) a small functional right ventricle and large atrialized right ventricle, (b) extreme displacement or absence of the septal leaflet, (c) degree of displacement or tethering of the anterior leaflet, and (d) the aneurysmal dilation of the right ventricular outflow tract were associated with reduced functional status, as measured by New York Heart Association (NYHA) classification.

Although the primary focus in patients with Ebstein anomaly has been on right-sided structures, there have been an increasing number of reports of left-sided abnormalities, specifically in left ventricular size, shape, and function (Benson et al., 1978; Monibi et al., 1978; Ng et al., 1979). In the past, these have been attributed to the degree of right heart enlargement (compromising the left ventricle) and to leftward diastolic bowing of the interventricular septum. Radionuclide scans and cineangiograms have shown impaired left ventricular function at rest in unoperated patients. During formal exercise testing, most unoperated patients show an appropriate increase in left ventricular ejection fraction due to a reduced end-systolic volume and unchanged end-diastolic volume (Benson et al., 1978). Recently however, Attenhofer and colleagues reported that 19 of 106 (18%) patients with Ebstein anomaly had a markedly abnormal echocardiographic appearance of the left ventricular myocardium (Attenhofer, in press; Attenhofer, 2004) These patients displayed segments of LV myocardium with multiple layers and deep intratrabecular recesses, consistent with myocardial noncompaction. An additional 11% had hypertrabeculated segments of left ventricular muscle reminiscent, but not diagnostic, of noncompacted myocardium. Although most patients had satisfactory left ventricular function, a small percentage showed severe systolic and diastolic dysfunction, even contributing to the need for transplantation in one young patient (Attenhofer et al., 2004). These left-sided myocardial abnormalities, although seen in only a fraction of patients, support the concept that Ebstein anomaly is actually a myocardial disorder that primarily manifests itself within the right ventricle and its derivative—the tricuspid valve.

The infant and fetus with Ebstein anomaly pose especially difficult clinical problems. Pulmonary vascular resistance is always high before and immediately after birth, and it usually decreases fairly rapidly in the first days of life. The infant with Ebstein anomaly is poorly prepared to deal with the transition to neonatal circulation. The combination of right ventricular myopathy, tricuspid regurgitation, and elevated pulmonary resistance can lead to poor pulmonary perfusion when the ductus arteriosus constricts or closes. Venous pressures rise, leading to right-heart failure and cyanosis due to right-to-left shunt across the foramen ovale. These infants present a diagnostic and therapeutic dilemma, until the pulmonary resistance decreases and the pulmonary flow increases. Patency of the pulmonary outflow tract and valve must be confirmed. This can be done by demonstrating valve opening on 2-D echocardiographic scans or by documenting flow across the valve by Doppler techniques (either ejection or more commonly regurgitation). In cases where echocardiographic findings are inconclusive, an angiogram (injecting from the ductus arteriosus) demonstrating pulmonary regurgitation or the ability to advance a catheter across the valve annulus are other methods that can confirm patency of the right ventricular outflow tract. When the outflow tract is open, support with prostaglandin infusion to maintain ductal patency (with or without ventilation) will often allow the baby to transition to postnatal circulation without the need for palliative surgery.

A fetus that displays significant cardiac enlargement before delivery due to Ebstein anomaly faces a very high risk of prenatal and/or infant mortality (Roberson and Silverman, 1989). The fetus with Ebstein anomaly and prenatal heart failure (hydrops fetalis) has the worst prognosis (Yetman et al., 1998). Conversely, an infant or fetus with incidentally noted Ebstein anomaly, normal overall heart size, and oxygen saturation may have a more favorable course.

CLINICAL FEATURES

Presentation and Natural History

Patients with Ebstein anomaly may present at any age. The most severe cases present prenatally or as newborns. Prenatal diagnosis is dependent upon ultrasonic screening examinations. Fetal presentation is accompanied by increased heart size, a significant incidence of hydrops fetalis, and in the most severe cases pulmonary parenchymal hypoplasia (secondary to marked cardiac enlargement). Interestingly, prenatal arrhythmia is not common. Newborns most often present with cyanosis and a very large heart (usually seen on chest x-ray). The newborn always has high resistance to blood flow through the lungs and high pulmonary vascular resistance. This physiology is normal for the fetus and needs to gradually transition to the low resistance pulmonary blood flow seen later in life. This transition is usually completed (or nearly completed) within 1–2 weeks of birth. When an infant with Ebstein anomaly has high resistance, the right ventricle will often be unable to produce normal or even adequate pulmonary blood flow. This can result in a situation called "functional pulmonary valve atresia." In these cases, the pulmonary valve never opens. All of the blood flow from the right heart must cross an atrial septal defect and enter the left heart/aortic circulation. These babies are dependent on the presence of a patent ductus arteriosus to provide pulmonary blood flow. The ductus can be maintained with intravenous prostaglandin infusion, while the pulmonary resistance decreases. Often, this process takes several days to weeks before the duct can be allowed to close. In the most severe cases, surgical intervention, such as a modified Blalock Taussig shunt, is required before prostaglandin support can be discontinued.

Slightly older infants present with a combination of desaturation and heart failure symptoms. Murmurs and arrhythmias become more frequent, presenting complaints in older patients. Although some patients remain asymptomatic, most will have some cardiovascular symptoms. Beyond infancy, the majority will display fatigue, dyspnea, or cyanosis with exertion or palpitations. Palpitations in a cyanotic child should raise the possibility of Ebstein anomaly (Table 15–1) (Bialostozky et al., 1972; Celermajer and Till, 1994; Giuliani et al., 1979).

Ultrasound technology has significantly influenced the age at which most patients with Ebstein anomaly are diagnosed. In 1979, Guiliani and colleagues found that 31% of Ebstein patients were diagnosed before 4 years of age. Another 38% were diagnosed before age 19, with remainder presenting in adulthood (up to 80 years of age) (Giuliani et al., 1979; Seward et al., 1979). In contrast, Celermajer et al. (1994) described a group of 220 patients with Ebstein anomaly in 1994 (Table 15–1). In this series, 50% were diagnosed prenatally or as newborns. Ten percent presented between 1 and 12 months of age. Another 30% presented as children or adolescents. Despite the increased availability of ultrasound examination in this more recent cohort, 10% remained undiagnosed until adulthood (Celermajer and Till, 1994).

Physical Findings

Growth and development are generally normal. Inspection may reveal cyanosis and digital clubbing in patients with associated right-to-left shunt. However, many older children and adults may have normal oxygenation. Those with cyanosis may have an unusual facial coloration, described as violaceous hue, flushed, florid, red-checked, or malar flush (Giuliani et al., 1979). These patients have an associated mild erythrocytosis secondary to the lower oxygen level associated with the right to left shunt. Prominence or asymmetry of the chest is a frequent finding secondary to the dilated right heart structures. Arterial and venous pulsations are usually normal, even in the presence of tricuspid insufficiency. The jugular venous pulsations may not have a large V wave because of poor transmission of the venous pulse wave in the presence of a dilated, compliant right atrium. The precordium is usually not overactive. Generally it is the heart sounds that first alert the physician to the diagnosis of Ebstein anomaly. Many patients have multiple sounds and murmurs present, especially those with mobile anterior tricuspid valve leaflets. These multiple sounds are

TABLE 15–1. *Presenting Features of Ebstein Anomaly in 220 Subjects*

Feature	Fetus (n – 21)	Neonate (n – 88)	Infant (n – 23)	Child (n – 50)	Adolescent (n – 15)	Adult (n – 23)	Total (%)
Cyanosis	0	65	8	7	2	1	83 (38)
Heart failure	0	9	10	4	2	6	31 (14)
Murmur	0	8	3	33	5	3	52 (24)
Arrhythmia	1	5	1	6	6	10	29 (13)
Fetal echo	18	0	0	0	0	0	18 (8)

Age groups at presentation are: neonate, 0–1 month; infant, ≤2 year; child, ≤10 years; adolescent, ≤18 years; and adult, 18 years.

Based on data from reference 27; Celermajer DS, Bull C, Till JA, et al. Ebstein anomaly: presentation and outcome from fetus to adult. *J Am Coll Cardiol*. 1994;23:170–176.

so characteristic as to stand out even to the untrained ear. Occasionally the heart sounds are soft, but usually they are of normal intensity. The first heart sound is widely split because of increased excursion of the anterior leaflet and subsequent delayed closure of the abnormal tricuspid valve. The second heart sound is also widely and persistently split owing to late closure of the pulmonic valve, believed to be due to right bundle branch block. Ventricular filling sounds (S_3 or S_4 or both) are common contributors to the multiplicity of heart sounds. In the presence of so many heart sounds, one perceives a gallop or quadruple rhythm or cadence quality, which is fairly easily recognized. A holosystolic murmur (grade 2–4 of 6) is found along the left sternal border—in those with an organized jet of tricuspid regurgitation. Low-intensity diastolic murmurs can be appreciated in the same location, as a result of anterograde flow across the tricuspid valve. All murmurs tend to vary with respiration, increasing during inspiration. In patients with very little functional tricuspid valve tissue, there may be few murmurs present, since the flows between right atrium and the ventricle are essentially unrestricted and not turbulent. The first heart sound is single in these cases.

Electrocardiography

The electrocardiogram is usually abnormal and helps to confirm the clinical diagnosis (Giuliani et al., 1979). Although sinus rhythm is usually present, atrioventricular dissociation or atrial fibrillation can be found in a few patients. In a large series, one-third to one-half of the patients have prolonged PR intervals, and one-fourth to three-fourths meet criteria for right atrial enlargement (Himalayan P waves, Figure 15–3). (Giuliani et al., 1979) The QRS axis in the frontal plane occasionally shows right-axis deviation. Most patients have right bundle branch block and many have low-voltage QRS complexes in the right precordial leads. Findings consistent with right ventricular hypertrophy are extremely uncommon.

Some 4%–26% of patients with Ebstein anomaly have the Wolff Parkinson White pattern (premature ventricular activation) (Giuliani et al., 1979; Soulie et al., 1970). This is due to accessory atrioventricular connections. Several resting or exercise electrocardiograms or 24-hour ambulatory electrocardiograms may have to be examined to find the characteristic pattern. Occasionally the pattern is transient or intermittent (Friedman et al., 1969; Klein and Gulamhusein, 1983; Schiebler et al., 1959). In addition, concealed accessory pathways (without manifest delta-waves) are not uncommon. Therefore, absence of anterograde preexcitation indicates neither that the accessory connection is no longer present nor that the patient is no longer susceptible to tachycardia. The patient may still have retrograde conduction, which allows for atrioventricular reciprocating tachycardia. Patients with Ebstein anomaly, a normal PR interval, and a delta-wave may still have Wolff Parkinson White syndrome but the PR interval is artificially lengthened by delayed conduction through the large right atrium. In those patients who

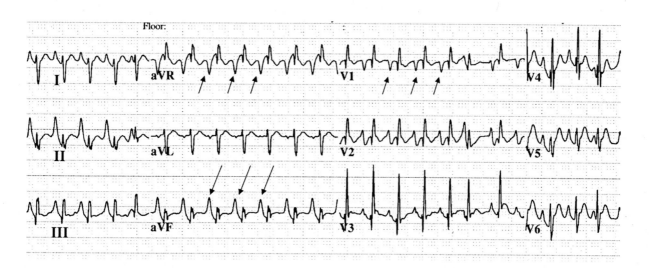

FIGURE 15–3. This is an image of a 12-lead electrocardiogram taken from an infant with Ebstein anomaly. The QRS axis is shifted to the right (175 degrees) and there is evidence of prominent atrial enlargement with large P waves that exceed the voltage achieved by ventricular QRS complexed in some leads (P waves are indicated by the series of three arrows in lead aVF). The rhythm in slightly irregular due to occasional premature contractions.

demonstrate left-axis deviation, there may be accessory nodoventricular connections present (Mahaim fibers) (Follath and Hallidie-Smith, 1972).

Arrhythmias in the unoperated patient with Ebstein anomaly are common (Oh et al., 1985). Forty-one of 52 preoperative patients (79%) had either documented arrhythmias or histories of palpitations, near-syncope, or syncope. In those with documented arrhythmias (34/52), 18 had paroxysmal supraventricular tachycardia, 10 had paroxysmal atrial fibrillation or flutter, 13 had ventricular arrhythmias (7 with frequent ventricular premature complexes and 6 with nonsustained ventricular tachycardia), and 3 had atrioventricular block (2 complete heart block and 1 Mobitz II second degree). Of the 13 patients with ventricular arrhythmias, 5 also had paroxysmal supraventricular tachycardia, 4 had paroxysmal atrial fibrillation or flutter, and 1 had complete heart block. The patients with arrhythmias or symptoms compatible with arrhythmia were significantly older than patients without symptoms or arrhythmias.

Surgical intervention appears to decrease the frequency of arrhythmias, at least in early, short-term follow up. Review of 167 patients before and after definitive repair of Ebstein anomaly revealed arrhythmias in 44% postoperatively compared with 61% preoperatively (Cordes et al., unpublished data). Supraventricular tachycardias decreased from 48%–26% postoperatively. Twenty-six patients underwent ablation of an accessory pathway at the time of operation for tricuspid valve repair or replacement and atrial septal defect closure with no late complete heart block. Early postoperative arrhythmia was associated with an increased risk of late sudden death. Introduction of more extensive arrhythmia surgery seems to improve results even further. Greason and colleagues (2003) reported the results of right atrial maze procedure for atrial arrhythmias in congenital

heart patients. Seventy percent of the series (31/44) had Ebstein anomaly. One patient with severe anatomic disease and multiple arrhythmias did not survive the operation. Most patients (85%) remained in sinus rhythm at a mean of 17 months postoperatively (range up to 5.5 years). Only 6% had recurrent atrial fibrillation/flutter, 8% were in junctional rhythm, and only one patient required long-term pacemaker therapy.

Chest Radiography

The cardiac size may vary from near normal to extreme cardiomegaly. When the heart is severely dilated, it takes on a globular shape that is similar to that seen with large pericardial effusions or severe dilated cardiomyopathy (Figure 15–4). There may be a dramatic change from the preoperative to the postoperative radiograph (Figure 15–4). The dilated right atrium is responsible for most of the enlarged cardiac silhouette. In the frontal view, the right atrium produces a significant convexity of the right heart border, and in the lateral view, the right atrium may fill the entire retrosternal space. The convex left border is primarily due to dilation of the right ventricular outflow tract. The convexities of both left and right heart borders produce the characteristic globular cardiac silhouette. In cyanotic patients with a right-to-left shunt, the pulmonary vascularity is decreased; otherwise, it is usually normal. In the asymptomatic patient, it is not unusual for the heart to have a normal size and shape. This may confuse the clinical diagnosis.

Echocardiography

Echocardiographic evaluation of Ebstein anomaly has evolved and has now become the procedure of choice for both the diagnosis and long-term assessment of

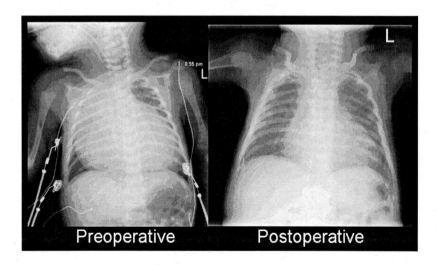

FIGURE 15–4. These two chest x-rays were taken from the same infant with severe Ebstein anomaly before (preoperative) and after (postoperative) tricuspid valve repair, right atrial reduction, closure of ductus arteriosus, and partial closure of the atrial septal defect. Preoperatively, the heart nearly fills the chest on this frontal view. Although the heart is still significantly enlarged after surgery, the cardiac volume has been markedly decreased, allowing improved cardiac and lung function.

patients with Ebstein anomaly. In the 1980s, 2-D echocardiography replaced M-mode as the clinical standard (Hirschklau et al., 1977; Matsumoto et al., 1976; Ports et al., 1978). In fact, as early as 1984 2-D echocardiographic imaging was reported to be comprehensive enough that angiography was no longer necessary to diagnose Ebstein anomaly (Shiina et al., 1984). Two-dimensional imaging of the internal cardiac crux, tricuspid valve structure, and right ventricular myocardium reveal several features that are reliably used to identify patients with Ebstein anomaly. The single most sensitive and specific diagnostic feature is the apical (downward) displacement of the annular insertion of the tricuspid septal leaflet (relative to the insertion of the anterior mitral leaflet, Figure 15–1). It should be noted that the septal leaflet of the normal tricuspid valve normally inserts at a position that is slightly apical to the insertion of the mitral valve. However, in patients with Ebstein anomaly, this displacement is exaggerated. The distance between septal mitral and septal tricuspid leaflet insertion can be easily measured in a standard apical four-chamber view. This distance, when divided by the patient's body surface area in square meters, is known as the displacement index. An index value greater than 8 mm/m^2 reliably distinguishes patients with Ebstein anomaly from both normals and from patients with other disorders associated with enlargement of the right ventricle (Gussenhoven et al., 1984; Shiina et al., 1984). Occasionally, the offset between the tricuspid and mitral valves at the internal crux can be difficult to assess. Other echocardiographic features

that may suggest the presence of Ebstein anomaly are: (a) elongation of the anterior leaflet of the tricuspid valve, (b) tethering any of the tricuspid leaflets to the underlying myocardium, (c) shortened tricuspid valve chordal support structures, (d) attachment of the leading edge of the anterior leaflet to the right ventricular myocardium, (e) apical displacement of the annular attachment of the anterior leaflet (uncommon), (f) absence of septal or posterior tricuspid leaflets (rare findings, Figure 15–5), and/or (g) congenital fenestration of the tricuspid valve leaflets, and (h) enlargement of the tricuspid valve annulus.

Echocardiography should also be used to define suitability for valve repair, associated cardiovascular features, and function. Anatomic features of the tricuspid valve that indicate good candidacy for repair include: (a) a freely mobile anterior leaflet within the right ventricular inflow tract—this assessment must be made in the apical four-chamber view. It is especially important that the mobile leaflet segments include the leading edge (Figure 15–6), (b) a single central jet of regurgitation, and (c) the lack of direct muscular insertions into the anterior leaflet (Figure 15–7).

The functional impact of the malformation of the right ventricle and tricuspid valve should be determined. Anatomical and functional severities are not necessarily related. For example, a patient can have a severe anatomical form of Ebstein anomaly and mild functional disease. Both aspects of severity play an important role in determining functional status, prognosis, and reparability of the tricuspid valve

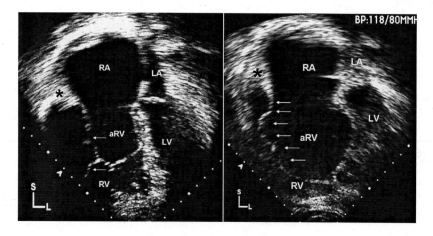

FIGURE 15–5. These apical four-chamber echocardiographic images demonstrate advanced forms of EA. The right heart is tremendously dilated in both (anulus diameters more than 50 mm). RV function was severely depressed. The anterior leaflet tissue was tethered at multiple levels in the inflow tract (arrows). Valve mobility was markedly reduced in the case to the left and complete absent on the right. The anatomic TV annulus is marked with an asterisk (*). No septal leaflet tissue can be seen in either patient. The native, mobile valve tissue was displaced to the entrance of the RVOT (the infundibular orifice). These valves were not suitable for repair. The TV remnants were resected to avoid RV outflow obstruction and a bioprosthesis was placed at the anatomic anulus, restoring the "functional" RV to an adequate volume to support the circulation.

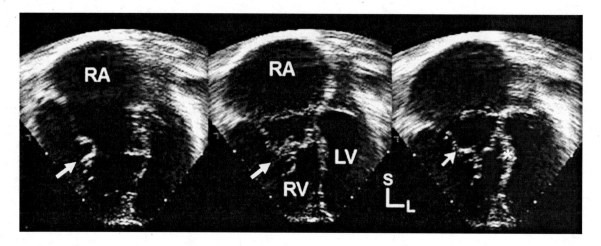

FIGURE 15–6. The three panels of this figure are all apical four–chamber inflow images. The left frame is from mid-diastole. The middle and right frames are from mid- and end-systole, respectively. Features that suggest favorable anatomy for repair are: the anterior leaflet in this patient is freely mobile, including its leading edge (arrows). There are no muscular insertions that limit or distort the motion of the valve. The regurgitant jet originated as a single jet from the gap in coaptation seen between the anterior leaflet and the remnant of the septal leaflet. The leading edge of the valve reaches a point near enough to the septum in systole, that an anuloplasty can "advance" it to a point where it will coapt with the septum, given the degree of anular dilation(*).

(Gussenhoven et al., 1984; Seward, 1993; Shiina et al., 1983, 1984). The degree of right atrial and ventricular volume enlargement and functional state of the right ventricular myocardium should be defined (Eidem et al.,

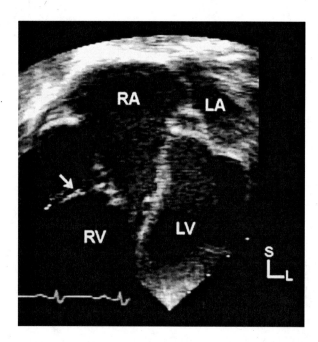

FIGURE 15–7. Although the anterior leaflet in this case has some mobility, there is a direct muscular insertion of a free wall papillary muscle into the anterior leaflet (arrow). This will limit the motion of the leaflet. More importantly, there were multiple fenestrations in the anterior leaflet, causing at least three separate regurgitant jets. The multiple points of regurgitation and limited systolic mobility made this patient a poor candidate for valve repair.

1998). Other important features include the degree of right ventricular outflow tract dilation, the presence and size of any atrial septal defect, and the degree of "transvalvular" tricuspid valve regurgitation (Seward, 1993; Shiina et al., 1984). The left ventricular myocardium has also been described as being abnormal in many patients with Ebstein anomaly (Celermajer et al., 1992; Hurwitz, 1994; Ng et al., 1979; Van Mierop and Gessner, 1972). Therefore, quantitative evaluation of left ventricular performance should also be a routine component of the echocardiographic evaluation of the patient with Ebstein anomaly. Abnormalities such as ventricular septal defects and pulmonary stenosis may also be found in association with Ebstein anomaly. Doppler and color flow echocardiographic assessment can help determine hemodynamic alterations such as valve regurgitation and intracardiac shunting.

Echocardiography also plays an important role intraoperatively and postoperatively in assessing adequacy of tricuspid valve repair or replacement (Hagler, 1993; Randolph et al., 2002). The most important use of intraoperative echocardiography in the patient with Ebstein anomaly is the immediate evaluation of the "repaired" tricuspid valve. A repair that is not functioning well can be immediately revised or converted to a valve replacement without the need for a second operation. The postoperative examination can also be used to assess prosthetic valve function, changes in right and left ventricular function, and to exclude significant residual atrial level shunting. Similarly, postoperative echocardiography is important not only to assess the adequacy of the surgical repair but also to exclude postoperative complications, including pericardial or pleural effusion, mediastinal hematoma, and intracardiac thrombus. Degree of residual tricuspid regurgitation or tricuspid stenosis should be determined. Assessment of ventricular function and regional wall abnormalities plays an important role. Rarely, right coronary artery flow can be compromised because of the proximity of the right coronary artery to the plicated portion of the atrialized right ventricle.

Echocardiography can accurately define the features of Ebstein anomaly in the fetus. Characteristics that have been identified with early neonatal mortality include marked right heart enlargement, severe tethering of the anterior tricuspid leaflet tissue, left ventricular compression, and associated lesions such as pulmonary atresia (Roberson and Silverman, 1989). Pulmonary hypoplasia develops secondary to severe cardiomegaly and hydrops with pleural and pericardial effusions. Detection of rhythm disturbances, such as supraventricular tachycardia, should be attempted at the time of fetal echocardiography because they can contribute to the development of hydrops. A Celermajer index >1 (the ratio of the combined right atrial and atrialized ventricular area to the combined area of the functional right ventricle and left heart) (Yetman et al., 1998) was associated with very poor fetal or neonatal outcome. Other fetal or neonatal findings that were associated with increased risk of mortality were a larger atrial septal defect, functional or anatomic pulmonary atresia, or reduced left ventricular function.

Exercise Testing

Exercise testing has become one of the routine noninvasive studies used to evaluate patients with Ebstein anomaly, both before and after surgical intervention. Studies performed before and after surgery have described several interesting findings (Barber et al., 1985; Driscoll et al., 1988; MacLellan-Tobert et al., 1997). In the largest of these series (MacLellan-Tobert et al., 1997), unoperated patients had indices of exercise tolerance (work, exercise duration, maximal oxygen uptake) that were significantly reduced (mean "maximum" oxygen uptake—20.5 mL/kg). However, in postoperative patients these indices all increased and approached the lower limits of normal (mean "maximum" oxygen uptake—25.3 mL/kg). Both rest and exercise arterial oxygen saturations were significantly lower in unoperated patients than in postoperative patients (undoubtedly due to atrial septal defect closure). In the unoperated patient, progressively lower oxygen saturations (both at rest and at maximum exercise) were associated with progressively reduced exercise tolerance (lower achieved maximum oxygen uptake). Preoperative resting and exercise cardiac output was assessed only in those patients without

cyanosis (acetylene-helium rebreathing technique). In this subgroup (12% of the total), cardiac outputs were reduced compared to expected norms, both at rest and at peak exercise. Surgical intervention improved exercise tolerance. Most postoperative patients had resting and exercise cardiac outputs that were similar to the normal population. Patients with an atrial septal defect and right-to-left shunting demonstrated excessive ventilation at rest and during exercise. In these patients, a right-to-left shunt is a strong stimulus to increased ventilation.

CARDIAC CATHETERIZATION

Electrophysiology

Echocardiographic evaluation of anatomy is so accurate that diagnosis of Ebstein anomaly no longer depends on catheterization and angiocardiography. However, invasive electrophysiologic testing and catheter ablation continue to and may actually be growing in importance. The Pediatric Electrophysiology Society reported 65 patients with Ebstein anomaly that had invasive studies and attempted radiofrequency ablations (Reich et al., 1998). Accessory pathway-mediated tachycardia was very common. Only 9% of the patients had nonaccessory pathway mechanism for their tachyarrhythmias. Right-sided free wall and septal accessory pathways were responsible for the majority of the re-entrant arrhythmias (only 4% were left sided pathways). Twenty-nine percent had more than one accessory conduction pathway. Radiofrequency ablation was able to temporarily eliminate the tachycardia in 75%–89% of cases (depending on the mechanism). However, recurrence of tachyarrhythmia was common. Only 27%–32% of patients were considered long-term successes.

More specific delineation of the anatomy of accessory conduction pathways in Ebstein anomaly was provided by Olson et al. (1991, 1993). They described 25 patients with Ebstein anomaly who electrophysiologically proven accessory pathway tachycardia. The accessory atrioventricular connections were localized to the right posterolateral free wall in 11 patients, to the posterior septum in nine, and to both the septum and right free wall in four. One patient had a right anterolateral connection. The mechanisms of arrhythmia included orthodromic reciprocating tachycardia in 15 patients, both orthodromic and antidromic reciprocating tachycardia in four, inducible atrial flutter or fibrillation in seven, atrioventricular nodal reentry in two, and ventricular tachycardia in one. All of these patients had surgical pathway ablations. None had recurrence of accessory pathway-mediated tachycardia over a

4-year follow up period. Early results of the right-sided atrial maze procedure have also been encouraging in patients with Ebstein anomaly and multiple mechanisms causing tachyarrhythmias (Greason et al., 2003; Smith et al., 1982; Theodoro et al., 1998).

Hemodynamics

In the early days of intracardiac investigation, it became evident that patients with Ebstein anomaly were at increased risk during catheter procedures. Some physicians stated that these patients should not be studied. However, concerns about the safety of cardiac catheterization in these patients have been dispelled by modern techniques of monitoring the patient's hemodynamic status during the study, more flexible catheter materials, and the availability of effective treatment for arrhythmias provoked by catheter manipulation. Even though patients with Ebstein anomaly can now be safely studied, the need to do so arises infrequently, such as when there are clinical questions regarding coexisting malformations or pulmonary arterial pressure and resistance.

Natural History

The outcome of Ebstein anomaly depends a great deal on the age of the patient at presentation, severity of the lesion, and associated defects (all of which are interrelated). Severely affected fetuses or neonates can easily be detected with echocardiography. However, as a result of their severe disease, they generally have a poor outcome (Celermajer and Till, 1994). In fact, one series observed universal mortality in those neonates that had a combined area of the right atrium and atrialized right ventricle greater than the combined area of the functional right ventricle, left atrium, and left ventricle (Yetman et al., 1998). Mild disease in neonates and young children has a relatively good outcome, depending primarily on the presence of associated lesions.

The "natural" history of Ebstein anomaly was first reviewed by Watson (1974). This international cooperative study described 505 patients from 61 centers in 28 countries. Only 35 patients were less than 1 year old, 403 were between 1 and 25 years, and 67 were over 25 years. Heart failure was common among the infants (72%). In contrast, 81% of the patients that presented at older ages were said to have had normal growth and development during infancy. Also, 71% of the patients aged 1–25 years and 60% of those over age 25 years had little or no disability at the time of diagnosis and were classified as NYHA class I or II. Cardiac catheterizations had been done on 363 patients, with 13 deaths and 6 cardiac arrests that were treated successfully.

A paroxysmal tachycardia occurred during the catheterization in 90 patients.

Seventy-seven (15.2%) of the 505 died secondary to medical complications of the disease. After an initial higher mortality risk in the neonatal time period, the hazard for death was similar among all age groups greater than 1 year. In those between the ages of 1 and 25 years, 50 (12.4%) of the 403 patients died of the disease. Half of the deaths were due to heart failure and 20% were sudden deaths, presumably due to an arrhythmia. In those over 25 years, there were 11 natural deaths (16.4%) in 67 patients, 2 from congestive heart failure, and 2 sudden.

Watson (1974) reported high mortalities with surgical treatment, with only 26 of the 57 (45%) surgical patients surviving. Patients between ages 1 and 15 years had 64% mortality for palliative procedures, such as Glenn or Blalock shunts. They reported a 56% mortality rate for definitive surgical treatment, such as insertion of a tricuspid prosthesis. In 15 patients over age 15 years who had definitive repair with a prosthesis, there was 33% mortality. Thus this early paper concluded that surgery was not beneficial, although more recent reports have proven otherwise. Certainly there have been patients with Ebstein anomaly who survived into their ninth decade without surgical intervention (Seward et al., 1979).

In 1994, Celermajer et al. described 220 cases of Ebstein anomaly presenting from fetus to adulthood (Table 15–1). The median age at time of presentation had decreased to less than 1 year, emphasizing the role echocardiography now plays in early diagnosis. Neonatal mortality was due to heart failure and pulmonary hypoplasia, secondary to cardiomegaly. Associated cardiac defects were more common in patients who presented early. However, those newborns with isolated Ebstein anomaly usually showed spontaneous improvement as the pulmonary vascular resistance decreased. Patients diagnosed in later in childhood tended to present with a cardiac murmur discovered incidentally. Arrhythmias and progressive right-to-left shunt (desaturation) were more common in the older child and adult.

Women with Ebstein anomaly can tolerate pregnancy, particularly when pregestational functional status is good (Littler, 1970; Mair et al., 1985; Waickman et al., 1984). However, as a group there is an increased risk of fetal demise and prematurity in mothers who had more significant disease (Copeland et al., 1963; Donnelly et al., 1991; Whittemore et al., 1982). In 1994, Connolly and Warnes (1994) reported a comprehensive review of pregnancy outcome in patients with Ebstein anomaly. The pregnancy histories of 72 couples, in which one member (44 women and 28 men) had Ebstein anomaly, were analyzed. Pregnancy seemed well tolerated by the affected mothers, but was associated with an increased risk of prematurity, fetal loss, and congenital heart disease in the offspring. The miscarriage and fetal loss rates were 18%, slightly higher than the expected age-matched rates of 10%–15%. Infants born to cyanotic women had significantly lower birth weights than were observed in infants of noncyanotic mothers. The incidence of congenital heart disease in the offspring of the women with Ebstein anomaly was 6%. Congenital heart disease was diagnosed in only 1 of the 75 children (1.3%) born to couples in whom the man had Ebstein anomaly. The incidence of Ebstein anomaly in the offspring was 0.6% (1 in 158 children). No significant maternal complications or death occurred in this series, suggesting that women with Ebstein anomaly tolerate pregnancy well. However, maternal arrhythmias and cyanosis warrant close observation during pregnancy.

THERAPY

In Ebstein anomaly, a wide spectrum of hemodynamic abnormalities and arrhythmias occur at various ages. Therefore, no dogmatic recommendations can be made; general guidelines can be presented and each case must be judged individually. At one end of the spectrum are patients with mild anatomic abnormalities, relatively normal hemodynamics, and no symptoms, who require only observation and normal precautions to prevent bacterial endocarditis. But beyond this, the anatomic and hemodynamic abnormalities may become important enough to cause symptoms and significantly alter the patient's lifestyle. For these patients, surgical therapy is often the most effective treatment.

Indications for Operation

Most patients in functional classes I and II, with mild or no cardiomegaly can be managed medically. Operative correction is generally reserved for those with progressing symptoms, increasing cyanosis, or if paradoxical embolism occurs. Operation should also be considered if there is objective evidence of deterioration such as decreasing exercise performance by exercise testing, progressive increase in heart size on chest x-ray, progressive right ventricular dilatation, or reduction of systolic function by echocardiography, or inadequate control of atrial or ventricular arrhythmias. In borderline situations, echocardiographic images demonstrating features favorable for valve repair make the decision to proceed with operation easier.

Once symptoms develop and progress to Classes III and IV, medical management has little to offer; operation then becomes the only chance for improvement. A biventricular repair is usually possible, but in some circumstances, such as when significant left ventricular dysfunction has developed, cardiac transplantation may be the best option.

Surgical Treatment: History

The surgical approach to Ebstein anomaly has evolved over the past 40 years. Attempts to treat Ebstein anomaly surgically began in the 1950s with the use of systemic-to-pulmonary artery shunts for relief of cyanosis. For the minority of patients with obstruction of blood flow at either the pulmonary or tricuspid valve level, a shunt in infancy can be lifesaving. In the absence of obstructing lesions, systemic-pulmonary shunts have usually not significantly benefited patients. Superior vena cava–right pulmonary artery (classic Glenn) anastomosis was somewhat more successful at providing effective palliation (Glenn et al., 1966) but does not address the intracardiac abnormalities.

In 1958, Hunter and Lillehei tried repositioning the septal and posterior tricuspid valve leaflets, but this and other early valve "repairs" had little or no apparent success (Hardy and Roe, 1969; Hunter and Lillehei, 1958; Lillehei et al., 1967). In 1963 Barnard and Schrire successfully replaced the tricuspid valve with a prosthesis; this patient was still alive and doing well 19 years after operation (Charles et al., 1981). Drawing from the pioneering efforts by other surgeons, Danielson et al. (1979) of the Mayo Clinic developed a valve repair that could be applied in cases of Ebstein anomaly. The repair consisted of plication of the free wall of the atrialized portion of the right ventricle, posterior tricuspid annuloplasty, and excision of redundant right atrial wall (right reduction arterioplasty). The repair is based on the construction of a functional valve in which the only mobile component is the native anterior leaflet of the tricuspid valve. The annuloplasty is designed to allow the anterior leaflet to coapt with the ventricular septum, a concept that has been described as creation of a "monocusp" valve. Since the initial report, modifications to the surgical technique have allowed application to many anatomic variants of Ebstein anomaly (Dearani and Danielson, 2003; Dearani J and Danielson, in press).

More recently, other types of valve reconstruction have been proposed (Carpentier et al., 1988; Schmidt-Habelmann et al., 1981; Quaegebeur et al., 1991). In selected neonatal cases, closure of the tricuspid valve, atrial septectomy, and an aorto-pulmonary shunt have been advocated, and the patient is subsequently managed as a single ventricle (Starnes et al., 1991). However, late results of these procedures in significant numbers of patients have not yet been reported.

Surgical Treatment: Results

Prosthetic valve replacement, although remaining the most frequent method used to repair Ebstein anomaly, has given less-than-ideal results for some patients. Mechanical valves in the tricuspid position are associated with a higher frequency of valve malfunction and thrombotic complications than they are in other cardiac positions (Sanfelippo et al., 1976). Tissue valves do not have the thromboembolic complications of mechanical valves, but they do have a limited life expectancy, particularly in growing infants and children.

Therefore, we believe repair is preferable to valve replacement whenever repair is feasible. However, if there is failure of delamination of more than 50% of the anterior leaflet or if the leading edge of the anterior leaflet has hyphenated or linear attachment to the right ventricle, a durable repair may not be obtainable with valvuloplasty techniques. In these cases, valve replacement is then preferred. When valve replacement is necessary, it must be performed in a manner that protects the conduction tissue and the right coronary artery.

The largest series of surgical therapy for Ebstein anomaly comes from Danielson and colleagues (1997). In 42.7% (138/323), a tricuspid valve reconstruction was possible, in 54.8% (177/323), a prosthetic valve was required (usually a bioprosthesis), and in 2.5% a modified Fontan or other procedure was performed. There were 21 early deaths (6.5%). Concomitant procedures included ablation of accessory conduction pathways in 45 patients, a right-sided maze procedure for atrial flutter/fibrillation in 14 patients, and ablation of AVNRT in eight patients. Mean postoperative follow up was 7 years (maximum—25 years). The valve reconstructions were durable. Only 23 (16.7%) of the 138 repairs subsequently required reoperation. In this subgroup, the mean interval between the initial and the subsequent operation was 9.4 years (range—1.5–17.7 years). At late follow-up, incidence of atrial arrhythmias was reduced and 92.1% of patients were in NYHA functional Class I or II. Postoperative reduction in heart size was usual and occasionally considerable (Figure 15–6).

A separate report described the late outcome of 158 patients treated with tricuspid valve replacement (Kiziltan et al., 1998). The freedom from bioprosthesis replacement was 97.5% + 1.9% at 5 years and 80.6% + 7.6% at 10 and 15 years. Interestingly, freedom from reoperation at 10 and 15 years after tricuspid replacement (both bioprosthetic and mechanical) was not significantly different from that seen in the group treated with tricuspid valve repair (81.9% vs. 83.1%). It was speculated that the favorable outcome of prosthetic valves in this series may have been related to the large size of the bioprosthesis that can be implanted in the prominently enlarged right heart of patients with Ebstein anomaly. The presence of low right ventricular systolic pressure after repair in patients with Ebstein anomaly was also thought to favorably influence the longevity of the prosthesis.

The best treatment for the neonate born with Ebstein anomaly is still debated. Our philosophy is to try to bring the infant through the first few weeks of life by maintaining ductal patency with prostaglandin infusion. This will often provide adequate pulmonary vasodilation as well, but in severe cases, the addition of nitric oxide may be beneficial. If this is not successful, we offer operation. Based on recent experience (Knott-Craig et al., 2002), and on our own recent success in infants, we prefer a biventricular repair to the single-ventricle approach. Adjunctive use of atrial fenestration and/or a bidirectional cavopulmonary shunt remain controversial. In our practice, we reserve bidirectional cavopulmonary shunts for those with severe right ventricular failure. Atrial fenestration is rarely employed.

ACKNOWLEDGMENTS

The authors gratefully acknowledge the tremendous contributions made by Dr. Gordon K. Danielson to our understanding of the anatomy, pathophysiology, and care of the patient with Ebstein anomaly.

REFERENCES

Abbott M. Atlas of congenital heart disease. New York. *Am Heart Assoc.* 1936:24.

Anderson K, Danielson G, McGoon D, Lie J. Ebstein anomaly of the left-sided tricuspid valve: pathological anatomy of the valvular formation. *Circulation.* 1978;58:187–191.

Anderson K, Zuberbuhler J, Anderson R, Becker A, Lie J. Morphologic spectrum of Ebstein anomaly of the heart: a review. *Mayo Clinic Proc.* 1979;54:174–180.

Arnstein A. Elne seltene Missbildung der Trikuspidalklappe ("Ebsteinsche Krankheif"). *Virchows Arch Pathol Anat Physiol.* 1927;266:247–254.

Attenhofer Jost C, Connolly H, O'Leary P, Warnes C, Tajik A, Seward J. Occurrence of left ventricular myocardial dysplasia/noncompaction in patients with Ebstein anomaly. *Mayo Clinic Proc.* in press.

Attenhofer Jost C, Connolly H, Warnes C, O'Leary P, Tajik A, Pellikka P. Noncompacted myocardium in Ebstein anomaly: initial description in three patients. *J Am Soc Echocardiogr.* 2004;17:677–680.

Barber G, Danielson G, Heise C, Driscoll D. Cardiorespiratory response to exercise in Ebstein anomaly. *Am J Cardiol.* 1985;56:509–514.

Barnard C, Schrire V. Surgical correction of Ebstein malformation with prosthetic tricuspid valve. *Surgery.* 1963;54:302–308.

Benson L, Child J, Schwaiger M. Left ventricular geometry and function in adults with Ebstein anomaly of the tricuspid valve. *Circulation.* 1978;75:353–359.

Bialostozky D, Horwitz S, SEspino-Vela J. Ebstein malformation of the tricuspid valve: a review of 65 cases. *Am J Cardiol.* 1972;29:826–836.

Carpentier A, Chauvaud S, Mace L. A new reconstructive operation for Ebstein anomaly of the tricuspid valve. *J Thorac Cardiovasc Surg.* 1988;96:92–101.

Celermajer D, Bull C, Till J. Ebstein anomaly: presentation and outcome from fetus to adult. *J Am Coll Cardiol.* 1994;23:170.

Celermajer D, Cullen S, Sullivan I. Outcome in neonates with Ebstein anomaly. *J Am Coll Cardiol.* 1992;19:1041–1046.

Charles R, Barnard C, Beck W. Tricuspid valve replacement for Ebstein anomaly: a 19 year review of the first case. *Br Heart J.* 1981;46:578–580.

Cohen L, Friedman J, Jefferson J, Johnson E, Weiner M. A reevaluation of risk of in utero exposure to lithium. *JAMA.* 1994;271:146–150.

Connolly H, Warnes C. Ebstein anomaly: outcome of pregnancy. *J Am Coll Cardiol.* 1994;23:1194–1198.

Copeland W, Wooley C, Ryan J. Pregnancy and congenital heart disease. *Am J Obstet Gynecol.* 1963;86:107–110.

Danielson G, Maloney J, Devloo R. Surgical repair of Ebstein anomaly. *Mayo Clinic Proc.* 1979;54:185–192.

Dearani J, Danielson G. Ebstein anomaly. In: *Sabiston & Spencer Surgery of The Chest* (in press). Chapter 127.

Dearani J, Danielson G. Tricuspid valve repair for Ebstein anomaly. *Oper Tech Thorac Cardiovasc Surg.* 2003;8:188–192.

Donnelly J, Brown J, Radford D. Pregnancy outcome and Ebstein anomaly. *Br Heart J.* 1991;66:368–71.

Driscoll D, Mottram C, Danielson G. Spectrum of exercise intolerance in 45 patients with Ebstein anomaly and observations on exercise tolerance in 11 patients after surgical repair. *J Am Coll Cardiol.* 1988;11:831–836.

Ebstein W. Ober einen sehr seltenen Fall von Insufficienz der Valvula tricuspidalis, bedingt durch elne angeborene hochgradige Missbildung derslben. *Arch Anat Physiol Wissensch Med.* 1866;33:238–254.

Eidem BW, Tei C, O'Leary PW, Cetta F, Seward JB. Nongeometric quantitative assessment of right and left ventricular function: myocardial performance index in normal children and patients with Ebstein anomaly. *J Am Soc Echocardiograp.* 1998;11:849–856.

Emanuel R, O'Brien K, Ng R. Ebstein anomaly: genetic study of 26 families. *Br Heart J.* 1976;38:5–7.

Follath F, Hallidie-Smith K. Unusual electrocardiographic changes in Ebstein anomaly. *Br Heart J.* 1972;34:513–519.

Friedman S, Wells R, Amiri S. The transient nature of Wolff-Parkinson White anomaly in childhood. *J Pediatr.* 1969;74:296–300.

Fyler D, Bernhard W. Report of the New England Regional Infant Cardiac Program. *Pediatrics.* 1980;65:375–461.

Giuliani E, Fuster V, Brandenburg R, Mair D. Ebstein anomaly: the clinical features and natural history of Ebstein anomaly of the tricuspid valve. *Mayo Clinic Proc.* 1979;54:163–173.

Glenn W, Browne M, Whittemore R. Circulatory bypass of the right-side of the heart: cavopulmonary artery shunt—indications and results (report of a collected series of 537 cases). In: Cassels DE, ed. *The Heart and Circulation in the Newborn and Infant.* New York: Grune & Stratton; 1966:345–357.

Greason K, Dearani J, Theodore D, Porter C, Warnes C, Danielson G. Surgical management of atrial tachyarrhythmias associated with congenital cardiac anomalies: Mayo Clinic experience. *Semin Thorac Cardiovasc Surg Pediatr Card Surg Annu.* 2003;6.

Gussenhoven E, Stewart P, Becker A. "Offsetting" of the septal tricuspid leaflet in normal hearts and in hearts with Ebstein anomaly: anatomic and echographic correlation. *Am J Cardiol.* 1984;54:172–176.

Gussenhoven W, de Villeneuve V, Hugenholtz P. The role of echocardiography in assessing the functional class of the patient with Ebstein anomaly. *Eur Heart J.* 1984;5:490–493.

Hagler D. Echocardiographic assessment of Ebstein anomaly. *Prog Pediatr Cardiol.* 1993;2:28–37.

Hardy K, Roe B. Ebstein anomaly: further experience with definitive repair. *J Thorac Cardiovasc Surg.* 1969;58:533–561.

Hirschklau M, Sahn D, Hagan A. Cross-sectional echocardiographic features of Ebstein anomaly of the tricuspid valve. *Am J Cardiol.* 1977;40:400–404.

Hunter S, Lillehei C. Ebstein malformation of the tricuspid valve: study of a case together with suggestion of a new form of surgical therapy. *Dis Chest.* 1958;33:297–304.

Hurwitz R. Left ventricular function in infants and children with symptomatic Ebstein anomaly. *J Am Coll Cardiol.* 1994;73:716–718.

Keith J, Rowe R, Vlad P. *Heart Disease in Infancy and Childhood.* New York: Macmillan; 1958:314.

Kiziltan HT, Theodoro DA, Warnes CA, O'Leary PW, Anderson BJ, Danielson GK. Late results of bioprosthetic tricuspid valve replacement in Ebstein anomaly. *Ann Thorac Surg.* 1998;66:1539–45.

Klein G, Gulamhusein S. Intermittent preexcitation in the Wolff Parkinson White syndrome. *Am J Cardiol.* 1983;1983:292–296.

Knott-Craig C, Overhold E, Ward K. Repair of Ebstein anomaly in the asymptomatic neonate: an evaluation of technique with 7 year follow-up. *Ann Thorac Surg.* 2002;73:1786–1793.

Lev M, Gibson S, Miller R. Ebstein disease with Wolff Parkinson White syndrome: report of a case with a histopathologic study of possible conduction pathways. *Am Heart J.* 1955;49:724–741.

Lillehei C, Kalke B, Carlson R. Evoluton of corrective surgery for Ebstein anomaly. *Circulation.* 1967;35–36:111–118.

Littler W. Successful pregnancy in a patient with Ebstein anomaly. *Br Heart J.* 1970;32:711–713.

MacCallum W. Congenital malformations of the heart as illustrated by the specimens in the pathological museum of the Johns Hopkins Hospital. *Johns Hopkins Hosp Bull.* 1900;11:6971.

MacLellan-Tobert S, Driscoll D, Mottram C, Mahoney D, Wollan P, Danielson G. Exercise tolerance in patients with Ebstein anomaly. *J Am Coll Cardiol.* 1997;29:1615–1622.

Mair D, Seward J, Driscoll D, Danielson G. Surgical repair of Ebstein anomaly: selection of patients and early and late operative results. *Circulation.* 1985;72:1170–1176.

Mann R, Lie J. The life story of Wilhelm Ebstein (1836–1912) and his almost overlooked description of a congenital heart disease. *Mayo Clinic Proc.* 1979;54:197–204.

Matsumoto M, Matsu H, Nagata S, Hamanaka Y, Fujita T. Visualization of Ebstein anomaly of the tricuspid valve by two-dimensional and standard echocardiography. *Circulation.* 1976;53:59–79.

Monibi A, Neches W, Lenox C. Left ventricular anomalies associated with Ebstein malformation of the tricuspid valve. *Circulation.* 1978;57:303–306.

Ng R, Somerville J, Ross D. Ebstein anomaly: late results of surgical correction. *Eur J Cardiol.* 1979;9:39–52.

Nora J, Nora A, Toews W. Lithium, Ebstein anomaly, and other congenital heart defects. *Lancet. (Letter)* 1974;4:594–595.

Oh J, Holmes D, Hayes D. Cardiac arrhythmias in patients with surgical repair of Ebstein anomaly. *J Am Coll Cardiol.* 1985;6:1351–1357.

Olson T, Porter C, Danielson G. Surgical treatment of Ebstein anomaly and preexcitation (abstract). *PACE.* 1991;14:645.

Olson T, Porter C. Electrocardiographic and electrophysiologic findings in Ebstein anomaly: pathophysiology, diagnosis, and management. *Prog Pediatr Cardiol.* 1993;2:38–50.

Ports T, Silverman N, Schiller N. Two-dimensional echocardiographic assessment of Ebstein anomaly. *Circulation.* 1978;58:336–343.

Quaegebeur J, Sreeram N, Fraser A. Surgery for Ebstein anomaly: the clinical and echocardiographic evaluation of a new technique. *J Am Coll Cardiol*. 1991;17:722–728.

Randolph G, Hagler D, Connolly H, et al. Intraoperative transesophageal echocardiography during surgery for congenita heart defects. *J Thorac Cardiovasc Surg*. 2002;124:1176–1182.

Reich J, Auld D, Hulse E, Sullivan K, Campbell R. The Pediatric Radiofrequency Ablation Registry's experience with Ebstein anomaly. Pediatric Electrophysiology Society. *J Cardiovasc Electrophysiol*. 1998;9:1370.

Roberson D, Silverman N. Ebstein anomaly: echocardiographic and clinical features in the fetus and neonate. *J Am Coll Cardiol*. 1989;14:1300–1307.

Rosenmann A, Arad I, Simcha A, Schaap T. Familial Ebstein anomaly. *J Med Genet*. 1976;13:532–535.

Sanfelippo P, Giuliani E, Danielson G. Tricuspid valve prosthetic replacement: early and late results with the Starr-Edwards prosthesis. *J Thorac Cardiovasc Surg*. 1976;71:441–445.

Schiebler G, Adams P, Anderson R. The Wolff Parkinson White syndrome in infants and children: a review and a report of 28 cases. *Pediatrics*. 1959;24:585–603.

Schmidt-Habelmann P, Meisner H, Struck E, Sebening F. Results of valvuloplasty for Ebstein anomaly. *Thorac Cardiovasc Surg*. 1981;29:155–157.

Seward J, Tajik A, Feist D, Smith H. Ebstein anomaly in an 85-year-old man. *Mayo Clinic Proc*. 1979;54:193–196.

Seward J. Ebstein anomaly: ultrasound imaging and hemodynamic evaluation. *Echocardiography*. 1993;10:641–664.

Shiina A, Seward J, Edwards W. Two-dimensional echocardiographic spectrum of Ebstein anomaly: detailed anatomic assessment. *J Am Coll Cardiol*. 1984;3:356–370.

Shiina A, Seward J, Tajik A, Hagler D, Danielson G. Two-dimensional echocardiographic-surgical correlation in Ebstein anomaly: preoperative determination of patients requiring tricuspid valve plication vs. replacement. *Circulation*. 1983;68:534–544.

Smith W, Gallagher J, Kerr C. The electrophysiologic basis and management of symptomatic recurrent tachycardia in patients with Ebstein anomaly of the tricuspid valve. *Am J Cardiol*. 1982;49:1223–1234.

Soulie P, Heulin A, Ualy-Laubry C, Degeorges M. Ebstein disease: clinical study and development (40 cases, 9 of which surgical). *(French) Arch Mal Coeur Vaiss*. 1970;63:615–637.

Starnes V, Pitlick P, Bernstein D, Griffin M, Choy M, Shumway N. Ebstein anomaly appearing in the neonate. *J Thorac Cardiovasc Surg*. 1991;101:1082–1087.

Theodoro D, Danielson G, Kiziltan H. Surgical management Ebstein anomaly: 25-year experience. *Circulation*. 1997;96:121.

Theodoro D, Danielson G, Porter C. Right-sided maze procedure for right and atrial arrhythmias in congenital heart disease. *Ann Thorac Surg*. 1998;65:149–154.

Uhl H. A previously undescribed congenital malformation of the heart: almost total absence of the myocardium of the right ventricle. *Johns Hopkins Hosp Bull*. 1952;91:197–205.

Van Mierop L, Gessner I. Pathogenetic mechanisms in congenital cardiovascular malformations. *Prog Cardiovasc Dis*. 1972;15:67–85.

Waickman L, Skorton D, Varner M. Ebstein anomaly and pregnancy. *Am J Cardiol*. 1984;53:357–358.

Watson H. Natural history of Ebstein anomaly of tricuspid valve in childhood and adolescence: an international co-operative study of 505 cases. *Br Heart J*. 1974;36:417–427.

Whittemore R, Hobbins J, Engle M. Pregnancy and its outcome in women with and without surgical treatment of congenital heart disease. *Am J Cardiol*. 1982;50:641–651.

Yetman A, Freedom R, McCrindle B. Outcome of cyanotic neonates with Ebstein anomaly. *Am J Cardiol*. 1998;81:749–754.

Yetman A, Freedom R, McGrindle B. Right-sided maze procedure for right atrial arrhythmias in congenital heart disease. *Am J Cardiol*. 1998;81:749–754.

III

Special Management Issues

16

Heart Transplantation

DEBRA A. DODD

INTRODUCTION

Heart transplantation was introduced to the public in 1967, when Dr. Christian Barnard performed the first heart transplant in an adult with ischemic cardiomyopathy (*The New York Times*, 1967). Just a few days later, Dr. Adrian Kantrowitz transplanted the heart from an anencephalic infant into an infant with a fatal congenital heart defect at Maimonides Medical Center in Brooklyn (Kantrowitz A, 1998). Thus, from its clinical inception, heart transplantation has been considered therapy for both types of end-stage heart disease, dilated cardiomyopathies, and congenital heart disease. These early heart transplant recipients often lived only hours or days. It became clear that the surgical technique was only the first hurdle, and that suppression of the immune system to prevent rejection of the new heart was crucial to meaningful survival. Approval of the new immunosuppressive agent, cyclosporine, in 1980 led to much improved survival and to a steady increase in number of heart transplants during the 1980s (Figure 16–1) (Boucek et al., 2007). Dr. Leonard Bailey pioneered infant heart transplantation for hypoplastic left heart syndrome beginning in 1985, and the majority of these infant transplants in the early years were performed at Loma Linda University (Bailey et al., 1986b). His results encouraged the growth of pediatric transplantation worldwide. Since 1991, the annual number of pediatric heart transplants has remained steady at approximately 400 per year and the annual number of adult heart transplants peaked at 4439 in the mid 1990s and now has settled out at about 3000 per year (Boucek et al., 2007; Taylor et al., 2007). Over the last two decades, approximately 50% of children underwent heart transplantation for the indication of congenital heart disease. In contrast, the primary indication for heart transplant in the adult population has remained dilated or ischemic cardiomyopathy, though the percent of adults being transplanted for end-stage congenital heart disease has been steadily increasing. Between 1995 and 2005, only 2.2% (790 of 336,197) of adults listed for transplantation in the United States were listed for congenital heart disease (Davies, et al., 2008b). However, this percentage increased annually almost threefold from 1.4% to 3.5% over that 10-year period. As more children survive into adulthood following palliative procedures for complex congenital heart disease, the number of adults requiring transplantation for this indication would be expected to continue to rise.

For now, the adult heart transplant experience reflects primarily results in patients in their later decades of life with cardiomyopathy. In the annual International Society for Heart and Lung Transplantation (ISHLT) registry report, the mean age for adults was 50.7 ± 12.5 years (Taylor et al., 2007). The focus of this chapter is congenital heart disease as an indication for heart transplantation, and as such, most discussions to follow will focus on the pediatric experience since it is more representative of the patient likely to undergo transplantation for congenital heart disease in the near future.

Survival after heart transplantation has improved significantly in each of the last three decades with advances in early postoperative care and use of new immunosuppressive medications (Figure 16–2) (Boucek et al., 2007; Chen et al., 2004). According to the latest ISHLT pediatric registry report, actuarial survival is presently 88% at 30 days, 81% at 1 year, 69% at 5 years, and 58% at 10 years (Boucek et al., 2007). The estimated half-live for infants is 15.8 years, 14.2 years for children 1–10 years of age, and 11.4 years for adolescents (Boucek et al., 2007). For those who survived the first year following transplantation, the respective

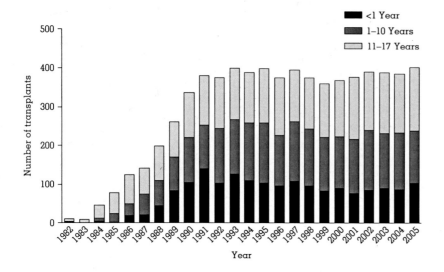

FIGURE 16–1. Age distribution for pediatric heart transplants by year of transplant. (Reprinted from Boucek et al., 2007, with permission of the publisher. Copyright © 2007, Elsevier Science Inc.)

estimated half-lives are 17.5 years for children 1–10 years of age, and 16.2 years for adolescents. The number of infant transplant patients who have died is too low to calculate 1 year conditional half-life at this time. These excellent survival outcomes have allowed transplant physicians to shift attention from short-term survival alone to improving quality of life and prevention of long-term complications of organ transplantation and immunosuppression.

SURGICAL TECHNIQUE

Orthotopic heart transplantation refers to the replacement of a diseased heart with a donor heart that then sits in the normal position in the chest. Despite 40 years of heart transplant experience, the optimal atrial anastomotic technique remains unclear (Schmid et al., 2004; Weiss et al., 2008). The two major techniques presently used are called biatrial and bicaval (Figures 16–3 and 16–4). A third technique, called total cardiac transplant, is used much less often. The biatrial technique leaves the back of both recipient atria intact including pulmonary veins and caval veins. The donor atria are sutured to the respective recipient atria, and the main pulmonary artery and ascending aorta are sutured end-to-end to their respective vessels. The bicaval technique leaves the back of the left atrium with pulmonary veins intact, but removes all of the right atrium, leaving only the inferior and superior cavae.

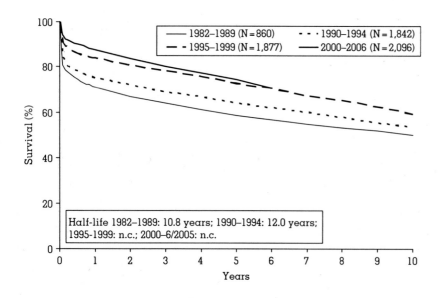

FIGURE 16–2. Kaplan-Meier survival stratified by era of transplant for pediatric heart transplants performed between January 1982 and June 2005. (Reprinted from Boucek et al., 2007, with permission of the publisher and the ISHLT. Copyright © 2007, Elsevier Science Inc.)

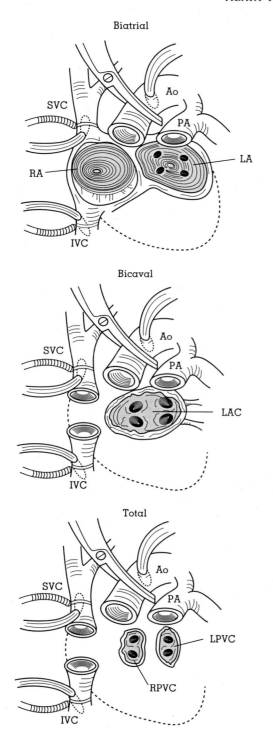

FIGURE 16–3. Illustration of the biatrial, bicaval, and total orthotopic cardiac transplantation techniques, depicted as the preparation of the recipient's mediastinum before transplantation. *Dotted lines*, original position of excised native heart. *Ao*, aorta; *IVC*, inferior vena cava; *LA*, left atrium; *LAC*, left atrial cuff; *LPVC*, left pulmonary vein cuff; *PA*, pulmonary artery; *RA*, right atrium; *RPVC*, right pulmonary vein cuff; *SVC*, superior vena cava. (Reprinted from Miniati and Robbins, 2001, as adapted from Aziz et al., 1999 with permission from Lippincott Williams & Wilkins, Inc, and Elsevier Science Inc, Copyright © 1999 Elsevier Science Inc.)

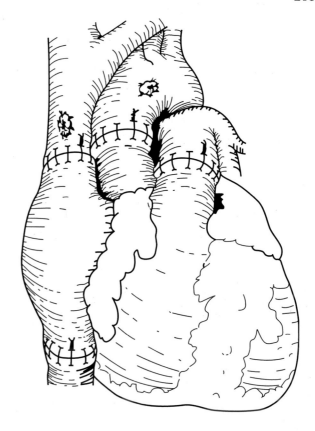

FIGURE 16–4. Bicaval orthotopic cardiac transplantation. (Reprinted from Morgan and Edward, 2005, with permission from the publisher. Copyright © 2005, Wiley-Blackwell Publishing.)

The donor caval veins are separately sutured end-to-end to the respective recipient cavae, while the left atrial and great artery anastamoses are done as with the biatrial technique. Both techniques have equivalent survival, but the bicaval method has slightly lower incidence of the need for pacemaker, usually placed for sinus node dysfunction (Weiss et al., 2008). The bicaval anastomosis may have more risk of caval obstruction, especially in small children (Sachdeva et al., 2007; Sze et al., 1998). Either technique is technically possible with most forms of congenital heart disease as long as the pulmonary veins are unobstructed and pulmonary arteries are not severely hypoplastic. If these structural abnormalities are present, combined heart/lung transplantation may be the only option. Additional donor vessel can be used to reconstruct the superior vena cava, innominate vein, main or branch pulmonary arteries, and ascending and transverse aortic arch as needed for repair of congenital heart disease. Extra donor vessel can be harvested and left attached to the heart at the donor explantation.

Complex congenital heart disease, often associated with heterotaxy, is frequently accompanied by anomalies of the systemic and pulmonary venous return, including partial or total anomalous pulmonary venous return, interrupted inferior vena cava, bilateral superior vena cavae, dextrocardia, and/or situs inversus. These abnormalities have not proven to be absolute contraindications to transplantation as the congenital heart surgeons have been very inventive in reestablishing functional connections (Bailey et al., 1986a; Del Riol, 2000; Razzouk et al., 1995; Vricella et al., 1998). However, these modified connections may make surveillance cardiac catheterizations and/or endomyocardial biopsies difficult or impossible.

Heterotopic transplantation refers to the placement of the donor heart in a position other than the normal position, often leaving the recipient heart in place and the donor heart as a "booster" heart. This was done more frequently in the early heart transplant experience in humans, but now is done rarely except in some animal models of heart transplantation (Chiu et al., 2006).

THE RECIPIENTS

In the mid-1980s, poor survival with the staged palliative surgery for hypoplastic left heart syndrome encouraged some children's hospitals to establish pediatric heart transplant programs and to pursue transplantation as the primary operative procedure for these infants. Success in these infants lead to consideration of heart transplantation as the primary surgery in rarer examples of lethal congenital heart disease such as pulmonary atresia with right ventricular-dependent coronary circulation, single ventricle with total anomalous pulmonary venous return, and complex unbalanced atrioventricular septal defect. During this early era, most infants underwent transplantation without a history of prior cardiac operation. As outcome for the staged palliative operations for hypoplastic left heart syndrome and other complex congenital heart disease has improved, today most infants being listed for transplantation have had one or more prior operative procedures. Also in the early era, transplantation was also recognized as the only option for children with end-stage congenital heart disease secondary to late onset ventricular failure following attempts at surgical repair or palliation early in life. This typically developed a decade or more following initial cardiac surgery, usually in adolescence or in early adulthood. Therefore, the pediatric experience in heart transplantation has been concentrated at each end of the age spectrum, less than 1 year of age and older than 12 years of age (Lamour et al., 2005). The congenital heart disease diagnoses for recipients of heart transplant beyond the infant age group (>6 months of age) in the Pediatric Heart Transplant Study Group (PHTSG) and Cardiac

Transplant Research Database (CTRD) are listed in Table 16–1 (Lamour et al., 2005). Single ventricle is the most common diagnosis transplanted. In a smaller study including infants, single ventricle morphology accounted for 67% of the children (<20 years of age) who were listed for transplantation (Mital et al., 2003). In this group of children listed for congenital heart disease, 29% died waiting, similar to that for all children listed. The most common reasons for referral for transplantation were ventricular dysfunction (78%), failed Fontan procedure (18%), and severe hypoxemia (4%). Even the "perfect" single ventricle candidate for Fontan procedure demonstrates significant late morbidity and mortality, with survival of 81% at 10 years and 73% at 15 years (Fontan et al., 1990). Now the Fontan procedure has been extended to many other "high-risk" Fontan candidates, with more morbidity and mortality. The age at which children with single ventricle come to listing for transplantation depends in part on the morphology of their single ventricle. The median age at transplantation is significantly older in those with left ventricular morphology (11.82 years) than those with right ventricular morphology (8.05 years) (Botha et al., 2008). Thirty-five percent of failed Fontan patients are listed urgently with acute postoperative failure. The recipients transplanted for single ventricle frequently have had multiple prior operations (mean 2.6 ± 1.6; range 1–8) (Jayakumar et al., 2004).

For children, the following risk factors have been linked with poorer survival after transplantation: complex congenital heart disease (especially following Fontan procedure), previous sternotomy, renal dysfunction, mechanical ventilation, extracorporeal membrane oxygenation (ECMO), pulmonary hypertension, pulmonary artery anatomy requiring reconstruction, and HLA sensitization (Boucek et al., 2007; Chen et al., 2004; Davies et al., 2008a). Complex congenital heart disease often requires significant reconstructive surgery

TABLE 16–1. *Congenital Heart Disease Diagnoses for Heart Transplant Recipients within the Pediatric Heart Transplant Study Group (1993–2002) and Cardiac Transplant Research Database (1990–2002) For Recipients Less Than 6 Months*

Diagnosis	N (N = 488)	%
Single ventricle	176	36
D-transposition of the great arteries	58	12
Right ventricular outflow tract lesions	49	10
L-transposition of the great arteries	39	8
Ventricular/atrial septal defect	38	8
Left ventricular outflow tract lesions	38	8
Other	53	18

Data from Lamour et al., 2005, with permission of the publisher. Copyright © 2005, Elsevier Science Inc.

at the time of transplantation with longer bypass and ischemic time accompanied by delayed graft recovery (Jayakumar et al., 2004). Renal dysfunction complicates postoperative fluid management and can be further worsened by cardiopulmonary bypass and the immunosuppressive medications used in the postoperative period. Mechanical ventilation and ECMO as risk factors probably represent the severity of the heart failure and risk of multiorgan dysfunction, infection, and longer postoperative recovery periods. The need for pulmonary artery reconstruction increased mortality both short- and long-term (Chen et al., 2004). This is likely secondary to a higher risk of residual pulmonary artery stenosis and/or unreactive pulmonary hypertension leading to early right heart failure (see discussion of pulmonary resistance below). For the first few decades of heart transplantation, discontinuous pulmonary arteries with unilateral pulmonary hypertension, or absence of one pulmonary artery, were considered an indication for heart/lung transplantation. However, heart transplant alone can be done in many of these patients with one healthy lung with good operative survival of 82% (Chen et al., 2004; Lamour et al., 2004). Pulmonary hypertension and HLA sensitization tend to be more clinically significant in patients with congenital heart disease referred for transplant compared to patients with dilated cardiomyopathy.

Pulmonary hypertension with elevated pulmonary vascular resistance was considered an absolute contraindication to heart transplantation for much of the early history of heart transplantation due to the rapid development of right ventricular failure in the donor heart. All neonates have higher pulmonary vascular resistance than adults, and this will persist in infants with hypoplastic left heart syndrome or other complex congenital heart disease maintained on prostaglandin for systemic output or pulmonary blood flow. This was thought to be a major contributor to perioperative deaths following transplantation for hypoplastic left heart disease during the early experience. Also, children with a history of surgical aortopulmonary shunts for treatment of cyanotic heart disease (Hofschire et al., 1977; Wauthy et al., 2003) or longstanding elevation of left atrial pressures due to left heart obstructive lesions will also frequently have elevated pulmonary vascular resistance (Brauner et al., 1997; Burch et al., 2004). If the pulmonary vascular bed can be shown to be reactive to vasodilators, such as nitroprusside, nitric oxide, or prostacyclin, in the cardiac catheterization laboratory, then these patients most commonly survive heart transplantation in the recent era (Addonizio et al., 1987; Webber et al., 2003b; Goland et al., 2007). These same vasodilators can be used to control the pulmonary hypertension in the intensive care unit following surgery as needed. Satisfactory outcomes can be obtained with pretransplant pulmonary vascular resistance as high as 10 IU (normal <3 IU) in children (Webber et al., 2003b). In cases of moderate pulmonary hypertension, pulmonary artery pressure will fall significantly within 1 week and will reach normal values by 2 weeks following transplantation (Bhatia et al., 1987). In transplant candidates with single ventricle morphology, accurate assessment of pulmonary vascular resistance prior to transplantation is impossible as the pulmonary blood flow cannot be measured. The primary assessment for vascular disease is measurement of the transpulmonary gradient, which has been demonstrated to increase by a mean of 6.8 mm following transplantation relative to pretransplantation (Mitchell et al., 2004). After transplantation, cardiac catheterization in this group of recipients has shown most had mild to moderate pulmonary vascular disease if the indication for transplantation was late failure (mean 7.4 years following Fontan procedure), but not if indication was early failure within 1 year following Fontan procedure (Mitchell et al., 2004). Survival was good despite this modest elevation in pulmonary vascular resistance at 93%, 82%, and 82% at 3, 5, and 7 years. This suggests that elevated pulmonary vascular resistance is common following the Fontan procedure and may contribute to Fontan failure, but that the severity is not usually associated with donor right ventricular failure and does not preclude successful heart transplantation.

The presence of anti-donor HLA antigens (and/or the presence of a positive crossmatch) has been considered an absolute contraindication to transplantation. Untreated, it leads to hyperacute rejection, often causing acute failure of the transplanted heart while still in the operating room. The degree of presensitization is often measured preoperatively as a panel reactive antibody (PRA), given as a percent of total HLA antigens against which the recipient has preformed antibodies. The higher this percentage, the less likely the crossmatch will be negative for a given donor. Pregnancy, blood transfusions, mechanical support, and prior organ transplant have been the major causes for elevated PRA in the adult population (Kobashigawa, 2007). In children with congenital heart disease, the incidence and severity of HLA sensitization has proven problematic as a result of the common use of allografts (cadaver tissue) and xenografts (porcine and bovine tissue) for enlargement of small vessels or re-recreation of absent connections. Most types of allografts (homovital, antibiotic-sterilized, and cryopreserved) and xenografts have stimulated strong immune responses and very high PRA levels (Breinholt et al., 2000; Meyer et al., 2005; Shaddy et al., 1996; Smith et al., 1995). Immunosuppression with mycophenolate mofetil started at allograft placement and continued for

3 months yielded a marked reduction in HLA sensitization in a majority of the patients that persisted for at least 2 years of follow-up (Anderson et al., 2005). For now, only modification of surgical technique to exclude use of allografts and xenografts may be fully effective at avoiding HLA sensitization in all patients. For the future, an excellent alternative would be tissue engineered autologous valves, perhaps created from the patient's own umbilical cord cells (Sodian et al., 2006), or by temporarily placing a "scaffold" subcutaneously to allow collagen deposition (Hayashida et al., 2007). These and other experimental methods may hold potential for optimal initial surgical outcome and lower risk of end-stage heart disease, while minimizing risk factors for later transplantation, if it is needed. The risk associated with an elevated PRA also seems to be evolving. Hyperacute rejection can now be prevented in most cases with one or more methods to reduce antibody load: plasmapheresis to remove antibody, cyclophosphamide, or mycophenolate mofetil or rituximab to reduce antibody production, or intravenous immunoglobulin to compete with harmful antibody (Pollock-BarZiv et al., 2007; Shaddy and Fuller, 2005). With elevated pretransplant PRA, there is still a higher risk of early rejection in the first 2–3 months following heart transplantation, but there is no consistent evidence of difference in survival or incidence of graft coronary artery disease (Almond et al., 2008; DiFilippo et al., 2005; Feingold et al., 2007; Holt et al., 2007; Mahle et al., 2004; Pollock-BarZiv et al., 2007).

Several morbidities rarely seen except in the patient with single ventricle physiology include aortopulmonary collateral vessels, protein losing enteropathy (PLE), and pulmonary arteriovenous malformations (AVMs). Aortopulmonary collaterals occur commonly in association with cyanotic congenital heart defects and can lead to congestive heart failure due to large left-to-right shunt following heart transplantation (Krishnan et al., 2004). Early recognition and coil embolization in the cardiac catheterization laboratory can significantly improve the postoperative course. Both protein-losing enteropathy and pulmonary ateriovenous malformations will resolve following transplantation, but may complicate postoperative care following transplantation. Protein-losing enteropathy is a poorly understood loss of protein from the gut that leads to ascites, diarrhea, pleural, and pericardial effusions, and peripheral edema with high mortality. This complication of Fontan procedure can be unrelenting with medical interventions and attempts at Fontan revision in the cardiac catheterization laboratory or operative suite. Following heart transplantation, it does resolve in the majority of patients, with normalization of the serum protein levels within 6–18 months (Bernstein

et al., 2006; Gamba et al., 2004; Mitchell et al., 2004). Another complication of the single ventricle palliative procedures is the development of pulmonary arteriovenous malformations. These are seen following either Glenn shunt or Fontan procedure, and are felt due to the lack of a hepatic factor reaching the lungs. Prior to transplantation, they can lead to severe cyanosis and exercise intolerance. Regression of the pulmonary arteriovenous malformations has been demonstrated with normalization of systemic saturations (>96%) by 14–180 days posttransplantation (Lamour et al., 2000; Mitchell et al., 2004).

In summary, congenital heart disease is a risk factor for increased morbidity and mortality following heart transplantation, primarily due to early postoperative risks. The 30-day mortality risk is 26% for congenital heart disease compared to 7% for dilated cardiomyopathy (Tjang et al., 2008). However, if the recipient survives the perioperative period, long-term survival for congenital heart disease patients is equivalent to those transplanted for cardiomyopathy (Figure 16–5) (Bernstein et al., 2006; Chen et al., 2004; Lamour et al., 1999 & 2005; Larsen et al., 2002). The major operation prior to transplant is more predictive of survival than the actual congenital diagnosis, with Fontan procedure for single ventricle having the highest early mortality (Botha et al., 2008; Lamour et al., 2005). Despite a higher early postoperative mortality, the long-term survival in the post-Fontan group is also similar to that in patients undergoing transplantation for cardiomyopathy (Figure 16–5) (Bernstein et al., 2006; Botha et al., 2008; Gamba et al., 2004). There are few absolute "structural" contraindications to heart transplantation in the present era with the most common being severe hypoplasia of the pulmonary arteries, pulmonary vein stenosis, or irreversible severe pulmonary hypertension (Canter et al., 2007).

THE DONORS

As noted in the introduction, the first pediatric heart donor was an anencephalic infant. This child could not legally be a donor today. With the medical community able to support respirations and heartbeat indefinitely after the brain ceased to function, and with the new potential of organ transplantation, concerns developed over which patients should ethically be a donor. This led to the development of formal definitions of "brain death" and the stipulation that organ donors must meet brain death criteria. In addition, the donors must be free of certain infections that would be transferred to the donor and lead to serious donor disease and/or death. Classically this excludes donors with HIV, active Hepatitis B or C, active tuberculosis (TB),

Greenfield Medical Library - Issue Receipt

Customer name: Granados Riveron, Javier Tadeo

Title: Congenital heart defects : from origin to treatment / edited by Diego F. Wyszynski, Adolfo Correa-Vi

ID: 1006084063
Due: 30/06/2011 23:59

Total items: 1
07/02/2011   14:00

All items must be returned before the due date and time.

The Loan period may be shortened if the item is requested.

WWW.nottingham.ac.uk/is

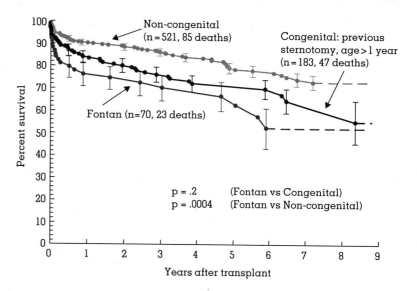

FIGURE 16–5. Survival after transplantation in Fontan patients compared with noncongenital heart disease (No-CHD) and patients with congenital heart disease and a previous sternotomy (CHD). There was no difference in survival between Fontan and congenital heart disease groups, although the survival of both of these groups was less than for patients without congenital heart disease. (Reprinted from Bernstein et al., 2006, with permission of the publisher. Copyright © 2006, Lippincott Williams & Wilkins.)

syphilis, viral encephalitis, or other active viral infections. Typically, most donor bacterial infections will not be transmitted to the recipient, especially if due to gram-positive bacteria or if treated with an appropriate course of antibiotics before transplantation (Bull et al., 1995; Lammermeier et al., 1990). The donor cardiac anatomy and function must be acceptable as assessed by history, vital signs, and echocardiography.

If the donor meets these criteria, they are matched by computer according to blood type, donor/recipient weight ratio, status of the recipient, and location of the recipient and donor. From the beginning, heart donors have been matched only for blood type (ABO-compatible) without the detailed HLA matching required for some other solid organ transplantations. HLA matching was initially not feasible due to the short ischemic time needed between explantation from the donor and implantation into the recipient, the relatively limited number of heart recipients listed at any given time, and the usual cardiac recipient instability allowing short wait times before death. Fortunately, for heart transplantation, the data has continued to demonstrate no or minimal benefit to HLA matched donors when reviewed retrospectively (Almenar et al., 2005; Hathout et al., 2005). HLA typing of the donor can now be done rapidly but matching is reserved for the presensitized recipient. The heart must be appropriate size to fit into the recipient's chest and to perform properly in the immediate postoperative period. It has been shown that outcomes are best if the donor/recipient weight ratio is between 0.8 and 2.5 (Boucek et al., 2007). The recipients are ranked according to clinical status as 1a, 1b, or 2, with 1a being the sickest patients in the intensive care unit and 2 being the most stable patients that are typically at home. Lastly,

the proximity of the donor and recipient are taken into account in order to minimize the ischemic time of the donor heart and optimize chances for good cardiac function following transplantation. Under these restrictions, there remain many more children awaiting a new heart than there are appropriate donors. Over the last 10 years, in children (0–10 years of age), there has been an average of 323 children listed annually to 200 donors annually (OPTN website, 2008). The mismatch is even larger in the infants under 1 year of age with 162 infants listed annually and 67 donors annually in that same time period.

Recently, it has been shown that in infants and young children who have not yet developed antibody to ABO blood antigens, ABO-incompatible transplantation can be done with good short-term survival and with long-term failure to develop the expected ABO antibodies (Roche et al., 2008; West et al., 2001; West, 2006). These antibodies typically arise between age 6 months and 2 years, so listing for ABO-incompatible heart transplantation is restricted to recipients under 2 years of age under UNOS listing in the United States. Older children and adults who do have ABO antibody will develop hyperacute rejection and immediate graft dysfunction following ABO-incompatible transplantation. ABO-incompatible transplantation has decreased time to heart transplant in infants in some regions.

Another new potential donor is the "DCD donor" or donor after cardiac death (Boucek, 2008; Koogler and Costarino, 1998). It has been recognized that many children with irreversible brain injury did not meet brain death criteria due to continued minor brain stem function. Although families frequently requested donation, this was not an option until now. The DCD donor has a terminal illness for which additional therapy only prolongs the dying process, the quality of life on support is felt by staff and family to be unsatisfactory, and the amount of support is high such that its withdrawal will be expected to lead to death within 30 minutes. Support is withdrawn and after the heart has stopped beating and the child/adult has been pronounced dead, the donor is resuscitated and the organs are recovered. It has been estimated that 35% of pediatric hospital deaths involve withdrawal of support, with 28% would qualify as pediatric DCD donors (Koogler et al., 1998). The Joint Commission on the Accreditation of Health Care Organizations (JCAHO) is mandating that all hospitals have a formal DCD protocol in place (JCAHO, 2004). It is estimated that this could increase the donor pool by a minimum of 40%–100% (Boucek, 2008; Koogler et al., 1998).

TABLE 16–2. *Posttransplant Morbidity Cumulative Prevalence in Survivors Within 5 Years Posttransplant (Follow-ups: April 1994 to June 2006)*

Outcome	Within 5 Years (%)	Total Number with Known Response
Hypertension	63.2	980
Renal dysfunction	9.3	1021
Abnormal creatinine <2.5 mg/dL	7.5	
Creatinine >2.5 mg/dL	1.0	
Long-term dialysis	0.6	
Renal transplant	0.2	
Hyperlipidemia	25.6	1062
Diabetes	5.0	981
Coronary artery vasculopathy	10.9	724

Reprinted Boucek et al., 2007, with permission of the publisher. Copyright © 2007, Elsevier Science Inc.

LIFE AFTER CARDIAC TRANSPLANTATION

The majority of pediatric heart transplant recipients today can be expected to do well during the first year following transplantation, with a good balance attained between under-immunosuppression with risk of rejection and over-immunosuppression with risk of infection. Beyond the immediate operative risks, the focus becomes prevention of long-term complications. Some of the long-term complications such as rejection, graft coronary artery disease, cancer, and renal failure can be life-threatening. Others, such as allergic conditions, may significantly alter quality of life, but they are rarely the cause of death following transplantation. Lastly, morbidities, such as hypertension, hyperlipidemia, and diabetes, can be managed with diet and medications, and are minimized on steroid-free maintenance immunosuppression. The prevalence of complications at 5 years following transplantation is listed in Table 16–2 (Boucek et al., 2007). In pediatric heart transplant recipients surviving greater than 10 years, cancers had occurred in 23%, graft coronary artery disease in 31%, retransplantation in 15%, and death in 23% (Ross et al., 2006). Graft coronary artery disease was the most common cause of death in these long-term survivors (Boucek et al., 2007).

Rejection

Rejection is a response of the recipient's immune system against a transplanted organ producing injury to that donor organ. Approximately 45%–50% of children have an episode of rejection during the first year following heart transplantation (Boucek et al., 2007). Isolated episodes during this time period do not appear to alter long-term survival. However, two or more episodes of rejection in the first year are associated with higher risk of graft coronary artery disease and death (Boucek et al., 2007; Pahl et al., 2005). Rejection rates do vary depending upon the immunosuppressive regimen used, and there is a wide variation in regimens used between transplant centers and within transplant centers. In 2006, approximately 60% of children received induction therapy, approximately one-third IL-2R antagonist, and two-thirds polyclonal antithymocyte globulin (Boucek et al., 2007). This was followed by a maintenance regimen including a calcineurin-inhibitor (cyclosporin or tacrolimus), an antiproliferative drug (azathioprine or mycophenolate mofetil) with or without steroids. Approximately half of the children received maintenance steroids. Children on the newer calcineurin-inhibitor, tacrolimus, had a significantly lower incidence of rejection during the first year than those on cyclopsorine. The choice of regimen is largely center-dependent, but many centers have also individualized therapy based on the recipient's risk factors and their side effects from medications.

Most rejection episodes are "cellular rejection" and are largely T-cell-mediated. However, as the incidence and morbidity of cellular rejection after heart transplantation has fallen with newer immunosuppressive regimens, the occurrence of "biopsy-negative" episodes of rejection has remained fairly constant, comprising a greater percent of all rejection episodes (Fishbein et al., 2004). The majority of these are felt to be antibody-mediated or humoral, and, therefore, also involve B-cell activation. Since the majority of antibody is intravascular, the injury seen with antibody-mediated rejection is primarily a vasculitis. Antibody-mediated rejection is more often associated with hemodynamic compromise, and is more difficult to treat, than classical acute cellular rejection (Fishbein et al., 2004; Kobashigawa, 2007; Pahl et al., 2001). Antibody-mediated rejection has been shown to significantly decrease survival and to predispose to transplant-associated coronary artery disease earlier and at an increased frequency compared to cellular rejection.

Late rejection episodes (more than 1 year after transplantation) with hemodynamic compromise occur in approximately 20%–25% of pediatric transplant patients with a subsequent higher risk of graft coronary artery disease and death (Mulla et al., 2001; Webber et al., 2003a). They are more frequently antibody-mediated with or without cellular rejection (McOmber et al., 2004; Pahl et al., 2001). It is thought that a majority of these late rejection episodes are precipitated by medication noncompliance (See later section on noncompliance). However, it is clear that some patients have recurrent and/or late rejection episodes despite good medication compliance, while others do well with poor compliance. Contributing to this are probably both donor and recipient factors that are not yet fully understood. Recent studies have suggested that the risk of rejection may vary based on gene polymorphisms (Girnita et al., in press). In pediatric transplant recipients, those with polymorphisms altering cytokine production that yield a high IL-6, low IL-10, high VEGF phenotype have high risk of rejection regardless of ethnic group. Late rejection episodes occur less frequently in infant heart transplant recipients than older children (8% vs. 28%), suggesting immaturity of the immune system at the time of transplantation may have a long-term benefit (Ibrahim et al., 2002). Late rejection significantly worsens long-term prognosis, with the risk of death rising from 1.2% in those without late rejection to 25% in those with late rejection during a median follow-up of 32.9 months (Webber et al., 2003a).

The "gold standard" for monitoring for rejection is the endomyocardial biopsy (Billingham et al., 1990). Despite this, it is well known that it is far from perfect. There are significant sampling errors with mild and moderate rejection episodes, leading to both under and over estimation of the level of rejection (Fishbein et al., 1994; Nakhleh et al., 1992). There is marked inconsistency between pathologists, even when they are experts in transplant pathology looking at the same slides (Marboe et al., 2005). Furthermore, antibody-mediated rejection may show no changes on the routine hematoxylin and eosin–stained pathology slides. A second method for monitoring for rejection, used more frequently in children as primary surveillance without endomyocardial biopsy than in adults, is echocardiography (Boucek et al., 1994). Echocardiography can demonstrate acute onset of cardiac dysfunction that recovers after enhanced immunosuppression, but gives no insight into the type of rejection, cellular or anti-body mediated. The newest method gaining favor

for surveillance of rejection is the gene array analysis of peripheral blood samples, monitoring profiles of genes up or downregulated with rejection (Deng et al., 2006). This is currently only approved for use in those 15 years or older. The IMAGE study is an ongoing comparison of outcome using a biopsy-based surveillance protocol compared to a gene array-based surveillance protocol (Pham et al., 2007). There seems to be real promise that this technology could replace the more invasive biopsy for monitoring of both cellular and antibody-mediated rejection.

Infections

Infectious complications are most likely early following transplantation, when the level of immunosuppression is highest and the recipients are in the hospital with intravenous lines, endotracheal tubes, and other predisposing factors. For pediatric heart transplant recipients, freedom from infection is 75% at 1 month, 64% at 3 months, and 46% at 2 years (Schowengerdt et al., 1997). Most infections are bacterial (60%), followed by cytomegalovirus (18%), and other viral (13%), and fungal (7%). The highest risk of fungal and bacterial infections is the immediate operative period and then tapers rapidly afterwards, reaching low rates beyond 1 month for fungal and 2 months for bacterial infections (see Figure 16–6) (Schowengerdt et al., 1997). Viral infections appear a little later, peaking at 6 weeks and falling to low rates after 3 months. Cytomegalovirus (CMV) acquired from the donor organ is one of the most common, and potentially life-threatening, infections occurring early after transplantation in the subgroup of CMV negative recipients who receive a CMV-positive donor. Suppressive or preemptive therapy for CMV infection is routine at most centers in this high-risk group. Pneumocystis pneumonia (PCP) occurred in 7% of infant transplant recipients not on prophylaxis (Janner et al., 1996). Most centers now use trimethoprim-sulfamethoxazole prophylaxis but the length of therapy is variable, typically 6 to 12 months for PCP prevention. Infections account for approximately 15% of the deaths in the first year following transplantation, and 1.9%–8.3% of the deaths after the first year (Boucek et al., 2007).

All live vaccines are contraindicated in solid organ transplants due to the increased risk of significant disease even with the attenuated viruses. Other vaccines are encouraged, though it is unclear that the response is protective with all vaccines. The level of response may also vary greatly depending on the maintenance immunosuppression, especially whether steroids are used. There have been anecdotal reports of rejection following vaccination, especially influenzae vaccine, suggesting vaccines may cause generalized stimulation

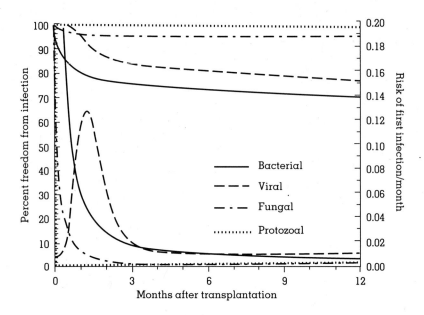

FIGURE 16–6. Freedom from infection according to causative agent. Upper family of curves depict parametric freedom from infection caused by indicated infectious agent. Lower family of curves represent associated hazard function (instantaneous risk). (Reprinted from Schowengerdt et al., 1997, with permission of the publisher. Copyright © 1997 Elsevier Science Inc.)

of the immune system. Several large studies have not supported an association between influenzae vaccine and rejection episodes, and the vaccine did appear effective despite immunosuppression (Kimball et al., 2001; Magnani et al., 2005; White-Williams et al., 2006).

Graft Coronary Artery Vasculopathy

Transplant graft coronary artery vasculopathy (GCAV) is the main cause of death in long-term heart transplant survivors and is the most common indication for retransplantation (Boucek et al., 2007). The pathogenesis is most likely an initial subclinical graft endothelial cell injury caused by a variety of inciting events (ischemia, rejection, viral infection, etc) that progresses to persistent immunologic attack on the donor organ, leading to the graft coronary artery vasculopathy (Moien-Afshari et al., 2003). Transplant vasculopathy is typically characterized by a diffuse thickening of the intima and luminal narrowing of all coronary vessels. It is usually detected on angiography during routine surveillance cardiac catheterization or at autopsy following sudden death. Coronary angiography is an insensitive method to monitor a process so diffuse, and the vasculopathy is often well advanced when first detected. Some pediatric centers screen with intracoronary ultrasound at cardiac catheterization, but this has not gained wide acceptance. Since transplant graft coronary vasculopathy is usually not associated with calcification, electron beam computed tomography used to monitor coronary atherosclerosis in the general population is not applicable (Ratliff et al., 2004).

The prevalence of graft coronary artery vasculopathy in children (21%–30% at 10 years) is low compared to adults (53% at 10 years) and is lower in infant recipients than adolescent recipients (Boucek et al., 2007; Hathout et al., 2005; Pahl et al., 2005; Taylor et al., 2007). The incidence does appear to be falling with newer immunosuppressive regimens and the decrease in rejection rates (Hathout et al., 2005). Risk factors for graft coronary artery vasculopathy in the pediatric population include: two or more episodes of rejection in the first year following transplantation; rejection with hemodynamic compromise beyond 1 year posttransplantation; older recipient (adolescent); and older donor (>30 years) (Hathout et al., 2005; Mulla et al., 2001; Pahl et al., 2005). Cytomegalovirus (CMV) infection, induction therapy, race, sex, cholesterol, or LDL levels have not proven significant risk factors for graft vasculopathy in the pediatric patients. Some studies have suggested that HLA mismatch and anti-HLA antibodies are correlated with graft coronary artery vasculopathy (Vasilescu et al., 2003) while others have shown no correlation with HLA mismatches (Almenar et al., 2005; Hathout et al., 2005). The presence of graft vasculopathy does carry a significant mortality risk. Upon the diagnosis of any graft coronary artery vasculopathy, 24% of recipients died within 2 years, and with moderate-to-severe graft coronary artery vasculopathy, 50% died within 2 years (Pahl et al., 2005). Severe coronary artery vasculopathy correlated with poor prognosis, with retransplantation the only effective therapy. The diffuse nature of the graft coronary artery vasculopathy makes balloon angioplasty or coronary stenting procedures at best palliative, and bypass surgery rarely worth the risk of surgery (Benza et al., 2004; Moien-Afshari et al., 2003). Methods for noninvasive diagnosis and monitoring of graft coronary artery vasculopathy are much needed.

Posttransplant Lymphoproliferative Disorder

The immune system is responsible for surveillance and prevention of malignancies. Consequently, solid organ transplant patients are at higher risk than the general population for all types of cancer. Posttransplant lymphoproliferative disease (PTLD) accounts for 94% of the cancers seen in children in the first 10 years after transplantation (Boucek et al., 2007). Freedom from malignancy up to the tenth year following pediatric heart transplantation is 91%. In children, the mean time to PTLD was 2 years, with the hazard curve peaking at 6 months posttransplant and progressively falling off (Webber et al., 2006). In adults, the risk of PTLD by 10 years is only 3.97%, but the risk of other cancers, especially skin cancer, is much higher at 33.3% (Taylor et al., 2007). In pediatric recipients, PTLD is almost always B-cell lymphoma (98%) and usually Epstein Barr virus (EBV) positive (87%), though T cell and EBV-negative B cell lymphomas do occur very rarely (Webber et al., 2006). The reason PTLD is more common in the pediatric population is that most pediatric patients are EBV seronegative at the time of transplantation, which is a known risk factor for development of PTLD. PTLD usually presents as either early polymorphic PTLD (65%) that is directly related the level of immunosuppression, late monoclonal PTLD (35%), or "true lymphoma" (Webber et al., 2006). Polymorphic PTLD is essentially a case of mononucleosis that is out of control due to the level of immunosuppression. Polymorphic PTLD may respond simply to lowering of immunosuppression, but monoclonal PTLD usually requires at least a low dose course of chemotherapy. The ability to monitor EBV loads by polymerase chain reaction (PCR) has proven helpful in identifying a subgroup of recipients at higher risk for PTLD, but it remains unclear if intervention prior to PTLD can alter outcome (Toyoda et al., 2008). Survival after the diagnosis of PTLD is 75% at 1 year and 67% at 5 years with almost all deaths during the first 2 years after its diagnosis (Webber et al., 2006).

Renal Insufficiency

Many heart transplant recipients may have significant renal dysfunction secondary to heart failure at the time of transplantation that improves following transplantation, but others will have irreversible renal insufficiency as a result of prolonged pretransplant heart failure and multiple prior operations. It is often impossible to ascertain how significant the irreversible component is prior to transplantation, so some patients begin their transplant years with renal function that is already below normal. In addition, almost all heart transplant recipients are maintained on immunosuppressive regimens containing one of the calcineurin inhibitors, cyclosporine or tacrolimus. This class of medication led to the marked improvement in posttransplant survival and reduced rejection incidence. However, both drugs are well known to have renal toxicity as a major side effect. Most patients on these drugs have a reversible 25% drop in glomerular filtration rate (GFR) due to afferent arteriolar constriction, but there is also an irreversible component to the renal toxicity perhaps mediated by TGF-beta induced renal interstitial fibrosis (Baran et al., 2004).

In a recent pediatric cohort followed serially with isotopic GFR measurements, at least mild renal insufficiency was present in 16% at 1 year and 67% by 5 years following transplantation (Bharat et al., 2007). Eight percent of pediatric heart transplant recipients developed end-stage renal dysfunction (GFR < 30 mL/min/1.73 m²) by 7 years following transplantation. This is similar to reports stating that by 10 years following heart transplantation, 8% of children have severe renal dysfunction defined as a serum creatinine >2.5 mg/dL, dialysis, or renal transplantation (Boucek et al., 2007; Ross et al., 2006). There seems to be a higher incidence of end-stage renal failure in the children transplanted as infants, possibly due to calcineurin interference with normal renal maturation in the first year of life (Pradhan et al., 2002). The estimation of GFR from the serum creatinine appears to significantly underestimate the prevalence of renal insufficiency in pediatric heart transplant recipients (Bharat et al., 2007). The Loma Linda group had a similar finding with a normal mean serum creatinine of 0.8 mg/dL (71 µmol/L) despite a reduced mean GFR of 77 mL/min/1.73m² at 10 years following infant heart transplantation (Chinnock et al., 2000). Transplantation prior to 1997 had the highest hazard ratio (27.6) of abnormal GFR over time, presumably due to higher target trough levels for medications early in their use (Bharat et al., 2007). The calcineurin-inhibitor levels within the first few months following transplantation do have a greater influence on the long-term risk of renal insufficiency than does late calcineurin inhibitor dose (Bharat et al., 2007; Pradhan et al., 2002). Hopefully, the trend toward lower tacrolimus and cyclosporine levels in the first few months following transplantation will manifest less in late renal failure for the new generation of pediatric heart transplant recipients.

Allergies and Eczema

Since allergies (eczema, rhinitis/sinusitis, asthma, eosinophilic enteritis) are immune-mediated, one might expect that immunosuppressive therapy following orthotopic heart transplant would lead to less allergic symptoms. In fact, food allergies, including infrequently serious manifestations such as anaphylaxis and eosinophilic gastroenteropathy, occur more commonly following organ transplantation. Eosinophilia is present in 39%–50% of children on tacrolimus or cyclosporine, and 40%–58% of those had clinical allergic symptoms, often food allergies (Asante-Korang et al., 1996; Granot et al., 2006). This may be multifactorial including innate atopy, tacrolimus-induced increased permeability of the gut to food allergens, and a tacrolimus-induced imbalance in Th1 and Th2 lymphocyte activity and cytokine profiles (Hinds and Dhawan, 2006; Özdemir et al., 2006; Saeed et al., 2006). Tacrolimus and cyclosporine inhibit interleukin-2, which may cause a selective suppression of Th1 lymphocytes, allowing promotion of the Th2 lymphocytes and an allergic immune response. This seems most prevalent with tacrolimus, though also reported with cyclosporine immunosuppression. While these are life-threatening in a small percent of transplant patients, allergic manifestations can be quite debilitating to a significant number of pediatric heart transplant recipients with eczema, recurrent allergic rhinitis, chronic noninfectious sinusitis, and diarrhea. When secondary to food allergy, the symptoms can be significantly improved with elimination diet (Özdemir et al., 2006).

Growth and Development

Growth retardation at the time of pediatric heart transplantation is common with mean Z-score ranging from −0.95 to −2.15 (Au et al., 1992; Chinnock and Baum, 1998; de Broux et al., 2000). Most studies with steroid maintenance immunosuppression following pediatric heart transplantation have shown normal growth rate, with no significant change in Z-score or catch-up growth (deBroux et al., 2000; Hirsch et al., 1996; Peterson et al., 2007). Other studies with steroid-free maintenance immunosuppression following pediatric heart transplantation did show catch-up growth (Au et al., 1992; Chinnock and Baum, 1998). Steroid dose did correlate with lack of growth (Baum et al., 1991; Peterson et al., 2007). Steroids have long been known to impair growth and have been eliminated from the maintenance immunosuppressive protocols at many pediatric centers, with only 58.7% of pediatric heart transplant patients on steroids at 1-year follow-up and 39.8% at 5-year follow-up (Boucek et al., 2007).

Using a steroid-free maintenance protocol in infant pediatric heart transplant recipients, somatic growth was normal in 88%, with only 12% having a most recent height less than the fifth percentile (Chinnock and Baum, 1998). In infant heart transplant patients, the donor heart is often oversized at implantation, but it adjusts to normal size during the first year and subsequently remains appropriate for recipient size (Hirsch et al., 1996).

In infants surviving heart transplantation, 89% were felt to be neurologically normal at an average of 14 months after surgery (Baum et al., 1991). In a 10-year follow-up of infant heart transplant patients from that same center, 66% were felt to be developmentally normal by the parents and were in regular classes at school, while 10% had severe developmental delay (Chinnock et al., 2000). For pediatric heart transplant recipients of all ages, functional status is good and very stable for at least the first 5 years following transplantation, with no activity limitations in 92% at 1 year and in 94% at 5 years (Boucek et al., 2007). The hospitalization rate following transplantation is 50% during the first year, 26% during the fourth year, and 24% during the ninth year (Boucek et al., 2007).

Exercise

Just like their well peers, pediatric heart transplant recipients are at risk for development of the cardiac risk factors that are increasingly common today, including obesity, hypertension, diabetes, and sedentary lifestyle. This can be promoted further by unnecessary restrictions on activity placed by family and physicians in the face of "heart disease." The heart following orthotopic heart transplantation is denervated, leading to diminished chronotropic response to exercise (70%–80% of age-matched controls), a mild resting tachycardia (about 10 ppm faster than age-matched controls), and reduced VO_{2max} (70% of age-matched controls) in some studies (Marconi and Marzorati, 2003). Other studies have shown that these measures of physical fitness can be altered with training following heart transplantation. In two small series, heart transplant recipients who maintained a "rigorous competitive schedule for training" or a "high-intensity endurance training program" were able to achieve both peak heart rate and VO_{2max} equivalent to or above age-matched controls (Pokan et al., 2004; Richard et al., 1999). This suggests that heart rate does not limit their exercise capacity. Richard et al. also pointed out that physical work can be sustained easily only when energy expenditure does not exceed 35% of the VO_{2max}. Consequently, sedentary heart transplant recipients are unable to carry out many routine daily activities. The reintegration of heart transplant recipients back into "the labor and leisure society" may be expedited and quality life may improve with exercise training.

The precedent has been set with patients with congestive heart failure secondary to ischemic or dilated cardiomyopathy. They used to be restricted by physicians due to concern of sudden death with exercise, but they are now encouraged to participate in routine exercise and conditioning with improved outcomes and sense of well-being as recommended in the ACC/AHA Practice Guidelines for Chronic Heart Failure Management (Hunt et al., 2001). Similar benefit has now been demonstrated in pediatric heart transplant recipients. Establishing a routine home exercise training program with treadmill or exercise bike for 20–30 min sessions three times a week, along with strength training twice a week, was found to be both safe and beneficial in stable transplant recipients without active rejection, documented coronary artery disease, uncontrolled hypertension, or significant arrhythmias (Patel et al., 2008). Participants demonstrated significant improvement in endurance time, peak oxygen consumption, and strength at the end of 12 weeks.

Improved quality of life and return to a normal lifestyle are the goals of heart transplantation. The normal lifestyle for many children, adolescents, and adults includes routine exercise and competitive sports. While the heart transplant recipient may have the substrate for lethal arrhythmias during exercise in the presence of graft coronary vasculopathy or active rejection, there are isolated reports of heart transplant patients engaging in mountain climbing or participating in a half-ironman triathlon a decade or two following heart transplant (MSNBC, 2007; Haykowsky and Tymchak, 2007). At present, there remains uncertainty in how much activity the physician should allow. Clearly one should encourage some routine exercise for conditioning and strength training in all recipients. The decision about more rigorous activity or competitive sports should be individualized based on the absence of known risk factors such as graft coronary vasculopathy, active rejection, or exercise-induced arrhythmias with periodic reassessment. Exercise may go a long way in improving their sense of well-being and compliance with long-term medical therapy.

Compliance

Late rejection is frequently attributed to patient medication noncompliance, with some studies confirming that most or all late episodes result from noncompliance (Ringewald et al., 2001; Di Filippo et al., 2003; Webber et al., 2003a). Improvements in immunosuppressive medications and posttransplant management are ineffective if the patient is not cooperative with the regimen. Noncompliance is higher in adolescents compared to adult transplant recipients and younger pediatric recipients across all organ types (Dobbels et al., 2005). Noncompliance is seen across all solid organ transplants, with prevalence in the adolescent population of 30%–32% for renal and liver transplant recipients, and 15.9% for heart transplant recipients. On clinical assessment, physicians and nursing staff often do not correctly identify the noncompliant patients (Blowley et al., 1997). Drug level variability (>20% too high or too low) is helpful in identifying noncompliance and risk for recurrent rejection (Flippin et al., 2000; Ringewald et al., 2001). In pediatric heart transplant recipients presenting with late rejection with hemodynamic compromise, at least 80% of the episodes were secondary to noncompliance (Pahl et al., 2001). Calculated from the literature, it is estimated that 73.3% of late rejection episodes and 34.6% of graft loss in pediatric heart transplant patients result from noncompliance (Dobbels et al., 2005). Several simple factors that improve compliance in adolescent transplant patients are: better knowledge of medication regimen; use of a pillbox to organize medications; and direct parental supervision of medication dosing (Zelikovsky et al., 2008).

TOLERANCE AND THE FUTURE OF PEDIATRIC HEART TRANSPLANTATION

Pediatric heart transplantation has made great strides in the last three decades. Survival has improved greatly, and the scope of congenital heart diagnoses amenable to transplantation has continued to expand. Many issues of anatomy or physiology once thought to be absolute contraindications to heart transplantation are now lower hurdles that can be surmounted. However, long-term survival is often limited today by issues that seem difficult to control, such as adolescent patient compliance with medications and the side effects of the immunosuppressive medications. The "holy grail" for the transplant physician is tolerance. Compliance and medication side effects would be irrelevant. While some have questioned whether this will ever be possible in humans, several recent reports have suggested we may be a lot closer to accomplishing this goal.

Tolerance is the absence of a destructive immune response against the donor organ without maintenance immunosuppression, and with normal response to other foreign antigens. Tolerance can be achieved by central mechanisms such as clonal deletion or peripheral mechanisms such as altered antigen expression (Petranyi, 2002). In animal models, tolerance has often been accompanied by mixed chimeric states where both donor and recipient hematopoietic cells exist together (Kean et al., 2006). Chimeric states have been generated in animal models by nonmyeloablative therapies combined with hematopoietic stem cell infusion. This has allowed prolonged rejection-free survival and withdrawal of immunosuppression, but it has been difficult to replicate in humans.

Tolerance most likely involves an active equilibrium between regulatory T cells (Foxp3) and effector T cells (Th1, Th2, Th17), rather than the absence of an immune response (Heslan et al., 2006; Koshiba et al., 2006). On rare occasions, solid organ transplant patients who have discontinued their medications have surprisingly remained free of rejection for prolonged periods, suggesting they may have developed some tolerance of the donor organ. To better understand this tolerant state, a group of renal transplant patients was divided by present clinical status into four groups and gene array analysis was performed: tolerant recipients (off medications greater than 2 years), chronic rejectors, stable recipients (on medication), and acute rejectors (Brouard et al., 2007). They found that the groups had very distinct profiles, the genes of T effector cells (Th1 and Th2) are upregulated in rejectors, while TGF-β is upregulated in the tolerant profile. However, these patient profiles appear to be "metastable" and intercurrent events such as infection may cause a patient to move from tolerant to rejector profile. In the future, it may be possible to monitor the patient gene activity profile to determine the likelihood of rejection, and to adjust immunosuppression up or down based on these gene profiles, or to use these findings as templates for future immunosuppressant medication development.

Finally, in an exciting recent report, tolerance appears to have been achieved *intentionally* for the first time in humans in a group of HLA-mismatched renal transplant recipients (Kawai et al., 2008). The patients were started on nonmyeloablative preparative regimens 7 days prior the transplantation followed by infusion of donor bone marrow at the time of renal transplantation. Transient chimerism developed in all recipients. Unlike the animal models, these renal transplant patients had no permanent chimerism established, but the effect on what was recognized as "self" appears to have been permanent. These patients were weaned from all immunosuppressive medications 9–14 months after transplantation without evidence of rejection for up to 5.3 years of follow-up to date. The T lymphocytes from these recipients show donor-specific nonreactivity when tested in vitro. All these renal patients received living donors, so that operative dates could be scheduled in advance. The protocols utilized for these renal patients all started 7 days prior to transplantation, so they are not directly applicable to heart transplantation where surgery cannot be electively scheduled. However, in nonhuman primates, it has been demonstrated that one can induce tolerance by performing renal transplantation first, followed by "conditioning therapy" and donor bone marrow infusion 4 months later (Koyama et al., 2007). In the future, this type of regimen where the solid organ and bone marrow transplant are performed in series may be applicable for induction of tolerance in heart transplant recipients.

REFERENCES

Addonizio LJ, Gersony WM, Robbins RC, et al. Elevated pulmonary vascular resistance and cardiac transplantation. *Circulation.* 1987;76 (suppl V):V-52–V-55.

Almenar L, Maeso MLC, Martinez-Dolz L, et al. Influence of HLA matching on survival in heart transplantation. *Transplant Proc.* 2005;37:4001–4005.

Almond CS, McElhinney DB, Piercey GE, et al. Class I and II HLA sensitization pre-transplant by solid-phase assay and early outcome after pediatric heart transplantation. *J Heart Lung Transplant.* 2008;27(2S):S173.

Anderson JB, Fuller TC, Hawkins JA, et al. Two-year reduction of panel reactive human leukocyte antigen antibodies in children receiving mycophenolate mofetil after valved allograft placement. *Transplantation.* 2005;80:414–416.

Asante-Korang A, Boyle GJ, Webber SA, Miller SA, Fricker FJ. Experience of FK506 immune suppression in pediatric heart transplantation: A study of long-term adverse effects. *J Heart Lung Transplant.* 1996;15:415–422.

Au J, Gregory JW, Colquhoun IW, et al. Paediatric cardiac transplantation with steroid-sparing maintenance immunosuppression. *Arch Dis Child.* 1992;67:1262–1266.

Aziz TM, Burgess MI, El-Gamel A, et al. Orthotopic cardiac transplantation technique: a survey of current practice. *Ann Thorac Surg.* 1999;68:1242–1246.

Bailey L, Concepcion W, Shattuck H, Huang L. Method of heart transplantation for treatment of hypoplastic left heart syndrome. *J Thorac Cardiovasc Surg.* 1986a;92:1–5.

Bailey LL, Nehlsen-Cannarella SL, Doroshow RW, et al. Cardiac allotransplantation in newborns as therapy for hypoplastic left heart syndrome. *N Engl J Med.* 1986b;315:949–951.

Baran DA, Galin ID, Gass AL. Calcineurin inhibitor-associated early renal insufficiency in cardiac transplant patients. *Am J Cardiovasc Drugs.* 2004;4:21–29.

Baum MF, Cutler DC, Fricker FJ, Trimm RF. Physiologic and psychological growth and development in pediatric heart transplant recipients. *J Heart Lung Transplant.* 1991;10:848–855.

Benza RL, Zoghbi GJ, Tallaj J, et al. Palliation of allograft vasculopathy with transluminal angioplasty. *J Am Coll Cardiol.* 2004;43:1973–1981.

Bernstein D, Naftel D, Chin C, et al. Outcome of listing for cardiac transplantation for failed Fontan: a multi-institutional study. *Circulation.* 2006;114:273–280.

Bharat W, Manlhiot C, McCrindle BW, Pollock-BarZiv S, Dipchand AI. The profile of renal function over time in a cohort of pediatric heart transplant recipients. *Pediatr Transplant.* 2009;13:111–118.

Bhatia SJ, Kirshenbaum JM, Shemin RJ, et al. Time course of resolution of pulmonary hypertension and right ventricular remodeling after orthotopic cardiac transplantation. *Circulation.* 1987;76:819–826.

Billingham ME, Cary NRB, Hammond ME, et al. A working formulation for the standardization of nomenclature in the diagnosis of heart and lung rejection: Heart Rejection Study Group. *J Heart Lung Transplant.* 1990;9(6):587–593.

Blowley DL, Hebert D, Arbus GS, Pool R, Korus M, Koren G. Compliance with cyclosporine in adolescent renal transplant recipients. *Pediatr Nephrol.* 1997;11:547–551.

Botha P, Chaudhari M, Wrightson N, et al. Cardiac transplantation for the failing Fontan circulation. *J Heart Lung Transplant.* 2008;27(2S):S237.

Boucek, MM. *Cardiac donation after cardiac death at Satellite Symposium: Strategies to improve donor availability in children.* Presented at ISHLT 28th Annual Meeting and Scientific Sessions, Boston April 9, 2008.

Boucek MM, Aurora P, Edwards LB, et al. Registry of the International Society for Heart and Lung Transplantation: Tenth Official Pediatric Heart Transplantation Report—2007. *J Heart Lung Transplant.* 2007;26:796–807.

Boucek MM, Mathis CM, Boucek RJ, et al. Prospective evaluation of echocardiolgraphy for primary rejection surveillance after infant heart transplantation: comparison with endomyocardial biopsy. *J Heart Lung Transplant.* 1994;13(1):66–73.

Brauner RA, Laks H, Drinkwater DC, Scholl F, McCaffery S. Multiple left heart obstructions (Shone's anomaly) with mitral valve involvement: long-term surgical outcome. *Ann Thorac Surg.* 1997;64:721–729.

Breinholt JP, Hawkins JA, Lambert LM, Fuller TC, Profaizer T, Shaddy RE. A Prospective analysis of the immunogenicity of cryopreserved nonvalved allografts used in pediatric heart surgery. *Circulation.* 2000;102:III-179–III-182.

Brouard S, Mansfiled E, Braud C, et al. Identification of a peripheral blood transcriptional biomarker panel associated with operational renal allograft tolerance. *PNAS.* 2007;104:15448–15453.

Bull DA, Stahl RD, McMahan DL, et al. The high risk heart donor: potential pitfalls. *J Heart Lung Transplant.* 1995;14:424–428.

Burch M, Kaufman L, Archer N, Sullivan I. Persistant pulmonary hypertension late after neonatal aortic valvotomy: a consequence of an expanded surgical cohort. *Heart.* 2004;90:918–920.

Canter CE, Shaddy RE, Bernstein D, et al. Indications for heart transplantation in pediatric heart disease: a scientific statement from the american heart association council on cardiovascular disease in the young; the councils on clinical cardiology, cardiovascular nursing, and cardiovascular surgery and anesthesia; and the quality of care and outcomes research interdisciplinary working group. *Circulation.* 2007;115:658–676.

Chen Jm, Davies RR, Mital SR, et al. Trends and outcomes in transplantation for complex congenital heart disease: 1984 to 2004. *Ann Thorac Surg.* 2004;78:1352–1361.

Chinnock R, Baum M. Somatic growth in infant heart transplant recipients. *Pediatr Transplant.* 1998;2:30–34.

Chinnock RE, Cutler D, Baum M. Clinical outcome 10 years after infant heart transplantation. *Prog Pediatr Cardiol.* 2000;11:165–169.

Chiu KM, Lin TY, Chu SH. Successful heterotopic heart transplant after cardiopulmonary bypass rescue of an arrested donor heart. *Transpl Proceed.* 2006;38:1514–1515.

Costanzo-Nordin MR, Heroux AL, Radvany R, Koch D, Robinson JA. Role of humoral immunity in acute cardiac allograft dysfunction. *J Heart Lung Transplant.* 1993;12:S143–S146.

Davies RR, Chen JM, Naftel DC, et al.The impact of high-risk criteria on mortality following heart transplantation in children: a multi-institutional study. *J Heart Lung Transplant.* 2008a;27(2S):S255–S256.

Davies RR, Russo MJ, Mital SR, et al. Listing for cardiac TXP among adults with congenital heart disease (CHD) in the UNOS database. *J Heart Lung Transplant.* 2008b;27(2S):S127.

DeBroux E, Huot CH, Chartrand S, Vobecky S, Chartrand C. Growth and pubertal development following pediatric heart transplantation: a 15 year experience at Ste-Justine Hospital. *J Heart Lung Transplant.* 2000;19:825–833.

Del Rio MJ. Transplantation in complex congenital heart disease. *Prog Pediatr Cardiol.* 2000;11:107–113.

Deng MC, Eisen HJ, Mehra MR, et al. Noninvasive discrimination of rejection in cardiac allograft recipients using gene expression profiling. *Am J Transplant.* 2006;6:150–160.

Di Filippo S, Boissonnat P, Sassolas F, et al. Rabbit antithymocyte globulin as induction immunotherapy in pediatric heart transplantation. *Transplantation.* 2003;75(3):354–358.

Di Filippo S, Girnita A, Webber SA, et al. Impact of ELISA-detected anti-HLA antibodies on pediatric cardiac allograft outcome. *Hum Immunol.* 2005;66:513–518.

Dobbels F, Van Damme-Lombaert R, Vanhaecke J, De Geest S. Growing pains: non-adherence with the immunosuppressive regimen in adolescent transplant recipients. *Pediatr Transplant.* 2005;9:381–390.

Feingold B, Bowman P, Zeevi A, et al. Suvival in allosensitized children after listing for cardiac transplantation. *J Heart Lung Transplant.* 2007;26:565–571.

Fishbein MC, Kobashigawa J.Biopsy-negative cardiac transplant rejection: etiology, diagnosis, and therapy. *Curr Opin Cardiol.* 2004;19:166–169.

Fishbein MC, Bell G, Lones MA, et al. Grade 2 cellular heart rejection: Does it exist? *J Heart Lung Transplant.* 1994;13:1051–1057.

Flippin MS, Canter CE, Balzer DT. Increased morbidity and high variability of cyclosporin levels in pediatric heart transplant recipients. *J Heart Lung Transplant.* 2000;9:343–349.

Fontan F, Kirklin JW, Fernandez G, et al. Outcome of a "perfect" Fontan operation. *Circulation.* 1990;81:1520–1536.

Gamba A, Merlo M, Giocchi R, et al. Heart transplantation in patients with previous Fontan operations. *J Thorac Cardiovasc Surg.* 2004;127(2):555–562.

Girnita D, Brooks M, Burckart G, et al. Genetic polymorphisms impact the risk of acute rejection in pediatric heart transplantation: a multi-institutional study. *Transplantation.* 2008;85(11):1632–1639.

Goland S, Czer LSC, Kass RM, et al. Pre-existing pulmonary hypertension in patients with end-stage heart failure: impact on clinical outcome and hemodynamic follow-up after orthotopic heart transplantation. *J Heart Lung Transplant.* 2007;26:312–318.

Granot E, Yakobovich E, Bardenstein R. Tacrolimus immunosupression—an association with asymptomatic eosinophilia and elevated total and specific IgE levels. *Pediatr Transplant.* 2006;10:647–649.

Hathout E, Beeson WL, Kuhn M, et al. Cardiac allograft vasculopathy in pediatric heart transplant recipients. *Transpl Int.* 2005;19:184–189.

Hayashida K, Kanda K, Yaku H, Ando J, Nakayama Y. Development of an in vivo tissue-engineered, autologous heart valve (the biovalve): preparation of a prototype model. *J Thorac Cardiovasc Surg.* 2007;134:152–159.

Haykowsky M, Tymchak W. Superior athletic performance two decades after cardiac transplantation. *N Engl J Med.* 2007;356:2007–2008.

Heslan JM, Renaudin K, Thebault P, Josien R, Cuturi MC, Chiffoleau E. New evidence for a role of allograft accomodation in long-term tolerance. *Transplantation.* 2006;82:1185–1193.

Hinds R, Dhawan A. Food allergy after liver transplantation—is it the result of T cell imbalance. *Pediatr Transplant.* 2006;10:647–648.

Hirsch R, Huddleston CB, Mendeloff EN, Sekarski TJ, Canter CE. Infant and donor organ growth after heart transplantation in neonates with hypoplastic left heart syndrome. *J Heart Lung Transplant.* 1996;15:1093–1100.

Hofschire PJ, Rosenquist GC, Ruckerman RN, Moller JH, Edwards JE. Pulmonary vascular disease complicating the Blalock-Taussig anastamosis. *Circulation.* 1977;56:124–126.

Holt DB, Lublin DM, Phelan DL, et al. Mortality and morbidity in pre-sensitized pediatric heart transplant recipients with a positive donor crossmatch utilizing peri-operative plasmapheresis and cytolytic therapy. *J Heart Lung Transplant*. 2007;26:876–882.

Hunt SA, Baker DW, Chin MH, et al. ACC/AHA guidelines for the evaluation and management of chronic heart failure in the adult: a report of the American College of Cardiology/American Heart Association Task Force on Practice Guidelines. American College of Cardiology Web site. http://www.acc.org/clinical/guidelines/failure/hf_index.htm. 2001.

Ibrahim JE, Sweet SC, Flippin M, et al. Rejection is reduced in thoracic organ recipients when tranpslanted in the first year of life. *J Heart Lung Transplant*. 2002;21:311–318.

Janner D, Bork J, Baum M, Chinnock R. *Pneumocystis Carinii* pneumonia in infants after heart transplantation. *J Hear Lung Transplant*. 1996;15:758–763.

Jayakumar KA, Addonizio LJ, Kichuk-Chrisant MR, et al. Cardiac transplantation after the Fontan or Glenn procedure. *J Am Coll Cardiol*. 2004;44:2065–2072.

Joint Commission on Accreditation of Healthcare Organizations (JACHO). Health care at the crossroads. http://www.jointcommission.org/NR/rdonlyres/E4E7DD3F-3FDF-4ACC-B69E-AEF3A1743AB0/0/organ_donation_white_paper.pdf. 2004.

Kabashigawa JA. Contemporary concepts in noncellular rejection. *Heart Failure Clin*. 2007;3:11–15.

Kantrowitz A. American's first human heart transplantation: the concept, the planning, and the furor. *ASAIO J*. 1998;44:244–252.

Kawai T, Cosimi B, Spitzer TR, et al. HLA-mismatched renal transplantation without maintenance immunosuppression. *N Engl J Med*. 2008;358:353–361.

Kean LS, Gangappa S, Pearson TC, Larsen CP. Transplant tolerance in non-human primates: progress, current challenges and unmet needs. *Am J Transplant*. 2006;6:884–893.

Kimball P, Verbeke S, Tolman D. Influenzae vaccination among heart transplant recipients. *Transplant Proc*. 2001;33:1785–1786.

Koogler T, Costarino AT Jr. The potential benefits of the pediatric nonheartbeating organ donor. Pediatrics. 1998;101:1049–1052.

Koshiba T, Li Y, Takemura M, et al. Clinical, immunological, and pathological aspects of operational tolerance after pediatric living-donor liver transplantation. *Transpl Immunol*. 2006;17:94–97.

Koyama I, Nadazdin O, Boskovic S, et al. Depletion of CD8 memory T cells for induction of tolerance of a previously transplanted kidney allograft. *Am J Transplant*. 2007;7:1055–1061.

Krishnan US, Lamour JM, Hsu DT, Kichuk MR, Donnelly CM, Addonizio LJ. Management of aortopulmonary collaterals in children following cardiac transplantation for complex congenital heart disease. *J Heart Lung Transplant*. 2004;23:564–569.

Lammermeier DE, Sweeney MS, Haupt HE, Radovancevic B, Duncan JM, Frazier OH. Use of potentially infected donor heart for cardiac transplantation. *Ann Thorac Surg*. 1990;50:222–225.

Lamour JM, Addonizio LJ, Galantowicz ME, et al. Outcome after orthotopic cardiac transplantation in adults with congenital heart disease. *Circulation*. 1999;100:II-200–II-205.

Lamour JM, Hsu D, Kichuk MR, Galantowicz ME, Quaegebuer JM, Addonizio LJ. Regression of pulmonary venous arteriovenous malformations following heart transplantation. *Pediatr Transpl*. 2000;4:280–284.

Lamour JM, Hsu DT, Quaegebuer JM, et al. Heart transplantation to a physiologic single lung in patients with congenital heart disease. *J Heart Lung Transplant*. 2004;23:948–953.

Lamour JM, Kanter KR, Naftel DC, et al. The effect of age, diagnosis and previous surgery in 488 children and adults who undergo heart transplantation for congenital heart disease. *J Am Coll Cardiol*. 2005;45:322A.

Larsen RL, Eguchi JH, Mulla NF, et al. Usefulness of cardiac transplantation in children with visceral heterotaxy (asplenic and polysplenic syndromes and single right-sided spleen with levocardia) and comparison of results with cardiac transplantation in children with dilated cardiomyopathy. *Am J Cardiol*. 2002;89:1275–1279.

Magnani G, Falchetti E, Pollini G, et al. Safety and efficacy of two types of influenza vaccination in heart transplant recipients: a prospective randomised controlled study. *J Heart Lung Transplant*. 2005;24:588–592.

Mahle WT, Naftel DC, Rusconi P, Edens RE, Shaddy RE. Pediatric Heart Transplant Study Group. Panel-reactive antibody cross-reactivity and outcomes in the pediatric heart transplant study group. *J Heart Lung Transplant*. 2004;23:S167.

Marboe CC, Billingham M, Eisen H, et al. Nodular endocardial infiltrates (quilty lesions) cause significant variability in diagnosis of ISHLT grade 2 and 3A rejection in cardiac allograft recipients. *J Heart Lung Transplant*. 2005;24:S219–S226.

Marconi C, Marzorati M. Exercise after heart transplantation. *Eur J Appl Physiol*. 2003;90:250–259.

McOmber D, Ibrahim J, Lublin DM. Non-ischemic left ventricular dysfunction after pediatric cardiac transplantation: treatment with plasmapheresis and OKT3. *J Heart Lung Transplant*. 2004;23:552–557.

Meyer SR, Campbell PM, Rutledge JM, et al. Use of an allograft patch in repair of hypoplastic left heart syndrome may complicate future transplantation. *Eur J Cardiothorac Surg*. 2005;27:554–560.

Miniati DN, Robbins RC. Techniques in orthotopic cardiac transplantatioin: A review. *Cardiol Rev*. 2001;9:131–136.

Mital S, Addonizio LJ, Lamour JM, Hsu D. Outcome of children with end-stage congenital heart disease waiting for cardiac transplantation. *J Heart Lung Transplant*. 2003;22:147–153.

Mitchell MB, Campbell DN, Ivy D, et al. Evidence of pulmonary vascular disease after heart transplantation for Fontan circulation failure. *J Thorac Surg*. 2004;128:693–702.

Moien-Afshari F, McManus BM, Laher I. Immunosuppression and transplant vascular disease: benefits and adverse effects. *Pharmacol Ther*. 2003;100:141–156.

Morgan JA, Edwards NM. Orthotopic cardiac transplantation: comparison of outcome using biatrial, bicaval, and total techniques. *J Card Surg*. 2005;20:102–106.

MSNBC. Heart transplant patient conquers Andes climb. http://www.msnbc.msn.com/id/17451843/2007.

Mulla NF, Johnston JK, Vander Dussen L, et al. Late rejection is a predictor of transplant coronary artery disease in children. *J Am Coll Cardiol*. 2001;37:243–250.

Nakhleh RE, Jones J, Goswitz JJ, Anderson EA, Titus J. Correlation of endomyocardial biopsy findings with autopsy findings in human cardiac allografts. *J Heart Lung Transplant*. 1992;11:479–485.

OPTN (Organ Procurement and Transplant Network Database) Available at http://www.OPTN.org. 2008.

Özdemir Ö, Arrey-Mensah A, Sorensen RU. Development of multiple food allergies in children taking tacrolimus after heart and liver transplantation. *Pediatr Transplant*. 2006;10:380–383.

Pahl E, Natfel DC, Canter CE, Frazier EA, Kirklin JK, Morrow WR, and the Pediatric Heart Transplant Study. Death after rejection with severe hemodyanmic compromise in pediatric heart transplant recipients: A multi-institutional study. *J Heart Lung Transplant*. 2001;20:279–287.

Pahl E, Naftel DC, Kuhn MA, et al. The impact and outcome of transplant coronary artery disease in a pediatric population: a 9-year multi-institutional study. *J Heart Lung Transplant*. 2005;24:645–651.

Patel JN, Kavey RE, Pophal SG, Trapp EE, Jellen G, Pahl E. Improved exercise performance in pediatric heart transplant recipients after home exercise training. *Pediatr Transplant.* 2008;12:336–340.

Peterson RE, Perens GS, Alejos JC, Wetzel GT, Chang RKR. Growth and weight gain of prepubertal children after cardiac transplantation. *Pediatr Transplant.* 2007;12(4):436–441.

Petranyi GG. The induction of active or peripheral tolerance in organ transplantation: Dream or reality. *Ann Transplant.* 2002;7:16–22.

Pham MX, Deng MC, Kfoury AG, Teuteberg JJ, Starling RC, Vanantine H. Molecular testing for long-term rejection surveillance in heart transplant recipients: design of the Invasive Monitoring Attenuation Through Gene Expression (IMAGE) trial. *J Heart Lung Transplant.* 2007;26:808–814.

Pokan R, von Duvillard SP, Ludwig J, Rohrer A, Hofmann P, Wonisch M, Smekal G, et al. (2004) Effect of high-volume and -intensity endurance training in heart transplant recipients. *Med Sci Sports Exerc.* 36:2011–2016.

Pollock-BarZiv SM, den Hollander N, Ngan BY, Kantor P, McCrindle B, Dipchand AI. Pediatric heart transplantation in human leukocyte antigen-sensitized patients. *Circulation.* 2007;116:I-172–I-178.

Pradhan M, Leonard MB, Bridges NC, Jabs KL. Decline in renal function following thoracic organ transplantation in children. *Am J Transplant.* 2002;2:652–657.

Ratliff N, Jorgensen CR, Gobel FL, Hodges M, Knickelbine T, Pritzker MR. Lack of usefulness of electron beam computed tomography for detecting coronary allograft vasculopathy. *Am J Cardiol.* 2004;93:202–206.

Razzouk AJ, Gundry SR, Chinnock RE, et al. Orthotopic transplantation for total anomalous pulmonary venous connection associated with complex congenital heart disease. *J Heart Lung Transplant.* 1995;14:713–717.

Richard R, Verdier JC, Duvallet A, et al. Chronotropic competence in endurance trained heart transplant recipients: Heart rate is not a limiting factor for exercise capacity. *J Am Coll Cardiol.* 1999;33:192–197.

Ringewald JM, Gidding SS, Crawford SE, Backer CL, Mavroudis C, Pahl E. Nonadherence is associated with late rejection in pediatric heart transplant recipients. *J Pediatr.* 2001;139:75–78.

Roche SL, Burch M, O'Sullivan J, et al. Multicenter experience of ABO-incompatible pediatric cardiac transplantation. *Am J Transplant.* 2008;8:208–215.

Ross M, Kouretas P, Gamberg P, et al. Ten- and 20-year survivors of pediatric orthotopic heart transplantation. *J Heart Lung Transplant.* 2006;25:261–270.

Sachdeva R, Seib PM, Burns SA, Fontenot EE, Frazier EA. Stenting for superior vena cava obstruction in pediatric heart transplant recipients. *Catheter Cardiovasc Interv.* 2007;70:888–892.

Saeed SA, Integlia MJ, Pleskow RG, et al. Tacrolimus-associated eosinophilic gastroenterocolitis in pediatric liver transplant recipients: role of potential food allergies in pathogenesis. *Pediatr Transplant.* 2006;10:731–735.

Schmid C, Tjan TDT, Scheld HH. Techniques of pediatric heart transplantation. *Thorac Cardiov Surg.* 2004;53(Suppl2):S141–S145.

Schowengerdt KO, Naftel DC, Seib PM, et al. Infection after pediatric heart transplantation: results of a multiinstitutional study. *J Heart Lung Transplant.* 1997;16:1207–1216.

Shaddy RE, Fuller TC. The sensitized pediatric heart transplant candidate: causes, consequences, and treatment options. *Pediatr Transplant.* 2005;9:208–214.

Shaddy RE, Hunter DD, Osborn KA, et al. Prospective analysis of HLA immunogenicity of cryopreserved valved allografts used in pediatric surgery. *Circulation.* 1996;94:1063–1067.

Smith JD, Ogino H, Hunt D, Laylor RM, Rose ML, Yacoub MH. Humoral immune response to human aortic valve homografts. *Ann Thorac Surg.* 1995;60:S127–S130.

Sodian R, Lueders C, Kraemer L, et al. Tissue engineering of autologous human heart valves using cryopreserved vascular umbilical cord cells. *Ann Thorac Surg.* 2006;81:2207–2216.

Sze DY, Robbins RC, Semba CP, Razavi MK, Dake MD. Superior vena cava syndrome after heart transplantation: Percutaneous treatment of a complication of bicaval anastomoses. *J Thorac Cardiovasc Surg.* 1998;116:253–261.

Taylor DO, Edwards LB, Boucek MM, et al. Registry of the International Society for Heart and Lung Transplantation: twenty-fourth official adult heart transplant report—2007. *J Heart Lung Transplant.* 2007;26:769–781.

Tjang YS, Stenlund H, Tenderich G, Hornik L, Bairaktaris A, Korfer R. Risk factor analysis in pediatric heart transplantation. *J Heart Lung Transplant.* 2008;27:408–415.

Toyoda M, Moudgil A, Warady BE, Puliyanda DP, Jorndan SC. Clinical significance of peripheral blood Epstein-Barr viral load monitoring using polymerase chain reaction in renal transplant recipients. *Pediatr Transpl.* 2008;12(7):778–784.

Transplanted the Heart—Christian Neething Barnard. *The New York Times*, December 6, 1967.

Vasilescu ER, Ho EK, de la Torre, et al. Anti-HLA antibodies in heart transplantation. *Tranpl Immunol.* 2003;12:177–183.

Vricella LA, Razzouk AJ, Gundry SR, Larsen RL, Kuhm MA, Bailey LL. Heart transplantation in infants and children with situs inversus. *J Thorac Cardiovasc Surg.* 1998;116:82–89.

Wauthy P, Kafi SA, Mooi WJ, Naeije R, Brimioulle S. Inhaled nitric oxide versus prostacyclin in chronic shunt-induced pulmonary hypertension. *J Thorac Cardiovasc Surg.* 2003;126:1434–1441.

Webber SA, Naftel DC, Parker J, et al. Late rejection episodes more than 1 year after pediatric heart transplantation: risk factors and outcomes. *J Heart Lung Transpl.* 2003a;22:869–875.

Webber SA, Pereira JR, Miller SA, et al. A re-evaluation of pre-transplant increased pulmonary vascular resistance as prognostic indicator after pediatric heart transplant. *Am J Transplant.* 2003b;3(suppl 5):157.

Webber SA, Naftel DC, Fricker FJ, et al. Lymphoproliferative disorders after paediatric heart transplantation: a multi-institutional study. *Lancet.* 2006;367:233–239.

Weiss ES, Nwakanma LU, Russell SB, Conte JV, Shah AS. Outcomes in bicaval versus biatrial techniques in heart transplantation: an analysis of the UNOS database. *J Heart Lung Transplant.* 2008;27:178–183.

West LJ, Pollack-Barziv SM, Dipchand AI, et al. ABO-incompatible heart transplantation in infants. *N Engl J Med.* 2001;344:793–800.

West LJ. B-cell tolerance following ABO-incombatible infant heart transplantation. *Transplantation.* 2006;81:301–307.

White-Williams C, Brown R, Kirklin J, et al. *J Heart Lung Transplant.* 2006;25:320–323.

Zelikovsky N, Schast AP, Palmer JA, Meyers KEC. Perceived barriers to adherence among adolescent renal transplant candidates. *Pediatr Transplant.* 2008;12:300–308.

17

Congenital Heart Defects in Adults

FRED M. WU

MICHAEL J. LANDZBERG

INTRODUCTION

Before the advent of cardiac surgery in the 1940s, fewer than 25% of infants born with complex congenital heart disease (CHD) survived past their first year of life. Today, in the beginning of the 21st century, over 90% of such infants are expected to live into adulthood, and the number of adults with CHD has surpassed the number of children with the disease. By rough estimates, some 800,000–1,500,000 American adults are now living with this most common class of birth defect, and 20,000 new patients reach adolescence annually (Marelli et al., 2007; Warnes et al., 2001). This shift in the demographic of CHD is the direct result of advanced diagnostic tools, medical therapies, and surgical techniques.

Despite improvements in life expectancy, however, few if any adult survivors of CHD are ever truly "cured" of their disease. For some patients, such as those with a single functional ventricle, complete repair is not possible, and our available palliative approaches alter the patient's anatomy in such a way that they create potential for an entirely new set of problems. Even when normal cardiac architecture has been apparently restored, subtle changes in structure and function can be expected to persist, setting the stage for future complications. For example, after uncomplicated surgical closure of simple secundum atrial septal defects, natriuretic peptide levels remain elevated over 20 years later (Groundstroem et al., 2003), and long-term functional ability is significantly altered in patients repaired in adulthood when compared with age-matched controls (Murphy et al., 1990).

This is borne out by statistical data showing that adult survivors of CHD, even those classified as having less-than-severe disease, have significantly higher rates of health care utilization than their age-matched peers (Figure 17–1) (Mackie et al., 2007). Furthermore, those with severe cardiac lesions have significantly higher rates of cardiology outpatient care, emergency department use, days in hospital, and days in critical care units than those with other lesions. The way in which this relates to noncardiac comorbidities, and the relationship of these comorbidities to the natural history of complex CHD, has yet to be fully explored.

As a handful of pioneers began to recognize the unique needs of the aging CHD population in the 1970s, the first units specifically geared to the care of adults with congenital cardiac disease were established. This paved the way for the identification of issues in the management of CHD that can be more apparent in, and at times unique to, the adult with CHD. This chapter will discuss broad categories of issues common to adults with varying forms of CHD: heart failure, arrhythmia, pulmonary vascular disease, and multiorgan dysfunction. The authors' intent is not to review the management of specific lesions in detail—this information is covered elsewhere in this volume—but to provide a general overview of the problems that are frequently faced when caring for the adult CHD population.

HEART FAILURE

In the past, the approach to heart failure in the adult with CHD focused largely on measures of ventricular systolic performance, typically emphasizing the effect of long-standing alterations in either volume or anatomic loading conditions on ventricular function (Graham, 1991; Perloff and Warnes, 2001). While these factors are clearly important, heart failure in the adult CHD population is often the result of a broad array of mechanisms related to alterations in preload, afterload, and contractility. Almost nowhere else in medicine does the

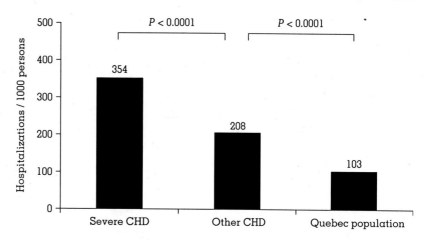

FIGURE 17–1. One-year hospitalization rate of patients with severe and other cardiac lesions compared with the adult population of Quebec (April 1, 1999–March 31, 2000). (Reproduced with permission. Mackie AS, et al. *Am J Cardiol.* 2007;99:839–843.)

categorization of a patient with "heart failure" carry so many pathophysiologic potentials as in the adult patient with CHD.

As Bolger and colleagues have noted, any CHD patient with symptoms could be considered, by some conventional definitions, to have "heart failure" (Bolger and Gatzoulis, 2004). Many adults with CHD are limited in aerobic functional capacity, sometimes profoundly so, when compared with normal controls. Maximal achievable peak oxygen consumption (peak VO$_2$) may be less than 50% of that for normal controls with important reductions seen even after repair of simple atrial level defects (Fredriksen et al., 2001). However, as we will discuss later in this chapter, adults with CHD often have pulmonary vascular disease or other organ dysfunction that may contribute to their clinical limitations. For the purposes of this section, we will focus on systemic ventricular dysfunction with the understanding that this represents only one aspect of a much more complex problem.

Alterations in Contractility

One of the common mechanisms of ventricular dysfunction in the adult with CHD is acquired alteration in myocardial contractility. Over a patient's lifetime, multiple insults may be sustained as a result of surgical interventions (in the form of postsurgical scar formation and cardiopulmonary bypass), acute or chronic ischemia, cyanosis, and chronic alterations in pressure and/or volume loads. Each of these can contribute to myocardial fibrosis, impaired contractility, decreased ventricular compliance, and impaired relaxation.

{S,L,L} transposition of the great arteries (L-TGA) is an instructive example of a congenital lesion highly prone to systemic ventricular dysfunction. Unoperated patients have consistently lower systemic ventricular ejection fractions when compared with age-matched controls (Beauchesne et al., 2002). The reasons for this are multifactorial. Ischemia due to coronary perfusion mismatch has been implicated as a contributing factor (Hornung et al., 1998). The combination of reduced perfusion and increased oxygen demand, resulting from hypertrophy and pressure overload, leads to progressive fibrosis and infarction. Perioperative insults and additional volume overload from systemic atrioventricular valve regurgitation (Prieto et al., 1998) and prior shunts (Warnes, 1996) further compromise cardiac reserve.

Similar issues are seen in patients who have undergone atrial switch palliation for {S,D,D} transposition of the great arteries (D-TGA), an operation which restores a physiologic direction of blood flow but leaves the morphologic right ventricle in the subaortic position. Excessive hypertrophy (Hornung et al., 2002), fibrosis due to pressure overload, volume overload due to AV valve regurgitation, and ischemia relating to coronary perfusion mismatch (Lubiszewska et al., 2000; Millane et al., 2000) lead to fibrosis and systolic heart failure. The reported incidence of systemic ventricular dysfunction ranges from 8% to 45% (Helbing et al., 1994; Hucin et al., 2000) and increases with age.

Abnormalities in myocardial contractility are not, however, restricted to fibrosis and myocyte loss. Recent studies have demonstrated limited cardiac contractile reserve in response to increased heart rates in asymptomatic patients with Fontan palliation despite preserved global ventricular contractile function at rest (Senzaki et al., 2006). This finding may be due, in part, to restriction of ventricular motion by the Fontan circuit itself (Fogel et al., 1996) as well as to the absence of a second pumping chamber, which plays an important role in the augmentation of systolic force generated by each ventricle (Fogel et al., 1995). This loss of ventricular–ventricular interaction is an excellent example of the unique considerations that can adversely affect myocardial performance in the adult CHD population.

Alterations in Preload

Abnormal increases in preload are characteristic of congenital heart lesions associated with intracardiac or aortopulmonary shunts. Over time, this chronic volume overload leads to progressive ventricular dilatation and, eventually, dysfunction. Furthermore, valvular regurgitant lesions, which are often the result of congenital heart defects (e.g., Ebstein's anomaly, L-TGA) and their associated surgeries (e.g., tetralogy of Fallot [TOF] repair with transannular patch), may impose an additional volume load on an already struggling ventricle.

In other situations, such as in patients who have undergone Fontan palliation, a low preload can result in poor ventricular filling and thus impaired cardiac output (Gewillig, 2005). Similarly, atrial switch patients in whom noncompliant baffles can restrict transatrial flow demonstrate impaired augmentation of stroke volume during stress, suggesting that the resulting decrease in ventricular filling may impair ventricular performance (Derrick et al., 2000).

Alterations in Afterload

Congenital heart lesions that involve either right ventricular or left ventricular outflow tract obstruction, semilunar valve stenosis or coarctation of the aorta, among others, all lead to an increase in cardiac afterload. Although the initial hypertrophic response is characterized by normal or even enhanced myocardial contractility, sustained pressure overload eventually leads to ventricular dysfunction through poorly understood mechanisms (Frey and Olson, 2003; MacLellan and Schneider, 2000; Molkentin and Dorn, 2001). Inadequate neovascularization may play a significant role in this functional deterioration. As ventricular mass increases, so too does oxygen utilization. However, limitations in coronary vascular reserve have been observed due to a disproportionate increase in ventricular mass compared to microvascular growth, abnormal coronary vascular resistance, and extravascular compression by the hypertrophied ventricle (Giordano et al., 2001; Sheridan, et al., 1993; Shiojima et al., 2005). This results in chronic ischemia, fibrosis and, as previously discussed, impairment in myocardial contractility (Weber and Brilla, 1991).

Abnormal increases in afterload are not limited to obstructive lesions, however. Several studies have demonstrated an increased afterload in certain Fontan patients and its role in the decreased cardiac index and shortening fraction observed in this population due to ventricular–vascular mismatch (Akagi et al., 1992; Senzaki et al., 2006). Afterload-reducing agents are currently being investigated to see whether they can improve Fontan hemodynamics, particularly in such patients with an increased ventricular afterload, by improving ventricular–vascular interaction.

Alterations in Ventricular–Vascular Coupling

Blood flow through the ventricular–arterial system is an extremely efficient process that both conserves energy and minimizes stress relationships between the heart, central and peripheral conduits, resistance vessels, and the microvasculature (Dell'Italial et al., 1992; O'Rourke, 1982; O'Rourke et al., 1993). Modern understanding of ventricular–vascular coupling suggests that determinants of systolic and diastolic ventricular performance and those of vascular function have direct and profound effects on one other, as well as on coronary perfusion (Smulyan and Safar, 1997). Measures of the pulsatile hemodynamics of such coupling in heart failure, including alterations in arterial stiffness and cushioning, pulse pressure, wave characteristics, and velocities, have been shown to correlate with patient morbidity and mortality (Chae et al., 1999; Domanski et al., 1999; Mitchell et al., 1997, 2001). Demonstration of abnormal brachial artery responsiveness to endothelium-dependent and -independent vasomediators in young adults after successful coarctation repair led to the use of conduit artery pulse wave velocity as a marker of arterial stiffness (de Divitiis et al., 2001; Gardiner et al., 1994). Delay of conduit artery pulse wave velocity correlated with alterations in vasodilatation, pulse pressure, and increase in left ventricular mass (de Divitiis et al., 2003). Further investigation of pulse wave abnormalities in other congenital heart lesions in the adult and of their relationship to heart failure is expected.

There is increasing recognition that adults with CHD have additional cardiovascular abnormalities that affect key determinants of ventricular–vascular coupling. Changes in intrinsic heart rate (e.g., postoperative patients [de Divitiis et al., 2003]), stroke volume (e.g., patients with intracardiac mixing and volume loading), pulse pressure (e.g., patients with nonpulsatile pulmonary blood flow, patients with systemic arterial diastolic runoff), systemic arterial impedance (e.g., patients with aortic coarctation [Gardiner et al., 1994; de Divitiis et al., 2001, 2003]), and neurohormonal or cardiac autonomic nervous system activity (Bolger et al., 2002; Ohuchi et al., 2003) seen in such patients may have real and substantive effects on the health and functional capacity of affected individuals. Compromise of effective circulation may also result from intrinsic factors not typically considered within the cardiopulmonary tree. For example, energy conservation within a high-pressure nonpulsatile systemic venous inflow may be markedly diminished due to anatomic veno-atrial connections, compromising forward output in patients with early atriopulmonary-type Fontan palliations (Be'eri et al., 1998).

Alterations in Autonomic Nervous System Activity and Neurohormonal Activation

Abnormalities of cardiac autonomic nervous activity and elevations in neurohormone levels are being increasingly recognized in the adult CHD population (Driscoll et al., 1986; Kondo et al., 1998). These changes have been shown in conventional heart failure cohorts to correlate with degree of LV dysfunction, functional capacity, and mortality, and have been incorporated into various definitions of heart failure syndromes (Cohn et al., 1984; Eichhorn, 2001; Gottlieb et al., 1989; Remme and Swedberg, 2001).

Ohuchi and colleagues first demonstrated that relatively severe postoperative sympathetic denervation of the ventricle was common in a series of young adults following RV outflow tract reconstruction (Ohuchi et al., 2000). They confirmed in this population that exercise-mediated changes in heart rate, largely a function of parasympathetic nervous tone and postsynaptic β sensitivity (shown to correlate with functional ability), could also be affected. Parasympathetic nervous activity early after surgical repair was inversely related to number of surgeries and had a tendency to recover in the first year, likely as a function of recovery from sinus node ischemia. Postoperative β sensitivity was maintained, allowing for adequate heart rate augmentation. This augmentation of heart rate correlated with maximal oxygen consumption (peak VO_2) for postoperative patients without residual outflow tract stenosis, in contrast to those with residual obstruction in whom there was no correlation. These results emphasize that surgically mediated changes in heart rate (parasympathetic nervous activity, baroreceptor sensitivity, postoperative β sensitivity) and their recovery are important determinants of functional ability.

A follow-up assessment of cardiac autonomic nervous activity in mostly teenage patients after Fontan palliation demonstrated similar global alteration in cardiac autonomic nervous activity with the preservation of postsynaptic β sensitivity (Ohuchi et al., 2001). In this series, cardiac autonomic nervous activity abnormalities correlated with reductions in heart rate augmentation, but not with the number of surgical procedures, age at the time of Fontan operation, or length of follow-up. Similar to the group with residual outflow tract obstruction in the previous study, heart rate augmentation in patients with Fontan physiology did not correlate with peak VO_2. The authors theorized that in older patients with Fontan circulation, with attendant higher central filling pressures, lower resting systemic cardiac index, and lower resting systemic arterial blood pressure, it was direct surgery-related or subclinical injury rather than specific hemodynamic abnormalities that led to changes in cardiac autonomic nervous activity.

These findings, in part, were challenged by Davos and colleagues who assessed cardiac autonomic nervous activity in 22 older adults after Fontan palliation (Davos et al., 2003). Global depression of baroreceptor sensitivity and both low- and high-frequency domains of heart rate variability were noted, with a greater reduction in the low-frequency (reduction in sympathetic modulation) range. In contrast to the findings in Ohuchi and colleagues' (2000) younger patient population, reduction in low-frequency heart rate variability correlated an increase in right atrial (RA) dimension, a marker of hemodynamic abnormality, and baroreceptor sensitivity was greater in patients with a history of sustained atrial tachyarrhythmia.

In a study of 53 adults with a wide spectrum of CHDs by Bolger and colleagues (2002), neurohormones were elevated in all patients and increased in stepwise fashion with worsening New York Heart Association (NYHA) functional class. Atrial natriuretic peptide, brain natriuretic peptide, endothelin-1, norepinephrine, and epinephrine correlated with each other and with increases in QT interval and cardiothoracic ratio, echocardiographically measured ventricular systolic function, and exercise peak VO_2. Aldosterone and renin correlated only with each other and with right and left atrial volumes, suggesting that control mechanisms other than central pressure–volume relationships may be instrumental in the control of natriuretic peptides and catecholamines. In a separate study, Bolger's group demonstrated a similar elevation in circulating inflammatory cytokines, again increasing stepwise with worsening functional class (Sharma et al., 2003).

Ohuchi and colleagues (2003) expanded on these results, assessing both neurohormones and measures of cardiac autonomic nervous activity in 297 patients (75% of pediatric age) with CHD. Neurohormonal activation correlated with worsening subjective functional class in both pediatric and adult patients, with significantly higher levels of natriuretic peptides seen in the pediatric cohort. Serum norepinephrine levels differentiated NYHA class II from class III and IV patients in adults, but not in children. Baroreceptor sensitivity, heart rate variability, and vital capacity were related to functional capacity in NYHA class I and II patients, but not in class III and IV patients. The authors suggested that assessing both neurohormonal activation and cardiac autonomic nervous activity is useful in categorizing patients with CHD, with measures of parasympathetic activity being more helpful in less symptomatic patients and neurohormone levels being more helpful in more symptomatic patients.

Other Considerations

The complex relationships between aging, ventricular function, and outcome in adults with CHD is highlighted by long-term survival data in patients with TOF and D-TGA where continuous mortality appears to take a steeper drop-off in survival after the second postoperative decade.

Abnormalities in diastolic ventricular function may correlate with functional capacity and survival. Most notable are those seen in patients after repair of TOF, in whom restrictive right ventricular physiology demonstrated in the early postoperative period correlates with later restrictive markers, small chamber sizes, and narrower QRS durations (Norgard et al., 1996, 1998). This physiology appears to limit the potentially detrimental effects of pulmonary regurgitation, thus improving survival.

Regional changes in not only systolic but also diastolic function have been shown in patients with TOF using echocardiographic tissue Doppler analyses (Vogel et al., 2001). Analysis of similar tissue Doppler characteristics in patients with D-TGA has shown regional variation and reduced early and late diastolic myocardial velocities as well, with prolonged isovolumic relaxation time and potential absence of A-wave myocardial velocities independent of systolic abnormalities of the systemic right ventricle (Vogel et al., 2004). These changes may reflect intrinsic muscle abnormalities, changes in electrical–mechanical coupling, or regional injury in affected patients (Chaturvedi et al., 1999).

Native and postoperative anatomic sequelae, aside from residual shunts and obstruction, can contribute to abnormalities in cardiac output, functional capacity, and survival. The presence of a right ventricular outflow aneurysm in patients with TOF is associated with right ventricular dysfunction assessed by magnetic resonance imaging. Furthermore, while there is no significant correlation between the presence of a right ventricular outflow aneurysm and left ventricular ejection fraction, LV systolic dysfunction does correlate with RV dysfunction, emphasizing the role of interventricular dependency in maintaining efficient ventricular systolic function (Davlouros et al., 2002).

Progressive aortic dilation or distortion, with or without associated aortic regurgitation, typically associated with bicuspid aortic valve disease and mixing lesions such as TOF and single ventricle physiologies, also carries potential for altering left ventricular, and ultimately right ventricular, contractile function and ventricular–vascular coupling. It has been shown on occasion to eventuate in obstruction of coronary artery ostia or coronary dissection (Niwa et al., 2002). Pulmonary arterial enlargement, as well, has been reported to encroach upon the coronary artery ostia, sometimes leading to acute ischemia or global myocardial stunning.

ARRHYTHMIAS

Arrhythmias are frequently an active, if not central, issue for adult CHD patients. The arrhythmogenic substrate in these individuals is quite complex. While some arrhythmias are inherent to the structural abnormalities of the lesion—for example, the accessory muscle bundles of Ebstein's anomaly form the substrate for ventricular preexcitation typical of the Wolff-Parkinson-White syndrome—the majority of CHD patients present with acquired arrhythmias that are born out of long-standing hypertrophy, fibrosis, cyanosis, hemodynamic overload, and postsurgical scarring. These arrhythmias include re-entrant atrial and ventricular tachycardias, heart block, and sinus node dysfunction. In this section, we will review some of these rhythm disturbances and the disease entities with which they tend to be associated.

Bradycardias

Gradual loss of sinus rhythm occurs after the Mustard, Senning, Glenn, and Fontan procedures and appears to increase the risk of sudden death (Duster et al., 1985; Flinn et al., 1984; Manning et al., 1996). Direct surgical trauma to the sinoatrial node or the SA nodal artery may be implicated in the early postoperative period. However, the continued progressive loss of sinus rhythm over subsequent decades suggests that ongoing processes, perhaps related to chronic hemodynamic abnormalities and ischemia, are likely to play a role as well.

Bradycardias in adult CHD patients can also occur as a result of block occurring at the level of the atrioventricular node. As with the sinoatrial node, the AV node may be injured directly during surgical repair or may suffer indirect damage due to local inflammation and scarring. In many cases, postoperative AV block is transient and recovers within 5–7 days as inflammation and edema improve (Weindling et al., 1998). However, AV block that persists beyond this window is typically considered an indication for permanent cardiac pacing (Gregoratos et al., 2002).

Complete heart block is also a recognized complication of certain lesions including L-TGA and AV canal defects (Thiene et al., 1981; Van Praagh et al., 1998). Both of these lesions are associated with displacement of the AV node and the Bundle of His. The aberrant anatomy does render these structures particularly vulnerable to mechanical injury, but additional abnormalities are commonly demonstrated on electrophysiologic testing as well (Walsh and Cecchin, 2007).

Permanent pacemaker implantation is a treatment of choice for bradycardia (Gregoratos et al., 2002) but presents unique challenges in the adult CHD population. Congenital and acquired cardiovascular abnormalities such as Fontan circuits may limit options for endocardial lead placement and may require an epicardial approach, although a few institutions have reported success in accessing the coronary sinus for ventricular lead placement (Ermis et al., 2002). In other situations, such as in the patient with a Mustard or Senning baffle, placement of intravascular leads may result in an increased risk of thrombosis or vascular obstruction (Khairy et al., 2004). Another consideration is the increased risk of stroke that has been observed in patients with transvenous pacing leads and an intracardiac shunt (Khairy et al., 2006). Due to these concerns, it is crucial that device implantation be performed by an adult or pediatric cardiologist familiar with the intricacies of the patient with CHD.

Atrial Tachyarrhythmias

Perhaps one of the most vexing issues faced by those caring for adults with CHD is intra-atrial reentrant tachycardia (IART). IART describes a macroreentrant atrial tachycardia, often distinct from atrial flutter, that is commonly seen late in many forms of repaired CHD that involved an atriotomy or other surgical manipulation of right atrial tissue, indicating a particular dependence on surgical injury (Garson et al., 1985). The reentrant pathway in IART varies depending on the specific defect and the location of the surgical suture line (Collins et al., 2000; Mandapati et al., 2003; Triedman et al., 2001). Often, multiple reentrant circuits can be identified in the same patient (Delacretaz et al., 2001).

IART is particularly problematic for patients who have undergone Mustard, Senning, or Fontan procedures, operations that involve extensive suture lines. Roughly 50% of those with the older atriopulmonary-type Fontan palliations will develop IART within 10 years of surgery (Fishberger et al., 1997) and those with greater arrhythmic burden are being increasingly referred for surgical conversion to lateral tunnel or extracardiac Fontan anastomoses (Kao et al., 1994; Kreutzer et al., 1996; Mavroudis et al., 1998;

McElhinney et al., 1996). However, while the incidence of IART in patients with lateral tunnel or extracardiac Fontans may be lower initially, it increases over time (Shirai et al., 1998; Stamm et al., 2001). IART also occurs more commonly than ventricular tachycardia in patients who have undergone TOF repair and is a greater cause of morbidity, affecting about one-third of this population (Roos-Hesselink et al., 1995).

Since it is functionally quite similar to atrial flutter and atrial fibrillation, IART is thought to impart a modestly increased risk of intravascular and intracardiac thromboses. The prevalence of intracardiac thrombi seen on echocardiography prior to cardioversion for IART is reportedly as high as 42% (Gelatt et al., 1997; Shirai et al., 1998). Thus, although there are few reports of stroke postcardioversion, it is generally felt that long-term anticoagulation with warfarin is reasonable, although no randomized controlled trial-based consensus exists in this regard.

Experience with antiarrhythmic drug therapies for the treatment of IART has been generally disappointing, and most specialists feel they are unlikely to suppress recurrent episodes over the long term (Garson et al., 1985). Class Ic and class III drugs have been used with varying degrees of success, but their proarrhythmic potential and adverse effects on ventricular and nodal function limit their usefulness. As a result, catheter ablation is increasingly used as an early treatment modality in adult CHD patients with IART (Triedman et al., 1997). Recent short-term success rates have been reported to be as high as 90% in some centers/populations (Collins et al., 2000). Long-term follow-up has revealed that symptoms and quality of life are improved for most patients, although recurrences are documented in as many as 40% of all cases (Triedman et al., 1997).

Atrial fibrillation is also common and is associated with residual left-sided obstructive lesions or unrepaired heart disease (Kirsh et al., 2002). Treatment principles for the general population apply, with the caveat that risk of thromboembolism is probably elevated in this patient population. Transcatheter pulmonary vein isolation and the use of internal atrial defibrillators have not been explored extensively in the adult CHD population.

Ventricular Arrhythmias

In general, the patients at greatest risk for ventricular arrhythmias are those who have undergone a ventriculotomy and/or patch repair of certain kinds of ventricular septal defects. As described in IART, the presence of these surgical suture lines sets up the potential for macroreentrant circuits (Downar et al., 1992). However, VT can also occur in the setting of chronic hemodynamic overload, resulting in hypertrophy, fibrosis, and ventricular dysfunction. Thus, ventricular arrhythmias may be observed in cases of aortic valve disease, L-TGA, severe Ebstein's anomaly, certain forms of single ventricle, Eisenmenger's syndrome, and unrepaired TOF (Walsh and Cecchin, 2007). Patients with Fontan circulation and those who have undergone Mustard or Senning procedures are prone to atrial tachycardias, but, in the absence of systemic ventricular dysfunction, appear to be at lesser risk of VT (Gelatt et al., 1997; Kammeraadn et al., 2004; Kirjavainen et al., 1999).

The classic example of the adult CHD patient at risk for serious ventricular arrhythmias is the individual with repaired TOF. Considerable data are available on the natural history of ventricular arrhythmias and clinical outcomes among this group of patients because of the relative prevalence of the lesion in the adult CHD population. Although clinical presentation of adult TOF patients with sustained VT is uncommon, programmed stimulation can elicit ventricular arrhythmias in 15%–30% of these patients (Chandar et al., 1990; Lucron et al., 1999). Sudden death occurs with an overall prevalence of 2%–3% over 25 years of follow-up (Nollert et al., 1997). Mapping studies in repaired TOF have shown that VT in this population involves a macroreentrant circuit dependent on the right ventricular outflow tract patch and/or the conal septum (Horton et al., 1997).

Risk stratifying patients with repaired TOF for serious ventricular arrhythmias has long been a subject of intense investigation. Although no consensus exists, several clinical features with varying prognostic value have been identified. These include older age at the time of surgical repair, poorer hemodynamic status, pronounced prolongation of QRS duration (>180 ms), and inducible sustained VT in the EP laboratory (Gatzoulis et al., 1997). Taken as a whole, these variables can help to identify the individual at higher risk, but no individual item has sufficient predictive accuracy.

Since the available risk stratification schemas are limited at best, current practice relies largely on the individual's symptoms. For example, in patients with repaired TOF, the presence of severe symptoms or inducible VT warrants consideration of aggressive antiarrhythmic drug therapy and AICD placement, which had demonstrated proven benefit for both primary and secondary prevention of sudden cardiac death in noncongenital cardiac patients. Those with syncope or nonsustained VT warrant comprehensive evaluation including right heart catheterization for hemodynamic assessment and EP study with programmed ventricular stimulation.

The best approach to patients with minimal symptoms and to those who are truly asymptomatic remains undefined. Those with negative studies and favorable hemodynamics are often followed annually or semiannually with ECG and periodic exercise testing, echocardiography or magnetic resonance imaging, and Holter monitoring. They may be managed without treatment or with beta-blockade to suppress symptomatic ectopy. If nonsustained VT or deterioration in RV function is identified with or without associated valvular regurgitation, further studies and more aggressive antiarrhythmic management or pulmonary valve replacement may be indicated, but again, no consensus guidelines yet exist due to the lack of robust, long-term multicenter data.

PULMONARY VASCULAR DISEASE

Endothelial, smooth muscle, and vascular matrix dysfunction of the pulmonary arterial bed contribute to nonanatomic pulmonary ventricular afterload and, as a result, potential for reduction in transpulmonary blood flow in patients with previous or current intracardiac mixing (Khambadkone et al., 2003). Since the presence of increased pulmonary pressures does not necessarily indicate the presence of disease in the pulmonary arterial bed, but may be indicative of any of a number of triggers for such (e.g., pulmonary venous hypertension, restrictive or hypoventilatory lung disease, thromboembolic pulmonary vascular occlusion), catheter-based hemodynamic assessment remains critical to the diagnosis and appropriate treatment of pulmonary hypertension associated with CHD. Pulmonary arterial hypertension (PAH) may also result from different mechanisms over the life span of an individual with CHD relating to flow and pressure from an open shunt early in life; in association with perioperative triggers; or late after surgical shunt correction, even if preoperative resistance changes were not noted.

Analyses of epidemiologic databases associated with PAH patients have suggested a nearly universal increase in the mortality of untreated patients with severe pulmonary hypertension, regardless of etiology. Correlation of survival with variables relating to right ventricular function (typically assessed by hemodynamic measure of systemic cardiac output, mixed venous oxygen saturation, and right atrial pressure) and physical capacity (typically measured by 6-minute walk distance) emphasizes the delicate balance and direct relationships between pulmonary afterload, cardiac function, physical capacity, and life (Oya et al., 2002). The improved survival outcomes seen in patients with severe PAH associated with Eisenmenger syndrome—a 10- to 20-year survival greater than 80% in contrast to a median survival of 2.8–3.4 years in other patients with CHD-PAH without open shunts—suggest the potential for improved response to increased pulmonary afterload when the burden is shared between the right and left ventricles (Oya et al., 2002).

During the past decade, the "vasoconstriction" monolayer model of primary pulmonary hypertension has been replaced by the current vascular wall inflammation paradigm, with therapies reflecting this change in pathophysiologic thought. Increasing evidence exists for genetically inherited abnormalities in endothelial cell apoptosis and growth potential, with links of familial and sporadic PAH to bone morphogenetic protein receptor type-2 (BMPR2) and activin-like kinase type-1 (ALK1), two receptors in the transforming growth factor β superfamily. In addition, increasing data suggest that the hallmark lesion of PAH, the plexiform lesion, occurs in response to local hypoxia or inflammation and, in certain individuals with PAH, may represent a tumor-like proliferation of endothelial cells (monoclonal in PPH and polyclonal in secondary forms of PAH). Markers of cellular inflammation, matrix stimulation and cellular growth, and platelets and coagulant activity, including fractalkine, RANTES (*r*egulated upon *a*ctivation, *n*ormal T-cell *e*xpressed and *s*ecreted), interleukin-1β, interleukin-6, soluble intracellular adhesion molecule, soluble vascular cell adhesion molecule, soluble P-selectin, soluble electin, vascular endothelial growth factor, serum elastase, von Willebrand factors, serotonin plasminogen activator inhibitor, fibrinopeptide A, and thrombomodulin, have all been found in tissue biopsies and blood tests of PAH patients.

For most affected patients, modern treatment, however indirectly, has begun to center on mediators of chemotaxis, cellular proliferation and differentiation, and regulation of vasoactive peptides and growth factors. These mediators currently include prostanoids (intravenous, inhaled, and oral), endothelin antagonists, nitroso compounds, and phosphodiesterase inhibitors. At present, although phase III randomized controlled trials for many of these agents have included small numbers of CHD patients, only one randomized controlled trial has been performed to, assess the safety and clinical benefit of PAH therapy in adults with rigorously defined PAH-CHD, in particular, those with Eisenmenger syndrome (Galiè et al., 2006). In this trial, short-term use of a combined endothelin A and B receptor antagonist over 4 months was associated with improved hemodynamics and with improved subjective and objective measures of functional capacity, without significant adverse effects as compared to placebo. Trials addressing the safety and efficacy of other treatments in specific forms of CHD-associated pulmonary hypertensive disorders are expected.

MULTIORGAN DYSFUNCTION

In patients with both corrected and uncorrected CHD, classic clinical definition of heart failure—"failure of the heart (in whatever form it may be) to keep up with the demands of the body"—is demonstrated by what may be considered premature senescence and not only decrement of cardiac function but abnormalities and increased demand of nearly every organ system (Table 17–1). Indeed, one could justifiably make the argument that CHD is truly a multisystem disease. Increased potential for endocrine dysfunction, gas-exchanging and nonparenchymal lung disease, abnormalities of renal or hepatic function, and altered skeleton and muscle metabolism all highlight the multitude of extracardiac conditions contributing to observed abnormalities in functional capacity.

The adult with CHD may be profoundly limited in aerobic functional capacity when compared with normal controls (Fredriksen et al., 2001). As noted earlier, maximal achievable peak oxygen consumption (peak VO_2) may be less than half that for normal controls. Restriction in ventilatory function (with respiratory volumes typically 75%–85% of normal predicted values),

TABLE 17–1. *Potential Noncardiac Morbidities in the Adult CHD Patient*

Endocrinologic/neurohormonal
Hypothyroidism
Diabetes
Loss of adrenergic and vagal responsiveness

Pulmonary
Restrictive lung disease
Hypoventilation/obstructive sleep apnea
Arterio-venous malformations
Pulmonary vascular disease
Chronic parenchymal infection

Liver
Chronic hepatitis
Portal hypertension
Cardic cirrhosis

Renal
Altered glomerular filtration
Altered water handling
Hyperuricemia

Hematologic
Iron deficiency
Erythrocytosis
Lymphopenia
Hemostatic abnormalities (prothrombosis, bleeding)

Skeletal
Metabolically dependent poor muscle training
Volitional/iatrogenic poor muscle training
Kyphoscoliosis

Infectious
Chronic infectious potential

Neurologic
Cerebrovascular injury

Pregnancy

whether due to developmental or acquired structural and physiologic changes, may contribute to fatigue and incapacity (Fredriksen et al., 2001). Hepatitis-induced cirrhosis and cardiac cirrhosis (felt by some to be diseases of past medical generations) have been recapitulated in a patient population plagued by chronically elevated central venous pressures, potential for low systemic cardiac output, and ongoing exposure to blood products. The neurohormonal activation triggered by portal hypertension may be profound and can exacerbate volume retention and curb functional ability.

CONCLUSIONS

The past few decades have seen an increase in the population of adults with CHD to numbers now surpassing their pediatric counterparts. Indeed, in the experience of Children's Hospital Boston, by the early 1990s, roughly 85% of all patients *including* those with hypoplastic left heart syndrome were alive at age 17 years. Patients with increasing anatomic complexity, greater numbers of surgical and catheter-based procedures, alteration in pulmonary and systemic arterial and venous function, neurohormonal activation, and abnormalities in rhythm, coupled with changes of myocardial, vascular, and multiorgan "premature" senescence, are alive, functioning, and demanding our protection and care for today and for their future. The past few years have seen enormous growth in the understanding of heart failure syndromes in these patients who, in their own existence, define a uniquely altered physiology. It is only through continued insights into these new paradigms of physiologic understanding, coupled with randomized clinical therapeutic trials in this growing population, that a future of optimal functioning can be guaranteed for the adult survivor of CHD.

REFERENCES

Akagi T, Benson LN, Green M, et al. Ventricular performance before and after Fontan repair for univentricular atrioventricular connection: angiographic and radionuclide assessment. *J Am Coll Cardiol.* 1992;20(4):920–926.

Be'eri E, Maier SE, Landzberg MJ, et al. In vivo evaluation of Fontan pathway flow dynamics by multidimensional phase-velocity magnetic resonance imaging. *Circulation.* 1998;98(25): 2873–2882.

Beauchesne LM, Warnes CA, Connolly HM, Ammash NM, Tajik AJ, Danielson GK. Outcome of the unoperated adult who presents with congenitally corrected transposition of the great arteries. *J Am Coll Cardiol.* 2002;40(2):285–90.

Bolger AP, Gatzoulis MA. Towards defining heart failure in adults with congenital heart disease. *Int J Cardiol.* 2004;97(suppl 1):15–23.

Bolger AP, Sharma R, Li W, et al. Neurohormonal activation and the chronic heart failure syndrome in adults with congenital heart disease. *Circulation.* 2002;106(1):92–99.

Chae CU, Pfeffer MA, Glynn RJ, Mitchell GF, Taylor JO, Hennekens CH. Increased pulse pressure and risk of heart failure in the elderly. *JAMA.* 1999;281(7):634–639.

Chandar JS, Wolff GS, Garson A Jr., et al. Ventricular arrhythmias in postoperative tetralogy of Fallot. *Am J Cardiol.* 1990;65(9):655–661.

Chaturvedi RR, Shore DF, Lincoln C, et al. Acute right ventricular restrictive physiology after repair of tetralogy of Fallot: association with myocardial injury and oxidative stress." *Circulation.* 1999;100(14):1540–1547.

Cohn JN, Levine TB, Olivari MT, et al. Plasma norepinephrine as a guide to prognosis in patients with chronic congestive heart failure. *N Engl J Med.* 1984;311(13):819–823.

Collins KK, Love BA, Walsh EP, Saul JP, Epstein MR, Triedman JK. Location of acutely successful radiofrequency catheter ablation of intraatrial reentrant tachycardia in patients with congenital heart disease. *Am J Cardiol.* 2000;86(9):969–974.

Davlouros PA, Kilner PJ, Hornung TS, et al. Right ventricular function in adults with repaired tetralogy of Fallot assessed with cardiovascular magnetic resonance imaging: detrimental role of right ventricular outflow aneurysms or akinesia and adverse right-to-left ventricular interaction. *J Am Coll Cardiol* 2002;40(11):2044–2052.

Davos CH., Francis DP, Leenarts MF, et al. Global impairment of cardiac autonomic nervous activity late after the Fontan operation. *Circulation.* 2003;108 Suppl 1:II180–II185.

de Divitiis M, Pilla C, Kattenhorn M, et al. Ambulatory blood pressure, left ventricular mass, and conduit artery function late after successful repair of coarctation of the aorta. *J Am Coll Cardiol.* 2003;41(12):2259–2265.

de Divitiis M, Pilla C, Kattenhorn M, et al. Vascular dysfunction after repair of coarctation of the aorta: impact of early surgery. *Circulation.* 2001;104(12 suppl 1):I165–I170.

Delacretaz E, Ganz LI, Soejima K, et al. Multi atrial maco-re-entry circuits in adults with repaired congenital heart disease: entrainment mapping combined with three-dimensional electroanatomic mapping. *J Am Coll Cardiol.* 2001;37(6):1665–1676.

Dell'Italia LJ, Blackwell GG, Blackwell GG , Thorn BT, Pearce DJ, Bishop SP, Pohost GM. Time-varying wall stress: an index of ventricular vascular coupling. *Am J Physiol.* 1992;263(2 Pt 2):H597–H605.

Derrick GP, Narang I, White PA, et al. Failure of stroke volume augmentation during exercise and dobutamine stress is unrelated to load-independent indexes of right ventricular performance after the Mustard operation. *Circulation.* 2000;102(19 suppl 3):III154–III159.

Domanski MJ., Mitchell GF, Norman J, Pitt B, Exener D, Pfeffer MA. Independent prognostic information provided by sphygmomanometrically determined pulse pressure and mean arterial pressure in patients with left ventricular dysfunction. *J Am Coll Cardiol.* 1999;33(4):951–958.

Downar E, Harris L, Kimber S, et al. Ventricular tachycardia after surgical repair of tetralogy of Fallot: results of intraoperative mapping studies. *J Am Coll Cardiol.* 1992;20(3):648–655.

Driscoll DJ, Danielson GK, Puga FJ, Schaff HV, Heise CT, Staats BA. Exercise tolerance and cardiorespiratory response to exercise after the Fontan operation for tricuspid atresia or functional single ventricle. *J Am Coll Cardiol.* 1986;7(5):1087–1094.

Duster MC, Bink-Boelkens MT, Wampler D, Gillette PC, McNamara DG, Cooley DA. Long-term follow-up of dysrhythmias following the Mustard procedure. *Am Heart J.* 1985;109(6):1323–1326.

Eichhorn EJ. Prognosis determination in heart failure. *Am J Med.* 2001;110 Suppl 7A:14S–36S.

Ermis C, Zadeii G, Gupta M, Benditt DG. Trans-aortic His bundle ablation with permanent ventricular pacing via the coronary sinus in L-transposition of great arteries with classic Fontan procedure. *J Interv Card Electrophysiol.* 2002;7(3):257–260.

Fishberger SB, Wernovsky G, Gentles TL, et al. Factors that influence the development of atrial flutter after the Fontan operation. *J Thorac Cardiovasc Surg.* 1997;113(1):80–86.

Flinn CJ, Wolff GS, Dick M II, et al. Cardiac rhythm after the Mustard operation for complete transposition of the great arteries. *N Engl J Med.* 1984;310(25):1635–1638.

Fogel MA, Weinberg PM, Chin AJ, Fellows KE, Hoffman EA. Late ventricular geometry and performance changes of functional single ventricle throughout staged Fontan reconstruction assessed by magnetic resonance imaging. *J Am Coll Cardiol.* 1996;28(1):212–221.

Fogel MA, Weinberg PM, Fellows KE, Hoffman EA. A study in ventricular-ventricular interaction. Single right ventricles compared with systemic right ventricles in a dual-chamber circulation. *Circulation.* 1995;92(2):219–230.

Fredriksen PM, Veldtman G, Hechter S, et al. Aerobic capacity in adults with various congenital heart diseases. *Am J Cardiol.* 2001;87(3):310–314.

Frey N, Olson EN. Cardiac hypertrophy: the good, the bad, and the ugly. *Annu Rev Physiol.* 2003;65:45–79.

Galiè N, Beghetti M, Gatzoulis MA, et al. Bosentan therapy in patients with Eisenmenger syndrome: a multicenter, double-blind, randomized, placebo-controlled study. *Circulation.* 2006;114(1):48–54.

Gardiner HM, Celermajer DS, Sorensen KE, et al. Arterial reactivity is significantly impaired in normotensive young adults after successful repair of aortic coarctation in childhood. *Circulation.* 1994;89(4):1745–1750.

Garson A Jr, Bink-Boelkens M, Hesslein PS, et al. Atrial flutter in the young: a collaborative study of 380 cases. *J Am Coll Cardiol.* 1985;6(4):871–878.

Gatzoulis MA, Till JA, Redington AN. Depolarization-repolarization inhomogeneity after repair of tetralogy of Fallot. The substrate for malignant ventricular tachycardia? *Circulation.* 1997;95(2):401–404.

Gelatt M, Hamilton TM, McCrindle BW, et al. Arrhythmia and mortality after the Mustard procedure: a 30-year single-center experience. *J Am Coll Cardiol.* 1997;29(1):194–201.

Gewillig M. Ventricular dysfunction of the functionally univentricular heart: management and outcomes. *Cardiol Young.* 2005;15 (suppl 3):31–34.

Giordano FJ, Gerber HP, Williams SP, et al. A cardiac myocyte vascular endothelial growth factor paracrine pathway is required to maintain cardiac function. *Proc Natl Acad Sci U S A.* 2001;98(10):5780–5785.

Gottlieb SS, Kukin ML, Ahern D, Packer M. Prognostic importance of atrial natriuretic peptide in patients with chronic heart failure. *J Am Coll Cardiol.* 1989;13(7):1534–1539.

Graham TP Jr. Ventricular performance in congenital heart disease. *Circulation.* 1991;84(6):2259–2274.

Gregoratos G, Abrams J, Epstein AE, et al. ACC/AHA/NASPE 2002 guideline update for implantation of cardiac pacemakers and antiarrhythmia devices: summary article: a report of the American College of Cardiology/American Heart Association Task Force on Practice Guidelines (ACC/AHA/NASPE Committee to Update the 1998 Pacemaker Guidelines). *Circulation.* 2002;106(16):2145–2161.

Groundstroem KW, Iivainen TE, Lahtela JT, et al. Natriuretic peptide and echocardiography after operation of atrial septal defect. *Int J Cardiol.* 2003;89(1):45–52.

Helbing WA, Hansen B, Ottenkamp J, et al. Long-term results of atrial correction for transposition of the great arteries. Comparison of Mustard and Senning operations. *J Thorac Cardiovasc Surg.* 1994;108(2):363–372.

Hornung TS, Bernard EJ, Jaeggi ET, Howman-Giles RB, Celermajer DS, Hawker RE. Myocardial perfusion defects and associated systemic ventricular dysfunction in congenitally corrected transposition of the great arteries. *Heart.* 1998;80(4):322–326.

Hornung TS, Kilner PJ, Davlouros PA, Grothues F, Li W, Gatzoulis MA. Excessive right ventricular hypertrophic response in adults with the mustard procedure for transposition of the great arteries. *Am J Cardiol.* 2002;90(7):800–803.

Horton RP, Canby RC, Kessler DJ, et al. Ablation of ventricular tachycardia associated with tetralogy of Fallot: demonstration of bidirectional block. *J Cardiovasc Electrophysiol.* 1997;8(4):432–435.

Hucin B, Voriskova M, Hruda J, et al. Late complications and quality of life after atrial correction of transposition of the great arteries in 12 to 18 year follow-up. *J Cardiovasc Surg (Torino).* 2000;41(2):233–239.

Kammeraad JA, van Deurzen CH, Sreeram N, et al. Predictors of sudden cardiac death after Mustard or Senning repair for transposition of the great arteries. *J Am Coll Cardiol.* 2004;44(5):1095–1102.

Kao JM, Alejos JC, Grant PW, Williams RG, Shannon KM, Laks H. Conversion of atriopulmonary to cavopulmonary anastomosis in management of late arrhythmias and atrial thrombosis. *Ann Thorac Surg.* 1994;58(5):1510–1514.

Khairy P, Landzberg MJ, Gatzoulis MA, et al. Transvenous pacing leads and systemic thromboemboli in patients with intracardiac shunts: a multicenter study. *Circulation.* 2006;113(20):2391–2397.

Khairy P, Landzberg MJ, Lambert J, O'Donnell CP. Long-term outcomes after the atrial switch for surgical correction of transposition: a meta-analysis comparing the Mustard and Senning procedures. *Cardiol Young.* 2004;14(3):284–292.

Khambadkone S, Li J, de Leval MR, Cullen S, Deanfield JE, Redington AN. Basal pulmonary vascular resistance and nitric oxide responsiveness late after Fontan-type operation. *Circulation.* 2003;107(25):3204–3208.

Kirjavainen M, Happonen JM, Louhimo I. Late results of Senning operation. *J Thorac Cardiovasc Surg.* 1999;117(3):488–495.

Kirsh JA, Walsh EP, Triedman JK. Prevalence of and risk factors for atrial fibrillation and intra-atrial reentrant tachycardia among patients with congenital heart disease. *Am J Cardiol.* 2002;90(3):338–340.

Kondo C, Nakazawa M, Momma K, Kusakabe K. Sympathetic denervation and reinnervation after arterial switch operation for complete transposition. *Circulation.* 1998;97(24):2414–2419.

Kreutzer J, Keane JF, Lock JE, et al. Conversion of modified Fontan procedure to lateral atrial tunnel cavopulmonary anastomosis. *J Thorac Cardiovasc Surg.* 1996;111(6):1169–1176.

Lubiszewska B, Gosiewska E, Hoffman P, et al. Myocardial perfusion and function of the systemic right ventricle in patients after atrial switch procedure for complete transposition: long-term follow-up. *J Am Coll Cardiol.* 2000;36(4):1365–1370.

Lucron H, Marcon F, Bosser G, Lethor JP, Marie PY, Brembilla-Perrot B. Induction of sustained ventricular tachycardia after surgical repair of tetralogy of Fallot. *Am J Cardiol.* 1999;83(9):1369–1373.

Mackie AS, Pilote L, Ionescu-Ittu R, Rahme E, Marelli AJ. Health care resource utilization in adults with congenital heart disease. *Am J Cardiol.* 2007;99(6):839–843.

MacLellan WR, Schneider MD. Genetic dissection of cardiac growth control pathways. *Annu Rev Physiol.* 2000;62:289–319.

Mandapati R, Walsh EP, Triedman JK. Pericaval and periannular intra-atrial reentrant tachycardias in patients with congenital heart disease. *J Cardiovasc Electrophysiol.* 2003;14(2):119–125.

Manning PB, Mayer JE Jr, Wernovsky G, Fishberger SB, Walsh EP. Staged operation to Fontan increases the incidence of sinoatrial node dysfunction. *J Thorac Cardiovasc Surg.* 1996;111(4):833–839; discussion 839–840.

Marelli AJ, Mackie AS, Ionescu-Ittu R, Rahme E, Pilote L. Congenital heart disease in the general population: changing prevalence and age distribution. *Circulation.* 2007;115(2):163–172.

Mavroudis C, Backer CL, Deal BJ, Johnsrude CL. Fontan conversion to cavopulmonary connection and arrhythmia circuit cryoblation. *J Thorac Cardiovasc Surg.* 1998;115(3):547–556.

McElhinney DB, Reddy VM, Moore P, Hanley FL. Revision of previous Fontan connections to extracardiac or intraatrial conduit cavopulmonary anastomosis. *Ann Thorac Surg.* 1996;62(5):1276–1282; discussion 1283.

Millane T, Bernard EJ, Jaeggi E, et al. Role of ischemia and infarction in late right ventricular dysfunction after atrial repair of transposition of the great arteries. *J Am Coll Cardiol.* 2000;35(6):1661–1668.

Mitchell GF, Moyé LA, Braunwald E, et al. Sphygmomanometrically determined pulse pressure is a powerful independent predictor of recurrent events after myocardial infarction in patients with impaired left ventricular function. SAVE investigators. Survival and Ventricular Enlargement. *Circulation.* 1997;96(12):4254–4260.

Mitchell GF, Tardif JC, Arnold JM, et al. Pulsatile hemodynamics in congestive heart failure. *Hypertension.* 2001;38(6):1433–1439.

Molkentin JD, Dorn IG II. Cytoplasmic signaling pathways that regulate cardiac hypertrophy. *Annu Rev Physiol.* 2001;63:391–426.

Murphy JG, Gersh BJ, McGoon MD, et al. Long-term outcome after surgical repair of isolated atrial septal defect. Follow-up at 27 to 32 years. *N Engl J Med.* 1990;323(24):1645–1650.

Niwa K, Siu SC, Webb GD, Gatzoulis MA. Progressive aortic root dilatation in adults late after repair of tetralogy of Fallot. *Circulation.* 2002;106(11):1374–1378.

Nollert G, Fischlein T, Bouterwek S, Böhmer C, Klinner W, Reichart B. Long-term survival in patients with repair of tetralogy of Fallot: 36-year follow-up of 490 survivors of the first year after surgical repair. *J Am Coll Cardiol.* 1997;30(5):1374–1383.

Norgard G, Gatzoulis MA, Moraes F, et al. Does restrictive right ventricular physiology in the early postoperative period predict subsequent right ventricular restriction after repair of tetralogy of Fallot? *Heart.* 1998;79(5):481–484.

Norgard G, Gatzoulis MA, Moraes F, et al. Relationship between type of outflow tract repair and postoperative right ventricular diastolic physiology in tetralogy of Fallot. Implications for long-term outcome. *Circulation.* 1996;94(12):3276–3280.

O'Rourke MF. *Arterial Function in Health and Disease.* Edinburgh: Churchill Livingstone; 1982.

O'Rourke MF, Safar ME, Dzau V. *Arterial Vasodilation: Mechanisms and Therapy.* Philadelphia: Lea & Febiger; 1993.

Ohuchi H, Hasegawa S, Yasuda K, Yamada O, Ono Y, Echigo S. Severely impaired cardiac autonomic nervous activity after the Fontan operation. *Circulation.* 2001;104(13):1513–1518.

Ohuchi H, Suzuki H, Toyohara K, et al. Abnormal cardiac autonomic nervous activity after right ventricular outflow tract reconstruction. *Circulation.* 2000;102(22):2732–2738.

Ohuchi H, Takasugi H, Ohashi H, et al. Stratification of pediatric heart failure on the basis of neurohormonal and cardiac autonomic nervous activities in patients with congenital heart disease. *Circulation.* 2003;108(19):2368–2376.

Oya H, Nagaya N, Uematsu M, et al. Poor prognosis and related factors in adults with Eisenmenger syndrome. *Am Heart J.* 2002;143(4):739–744.

Perloff JK, Warnes CA. Challenges posed by adults with repaired congenital heart disease. *Circulation.* 2001;103(21):2637–2643.

Prieto LR, Hordof AJ, Secic M, Rosenbaum MS, Gersony WM. Progressive tricuspid valve disease in patients with congenitally corrected transposition of the great arteries. *Circulation.* 1998;98(10):997–1005.

Remme WJ, Swedberg K. Guidelines for the diagnosis and treatment of chronic heart failure. *Eur Heart J.* 2001;22(17):1527–1560.

Roos-Hesselink J, Perlroth MG, McGhie J, Spitaels S. Atrial arrhythmias in adults after repair of tetralogy of Fallot. Correlations with clinical, exercise, and echocardiographic findings. *Circulation.* 1995;91(8):2214–2219.

Senzaki H, Masutani S, Ishido H, et al. Cardiac rest and reserve function in patients with Fontan circulation. *J Am Coll Cardiol.* 2006;47(12):2528–2535.

Sharma R, Bolger AP, Li W, et al. Elevated circulating levels of inflammatory cytokines and bacterial endotoxin in adults with congenital heart disease. *Am J Cardiol.* 2003;92(2):188–193.

Sheridan DJ, McAinsh A, O'Gorman DJ. The coronary circulation in cardiac hypertrophy. *J Cardiovasc Pharmacol.* 1993;22 (suppl 6): S18–28.

Shiojima I, Sato K, Izumiya Y, et al. Disruption of coordinated cardiac hypertrophy and angiogenesis contributes to the transition to heart failure. *J Clin Invest.* 2005;115(8):2108–2118.

Shirai LK, Rosenthal DN, Reitz BA, Robbins RC, Dubin AM. Arrhythmias and thromboembolic complications after the extracardiac Fontan operation. *J Thorac Cardiovasc Surg.* 1998;115(3):499–505.

Smulyan H, Safar ME. Systolic blood pressure revisited. *J Am Coll Cardiol.* 1997;29(7):1407–1413.

Stamm C, Friehs I, Mayer JE Jr, et al. Long-term results of the lateral tunnel Fontan operation. *J Thorac Cardiovasc Surg.* 2001;121(1):28–41.

Thiene G, Wenink AC, Frescura C, et al. Surgical anatomy and pathology of the conduction tissues in atrioventricular defects. *J Thorac Cardiovasc Surg.* 1981;82(6):928–937.

Triedman JK, Alexander ME, Berul CI, Bevilacqua LM, Walsh EP. Electroanatomic mapping of entrained and exit zones in patients with repaired congenital heart disease and intra-atrial reentrant tachycardia. *Circulation.* 2001;103(16):2060–2065.

Triedman JK, Bergau DM, Saul JP, Epstein MR, Walsh EP. Efficacy of radiofrequency ablation for control of intraatrial reentrant tachycardia in patients with congenital heart disease. *J Am Coll Cardiol.* 1997;30(4):1032–1038.

Van Praagh, R, Papagiannis J, Grünenfelder J, Bartram U, Martanovic P. Pathologic anatomy of corrected transposition of the great arteries: medical and surgical implications. *Am Heart J.* 1998;135(5 Pt 1):772–785.

Vogel M, Derrick G, White PA, et al. Systemic ventricular function in patients with transposition of the great arteries after atrial repair: a tissue Doppler and conductance catheter study. *J Am Coll Cardiol.* 2004;43(1):100–106.

Vogel M, Sponring J, Cullen S, Deanfield JE, Redington AN. Regional wall motion and abnormalities of electrical depolarization and repolarization in patients after surgical repair of tetralogy of Fallot. *Circulation.* 2001;103(12):1669–1673.

Walsh EP, Cecchin F. Arrhythmias in adult patients with congenital heart disease. *Circulation.* 2007;115(4):534–545.

Warnes CA. Congenitally corrected transposition: the uncorrected misnomer. *J Am Coll Cardiol.* 1996;27(5):1244–1245.

Warnes CA, Liberthson R, Danielson GK, et al. Task force 1: the changing profile of congenital heart disease in adult life. *J Am Coll Cardiol.* 2001;37(5):1170–1175.

Weber KT, Brilla CG. Pathological hypertrophy and cardiac interstitium. Fibrosis and renin-angiotensin-aldosterone system. *Circulation.* 1991;83(6):1849–1865.

Weindling SN, Saul JP, Gamble WJ, et al. Duration of complete atrioventricular block after congenital heart disease surgery. *Am J Cardiol.* 1998;82(4):525–527.

18

Pregnancy and Congenital Heart Disease

MARY M. CANOBBIO

REEMA CHUGH

INTRODUCTION

Given the dramatic advances in diagnostic techniques, medical interventions, and early surgical interventions, increasing number of females born with congenital heart disease will be reaching childbearing age. For the majority, the ability to conceive and care a pregnancy to terms will present little problem, however a large percent, while clinically stable, face a higher risk of morbidity given the residua often associated with defects.

This chapter provides an overview of the effects of pregnancy on CHD.

Physiologic Changes Associated with Normal Pregnancy

A variety of major physiologic and biochemical changes are known to occur as a characteristic of normal pregnancy. Because of the increased burden on the cardiovascular system, it is important to understand these normal changes in order to determine their significance in the setting of maternal heart diseases. While the majority of hemodynamic changes associated with pregnancy are well tolerated, the increase circulatory demands can precipitate serious complications in certain patients. Accordingly, a comprehensive understanding of the expected hemodynamic adjustments of pregnancy labor and delivery is essential for rational management of any pregnant patient with underlying cardiac disease.

Pregnancy has profound effects on the maternal cardiovascular system (Table 18–1). Thus, a key question is whether a woman with CHD has the cardiovascular reserve to withstand the increase in blood volume, cardiac output, stroke volume, and the additional hemodynamic stress associated with labor and delivery.

Blood Volume. Maternal plasma volume increases progressively during pregnancy, reaching peak levels of about 50% by 32 weeks gestation, which represents a ~40%–50% increase in blood volume over nonpregnant values. This increment is higher in multigravidas than primigravidas, and is greater in twin pregnancies (67%) than in a singleton pregnancy (Metcalfe and Ueland, 1974; Ueland, 1976). While the rise in total red cell volume parallels the rise in plasma blood volume, the increase is not as great, averaging only 20%–40% of nonpregnant values. Most of the expansion in blood volume is due to the increase in plasma volume, resulting in a reduction of the maternal hemoglobin concentration, a condition known as dilutional anemia or physiological anemia of pregnancy (Pritchard, 1965). Maternal hematocrit levels have been reported to be as low as 33%–38% with hemoglobin levels of falling to levels of 11–12 g/100 mL during the second trimester (Kaneshige, 1981; Pritchard, 1965).

Heart Rate. Maternal heart rate progressively rises 10–20 bpm or 17% over pregestational rates. Mean values range from 78 to 89 beats per minute. Changes in body position from supine to lateral recumbency may decrease heart rate (Ueland and Hansen, 1969a).

Cardiac Output. The product of an increased in stroke volume and increased heart rate is an increase in cardiac output of 30%–50% over nonpregnant levels. A rapid rise occurs late in the first trimester with peak levels reached by the 20th to 24th weeks where

TABLE 18–1. *Cardiovascular Changes Associated with Normal Pregnancy*

Blood volume	Increased	40–50
Cardiac output	Increased	30–50
Stroke volume	Increased	18–25
Heart rate	Increased	20% (10–20 beats/min)
Systemic blood pressure		
Systolic	Slightly decreased	
Diastolic	Decreased	
Pulse pressure	Increased	
Systemic vascular resistance	Decreased	
Pulmonary vascular resistance	Decreased	

TABLE 18–2. *Hematologic Changes in Normal Pregnancy*

Plasma volume	↑	40–50
Red cell mass	↑	20–30
Hematocrit	↓	Hct ≥ 33%
Hemoglobin	↓	Hgb ≥ 11g/dL
Red blood cells		Thicker, more spheric
Clotting		Hypercoagulable state

it is maintained until late in pregnancy (Ueland and Metcalfe, 1975). Between the 38th and 40th week, a decline in cardiac output is dependent on maternal position, however little or no change is observed when cardiac output is measured with the patient in the lateral recumbent position (Ueland et al., 1969; Ueland and Hansen, 1969). Maternal position exerts a profound mechanical effect on cardiovascular hemodynamics, particularly toward the end of gestation. Compression of the inferior vena cava by the gravid uterus when in the supine position can decrease venous return, stroke volume, and cardiac output. In the last trimester of gestation, approximately 8% of women will experience feel light headedness and nausea. This "supine hypotensive syndrome," can be relieved by placing the patient in lateral recumbency (Kinsella and Lohmann, 1994).

This effect is attributed to the mechanical compression of the inferior vena cava produced by the enlarging uterus. Kerr (1965) demonstrated that in approximately 90% of women studied, complete obstruction of the inferior vena cava occurred in the supine position. Ueland et al. (1969) found an average rise in resting cardiac output of 27%–31% rise in stroke volume and decline of 7% in heart rate when the position of the mother changes from supine to lateral recumbent.

Vascular Resistance. Paralleling the increase in blood volume mentioned earlier is a decrease in systemic vascular resistance (SVR), which reduces preload and afterload. Attributed to hormonal influence that interrupts uterine perfusion by creating a low resistance circuit in the pregnant uterus, SVR declines within the first 8 weeks of pregnancy (Metcalfe and Ueland, 1974).

Similarly pulmonary vascular resistance decreases during pregnancy in association with the increase in flow. As a result, mean pulmonary artery pressure (14 mmHg) is similar to nonpregnant values. Postpartum pulmonary vascular resistance normally remains slightly reduced until about 8 weeks after delivery.

Arterial Blood Pressure. Systemic arterial blood pressure declines early in the first trimester. A modest decrease in systolic pressure of 10–15 mmHg, and a somewhat greater reduction of the diastolic pressure of 20–25 mmHg results in a widened pulse pressure and reflects the gestational decrease in vascular resistance (Christianson, 1976; Elkayam and Gleicher, 1998). This change is maximized by midpregnancy, but both systolic and diastolic pressures return to nonpregnant levels before term. A variety of factors may influence arterial blood pressure during pregnancy including increasing maternal age (age 35 and older) and parity (Christianson, 1976). Maternal position at time of measurement also has an effect on blood pressure values. In most pregnant patients, the blood pressure taken in supine position will be higher than when taken in the left lateral position (Ueland and Hansen, 1969a).

Hematologic Changes. Apart from circulatory overload, a state of physiologic hypercoagulability is present throughout the pregnancy characterized by increase in clotting factors, decreased fibrinolysis, and increased venous stasis. This hypercoagulable state predisposes to venous thromboembolism, particularly with bed rest or surgery. The erythrocyte volume also expands, and because of the disproportionate increase in plasma volume, there is a decrease in hematocrit and hemoglobin as outlined in Table 18–2.

Extravascular fluid also increases. Due chiefly to the increase in body water and total exchangeable sodium with the additive effect of elevated venous pressure in the lower extremities, peripheral and generalized edema in late term is considered normal.

Regional Blood Flow. As previously discussed, both estrogen and prolactin significantly effect the vascular resistance (Ueland and Parer, 1966). The net effect not only augments uterine blood flow, but also increases the regional blood flow to other organs and tissues such as the kidneys, the skin, extremities, and breast (Katz and Sokal, 1980). In addition to their effect on vascular reactivity, estrogens are thought to increase myocardial contractility by altering the actomyosin–ATPase relationship in the myocardium (Csapo, 1950; Little, 1965). While the reason for the dramatic expansion of maternal blood volume is not clearly understood, it is probably related to the estrogenic effect on maternal vascular capacity as well as to the increased levels of progesterone. Both, which rise progressively during gestation, act to increase plasma aldosterone levels, thereby promoting sodium retention and increase in total body water (Hytten and Chamberlain, 1991; Landau and Lugibihl, 1958; Ueland, 1976). Aldosterone production is also stimulated by the rise in plasma renin activity that occurs during normal pregnancy, thereby contributing further to the reabsorption of sodium from the renal tubule and therefore the retention of fluid (Seitchik, 1955).

Renal Blood Flow. Early in the first trimester, blood flow to the kidney is significantly increased reaching levels of 30% higher than nonpregnant levels (Chesley, 1960). Renal blood flow is particularly sensitive to changes in body position. In women, at term, in the supine position, the flow may fall to the nonpregnant level or even below it. The glomerular filtration rate is increased by about 50% during pregnancy. A delicate balance exists throughout pregnancy between glomerular filtration and renal tubular function and also between sodium retention and excretion. Utilized for the expansion of intravascular and extravascular fluid volume, retention of about 1000 meq of sodium has been reported (Elkayam and Gleicher, 1998).

Pulmonary Blood Flow. By the 38th week of pregnancy, pulmonary blood flow increases by more than 32%. But despite the increase in flow, there is only a small decreased in pulmonary vascular resistance. However the mean pulmonary artery pressure (~14 mmHg) does not significantly change during pregnancy.

HEMODYNAMIC CHANGES DURING LABOR, DELIVERY, AND PUERPERIUM

Additional demands are imposed on the cardiovascular system during labor and delivery. These hemodynamic responses to uterine contractions will vary throughout labor and depend on factors such as the stage of labor, intensity and frequency of uterine contraction, the maternal posture, the type and amount of anesthesia employed, and the type of delivery. With each uterine contraction, an additional 300–500 cc of blood is squeezed out of the uterus into the maternal circulation. As a result of this increase in circulating blood volume, there is a rise in right atrial pressure, an increase in cardiac output on the order of 20%–30% during contractions over that during the relaxed state (Pritchard, 1965; Ueland and Hansen, 1969b), and a rise of the mean systemic arterial pressure by about 10%. This rise in blood pressure, which returns to

resting levels between contractions, is attributed to the rise in cardiac output since the peripheral resistance changes only slightly during labor. The effect of uterine contractions on heart rate is less pronounced. Variations have been reported, but it appears that while the heart rate during contraction may increase slightly or remain the same, it is followed by a reflex bradycardia. The hemodynamic response to pain and anxiety, particularly in the primipara also has been found to contribute as much as 40%–50% to the rise in cardiac output during active labor (Ueland and Metcalfe, 1975). Since this rise in cardiac output is accompanied by an increase in blood pressure and tachycardia, it is thought to be due to increased serum catecholamine and myocardial contractility.

Throughout pregnancy, particularly during labor, maternal position continues to exert a significant influence on cardiovascular hemodynamics. In the lateral recumbent position, there is a 15%–20% increase in cardiac output above the values observed between contractions. In contrast, when the patient is placed in the lateral position, the hemodynamic effect is more stable, making this the preferred position for labor.

Immediately following delivery, there is a dramatic rise in cardiac output on the order of 20%–60% over predelivery values depending on the type of anesthesia and method of delivery (Ueland and Hansen, 1969b). These abrupt changes are the result of an increase in venous return to heart due to the relief of caval obstruction by the uterus and a shift of blood from the emptied uterus into the systemic circulation. Peak values last for less than an hour, and within a week, cardiac output returns to near prepregnant values. A sustained bradycardia ranging from 4–17 bpm, a normal postpartum event, can persist for up to 2 weeks, but by 6–12 weeks, the heart rate returns to normal. In addition, it has been found that women can have up to a 30% decrease in blood volume at time of delivery depending on mode of delivery and blood loss. On average, blood loss from vaginal delivery is 500 mL compared with up to 1000 mL with a cesarean section. The cardiovascular status generally returns to normal nonpregnant levels with 1–2 weeks postdelivery. Blood volume declines by 16% of the predelivery value by the third postpartum day regardless of type of delivery. The stroke volume and left ventricular end-diastolic volume, however, remain higher than preconception values, and SVR remains lower than preconception values. All of these circulatory adjustments present a potential hazard to the mother with significant cardiac disease. About two-thirds of all deaths recorded in patients with heart disease occur around delivery (Conradsson and Werko, 1974) and therefore warrant close monitoring.

PHYSICAL SIGNS AND SYMPTOMS IN NORMAL PREGNANCY

The normal physiologic alterations imposed by pregnancy induce signs and symptoms that may closely resemble a cardiopulmonary disease state. For example, during pregnancy, hyperventilation, a normal finding, is described as breathlessness and may be misinterpreted as dyspnea. Fatigue, exercise intolerance, and orthopnea are other common complaints associated with an advancing pregnancy. Dependent lower-extremity edema results from an enlarging uterus and high venous pressure in the legs caused by increase in total body sodium. Palpitations or the sensation of the heart "beating faster or stronger" particularly when the woman is in the supine position are not uncommon and represent a normal sinus tachycardia (Perloff and Koos, 1998). The carotid pulse is generally brisk and full. Jugular venous pressure is normal but as pregnancy continues the "a" and "v' waves become more prominent. The apical pulse, while easily palpated, may be diffuse and often displaced laterally. Normal pregnancy is also associated with a number of auscultatory changes including a loud first heart sound that may be widely split, representing early closure of mitral valve. The second heart sound may be persistently split. A physiologic third heart sound, which can be heard in up to 90% of women, reflects the normal volume overloaded state in pregnancy. Clinical signs and symptoms associated with a normal pregnancy are summarized in Table 18–3.

ASSESSMENT AND DIAGNOSTIC EVALUATION

All females of reproductive age with CHD should be counseled early in their medical care about pregnancy and contraception. It should be explained that while pregnancy is possible for the majority of patients, it is important to stress the need to plan their pregnancy and to undergo a thorough preconception evaluation that is based on their clinical status *at the time* pregnancy is being contemplated. In this way, correction of any unrepaired or residual heart defects and/or treatment of sequelae associated with postoperative repair may be corrected prior to conception. Furthermore, depending on the complexity of the underlying cardiac defect and functional status of the patient, the decision to permit pregnancy must be a collaborative effort, which includes input from a multidisciplinary effort that includes the cardiologist, obstetrician, and a genetic counselor all who have knowledge and experience of CHD as well as the patient and her spouse/partner. A team approach from the beginning ensures an informed decision from the prospective parent(s).

Estimating Maternal and Fetal Risk. While the information regarding pregnancy outcomes across the spectrum of CHD has grown, it is still difficult to categorize patients and assign risk solely on the cardiac lesion. Therefore, in order to determine maternal risk, individual patients must be evaluated against a number of parameters (Table 18–4) that include maternal functional capacity, identification of any residue associated with the primary defect, and any prior surgical interventions. A thorough review of the past medical history should also include the presence of any noncardiac comorbidities that may influence pregnancy such as thyroid disease, diabetes, previous use of recreational drugs, and alcohol abuse. The history must also consider the socioeconomic status of the

TABLE 18–3. *Clinical Signs and Symptoms Observed Throughout Normal Pregnancy*

Respiratory	Hyperventilation causing shortness of breath, dyspnea
Cardiac	Distended neck veins with prominent A and V waves
	Diffuse, and displaced left ventricular impulse palpable right ventricular impulse
	Increased first heart sound; persistent splitting of second heart sound
	Early and midsystolic ejection-type murmurs at the lower left sternal edge over pulmonary area
	Continuous murmurs (venous hum, mammary soufflé)
	Diastolic murmurs

TABLE 18–4. *Preconception Maternal Factors to Assess in Estimating Pregnancy Risk*

Medical
  Primary Cardiac Lesion(s)
  Surgical Interventions
    Palliative
    Corrective
    Integrity of prosthetic valves
    Patency of baffles/conduits
  Co-Morbidities (e.g. thyroid disease; diabetes)
  Medications (e.g. Ace inhibitors, anticoagulants)
  Presence of devices: pacemaker, internal defibrillator
  Residua and/or Sequelae associated with lesion or surgery
    Cyanosis
    Pulmonary hypertension
    Obstruction
    Arrhythmias
    Systemic hypertension
    Ventricular dysfunction

Social
  Family/social support
  Ability to care for infant

From Canobbio MM. Estimating Maternal Risk. *Prog Pediat Cardiol.* 2004;19:1–3.

patient, which also includes the patient's spousal and extended family support. This is of particular concern for the patient considered to be at moderate to high risk in the event that postdelivery clinical problems arise, making it difficult for the patient to care for her infant. Finally, counseling the prospective mother who is at high or at an unknown risk, it is important that she be made aware not only of the immediate risks of a pregnancy on the cardiovascular system, but also she must have a clear understanding about the uncertainty of her functional capacity that may be incurred as a result of the pregnancy as well as a potentially shortened life span.

Assigning Risk. Maternal functional capacity using the New York Heart Association (NYHA) classification has traditionally been used as a predictor of maternal and fetal prognosis. Thus women who enter the pregnancy in NYHA Class I and II will having maternal mortality rate of less than 1% (0.4%) while Class III–IV patients have a rate that ranges from 5%–15%. A major limitation of this system, however, is that assessments are based upon subjective assessment rather than clinical data.

Similarly the 2008 guidelines on Adult Congenital Heart Disease have assigned a "C" Level of Evidence for pregnancy in the majority of congenital heart lesions, indicating that much of the data on pregnancy outcomes remain at a consensus or expert opinion level rather than being derived from multiple clinical trials (Warnes et al., 2008).

One risk index scoring system (Siu et al., 1997), however, has been developed to predict the risk of an adverse maternal event. The risk index awards one point each for poor functional status (NYHA >II), cyanosis (<90%), left ventricular (LV) systolic dysfunction, left heart obstruction, and history of cardiac events prior to pregnancy including arrhythmias, stroke, or pulmonary edema (Siu et al., 1997, 2001). Thus a risk index score of 0 is approximately 5%, whereas a risk index of 1 rises to 27% and a risk index >1 the likelihood of adverse event 75% (Table 18–5). In addition, there is a growing body of evidence that permits us to advise patients on the safety of pregnancy in women with operated and unoperated CHD (Table 18–6).

Risk to Infant. Maternal functional class is a major determinant of fetal mortality with an incremental risk ranging from zero for gravidas who are asymptomatic to a 20%–30% fetal mortality rate in women who fall into Class III and IV (Wada et al., 1996). Maternal cyanosis threatens the growth development and viability of the fetus. Infants born to cyanotic mothers are typically small for gestational age and premature (see later). The rate of spontaneous abortion is high, and

the rate increases roughly in parallel to maternal hypoxemia (Presbitero et al., 1994).

Additional risk takes the form of recurrence of CHD in the offspring. It is generally agreed that the risk for CHD increases 10-fold over the general population if the mother is affected (Siu and Colman, 2001). The exact risk of inheritance varies, but it is generally agreed that recurrent risk of any defect is between 3% and 7% (Driscoll et al., 1993; Nora and Nora, 1987; Taussig et al., 1975; Whittemore et al., 1982) however, patients with left heart obstructive lesions have a reportedly higher rates (Whittemore et al., 1982). Autosomal dominant conditions including 22q11 deletion syndrome confer a 50% risk of recurrence. Genetic counseling, particularly in those patients with a history of multiple cases of congenital heart lesions, should be offered to ensure a fully informed decision to proceed with pregnancy.

Preconception genetic counseling and fetal echocardiography, beginning at 14–16 weeks of pregnancy, can provide parents with further guidance in deciding on whether or not to proceed with a pregnancy. Screening for fetal chromosomal abnormalities may also be performed between 12 and 13 weeks ("ACOG Practice Bulletin No. 77: screening for fetal chromosomal abnormalities," 2007). The maternal serum markers, alpha-fetoprotein, along with the human chorionic gonadotropin (HCG) and unconjugated estriol (triple test) have improved detection rates of Down syndrome and trisomy 18 and amniocentesis can more specifically detect chromosomal defects but carries a procedure-related fetal loss of 0.06% (Eddleman et al., 2006).

Diagnostic Testing

Ideally, a full cardiovascular examination should occur just prior to conception but as is often the case, it is an unplanned pregnancy that brings the patient with CHD back to the cardiologist for evaluation. Once pregnant, diagnostic testing must be individualized

TABLE 18–5. *Predictors of Maternal Risk for Cardiac Complications*

History of prior cardiac events (arrhythmias, heart failure, transient ischemic attack, stroke, pulmonary edema)
Prior arrhythmia (symptomatic sustained tachyarrhythmia or bradyarrhythmia requiring treatment)
Poor NYHA functional class (>2)
Cyanosis (oxygen saturation <90% on room air)
Valvular and outflow tract obstruction (aortic valve area <1.5 cm², mitral valve area <2 cm², or left ventricular outflow tract peak gradient >30 mm Hg)
Systemic ventricular ejection fraction <40%

NYHA = New York Heart Association

TABLE 18–6. *Common Congenital Heart Defects and Pregnancy by Pregnancy Risk**

Category A Low	Category B Intermediate	Category C Moderate to High	Category D High
Pregnancy Well tolerated	Pregnancy tolerated well	Pregnancy well tolerated if clinically stable	Pregnancy poorly tolerated
Risk similar to general population	Risk mild to moderate	Risk intermediate	Risk High; pregnancy contraindicated
Surgically repaired Atrial septal defect (ASD) Ventricular septal (severe) Defect (VSD) Patent ductus arteriosus Pulmonic stenosis (PS) Congenital complete heart block Aortic valve stenosis (gradient <25 mm Hg)	**Surgically Unrepaired** ASD, VSD (large left to right shunts) Coarctation of aorta PS (moderate) Ebstein's anomaly (without cyanosis); Congenitally corrected TGA	**Surgically repaired** Fontan for SV, TA Atrial repair for D-TGA Rastelli for PA Ventricular dysfunction	Cyanotic CHD Pul. hypertension Eisenmenger syndrome
Unoperated Bicuspid AV valve with no obstruction ASD/VSD (small left to right shunts) Mild PS	**Operated** Coarctation of aorta Tetralogy of Fallot Ebstein's Anomaly		

Abbreviations: PA: Pulmonary atresia; SV: single ventricle; TA: tricuspid atriesia; TGA: transposition of great; Pul: pulmonary
From Canobbio MM 2004 Estimating Maternal Risk. Prog Pediat Cardiol 19:1–3.
Note: *Risk is based upon published reports:
- Low risk: No residual effects; carries no additional risk; may be managed as general population;
- Intermediate risk: Clinically stable at time of conception; poses a potential risk for endocarditis, embolization, arrhythmias, hypertension; ventricular dysfunction.If residual effects after operation are present, it should be managed in high-risk obstetrical team
- Moderate to high risk: Reported data is limited; risk mild to moderate if clinically stable at time of conception; but has potential for serious complications; should be managed in high risk tertiary care center
- High risk: High maternal and fetal morbidity and mortality; Pregnancy is contra-indicated

with special consideration of the risk to both mother and her fetus.

Laboratory Testing. In addition to routine laboratory assays (complete blood count, serum electrolytes, and urinalysis), calcium and magnesium levels, renal and liver function test, thyroid function tests (thyroid stimulating hormone) should be measured in patients suspected of depressed ventricular function, because hypothyroidism as well as hyperthyroidism can cause or contribute further to systemic ventricular dysfunction (Hamilton and Stevenson, 1996).

12-Lead Electrocardiogram. Normal electrocardiographic (ECG) changes associated with pregnancy include a leftward shift of the QRS axis with the greatest shift in the third trimester due to elevation of the diaphragm. A shortening of the PR, QRS, and QT intervals may accompany the increase in resting heart rate. Nonspecific ST abnormalities including segment depression, flattened and inverted T waves in lead III occur frequently (Perloff and Koos, 1998). Rhythm disturbances are not uncommon during pregnancy particularly during labor in the early puerperium. The ECG may show occasional premature atrial and ventricular beats, short paroxysms of supraventricular tachycardia, and sinus arrhythmia.

Chest Radiography. While sometimes valuable in assessment of pulmonary congestion, chest radiography is generally not advocated during pregnancy. If necessary, however, the film should be compared with the one taken before pregnancy since the normal heart may often appear to be increased in size during pregnancy (Perloff and Koos, 1998).

Echocardiogram. Normal echocardiographic and Doppler findings in pregnancy include increased systolic and diastolic left ventricular dimensions (in left lateral position), moderate increase in size of right atrium, right ventricle, and left atrium. There is also progressive dilatation of the valve annuli and functional regurgitation in all but the aortic valve. Some studies have also shown a gradual improvement in left ventricular systolic function from the first trimester until the 20th week of gestation that may be due to the physiologic afterload reduction from a drop in systemic vascular resistance. In addition to these changes, small pericardial effusions have been reported during pregnancy but are generally resolved by 6 weeks postdelivery (Elkayam, 1998). An echocardiogram taken before the pregnancy is, therefore, useful in establishing the baseline status and because of lack of radiation exposure to the mother or the fetus associated with the procedure, may be repeated safely throughout pregnancy.

Two-dimensional echocardiogram with Doppler is the test of choice for evaluation and monitoring of the morphologic left ventricular function before, during and after pregnancy. The Simpson's rule, used to quantify the morphologic left ventricular function, has its limitations and may not be as accurate in assessment of a morphologic right ventricle because of its nonellipsoid and crescenteric shape. In patients with good echocardiographic windows, transthoracic echocardiogram is adequate for the assessment of ventricular function as well as for identifying residua or sequela of unrepaired or repaired congenital heart defects. In those with limited echocardiographic windows, transesophageal echocardiography can be safely used during pregnancy (Campos, 1996).

Exercise Stress Testing with Echocardiographic Imaging. Exercise stress testing may help in better risk stratification. In patients with preexisting ventricular dysfunction, symptom-limited supine bicycle exercise test or a symptom-limited exercise treadmill test using the standard modified Bruce protocol aids not only in objective assessment of prepregnancy functional capacity and symptoms elicited by exertion- or exercise-induced arrhythmias, but also predicts the likelihood of systemic ventricular adaptation to hemodynamic changes of pregnancy and to the stress of labor and delivery.

In the pregnant female, a submaximal stress test with echocardiographic imaging is preferred because of reported concern of fetal bradycardia with maximal exercise testing. A low-level exercise protocol (70% of the maximal predicted heart rate) with concomitant fetal monitoring is recommended (van Doorn et al., 1992).

Maximal Oxygen Consumption. The measurement of maximal oxygen consumption (VO_{2max}) during exercise can also be used as in evaluating cardiopulmonary reserve and functional status during pregnancy (Piran et al., 2002). While data on normal parameters for maximum oxygen consumption during pregnancy is limited, there should be no change in normal pregnancy. Specific parameters for CHD are not yet established (Spatling et al., 1992).

Magnetic Resonance Imaging. Magnetic resonance imaging is increasingly used as a quantitative measure of the morphologic right ventricular function. It is more accurate than echocardiography in this respect especially in centers where the likelihood of interobserver variability during echocardiographic assessment is higher. It also provides additional information about the extracardiac structures.

While majority of studies evaluating MRI safety during pregnancy have shown no ill effect to fetus, because of the limited experience in pregnant women, the current FDA guidelines require labeling of the MRI devices to inform patients that safety of MRI with respect to the fetus has not been established (Shellock and Kanal, 1991). Fetal concerns center on potential teratogenic effects, spontaneous abortion, and to lesser degree the possibility of acoustic damage. If required, it is recommended to wait until the second or third trimester after organogenesis is completed.

Radionuclide Ventriculography. Radionuclide ventriculography has limited use in congenital heart disease, but it is accurate in estimating the ventricular function and in measurement of global and regional function. Because of the associated radiation risks, radionuclide ventriculography is reserved for use before and after pregnancy.

Cardiac Catheterization. Due to high dose of radiation, cardiac catheterization is limited to rare cases where sufficient information cannot be obtained through noninvasive measures or hemodynamic compromise requires an emergent intervention. Where possible, the procedure should be avoided in the first trimester. Radiation exposure less than 5 rad have very low likelihood of fetal risk, while 15 rad or greater is considered high-risk for fetal abnormalities and termination of pregnancy is recommended (Elkayam, 1998).

SPECIFIC LESIONS

Shunts

The common shunt lesions include secundum atrial septal defect, ventricular defect, and patent ductus arteriosus. In the absence of increased pulmonary hypertension, women with unrepaired shunt lesions usually tolerate pregnancy well because left-to-right shunting tends to be diminished as result of the drop in systemic vascular resistance that normally occurs in pregnancy. Once repaired and in the absence of any residual effects, pregnancy outcomes are well tolerated (Drenthen et al., 2005).

Atrial Septal Defect. Atrial septal defect (ASD) is a direct communication between the atrial chambers that permits shunting of the blood. ASD is the most common defect to be seen in pregnancy. In unrepaired secundum ASD, the increased volume of pregnancy can stress the right ventricle; however, in the absence of pulmonary hypertension, the pulmonary vasculature can accommodate this volume overload. While pregnancy is generally tolerated, symptoms of effort intolerance, palpitations secondary to right ventricular failure or supraventricular tachyarrhythmias may develop. Paradoxical emboli, while rare in left-to-right shunts, may occur if shunt reversal occurs as result of a sudden rise in pulmonary pressure. This may occur with maneuvers that transiently elevate right atrial pressure such as Valsava, or a sudden drop in systemic pressures brought on by hypotension, secondary to hemorrhage during delivery, which can then result in augmentation of a left-to-right shunt (Effeney and Krupski, 1984; Loscalzo, 1986). During labor, avoidance of fluid overload, use of air bubble filters, and attention to leg care to minimize venous stasis during delivery are important considerations. Transcatheter device closure is possible during pregnancy using transesophageal echocardiography as the imaging technique (Soydemir et al., 2005). However, unless the patient is markedly symptomatic, it is best to defer closure until after delivery.

Women who have undergone ASD closure (surgical or by percutaneous device) carry little to no risk as long as they have no significant residual pulmonary hypertension, ventricular dysfunction, or supraventricular arrhythmias, which are often associated with a large defect or late repair (Warnes et al., 2008; Webb and Gatzoulis, 2006). In some cases, sinus node dysfunction including complete heart block may develop, particularly in those who have undergone repair for ostium primum. Patients with slow baseline heart rates, therefore, should be evaluated for chronotropic response to exercise to see whether they can raise their heart rate to accommodate the demands of pregnancy.

Ventricular Septal Defect. The ventricular septal defect (VSD) is a communication between the two ventricles resulting from failure of the components of the interventricular septum to fuse. The perimembranous ventricular septal defect is the most common form.

The size rather than location of the defect is the important determinant of pregnancy outcome. Women with small isolated VSD tolerate pregnancy well and carry no additional risk. Women with a large unrepaired ventricular septal defect carry the risk of developing pulmonary vascular disease followed by pulmonary hypertension. In large uncorrected VSD, the pregnancy-induced increase in blood volume further predisposes the patient to develop heart failure.

Patients who developed pulmonary hypertension increase their risk of shunt reversal, resulting in decreased oxygen saturation and cyanosis, particularly in cases of sudden hypotension that may occur as result of postpartum hemorrhage or incorrect management of epidural anesthesia. They are also at increased risk for infective endocarditis. Once completely repaired, pregnancy outcomes are similar to that of the general population (Warnes et al.2008). The exceptions are those

left with residual left ventricular dysfunction or a post-ventriculotomy scar, which will increase their predisposition for arrhythmias such ventricular tachycardia.

Patent Ductus Arteriosus. Patent ductus arteriosus (PDA) is a residual fetal communication between the proximal left pulmonary artery and the descending aorta distal to the left subclavian artery. During fetal life, it allows the diversion of blood from the right ventricle to the descending aorta, thus bypassing the pulmonary circulation. Maternal mortality in unrepaired patent ductus arteriosus is low, but depending on the size of the ductus and degree of shunt, there is an increased risk for developing pulmonary hypertension or congestive heart failure. They are also at risk for bacterial endocarditis/endarteritis. Women with a ligated or divided patent ductus arteriosus carry no risk if pulmonary artery pressure and ventricular function remain normal (Actis Dato et al., 1999).

Valve Defects

Pulmonic Stenosis. Isolated pulmonic stenosis (PS) is usually well tolerated during pregnancy.(Hameed et al., 2001; Neilson et al., 1970). Previous reports indicate that patients with milder PS (mean gradient 25–34 mmHg to severe PS (peak gradient >50 mmHg) show no difference in outcomes, indicating that pregnancy with PS is tolerated well throughout pregnancy and delivery, and that, in contrast to aortic stenosis, the severity of PS does not adversely impact maternal or fetal outcomes. However, a more recent study (Drenthen et al., 2006) reported that women with isolated PS may be at higher risk for noncardiac complications such as gestational hypertension, preeclampsia, and eclampsia even after correction of the defect. There is a 17% incidence of prematurity and fetal mortality of 4.9%.

Prepregnancy balloon valvuloplasty is recommended when the gradient across the right ventricular outflow track is >50 mmHg at rest (Therrien et al., 2001) or when the patient is symptomatic. Once pregnant, balloon valvuloplasty can be safely performed but is recommended only in patients with severe PS who are symptomatic (Elkayam and Bitar, 2005; Warnes et al., 2008). Patients with mild PS may be managed as general population but those females with moderate to severe PS, management by high risk obstetrical team is advised.

Bicuspid Aortic Valve/Aortic Stenosis

Isolated bicuspid aortic valve without stenosis or without aortic root dilatation carries little to no risk. In the setting, however, of root enlargement, or increased pressure gradient across the valve area the level of risk increases. An aortic root dimension greater that >4 cm should be carefully monitoring by echocardiogram throughout pregnancy and prior to delivery as they are at increased risk for dissection (Immer et al., 2003). It has been suggested that these patients may benefit from beta blockade throughout pregnancy (Head and Thorne, 2005). The risk of dissection and/or rupture increases when the diameter reaches 5–5.5 cm or if growth is 1 cm or greater per year (Elefteriades, 2002; Lobato and Puech-Leão, 1996) Elective surgery prior to conception may be offered to asymptomatic women.

Mild to moderate aortic valve stenosis with valve are >1.0 cm² is well tolerated during pregnancy. If, however, the valve area is less than 1.0 cm (peak >64 mm Hg), severe stenosis begins to encroach upon circulatory reserve as the cardiac output is relatively fixed and during exertion, it may be inadequate to maintain coronary artery or cerebral perfusion (Elkayam and Bitar, 2005; Head and Thorne, 2005). A woman with severe aortic stenosis (AS) presenting for preconception counseling should be advised to undergo valve replacement prior to pregnancy, explaining that the valve gradient will increase as the pregnancy progresses. Once pregnant, a woman with severe AS should be closely watched for dyspnea, angina, syncope and cerebral symptoms. Her physical activity should also be markedly limited. If severe symptoms persist, balloon dilatation may be an option as a bridge to surgery that can be performed after delivery. Endocarditis prophylaxis is generally not recommended during labor unless there has been a history of previous infection (Wilson, 2007). ·

Coarctation of Aorta. Coarctation of the aorta (COA) represents about 10% of all congenital cardiac defects. The most common site of coarctation is at the junction of the distal aortic arch and the descending aorta, below the origin of the left subclavian artery. COA may occur as an isolated defect, but is often associated with a number of additional anomalies including bicuspid aortic valve, VSD, PDA, and intracranial aneurysm in the circle of Willis (Mendelson, 2004). While majority of cases are identified and repaired in childhood, a number may go undetected into adulthood. If unrepaired, there is an increased risk of hypertension, arteritis and paracoarctation aortic dissection in the third trimester of pregnancy or postpartum period. The latter is associated with the increased estrogen levels that contribute to changes in the connective tissue of the arterial walls and along with the increase in cardiac output, there may be an increased risk for dissection or rupture (Beauchesne et al., 2001; Mendelson, 2004; Vriend et al., 2005). In the postpartum period, the risk of dissection remains high because of estrogen withdrawal. The mortality rate in unrepaired COA is 3% with the risk being higher in women with associated defects, aortopathy, or hypertension (Deal and Wooley, 1973; Siu and Colman, 2001).

The risk of aortic dissection and rupture is reduced with surgical repair, and therefore women with paracoarctation aneurysm or significant coarctation presenting for preconception counseling should be advised to undergo surgical resection prior to pregnancy.

Once repaired, maternal outcomes are good, however, the risks of systemic hypertension prevails (Beauchesne et al., 2001; Vriend et al., 2005). Women, therefore, who present with prepregnancy hypertension should also be evaluated for possible recoarctation, particularly if they had a primary repair of end-to-end anastomosis, which tend to carry a higher risk of restenosis later in life (Dodge-Khatami et al., 2000; Mendelson, 2004). There has been one reported maternal death due to a type A aortic dissection at 36 weeks in a woman with Turners syndrome carrying a twin pregnancy, who had undergone an end-to-end repair at 4 years of age. While residual gradients of less than 20 mmHg across the coarctation have been reported to be well tolerated during pregnancy, they should be carefully evaluated and where possible relieved or repaired prior to conception (Dodge-Khatami et al., 2000; Mendelson, 2004; Saidi et al., 1998). In the presence of systemic hypertension, regular blood pressure monitoring and control with beta blockers and hydrazine may be used. However, use of vasodilating agents must be cautiously administered because of the risk of hypotension distal to the site of the native coarctation or restenosis, which can compromise uteroplacental perfusion. Vaginal delivery with a shortened second stage labor is preferred mode of delivery with epidural analgesia. Endocarditis prophylaxis is recommended for patients who have had a conduit inserted or have prior history of infective endocarditis (Warnes et al., 2008). Fetal mortality has been reported to be 9% in one series to 19% in a second series (Beauchesne et al., 2001; Vriend et al., 2005). It may be that a compromised blood supply to the fetoplacental unit in the setting of significant stenosis or hypertension accounts for the wide range reported in fetal mortality. The incidence of recurrence of CHD in offspring is 4%.

Ebstein's Anomaly. Ebstein's anomaly is characterized by downward displacement of the septal leaflet tricuspid valve into the right ventricle, resulting in the "atrialized right ventricle," An atrial septal defect (ASD) or patent foramen ovale often coexists. A right ventricular outflow tract obstruction due to fixed anterior leaflet of the tricuspid valve then contributes to the right to left shift through the ASD. As a result, the clinical presentation may vary from asymptomatic to those who present as cyanotic (Donnelly et al., 1991). Ten to twenty-five percent also may have an accessory pathway such as Wolff-Parkinson-White, making these patients prone to supraventricular tachycardia.

In two large series, pregnancies have been reported to be well tolerated but at additional risk for heart failure (Connolly and Warnes, 1994; Donnelly et al., 1991). In one series of 111 pregnancies in 44 women, there was an increased risk of fetal loss and prematurity, and a significantly lower birth weight was reported in the offspring of cyanotic (2.53 kg) versus acyanotic (3.14 kg) women, with a recurrence rate of 6% of congenital heart defects in the mother's offspring has been reported (Connolly and Warnes, 1994).

In the female with Ebstein's anomaly and an unrepaired ASD, the risk of maternal mortality is related to the degree of cyanosis to potential deterioration of right ventricular function due to the increase in blood volume as well as the threat of paradoxical cerebral embolism through the shunt (Groves and Groves, 1995; Littler, 1970; Waickman et al., 1984).

In the absence of an ASD, the risk of pregnancy depends on baseline functional NYHA class, adequacy of tricuspid valve repair or replacement, and the presence of arrhythmias related to an accessory pathway.

Tetralogy of Fallot. Tetralogy of Fallot (TOF) is the most common complex congenital heart defect. Included in this tetrad is a large nonrestrictive misaligned ventricular septal defect, an overriding aorta, a right ventricular outflow tract obstruction and right ventricular hypertrophy.

Today the majority of females with tetralogy of Fallot are repaired in infancy or childhood. If definitive repair escapes them, palliative procedures usually permit survival to adulthood. Women who remain uncorrected are cyanotic and with pregnancy may become more desaturated as the systemic vascular resistance decreases causing an increase right-to-left shunting. As result, they become at risk for right ventricular failure and paradoxical emboli. In a series of studies, maternal and fetal mortality was related to the degree of shunting and hypoxia ranging from 4%–15% for the mother and as high as 30% for the fetus (Meyer et al., 1964; Shime et al., 1987).

From previous series, pregnancy outcomes in women with corrected tetralogy of Fallot with no significant residua have been favorable ((Nissenkorn et al., 1984; Ralstin and Dunn, 1976; Singh et al., 1982; Taussig et al., 1975). More recently however, a series of 112 pregnancies in 43 women reported pregnancies were well tolerated among those who had a reasonably good repair with normal or mildly decreased right ventricular function, and mild-to-moderate pulmonary regurgitation and/or pulmonary stenosis (Veldtman et al., 2004).

Pregnancy complications, while rare, were related to left ventricular dysfunction, severe pulmonary hypertension, and severe pulmonic regurgitation with RV dysfunction. Additionally, patients with residual right heart enlargement with moderate to severe pulmonary regurgitation are predisposed to postventriculotomy, monomorphic ventricular tachycardia, and therefore would benefit from alleviating the significant residual hemodynamic burden prior to pregnancy by pulmonary valve repair or replacement. A QRS duration of 180 ms or more is a sensitive marker for sustained ventricular tachycardia and sudden death in adult who have had previous repair of tetralogy can help to identify patients at risk. In the setting of tricuspid regurgitation, there is an increased risk of atrial arrhythmias (Gatzoulis et al., 2000).

Patients with TOF have an increased risk of fetal loss (24%), low birth weight, and a higher incidence (6%) of congenital heart anomalies than previously reported (Singh et al., 1982; Veldtman et al., 2004).

D Transposition of the Great Arteries

In dextro or D transposition of the great arteries, there is discordant connection between the ventricles and the great arteries (left ventricle to pulmonary artery, right ventricle to aorta). The morphologic right ventricle is in the systemic position and the morphologic left ventricle is in the pulmonic position. The majority of women born with d transposition of the great arteries, who are currently in their reproductive age, have previously undergone atrial switch (Mustard or Senning) procedure introduced in the 1960s, which converts the morphological right ventricle to into the systemic ventricle (Mustard et al., 1964).

Over the past decade, data regarding pregnancy outcomes has been emerging (Canobbio et al., 2006; Clarkson et al., 1994; Drenthen et al., 2005; Genoni et al., 1991). While it would appear that patients with good ventricular function and no history of arrhythmias prior to pregnancy can expect good maternal and fetal outcomes, recent multicenter studies reported that females with atrial repair D-TGA carry the potential risk for development of cardiac complications in late pregnancy and immediately following delivery, thus requiring careful monitoring throughout pregnancy (Canobbio et al., 2006; Drenthen et al., 2005). Atrial arrhythmias tend to be the most significant complication occurring in 22% in one series, particularly if there was a previous history of arrhythmia (Drenthen et al., 2005). In one series, there were two maternal deaths after delivery (Canobbio et al., 2006) There is a higher rate of miscarriage, as well as prematurity and low birth weight of the infant reported in all series. Drenthen also reported a high incidence of obstetrical complication (65%) that included premature labor (24.4%), premature rupture of membranes (14.3%), preeclampsia (10.2%), and thromboembolic complication (4.1%) (Drenthen et al., 2005).

Congenitally Corrected Transposition of the Great Arteries

Congenitally corrected transposition of the great arteries (CCTGA) is characterized by atrioventricular (AV) and ventricular–arterial discordance. Therefore, the morphological right ventricle serves as the systemic ventricle. In the majority of cases, CCTGA is associated with other anomalies including ventricular septal defect with pulmonary outflow tract obstruction and abnormalities of the systemic AV valve and complete heart block (Connolly, 1999). Symptoms and long-term survival is dependent on presence of any associated defects, and the function of the systemic right ventricle. While many patients will have undergone repair of the VSD and relief of the pulmonic stenosis, a number of them may remain unpalliated and their condition should be corrected prior to conception. Patients with CCTGA are subject to progressive systemic ventricular dysfunction and clinical congestive heart failure (CHF) with advancing age, particularly by fourth and fifth decade, with the degree of tricuspid regurgitation being strongly associated with progressive systemic right ventricular dysfunction and CHF (Graham et al., 2000). In patients with previous surgery for associated anomalies, potential complications are heart failure, atrial arrhythmias, AV block, and stroke.

During pregnancy, the primary concern is whether the right systemic ventricle will be able to support the additional hemodynamic burden pregnancy. While successful pregnancy can be achieved, in two series of 19 and 22 patients with a total of 105 pregnancies, there were substantial maternal complications including CHF, stroke, endocarditis, and myocardial infarction (Connolly et al., 1999; Therrien et al., 1999). There were no maternal mortalities but fetal loss was high ranging from 16%–27%, which is two to three times higher than the national average heart failure is more likely to occur in later stage of pregnancy from systemic right ventricular dysfunction and/or worsening left atrioventricular (tricuspid) regurgitation.

Univentricular Heart

Univentricular heart ("single ventricle") is characterized by a large dominant ventricle while the other ventricle is a small rudimentary chamber. Most commonly, the large dominant ventricle is a morphologic left ventricle, with the rudimentary right ventricle located anterosuperiorly. A common presentation is right ventricular hypoplasia with tricuspid atresia. Patients with single ventricle physiology are at risk for heart failure since the dominant ventricle (either morphologic left or right) receives blood from both the mitral and tricuspid valves or from one large atrioventricular valve

(AVV) and may face volume and pressure overload. The majority of the women in the childbearing age have undergone either a bidirectional Glenn procedures performed as part of a staged procedure prior to the definitive surgical correction, the Fontan repair (Fontan and Baudet, 1971). Survival to adulthood in patients palliated with an aortopulmonary shunt is possible, but progressive systemic ventricular failure, as well as the development of arrhythmias (mainly atrial fibrillation/flutter) and cyanosis are common.

The Fontan procedure, a right atrium to pulmonary artery conduit, or one of its modifications permits systemic venous return to enter directly into the pulmonary circulation, bypassing the pulmonic ventricle or outlet chamber. Long-term concerns centers on the ability of systemic ventricle to increase cardiac output and the development of atrial arrhythmias (SVT, atrial fibrillation) with some of the Fontan connections.

Pregnancy in patients with a palliated bidirectional shunt can be well tolerated if ventricular function is good and the oxygen saturation is >85%, but the risk of paradoxical emboli remains high and meticulous attention should be paid to avoid deep venous thrombosis in these patients.

Pregnancy following the Fontan operation without clinically significant complications is well tolerated. In two reported series with various types of univentricular heart disease, there were a total of 39 pregnancies from 31 women that resulted in 20 live births (Canobbio et al., 1996; Drenthen et al., 2006). There were no maternal mortalities, but there was a higher than normal first trimester miscarriage rate of 39% as well as prematurity (gestational age 36.5 weeks) and low birth weight of the infant (2.3 kg) (Canobbio et al., 1996). The most common problems reported in these and other case reports is the development of atrial arrhythmias (SVT, atrial fibrillation) and ventricular dysfunction particularly if there was a prepregnancy history of cardiovascular problems.

Pulmonary Atresia with an Intact Septum Post Biventricular Repair

Patients with pulmonary atresia with an intact septum (PAIVS) have complete obstruction of their right ventricular outflow tract, leading to lack of blood flow from the right ventricle into the lungs. Surgical intervention is essential since early survival is dependent upon the patent ductus. There is very limited data on pregnancy in women with PAIVS and a biventricular repair.

In one study of five pregnancies in three women with repaired PAIVS, all of the women were in NYHA class I and II at time of pregnancy (Drenthen et al., 2006). Complications during pregnancy included supraventricular arrhythmia in the first pregnancy and worsening pulmonary regurgitation during the second pregnancy in the same woman. There were three live births at term with average birth weight of 3400 g. There was one therapeutic termination of pregnancy in a woman with symptomatic heart failure with pulmonary regurgitation as well as psychological difficulties and one ectopic pregnancy. Findings based on this small series suggest that pregnancy in these women is high with probable maternal morbidity and adverse fetal outcomes.

Cyanotic Congenital Heart Disease

Patients with unrepaired or palliated defects associated with right to left shunts are prone to increased maternal hypoxemia, increased desaturation brought on by the normal drop in systemic vascular resistance associated with pregnancy, which in turn increases the right-to-left shunting. Maternal fetal prognosis is less favorable in a woman with a prepregnancy hemoglobin of less than 20 g/dL and an arterial oxygen saturation of <85% (Presbitero et al., 1994). In women with unrepaired complex cyanotic CHD, pregnancy carries the additional risk of cardiovascular complications such as heart failure, hemoptysis, thrombotic complications, supraventricular tachycardia, and endocarditis (Presbitero et al., 1994; Weiss and Atanassoff, 1993). The incidence of spontaneous fetal loss is up to 50% during the first trimester and 6% later in pregnancy. Infant survivors have high rate of prematurity (43%) are small for gestational age (mean 2576 g) and carry a 5% at risk of having a congenital heart defect (Koos, 2004; Presbitero et al., 1994; Whittemore et al., 1982). Additionally, due to the hypercoaguable state present in pregnancy, which predisposes patients to venous thromboembolism, patients with cyanotic heart disease have an increased bleeding tendency that can increase the risk of hemorrhage during delivery.

Eisenmenger Syndrome

Eisenmenger syndrome exists when there is a congenital communication between the systemic and pulmonary circulation, resulting in severe pulmonary hypertension due to high pulmonary vascular resistance with reversed or bidirectional shunts at the aortic-pulmonary, ventricular, and to lesser degree at the atrial level. It is associated with decreased systemic oxygen saturation, cyanosis, erythrocytosis, and thromboembolism. Maternal mortality is reported to be between 41% and 67% (Avila et al., 1995; Gleicher and Jaffin, 1980; Yentis et al., 1998) with the greatest risk of death being in the peripartum period. Death has been attributed

to hemorrhage, which decreases blood volume and increases right to left shunting due to drop in systemic vascular resistance, which in turn increases cyanosis and tissue hypoxia (Pitts et al., 1977) Fetal wastage in this group is estimated to be as high as 50%.

While pregnancy is clearly ill advised, patients who choose to continue their pregnancy should be admitted to hospital for the duration of their pregnancy. Continuous administration of oxygen, with attention to fluid levels, and prevention of thromboembolism is essential. While there is some risk associated with heparin therapy (Pitts et al., 1977), prophylactic anticoagulation with subcutaneous heparin is recommended along with use of thromboembolic stocking, and bubble-filters with intravenous therapy because of the risk of thromboembolism (Kansaria and Salvi, 2000). Maternal oxygen saturation should be maintained at a level of 70% or above (Sobrevilla et al., 1971). Fetal surveillance with ultrasound is important because of the 30% of the fetal growth retardation reported (Gleicher and Jaffin, 1980).

While traditional medical management has had little to offer these patients, recent attention has been give the use of pulmonary vasodilators during pregnancy (Gleicher et al., 1979; Goodwin et al., 1999; Geohas and McLaughlin, 2003; Lust et al., 1999). It has been suggested that inhaled nitric oxide may improve oxygenation by decreasing pulmonary resistance. There have been two case reports, one in which the patient was given inhaled nitric oxide during the second stage of labor and the postpartum period (Goodwin et al., 1999) and in the second case, the patient received nitric oxide in postpartum period. While there was immediate improvement of oxygenation and lowering of pulmonary artery pressures, both patients died in the postpartum period, one at 6 days and one at postpartum day 22 (Lust et al., 1999). More recently, two case reports, one using Epoprostenol (Geohas and McLaughlin, 2003) and sildenafil with L-arginine (Lacassie et al., 2004) have proven to have more successful outcomes.

COMPLICATIONS

Arrhythmias

Women with structural heart disease, particularly those with history of arrhythmias, are at greater risk for development of arrhythmias during pregnancy (Silversides et al., 2006; Siu et al., 1997; Tateno et al., 2003). Owing to hormonal, and hemodynamic changes and increased catecholamine sensitivity associated with pregnancy, arrhythmias may occur de novo or can trigger a recurrence in women with previous history of tachyarrhythmias (Ekholm et al., 1994; Silversides et al., 2006). Increased levels of estrogens and changes in ion channels may alter refractoriness and increase excitability (Nakajima et al., 1999), which can exacerbate or contribute to arrhythmogenesis (Mark and Harris, 2002), particularly during labor and delivery (Upshaw, 1970).

Palpitations are a common concern during pregnancy but are generally due to sinus tachycardia associated with circulatory adaptations (Ostrezega, 1992). Women with structural heart disease, particularly those with known history of rhythm disturbances, are, however, at increased risk for recurrence. Silversides et al. found that tachyarrhythmias reoccurred in 44% of pregnancies in women who began their pregnancies in normal sinus rhythm (Silversides et al., 2006). Similarly Tateno et al. found that prior surgical repair of congenital heart defects did not protect against the subsequent occurrence of symptomatic arrhythmias during pregnancy (Tateno et al., 2003). Reentrant supraventricular tachycardia and atrial fibrillation are the most common causes of sustained tachycardia reported in congenital heart literature, particularly those who have undergone surgical correction such as intra-atrial repair, as in Mustard and Senning for d-transposition of great arteries, Fontan or modified Fontan, or tetralogy of Fallot. Conventional treatment includes use of beta blockers, digoxin, and adenosine. If refractory to standard drug therapy, cardioversion can be safely used without significant maternal or fetal adverse effects (Lee et al., 2004; Rosemond, 1993).

New onset ventricular arrhythmias, while uncommon in pregnancy, generally are monomorphic, originating from the right ventricular outflow tract and respond well to beta blockers (Brodsky et al., 1992). In the setting of structural heart disease, ventricular ectopy must be carefully evaluated and, ideally, treated prior to pregnancy. Once pregnant, patients with stable ventricular tachycardia may be safely treated with beta blockers. In hemodynamically unstable patients, electrical cardioversion and/or an implantable defibrillator is indicated.

Ventricular Dysfunction

Women with decreased systemic ventricular function and/or decreased functional capacity are at higher risk for cardiovascular complications with the risk for developing heart failure being highest during the second and third trimesters of pregnancy, and in the immediate postpartum period (Canobbio et al., 2006; Drenthen et al., 2005; Khairy et al., 2006). Therefore, females with depressed ventricular dysfunction should undergo careful prepregnancy evaluation that includes stress echocardiogram to assess baseline systemic ventricular function and the contractile reserve in response to exercise.

Current therapeutic options for the patient who develop heart failure during pregnancy consist of conventional supportive therapies, which include diuretics to decrease pulmonary congestion and volume overload, sodium restriction, and afterload reduction. Angiotensin-converting enzyme inhibitors, while contraindicated during pregnancy, may be used in postpartum period. Hydralazine and nitrates are preferred options during the pregnancy (Chugh, 2004). Beta blockers may be used but because long-term use has been associated with low-birth-weight and fetal bradycardia, care should be exercised when prescribing throughout the entire gestational period. If medically necessary, treatment of the symptomatic patient should consider the use intravenous preload and afterload reducing agents (nitroprusside, nitroglycerin) or inotropic agents (dobutamine, dopamine). Invasive hemodynamic monitoring may be used in selected cases to guide the acute phase of this therapy.

MANAGEMENT

Antepartum Care

Once pregnancy is confirmed in women with CHD that is considered low risk, the condition may be managed as noncardiac gravidas. Women who are clinically symptomatic and/or are considered as intermediate to high risk women should be seen each trimester or more often particularly if signs of cardiovascular decompensation develop. Women considered at high risk should be referred to high-risk obstetrical team that includes cardiac anesthesiologist as well as neonatologist for continuous monitoring of the mother and the fetus.

Activity allowances and limitations must be individualized. Patients are generally encouraged to exercise as before pregnancy, but are advised to avoid sudden strenuous or isometric exercises, avoid extremes in temperatures, and allow for frequent rest periods during the day, instructing the patient to lie on her left side. Cyanotic patients with or without pulmonary hypertension should restrict activities throughout the pregnancy and because excessive heat produces peripheral vasodilatation and promotes venous pooling, hot baths, showers, or use of hot tubs/Jacuzzis should be discouraged (Perloff and Koos, 1998).

The gestational tendency for lower extremity venous stasis and potential risk for thromboembolism due to the hypercoagulable state of pregnancy may be reduced by advising women to avoid positions that impede venous return such as standing or sitting with knees flexed for extended periods of times, by avoiding

TABLE 18–7. *Common Cardiovascular Drugs Used in Pregnancy*

Drug	Placenta Transfer	Adverse Effects in Pregnancy, Fetal, and Neonatal	Secreted in Breast Milk	FDA Class
Digitalis	+	Low birthweight	+	A
Thaizides	+	May cause neonatal hyponatremia, hypokalemia	+	B
Antiarrhythmics				
Quinidine	+	No known terotogenic effect; toxic levels may cause thrombocytopena	+	C
Procainamide	+	Fetal bradycardia, fetal growth retardation (chronic use)	+	B
Lidocaine	+	Toxic levels may cause CNS/CV depression in neonate	+	B
Disopyramide	+	May stimlate uterine contractions and cause premature labor	+	C
Flecanide	+	May stimulate uterine contractions and cause premature labor	+	C
Sotalol	+	Torsadas de pointes; fetal bracycardia, hypotension	+	C
Verapamil	+	No evidence of birth defects	+	C
Adenosine	+	May cause maternal and fetal bradycardia,; may stimulate uterine activity	No clear data	C
Beta Blockers	+	Growth retardation, prematurity hypoglycemia, respiratory depression, oxytoxic effect on uterus	+	C
Vasodilators				
Hydralzaine	+	Reduced uteroplacental blood flow; thrombocytopenia	+	C
Anticoagulants				
Heparin	–	No terotogenic effect	–	C

U.S. Food and Drug Administration (FDA) Classes: **A.** Studies fail to demonstrate risk to fetus in any trimester; **B.** No adverse effects in animal reproduction studies; no human studies available; **C.** Only given if potential benefit justifies risks to fetus; animal studies have revealed adverse effects on the fetus, but no studies in women; **D.** Evidence of human fetal risk,, may be given in spite of risk if drug is needed in a life-threatening situation; **X.** Absolute fetal abnormalities. Drug is contraindicated in women who are or may become pregnant.

* Considered compatible with breast feeding by American Academy of Pediatrics

dehydration, and use of support stockings while walking or standing. Moderate sodium restriction is also advised because of the tendency to retain sodium and increase total body water. To reduce the incidence of neural tube defects, a daily folic acid intake of over 400 μg is recommended (Bailey, 2005).

Medications. The hazard posed by cardiovascular drugs used by the mother must be evaluated relative to the risk to the mother and her unborn child. The majority of drugs used to treat cardiac-related disorders can safely be used throughout pregnancy after 8–10 weeks of gestation as the likelihood of embryopathy risk is reduced (Table 18–7, 18–8).

Currently there are few cardiac drugs clearly proven to be tetratogenic and therefore contraindicated during pregnancy (Table 18–8) including angiotensin-converting enzyme (ACE) inhibitors, which have been linked to fetal loss and neonatal renal failure, and warfarin, which is associated with fetal embyropathy (Cotrufo et al., 2002). Although not clearly associated with teratogenesis, amiodarone has been associated with a 9% incidence of fetal hypothyroidism and a 21% incidence of intrauterine growth retardation and should be reserved for cases of refractory ventricular arrhythmias (McKenna et al., 1983). Atenolol has been associated with low birth weight and therefore is not the beta blocker of choice during pregnancy (Lip et al., 1997). Propanolol is preferred since it has the longest standing safety data. Diuretics in late pregnancy produce no apparent effects but routine use of diuretics is discouraged because of the potentially reduction in maternal plasma volume early in gestation, which is undesirable and potential harmful to the fetus (Lindheimer and Katz, 1973). In addition, thiazides have been associated with maternal and fetal thrombocytopenia, and given during lactation, they may interfere with milk production (Perloff and Koos, 1998).

TABLE 18–8. *Drugs Contraindicated in Pregnancy*

Coumadin	Known teratogenic when exposure occurs during first trimester
Phenytoin	Mental and growth retardation; fetal hydantoin syndrome
Amiodarone	Fetal and neonatal hypothyroidism, growth retardation
Ace inhibitors	Oligohydraminios, fetal calvaria, hypoplasia, fetal growth retardation, and death can occur with second and third trimester exposure (also dangerous in first trimester)

Endocarditis Prophylaxis

Routine prophylaxis is not recommended in normal delivery, but in selected patients who are susceptible to infective endocarditis is an important consideration in the management of the patient with congenital heart disease. Patients must be carefully evaluated for the presence of residual lesions that will necessitate preventive measures for endocarditis during delivery (Warnes

TABLE 18–9. *Recommendations for Anticoagulation During Pregnancy*

Weeks 1 through 35 in patients with mechanical prosthetic valves

The decision whether to use heparin during the first trimester or to continue oral anticoagulation throughout pregnancy should be made after full discussion with the patient and her partner; if she chooses to change to heparin for the first trimester, she should be made aware that heparin is less safe for her, with a higher risk of both thrombosis and bleeding, and that any risk to the mother also jeopardizes the baby.*

High-risk women (a history of thromboembolism or an older-generation mechanical prosthesis in the mitral position) who choose *not* to take warfarin during the first trimester should receive continuous unfractionated heparin intravenously in a dose to prolong the midinterval (6 hours after dosing) aPTT to 2–3 times control. Transition to warfarin can occur thereafter.

In patients receiving warfarin, INR should be maintained between 2.0 and 3.0 with the lowest possible dose of warfarin, and low-dose aspirin should be added. Women at low risk (no history of thromboembolism, newer low-profile prosthesis) may be managed with adjusted-dose subcutaneous heparin (17 500 to 20 000 U BID) to prolong the midinterval (6 hours after dosing) aPTT to 2–3 times control.

After the 36th week in patients with mechanical prosthetic valves

Warfarin should be stopped no later than week 36 and heparin substituted in anticipation of labor. If labor begins during treatment with warfarin, a cesarean delivery should be performed. In the absence of significant bleeding, heparin can be resumed 4 to 6 hours after delivery and warfarin begun orally.

Adapted from Bonow WO, et al. *Circulation.* 1998;98:1949–1984.

TABLE 18–10. *Recommendations of the Seventh ACCP Consensus Conference on Antithrombotic Therapy for Prophylaxis in Patients with Mechanical Heart Valves*

Aggressive adjusted-dose UFH, given every 12 hr subcutaneously throughout pregnancy, mid-interval activated partial thromboplastin time maintained at $\geq 2 \times$ control levels, or anti-Xa heparin level maintained at 0.35 to 0.70 IU/ml

OR

LMWH throughout pregnancy in doses adjusted according to weight or as necessary to maintain a 4-h postinjection anti-Xa heparin level of about 1.0 IU/ml

OR

UFH or LMWH, as above, until the 13th week, change to warfarin until the middle of the third trimester, then restart UFH or LMWH therapy until delivery.

Reprinted with permission, from (Bates et al., 2004)
ACCP, American College of Chest Physicians; LMWH, low molecular weight heparin; UFH, unfractionated heparin.

et al., 2008). The 2007 American Heart Association's guidelines recommends antibiotic prophylaxis only in patients with prosthetic valves, with a history previous infective endocarditis, and with complex cyanotic congenital heart disease or surgically constructed systemic pulmonary shunts or conduits (Wilson et al., 2007). Intravenous (IV) prophylaxis should be given at the time of the rupture of the membranes. The standard dosage is 2 g of ampicillin and gentamicin 1.5 mg/kg given by IV or by intramuscular (IM) injection initially followed by another dose of ampicillin 1 g by IV/IM or orally 6 hours later. Vancomycin, 1 g IV, over 1–2 hours plus gentamicin is also recommended.

Anticoagulation

Management of the pregnant patient on anticoagulation for mechanical prosthetic valves or atrial fibrillation is challenging and controversial with no method free from maternal or fetal risks. Warfarin is relatively contraindicated in all stages of gestation because of the fetal embryopathy that occurs with exposure between weeks 6 and 13, as well as the intracerebral bleeding events that can occur later in pregnancy (Cotrufo et al., 2002). Unfractionated heparin, an alternative choice, is however not without complications as it has been associated with maternal osteopenia and more recently, the risk of thrombotic complications has been reported in women who were using heparin alone (Dahlman, 1993; Elkayam and Bitar, 2005).

Published guidelines on the management of patients with prosthetic valves (PV) recommend use of warfarin in women considered high risk (older generation mechanical valve in mitral position, history previous thromboembolism) through week 35, when it should be substituted with unfractionated heparin (UFH) in preparation for delivery (Table 18–9) (Bonow et al., 1998). Two alternative methods suggest use of low molecular weight heparin (LMWH) throughout pregnancy, subcutaneously adjusted to weight and creatinine clearance, to achieve anti-Factor Xa levels of 1.0–1.2 U/mL, 4–6 hours after injection, tested biweekly or the use of adjusted-dose of UFH throughout pregnancy (Table 18–10) (Bates et al., 2004; Elkayam and Bitar, 2005).

Women with prosthetic valves should be advised that no anticoagulation regimen provides complete protection from thromboembolic phenomena in pregnancy (Nassar et al., 2004). The anticoagulation protocol should be individualized, taking into consideration not only the risk profile and patient preference but also the ease and compliance of the patient in getting frequent laboratory tests required to maintain dose adjustments accordingly.

Labor, Delivery, and Anesthesia. Women with successfully repaired CHD, as well as those with functionally mild unoperated CHD (Class I, II), management of labor and delivery should proceed as for normal gravidas. For gravidas considered moderate to high risk or with functionally significant CHD (Class III, IV), a coordinated plan of care must be developed as she approaches her due date. For the latter, elective induction of labor under controlled conditions is recommended. The timing of induction must take into account the woman's cardiac status, the inducibility of the cervix, and fetal lung maturity. Induction should be scheduled so that the delivery occurs when all members of multidisciplinary team (obstetrical, perinatologist, anesthesia, and cardiologist) are readily available. Additionally, the labor and delivery nursing staff must be included in the plan so they can prepare not only necessary monitoring equipment but to arrange for appropriate cardiac care nursing coverage if required.

Intrapartum management is to minimize the marked fluctuations in cardiac output that normally occur during labor and delivery. These include laboring in the lateral position, vaginal delivery with a shortened second stage, and pain control with repeated doses of intramuscular or intravenous narcotic (e.g., meperidine) during the early stages of labor. A forcep or vacuum-assisted delivery at a low station should be performed to reduce the voluntary expulsive efforts and to avoid Valsalva maneuvers, which increase the risk of syncope (Koos, 2004) Epidural analgesia is generally the preferred choice of management for pain as it promotes hemodynamic stability by reducing pain-related increases in sympathetic activity. Epidural anesthesia should, however, be used cautiously, or not at all if cardiac output is suspected to be unusually sensitive to decreases in preload. In such cases, epidural narcotic may be a more appropriate alternative.

Cesarean delivery is generally reserved for obstetrical reasons (Metcalfe and Ueland, 1974; Perloff and Koos, 1998), however, cesarean delivery is indicated in certain cardiac conditions including a significant dilated aortic root (>4 cm), aneurysm or dissection, acute cardiac decompensation, or when patient is on warfarin at time of delivery (Elkayam and Bitar, 2005; Gatzoulis et al., 2000; Yentis et al., 2003).

For the cyanotic or unpalliated patient with significant residual shunts, care must be taken to ensure adequate hydration to avoid hypovolemia, antiembolic stockings to reduce risk of thromboembolism, and bubble filters to prevent paradoxical embolization.

Patients considered high risk should have continuous electrocardiogram monitoring and systemic arterial oxygen saturation by pulse oximetry throughout labor, delivery, and immediate postdelivery. The use of systemic arterial pressure (with an intra-arterial line) or other invasive hemodynamic monitoring is reserved for selected cases such as women with obstructive left ventricular lesions such as severe aortic stenosis or coarctation of the aorta in whom large fluid shifts may not be tolerated. In these cases, maintenance of the cardiac output is crucial as are any factors, such as

hypotension that diminish venous return, which causes increase in gradient and decrease the cardiac output (Lao et al., 1993).

Puerperium. After expulsion of the placenta, bleeding is reduced by uterine massage and intravenous oxytocin administration. Oxytocin should be infused slowly (less than 2 units/min) to avoid hypotensive effects. In the postpartum period, meticulous leg care, elastic support stockings, and early ambulation are important preventive measures that reduce the risk of deep vein thrombosis and thromboembolism as well as the possibility of paradoxical embolism in patients with right to left shunts.

Patients with pulmonary hypertension are at particular risk for mortality during the immediate postpartum period and up to within 1 week or more after delivery (Avila et al., 1995). Similarly, due to the dramatic hemodynamic shift following delivery, patients considered at high risk should be closely monitored for the first 24–48 hours in a cardiac care unit equipped for continuous monitoring.

Other Cardiac Therapies

Pacemakers. Permanent pacemakers are well tolerated and do not require special management during pregnancy. However, in females with sinus node dysfunction, it is necessary to increase the baseline heart rate usually by end of first trimester to parallel the normal physiologic heart rate increase associated with pregnancy. For patients diagnosed with complete heart block during pregnancy, permanent pacemaker should be considered. Insertion of cardiac pacemaker during pregnancy has been reported and may be safely performed under guidance of ECG and 2-D transthoracic echocardiography without use of fluoroscopy. If fluoroscopy is used, a protective lead shield covering the gravid uterus should be used to avoid risk of fetal teratogenicity. If the patient is at term, then temporary pacing may be initiated just prior to induction of labor.

Cardioversion

Cardioversion can be performed safely during pregnancy without affecting the rhythm of the fetus because the fetal heart appears to have a high fibrillatory threshold and fetal arrhythmias are uncommon. Currently ACLS guidelines recommend synchronized monophasic energy doses of 100, 200, and 300 joules for the general population (Blomström-Lundqvist et al., 2003). Because pregnancy does not change the transthoracic impedance, there is no evidence that cardioversion or defibrillation output should be increased in pregnancy (Nanson et al., 2001). Certain precautions, however, should be taken to prevent maternal complications. For example, careful monitoring of digitalis levels is important in order to avoid toxicity, which can cause maternal and possibly fetal arrhythmias. Because the risk of embolism is increased immediately following cardioversion, some may elect to anticoagulate their patients prior to cardioversion, and continue for a month particularly in setting of atrial flutter or fibrillation. However, attention and care must be given in the selection of anticoagulant agent and its associated risk to the fetus during pregnancy.

Implantable Defibrillators. Implantable defibrillators are becoming part of standard treatment for life-threatening arrhythmias. While the data is limited, it appears that in majority of cases, women with ICDs can complete and tolerate pregnancy without complications. In one multicenter study, 33 (75%) of 44 women with ICDs had no shocks during their pregnancy. Of those who did receive shocks, there were no device-related complications reported nor were there any adverse fetal events (Natale et al., 1997).

Cardiopulmonary Resuscitation. Cardiac arrest occurs in 1:30,000 pregnancies (Kloeck et al., 1997). Women with CHD who are at higher risk of sudden death are those with tetralogy of Fallot postventriculotomy since they can have monomorphic ventricular tachycardia. Women with severe cardiomyopathy (ejection fraction less than 30%) are also at high risk for ventricular arrhythmias. Aortic dissection in women with dilated aortic root can present as a catastrophic event. Other general medical causes of cardiopulmonary arrest that can occur include amniotic fluid embolism, eclampsia, drug toxicity, massive pulmonary embolism, and hemorrhage.

Cardiopulmonary resuscitation should follow standard ACLS algorithms for medications, intubation, and defibrillation, however, after 20 weeks, the gravid uterus can press against the inferior vena cava and aorta impeding venous return and cardiac output, thus limiting the effectiveness of chest compressions. ("American Heart Association Guidelines for Cardiopulmonary Resuscitation and Emergency Cardiovascular Care," 2005). Therefore, the pregnant woman should be turned to the left lateral position, or the gravid uterus should be pulled to the left side (Goodwin and Pearce, 1992). Chest compressions should be performed higher on the sternum to adjust for elevation of the diaphragm and abdominal contents caused by the gravid uterus. Defibrillation may be used using standard ACLS defibrillation doses without causing adverse effect to the fetal heart (Nanson et al., 2001). Delivering the fetus will ensure improved maternal venous return, but

emergency hysterotomy should be performed only if the fetus is older than 25 weeks gestation and within 4 minutes of the arrest. Maternal resuscitation is the key to fetus resuscitation and one may lose both if maternal blood flow is not restored promptly.

CONTRACEPTION

Contraception counseling should be an integral part of any adolescent or adult congenital heart disease program regardless of whether or not the patient is known to be sexually active. There is no contraceptive that is both completely effective and completely free from side effects in females with CHD. Therefore the selection of a contraceptive method for the female with CHD must be individualized, taking into account the primary cardiac defect, related surgical interventions, and postoperative residua and sequelae.

Oral Contraceptives

The contraceptive effect of oral contraception is based on the suppression of the follicle-stimulating hormone (FSH) and the luteinizing hormone (LH), the alteration of cervical mucus that renders it less penetrable by sperm, and by changes of the endometrium that render it less conducive to implantation. There are two categories of oral contraceptives in use: agents with low-dose estrogen combined with varying amounts of progestin referred to as combined oral contraceptives (COC) and the progestin-only preparations.

Unlike earlier forms that contained dosage levels considered high risk for thromboembolic disease, current COCs contain much lower dose of estrogen combined with varying amounts of progestin (Beller and Ebert, 1985; Borgelt-Hansen, 2001; Nanson et al., 2001). The dose of estrogen in current multiphasic preparation ranges between 20 and 35 µg of synthetic ethinyl estradiol per tablet. Patients at highest thrombotic risk are those with history of previous thromboembolism, clotting or liver disorders, persistent systemic hypertension, pulmonary hypertension with or without the Eisenmenger physiology, patients with dilated cardiac changes at risk of atrial fibrillation, diabetes, and hyperlipidemia (Hatcher et al., 1998; WHO, 2004; Warnes et al., 2008).

The progestin only "Mini Pill" containing 0.35 mg of norethindrone acetate taken daily offers a good alternative when estrogen is contraindicated. Progestin-only pills act by suppression of ovulation. Untoward side effects include breakthrough vaginal bleeding, and amenorrhea (Hatcher et al., 1998). Failure rates tend to be higher than with the COC, because the mini pill must be taken regularly at the same time each day because effectiveness diminishes within 24 hours after administration.

Injectable Contraceptive

Depomedroxyprogesterone acetate (DMPA), known as DepoProvera, is a highly effective long-acting progesterone-only injectable contraceptive that is administered in a dosage of 150 mg every 3 months deep in the gluteal or deltoid muscle. There are a number of side effects including breakthrough bleeding, weight gain due to fluid retention, and headache. Because of the potential for fluid retention, caution should be exercised in females with ventricular dysfunction. Depomedroxyprogesterone acetate is associated with a delay return to fertility often requiring between 12–18 months before baseline fertility is returned. The risk of osteoporosis associated with amenorrhea in long-term users is an additional concern particularly for small thin adults and adolescents (Cromer et al., 1996).

Implantable Contraceptive

Subcutaneous implants prevent pregnancy by inhibiting ovulation and by increasing viscosity of the cervical mucus, thereby producing an unfavorable endometrial lining. Etonogestrel (Implanon), a progestogen only implant, consists of a single small plastic rod, which is inserted just under the skin on the inside of the upper arm. Each rod contains 68 mg etonorgestrel and is effective for 3 years. Once removed, the female baseline fertility level returns usually within 3 months (Croxatto and Mäkäräinen, 1998).

Transdermal Patch

The "Patch" (Evra), another progestrin/estrogen contraceptive combination, releases 0.6 mg norelgestromin, the active metabolite of norgestimate and 0.75 mg ethinyl estradiol every 24 hours. The patch is applied every week for a 3-week period followed by one "patch-free" week during which breakthrough bleeding may occur. Side effects include breast tenderness, which resolves with subsequent cycle use, headache, and local skin irritation.

Vaginal Ring

Vaginal rings are designed to release progestin alone or in combination with estrogen. Available in the United States as NuvaRing, it releases 15 μg of ethinyl estradiol and 120 μg of etonogestrel daily, and is worn for 3 weeks followed by one "ring-free" week. During the "ring-free" week, withdrawal bleeding usually occurs lasting about 4–5 days.

Intrauterine Devices

The intrauterine device (IUD) is a long-term birth control method and unlike IUDs used in the 1970s, present-day IUDs are small, safe, and highly effective. IUD-related infections have been attributed to transient microbiologic contamination of the endometrium at the time of insertion (Farley et al., 1992; Hatcher et al., 1998), a risk that is incurred within the first 20–30 days. Infections occurring 3–4 months after insertion are believed to be due to acquired sexually transmitted disease (STD) rather than the direct result of the IUD. Infective endocarditis associated with IUD's is rare, occurring less than once per million patient-years, but remains a consideration in women with high-risk substrates. IUDs should be inserted with caution in women with bradycardia or conduction defects because of the potential for vasovagal response that can occur at the time of implantation (Lee et al., 1988). Other side effects include increased menstrual cramps and pain, and iron deficiency anemia from increased menstrual blood loss. IUDs probably should also be avoided in women at risk for endometriosis and (Seaworth and Durack, 1986) are generally not recommended for adolescents, or in nulliparous females as they are more likely to expel the IUD or have more pain and cramping after insertion.

There are three models of IUDs, the ParaGard T380A, a copper bearing device, and the hormone-releasing IUDs, Progestasert and Mirena. The ParaGard model is effective for 10 years. Reasons for early removal are bleeding or pain, which occurs in 3%–12% of women usually within the first 3 years. The Progestasert, which releases 65 μg of progesterone per day, causes less cramping and blood loss than ParaGard, but its utility is limited by the need for yearly reinsertions. The newer progestin-containing IUD "Mirena" releases 20 μg per day of levonorgestrel and is effective for 5 years (French et al., 2000). Mirena can initially cause abnormal bleeding or spotting, but after 3–6 months, hypomenorrhea or amenorrhea usually occurs.

Barrier Methods

Conventional barrier methods are safe for all patients with CHD but unfortunately these methods carry a greater risk of an unwanted pregnancy. Vaginal barrier contraceptives include the diaphragm, cervical cap, and female condom. Used with spermicide, clinical trials have demonstrated an effectiveness rate of approximately 80% (Hatcher et al., 1998).

Regardless of the contraceptive method selected, the added use of a male synthetic latex condom with spermicide must be stressed to ensure protection against sexually transmitted diseases, HIV and hepatitis B.

Emergency Contraception

Emergency contraception is used to reduce the risk of pregnancy after an unprotected coital act. Often referred to as the "morning-after pill" or postcoital contraception, the two most commonly used emergency contraceptive methods are the combined estrogen–progestin (Preven), referred to as the Yuzpe regimen, and the progestin-only regimens of oral contraceptive pills, referred to as Plan B (Ho and Kwan, 1993). Both consist of two doses of contraceptive steroids taken in two doses, 12 hours apart. They can reduce the risk of pregnancy up to 120 hours after unprotected vaginal intercourse, but are more effective when the first dose is taken within 72 hours. Of the two regimens, the progestin-only (Plan B) is considered theoretically safer for women with cardiac disease and those at risk of thrombosis.

Tubal Occlusion

Permanent sterilization is clinically indicated for females in whom pregnancy is contraindicated or by personal choice. Two procedures are now available in the United States: the traditional tubal ligation, which is an invasive surgical procedure requiring anesthesia and a transcervical procedure known as the Essure method. Essure is a nonincisional procedure in which a transcervical access device, carrying a microinsert, is implanted into the fallopian tubes. Once in place, the device expands causing scar tissue to form over the implant and block the fallopian tube. Clinical trials report the fallopian tubes are closed in 96.5% of the women within 3 months and in 100% of the women within 6 months of the procedure (Cooper et al., 2003).

Termination of Pregnancy

Once a decision to terminate a pregnancy is reached, it is important to act swiftly because the choice of procedure is determined by the duration of pregnancy. If there is discrepancy between dates and uterine size, ultrasound should be performed. Abortion at 12 weeks of gestation or earlier is preferred because cardiac output begins to increase by 8 weeks. Dilation and suction curettage under local anesthesia is the method employed for first trimester termination. Medical abortion utilizing oral antiprogesterone agents such as RU486 (Mefipristone) and vaginally administered Misoprostol (prostaglandin E1 analog) are as effective as suction curettage if performed within the first 7 weeks of gestation (Spitz et al., 1998). Because expulsion and bleeding occur at home, the process is not controlled, so the systemic vasodilation afforded by the PGE could potentially be

risky for women with Eisenmenger syndrome or primary pulmonary hypertension.

Second trimester termination methods include medical and surgical procedures. Intrauterine instillation of prostaglandin (E2 or F) and hypertonic urea results in uterine contractions and expulsion of the fetus, but labor can take up to 20 hours, is painful, requires in-patient care, and there is the risk of retention of the placenta, hemorrhage, and infection. Accordingly, dilatation and evacuation of fetus and placenta are more frequently used for termination of second-trimester pregnancies. With introduction of a small dilator, called Laminaria, the cervix is slowly dilated, most of which occurs in the first 6 hours, with maximum dilation usually occurring 12–24 hours followed by evacuation.

REFERENCES

ACOG Practice Bulletin No. 77: screening for fetal chromosomal abnormalities. *Obstet Gynecol.* 2007;109(1):217–227.

Actis Dato G, Cavaglia M, Aidala E, et al. Patent ductus arteriosus. Follow-up of 677 operated cases 40 years later. *Minerva Cardioangiol.* 1999;47(7–8):245–254.

American Heart Association. Guidelines for cardiopulmonary resuscitation and emergency cardiovascular care. *Circulation.* 2005;112(24 Suppl):IV1–IV153.

Avila W, Grinberg M, Snitcowsky R, et al. Maternal and fetal outcome in pregnant women with Eisenmenger's syndrome. *Eur Heart J.* 1995;16(4):460–464.

Bailey LB. Do low doses of folic acid result in maximum lowering of homocysteine? *Am J Clin Nutr.* 2005;82(4):717–718.

Bates S, Greer I, Hirsh J, Ginsberg J. Use of antithrombotic agents during pregnancy: the Seventh ACCP Conference on Antithrombotic and Thrombolytic Therapy. *Chest.* 2004;126(3 Suppl):627S–644S.

Beauchesne L, Connolly H, Ammash N, Warnes C. Coarctation of the aorta: outcome of pregnancy. *J Am Coll Cardiol.* 2001;38(6):1728–1733.

Beller F, Ebert C. Effects of oral contraceptives on blood coagulation. A review. *Obstet Gynecol Surv.* 1985;40(7):425–436.

Blomström-Lundqvist C, Scheinman M, Aliot E, et al. ACC/AHA/ESC guidelines for the management of patients with supraventricular arrhythmias—executive summary. A report of the American college of cardiology/American heart association task force on practice guidelines and the European society of cardiology committee for practice guidelines (writing committee to develop guidelines for the management of patients with supraventricular arrhythmias) developed in collaboration with NASPE-Heart Rhythm Society. *J Am Coll Cardiol.* 2003;42(8):1493–1531.

Bonow R, Carabello B, de Leon AJ, et al. Guidelines for the management of patients with valvular heart disease: executive summary. A report of the American College of Cardiology/American Heart Association Task Force on Practice Guidelines (Committee on Management of Patients with Valvular Heart Disease). *Circulation.* 1998;98(18):1949–1984.

Borgelt-Hansen L. Oral contraceptives: an update on health benefits and risks. *J Am Pharm Assoc (Wash).* 2001;41(6):875–886; quiz 925–926.

Brodsky M, Doria R, Allen B, Sato D, Thomas G, Sada M. New-onset ventricular tachycardia during pregnancy. *Am Heart J.* 1992;123(4 Pt 1):933–941.

Campos O. Doppler echocardiography during pregnancy: physiological and abnormal findings. *Echocardiograph.* 1996;13(2):135–146.

Canobbio M, Mair D, van der Velde M, Koos B. Pregnancy outcomes after the Fontan repair. *J Am Coll Cardiol.* 1996;28(3):763–767.

Canobbio M, Morris C, Graham T, Landzberg M. Pregnancy outcomes after atrial repair for transposition of the great arteries. *Am J Cardiol.* 2006;98(5):668–672.

Chesley L. Renal functional changes in normal pregnancy. *Clinical Obstet Gynecol.* 1960;3:349–363.

Christianson R. Studies on blood pressure during pregnancy. I. Influence of parity and age. *Am J Obstet Gynecol.* 1976;125(4):509–513.

Chugh R. Management of pregnancy in patients with congenital heart disease and systemic ventriuclar failure. *Prog Pediat Cardiol.* 2004;19:47–60.

Clarkson P, Wilson N, Neutze J, North R, Calder A, Barratt-Boyes B. Outcome of pregnancy after the mustard operation for transposition of great arteries with intact ventricular septum. *J Am Coll Cardiol.* 1994;24(1):190–193.

Connolly H, Grogan M, Warnes C. Pregnancy among women with congenitally corrected transposition of great arteries. *J Am Coll Cardiol.* 1999;33(6):1692–1695.

Connolly H, Warnes C. Ebstein's anomaly: outcome of pregnancy. *J Am Coll Cardiol.* 1994;23(5):1194–1198.

Conradsson TB, Werko L. Management of heart disease in pregnancy. *Prog Cardiovasc Dis.* 1974;16(4):407–419.

Cooper J, Carignan C, Cher D, Kerin J, Group STOPI. Microinsert nonincisional hysteroscopic sterilization. *Obstet Gynecol.* 2003;102(1):59–67.

Cotrufo M, De Feo M, De Santo L, et al. Risk of warfarin during pregnancy with mechanical valve prostheses. *Obstet Gynecol.* 2002;99(1):35–40.

Cromer B, Blair J, Mahan J, Zibners L, Naumovski Z. A prospective comparison of bone density in adolescent girls receiving depot medroxyprogesterone acetate (Depo-Provera), levonorgestrel (Norplant), or oral contraceptives. *J Pediatr.* 1996;129(5):671–676.

Croxatto H, Mäkäräinen L. The pharmacodynamics and efficacy of Implanon. An overview of the data. *Contraception.* 1998;58(6 Suppl):91S–97S.

Csapo A. Actomyosin formation by estrogen action. *Am J Physiol.* 1950;162(2):406–410.

Dahlman TC. Osteoporotic fractures and the recurrence of thromboembolism during pregnancy and the puerperium in 184 women undergoing thromboprophylaxis with heparin. *Am J Obstet Gynecol.* 1993;168(4):1265–1270.

Deal K, Wooley CF. Coarctation of the aorta and pregnancy. *Ann Intern Med.* 1973;78(5):706–710.

Dodge-Khatami A, Backer C, Mavroudis C. Risk factors for recoarctation and results of reoperation: a 40-year review. *J Card Surg.* 2000;15(6):369–377.

Donnelly J, Brown J, Radford D. Pregnancy outcome and Ebstein's anomaly. *Br Heart J.* 1991;66(5):368–371.

Drenthen W, Pieper P, Ploeg M, et al. Risk of complications during pregnancy after Senning or Mustard (atrial) repair of complete transposition of the great arteries. *Eur Heart J.* 2005;26(23):2588–2595.

Drenthen W, Pieper P, Roos-Hesselink J, et al. Non-cardiac complications during pregnancy in women with isolated pulmonary valvar stensosis. *Heart.* 2006;92(12):1838–1843.

Drenthen W, Pieper P, Roos-Hesselink J, et al. Pregnancy and delivery in women after Fontan palliation. *Heart.* 2006;92(9):1290–1294.

Drenthen W, Pieper P, Roos-Hesselink J, et al. Fertility, pregnancy, and delivery after biventricular repair for pulmonary atresia with an intact ventricular septum. *Am J Cardiol.* 2006;98(2):259–261.

Drenthen W, Pieper P, van der Tuuk K, et al. Cardiac complications relating to pregnancy and recurrence of disease in the offspring of women with atrioventricular septal defects. *Eur Heart J.* 2005;26(23):2581–2587.

Driscoll D, Michels V, Gersony W, et al. Occurrence risk for congenital heart defects in relatives of patients with aortic stenosis, pulmonary stenosis, or ventricular septal defect. *Circulation.* 1993;87(suppl 2):I114–120.

Eddleman KA, Malone FD, Sullivan L, et al. Pregnancy loss rates after midtrimester amniocentesis. *Obstet Gynecol.* 2006;108(5):1067–1072.

Effeney D, Krupski W. Paradoxical embolus in pregnancy. An unusual thromboembolic event. *West J Med.* 1984;140(2):287–288.

Ekholm E, Piha S, Erkkola R, Antila K. Autonomic cardiovascular reflexes in pregnancy. A longitudinal study. *Clin Auton Res.* 1994;4(4):161–165.

Elefteriades J. Natural history of thoracic aortic aneurysms: indications for surgery, and surgical versus nonsurgical risks. *Ann Thorac Surg.* 2002;74(5):S1877–1880; discussion S1892–1878.

Elkayam U, Bitar F. Valvular heart disease and pregnancy: part II: prosthetic valves. *J Am Coll Cardiol.* 2005;46(3):403–410.

Elkayam U, Bitar F. Valvular heart disease and pregnancy part I: native valves. *J Am Coll Cardiol.* 2005;46(2):223–230.

Elkayam U, Gleicher N. *Hemodynamics and Cardiac Function during Normal Pregnancy and the Puerperium.* 4th ed. New York: Alan R Wiley-Liss Inc; 1998.

Elkayam UGN. Evaluating the cardiac patient. In Gleicher N, ed. *Principles and Practice of Medical Therapy in Pregnancy.* 3rd ed. Stamford: Appleton & Lange; 1998:908–911.

Farley T, Rosenberg MJ, Rowe P, Chen J, Meirik O. Intrauterine devices and pelvic inflammatory disease: an international perspective. *Lancet.* 1992;339:785–788.

Fontan F, Baudet E. Surgical repair of tricuspid atresia. *Thorax.* 1971;26(3):240–248.

French R, Cowan F, Mansour D, et al. Levonorgestrel-releasing (20 microgram/day) intrauterine systems (Mirena) compared with other methods of reversible contraceptives. *BJOG.* 2000;107(10):1218–1225.

Gatzoulis M, Balaji S, Webber S, Siu S, et al. Risk factors for arrhythmias and sudden cardiac death late after repair of tetralogy of Fallot: a multicentre study. *Lancet.* 2000;356(9234):975–981.

Genoni M, Jenni R, Hoerstrup S, Vogt P, Turina M. Pregnancy after atrial repair for transposition of the great arteries. *Heart.* 1991;81(3):276–277.

Geohas C, McLaughlin V. Successful management of pregnancy in a patient with eisenmenger syndrome with epoprostenol. *Chest.* 2003;124(3):1170–1173.

Gleicher N, Jaffin N. Eisenmenger's syndrome and pregnancy. *N Engl J Med.* 1980;302(13):751–752.

Gleicher N, Midwall J, Hochberger D, Jaffin H. Eisenmenger's syndrome and pregnancy. *Obstet Gynecol Surv.* 1979;34(10):721–741.

Goodwin A, Pearce A. The human wedge. A manoeuvre to relieve aortocaval compression during resuscitation in late pregnancy. *Anaesthesia.* 1992;47(5):433–434.

Goodwin T, Gherman R, Hameed A, Elkayam U. Favorable response of Eisenmenger syndrome to inhaled nitric oxide during pregnancy. *Am J Obstet Gynecol.* 1999;180(1 Pt 1):64–67.

Graham TJ, Bernard Y, Mellen B, et al. Long-term outcome in congenitally corrected transposition of the great arteries. *J Am Coll Cardiol.* 2000;36(1):255–261.

Groves ER, Groves JB. Epidural analgesia for labour in a patient with Ebstein's anomaly. *Can J Anesth.* 1995;42(1):77–79.

Hameed A, Karaalp IS, Tummala PP, et al. The effect of valvular heart disease on maternal and fetal outcome of pregnancy. *J Am Coll Cardiol.* 2001;37(3):893–899.

Hamilton MA, Stevenson LW. Thyroid hormone abnormalities in heart failure: possibilities for therapy. *Thyroid.* 1996;6(5):527–529.

Hatcher R, Trussell J, Stewart F, et al. *Contraception Technology.* 17th ed. New York: Ardent Media; 1998.

Head C, Thorne S. Congenital heart disease in pregnancy. *Postgrad Med J.* 2005;81(955):292–298.

Ho PC, Kwan MS. A prospective randomized comparison of levonorgestrel with the Yuzpe regimen in post-coital contraception. *Hum Reprod.* 1993;8(3):389–392.

Hytten F, Chamberlain G. *Clinical Physiology in Obstetrics.* Oxford: Blackwell Scientific; 1991.

Immer F, Bansi A, Immer-Bansi A, et al. Aortic dissection in pregnancy: analysis of risk factors and outcome. *Ann Thorac Surg.* 2003;76(1):309–314.

Kaneshige E. Serum ferritin as an assessment of iron stores and other hematologic parameters during pregnancy. *Obstet Gynecol.* 1981;57(2):238–242.

Kansaria J, Salvi V. Eisenmenger syndrome in pregnancy. *J Postgrad Med.* 2000;46(2):101–103.

Katz M, Sokal M. Skin perfusion in pregnancy. *Am J Obstet Gynecol.* 1980;137(1):30–33.

Kerr M. The mechanical effects of the gravid uterus in late pregnancy. *J Obstet Gynaecol Br Commonw.* 1965;72:513–529.

Khairy P, Ouyang DW, Fernandes SM, Lee-Parritz A, Economy KE, Landzberg MJ. Pregnancy outcomes in women with congenital heart disease. *Circulation.* 2006;113(4):517–524.

Kinsella S, Lohmann G. Supine hypotensive syndrome. *Obstet Gynecol.* 1994;83(5 Pt 1):774–788.

Kloeck W, Cummins RO, Chamberlain D, et al. Special resuscitation situations: an advisory statement from the International Liaison Committee on Resuscitation. *Circulation.* 1997;95(8):2196–2210.

Koos B. Management of uncorrected, palliated, and repaired cyanotic congenital heart disease in pregnancy. *Prog Pediat Cardiol.* 2004;19:25–45.

Lacassie H, Germain A, Valdés G, Fernández M, Allamand F, López H. Management of Eisenmenger syndrome in pregnancy with sildenafil and L-arginine. *Obstet Gynecol.* 2004;103(5 Pt 2):1118–1120.

Landau R, Lugibihl K. Inhibition of the sodium-retaining influence of aldosterone by progesterone. *J Clin Endocrinol Metab.* 1958;18(11):1237–1245.

Lao T, Sermer M, MaGee L, Farine D, Colman J. Congenital aortic stenosis and pregnancy: a reappraisal. *Am J Obstet Gynecol.* 1993;169(3):540–545.

Lee J, Wetzel G, Shannon K. Maternal arrhythmia management during pregnancy in patients with structural heart disease. *Prog Pediat Cardiol.* 2004;19:71–82.

Lee NC, Rubin GL, Borucki R. The intrauterine device and pelvic inflammatory disease revisited: new results from the Women's Health Study. *Obstet Gynecol.* 1988;72(1):1–6.

Lindheimer M, Katz A. Sodium and diuretics in pregnancy. *N Engl J Med.* 1973;288(17):891–894.

Lip GY Beevers M Churchill D, Shaffer LM, Beevers DG. Effect of atenolol on birth weight. *Am J Cardiol.* 1997;79(10):1436–1438.

Little B. Water and electrolyte balance during pregnancy. *Anesthesiology.* 1965;26:400–408.

Littler W. Successful pregnancy in patient with Ebstein's Anomaly. *Br Heart J.* 1970;32(5):711–713.

Lobato A, Puech-Leão P. Predictive factors for rupture of thoracoabdominal aortic aneurysm. *J Vasc Surg.* 1996;27(3):446–453.

Loscalzo J. Paradoxical embolism: clinical presentation, diagnostic strategies, and therapeutic options. *Am Heart J.* 1986;112(1):141–145.

Lust K Boots R, Dooris M, Wilson J. Management of labor in Eisenmenger syndrome with inhaled nitric oxide. *Am J Obstet Gynecol.* 1999;181(2):419–423.

Mark S, Harris L. Arrhythmias in pregnancy. In: Wilansky S, Willerson J, eds. *Heart Disease in Women.* Philadelphia: Churchill Livingstone; 2002:497–514.

McKenna W, Harris L, Rowland E, Whitelaw A, Storey G, Holt D. Amiodarone therapy during pregnancy. *Am J Cardiol.* 1983;51(7):1231–1233.

Mendelson M. Pregnancy in patients with obstructive lesions: aortic stenosis, coarctation of the aorta and mitral stenosis. *Prog Pediat Cardiol.* 2004;19:61–70.

Metcalfe J, Ueland K. Maternal cardiovascular adjustments to pregnancy. *Prog Cardiovasc Dis.* 1974;16(4):363–374.

Meyer E, Tulsky A, Sigmann P, Silber E. Pregnancy in the presence of tetralogy of Fallot. Observations on two patients. *Am J Cardiol.* 1964;14:874–879.

Mustard W, Keith J, Trusler G, Fowler R, Kidd L. The surgical management of the transposition of the great vessels. *J Thorac Cardiovasc Surg.* 1964;48:953–958.

Nakajima T, Iwasawa K, Oonuma H, et al. Antiarrhythmic effect and its underlying ionic mechanism of 17beta-estradiol in cardiac myocytes. *Br J Pharmacol.* 1999;127(2):429–440.

Nanson J, Elcock D, Williams M, Deakin C. Do physiological changes in pregnancy change defibrillation energy requirements? *Br J Anaesth.* 2001;87(2):237–239.

Nassar A, Hobeika E, Abd Essamad H, Taher A, Khalil A, Usta I. Pregnancy outcome in women with prosthetic heart valves. *Am J Obstet Gynecol.* 2004;191(3):1009–1013.

Natale A, Davidson T, Geiger MJ, Newby K. Implantable cardioverter-defibrillators and pregnancy: a safe combination? *Circulation.* 1997;96(9):2808–2812.

Neilson G, Galea E, Blunt A. Congenital heart disease and pregnancy. *Med J Aust.* 1970;1(22):1086–1088.

Nissenkorn A, Friedman S, Schonfeld A, Ovadia J. Fetomaternal outcome in pregnancies after total Correction of tetralogy of Fallot. *Int Surg.* 1984;69(2):125–128.

Nora J, Nora A. Maternal transmission of congenital heart disease: new recurrent risk figures and the questions cytoplasmic inheritance and vulnerability to tetatogens. *Am J Cardiol.* 1987;59(5):459–463.

Ostrezega E. Evidence for increased incidence of arrhythmias during pregnancy: a study of 104 pregnant women with symptoms of palpitations, dizziness or syncope. *JACC.* 1992;19:125.

Perloff J, Koos B. Pregnancy and Congenital heart disease. In: Perloff J, Child J, eds. *Congenital Heart Disease in Adults.* 2nd ed. Philadelphia, PA: W.B. Saunders; 1998:144–164.

Piran S, Veldtman G, Siu S, Webb G, Liu P. Heart failure and ventricular dysfunction in patients with single or systemic right ventricles. *Circulation.* 2002;105(10):1189–1194.

Pitts J, Crosby W, Basta L. Eisenmenger's syndrome in pregnancy: does heparin prophylaxis improve the maternal mortality rate? *Am Heart J.* 1977;93(3):321–326.

Presbitero P, Somerville J, Stone S, Aruta E, Spiegelhalter D, Rabajoli F. Pregnancy in cyanotic congenital heart disease: outcome of mother and fetus. *Circulation.* 1994;89:2673–2676.

Pritchard J. Changes in the blood volume during pregnancy and delivery. *Anesthesiology.* 1965;26:393.

Ralstin J, Dunn M. Pregnancies after surgical correction of tetralogy of Fallot. *J Am Med Assoc.* 1976;235:2627–2628.

Rosemond, R. L. Cardioversion during pregnancy. *JAMA.* 1993;269(24):3167.

Saidi A, Bezold L, Altman C, Ayres N, Bricker J. Outcome of pregnancy following intervention for coarctation of the aorta. *Am J Cardiol.* 1998;82(6):786–788.

Seaworth BJ, Durack DT. Infective endocarditis in obstetric and gynecologic practice. *Am J Obstet Gynecol.* 1986;154(1):180–188.

Seitchik J. Total body water and total body density of pregnant women. *Obstet Gynecol.* 1955;29:155.

Shellock FG, Kanal E. Policies, guidelines, and recommendations for MR imaging safety and patient management. SMRI Safety Committee. *J Magn Reson Imaging.* 1991;1(1):97–101.

Shime J, Mocarski EJ, Hastings D, Webb GD, McLaughlin PR. Congenital heart disease in pregnancy: short- and long-term implications. *Am J Obstet Gynecol.* 1987;156(2):313–322.

Silversides C, Harris L, Haberer K, Sermer M, Colman J, Siu S. Recurrence rates of arrhythmias during pregnancy in women with previous tachyarrhythmia and impact on fetal and neonatal outcomes. *Am J Cardiol.* 2006;97(8):1206–1212.

Singh H, Bolton P, Oakley C. Pregnancy after surgical correction of tetralogy of Fallot. *Br Med J (Cl Res Ed).* 1982;285:168–170.

Siu S, Sermer M, Colman J, et al. Prospective multi-center study of pregnancy outcomes in women with heart disease. *Circulation.* 2001;104(5):515–521.

Siu S, Sermer M, Harrison D, et al. Risk and predictors for pregnancy-related complications in women with heart disease. *Circulation.* 1997;96:2789–2794.

Siu SC, Colman JM. Heart disease and pregnancy. *Heart.* 2001;85(6):710–715.

Sobrevilla L, Cassinelli M, Carcelen A, Malaga J. Human fetal and maternal oxygen tension and acid-base status during delivery at high altitude. *Am J Obstet Gynecol.* 1971;111(8):1111–1118.

Soydemir D, Johnston T, Clarke B. Percutaneous closure of an atrial septal defect during pregnancy using an Amplatzer occlusion device. *J Obstetr Gynaecol.* 2005;25(7):715–716.

Spatling L, Fallenstein F, Huch A, Huch R, Rooth G. The variability of cardiopulmonary adaptation to pregnancy at rest and during exercise. *Br J Obstet Gynaecol.* 1992;99 (Suppl. 8):1–40.

Spitz IM, Bardin CW, Benton L, Robbins A. Early pregnancy termination with mifepristone and misoprostol in the United States. *N Engl J Med.* 1998;338(18):1241–1247.

Tateno S, Niwa K, Nakazawa M, Akagi T, Shinohara T, Yasuda T. Arrhythmia and conduction disturbances in patients with congenital heart disease during pregnancy: multicenter study. *Circ J.* 2003;67(12):992–997.

Taussig H, Kallman C, Nagel D, Baumgardner R, Momberger N, Kirk H. Long-time observations on the Blalock-Taussig operation VIII. 20 to 28 year follow-up on patients with a tetralogy of Fallot. *John Hopkins Med J.* 1975;137:13.

Therrien J, Barnes I, Somerville J. Outcome of pregnancy in patients with congenitally corrected transposition of the great arteries. *Am J Cardiol.* 1999;84, 820–824.

Therrien J, Gatzoulis M, Graham T, et al. Canadian Cardiovascular Society Consensus Conference 2001 update: Recommendations for the Management of Adults with Congenital Heart Disease—Part II. *Can J Cardiol.* 2001;17(10):1029–1050.

Ueland K. Maternal cardiovascular dynamics VII: intrapartum blood volume changes. *Am J Obstet Gynecol.* 1976;126:671–677.

Ueland K, Hansen J. Maternal cardiovascular dynamics II: posture and uterine contractions. *Am J Obstet Gynecol.* 1969a;101:1–7.

Ueland K, Hansen J. Maternal cardiovascular dynamics III: labor and delivery under local and caudal anesthesia. *Am J Obstet Gynecol.* 1969b;103:8–18.

Ueland K, Metcalfe J. Circulatory changes in pregnancy. *Clinical Obstet Gynecol.* 1975;18:41–50.

Ueland K, Novy M, Peterson E, Metcalfe J. Maternal cardiovascular dynamics IV: the influence of gestational age on the maternal cardiovascular response to posture and exercise. *Am J Obstet Gynecol.* 1969;104:856–858.

Ueland K, Parer J. Effects of estrogens on the cardiovascular system of the ewe. *Am J Obstet Gynecol.* 1966;96:400–404.

Upshaw CJ. A study of maternal electrocardiograms recorded during labor and delivery. *Am J Obstet Gynecol.* 1970;107(1):17–27.

van Doorn M, Lotgering F, Struijk P, Pool J, Wallenburg H. Maternal and fetal cardiovascular responses to strenuous bicycle exercise. *Am J Obstet Gynecol.* 1992;166:854–859.

Veldtman G, Connolly H, Grogan M, Ammash N, Warne C. Outcomes of pregnancy in women with tetralogy of Fallot. *Am Coll Cardiol.* 2004;44:174–180.

Vriend J, Drenthen W, Pieper P, et al. Outcome of pregnancy in patients after repair of aortic coarctation. *Eur Heart J.* 2005;26(20):2173–2178.

Wada H, Chiba Y, Murakami M, Kawaguchi H, Kobayashi H, Kanzaki T. Analysis of maternal and fetal risk in 594 pregnancies with heart disease. *Nippon Sanka Fujinka Gakkai Zasshi.* 1996;48:255–262.

Waickman L, Skorton D, Varner M, Ehmke D, Goplerud C. Ebstein's anomaly and pregnancy. *Am J Cardiol.* 1984;53:357–358.

Warnes CA, Williams RG, Bashore TM, et al. ACC/AHA 2008 Guidelines for management of adults with congenital heart disease. A report of the American College of Cardiology/American Heart Association Task Force on Practice Guidelines. (writing committee to develop guidelines for the management of adults with congenital heart disease). *J Am Coll Cardiol.* 2008;52(23):143–263.

Webb G, Gatzoulis M. Atrial septal defects in the adult: recent progress and overview. *Circulation.* 2006;114(15):1645–1653.

Weiss B, Atanassoff P. Cyanotic congenital heart disease and pregnancy: natural selection, pulmonary hypertension and anesthesia. *K Clin Anesth.* 1993;5:332–341.

Whittemore R, Hobbins J, Engle M. Pregnancy and its outcome in women with and without surgical treatment of congenital heart disease. *Am J Cardiol.* 1982;50(3):641–651.

WHO. *Medical Eligibility Criteria for Contraceptive Use.* 3rd ed. Geneva: WHO; 2004.

Wilson W, Taubert KA, Gewitz M, et al. Prevention of Infective Endocarditis. Guidelines From the American Heart Association. A Guideline From the American Heart Association Rheumatic Fever, Endocarditis, and Kawasaki Disease Committee, Council on Cardiovascular Disease in the Young, and the Council on Clinical Cardiology, Council on Cardiovascular Surgery and Anesthesia, and the Quality of Care and Outcomes Research Interdisciplinary Working Group. *Circulation.* 2007.

Yentis S, Gatzoulis MA, Steer P. Pregnancy and coarctation of the aorta. *J R Soc Med.* 2003;96(9):471.

Yentis S, Steer P, Plaat F. Eisenmenger's syndrome in pregnancy: maternal and fetal mortality in the 1990s. *Br J Obstet Gynaecol.* 1998;105(8):921–922.

19

Neurodevelopmental Aspects of Congenital Heart Defects

WILLIAM T. MAHLE

Each year, over 40,000 infants with congenital heart disease (CHD) are born in the United States. One-third of these children will require surgery in the first year of life. Fortunately, surgical mortality has decreased dramatically in the last several decades. With more children surviving and growing into adolescence and adulthood, there is an increased interest in the long-term outcome. It is being recognized that in addition to medical complications, a significant number of individuals with CHD may have developmental impairment and issues related to school performance. These issues will later be of great import as more CHD survivors enter the workforce. Therefore, an understanding of the factors that lead to developmental impairment and expected outcome for individuals with CHD is critical.

STRUCTURAL CNS ABNORMALITIES

Newborns with CHD have a substantially higher incidence of brain abnormalities such as overt cerebral dysgenesis than the general population. Microcephaly has been reported in up to 36% of neonates with CHD (Limperopoulos et al., 2000). Pathologic and neuroimaging studies performed in neonates with CHD have also demonstrated an increased incidence of structural brain abnormalities. Glauser et al. (1990) reported postmortem examinations in 39 infants with CHD and found increased operculum in eight (20%) and absent corpus callosum in three (8%). Neuroimaging studies have demonstrated callosal agenesis, abnormal neuronal migration, temporal lobar hypoplasia, and Chiari I malformations. Microcephaly has also been reported in many patients with CHD.

FUNCTIONAL CNS ABNORMALITIES

While the association of genetic syndromes or associations with CHD was once thought to be a contraindication to undertaking complex neonatal repairs or palliations, many centers now routinely perform neonatal surgery in such patients. In fact, upon careful examination by a trained geneticist, 24% of infants with complex heart disease are found to have a genetic anomaly (Gaynor et al., 2003). An understanding of the expected long-term neurocognitive outcome for these patients is essential for management and appropriate counseling. The potential interactions of underlying CNS abnormalities, the hemodynamic effects of complex CHD, and the sequelae of cardiac surgery are incompletely understood.

GENETIC SYNDROMES AND ASSOCIATIONS WITH CONGENITAL HEART DISEASE

Knowledge of the most common congenital heart lesions in various genetic syndromes is essential in caring for these patients and counseling the families. Some of the more common genetic syndromes and associations found in patients with CHD are shown in Table 19–1.

Trisomy 21 (Down syndrome) has an incidence of 1 in 660 newborns. Approximately 40% of patients with trisomy 21 have CHD (Marino and de Zorzi, 1993). Of those with CHD approximately 40% have AV canal defects. Others lesions frequently associated with trisomy 21 include ventricular septal defect (VSD), tetralogy of Fallot (TOF), and patent ductus arteriosus.

TABLE 19–1. *Genetic Syndromes Associated with CHD and Neurodevelopmental Risks*

Syndrome		% of patients with CHD	Most common lesions	Neurocognitive deficits
Down	Trisomy 21	40	Endocardial cushion, VSD, TOF, PDA	Mental retardation (median IQ 25–50) (Byrne et al., 2002; Brugge et al., 1994)
DiGeorge	Microdeletion 22q11 or 10p13–p14	60	IAA, TOF, Truncus Arteriosus	Mean IQ 70–80, ADHD (Brugge et al., 1994)
Turner	Monosomy of chromosome 23	30	Bicuspid aortic valve, coarctation of the aorta	Mean IQ 90 (Temple and Carney, 1993; Swillen et al., 1993)
Williams	7q11 mutation	60	Supravalvar AS, PPS	Mean IQ 56, mild spasticity
Alagille	20p12 mutation	85	PPS	Majority with normal intelligence
Jacobsen	11q deletion	56	Left heart obstructive	Half with mental retardation (Grossfeld et al., 2004)
Cri du chart	5p deletion	30	VSD, ASD	Mental retardation
Associations				
VACTERL		53	VSD, ASD	Majority with normal brain function
CHARGE		>50	TOF, PDA, VSD, ASD	Mental retardation in almost all cases (Raqbi et al., 2003)

Abbreviations: ADHD, attention deficit hyperactivity disorder; ASD, atrial septal defect; DORV, double outlet right ventricle; IAA, interrupted aortic arch; PDA, patent ductus arteriosus; PPS, peripheral pulmonary stenosis; TOF, tetralogy of Fallot; VSD, ventricular septal defect

Neurodevelopmental delay is found in all patients (Brugge et al., 1994; Parikh and Goyel, 1990).

Another chromosomal defect found in a significant proportion of patients with CHD is microdeletion of 22q11.2. Also known by the eponyms, DiGeorge syndrome or velo-cardio-facial syndrome, 22q11.2 is associated with conotruncal defects. Of note, the 22q phenotype has also been localized to 10p13–14 deletion as well and approximately 15% of patients with this phenotype have neither 22q11.2 nor 10p13-p14 deletions. 22q11.2 has been found in over 50% of patients with interrupted aortic arch (type B) and in at least 15% of patients with TOF. In most cases, the identification of the CHD precedes the genetic diagnosis of microdeletion of 22q11.2. The presence of microdeletion of 22q11.2 puts these patients at higher risk following an open heart surgery. The risk appears to be more related to the severity of heart disease than to other factors such as predisposition to infection. It has now become routine to screen patients with certain high-risk lesions such as interrupted aortic arch, TOF and truncus arteriosus with flourescence in situ hybridization techniques. However, some lesions such as abnormalities of the aortic arch—for example, right-sided aortic arch—may not be clinically evident. While the presence of a perimembranous VSD is also associated with microdeletion of 22q11.2, the association is not as strong and routine screening is not always undertaken. Unlike AV canal in which the majority of patients will require only one operation in their lifetime, the patients with microdeletion of 22q11.2 often require close follow-up.

Neurocognitive deficits are common in the microdeletion of 22q11.2 population. Moss et al. (1999) reported a mean full-scale IQ of 71.2 in patients with microdeletion of 22q11.2. Other investigators have also found mean full-scale IQ scores in the 70s (Bearden et al., 2001). Patients with 22q11.2- demonstrate a unique profile of neurocognitive deficits. Both expressive and receptive language deficits are common in these patients. In addition, patients with 22q11.2- have a high incidence of attention deficit hyperactivity disorder (ADHD) and an increased risk for developing bipolar disorder.

Williams syndrome is a rare, congenital (present at birth) disorder characterized by physical and developmental problems including an impulsive and outgoing (excessively social) personality, limited spatial skills and motor control, and intellectual disability (i.e., developmental delay, learning disabilities, mental retardation, or attention deficit disorder). The prevalence is in 1/2000 livebirths. The most common congenital heart defect associated with Williams syndrome include supravalvar aortic stenosis.

CHARGE syndrome refers to children with a specific set of birth defects. "CHARGE" originally came from the first letter of some of the most common features seen in these children: C = coloboma, H = heart defects, A = atresia of the choanae, R = retardation of growth and development, G = genital and urinary abnormalities, E = ear abnormalities and/or hearing loss. The diagnosis of CHARGE is based on finding several of these features and possibly other features also in a child. The diagnosis should be made by a medical geneticist who has ruled out other disorders with overlapping findings. Heart defects are present in 80% of affected individuals. The most common CHD lesion in CHARGE is TOF. Other lesions include patent ductus arteriosus, double outlet right ventricle with an atrioventricular canal, ventricular septal/atrial septal defect, and right-sided aortic arch. As the microdeletion 22q11.2 patients, those with TOF and CHARGE will require annual cardiac follow-up and replacement of the pulmonary valve in adolescence or early adulthood is common. Most patients with CHARGE have profound developmental delay. The key to management of a child with CHARGE association is early identification, evaluation of the specific defects and needs, comprehensive intervention, and ongoing monitoring. A multidisciplinary approach involving specialists from different fields with a pediatrician leading and coordinating them is often helpful in proper management of these children.

GENETIC PREDISPOSITION TO NEUROLOGIC INJURY

Recently there has been considerable interest in the role that genetic polymorphisms might play in outcome of disease status. Polymorphisms are changes in the genetic code (like mutations) that occur commonly enough in the population such that they are considered a variation on normal. These may be harmful or helpful or neither to the persons who have a polymorphism. The protein Apolipoprotein ε (APOE) that is coded by the APOE gene is produced in the brain, where it plays multiple roles, including protecting against injury. It has been shown that infants with the ε2 allele who undergo open heart surgery in the first year of life have lower developmental tests and a smaller head circumference at 1 year of age (Gaynor et al., 2003). A similar association has been reported in children who had a history of birth asphyxia. These data may allow clinicians to identify children with greatest risk of later developmental deficits.

RISKS OF DEVELOPMENT IN CONGENITAL HEART DISEASE—BEYOND GENETIC DEFECTS

In addition to named genetic disorders, patients with unrepaired CHD have a higher incidence of neurologic deficits compared to the normal population. Several studies have identified neurologic abnormalities in patients with CHD prior to any surgical intervention. A recent study of newborns with a variety of CHDs demonstrated that over 50% had at least one abnormal finding on preoperative neurologic examination (Limperopoulos et al., 2000). Some of the more common abnormalities noted in neonates with CHD were abnormalities in tone, jitteriness, and poor oromotor coordination. Feeding difficulties were noted in more than one-third of patients. Similarly, Brunberg and associates found abnormalities on neurologic examination in 15 of 21 patients with CHD prior to surgical intervention (Brunberg et al., 1974). The reasons why children with CHD be hardwired for neurodevelopmental compromise are varied. Recently, a number of investigators have shown that before birth, brain perfusion is compromised in many complex heart lesions (Donofrio et al., 2003; Kochilas et al., 2001).

ABNORMAL HEMODYNAMICS AND THE CNS

In addition to congenital neurologic abnormalities, infants with complex CHD are at risk for preoperative neurologic insult. Factors that can impact preoperative neurologic status include hypoxemia, poor feeding, and congestive heart failure. In particular, newborns with ductal-dependent systemic blood may present with profound acidosis, hypoxic-ischemic injury, and/or shock upon closure of the ductus arteriosus. Preoperative seizures, intraventricluar hemorrhage, and periventricular leukomalacia (PVL) are known consequences of hypoperfusion in these ductal-dependent lesions (Mahle et al., 2000). Postnatal brain injury in these patients primarily involves the white matter and is more likely due to ischemic rather than hypoxic insult (Mahle et al., 2002). In one study, intraventricular hemorrhage (IVH) has also been documented in neonates with CHD occurring in up to 25% of neonates (van Houten et al., 1996). The risk of IVH increases when hemodynamic instability is superimposed on the delicate microvasculature of the immature brain. The incidence of IVH in premature infants with CHD is not well described, though presumably the risk would be even higher.

Congestive heart failure (CHF) also contributes to a poor neurodevelopmental outcome. The association between CHF and developmental outcome may be related to physical inactivity and failure to thrive. Children with CHD may not receive sufficient nutrient and caloric intake because of fatigue, recurrent infection or cardiac decompensation. Since 50% of the normal postnatal brain growth occurs during the first year of life, poor growth and nutrition during this critical period can put the infant at risk. It has been shown that infants with cyanotic heart lesions have significantly impaired growth in the first year of life. Generally, these infants are almost 1 standard deviation below normal in both length and weight in early childhood (Kelleher et al., 2006; Nydegger and Bines, 2006). In addition, studies in adults have shown that heart failure results in impaired cerebral blood flow. Gruhn and colleagues showed that cerebral blood flow is substantially, but reversibly, reduced in patients with NYHA class III/IV heart failure (Gruhn et al., 2001). This phenomenon suggests that redistribution of cardiac output inadequately secures brain perfusion in patients with severe CHF.

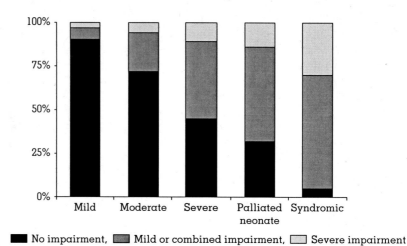

FIGURE 19–1. Schema of probable neurodevelopmental outcome based on severity of heart lesion and presence of genetic syndrome.

■ No impairment,   ■ Mild or combined impairment,   ☐ Severe impairment

Thus, even before the newborn or infant undergoes cardiac surgery, a number of factors—individually or in combination—place the child at an increased risk for abnormal neurologic and cognitive development. The interactions between genetic predisposition, acquired or congenital structural abnormalities, hypoxemia, low cardiac output, and nutrition must be considered in the overall risk assessment of the patient. In discussing the potential impact of CHD on developmental outcome, with parents or other caregivers, one can think of a schema of increasing risk with increasing complexity of heart disease and the presence of genetic syndromes (Figure 19–1).

CARDIOPULMONARY BYPASS AND CIRCULATORY ARREST

Cardiopulmonary bypass (CPB) is utilized in many neonatal and infant cardiac surgical procedures. CPB allows for perfusion of vital organs by providing oxygenated blood via a mechanical pump. During procedures using CPB, especially at low-flow rates, neuroprotection may be achieved with concomitant use of hypothermia. Hypothermia protects the brain by decreasing cerebral metabolism. Cardiovascular surgery with CPB leads to activation of a variety of inflammatory pathways. Cerebral edema has been noted in postoperative neuroimaging of adults. In addition, investigators have shown that microemboli can be detected in the carotid arteries of children undergoing repair of CHD—and are especially prevalent immediately after the release of the aortic cross-clamp.

In some procedures, it is necessary to stop blood flow altogether through a process known as deep hypothermic circulatory arrest (DHCA). Those procedures that require deep hypothermia are thought to pose a great risk to the infant brain. The infant is

cooled to 16°C–18°C by CPB; blood is drained into the venous reservoir and circulation arrested. Upon completion of surgery, the heart is de-aired, the circulation is restored, and the patient is rewarmed on CPB. Consequently, DHCA represents a clinical situation of *planned*, total-body ischemia-reperfusion. The relationship between the use and duration of DHCA and the risk for neurologic injury has been a matter of considerable controversy. Data obtained from animal studies have suggested that a total DHCA duration of less than 30 minutes is likely to be safe with respect to significant damage to the CNS, though longer periods of DHCA have been shown to have deleterious long-term effects on the neurodevelopment.

POSTOPERATIVE PERIOD

It has recently been recognized that immediately following heart surgery. The brain is particularly vulnerable to injury. As such, many centers now monitor cardiac function—and indirectly brain perfusion—in this critical period. Caregivers can monitor the same using indwelling vascular catheters or using a technique known as near infrared spectroscopy (NIRS). A number of contemporary studies have found that when brain perfusion is marginal in the days immediately following heart surgery, the children are at risk for later developmental delay (Hoffman et al., 2005; Dent et al., 2005).

NEUROLOGIC EXAMINATION AND NEUROIMAGING AFTER SURGERY

Neurologic examinations performed in the postoperative period have identified a variety of abnormalities including hypotonia, pyramidal findings, and asymmetry of tone. Miller and colleagues performed neurologic examinations on 91 young infants undergoing congenital heart surgery (Miller et al., 1994). In addition to clinical seizures in 15% of patients, the authors found hypotonia in 34% of patients at hospital discharge. Hypertonia was noted in 7% of infants and asymmetry of tone in 5%. A decreased level of alertness was noted in 19% of patients at hospital discharge. In the analysis of children with transposition of the great arteries who had undergone the arterial switch procedure, diffuse motor abnormalities were noted in 45% and cranial nerve abnormalities in 4% of patients at hospital discharge (Newburger et al., 1993).

Neuroimaging studies performed in the early postoperative period have demonstrated a high incidence of abnormalities. Galli et al. studied 105 infants who had undergone heart surgery with CPB—most as neonates—and found that over 50% had PVL on MRI imaging of the brain. The cysts are often replaced by an astroglial scar, resulting in PVL, which is characterized by a marked deficiency of cerebral white matter. Figure 19–2 demonstrates PVL in an infant who had undergone newborn surgery for hypoplastic left heart syndrome (HLHS). The factors that lead to the development of PVL after complex CHD surgery in the neonates appear to be related to younger age at operation and hypotension in the postoperative period (Galli et al., 2004). The white matter appears particularly susceptible to injury when cerebral blood flow auto-

regulation is compromised, such as after a period of circulatory arrest. The subsequent neurologic features of PVL relate to the topography of this lesion. Spastic diplegia, affecting the lower extremities more than the upper extremities, is the most common manifestation of clinical PVL.

NEUROLOGIC OUTCOMES IN SPECIFIC CHD

There have been several investigations that address the neurocognitive outcome for survivors of complex heart surgery; some are parts of prospective clinical trials, while others are retrospective or cross-sectional reviews. The results of some of these studies are summarized in Table 19–2. Results of these studies are influenced by many factors including the era in which patients underwent surgery, the outcome measures used, and the age at testing. Most standardized tests such as the Bayley scales of Infant Development and the Weschler scales are scored according to the population norms with a mean of 100 and a standard deviation of 15.

Transposition of the Great Arteries

The most extensively studied subgroup of patients is the transposition of the great arteries (TGA) population. This is likely due to the high prevalence of TGA (1/5000), the low mortality of surgical intervention, the long duration of follow-up (early repair was possible in the 1960s), and the low incidence of associated genetic syndromes. At presentation, many of these patients are profoundly hypoxemic until mixing of oxygenated and deoxygenated blood can be increased by procedures such as balloon atrial septostomy or the institution of prostaglandin E_1. Recent data suggest that those neonates requiring atrial septostomy may be at increased risk for ischemic injury (McQuillen et al., 2006). In the current era, the approach to TGA is early reparative surgery with the arterial switch procedure. Hesz and Clark studied 10 patients with TGA after arterial switch and found significantly lower developmental scores when compared to siblings (Hesz and Clark, 1988). In a randomized trial comparing two support techniques during the arterial switch, investigators reported a mean full scale IQ of 94 at 8 years of age, which was mildly, but significantly lower than the normal population. Deficits were most commonly noted in visual-spatial and visual-motor integration. Definite neurologic abnormalities were noted in 30% of patients. The incidence of speech abnormalities was also higher than the general population. Risk factors for lower full-scale IQ included perioperative seizures and the presence of a coexisting VSD.

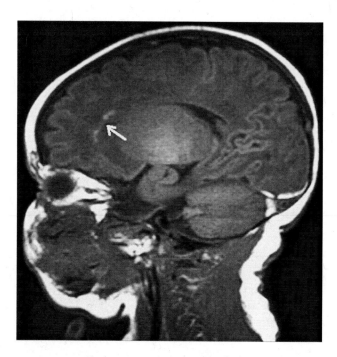

FIGURE 19–2. Early postoperative scan of the same subject. Hyperintense signal is noted in the frontal white matter (arrow) consistent with periventricular leukomalacia. Small amount of subdural blood noted are above and below the tentorium.

TABLE 19–2. *Reported Outcomes after Complex Infant Heart Surgery*

Lesion	Full scale IQ	Comments
TGA	92–101	Visual motor deficits, expressive language deficits
TOF	89–100	Significant limitations for 22q11.2- patients
TAPVC	95	Attention problems, poor visual motor integration (Kirshbom et al., 2005)
Single ventricle	95	Neurologic risk related to need for neonatal surgery
HLHS	86–88	Attention problems common
Heart transplantation	91	Infant recipients at greater risk
Ventricular septal defect	93*	Genetic syndromes higher risk

Notes: *Mental developmental index of Bayley's scales
Abbreviations: CPB, cardiopulmonary bypass; DHCA, deep hypothermic circulatory arrest; HLHS, hypoplastic left heart syndrome; TAPVC, total anomalous pulmonary venous return; TGA, transposition of the great arteries; TOF, tetralogy of Fallot.

Tetralogy of Fallot

Patients with TOF have previously been noted to have lower scores on standardized cognitive testing and poorer overall psychological functioning than the normal population. In a study of patients with TOF, the majority of whom had undergone complete repair, DeMaso et al. (1990) found that 22% of patients scored <80% on IQ testing versus 2.8% of the control population without CHD. However, a more recent study by Oates et al. (1995) found IQ scores within the normal range for 51 patients with TOF (100 ± 13). Potential risk factors in this population include prolonged hypoxemia, CHF, and thromboembolic events. An additional risk factor is the association of TOF and microdeletion of 22q11.2, which is found in over 15% of patients with TOF. In the current era, patients with TOF usually undergo complete repair within the first year of life. This strategy reduces the risk of right to left shunting, hypercyanotic spells, and CNS damage. Interestingly, preliminary data would suggest that developmental deficits are significant in infants who undergo early complete repair of TOF. Zeltser and colleagues presented data from 45 infants with TOF who had undergone complete repair in the first year of life. This study found a mean Mental Developmental Index of 89 ± 13 and a mean Psychomotor Developmental Index of 80 ± 12 (Zeltser et al., 2004). In this study, 10% of the infants examined had microdeletion of 22q11.2. Even after excluding the infants with known genetic syndromes, test scores were significantly below the normal range.

Single Ventricle Lesions

Patients with single ventricle who are palliated with the Fontan operation are at considerable risk for neurocognitive impairment. Risk factors in this population include multiple operations requiring CPB, prolonged hypoxemia, and failure to thrive. Patients palliated with the Fontan procedure appear to be at particular risk for a cerebrovascular accident (CVA). The risk of CVA late after Fontan procedure has been reported to be 2.7%–8.8% (Rosti et al., 1997).

Recent studies have investigated the long-term neurocognitive outcome of patients palliated with the Fontan operation. Wernovsky and colleagues (2000) evaluated 133 patients palliated with Fontan surgery at a median age of 11.1 years. The mean full-scale IQ in this cohort (95.7 ± 17.4) was lower than that in the general population. Mental retardation, defined as full scale IQ < 70, was noted in 7.8% of the population. Additional risk factors for lower scores on cognitive testing included lower socioeconomic status and the use of circulatory arrest prior to the Fontan procedure, and anatomic diagnosis. In particular, patients with HLHS scored significantly lower on standardized testing. Similarly, Uzark et al. (1998) reported a mean IQ of 97.5 ± 12.1 for 32 children with single ventricle palliated with the Fontan procedure. The diagnosis of HLHS was associated with lower scores.

Hypoplastic Left Heart Syndrome

There are several reasons why patients with HLHS may be at higher risk than patients with other forms of single ventricle. Previous investigations have demonstrated a relatively high incidence of congenital brain abnormalities in neonates with HLHS. In addition, these patients have ductal-dependent systemic blood flow; severe acidosis and end organ injury at the time of presentation are not uncommon. Circulatory arrest may be used for surgical palliation. In addition, maintaining adequate systemic blood flow and cerebral perfusion in the postoperative period can be unpredictable. The risk of postoperative seizures is significant, up to 18% after stage I reconstruction (Clancy et al., 2001).

In 1995, Rogers and colleagues reported the neurodevelopmental outcome of 11 preschool survivors of reconstructive surgery for HLHS at various stages of palliation. The study documented an alarmingly high incidence of neurodevelopmental deficits. Of the 11 children studied, seven (64%) were found to have mental retardation. Substantial functional disabilities were present in eight children (73%). Gross motor abnormalities were noted in five children (45%). In a study of 115 school age children with HLHS who had undergone staged palliation before 1992 (Kochilas et al., 2001), a questionnaire revealed that over 30% of patients were receiving some form of special education. While the majority of these patients scored within the normal range, the median full scale IQ of 86, was significantly lower than the general population. In addition, 18% of subjects had IQ scores in the mentally retarded range. Minor neurologic abnormalities were present in 55% of patients. These abnormalities included microcephaly in 13%, fine motor abnormalities in 48%, and gross motor abnormalities in 39%. Cerebral palsy was present in 17% of the patients. Over 60% of patients were thought to have problems with attention and 9% had mood disturbances. A number of other centers have reported quite similar findings, even for patients operated in a more recent era (Goldberg et al., 2000; Hoffman et al., 2005).

Heart Transplantation

Infant heart transplantation has been undertaken in many centers as an alternative management approach to complex CHD in which reconstructive surgery is associated with a high mortality. The most common lesion for which infant heart transplantation is undertaken is HLHS. As with patients who undergo reconstructive surgery, neonates with HLHS who undergo heart transplantation are at significant risk of preoperative, operative, and postoperative insult (Fleisher et al., 2002). Postoperatively patients are at risk for low cardiac output and have an increased risk of seizures, possibly related to immunosuppressive medications. One study of neurologic outcome in patients who had undergone infant heart transplantation evaluated 38 infants at 12–30 months of age. The mean scores of both the mental developmental index and psychomotor developmental index, 91 and 88, respectively, were lower than the scores for the normal population (Baum et al., 2000). Another study compared the developmental outcome of school-age children with HLHS who had undergone one of the two management strategies, palliative surgery or heart transplantation (Mahle et al., 2006). This study reported that mild to moderate developmental deficits were common and did not differ because of treatment strategy. These findings support the notion that children with some forms of CHD may be predisposed to neurologic injury regardless of management strategy.

Neuropsychiatric Issues

While much has been written about the cognitive outcome after complex CHD surgery, less is known about the neurobehavioral sequelae in this patient population. Several investigators have identified neurobehavioral issues that may contribute significantly to long-term morbidity in patients with CHD. Attention deficit disorder has been described in several evaluations of school-age children who underwent surgical repair after CHD (Clarkson et al., 1980; Haka-Ikse et al., 1978). In the evaluation of school-age survivors of staged palliation for HLHS, a high prevalence of attention problems was detected (Kochilas et al., 2001). Both neurologic evaluation and use of standardized behavior batteries suggested a high degree of attention and hyperactivity problems. While the incidence of ADHD in the general population is a matter of debate, several large series have reported ADHD to be present in 2%–5% of the normal population. Why ADHD may be more common in the CHD population is not known. Previous investigators have demonstrated an increased incidence of ADHD in populations with developmental delay. Further analysis will be needed to determine what perioperative factors are associated with attention problems.

In addition to ADHD, other behavioral problems have been identified. In our retrospective analysis, 18% of patients with HLHS had clinically significant anxiety problems (versus 2% in the normal population) as measured by the Achenbach Child Behavior Checklist (Kochilas et al., 2001). DeMaso and colleagues (1990) also used a standardized instrument to characterize psychological function in patients who had undergone repair of TOF and TGA. They demonstrated marked psychological impairment such as obsessive compulsive traits and disabling anxiety in over 15% of patients. An increased incidence of aggressive behavior was noted among patients with TGA who had undergone the arterial switch under DHCA (Hesz and Clark, 1988).

Brandhagen et al. (1991) used standardized psychologic instruments in the follow-up evaluation of 168 adults with CHD. They found that adults with CHD have significantly higher anxiety, hostility, and symptom distress than the normal population. Interestingly, the degree of psychological distress was not correlated to the clinical severity of the cardiac lesions, and did not seem to be related to all areas of social function, such as job stability, education attainment and other factors. A number of studies have suggested that adults with CHD are at increased risk of psychiatric conditions. Bromberg and colleagues reported that over one-third of adults with CHD had a "diagnosable psychiatric condition" with depression being the most common diagnosis.

Relationship between Neurodevelopmental and Behavioral Outcomes and Quality of Life

In light of the improved survival of children with CHD, caregivers are now focused on improving the quality of life (QOL) of these patients. Newer instruments are being developed to best measure outcomes such as QOL and health status. As with many other chronic disease states, CHD can significantly impact QOL. There are a variety of factors that influence QOL in the CHD population. The factors are sometimes directly related to cardiovascular impairment. For example, impaired exercise performance has been shown to correlate with lower measures of physical health (DeMaso et al., 1990). Developmental deficits and psychiatric condition also have a significant impact on a child's perceived health status. In a cohort of school-age children with HLHS, Jenkins and colleagues reported that visual motor impairments were significantly correlated with general behavior, impact on the parents' time, and social limitations, as assessed by the Child Health Questionnaire (CHQ-50). McCrindle et al. (2006) found in a cohort of over 500 children with forms of functional single ventricle that attention problems also had a strong correlation with parental perception of poor QOL.

IMPLICATIONS FOR HEALTH POLICY

The developmental deficits that occur in association with CHD result in an increased need for special educational services. In an analysis of over 200 school-age children with CHD who required surgery in infancy, Schillingford and colleagues reported that 38% of these children received special education services in school as compared to over 15% of general school-age population. As increasing numbers of these patients reach adulthood the developmental deficits are likely to have significant impact on employment opportunities. There are now a number of studies that have found that unemployment is relatively high among adults with CHD. This may be related in part to physical limitations for some. However, developmental deficits most likely play an important role. Previous studies have suggested that an intervention that increases cognition by 1 IQ point results in an increase in worker productivity of 2% (Grosse et al., 2002). This results in an increase in income of US$14,500 over a lifetime. While the present review demonstrates that the neurodevelopmental profile of children and adults is complex—with speech and visual motor impairments being more significant than deficits in cognition—the potential societal benefit of limiting neurologic injury in this population seems quite a worthy endeavor.

SUMMARY

Each year, there are more adult survivors of CHD a significant number of whom have neurocognitive sequelae. An understanding of the patients at greater risk and the unique profile of cognitive and behavioral impairments is needed to adequately address their long-term care.

REFERENCES

Baum M, Freier MC, Freeman KR, Chinnock RE. Developmental outcomes and cognitive functioning in infant and child heart transplant recipients. *Prog Pediatr Cardiol.* 2000; 11(2):159–163.

Bearden CE, Woodin MF, Wang PP, et al. The neurocognitive phenotype of the 22q11.2 deletion syndrome: selective deficit in visual-spatial memory. *J Clin Exp Neuropsychol.* 2001;23(4):447–464.

Brandhagen DJ, Feldt RH, Williams DE. Long-term psychologic implications of congenital heart disease: a 25-year follow-up. *Mayo Clin Proc.* 1991;66(5):474–479.

Brugge KL, Nichols SL, Salmon DP, et al. Cognitive impairment in adults with Down's syndrome: similarities to early cognitive changes in Alzheimer's disease. *Neurology.* 1994;44(2):232–238.

Brunberg JA, Reilly EL, Doty DB. Central nervous system consequences in infants of cardiac surgery using deep hypothermia and circulatory arrest. *Circulation.* 1974;50(Suppl 2):II60–II68.

Byrne A, MacDonald J, Buckley S. Reading, language and memory skills: a comparative longitudinal study of children with Down syndrome and their mainstream peers. *Br J Educ Psychol.* 2002;72(Pt 4):513–529.

Clancy RR, McGaurn SA, Goin JE, et al. Allopurinol neurocardiac protection trial in infants undergoing heart surgery using deep hypothermic circulatory arrest. *Pediatrics.* 2001;108(1):61–70.

Clarkson PM, MacArthur BA, Barratt-Boyes BG, Whitlock RM, Neutze JM. Developmental progress after cardiac surgery in infancy using hypothermia and circulatory arrest. *Circulation.* 1980;62(4):855–61.

DeMaso DR, Beardslee WR, Silbert AR, Fyler DC. Psychological functioning in children with cyanotic heart defects. *J Dev Behav Pediatr.* 1990;11(6):289–294.

Dent CL, Spaeth JP, Jones BV, et al. Brain magnetic resonance imaging abnormalities after the Norwood procedure using regional cerebral perfusion. *J Thorac Cardiovasc Surg.* 2005;130(6):1523–1530.

Donofrio MT, Bremer YA, Schieken RM, et al. Autoregulation of cerebral blood flow in fetuses with congenital heart disease: the brain sparing effect. *Pediatr Cardiol.* 2003;24:436–444.

Fleisher BE, Baum D, Brudos G, et al. Infant heart transplantation at Stanford: growth and neurodevelopmental outcome. *Pediatrics.* 2002;109(1):1–7.

Galli KK, Zimmerman RA, Jarvik GP, et al. Periventricular leukomalacia is common after neonatal cardiac surgery. *J Thorac Cardiovasc Surg.* 2004;127(3):692–704.

Gaynor JW, Gerdes M, Zackai EH, et al. Apolipoprotein E genotype and neurodevelopmental sequelae of infant cardiac surgery. *J Thorac Cardiovasc Surg.* 2003;126(6):1736–1745.

Glauser TA, Rorke LB, Weinberg PM, Clancy RR. Congenital brain anomalies associated with the hypoplastic left heart syndrome. *Pediatrics.* 1990;85(6):984–990.

Goldberg CS, Schwartz EM, Brunberg JA, et al. Neurodevelopmental outcome of patients after the fontan operation: a comparison between children with hypoplastic left heart syndrome and other functional single ventricle lesions. *J Pediatr.* 2000;137(5):646–652.

Grosse SD, Matte TD, Schwartz J, Jackson RJ. Economic gains resulting from the reduction in children's exposure to lead in the United States. *Environ Health Perspect.* 2002;110(6):563–569.

Grossfeld PD, Mattina T, Lai Z, et al. The 11q terminal deletion disorder: a prospective study of 110 cases. *Am J Med Genet A.* 2004;129(1):51–61.

Gruhn N, Larsen FS, Boesgaard S, et al. Cerebral blood flow in patients with chronic heart failure before and after heart transplantation. *Stroke.* 2001;32(11):2530–2533.

Haka-Ikse K, Blackwood MJ, Steward DJ. Psychomotor development of infants and children after profound hypothermia during surgery for congenital heart disease. *Dev Med Child Neurol.* 1978;20(1):62–70.

Hesz N, Clark EB. Cognitive development in transposition of the great vessels. *Arch Dis Child.* 1988;63(2):198–200.

Hoffman GM, Mussatto KA, Brosig CL, et al. Systemic venous oxygen saturation after the Norwood procedure and childhood neurodevelopmental outcome. *J Thorac Cardiovasc Surg.* 2005 October;130(4):1094–1100.

Kelleher DK, Laussen P, Teixeira-Pinto A, Duggan C. Growth and correlates of nutritional status among infants with hypoplastic left heart syndrome (HLHS) after stage 1 Norwood procedure. *Nutrition.* 2006;22(3):237–244.

Kirshbom PM, Flynn TB, Clancy RR, et al. Late neurodevelopmental outcome after repair of total anomalous pulmonary venous connection. *J Thorac Cardiovasc Surg.* 2005;129(5):1091–1097.

Kochilas L, Shores JC, Novello RT, Clancy RR, Rychik J. Aortic morphometry and microcephaly in the hypoplastic left heart syndrome. *J Am Coll Cardiol.* 2001;37:470A.

Limperopoulos C, Majnemer A, Shevell MI, Rosenblatt B, Rohlicek C, Tchervenkov C. Neurodevelopmental status of newborns and infants with congenital heart defects before and after open heart surgery. *J Pediatr.* 2000;137(5):638–645.

Mahle WT, Clancy RR, Moss EM, Gerdes M, Jobes DR, Wernovsky G. Neurodevelopmental outcome and lifestyle assessment in school-aged and adolescent children with hypoplastic left heart syndrome. *Pediatrics.* 2000;105(5):1082–1089.

Mahle WT, Tavani F, Zimmerman RA, et al. An MRI study of neurological injury before and after congenital heart surgery. *Circulation.* 2002;106(12 Suppl 1):I109–I114.

Mahle WT, Visconti KJ, Freier MC, et al. Relationship of surgical approach to neurodevelopmental outcomes in hypoplastic left heart syndrome. *Pediatrics.* 2006;117(1):e90–e97.

Marino B, de Zorzi A. Congenital heart disease in trisomy 21 mosaicism. *J Pediatr.* 1993;122(3):500–501.

McCrindle BW, Williams RV, Mitchell PD, et al. Relationship of patient and medical characteristics to health status in children and adolescents after the Fontan procedure. *Circulation.* 2006;113(8):1123–1129.

McQuillen PS, Hamrick SE, Perez MJ, et al. Balloon atrial septostomy is associated with preoperative stroke in neonates with transposition of the great arteries. *Circulation.* 2006;113(2):280–285.

Miller G, Mamourian AC, Tesman JR, Baylen BG, Myers JL. Long-term MRI changes in brain after pediatric open heart surgery. *J Child Neurol.* 1994;9(4):390–397.

Moss EM, Batshaw ML, Solot CB, et al. Psychoeducational profile of the 22q11.2 microdeletion: a complex pattern. *J Pediatr.* 1999;134(2):193–198.

Newburger JW, Jonas RA, Wernovsky G, et al. A comparison of the perioperative neurologic effects of hypothermic circulatory arrest versus low-flow cardiopulmonary bypass in infant heart surgery. *N Engl J Med.* 1993;329(15):1057–1064.

Nydegger A, Bines JE. Energy metabolism in infants with congenital heart disease. *Nutrition.* 2006;22(7–8):697–704.

Oates RK, Simpson JM, Turnbull JA, Cartmill TB. The relationship between intelligence and duration of circulatory arrest with deep hypothermia. *J Thorac Cardiovasc Surg.* 1995;110(3):786–792.

Parikh AP, Goyel NA. Mental performance in Down syndrome. *Indian J Pediatr.* 1990;57(2):261–263.

Raqbi F, Le Bihan C, Morisseau-Durand MP, Dureau P, Lyonnet S, Abadie V. Early prognostic factors for intellectual outcome in CHARGE syndrome. *Dev Med Child Neurol.* 2003;45(7):483–488.

Rogers BT, Msall ME, Buck GM, et al. Neurodevelopmental outcome of infants with hypoplastic left heart syndrome. *J Pediatr.* 1995;126(3):496–498.

Rosti L, Colli AM, Frigiola A. Stroke and the Fontan procedure. *Pediatr Cardiol.* 1997;18(2):159.

Swillen A, Fryns JP, Kleczkowska A, Massa G, Vanderschueren-Lodeweyckx M, Van den BH. Intelligence, behaviour and psychosocial development in Turner syndrome. A cross-sectional study of 50 pre-adolescent and adolescent girls (4–20 years). *Genet Couns.* 1993;4(1):7–18.

Temple CM, Carney RA. Intellectual functioning of children with Turner syndrome: a comparison of behavioural phenotypes. *Dev Med Child Neurol.* 1993;35(8):691–698.

Uzark K, Lincoln A, Lamberti JJ, Mainwaring RD, Spicer RL, Moore JW. Neurodevelopmental outcomes in children with Fontan repair of functional single ventricle. *Pediatrics.* 1998;101(4 Pt 1):630–633.

van Houten JP, Rothman A, Bejar R. High incidence of cranial ultrasound abnormalities in full-term infants with congenital heart disease. *Am J Perinatol.* 1996;13(1):47–53.

Wernovsky G, Stiles KM, Gauvreau K, et al. Cognitive development after the Fontan operation. *Circulation.* 2000;102(8):883–889.

Zeltser I, Jarvik GP, Bernbaum J, et al. Genetics factors are important determinants of neurodevelopmental outcome of tetralogy of Fallot. *Circulation.* 2004;110(17):iii–498.

20

Psychological Aspects of Congenital Heart Disease in Children

ELISABETH H.M. VAN RIJEN

ELISABETH M.W.J. UTENS

Over the last decades, major advances in diagnostic and surgical techniques and medical treatment of congenital heart disease (CHD) have led to dramatically lower mortality rates in children with CHD (Boneva et al., 2001). Despite improved survival, children with CHD may still have cardiac residua and sequelae after surgical or interventional treatment and medical follow-up may be required (Wren and O'Sullivan, 2001). Morbidity may result in reduced stamina (Fredriksen et al., 2004) and physical limitations (Spijkerboer et al., 2006), which in turn may negatively influence participation in social activities (e.g., performing sports). Limitations in daily activities can lead to increased distress and psychological maladjustment (Wallander and Varni, 1998), which have frequently been observed in children with CHD (Karsdorp et al., 2007). Moreover, difficulties with intellectual and academic performance have been reported in children with CHD (Wright and Nolan, 1994). In sum, children with CHD may be hampered in their emotional, social, as well as intellectual development.

Children with CHD constitute a heterogeneous group, in which mild as well as severe cardiac diagnoses are represented. The dramatic development of medical and surgical treatment for children with CHD has led to increasing survival rates during the last decades, also for children with the most severe conditions. For these reasons, results from different studies, performed across patient samples with different cardiac defects and performed in different periods of time, may be hard to compare. Therefore, in this chapter, studies performed before the mid-1990s will be referred to as "early studies" and studies performed after the mid-1990s will be referred to as "recent studies."

The focus of this chapter will be on empirical research findings regarding various psychological aspects of CHD in children. Results of studies into (1) emotional and behavioral problems, (2) self-concept, (3) academic functioning, and (4) quality of life will be presented.

In the first part, results on (1) emotional and behavioral problems from

(1a) studies using the Child Behavior Checklist (CBCL) and
(1b) studies using more specific instruments will be discussed as well as
(1c) the role of gender and age,
(1d) the role of cardiac diagnosis,
(1e) predictors and correlates, and
(1f) longitudinal development.

The second part on (2) self-concept, focuses on

(2a) self-concept and the related concept of
(2b) body-image.

In the third part on (3) academic functioning, the topics

(3a) emotional and behavioral problems at school,
(3b) academic achievement,
(3c) learning disabilities, and
(3d) repeating of classes and attendance of special education will be discussed.

The fourth part on (4) quality of life, will focus on
(4a) the concept of quality of life,
(4b) empirical studies into health-related quality of life,

(4c) the role of gender and age,

(4d) the role of cardiac diagnosis,

(4e) predictors and correlates, and

(4f) the agreement between parent and child reports.

Each of the four parts will be ended by conclusions and practical implications. For a more clinical, qualitative description of the impact of CHD at various stages of childhood and adolescence, we refer to Garson (1998). In the appendix, an overview will be provided of the different instruments used to assess psychological functioning in patients with CHD in the studies discussed in this chapter.

EMOTIONAL AND BEHAVIORAL PROBLEMS

Children with chronic physical disorders, such as CHD, are at risk for emotional and behavioral maladjustment (Wallander and Varni, 1998). In an early study, DeMaso et al. (1990) reported impaired psychological functioning in children with cyanotic CHD, compared to a group of children who spontaneously recovered from a mild CHD without medical intervention. DeMaso et al. (1990) used a rather global measurement of psychological problems, namely the Global Psychological Functional Scale, which distinguishes five levels of psychological impairment. Since then, the need to use psychometrically sound, cross-culturally well-known instruments to assess emotional and behavioral functioning in children with CHD was recognized. In most studies, the Child Behavior Checklist (CBCL) (Achenbach, 1991a; Achenbach and Rescorla, 2001) was used to assess a broad range of emotional and behavioral problems. In several other studies, more specific standardized instruments were used to assess medical-related fears, anxiety, or depression. Results of studies executed with (a) the CBCL and (b) more specific instruments will be discussed below.

Studies Using the Child Behavior Checklist

The CBCL (Achenbach, 1991a; Achenbach and Rescorla, 2001) has been used most often to assess emotional and behavioral problems in children with CHD in early studies (Oates et al., 1994; Utens et al., 1993), as well as recent studies (Casey et al., 1996; Fredriksen et al., 2004; Gupta et al., 2001; Hövels-Gürich et al., 2002; Karl et al., 2004; Miatton et al., 2007; Spijkerboer et al., 2007; Utens et al., 2001; Van der Rijken et al., 2007). This instrument is a standardized parent report measure, which covers a wide range of emotional and behavioral problems in children aged 6–18 years. The CBCL consists of eight specific syndrome scales, two broad problem areas (internalizing and externalizing), and an overall rating of emotional and behavior problems (total problem score). Internalizing consists of the syndrome scales: anxiety/depression, withdrawal and somatic complaints. Externalizing consists of the syndrome scales: rule-breaking (delinquent) and aggressive behavior. The syndrome scales social problems, thought problems, and attention problems belong neither to the internalizing, nor to the externalizing scale.

In a number of studies using the CBCL, parents of children with CHD reported more total problems in their children compared to normative groups (Gupta et al., 2001; Hövels-Gürich et al., 2002; Karl et al., 2004; Miatton et al., 2007; Oates et al., 1994; Spijkerboer et al., 2007; Utens et al., 1993). A recent meta-analysis concerning several of these studies yielded a medium estimate of effect size for total problems in children with CHD (unbiased estimate effect size: 0.47; Karsdorp et al., 2007). In a Dutch sample of 2–3-year-old children awaiting elective cardiac surgery or catheter intervention, increased levels of total emotional and behavioral problems were found using a preschool version of the CBCL (Utens et al., 2001).

Several studies showed significant higher levels of internalizing problems in children with CHD in comparison to normative samples (Fredriksen et al., 2004; Gupta et al., 2001; Hövels-Gürich et al., 2002; Oates et al., 1994). Increased levels of withdrawn behavior (Casey et al., 1996; Utens et al., 1993; Van der Rijken et al., 2007), somatic complaints (Casey et al., 1996; Fredriksen et al., 2004; Utens et al., 1993; Van der Rijken et al., 2007) as well as anxiety and depression (Gupta et al., 2001; Utens et al., 1993) were reported for children with CHD.

Externalizing problems have also been found in children with CHD (Hövels-Gürich et al., 2002; Utens et al., 1993). Increased scores were found on both delinquent and aggressive behaviors in comparison to normative groups (Utens et al., 1993).

Internalizing problems have been reported to occur more often in children with CHD than externalizing problems (Utens et al., 1993). The meta-analysis of Karsdorp et al. (2007) revealed a medium estimate of effect size for internalizing problems (unbiased estimate effect size: 0.47), and only a small estimate of effect size for externalizing problems in children with CHD (unbiased estimate effect size: 0.19).

Besides internalizing and externalizing problems, elevated levels of attention problems (Miatton et al., 2007; Utens et al., 1993; Van der Rijken et al., 2007), social problems (Casey et al., 1996, Fredriksen et al., 2004; Utens et al., 1993), and thought problems (Fredriksen et al., 2004; Utens et al., 1993) were also reported in children with CHD, when assessed with the CBCL.

A recent meta-analysis by Karsdorp et al. (2007), which includes most of the above mentioned studies, confirms that children with CHD exhibit more total, internalizing and externalizing problems, compared to children from normal populations. However, it is important to note that early studies (Oates et al., 1994; Utens et al., 1993) include patients who were operated for CHD in the 1970s, whereas, the most recent studies (Miatton et al., 2007; Van der Rijken et al., 2007) include patients who received operation for CHD in the 1990s. Since major advances took place in the treatment of congenital heart disease since the 1990s, the chronological aspects of these studies should be considered. A recent study of Spijkerboer et al. (2008), in which emotional and behavioral outcomes of children treated recently were compared to those of *same-age patients*, operated before 1980 ("historical sample"), revealed that the level of emotional and behavioral problems of the recent sample was comparable to that of the historical sample. The recent and historical sample both consisted of four diagnostic groups: atrial septal defect, ventricular septal defect, transposition of the great arteries, and pulmonary stenosis. Despite the major advances in medical treatment, children with CHD who were treated recently thus still seem to experience the same level of emotional and behavioral problems compared to their counterparts who were operated a few decades ago.

Regarding the generalization of the above discussed study results, it is also important to note that samples are generally heterogeneous as to age and cardiac diagnosis. Therefore, the role of gender, age, and cardiac diagnosis will be further discussed in later sections.

Critical Remark Regarding Use of the CBCL

The CBCL is a psychometrically sound, internationally well-known instrument to assess emotional and behavioral problems in children, but a critical remark can be made regarding its use for children with CHD. Problems arise with the syndrome scales Withdrawn and Somatic complaints, which both load on the broad area of internalizing problems. Withdrawn comprises the item "underactive," and the scale Somatic complaints contains the items "dizzy," "tired," and "headaches." These items resemble potential, actual somatic symptoms in children with CHD, and may therefore represent the children's medical condition, rather than internalizing problems. This problem can be dealt with by executing statistical analyses with and without these "difficult" items. In two studies (Casey et al.,1996; Utens et al., 1993), efforts were made to correct for this problem. Casey et al. (1996) found that, after adjusting, the parents' reports of somatic complaints in children with CHD were no longer significantly higher than those in the group of controls. The higher reports of withdrawn behavior in children with CHD, compared

to those of the controls, were reduced to borderline significance. In contrast, Utens et al. (1993), comparing the results of analyses with inclusion versus exclusion of all somatic items, found that differences in emotional and behavioral problems between the sample of children with CHD and the normative group were slightly smaller after exclusion of somatic items, but still remained significant. One difference between both studies is that Casey et al. (1996) studied the effect of omitting somatic items on the two scales Withdrawn and Somatic complaints, whereas Utens et al. (1993) did so for the overall rating, the total problem score. Another difference is that the sample studied by Casey et al. (1996) consisted of children with severe CHD, while in the sample studied by Utens et al. (1993) less severe diagnoses were also included.

In conclusion, when using the CBCL for children with symptomatic CHD, results on the Internalizing, Withdrawn and Somatic complaints scales must be interpreted carefully.

Studies Using Specific Instruments: Medical-Related Fears, Anxiety, and Depression

Some studies used instruments to focus more specifically on medical-related fears, anxiety. or depression. In an early study, Kramer et al. (1989) reported an elevated level of basic anxiety, using the Personality Questionnaire for Children (Seitz and Rausche, 1976) in children with CHD and additional physical limitations. In a recent study, Gupta et al. (2001), using the Fear Survey Schedule Revised (Ollendick, 1983), reported more fears of injury and more medical fears in children with CHD in comparison to normative groups. Furthermore, when using the Revised Child Manifest Anxiety Scale (Reynolds and Richmond, 1990), they found that their CHD sample reported higher levels of physiological anxiety. This indicates that the children with CHD showed more expression of physical manifestations of anxiety, such as sweating and nausea, compared to normative groups. In another study (Gupta et al., 1998) results on the Child Depression Inventory (Kovacs, 1992) indicated symptoms of anhedonia (inability to experience pleasure in daily life) and interpersonal problems in children with CHD.

In conclusion, in line with the previously described studies using the CBCL, results of studies with specific instruments also showed elevated levels of internalizing problems (e.g., anxiety and depression) for children with CHD.

Role of Gender and Age

The role of gender in the occurrence of emotional and behavioral problems in children with CHD has rarely been examined. All studies, which studied the role of gender (Fredriksen et al., 2004; Spijkerboer et al., 2007; Utens et al., 1993, 2001; Van der Rijken et al., 2007), used the CBCL (except for one early study: DeMaso et al., 1990). In most of these studies, no effect of gender was found (DeMaso et al., 1990; Spijkerboer et al., 2007; Utens et al., 1993, 2001; Van der Rijken et al., 2007). Fredriksen et al. (2004) reported higher levels of total problems, externalizing problems, attention problems, delinquency, and aggression on the CBCL for boys with CHD compared to girls with CHD, indicating better outcomes for young female patients. Although these results might reflect trends in the general population as to differences between boys and girls, the CHD boys in the sample of Fredriksen et al. (2004) showed higher levels of mainly externalizing problems, compared to normative groups, while the CHD girls did not.

As to the influence of age, in an early Dutch cohort study, no effect of age was found, comparing emotional and behavioral problems of 10- to 12-year-old versus those of 13- to 15-year-old CHD children, assessed with the CBCL (Utens et al., 1993). Within a recent sample of patients awaiting elective cardiac surgery or catheter intervention, again no differences were found in the level of emotional and behavioral problems of two age categories: 2- to 3-year-old versus 4- to 7-year-old CHD patients (Utens et al., 2001). Neither differences were found comparing emotional and behavioral problems reported on the CBCL of 7- to 12-year-old versus 13- to 17-year-old CHD patients treated between 1990 and 1995 (Spijkerboer et al., 2007). In a sample of 8- to 14-year-old patients with transposition of the great arteries (operated with the arterial switch procedure), Hövels-Gürich et al. (2002) reported that older age was associated with more externalizing problems on the CBCL. Fredriksen et al. (2004) found higher levels of social problems in 11- to 13-year-old patients with various types of CHD, compared to 14- to 16-year-old patients from the same sample. Possibly, more emotional and behavior problems occur when puberty sets in. In accordance with these previous findings, a meta-analysis by Karsdorp et al. (2007) revealed that older children (ages 10 years or older), show more total, internalizing and to a lesser extent externalizing problems compared to normative groups, whereas for younger children with CHD, this is less the case.

Overall, the results concerning the effect of gender on emotional and behavioral problems seem ambiguous and should be further investigated. Regarding the role of age, emotional and behavioral problems may increase as puberty sets in. Several explanations for this effect of age can be provided. It has been reported that the normal developmental milestones or barriers in life may result in more emotional struggle for children

with CHD than for healthy children (Garson, 1998; Utens, 1992). During adolescence, young patients with CHD might be hampered in fulfilling the developmental tasks of striving for independence and finding an own identity. An overprotective parenting style (Carey et al., 2002) and difficulties with letting go (Sparacino et al., 1997), which have been reported for parents of children with CHD, might interfere with a child's strive for independence during this period. Furthermore, hormonal changes during adolescence might make a child with CHD more vulnerable for stressful disease experiences (Walker et al., 2004).

Role of Cardiac Diagnosis

Differences in emotional and behavioral problems between different cardiac groups are rarely found. Two early studies, DeMaso et al. (1990) and Utens et al. (1993), included different diagnostic groups with variation in complexity in their studies. They did not find any differences in emotional and behavioral outcomes between the diagnostic groups. In a recent study, Miatton et al. (2007) found no differences in emotional and behavioral problems of children with tetralogy of Fallot who underwent a cardiac procedure, compared to children with acyanotic CHD (ventricular septal defect, atrial septal defect, aortic stenosis, or pulmonic stenosis). Fredriksen et al. (2004) neither found a significant effect of cardiac diagnosis on the level of total, internalizing and externalizing problems on the CBCL, but did find such an effect on somatic complaints. This effect of diagnosis could be attributed to the low scores of the patients with obstruction of the right ventricular outflow tract, which constituted only a small proportion of the total sample (about 10%). It should be considered that this finding might reflect actual somatic instead of psychological symptoms (see previous section on critical remark regarding use of the CBCL).

It could be argued that, in most of the previous studies, the numbers of children in the different diagnostic groups were too small to reveal significant differences between them. However, Fredriksen et al. (2004) found, in a sample of 326 CHD patients, that cardiac diagnosis did not predict emotional and behavioral problems, even when patients were divided into two groups of simple and complex disease. In correspondence with previous findings, the meta-analysis of Karsdorp et al. (2007) showed that disease severity was unrelated to the level of emotional and behavioral problems in children with CHD.

In conclusion, in studies using the CBCL, which measures a broad range of problems to detect psychopathology, hardly any differences between cardiac diagnoses were found. One study that used more specific instruments, however, did report such differences.

Gupta et al. (1998) found that cyanotic CHD children showed more fears of the unknown (e.g., death or dead people, being alone, dark places), more physiological anxiety, and more depression than acyanotic CHD children. This might indicate that, although there seem to be no apparent differences in emotional and behavioral problems between different cardiac diagnostic groups, children with a severe CHD might experience covert specific fears and depressive feelings, which might be related to their medical condition.

Predictors and Correlates

Several studies have tried to unravel predictors and correlates of (long-term) emotional and behavioral problems for children with CHD. The predictors and correlates can be categorized into five different categories. The first and second category of pre- and perioperative variables mainly contain objective medical variables from before and around the time of the heart surgery, which can be considered as *predictors* of long-term psychological outcome. The third, fourth, and fifth categories respectively of physical condition, neuropsychological functioning, and parental functioning contain (postoperative) variables from the present lives of children with CHD. These variables can thus be considered as *correlates* of long-term emotional and behavioral functioning.

(1) *Preoperative variables.* Hövels-Gürich et al. (2002) found that preoperative hypoxia predicted social problems in 8- to 14-year-old children who underwent arterial switch procedure for transposition of the great arteries ($n = 60$). In line with these findings, Utens et al. (1998) reported that low systemic oxygen saturation predicted internalizing problems in 10- to 15-year-old children with CHD ($n = 125$). In addition, a relatively short duration of pregnancy put these children at a greater risk for internalizing problems.

(2) *Perioperative variables.* Bellinger et al. (1997) investigated 171 children with transposition of the great arteries who underwent an arterial switch operation with either predominantly total circulatory arrest or predominantly continuous low-flow cardiopulmonary bypass. They found that, according to parents' reports (CBCL), children in the circulatory arrest group showed higher internalizing and depressive problems compared to those from the low-flow bypass group (at 2.5 years of age). Likewise, Utens et al. (1998) reported that the use of deep hypothermic circulatory arrest during the first heart operation predicted both total and internalizing problems in a cohort of CHD children, at least 9 years after cardiac surgery. Hövels-Gürich et al. (2002) found that peri- and postoperative cardio-circulatory insufficiency predicted total, internalizing, externalizing, and attention problems, 8–14 years after

neonatal arterial switch operation for transposition of the great arteries. The number of heart operations was found to predict total, internalizing, as well as externalizing problems in 10- to 15-year-old CHD children (Utens et al., 1998). Children with an older age at surgical repair appeared to have a greater risk to developing internalizing problems (Utens et al., 1998). Van der Rijken et al. (2007) found that children with the highest level of complexity of cardiac surgery showed more withdrawn behavior, somatic complaints, and attention problems compared to children with lower levels of surgical complexity ($n = 101$).

(3) *Physical condition of CHD children.* Fredriksen et al. (2000) found a decrease of internalizing problems in children and adolescents with CHD after they were submitted to a physical training intervention and improved their physical condition ($n = 129$). Fredriksen et al. (2004) reported that the parents' estimation of how far their CHD children ($n = 326$) could run, predicted the level of total, internalizing, and externalizing problems in their children.

(4) *Neuropsychological functioning of CHD children.* In an early study, DeMaso et al. (1990) found that lower intelligence and impairment of the central nervous system predicted worse psychological functioning in children with cyanotic CHD ($n = 140$). Bellinger et al. (1997) reported that 2.5-year-old CHD children with an additional expressive language delay demonstrated increased internalizing problems, social withdrawal, depression, and destructive behavior, according to their parents' reports (CBCL). Similarly, Hövels-Gürich et al. (2002) reported that reduced expressive language capacity was a significant predictor for total emotional and behavioral problems in 8- to 14-year-old children with transposition of the great arteries (operated with the arterial switch procedure).

(5) *Parental functioning.* Gupta et al. (1998) reported that maternal anxiety was associated with higher fears of the unknown, fears of injury, medical fears, and emotional and behavioral problems in general in children with CHD ($n = 39$). Goldberg et al. (1997), in a study of pediatric samples, found that parental stress during the first 3 years of life of their children with CHD ($n = 48$) predicted behavioral problems in their children at 4 years of age. Similarly, Visconti et al. (2002), in a study of children who underwent arterial switch procedure for transposition of the great arteries ($n = 153$), found that parents, who reported higher levels of stress when their child was 1 and 4 years old, also reported more behavioral problems in their child at the age of 4.

To summarize, a wide range of pre- and perioperative medical predictors (preoperative hypoxia, circulatory arrest during heart surgery, number of heart operations, etc.) appear to be associated with elevated levels of emotional and behavioral problems in children with

CHD. Furthermore, postoperative, present variables (physical condition and neuropsychological problems) form a risk factor for emotional and behavioral problems. Finally, parental anxiety and distress have been found to be associated with psychological maladjustment in children with CHD.

Although the above mentioned variables from the pre-, peri-, and postoperative course have been found to either predict or be associated with emotional and behavioral problems in children with CHD, their enduring influence on the patients' adult lives can be questioned. Van Rijen et al. (2004) studied the predictive value of medical variables, covering the complete medical course from birth up till adulthood, for long-term behavioral and emotional problems in adulthood, in a sample of 362 patients who were operated for CHD in childhood. Remarkably, they found that predictor variables from these patients' childhood, such as early hospitalizations with reoperations, were still predictive for emotional and behavioral problems in adulthood, as reported by informants familiar to the patient (e.g., the patients' parents or partners). These variables, however, were unrelated to the adult patients' functioning, according to patients' self-reports. Emotional and behavioral problems as reported by the adult patients themselves instead were predicted by variables from the patients' current lives and recent medical experiences. Patients who felt restricted by the surgical scar, who were found to have a low maximum exercise capacity on the bicycle ergometry test, or who had to deal with restrictions imposed by their physicians, were at risk for self-reported emotional and behavioral problems. Predictors and correlates of emotional and behavioral problems may thus be different for children versus adults with CHD. It is important that health care professionals, who work with upgrowing patients with CHD, keep up with the experiences and different life events that are relevant to their patients and may possibly lead to emotional and behavioral problems.

Longitudinal Development

Follow-up studies, with repeated measures of emotional and behavioral problems in children, adolescents and young adults with CHD over a long time period, have rarely been performed. In the Netherlands, longitudinal assessments of psychological functioning have been performed (Utens et al., 1993, 1998; Van Rijen, 2003; Van Rijen et al., 2004, 2005) in a cohort of patients with CHD, respectively 10–20 years (first follow-up) and 20–30 years (second follow-up) after the first open heart surgery in childhood. For assessment in childhood and adolescence (first follow-up), the CBCL, the parent report, and the Youth Self-Report (YSR; Achenbach, 1991b), a self-report for 11- to 17-year-olds with parallel items as in the CBCL, were used (Utens et al., 1993). In young adulthood (second follow-up), parallel versions of these instruments were used: the Young Adult Behavior Checklist (YABCL) (Achenbach, 1997) was filled in by either a parent or the partner of the patient, and the Young Adult Self-Report (YASR) (Achenbach, 1997) was filled in by the patients themselves (Van Rijen, 2003; Van Rijen et al., 2005). These longitudinal data provided the unique opportunity to compare levels of emotional and behavioral problems from childhood to young adulthood (Van Rijen, 2003) and from adolescence to young adulthood (Van Rijen et al., 2005). Only comparisons were made using the same type of informant (self or other) at the first and second follow-up (reports by parents or partners: CBCL, YABCL; self-reports: YSR-YASR). Table 20–1 shows the odds ratios for the longitudinal comparison of scoring in the deviant (psychopathological) range of total problems, from childhood (CBCL) to young adulthood (YABCL), for both gender groups, as well as for the total sample. The results showed that children who fell in the deviant range of emotional and behavioral problems during childhood, had a 3.1 time higher change of still falling into this deviant range during young adulthood ($n = 93$) (Van Rijen, 2003). Especially boys with emotional and behavioral problems were at risk for still having these problems in young adulthood. Similar results were found for the comparison from adolescence (YSR) to young adulthood (YASR) (Van Rijen et al., 2005). Adolescents who fell in the deviant range of emotional and behavioral problems during adolescence, had a 3.4 time higher chance of still falling into this deviant range during young adulthood

TABLE 20–1. *Odds Ratios for the Longitudinal Comparison of Scoring in the Deviant Range from Childhood to Young Adulthood Total Problems*

Childhood CBCL—Young Adulthood YABCL	Odds Ratios	95% Confidence Interval
Males	6.2	1.4–27.9
Females	1.6	0.4–6.9
Total sample	3.1	1.1–8.8

Abbreviations: CBCL, Child Behavior Checklist; YABCL, Young Adult Behavior Checklist.

($n = 127$). Again, adolescent males had the highest risk of maintaining their problem level into adulthood.

Conclusions and Practical Implications for Emotional and Behavioral Problems

Emotional and behavioral problems have frequently been observed in children with severe CHD, as well as in children with mild cardiac diagnoses. These problems are often related to the course of medical events or the subsequent consequences for the young patients' lives. The chances that emotional and behavioral problems in children with CHD persist into adulthood are considerable. Emotional and behavioral problems in children with CHD should therefore be taken seriously. Special attention should be given to screening and identifying children with emotional and/or behavioral problems at an early age, in order to provide them with adequate services and prevent the development of additional psychosocial problems into adolescence and adulthood.

Especially adolescents with CHD should be carefully monitored during their cardiac consultations, since the problem level seems to peak in the early teenage years. Moreover, during adolescence, CHD patients may experience difficulties with the transition from the child cardiologist to the adult cardiologist (Tong and Kools, 2004). This process should be carefully guided (Fernandes and Landzberg, 2004), moreover since adolescent and young adult patients with CHD often seem to lack information concerning their medical condition (Moons et al., 2001; Van Deyk et al., 2004). In order to achieve a successful transition, in which the adolescent learns to take responsibility for his or her health, it is important that the cardiologist addresses the young patient directly (instead of focusing on the parents when discussing the patient's health) (Van Deyk et al., 2004) and that the adolescent patient is given the feeling that he or she is taken seriously (Tong and Kools, 2004). Young patients with CHD should be provided with an environment, which enables them to become autonomic and self-reliant adults.

Overall, internalizing problems seem to be more prominently present in children with CHD, compared to externalizing problems. These internalizing problems might include anxiety and depression, but also specific medical-related fears (e.g., for somatic symptoms or death). These problems often are difficult to detect since they usually are not overtly expressed or reported by the patient. Therefore, health care professionals should be alert to symptoms that might indicate such feelings. Especially for shy and timid young patients, it may be easier to express feelings of anxiety and depression on a short screening questionnaire.

SELF-CONCEPT

Regarding the psychological well-being of children with CHD, not only emotional and behavioral problems are of interest, but also how these children perceive and judge themselves. Self-concept refers to the composite of beliefs and feelings that a person holds about him- or herself (Salzer-Muhar et al., 2002). Self-concept can consist of various physical, psychological, or social attributes, which generally constitute a very persistent mental conceptualization about oneself. To give two widely differing examples, one child might view him- or herself as a good-looking, intelligent child with lots of friends, another child might think of him- or self as a skinny, nervous child with whom nobody wants to play.

Several authors have studied self-concepts of children with CHD (Chen et al., 2005; Kramer et al., 1989; Salzer-Muhar et al., 2002; Wray and Sensky, 1998). Unlike the area of emotional and behavioral problems, which is dominated by a cross-culturally widely used standardized instrument (CBCL), there is a lot of variation in methods used to assess self-concepts of children with CHD. In an early study, Kramer et al. (1989) used a German list, the Personality Questionnaire for Children (Seitz and Rausche, 1976), in a sample of 77 CHD children (age range: 4–14 years). They found that patients with additional physical limitations experienced more feelings of impulsiveness and inferiority compared to healthy controls. Patients without additional physical limitations, however, did not show differences in self-concepts compared to their healthy peers. More recently, Wray and Sensky (1998) used a visual analogue scale to study the perception of actual versus ideal self in 5- to 15-year-old CHD patients, prior to and one year after cardiac surgery. Preoperatively, children with CHD rated themselves as weaker, more frightened and more ill, compared to a healthy group. Postoperatively, no differences were found between self-perceptions of the CHD group and the healthy children. Differences between self and ideal self ratings were similar for the CHD and healthy children, both pre- as postoperatively. Salzer-Muhar et al. (2002) studied different dimensions of self-concepts with the Frankfurter Selbstkonzept Skalen (Deusinger, 1986) in 12- to 16-year-old CHD patients ($n = 48$). In this study, boys with CHD showed impaired self-concepts regarding achievement (e.g., overall capability), whereas girls with CHD presented with self-concepts, which were comparable to normative groups. It was argued that reduced physical abilities interfere with the peer relationships of boys, and not so much with those of girls. Chen et al. (2005) used another questionnaire with a special focus on self-concepts, the Self-Concept Scale (Hou, 2001), in 64 9- to 12-year-old

CHD patients. They found that children with CHD showed lower self-concepts as to physical functioning compared to healthy peers, but otherwise had normal self-concepts regarding the family, school, appearance, and emotional functioning.

Body Image

Body image refers to perception of one's own physical appearance. This concept thus partly overlaps with self-concept. Aldén et al. (1998) studied the body-images of 31 children with transposition of the great arteries (mean age: 13 years) who were operated with the Senning or Mustard procedure, by a test in which children were requested to draw a person, the Machover Draw A Person Test (Kälvesten, 1965). The boys were found to perform significantly worse than the girls on this test, indicating poor body images in the boys. Vessey and O'Sullivan (2000) studied the knowledge that children with CHD had regarding their internal bodies, and the monetary values that children placed on their body parts. The children with CHD did not differ from their healthy peers in their knowledge of body parts and body part functions. Nor did the children with CHD differ from the control group in the values they assigned to the heart.

Conclusions and Practical Implications for Self-Concept

Overall, it may be concluded that problems with achievement and physical abilities are reflected in the self-concepts of children with CHD. The large variation in methods, however, makes it difficult to compare the results from various studies into self-concepts. International consensus regarding assessment of self-concept in children with CHD is therefore desirable.

Physical limitations may harm self-concepts of children with CHD. Kramer et al. (1989) found that CHD children with additional physical limitations showed feelings of inferiority. Self-concepts of children with CHD have been reported to improve after cardiac surgery (Wray and Sensky, 1998). Some investigators (Aldén et al., 1998; Salzer-Muhar et al., 2002) found that particularly boys with CHD appeared to have reduced self-concepts as to physical functioning and impaired body-images. As suggested by Salzer-Muhar et al. (2002), it might be that, regarding their peer group activities at school as well as during leisure time, boys are far more dependent from their physical performance and physical capacity compared to girls.

In order to reduce the negative effects of physical limitations on the self-concepts of children with CHD, Garson (1998) advises to find compensatory activities for the child, at which he or she is good at, such as music, writing, etc. When a child is unable to participate in a strenuous competitive sports activity, he or she could be offered the special task of referee. It is essential that parents encourage their older children to participate in daily peer activities and relationships to strengthen their self-esteem.

Moreover, it is also important that young CHD patients are well-informed about their physical abilities. A study of Moons et al. (2001) found that 20%–30% of a sample of young CHD patients did not know whether or not physical activities were contraindicated. This might lead to inappropriate restrictions. Monitored physical training might help children with CHD to overcome feelings of insecurity about their bodily functioning (Fredriksen et al., 2000).

ACADEMIC FUNCTIONING

Parents of children with CHD have reported poorer school performance in their offspring compared to parents of healthy children (Hövels-Gürich et al., 2002; Miatton et al., 2007). Teacher reports regarding school functioning and results on psychological tests for academic achievement provide additional insight into the actual academic functioning of children with CHD. The focus of this section will not be on intellectual functioning (intelligence or neuropsychological functioning) of children with CHD, but will specifically discuss the following aspects of their academic functioning: (a) emotional and behavioral problems at school, (b) academic achievement, (c) learning difficulties, and (d) rates of children who have repeated classes or attend special education.

Emotional and Behavioral Problems at School

To assess emotional and behavioral problems in the school context, a parallel version of the parent-report CBCL (see previous section on the CBCL), the Teacher Report Form (TRF; Achenbach, 1991c; Achenbach and Rescorla, 2001) is available. The TRF is a standardized report on children's or adolescents' emotional and behavioral problems during the previous 2 months, to be completed by teachers. The items and scales of the TRF are similar to those of the CBCL.

Several studies have used the TRF to assess emotional and behavioral problems that CHD children demonstrate at school. Oates et al. (1994) found that teachers of 7- to 15-year-old CHD patients with either transposition of the great arteries, tetralogy of Fallot, ventricular septal defect, or atrial septal defect did not report more internalizing, externalizing, or total problems for their pupils, compared to teachers of healthy controls. Wright and Nolan (1994) neither found any significant differences between teacher reports regarding 7- to 12-year-old children with transposition of the great arteries (operated with the Senning procedure) or tetralogy of Fallot and those regarding control children with innocent heart murmurs. Casey et al. (1996) found higher teacher reports of withdrawn behavior, somatic complaints, and internalizing problems in children with surgically palliated complex CHD, compared to children with innocent heart murmurs. However, after adjusting for items with a somatic content (see previous section on critical remark regarding use of the CBCL), significant differences between both groups were no longer found. Karl et al. (2004), who used a self-designed list based on the TRF, reported that teachers reported more withdrawn, restless, and inattentive behavior in 4- to 13-year-old children with transposition of the great arteries (operated with the arterial switch procedure), compared to teacher reports of the patients' best friends.

The TRF also contains additional competence scales. On these scales, no significant differences were found between social competence (Oates et al., 1994) and school adjustment (Casey et al., 1996) of CHD children, and those of healthy controls.

In an early study, the severity of the CHD and the intelligence level of CHD children (Youssef, 1988) appeared to be associated with teacher reports regarding emotional and behavioral problems in these children. Casey et al. (1996) found that family strain (impact of the child's chronic condition on the family's functioning) and exercise tolerance (functional physical ability) were strong predictors of school adjustment in CHD children, as reported by the teachers on the TRF. Children with more severe CHD, poorer physical abilities, and higher levels of family strains as a result of CHD might thus be at risk for emotional and behavioral maladjustment at school. Higher intelligence might be a protective factor.

Overall, teacher reports of emotional and behavioral problems in children with CHD appear to be similar to those of healthy peers or those with innocent heart murmurs. Withdrawn behavior or somatic complaints have been reported by teachers of CHD children. Those reports may reflect children's medical symptoms. Oates et al. (1994) and Wright and Nolan (1994) both found that parents reported higher degrees of emotional and behavioral problems in CHD children, compared to the children's teachers, whose reports were comparable to reference groups. Different explanations for these findings could be provided. CHD children might actually demonstrate different behaviors at home and at school. Parents may be more sensitive and alert to problems of the child compared to teachers. Children with CHD mostly show internalizing problems (see previous section on emotional and behavioral problems), which are often difficult to detect and nonintrusive in the classroom. Finally an explanation might be that parental overprotection and stress (Carey et al., 2002; Visconti et al., 2002) can play a role in high parents' reports of problem behavior in CHD children.

Academic Achievement

Studies on the academic achievement of children with CHD have largely used internationally well-known instruments, such as the Wide Range Achievement Test—Revised (Jastak and Wilkinson, 1984), used by Wright and Nolan (1994) and Wernovsky et al. (2000); the Kaufman Assessment Battery for Children (Kaufman and Kaufman, 1983), used by Wernovsky et al. (2000) and Hövels-Gürich et al. (2006); the Wechsler Individual Achievement Test (Wechsler, 1992), used by Bellinger et al. (2003) and McGrath et al. (2004), and the British Ability Scales (Elliott, 1983), used by Wray and Sensky (2001). These tests for academic achievement cover (pre-)academic abilities in the areas of arithmetic, reading, and spelling.

Wernovsky et al. (2000) studied academic performance of patients with single ventricles (mean age: 11 years), who were palliated with the Fontan procedure. Compared with normative data, younger (5 years or younger) as well as older (older than 5 years) children from the patient sample obtained a significantly worse composite achievement score. Wright and Nolan (1994) reported significantly worse performances in arithmetic, reading, and spelling in 7- to 12-year-old children with transposition of the great arteries (operated with the Senning procedure) or tetralogy of Fallot, compared to control children with innocent murmurs. In a sample of 4- to 12-year-old children with tetralogy of Fallot or ventricular septal defect, Hövels-Gürich et al. (2006) found a dysfunction in academic knowledge in 30% of the children, which was higher compared to normative groups. Bellinger et al. (2003) reported significantly poorer performance in 8-year-old children who underwent arterial switch procedure for transposition of the great arteries, on reading and mathematics composite scores, as well as on the subabilities basic reading, reading comprehension, spelling, and numerical operations, compared to a normative group. Wray and Sensky (2001) studied arithmetic, reading, and spelling abilities in 3- to 14-year-old CHD children, with cyanotic as well as acyanotic lesions. Pre- as well as postoperatively, the academic attainments of the CHD sample were comparable to those of healthy peers.

Complex and cyanotic CHD has been reported to be associated with poor academic achievement (Wernovsky et al., 2000; Wray and Sensky, 2001). Mental and psychomotor development at the age of one has been found to predict academic achievement at the age of eight in children with transposition of the great arteries who were operated with the arterial switch procedure (McGrath et al., 2004). Prior use of circulatory arrest during cardiac surgery or reoperation with cardiopulmonary bypass within 30 days after Fontan procedure have been reported to be risk factors for low academic achievement in patient with single ventricles (Wernovsky et al., 2000). Wray and Sensky (2001) found a significant negative correlation between age at surgical repair and arithmetic ability in children with cyanotic as well as in children with acyanotic lesions. Bellinger et al. (2003) found no differences between academic achievements of children with transposition of the great arteries who were either operated with predominantly circulatory arrest or predominantly low-flow cardiopulmonary bypass. Wright and Nolan (1994) found no significant association for academic achievement with several medical and surgical parameters, including age at operation, duration of cardiac arrest, or bypass and hypoxia.

In sum, most studies of academic achievement in CHD children report poorer performance compared to control groups in various areas (arithmetic, reading, and spelling). One exception is the study of Wray and Sensky (2001) who reported academic abilities similar to those of normative groups. In their study, the majority of the sample had acyanotic lesions, whereas most other studies encompassed children with more severe CHD. Besides severity of the cardiac diagnosis, several surgical variables (circulatory arrest, early reoperation, age at surgical repair) have been reported to be associated with poor academic achievement in CHD children (Wernovsky et al., 2000; Wray and Sensky, 2001). However, based on the current results, no uniform conclusions regarding predictors and correlates of academic achievement in CHD children can be drawn.

Learning Disabilities

Several studies (Bellinger et al., 2003; Ellerbeck et al., 1998; Wernovsky et al., 2000; Wray and Sensky, 2001) have investigated the occurrence of learning disabilities in children with CHD. Learning disabilities were generally defined as discrepancies between intelligence and academic achievement. That is, children whose academic achievements were significantly worse compared to what might have been expected given their intellectual functioning and were considered to have a learning disability. Ellerbeck et al. (1998) reported that 31% of a sample of preschool children with transposition of the great arteries, who had undergone atrial correction or arterial switch procedure, showed deficient early skill acquisition in letter-word identification, applied problems, and dictation, and were therefore at

high risk for developing learning disabilities. Among school-age children with the same cardiac diagnosis, 47% showed learning disabilities in the same areas. These rates were higher compared to those among the children's siblings. Wernovsky et al. (2000) found a lower rate: 5.5% of their sample of patients with single ventricles were reported to have a learning disability, considering their composite scores of (pre) academic abilities of reading, spelling, and arithmetic. In the study of Wray and Sensky (2001), rates of learning disabilities concerning arithmetic and reading in the total sample of children with CHD were comparable to those found in healthy peers. However, reading problems were more frequent in cyanotic than in acyanotic patients. Bellinger et al. (2003) reported that their sample of 8-year-old children with transposition of the great arteries showed learning deficits in the areas of reading, arithmetic, as well as spelling. Overall 37% of the children had at least one academic achievement score that was significantly lower than expected, given their intelligence. Children who were operated with predominantly total circulatory arrest demonstrated more learning difficulties as to reading comprehension, compared to children who were operated with predominantly low-flow cardiopulmonary bypass.

Repeating Classes and Attendance of Special Education

Miatton et al. (2007) found that significantly more school-age children with tetralogy of Fallot (mean age: 8 years) had to repeat a school year, compared to healthy peers (16.7% versus 5.6%). Bellinger et al. (2003) reported that 10% of their sample of 8-year-old children with transposition of the great arteries had repeated a grade in the past. Among children with single ventricles, palliated with the Fontan procedure, aged 6–17 years, 21.6% was reported to be held back in school at some time (Wernovsky et al., 2000). Problems in academic achievement and absence from school due to medical treatment and hospitalizations might play a role in the high rates of CHD children who have to repeat a class.

In a very early study, O'Dougherty et al. (1983) reported that 42% of a sample of children with transposition of the great arteries required special education services. In a recent study, Bellinger et al. (2003) reported that 37% of children with transposition of the great arteries (operated with the arterial switch procedure) needed remedial services in school. Wright and Nolan (1994) reported that 28% of children with transposition of the great arteries (operated with the Senning procedure) or tetralogy of Fallot had been referred for extra assistance at school. Van Rijen et al. (2003) reported that 27% of adult patients (age range: 20–46 years) with CHD had followed some sort of special education during childhood or adolescence. Of these patients, 85% attended schools for learning-disabled or mentally handicapped children and 15% for chronically ill children.

In conclusion, research findings show that CHD children are at risk for repeating a grade at school. A substantial part of the children with transposition of the great arteries appears to be in need of special education or remedial teaching services. Further research should focus on identifying whether such needs (and if which special needs) exist in CHD children with other diagnoses.

Conclusions and Practical Implications for Academic Functioning

Although emotional and behavioral problems at school are not so prevalent in children with CHD, these children are at risk for poor academic achievement and learning difficulties. In accordance with the predictors and correlates found for emotional and behavioral problems as reported by parents (see first section of the chapter), surgical and neuropsychological variables, as well as variables regarding physical condition and parental (family) functioning have been reported to be associated with either emotional and behavioral problems at school and/or academic achievement in children with CHD. Correlates and predictors of academic functioning, however, have not been studied as thoroughly as those of emotional and behavioral problems. Delays in academic achievement and learning difficulties are nevertheless clearly demonstrated in CHD children, especially in those with severe CHD, and deserve appropriate attention.

Teacher reports can provide additional and valuable information on how children with CHD are functioning, not only regarding their academic achievements, but also regarding their behavior at school. Remedial services should be offered when children with CHD get in danger of lagging behind their classmates, or when learning disabilities occur. Since neuropsychological deficits can contribute to a lowered school competency in CHD children (Miatton et al., 2007), early neuropsychological screening is useful to detect academic difficulties in children with CHD at an early stage.

QUALITY OF LIFE

Mortality and morbidity have traditionally been considered the main outcomes when studying the (long-term) results of surgical interventions for CHD in childhood. It has become increasingly clear that improved long-term survival may result in long-term morbidity and consequently quality of life has also become an important outcome measure (Spijkerboer et al., 2006). There is, however, no international consensus yet concerning the definition and measurement of quality of life (Moons et al., 2004). This section will discuss (a) the concept of quality of life, (b) results of empirical studies into health-related quality of life in children with CHD, (c) the role of gender and age, (d) the role of cardiac diagnosis, (e) predictors and correlates, and (f) agreement between informants on health-related quality of life.

The Concept of Quality of Life

Young CHD patients and their cardiologists may have different perceptions of the severity of the patients' condition (Falk et al., 2006; Kendall et al., 2001). The way CHD children experience and subjectively evaluate their health can be very determining for their well-being. This phenomenon is generally referred to as "quality of life."

In the literature on the concept of quality of life, the terms health status and health-related quality of life are sometimes used as equivalents, but should instead be clearly distinguished (Kamphuis et al., 2002). Health status refers to the patient's perception of his or her actual, more objective problems and limitations in functioning, whereas health-related quality of life includes the patient's subjective, emotional evaluation, and reaction to such problems and limitations.

Since assessment of health-related quality of life provides a more overall image of how CHD children experience and evaluate their health and limitations due to CHD subjectively, the next section will focus on studies into this area.

Empirical Studies into Health-Related Quality of Life

Only a few studies have explicitly studied health-related quality of life in children with CHD. There is little variation in instruments that have been applied to assess health-related quality of life in children with CHD.

Culbert et al. (2003), Dunbar-Masterson et al. (2001), Majnemer et al. (2006), and McCrindle et al. (2006) all used the Child Health Questionnaire (Landgraf et al., 1996). This questionnaire is a generic instrument that mainly assesses the perceived physical and psychosocial health status (and not the patient's subjective emotional evaluation and reaction to actual physical limitations and problems). In most studies, the results on the Child Health Questionnaire are correctly referred to as "health status," however, incorrect references to "health-related quality of life" have occasionally been made. Anyhow, the concept health-related quality of life is not adequately covered by the Child Health Questionnaire. In this section, results of studies that used this instrument will therefore be referred to as "perceived physical and psychosocial health status." Besides summary scores for physical and psychosocial health status, the Child Health Questionnaire provides information on more specific domains. Domains that contribute to physical health status include physical functioning, role/social limitations due to physical functioning, bodily pain, and general health perceptions. Domains that contribute to psychosocial health status include mental health, role/social limitations due to emotional and behavioral problems, general behavior, and self-esteem.

Uzark et al. (2003) developed the Pediatric Quality of Life Inventory Cardiac Module (a disease-specific instrument). This instrument consists of the Pediatric Quality of Life Inventory generic scales with additional cardiac items appended to it. The generic scales encompass physical and psychosocial health, emotional, social, and school functioning. The cardiac module measures heart problems or symptoms, appearance, treatment anxiety, cognitive problems, and communication.

Spijkerboer et al. (2006) used the TNO-AZL Child Quality of Life Questionnaire (Vogels et al., 2000), a generic instrument. The surplus value of this instrument is that it assesses the occurrence of functional problems on several domains of health-related quality of life (pain and physical symptoms, motor functioning, autonomy, cognitive functioning, and social functioning). If such problems do occur, the (negative) emotional reactions to these problems are assessed too. Furthermore, the questionnaire contains separate items regarding positive and negative emotional functioning.

The instruments used have in common in that they cover physical, social, and emotional domains of a child's functioning. Moreover, all three instruments have parents and child versions and can be used for assessment of both children and adolescents.

Dunbar-Masterson et al. (2001) reported that, according to parents' reports, the physical and psychosocial health status of a sample of 7- to 10-year-old children with transposition of the great arteries (operated with the arterial switch procedure) was similar to that in the general population. Culbert et al. (2003) even found better self-reported (physical and psychosocial) health status on nearly all domains in adolescents with transposition of the great arteries (mean age: 13 years, operated with either arterial switch, Senning, Mustard, or Rastelli procedure), compared to the normative population. Majnemer et al. (2006) found so called normal parent-reported levels of psychosocial and physical health status in 5-year-old CHD children with different cardiac diagnoses. In comparison to a normative group, significantly more unfavorable

parents' reports of psychosocial and physical health status were reported by McCrindle et al. (2006), for a sample of 6- to 18-year-old patients with single ventricles, who were palliated with the Fontan procedure. Except for bodily pain, on which the patient sample obtained better scores compared to the normative group, and behavior, for which no differences were found, the patients' parents reported worse health status in their children on all other domains. Uzark et al. (2003) studied both self- and parents' reports on health-related quality of life in a heterogeneous sample of 2- to 18-year-old patients, with CHDs that varied from mild to severe or complex. On all domains, the CHD sample showed poorer health-related quality of life compared to a healthy sample (except for physical functioning according to the self-reports). In a sample of 8- to 15-year-old children with atrial septal defect, ventricular septal defect, transposition of the great arteries (operated with arterial switch procedure). or pulmonary stenosis, Spijkerboer et al. (2006) found poorer self-reports of patients regarding motor functioning, cognitive functioning, and positive emotional functioning, compared to those of reference peers.

In sum, studies that used the Child Health Questionnaire show a favorable physical and psychosocial health status in the normal range or even better than the normative population for children with CHD. One exception is the study of McCrindle et al. (2006), who found unfavorable parents' reports of psychosocial and physical health status. However, their sample consisted of patients with complex CHD (single ventricles). Uzark et al. (2003) and Spijkerboer et al. (2006) used different instruments than the Child Health Questionnaire, which were more attuned to health-related quality of life. In both studies, more unfavorable findings were reported for children from varying cardiac diagnostic groups. Future research should be enhanced by the use of an internationally accepted definition of the concept of health-related quality of life and the use of a cross-culturally applicable and disease-specific CHD health-related quality of life questionnaire.

Role of Gender and Age

As for gender effects, Dunbar-Masterson et al. (2001) found no association between gender and (physical and psychosocial) health status. Culbert et al. (2003) reported that male gender was associated with more unfavorable self-reports on emotional and behavioral aspects of perceived health status and female gender was associated with more unfavorable general health perceptions. Spijkerboer et al. (2006) found that girls with CHD reported poorer health-related quality of life on motor functioning, cognitive functioning, and positive emotional functioning compared to same-sex reference peers, while CHD boys only did so for motor functioning and cognitive functioning. No significant differences were found between health-related quality of life of CHD boys and CHD girls, neither on the self reports nor on the parents' reports.

As for effects of age, Spijkerboer et al. (2006) found poorer child self-reports on motor functioning, cognitive functioning, social functioning, and positive emotional functioning in 8- to 11-year-old CHD children compared to same-aged reference peers, whereas for 12- to 15-year-old CHD children, only poorer child reports on motor functioning were found in comparison to same-aged reference groups. According to the parents' reports, 8- to 11-year-old CHD children showed poorer health-related quality of life in the domains of cognitive and emotional functioning compared to reference peers, while 12- to 15-year-old CHD children were comparable to the norm. Within the CHD sample, comparison of the two age categories revealed worse health-related quality of life on positive emotional functioning according to self-reports, and also worse cognitive functioning according to parents' reports for 8- to 11-year-old children, compared to 12- to 15-year-olds.

In conclusion, since only few studies have studied the role of gender on health-related quality of life in children with CHD and since results are indecisive, no firm conclusions can be drawn. One study compared different age categories within a CHD sample (Spijkerboer et al., 2006), indicating poorer health-related quality of life in younger children (11 years or younger) compared to older children.

Role of Cardiac Diagnosis

Dunbar-Masterson et al. (2001) found no association between cardiac diagnosis (transposition of the great arteries with intact ventricular septum versus with ventricular septal defect) and (physical and psychosocial) health status. Culbert et al. (2003) reported that children with simple transposition of the great arteries or children with transposition of the great arteries and ventricular septal defects reported better functioning on the domains physical functioning, general health perceptions, and mental health compared to children with transposition of the great arteries with additional ventricular septal defect and pulmonary stenosis. Uzark et al. (2003) reported that severity of the heart disease was related to cardiac symptom scores on both the self- and parents' reports. Spijkerboer et al. (2006) found no differences in health-related quality of life between children of four cardiac diagnostic groups (arterial septal defect, ventricular septal defect, transposition of the great arteries or pulmonary stenosis), neither on the parents' nor on the children's self-reports.

In sum, results regarding the influence of cardiac diagnoses on health-related quality of life are inconclusive due to different assessment instruments and age ranges. Further research on this topic is needed.

Predictors and Correlates

Some studies have tried to identify predictors and correlates of health-related quality of life for children with CHD. The predictors and correlates are categorized here in a way similar to the previous section regarding predictors and correlates (see section on emotional an behavioral problems). The pre- and perioperative variables can be considered as *predictors* of health-related quality of life. The other categories represent variables from the current lives of patients and should therefore be considered as *correlates* of health-related quality of life.

(1) *Preoperative variables.* In a follow-up study of CHD children with various diagnoses, who had undergone open heart surgery during infancy, Majnemer et al. (2006) reported that results from the preoperative neurological examination (which included reflexes, activity level, etc.; Limperopoulos et al., 2000) significantly predicted physical health status at 5 years of age. Arterial oxygen saturation levels below 85% prior to surgery significantly predicted psychosocial health status in these children at follow-up.

(2) *Perioperative variables.* In a sample of children with transposition of the great arteries, Culbert et al. (2003) reported that repair type (arterial switch operation versus atrial repair [Mustard or Senning]) was related to functioning on nearly all domains of physical and psychosocial health status during follow-up at a mean age of 13 years. Children who had undergone arterial switch operation reported better health status compared to children who had undergone atrial repair. Furthermore, perfusion parameters such as circulatory arrest, ischemic time, duration of cardiopulmonary bypass, and cooling temperature were associated with poorer social and behavioral functioning. In children and adolescents who had undergone Fontan procedure for single ventricles, McCrindle et al. (2006) found that higher patient weight at Fontan procedure, fenestration not performed at Fontan procedure, other surgical procedures performed at Fontan procedure, and arrhythmias occurring during follow-up predicted lower physical health status at follow-up at a mean age of 11 years. Dunbar-Masterson et al. (2001) reported that longer hospital stay after arterial switch operation for transposition of the great arteries during infancy was associated with poorer reports of physical health status at follow-up at a mean age of 8 years. Majnemer et al. (2006) reported that acute postoperative neurological functioning significantly predicted physical

health status at 5 years of age, in children with various CHD diagnoses. Spijkerboer et al. (2006) found no significant differences in self and parent reported health-related quality of life between children treated by surgical intervention (atrial septal defect, ventricular septal defect, transposition of the great arteries) and children treated by catheter intervention (pulmonary stenosis). The age range of the four diagnostic groups was 8–15 years.

(3) *Current medical functioning.* In a sample of children with transposition of the great arteries, Dunbar-Masterson et al. (2001) found an association between other medical conditions (e.g., asthma, diabetes) and psychosocial health status indicated that the presence of more medical conditions was related to worse health status. McCrindle et al. (2006) found similar results for young patients who had undergone Fontan procedure. The presence of additional asthma, nonasthma respiratory problems, and orthopedic problems was associated with lower physical health status. Furthermore, a higher number of currently used medications was also related to lower physical health status.

(4) *Current emotional and behavioral problems and academic achievement.* Dunbar-Masterson et al. (2001) found lower intelligence and lower academic achievement to be related to worse psychosocial health status in children who underwent arterial switch procedure for transposition of the great arteries. McCrindle et al. (2006) reported an association between behavioral problems, anxiety, depression, learning problems, and attention problems on the one hand, and psychosocial health status on the other hand. In this study, learning problems were also found to be related to poorer physical health status.

(5) *Current family situation.* McCrindle et al. (2006) reported lower family income to be related to poorer physical as well as psychosocial health status. Goldbeck and Melches (2006), using a self-designed instrument to assess health-related quality of life (Goldbeck and Braun, 2003) in a heterogeneous sample of CHD children (mean age: 8 years), found an interactive effect between severity of the CHD and social disadvantage. Social disadvantage (regarding family constitution, ethnicity, parental education, and employment) did not affect the health-related quality of life of children with mild CHD, but in children with moderate or severe CHD, social disadvantage appeared to be an additional risk factor for poor health-related quality of life.

In summary, different pre- and perioperative variables seem to predict health-related quality of life in children with CHD. Current medical functioning (e.g., other medical conditions, medication) also appeared to be associated with health-related quality of life. Familial factors should not be overlooked. Social disadvantage of the family puts children with severe CHD at higher risk for poor health-related quality of life. Finally, emotional and behavioral problems and academic achievement in CHD children appeared to be related to psychosocial health status in CHD children.

Agreement between Parent and Child Reports

Only a few studies in this area allowed comparison between parents' reports and children's self-reports using the same instrument. Uzark et al. (2003) reported medium to large correlations between children's and parents' reports of health-related quality of life. Goldbeck and Melches (2005) also found moderate correlations on almost every domain of health-related quality of life. Spijkerboer et al. (2006) reported that CHD children showed poorer self-reports of health-related quality of life on the domains pain and physical symptoms, motor functioning, autonomy and positive emotional functioning, compared to the parents' reports of their functioning.

Conclusions and Practical Implications for Quality of Life

More consensus regarding the definition and instruments used to assess health-related quality of life in CHD children is required. Particularly the concepts health status and health-related quality of life should be clearly distinguished. Differences in results on the Child Health Questionnaire and other instruments that more specifically measure health-related quality of life underline the importance of proper conceptualization.

Predictors and correlates of health-related quality of life are in line with those identified for emotional and behavioral problems and academic functioning. Besides pre- and postoperative variables, variables from the current lives of CHD children (medical functioning, family functioning) are also associated with their health-related quality of life. The previously discussed areas of emotional and behavioral problems and academic functioning were also found to be related to health-related quality of life.

In our opinion, it would be useful to implement in clinical practice a brief, disease-specific, cross-culturally widely applicable screening instrument to assess health-related quality of life of young CHD patients. Patients could complete such a brief screening list just before their medical check-ups at the outpatient pediatric cardiology department. If necessary and indicated, CHD children with poor health-related quality of life could then be adequately referred for counseling, preferably to a health professional (e.g., psychologist) who is specialized in the field of psychological functioning of children with CHD.

FINAL NOTES

Despite major advances in medical treatment for CHD, results from recent studies show that children with CHD may still have emotional and behavioral problems, a negative self-concept, impaired academic functioning and reduced health-related quality of life. It appears that having a CHD in itself, and to a lesser extent the level of severity of the CHD, makes children more vulnerable for psychological problems. Several studies have reported medical and physical factors (pre-, peri-, or postoperative variables) that either predicted or were associated with psychological functioning in CHD children. Although some predictors and correlates were frequently mentioned, their relation to (long-term) psychological outcome is very complex and still a lot remains to be explored. It is however clear that, besides medical and physical variables, environmental factors (e.g., parental stress and anxiety) also play an important role in a child's psychological functioning. When evaluating a child's risk for (long-term) psychological problems, positive as well as negative parental attitudes toward the child's disease should therefore be taken into account. Since psychological problems in childhood may result in problems with psychosocial functioning later in adult life, psychosocial problems should be screened and treated at an early age.

This chapter has focused on research findings regarding psychological aspects of CHD in children. An overview was provided on the methods, more specifically the instruments and definitions that various studies used to assess psychological functioning. Whereas results of research in some domains (emotional and behavioral problems and academic functioning) are fairly consistent, future research should focus on reaching international consensus on methodology in other domains (self-concept and health-related quality of life).

ACKNOWLEDGMENTS

We gratefully acknowledge Dr. J.W. Roos-Hesselink for her advice and constructive comments regarding this chapter.

REFERENCES

Achenbach TM. *Manual for the Child Behavior Checklist/4–18 and 1991 Profile.* Burlington: University of Vermont, Department of Psychiatry; 1991a.

Achenbach TM. *Manual for the Youth Self-Report and 1991 Profile.* Burlington: University of Vermont, Department of Psychiatry; 1991b.

Achenbach TM. *Manual for the Teacher's Report Form and 1991 Profiles.* Burlington: University of Vermont, Department of Psychiatry; 1991c.

Achenbach TM. *Manual for the Young Adult Self-Report and Young Adult Behavior Checklist.* Burlington: University of Vermont, Department of Psychiatry; 1997.

Achenbach TM, Rescorla LA. *Manual for the ASEBA School-Age Forms and Profiles.* Burlington: University of Vermont, Research Center for Children, Youth & Families; 2001.

Aldén B, Gilljam T, Gillberg C. Long-term psychological outcome of children after surgery for transposition of the great arteries. *Acta Paediatr.* 1998;87:405–410.

Bellinger DC, Rappaport LA, Wypij D, Wernovsky G, Newburger JW. Patterns of developmental dysfunction after surgery during infancy to correct transposition of the great arteries. *J Dev Beh Pediatr.* 1997;18:75–83.

Bellinger DC, Wypij D, DuPlessis AJ, et al. Neurodevelopmental status at eight years in children with dextro-transposition of the great arteries: the Boston Circulatory Arrest Trial. *J Thorac Cardiovasc Surg.* 2003;126:1385–1396.

Boneva RS, Botto LD, Moore CA, Yang Q, Correa A, Erickson JD. Mortality associated with congenital heart defects in the United States: trends and racial disparities, 1979–1997. *Circulation.* 2001;103:2376–2381.

Carey LK, Nicholson BC, Fox RA. Maternal factors related to parenting young children with congenial heart disease. *J Pediatr Nurs.* 2002;17:174–183.

Casey FA, Sykes DH, Craig BG, Power R, Mulholland HC. Behavioral adjustment of children with surgically palliated complex congenital heart disease. *J Pediatr Psychol.* 1996;21:335–352.

Chen CW, Li CY, Wang JK. Self-concept: comparison between school-aged children with congenital heart disease and normal school-aged children. *J Clin Nurs.* 2005;14:394–402.

Culbert EL, Ashburn DA, Cullen-Dean G, et al. Quality of life of children after repair of transposition of the great arteries. *Circulation.* 2003;108:857–862.

DeMaso DR, Beardslee WR, Silbert AR, Fyler DC. Psychological functioning in children with cyanotic heart defects. *J Dev Beh Pediatr.* 1990;11:289–294.

Deusinger IM. *Die Frankfurter Selbstkonzeptskalen.* Göttingen: Hogrefe; 1986.

Dunbar-Masterson C, Wypij D, Bellinger DC, et al. General health status of children with d-transposition of the great arteries after the arterial switch operation. *Circulation.* 2001;104:I-138–I-142.

Ellerbeck KA, Smith ML, Holden EW, et al. Neurodevelopmental outcomes in children surviving d-transposition of the great arteries. *J Dev Beh Pediatr.* 1998;19:335–341.

Elliott CD. *The British Ability Scales: Introductory Handbook, Technical Handbook and Manuals for Administration and Scoring.* Windsor: NFER-Nelson; 1983.

Falk B, Bar-Mor G, Zigel L, Yaaron M, Beniamini Y, Zeevi B. Daily physical activity and perception of condition severity among male and female adolescents with congenital heart malformation. *J Pediatr Nurs.* 2006;21:244–249.

Fernandes SM, Landzberg MJ. Transitioning the young adult with congenital heart disease for life-long medical care. *Pediatr Clin North Am.* 2004;51:1739–1748.

Fredriksen PM, Kahrs N, Blaasvaer S, et al. Effect of physical training in children and adolescents with congenital heart disease. *Cardiol Young.* 2000;10:107–114.

Fredriksen PM, Mengshoel AM, Frydenlund A, Sørbye Ø, Thaulow E. Follow-up in patients with congenital heart disease more complex than haemodynamic assessment. *Cardiol Young.* 2004;14:373–379.

Garson SL. Psychological aspects of heart disease in childhood. In: Garson A Jr, Bricker JT, Fishes DT, Neishe SR, eds. *The Science and Practice of Pediatric Cardiology.* 2nd ed. Baltimore: Williams & Wilkins; 1998;2929–2937.

Goldbeck L, Braun R. Ulm Inventory (LQ-KID)—Ein computergestütztes Verfahren zur Erfassung der Lebensqualität chronisch kranker Kinder und Jugendlicher. *Prävention und Rehabilitation.* 2003;15:117–126.

Goldbeck L, Melches J. Quality of life in families of children with congenital heart disease. *Qual Life Res*. 2005;14:1915–1924.

Goldbeck L, Melches J. The impact of the severity of disease and social disadvantage on quality of life in families with congenital cardiac disease. *Cardiol Young*. 2006;16:67–75.

Goldberg S, Janus M, Washington J, Simmons RJ, MacLusky I, Fowler RS. Prediction of preschool behavioral problems in healthy and pediatric samples. *J Dev Behav Pediatr*. 1997;18:304–313.

Gupta S, Giuffre RM, Crawford S, Waters J. Covert fears, anxiety and depression in congenital heart disease. *Cardiol Young*. 1998;8:491–499.

Gupta S, Mitchell I, Giuffre RM, Crawford S. Covert fears and anxiety in asthma and congenital heart disease. *Child Care Health Dev*. 2001;27:335–348.

Hou YL. The development of the self-concept scale for elementary school children. *Psychol Test*. 2001;48:141–166.

Hövels-Gürich HH, Konrad K, Skorzenski D, et al. Long-term neurodevelopmental outcome and exercise capacity after corrective surgery for tetralogy of Fallot or ventricular septal defect in infancy. *Ann Thorac Surg*. 2006;81:958–967.

Hövels-Gürich HH, Konrad K, Wiesner M, et al. Long term behavioural outcome after neonatal arterial switch operation for transposition of the great arteries. *Arch Dis Child*. 2002;87:506–510.

Jastak S, Wilkinson GS. *Wide Range Achievement Test—Revised*. Wilmington: Jastak Associates Inc; 1984.

Kälvesten AL. Machover Teckningstest. In: Jonsson G, Kälvesten AL, eds. 222 *Stockholmspojkar*. Uppsala: Almqvist & Wiksell; 1965.

Kamphuis M, Ottenkamp J, Vliegen HW, et al. Health related quality of life and health status in adult survivors with previously operated complex congenital heart disease. *Heart*. 2002;87:356–362.

Karl TR, Hall S, Ford G, et al. Arterial switch with full-flow cardiopulmonary bypass and limited circulatory arrest: neurodevelopmental outcome. *J Thorac Cardiovasc Surg*. 2004;127:213–222.

Karsdorp PA, Everaerd W, Kindt M, Mulder BJM. Psychological and cognitive functioning in children and adolescents with congenital heart disease: a meta-analysis. *J Pediatr Psycho*. 2007;32:527–541.

Kaufman AS, Kaufman NL. *Kaufman Assessment Battery for Children*. Circle Pines: Kaufman American Guidance Service Inc; 1983.

Kendall L, Lewin RJP, Parsons JM, Gruschen R, Veldtman JQ, Hardman GF. Factors associated with self-perceived state of health in adolescents with congenital cardiac disease attending paediatric cardiologic clinics. *Cardiol Young*. 2001;11:431–438.

Kovacs M. *Children's Depression Inventory*. Toronto: Multi-Health Systems; 1992.

Kramer HH, Awiszus D, Sterzel U, Van Halteren A, Claßen R. Development of personality and intelligence in children with congenital heart disease. *J Child Psychol Psychiat*. 1989;30:299–308.

Landgraf JM, Abetz L, Ware JE Jr. *Child Health Questionnaire*. Boston: The Health Institute, New England Medical Center; 1996.

Limperopoulos C, Majnemer A, Shevell MI, Rosenblatt B, Rohlicek C, Tchervenkov C. Neurodevelopmental status of newborns and infants with congenital heart defects before and after open heart surgery. *J Pediatr*. 2000;137:638–645.

Majnemer A, Limperopoulos C, Shevell M, Rohlicek C, Rosenblatt B, Tchervenkov C. Health and well-being of children with congenital cardiac malformations, and their families, following open-heart surgery. *Cardiol Young*. 2006;16:157–164.

McCrindle BW, Williams RV, Mitchell PD, et al. Relationship of patient and medical characteristics to health status in children and adolescents after the Fontan procedure. *Circulation*. 2006;113:1123–1129.

McGrath E, Wypij D, Rappaport LA, Newburger JW, Bellinger DC. Prediction of IQ and achievement at age 8 years from neurodevelopmental status at age 1 year in children with D-transposition of the great arteries. *Pediatrics*. 2004;114:572–576.

Miatton M, De Wolf D, François K, Thiery E, Vingerhoets G. Intellectual, neuropsychological, and behavioral functioning in children with tetralogy of Fallot. *J Thorac Cardiovasc Surg*. 2007;133:449–455.

Moons P, De Volder E, Budts W, et al. What do adult patients with congenital heart disease know about their disease, treatment, and prevention of complications? A call for structured patient education. *Heart*. 2001;86:74–80.

Moons P, Van Deyk K, Budts W, De Geest S. Caliber of quality-of-life assessments in congenital heart disease. A plea for more conceptual and methodological rigor. *Arch Pediatr Adolesc Med*. 2004;158:1062–1069.

O'Dougherty M, Wright FS, Garmezy N, Loewenson RB, Torres F. Later competence and adaptation in infants who survive heart defects. *Child Dev*. 1983;54:1129–1142.

Oates RK, Turnbull JAB, Simpson JM, Cartmill TB. Parent and teacher perceptions of child behaviour following cardiac surgery. *Acta Paediatr*. 1994;83:1303–1307.

Ollendick TH. Reliability and validity of the Revised Fear Survey Schedule for Children (FSSC-R). *Beh Res Ther*. 1983;21:685–692.

Reynolds CR, Richmond BO. *Revised Children's Manifest Anxiety Scale*. Los Angeles: Western Psychological Services; 1990.

Salzer-Muhar U, Herle M, Floquet P, et al. Self-concept in male and female adolescents with congenital heart disease. *Clin Pediatr*. 2002;41:17–24.

Seitz W, Rausche P. *Persönlichkeitsfragebogen für Kinder 9–14 (PFK)*. Braunschweig: Georg Westermann; 1976.

Sparacino PSA, Tong EM, Messias DKH, Foote D, Chesla CA, Gillis CL. The dilemmas of parents of adolescents and young adults with congenital heart disease. *Heart Lung*. 1997;26:187–195.

Spijkerboer AW, Utens EMWJ, Bogers AJJC, Verhulst FC, Helbing WA. Long-term behavioural and emotional problems in four cardiac diagnostic groups of children and adolescents after invasive treatment for congenital heart disease. *Int J Cardiol*, doi:10.1016/j.ijcard.2007.02.025; 2007.

Spijkerboer AW, Utens EMWJ, Bogers AJJC, Helbing WA, Verhulst FC. A historical comparison of long-term behavioural and emotional outcomes in children and adolescents after invasive treatment for congenital heart disease. *J Pediatr Surg*. 2008;43:534–539.

Spijkerboer AW, Utens EMWJ, De Koning WB, Bogers AJJC, Helbing WA, Verhulst FC. Health-related quality of life in children and adolescents after invasive treatment for congenital heart disease. *Qual Life Res*. 2006;15:663–673.

Tong EM, Kools S. Health care transitions for adolescents with congenital heart disease: patient and family perspectives. *Nurs Clin North Am*. 2004;39:727–740.

Utens EMWJ. Psychosocial aspects of congenital heart disease in children, adolescents and adults. In: Walter PJ, ed. *Quality of Life After Open Heart Surgery*. Netherlands: Kluwer Academic Publishers; 1992;325–331.

Utens EMWJ, Verhulst FC, Meijboom FJ, et al. Behavioural and emotional problems in children and adolescents with congenital heart disease. *Psychol Med*. 1993;23:415–424.

Utens EMWJ, Versluis-Den Bieman HJ, Witsenburg M, Bogers AJJC, Verhulst FC, Hess J. Cognitive, and behavioural and emotional functioning of young children awaiting elective cardiac surgery or catheter intervention. *Cardiol Young*. 2001;11:153–160.

Utens EM, Verhulst FC, Duivenvoorden HJ, Meijboom FJ, Erdman RA, Hess J. Prediction of behavioural and emotional problems in children and adolescents with operated congenital heart disease. *Eur Heart J.* 1998;19:801–807.

Uzark K, Jones K, Burwinkle TM, Varni JW. The pediatric quality of life inventory in children with heart disease. *Progr Pediatr Cardiol.* 2003;18:141–148.

Van der Rijken REA, Maassen BAM, Walk TLM, Daniëls O, Hulstijn-Dirkmaat GM. Outcome after surgical repair of congenital cardiac malformations at school age. *Cardiol Young.* 2007;17:64–71.

Van Deyk K, Moons P, Gewillig M, Budts W. Educational and behavioral issues in transitioning from pediatric cardiology to adult-centered health care. *Nurs Clin North Am.* 2004;39:755–768.

Van Rijen EHM. Psychosocial aspects of congenital heart disease in adulthood. A longitudinal cohort study of 20–33 years follow-up. PhD thesis, Erasmus University Rotterdam, Rotterdam; 2003.

Van Rijen EHM, Utens EMWJ, Roos-Hesselink JW, et al. Psychosocial functioning of the adult with congenital heart disease: a 20–33 years follow-up. *Eur Heart J.* 2003;24:673–683.

Van Rijen EHM, Utens EMWJ, Roos-Hesselink JW, et al. Medical predictors for psychopathology in adults with operated congenital heart disease. *Eur Heart J.* 2004;25:1605–1613.

Van Rijen EHM, Utens EMWJ, Roos-Hesselink JW et al. Longitudinal development of psychopathology in an adult congenital heart disease cohort. *Int J Cardiol.* 2005;99:315–323.

Vessey JA, O'Sullivan P. A study of children's concepts of their internal bodies: a comparison of children with and without congenital heart disease. *J Pediatr Nurs.* 2000;15:292–298.

Visconti K, Saudino KJ, Rappaport LA, Newburger JW, Bellinger DC. Influence of parental stress and social support on the behavioral adjustment of children with transposition of the great arteries. *J Dev Beh Pediatr.* 2002;23:314–321.

Vogels T, Verrips GHW, Koopman HM, Theunissen NCM, Fekkes M, Kamphuis RP. *TACQOL Manual Parent Form and Child Form.* Leiden: LUMC-TNO; 2000.

Walker EF, Sabuwalla Z, Huot R. Pubertal neuromaturation, stress sensitivity, and psychopathology. *Dev Psychopath.* 2004;16:807–824.

Wallander JL, Varni JW. Effects of pediatric chronic physical disorders on child and family adjustment. *J Child Psychol and Psychiat.* 1998;39:29–46.

Wechsler D. *Wechsler Individual Achievement Test Manual.* San Antonio: The Psychological Corporation; 1992.

Wernovsky G, Stiles KM, Gauvreau K, et al. Cognitive development after the Fontan operation. *Circulation.* 2000;102:883–889.

Wray J, Sensky T. How does the intervention of cardiac surgery affect the self-perception of children with congenital heart disease? *Child Care Health Dev.* 1998;24:57–72.

Wray J, Sensky T. Congenital heart disease and cardiac surgery in childhood: effects on cognitive function and academic ability. *Heart.* 2001;85:687–691.

Wren C, O'Sullivan JJ. Survival with congenital heart disease and need for follow-up in adult life. *Heart.* 2001;85:438–443.

Wright M, Nolan T. Impact of cyanotic heart disease on school performance. *Arch Dis Child.* 1994;71:64–70.

Youssef NM. School adjustment of children with congenital heart disease. *Matern Child Nurs J.* 1988;17:217–302.

APPENDIX

Overview of Instruments to Assess Psychological Functioning in Patients with CHD, Applied by Studies Discussed in This Chapter

Instrument	Used by	Specific domains of assessment (as reported in this chapter)
Emotional and behavioral problems		
Child Behavior Checklist (Achenbach, 1991a; Achenbach and Rescorla, 2001)	Bellinger et al. (1997) Casey et al. (1996) Fredriksen et al. (2000) Fredriksen et al. (2004) Gupta et al. (2001) Hövels-Gürich et al. (2002) Karl et al. (2004) Miatton et al. (2007) Oates et al. (1994) Spijkerboer et al. (2007) Spijkerboer et al. (2008) Utens et al. (1993) Utens et al. (1998) Utens et al. (2001) Van der Rijken et al. (2007) Van Rijen (2003)	Internalizing, Externalizing, and Total problems
Child Depression Inventory (Kovacs, 1992)	Gupta et al. (1998)	Depression
Fear Survey Schedule Revised (Ollendick, 1983)	Gupta et al. (1998) Gupta et al. (2001)	Fears of injury Medical fears Fears of unknown
Personality Questionnaire for Children (Seitz and Rausche, 1976)	Kramer et al. (1989)	Basic anxiety
Revised Child Manifest Anxiety Scale (Reynolds and Richmond, 1990)	Gupta et al. (1998) Gupta et al. (2001)	Physiological anxiety
Young Adult Behavior Checklist (Achenbach, 1997)	Van Rijen (2003) Van Rijen et al. (2004) Van Rijen et al. (2005)	Internalizing, Externalizing, and Total problems

Instrument	Used by	Specific domains of assessment (as reported in this chapter)
Young Adult Self-Report (Achenbach, 1997)	Van Rijen (2003) Van Rijen et al. (2004) Van Rijen et al. (2005)	Internalizing, Externalizing, and Total problems
Youth Self-Report (Achenbach, 1991b)	Utens et al. (1993) Van Rijen et al. (2005) Spijkerboer et al. (2007) Spijkerboer et al. (in press)	Internalizing, Externalizing, and Total problems
Self-concepts		
Frankfurter Selbstkonzept Skalen (Deusinger, 1986)	Salzer-Muhar et al. (2002)	Self-concepts (achievement)
Machover Draw A Person Test (Kälvesten, 1965)	Aldén et al. (1998)	Body-image
Personality Questionnaire for Children (Seitz and Rausche, 1976)	Kramer et al. (1989)	Impulsiveness Feelings of inferiority
Self-Concept Scale (Hou, 2001)	Chen et al. (2005)	Self-concepts (physical functioning)
Academic functioning		
British Ability Scales (Elliott, 1983)	Wray and Sensky (2001)	Academic achievement: Arithmetic Reading
Kaufman Assessment Battery for Children (Kaufman and Kaufman, 1983)	Hövels-Gürich et al. (2006) Wernovsky et al. (2000)	Academic achievement
Teacher Report Form (Achenbach, 1991c; Achenbach and Rescorla, 2001)	Casey et al. (1996) Karl et al. (2004) Oates et al. (1994) Wright and Nolan (1994) Youssef (1988)	Internalizing, Externalizing, and Total problems Competence
Wechsler Individual Achievement Test (Wechsler, 1992)	Bellinger et al. (2003) McGrath et al. (2004)	Academic achievement: Arithmetic Reading Spelling
Wide Range Achievement Test – Revised (Jastak and Wilkinson, 1984)	Wernovsky et al. (2000) Wright and Nolan (1994)	Academic achievement: Arithmetic Reading Spelling
Quality of life		
Child Health Questionnaire (Landgraf et al., 1996)	Culbert et al. (2003) Dunbar-Masterson et al. (2001) Majnemer et al. (2006) McCrindle et al. (2006)	Perceived physical and psychosocial health status
Pediatric Quality of Life Inventory Cardiac Module (Uzark et al., 2003)	Uzark et al. (2003)	Health-related quality of life
TNO-AZL Child Quality of Life Questionnaire (Vogels et al., 2000)	Spijkerboer et al. (2006)	Health-related quality of life
Ulm Inventory (LQ-KID) (Goldbeck and Braun, 2003)	Goldbeck and Melches (2006)	Health-related quality of life

Note: Besides the instruments mentioned in this overview, most studies have used other instruments as well. In this overview, only the instruments and domains discussed in this chapter are mentioned.

21

Psychological Aspects of Adults with Complex Congenital Heart Defects

GRAHAM J. REID

ADRIENNE H. KOVACS

Adults with complex congenital heart disease (CHD) often live life on the edge—balancing hope, despair, and uncertainty. They are the first cohorts of individuals with CHD living to adulthood. They have experienced first hand the benefits of advances in medical technologies. Their survival creates the hope that continuing advances will help them maintain the quality and longevity of their lives. However, adults with complex CHD are at risk for arrhythmias and sudden death, operation or reoperation(s), premature decreases in physical functioning, and early mortality. Current and expected limitations and losses in their social lives, educational or occupational attainment, and physical functioning may be additional sources of despair. In order to maintain healthy psychological functioning, they must cope with this uncertainty and maintain a positive, but realistic, appraisal of their health and future. Adults with CHD face general developmental tasks common to individuals regardless of their health. In addition, they face a number of CHD-specific tasks. There are large variations in both physical and psychosocial risks for adults with simple lesions (e.g., postoperative atrial septal defect, small ventricular septal defect) compared to those with intermediate (e.g., postoperative atrioventricular canal defects) or complex lesions (e.g., single ventricle physiology) (Connelly et al., 1998a). Psychosocial issues for patients with intermediate or complex CHD encompass those of patients with simple CHD lesions. As the specific issues and their intensity will vary depending on lesion severity, visibility (e.g., cyanosis, clubbing), and functional disability, the present review will discuss issues based primarily on patients with intermediate/complex CHD.

CONGENITAL HEART DISEASE AND LIFE-SPAN DEVELOPMENTAL TASKS

Table 21–1 outlines major developmental tasks for healthy individuals from adolescence on (Kennedy, 1990; Remschmidt, 1994; Thomas, 1990; Wilson and Klein, 2000) and is based on theories of life-span development (Erikson, 1963; Havighurst, 1953). A report from the Bethesda conference on adults with CHD summarized the developmental tasks for adolescents and young adults with CHD (see Table 21–2) (Warnes et al., 2001). The psychosocial outcomes of adults with CHD born in the 1960s are likely different from those born in the 1980s, due in part to dramatic improvements in life expectancy and advances in medical technology (Warnes et al., 2001). Because of these cohort effects, data from older studies should be considered cautiously. Also, given the shortened, but increasing, life expectancy for adults with CHD, greater attention needs to be given to understanding how developmental tasks may change for adults with CHD as they age, compared to individuals without chronic illness.

EMOTIONAL HEALTH AND PSYCHOLOGICAL ADJUSTMENT

Concurrent with an increase in the number of individuals with CHD reaching adulthood, there has been an increase in the number of studies examining the emotional status and psychological adjustment of this growing patient population. Table 21–3 provides a list of 15 of these studies published since 1990. As

TABLE 21–1. *Typical Life-Span Developmental Tasks after Childhood for Individuals Without a Chronic Illness*

Domains	Developmental tasks by age-group					
	Mid Adolescence (14–16 yrs)	Late Adolescence (16–19 yrs)	Young Adulthood (19–35 yrs)	Middle Adulthood (mid 30s–mid 40s)	Maturity (mid 40s–mid 60s)	Old Age (mid 60s+)
Physical	Completing puberty Positive body-image	Maintaining physical health Positive body-image	Maintaining physical health	Accepting physiological changes	Accepting physiological changes and onset of common illnesses of adulthood	Adjusting to decreased physical health and/or illness
Social and family relations	Dating Establishing peer relationships Increasing independence from family		Separation from family of origin Selecting a mate/ partner Starting a family Finding a social group	Childrearing	Assisting teen-age children in developing independence Adjusting to aging parents	Grandparenting Coping with loss of peers
Emotional	Competence in emotional self-regulation		Maintaining emotional/mental health			
Education and vocation	Completing high school	Higher education and/or entering work force	Establishing and/ or maintaining an occupation	Maintaining standard of living	Satisfaction with occupational productivity	Retirement
Health behaviors	Appropriate exercise and diet Avoiding health-risk behaviors Maintaining appropriate weight			Appropriate exercise and diet Maintaining appropriate weight Obtaining screening for health problems as recommended for age and sex		
Personality and identity	Sex-role development	Increasing independence	Balancing independence and interdependence with family and friends			Acceptance of one's life history Acceptance of death

presented in this table, the majority of adolescents and adults with CHD are free of emotional pathology. Nevertheless, several teams of researchers have concluded that on average, the psychological functioning of adults with CHD is lower than that of the general population. In a 25-year follow-up of adults with CHD who received treatment from the Mayo Clinic, higher levels of psychological symptoms were observed among patients compared to normative data (Brandhagen et al., 1991). In a sample of 32 Czech adults with complex CHD and chronic cyanosis, 34% of the sample received scores indicative of depression (Popelova et al., 2001). Two American studies conducted clinical interviews with adults with CHD in order to determine incidence rates of psychiatric diagnoses. Horner et al. (2000) conducted interviews with 29 adults with CHD between the ages of 26 and 56 years in Massachusetts. Approximately three quarters met full or partial diagnostic criteria for one or more psychiatric disorders including major depressive disorder, panic disorder, posttraumatic stress disorder, dysthymia, and adjustment disorder; none had received psychiatric treatment. Regular health care providers do not always know of, or recognize, psychological disturbance in their patients. Specifically, 8 (36%) of 22 interviewed adults with CHD who were considered "well adjusted"

by their medical team met diagnostic criteria for a psychiatric diagnosis (Bromberg et al., 2003).

The data, however, are equivocal, and there are published studies indicating that the psychological functioning of adults with CHD is comparable to that of healthy peers. A Dutch research team has published a number of cohort studies examining the emotional functioning among young adults with CHD (Utens et al., 1994; van Rijen et al., 2003). At multiple follow-up intervals, adults with CHD earned more desirable scores in characteristics of hostility, self-esteem, and neuroticism compared to reference norms (Utens et al., 1994; van Rijen et al., 2003). Compared to reference peers, there were few differences between young Dutch adults who underwent open heart surgery before the age of 15 years (Utens et al., 1998). Predictors of psychological disturbance in this Dutch cohort include being female, low exercise capacity, restrictions placed by physicians, and patient perceptions of scarring (van Rijen et al., 2004).

Similarly, some studies of children and adolescents have found elevated levels of emotional and/or behavioral problems among patients with CHD (DeMaso et al., 1990; Gupta et al., 1998; Oates et al., 1994; Utens et al., 1993) compared to health controls. However, other studies found no differences between these

TABLE 21–2. *Life-Span Developmental Tasks and Issues for the Adolescent and Adult with Congenital Heart Defects*

Domains	Developmental tasks by age-group			
	Mid Adolescence (14–16 years)	Late Adolescence (16–19 years)	Young Adulthood (19–35 years)	Middle Adulthood (mid 30s +)*
Physical	Coping with body image and limitations in physical functioning		Gradual or acute decreases in physical functioning; burden/ complications with onset of common illness of adulthood	
Social and family relations	Peer acceptance of physical appearance/ limitations; coping with stigmatization; lack of social support for CHD issues	Decisions about dating; increasing independence from family; lack of social support for CHD issues	Decisions regarding life partner and reproduction; coping with loss of normative family life cycle; finding a social group/network	Addressing the impact of premature death on partner, any children, and extended family
Emotional	Managing anxiety-provoking medical procedures; maintaining emotional adjustment during period of critical transitions		Managing anxiety-provoking medical procedures; avoiding arrhythmia-related anxiety/ phobic reactions; avoiding despair, depression, or anxiety; maintaining emotional/mental health	
Education and vocation	Coping with possible intellectual and/or learning disabilities	Selecting educational and vocational goals appropriate to present/future abilities	Stigmatization/discrimination in obtaining employment; maintaining employment during medical crises	Maintaining/changing employment and/or career goals with decreases in physical functioning
Medical	Taking some responsibility for medical care; learning appropriate health behaviors	Increasing responsibility for medical care; transition to adult care; knowledge of diagnosis, prognosis, and associated health behaviors	Primary responsibility for medical care; knowledge of prognosis; reoperation(s); CHD complications; coping with medical procedures and hospitalization; coping with procedure-related pain	
Health behaviors	Avoiding initiation of risky health behaviors; maintaining appropriate weight and getting exercise; maintaining oral hygiene and preventing endocarditis	Regular medical follow-up; avoiding risky health behaviors; maintaining appropriate weight; getting appropriate exercise; maintaining oral hygiene and preventing endocarditis		
Personality and identity	Integration of CHD into self; acceptance of being different and unique	Lack of control over health outcomes; increasing independence	Balancing independence and interdependence with family and friends	Resolving loss of typical life achievements; facing prospect of premature death

* Life expectancy varies with lesion severity and increases with improved medical care.
Source: Reprinted from the Journal of the American College of Cardiology, Foster E, Graham TP, Jr, Driscoll DJ, et al. Task force 2: Special health care needs of adults with congenital heart disease. *Journal of the American College of Cardiology.* 37(5):1176–1183, Copyright (2001), with permission from the American College of Cardiology Foundation.

groups (Kramer et al., 1989) and one study found that when items likely reflecting CHD symptoms (e.g., dizziness) were removed from the analyses, group differences were no longer significant (Casey et al., 1996).

The link between defect complexity and psychosocial functioning is unclear, as data regarding the impact of disease severity on psychosocial status and quality of life (QOL) are equivocal. There are data that suggest an absent or weak relationship between disease severity and well-being (Brandhagen et al., 1991; Kamphuis et al., 2002a; Rietveld et al., 2002; Utens et al., 1994, 1998). However, other data suggest that there are differences between cardiac defect diagnostic categories (Bromberg et al., 2003; Ternestedt et al., 2001; van Rijen et al., 2004). In contrast, there is increasing empirical support for the impact

of functional impairment on psychosocial outcomes among adults with CHD. For example, psychological difficulties have been associated with poorer functional status and lower exercise capacity (Popelova et al., 2001; van Rijen et al., 2004). Similarly, cardiopulmonary functioning has been observed to impact the physical component of health-related QOL (Rose et al., 2005).

Although emotional pathology and psychological maladjustment do not appear to be major issues for all patients with CHD, their importance should not be underestimated. First, there are too few studies of adults with CHD and results to date are too inconsistent to make definitive conclusions. Second, depression is a significant predictor of cardiac and all-cause mortality in patients with coronary artery disease

TABLE 21–3. *Quantitative Psychological Assessment of Adults with Congenital Heart Defects*

Reference	Patients	Cardiac History	Assessment Instruments	Conclusions
Brandhagen et al. (1991)	N = 168; American; median age = 31 years	Received treatment at the Mayo Clinic 25 years before; 20% had cyanosis at time of study	Symptom Checklist-90-R (SCL-90-R)	Compared to standardized normative data, adult CHD patients reported greater psychological distress on almost all SCL-90-R subscales. Psychological symptoms were not related to severity of cardiac defect (e.g., cyanotic vs. acyanotic, surgery vs. none).
Utens et al. (1994)	N = 288; Dutch; mean age = 23 years	Mean follow-up of 16 years after surgical correction in childhood	Dutch Personality Questionnaire	Adults with CHD reported better self-esteem and lower hostility and neuroticism than reference norms. Scores did not differ between five cardiac diagnostic categories.
Utens et al. (1998)	N = 166; Dutch; mean age = 22 years	Five diagnostic groups: atrial septal defect, ventricular septal defect, tetralogy of Fallot, transposition of the great arteries, pulmonary stenosis; all had open heart surgery before the age of 15 years	Young Adult Self-Report (YASP)	Compared to a normative reference group, adults with CHD had comparable scores on the majority (7/9) of YASP subscales. Scores did not differ between the five cardiac diagnostic categories.
Horner et al. (2000)	N = 29; American; mean age = 38 years	Complex CHD (tetralogy of Fallot, transposition of the great arteries, Eisenmenger syndrome, Ebstein anomaly)	Clinical interview	28% (8/29) of adults with CHD met diagnostic criteria for major depressive disorder or panic disorder.
Popelova et al. (2001)	N = 32; Czech; 19–64 years	Complex CHD and chronic cyanosis	Clinical interview Zung's Questionnaire	34% received scores indicative of depression on Zung's questionnaire. Depression was associated with older age, poorer functional status, and unemployment, but not with the number of previous surgical procedures.
Cox, Lewis, Stuart, and Murphy (2002)	N = 87; American; mean age = 32 years	Heterogeneity of cardiac defects	General Health Questionnaire 30 (GHQ30) Hospital Anxiety and Depression Scale (HADS)	Fewer psychological symptoms were reported by adults with CHD than a comparison sample of orthopedic outpatients.
Rietveld et al. (2002)	N = 82; Dutch; mean age = 30 years	16% had mild CHD; 54% had moderate CHD; 30% had severe CHD	Negative Affectivity Self-Statement Questionnaire State-Trait Anxiety Instrument Toronto Alexithymia Scale SF-36	Patients with many negative thoughts reported poorer psychosocial adjustment than adults, with few or moderate negative self-statements. Medical variables were not significantly correlated with psychological adjustment or quality of life.
Bromberg et al. (2003)	N = 22; American; mean age = 34 years	14 cyanotic and 8 acyanotic patients; all considered "well adjusted" by their medical teams	Clinical interview Brief Symptom Inventory	36% (8/22) met criteria for a mood or anxiety disorder. Patients diagnosed with depression had greater medical severity. There was a positive association between BSI symptoms and disease severity.
van Rijen et al. (2003)	N = 362; Dutch; mean age = 30 years	Followed up 20–33 years after first open-heart surgery; five diagnostic groups: atrial septal defect, ventricular septal defect, tetralogy of Fallot, transposition of the great arteries, pulmonary stenosis	Dutch Personality Questionnaire	Adults with CHD reported better self-esteem and lower hostility and neuroticism than reference norms.
van Rijen et al. (2004)	N = 362; Dutch; mean age = 30 years	Followed up 20–33 years after first open-heart surgery; five diagnostic groups: atrial septal defect, ventricular septal defect, tetralogy of Fallot, transposition of the great arteries, pulmonary stenosis	Young Adult Self-Report Young Adult Behavior Checklist	The following were significant predictors of emotional and behavioral problems: female sex, low exercise capacity, restrictions placed by physicians, and patient perceptions of scarring. Patients with VSDs or TGA reported more behavioral/emotional problems than patients with ASDs, TOF, or PS.

(Continued)

TABLE 21–3. *Continued*

Reference	Patients	Cardiac History	Assessment Instruments	Conclusions
van Rijen et al. (2003)	N = 362; Dutch; mean age = 30 years	Followed up 20–33 years after first open-heart surgery; five diagnostic groups: atrial septal defect, ventricular septal defect, tetralogy of Fallot, transposition of the great arteries, pulmonary stenosis	SF-36 Heart Patients Psychological Questionnaire	Compared to reference norms, adults with CHD reported poorer physical functioning but better social functioning and less bodily pain and role limitations due to emotional problems. Younger females reported more limitations due to physical limitations than older females.
van Rijen et al. (2005)	N = 251; Dutch; mean age = 27 years	Followed up 20–32 years after first open-heart surgery; five diagnostic groups: atrial septal defect, ventricular septal defect, tetralogy of Fallot, transposition of the great arteries, pulmonary stenosis	Young Adult Self-Report Young Adult Behavior Checklist	Younger patients (20–27 years) reported more emotional and behavioral problems than older patients (28–32 years). Compared to reference norms, females reported more problems than males.
Daliento et al. (2005)	N = 54; Italian; mean age = 32 years	Underwent surgery for tetralogy of Fallot at mean age of 8 years	Clinical Interview Minnesota Multiphasic Personality Inventory-2 SF-36 Neurocognitive assessment	With exception of physical functioning subscale, adults with CHD did not differ from normal population in SF-36 subscales. No pathological traits were observed in MMPI-2 results. Most common neurocognitive deficits were with executive functioning, problem solving, and planning.
Geyer et al. (2006)	N = 343; German; 14–45 years	Heterogeneity in diagnoses	Brief Symptom Inventory (BSI) Body Image Questionnaire	There was minimal impact of functional status on psychological symptoms. Body image impacted psychological status.
Norozi, Zoege, Buchhorn, Wessel, and Geyer (2006)	N = 361; German; 14–45 years	Heterogeneity in diagnoses; all had undergone previous surgery (61% reparative)	Brief Symptom Inventory (BSI)	Higher psychiatric symptoms were associated with poorer NYHA class.

(Glassman and Shapiro, 1998; Shapiro et al., 1997) and post–myocardial infarction patients (Ahern et al., 1990; Barefoot and Schroll, 1996; Carinci et al., 1997; Denollet and Brutsaert, 1998; Frasure-Smith et al., 1993, 1995a; Ladwig et al., 1991; Pratt et al., 1996). Similarly, there is some evidence linking anxiety and sudden cardiac death (Denollet et al., 1998; Frasure-Smith et al., 1995b; Kawachi et al., 1994; Moser and Dracup, 1996). Enhanced arrhythmogenic potential is hypothesized as one mechanism linking anxiety and depression to cardiac death (Kamarck and Jennings, 1991; Rozanski et al., 1999). Given the high prevalence of arrhythmias among adults with CHD, this relation is worthy of consideration. Finally, 20% of adults have a psychiatric disorder (U.S. Department of Health and Human Services, 1999). Even if adults with CHD are not at risk for psychopathology, one in five patients would be expected to have a significant mental health problem. Surgery, hospitalization, invasive medical procedures (e.g., catheterization, transesophageal echocardiogram), and for some patients, routine cardiac appointments may trigger acute emotional distress, especially in individuals with a preexisting emotional disorder.

SOCIAL AND FAMILY RELATIONS

Dating, being separated from one's family of origin, selecting a life partner, and establishing a family are typical developmental tasks for adolescents and young adults. The limited information available suggests that adolescents with chronic illness may be slightly less sexually active and have more concerns regarding sexuality than their peers (Alderman et al., 1995; Lock, 1998; Suris et al., 1996). One study reported that young adults with CHD were less sexually active than healthy peers but adolescents with CHD did not differ from their peers (Uzark et al., 1989). A recent study found fewer older adolescents (14%) and young adults (48%) to be sexually active compared to peers at the same age (33%–42% for adolescents; 58%–74% for young adults) (Reid et al., 2008). Many individuals with CHD who were sexually active (36% of young adults; 72% of adolescents) engaged in potentially risky behavior (i.e., two or more sexual partners in the past 3 months, questionable birth control, using drugs or alcohol before sex at least sometimes). Patients who had surgeries were less likely to engage in these risky sexual behaviors. Patients with CHD are often self-conscious and have a poor body image, particularly related to scars, which may be a factor in their sexual behavior (Kovacs et al., 2005; Swift and Balzano, 2004). More research is needed to understand how patterns of healthy and risky sexual behavior develop in this population. In the absence of such data, it is reasonable for clinicians to inquire about such concerns.

Individuals with CHD must make decisions about telling acquaintances or school/work staff about their condition and may have difficulty in talking to family or friends about CHD-specific issues (Horner et al., 2000; Sparacino et al., 1997; Tong et al., 1998). In families where parents rarely talked to the child about his/her condition, it may be particularly difficult for the patient to initiate conversations regarding CHD issues (Dhont et al., 1992; Horner et al., 2000). In families that do not discuss CHD issues, parents whose children die prematurely may have a particularly difficult time in coping with their adult child's death. Parents continue to be an important source of information for young people with CHD (Reid et al., 2006), many young adults continue to live with their parents, and parents frequently attend appointments with patients (Reid et al., 2004). It is important that both patients and their parents have accurate knowledge to minimize excessive avoidance or unnecessary self-imposed limitations.

Adults with CHD are less likely to be married/cohabiting or have children, and are more likely to live with their parents, compared to their healthy peers (Kokkonen and Paavilainen, 1992; Utens et al., 1994). These differences may reflect lifestyle decisions given a shortened life expectancy, concerns about genetic transmission of CHD, and risks associated with pregnancy for women with CHD (Alden et al., 1998; Clarke et al., 1991; Perloff, 1991; Van Tongerloo and De Paepe, 1998). Among single, young people with CHD, concerns about fertility or genetic transmission of CHD are few (Reid et al., 2008). Women with CHD and their children can be at risk during pregnancy, and thus there is a need for appropriate planning (Foster et al., 2001; Siu et al., 1997, 2001, 2002). Young women with CHD are knowledgeable about pregnancy risks and contraception (Moons et al., 2001) but still desire more information (Kamphuis et al., 2002). A study of 123 women with CHD, including 23 pregnant women, revealed that approximately one third were unaware that they were at increased risk of pregnancy complications and 40% were unaware that their offspring were

at greater risk of inheriting a cardiac lesion (Kovacs et al., 2006b). Concerns about fertility and the risk of pregnancy are much more relevant to married adults. Future research is needed to better understand their concerns and ways to help individuals for whom pregnancy is not recommended. If patients are basing decisions about dating and family planning on fears or misinformation, clinical intervention is warranted.

EDUCATION AND VOCATION

Adults with CHD seem to be less likely to complete high school or pursue higher education than their healthy peers (Doucet, 1981; Foster et al., 2001; Kokkonen et al., 1992; van Rijen et al., 2003), although some studies find comparable educational attainment (Ternestedt et al., 2001). Some data indicate that, among adults with tetralogy of Fallot or transposition of the great arteries, educational achievement was related to achievement expectations and anxiety, even after controlling for intelligence (Irvine, 1997). Selection of an education and vocation suitable to the individual's intelligence, interests, and functional abilities is best achieved with appropriate counseling (Kaemmerer et al., 1994). Deciding where to pursue education and occupational opportunities in light of factors such as whether to stay close to family and a suitable health care facility is particularly relevant for the adult with CHD. These discussions are most relevant to the older adolescent or young adult. Among older adults, changes in physical functioning may require job retraining or adjustment to unemployment or reduced workload. The emergence of debilitating symptoms, such as significant shortness of breath, and in many cases (re)operation, may mean that a patient is no longer able to engage in his/her previous occupation. Loss of employment, or a change in occupation, can force patients to redefine their identity. In the United States where medical insurance is covered by employers, loss of employment can have an added impact on access to medical care. Many patients could benefit from a discussion of careers in light of anticipated changes in physical functioning during adolescence or young adulthood, before educational and vocational decisions are made.

PHYSICAL DEVELOPMENT

Adults with CHD may struggle with their physical appearance (scars, smaller body size, cyanosis, clubbing), physical limitations, and either acute or gradual decreases in physical functioning (Gantt, 1992; Schneider et al., 1990; Tong et al., 1998). Decreases in physical abilities are normal parts of aging. For the adult with CHD, these changes occur prematurely. Physical declines may be particularly difficult for the young adult with CHD to deal with as his/her peers are likely unable to understand and empathize with these changes. Acute changes in functioning related to complications (e.g., arrhythmia) or surgery (e.g., valve replacement) may also require reestablishing one's identity to incorporate decreased physical capacity, and may trigger sadness and mourning for lost life opportunities.

MEDICAL

Becoming knowledgeable about their diagnosis, prognosis, and related health behaviors; assuming responsibility for medical care; making the transition to adult care; and coping with CHD-related complications, operation(s)/reoperation(s), and hospitalizations are tasks facing adolescents and adults with CHD (Moons et al., 2001; Reid et al., 2004). Only half to three quarters of adults with CHD can correctly state and/or describe their diagnosis (Cetta and Warnes, 1995; Ferencz et al., 1980; Kantoch et al., 1997). Knowing one's diagnosis would intuitively seem to be important. However, it has not been demonstrated that this knowledge is related to health outcomes. Given the complex anatomies of these patients and the surgical repairs they undergo, the relevance of ensuring that patients have this knowledge should be questioned. Knowing a diagnosis is likely far less important than knowing appropriate health behaviors and understanding the meaning and appropriate response to symptoms. A pocket health passport with diagnostic and surgical information is probably more efficient than trying to teach *all* patients this information (Foster et al., 2001).

Patients' appraisal of their risk for future adverse outcomes related to their CHD appears to underlie accessing appropriate medical care and their health behaviors, and it is likely a factor in their motivation to acquire knowledge related to their CHD. Unfortunately, many older adolescents and young adults seem to underestimate their risks. A recent study found that 16–20-year-olds with CHD expected to live to the age of 75 ± 11 years, which was only 4 years less than what they thought their healthy peers' life expectancy would be (Reid et al., 2006). These beliefs are not congruent with the best data we currently have on longevity in this population (Nieminen et al., 2001; Oechslin et al., 2000; Siu et al., 1997, 2001, 2002). One study from a CHD clinic found that among patients with moderate to complex CHD who had died the mean age of death was 37 ± 15 years (range 18–80) (Oechslin et al., 2000). More than 85% of 16–20-year-olds with CHD expected to live longer than the authors' estimates of

their life expectancy (Reid et al., 2006). Patients need to have discussions regarding their risks for decreased functioning as well as surgery, arrhythmias, and other information related to future health risks.

Repeated hospitalizations, surgeries, and other painful medical procedures may be particularly difficult for adults with CHD to cope with. Today's adults with CHD underwent childhood surgeries during an era of inadequate pain control (Anand and Hickey, 1992; Anand and McGrath, 1993; Anand et al., 1987). Suboptimal pain management during medical procedures as children, combined with repeated painful procedures, may result in centrally mediated pain sensitization effects among adults (Anand, 2000; Porter et al., 1999; Taddio et al., 1995, 1997). Thus, adults with CHD may be particularly sensitive to pain, and steps should be taken to ensure patients' understanding of pain and optimal medication/management of procedure-related pain (e.g., Acute Pain Management Guideline Panel, 1992a, 1992b; Howard, 2003; Rosenquist and Rosenberg, 2003).

Transition to adult care is another critical issue in this population. Factors such as underestimation of future health risks, lack of symptoms, and strong attachments to a pediatric health care team may result in the failure of patients to successfully transfer to adult cardiac services. A programmatic approach to transition beginning in early adolescence is needed. A comprehensive program taking a developmental approach should achieve better results than programs that focus only on the transfer to adult care (i.e., focus on the final adolescent and first adult appointments) (see Chapter 33).

PERSONALITY AND IDENTITY

Establishing one's identity, balancing independence and interdependence with family and friends, and acceptance of death are tasks of normal development. In addition, the adult with CHD must incorporate his/her condition into his/her identity, deal with the lack of control over changes in physical functioning, resolve the loss or disruption of typical developmental achievements (e.g., surgery results in loss of academic year), and face the prospect of premature mortality. These issues may have to be faced repeatedly throughout adulthood as new events, such as an unexpected surgery or having to leave work because of declining physical abilities, force reexamination of oneself and one's future.

HEALTH BEHAVIORS

Maintaining excellent oral hygiene, practicing endocarditis prophylaxis, engaging in appropriate levels of exercise, avoiding health-risk behaviors (e.g., smoking, substance abuse), maintaining appropriate weight, and having regular medical follow-up are the key health behaviors for adults with CHD. Poor knowledge and behaviors related to endocarditis and its prevention are too common among adults with CHD (Cetta et al., 1995; Ferencz et al., 1980; Kantoch et al., 1997; Moons et al., 2001; Otterstad, Tjore, and Sundby, 1986). A recent study found that among older adolescents and young adults with moderate to complex CHD, only about 15% had "excellent" oral hygiene (i.e., annual teeth cleaning by dentist, brushing and floss daily); nevertheless, virtually all patients (>95%) brushed daily and patients with CHD generally had comparable oral hygiene to comparison samples (Reid et al., 2008b).

Adults with CHD tend to be more sedentary than their peers (Fredriksen et al., 2000; van Rijen et al., 2003; Wright et al., 1985). Unrealistic fears (e.g., fear of damaging the heart, having a cardiac arrest) may be a factor in their lack of activity. However, some adolescents and young adults who have been advised against it will engage in excessive or inappropriate exercise (e.g., contact sports) (Schneider et al., 1990). Adults with CHD are less likely to engage in health-risk behaviors than their peers (Alderman et al., 1995; Wright et al., 1985). High-risk weight loss behavior occurs among some adolescents with chronic illness (Neumark-Sztainer et al., 1995) but has not been examined among patients with CHD. Most adults with CHD will know about the relation between a high-fat diet and coronary artery disease (Ferencz et al., 1980). Given early mortality, maintaining a low-fat diet to avoid coronary artery disease should not be a priority compared to other CHD-specific heath behaviors that would have more immediate impact on health outcomes. In fact, many young adults with CHD mistakenly view their risk for negative outcomes due to their CHD in terms of health behaviors related to coronary artery disease (Reid et al., 2006). Few studies have examined health-risk behaviors in this population. The study by Reid et al. (2008b) examined substance use in addition to oral hygiene. The overall rates of substance use among the patients were either comparable to or lower than similar-aged peers without CHD. However, more than one quarter of older adolescents (16–18 years old) had reported engaging in significant substance use (i.e., smoking cigarettes on more than 2 days, using marijuana or other illegal drugs at least once, or binge drinking) during the previous month. We do not know if substance use is more detrimental to the health of individuals with CHD compared to their peers. Nevertheless, in absence of these data, a prudent approach would be to counsel patients to avoid illicit substances (e.g., cocaine) and

smoking, and similar to any adult, to use alcohol in moderation.

Little is known about adherence to medical appointments in this population or the relation between attending medical appointments and health outcomes. Consensus (Connelly et al., 1998a) and common sense suggests that regular medical follow-up should result in better outcomes in this high-risk population compared to nonattendance. Patients' belief in a treatment's effectiveness or that engaging in health behaviors will relate to positive health outcomes is a significant predictor of compliance (Irvine et al., 1994; Lynch et al., 1992). There is a need to demonstrate that regular clinic attendance and engaging in other CHD-related health behaviors will result in better health outcomes in this population. Given the potential risks faced by these patients, clinicians should strive to ensure ongoing and regular follow-up for these patients (Reid et al., 2004).

QUALITY OF LIFE

Health-related QOL has traditionally focused on overall patient well-being including the impact of physical illness and treatment on a person's physical functioning, disease- and treatment-related symptoms, and physical and social functioning (Aaronson, 1991). Similar to data investigating emotional functioning, data comparing the health-related QOL of adults with CHD to that of healthy peers are equivocal (Fekkes et al., 2001; Gersony et al., 1993; Immer et al., 2005; Kamphuis et al., 2002b; Lane et al., 2002; Saliba et al., 2001; Simko and McGinnis, 2003; Rose et al., 2005). When subgroups of adults have been compared, poorer QOL has been observed among patients with tetralogy of Fallot compared to those with atrial septal defects (Ternestedt et al., 2001). In addition, it appears that cyanotic patients experience poorer QOL than other subgroups (Saliba et al., 2001). The experience of arrhythmias in the adult CHD populations has also been associated with poorer QOL (Irtel et al., 2005).

Historically, the majority of QOL research has included indices of QOL or health status selected by investigators. Moons et al. (2005), however, argued for a paradigm shift with regard to the conceptualization of the QOL of adults with CHD, such that it should be understood from the patient's perspective. Moreover, QOL should not be equated with health status (Kamphuis et al., 2004; Moons et al., 2005). QOL reflects overall life satisfaction that is impacted by "individuals' perception of certain aspects of life important to them, including matters both related and unrelated to health" (Moons et al., 2004). In contrast, health status typically refers to patients' ratings of their overall health, often assessed using a global scale ranging from "excellent" to "poor." In their investigation of the QOL of adults with CHD, Moons et al. (2005) found that these individuals placed less emphasis on financial and material well-being and greater emphasis on family, education and job, friends, health, and leisure time.

FACTORS CONTRIBUTING TO PSYCHOLOGICAL MALADJUSTMENT

The challenges common to all individuals as they progress through adolescence and adulthood are summarized in Table 21–1. There are, however, additional challenges for those managing a chronic illness (Geist et al., 2003) and Table 21–2 summarizes issues specific to individuals with CHD. The process and the statement, "it's hard," capture the sentiment of many adolescents with chronic disease (Woodgate, 1998). We now review some of the specific factors that are experienced by many adults with CHD and are thought to contribute to psychological difficulties.

(1) Neurodevelopmental Factors. There is a higher incidence of neurodevelopmental complications among individuals with CHD due to factors including cyanosis, surgical contributions, chromosomal abnormalities, and genetic syndromes (See Chapter 19). As Wernovsky (2006) explained, increased survival of individuals with CHD has produced a greater number of individuals at increased risk of academic difficulties. In addition to the impact of neurodevelopmental abnormalities on academic achievement, intellectual disability is associated with a three- to four-fold increase in comorbid psychiatric disorders (American Psychiatric Association, 1994).

(2) Sense of "Being Different." "Feeling different" is a central theme in adolescence and adulthood for many patients with CHD (Claessens et al., 2005; Horner et al., 2000; Tong et al., 1998). This is likely a reflection of a number of factors including body image concerns, physical limitations, school absences, and restricted interactions with others. Claessens et al. (2005) reported that a sense of being different was associated with visible signs including scarring, cyanosis, or digit clubbing. Many adolescents with CHD report social exclusion, isolation and embarrassment, and teasing; incidents of bullying are not uncommon (Horner et al., 2000; McMurray et al., 2001). Such negative social interactions may understandably contribute to psychological distress. Positive peer relationships, however, can enhance psychological adjustments. In fact, the results of one study indicate that friendships are one of the strongest components of QOL for adults with CHD (Moons et al., 2005).

(3) Body Image. Body image concerns have been linked to greater anxiety and depression and poorer self-esteem among healthy and chronically ill individuals (Kostanski et al., 1998; Wenninger et al., 2003). Although adolescence and young adulthood are developmental stages for which body image issues routinely occur for many individuals, the situation can be particularly precarious for those with atypical physical features. Depending upon the specific cardiac defect(s) and subsequent treatment history, adults with CHD have higher incidence rates of surgical scarring, clubbed digits, thoracic scoliosis, poor complexion, and smaller stature. Some genetic syndromes are also associated with facial dysmorphism. Many adults with CHD recall feeling self-conscious about their appearance in adolescence (Horner et al., 2000). In a qualitative study, over one third of the interviewed women reported long-standing dissatisfaction with their shape and size (Gantt, 1992).

(4) Family Matters. Many individuals with CHD were labeled "miracle babies" and their parents recall being informed that they were not expected to live beyond a young age. Therefore, for children and adolescents with CHD, it is understandable, perhaps even expected, that their parents will provide a strong degree of involvement and watchfulness. Parents are typically encouraged to shoulder great responsibility for their child's overall health care (e.g., accompany the child to medical visits and answer questions in the examination room, maintain health records, remain vigilant to changes in cardiac symptoms). Children and adolescents with a chronic illness like CHD are thus quite dependent on their parents, and likely more so than their healthy peers. For this reason, the transition from adolescence to adulthood, a change traditionally associated with growing independence, may be more complicated for individuals with CHD. Tong et al. (1998) referred to this as a "challenge of dependence versus independence" for adolescents and young adults with CHD. Approximately 25% of adults with CHD recall parental overprotection during childhood and adolescence (Brandhagen et al., 1991; McMurray et al., 2001). There is evidence suggesting that adults with CHD are more likely to live with their parents than are their healthy peers (Kokkonen et al., 1992). Claessens et al. (2005, p. 7) reported that some parents tend to "create a protected world by minimizing or compensating the limitations," which interferes with appropriate integration of the condition with one's lifestyle. In contrast, children of parents who provide more realistic views tend to learn to cope better with their limitations and feel less different from healthier peers. Therefore, the degree to which parents of children with CHD provide realistic expectations and foster increasing independence should positively impact the children's psychological adjustment.

(5) **Employment and Insurance.** Adults with CHD often experience difficulties with educational and occupational achievement (van Rijen et al., 2003). Difficulties securing employment and health insurance are not uncommon (Fekkes et al., 2001; Hart and Garson, 1993; Janus and Goldberg, 1997; Kamphuis et al., 2002a; Popelova et al., 2001). For example, in a sample of young adults with defects of lower complexity, 19% reported complications with preemployment and insurance medical exams (Fekkes et al., 2001). Almost 30% of Swiss adults with CHD report difficulties obtaining insurance (Immer et al., 2005). Crossland et al. (2005) found higher rates of unemployment among adults with CHD, irrespective of defect severity. Unemployment is of particular concern within the CHD population, in part, because it has been associated with higher levels of depression (Popelova et al., 2001). As noted in the preceding text, changes in employment and occupation may cause individuals to reexamine their identity. These psychological struggles and tangible difficulties (e.g., struggles with paying rent, difficulties accessing medical care) that may occur from loss of employment and/or insurance can be factors in the development of psychological disturbance.

(6) **Health Expectations.** In their qualitative study, Berghammer et al. (2006) described the ambivalence that many young adults with CHD experience. Specifically, these individuals balanced being different, being sick, and revealing their CHD, with not being different, being healthy, and concealing their CHD. Perhaps it is this ambivalence that contributes to the finding that many individuals with CHD have unrealistic health expectations. It is somewhat curious as to why the first cohorts of individuals with CHD reaching adulthood severely overestimate their life expectancy (Reid et al., 2006). In a similar fashion, adults with CHD often overestimate their exercise capacity (Hager and Hess, 2005), despite the fact that they are generally more sedentary than their peers (Fredriksen et al., 2000; Wright et al., 1985). There are implications of activity level on psychological well-being. A strong link between physical activity and psychological adjustment has been identified in the general population (North et al., 1990) and low exercise capacity is a predictor of psychological disturbance among individuals with CHD (van Rijen et al., 2004). Overestimation of life expectancy and exercise capacity might lead to further psychological difficulties for patients who unexpectedly experience a decline in health status or are referred for surgical (re)operation. Horner et al. (2000) noted that some individuals with CHD become angry when confronted with medical complications in adulthood. These individuals need to be assisted with the difficult and ongoing challenge of balancing uncertainty while maintaining a positive, realistic appraisal of their health and future.

SCREENING AND PREVENTION

Routine screening for psychosocial, or physical, problems is not without risk (Feldman, 1990; Hall et al., 2000; Perrin, 1998) and should only be undertaken if there are (a) accurate measures, (b) appropriate resources and mechanisms to provide feedback of results, and (c) appropriate resources for treatment. Both general and CHD-specific issues should be considered. Questionnaires to assess mental health (e.g., depression, anxiety) and health/risk behaviors (e.g., substance use, exercise) may be appropriate (Berwick et al., 1991; Brown et al., 1997; Leon et al., 1996; Madlon-Kay et al., 1995; Rost et al., 1993; Weinstein et al., 1989). Validated measures of CHD-specific psychosocial issues do not exist. Measures of perceived risk of CHD complications and CHD-health behaviors are needed. The timing and manner of asking patients about psychosocial issues is critical. Onset of sexual and health risk behaviors occurs during adolescence (Kann et al., 1996) or early adulthood (Reid et al., 2008a) and engagement in risk behaviors is often interrelated (Bolig and Weddle, 1988; Vingilis and Adlaf, 1990). Discussion of these issues is best started during adolescence but should also occur for adults.

Many adults with CHD, especially young adults, may have the impression that childhood surgery was a "cure" and/or they may be unaware of their prognosis (Horner et al., 2000). Patients who do not believe they are at risk of future complications will be less likely to see the need for regular medical follow-up (Irvine and Ritvo, 1998). Discussing reoperation, CHD complications, pregnancy, health risk behaviors, and early mortality during a single clinic appointment is too overwhelming. Such a discussion, especially if it occurs during the first or second visit after transfer from pediatric to adult care, may send the patient into despair. When patients are overwhelmed, they are more likely to avoid future medical encounters and potentially endanger their health (Sherbourne et al., 1992). Ideally, by early adulthood all relevant psychosocial issues would have been discussed with all patients at least once. A variety of options should be considered including group information/discussion sessions, multiple visits during the first few years after transfer to adult care, information booklets, and other options. Including a checklist of the relevant psychosocial issues that have been discussed in the patient's medical record may be useful. However, discussions will have to be repeated as patients at different phases of development may view the same issue very differently (e.g., sexual behavior during adolescence is mainly concerned with avoiding pregnancy but concerns about having a family will predominate during adulthood).

TREATMENT FOR PSYCHOSOCIAL PROBLEMS

Validated psychosocial and pharmacological treatments exist for many disorders (e.g., anxiety, depression, phobia) in case of both adults and children (Chambless et al., 1996; Roth and Fonagy, 2006; U.S. Department of Health and Human Services, 1999). Validated interventions addressing psychosocial issues for medical disorders (e.g., cancer) also exist (Devins et al., 1996). Treatment effectiveness could be enhanced if interventions were adapted to deal with CHD-specific issues. CHD-specific treatments should focus on enhancing knowledge, modifying maladaptive beliefs, and dealing with periods of transition and acute stress (e.g., transition from pediatric to adult care, moving away from home, entering into a marital or common-in-law relationship, family planning, unexpected surgery). Counseling for parents of CHD patients in relation to their child leaving home and end-of-life issues is also relevant. Educational and vocational interventions could include psychoeducational assessment and remediation for learning disabilities or academic underachievement, counseling related to interests and suitability for postsecondary education, assessment of vocational aptitude and interest, and assistance in matching intellectual and physical abilities to vocations. As noted earlier, this counseling is most appropriate for adolescents and young adults.

Limited numbers of qualified professionals, high frequency of treatment sessions, and significant geographic distances to specialty treatment centers limit access to psychosocial interventions, particularly in this population. Ideally, psychosocial interventions should have proven effectiveness, be able to reach the largest number of individuals in need, be cost effective, be responsive to individual patient differences and levels of distress, and be congruent with patients' cardiac conditions. Meeting the these conditions is best achieved through multiple types and levels of intervention. Individuals with mild psychosocial problems may be served through self-help materials that provide information (e.g., booklets, Internet-based resources). Individuals with moderate problems may be served by a combination of detailed self-help manuals and telephone support and counseling. Similar programs for patients with ischemic heart disease (Frasure-Smith and Prince, 1985), heart failure (Fonarow et al., 1997), and multiple sclerosis (Mohr et al., 2000) have proven effective in lowering patient distress, mortality, and hospital readmission. Individuals with severe psychological or psychiatric problems will require individual or group treatments. Most educational and vocational counseling will need to be individualized. Providing individual counseling to patients at a distance from medical centers could be overcome by providing professional consultation services to local practitioners and/or via video- or tele-conferencing. Patient discussion/support groups, either in person or via the Internet, are also useful in addressing problems of isolation and difficulty discussing CHD issues with family or friends. Provision of psychosocial services for adults with CHD cannot be limited to a specific profession. To address the complexity of psychosocial needs in this population, an interdisciplinary approach is required including clinical health psychology, neuropsychology, psychiatry, vocational rehabilitation, social work, and nursing (Child et al., 2001; Connelly et al., 1998b; Deanfield et al., 2003; Kovacs et al., 2006a; Moons et al., 2002; Report of the British Cardiac Society Working Party, 2002; Salzer, 2005). As interventions are developed, it is critical that procedures are documented and effectiveness evaluated so centers can share and build on each other's experiences.

CONCLUSIONS

There is a growing number of individuals with CHD reaching adulthood. Adults with CHD face a number of unique psychosocial challenges in addition to those associated with normal developmental tasks. Adults with CHD often engage in a tricky balancing act. On one hand, they strive to live full lives similar to their healthy peers and have overly favorable perceptions of their health status and life expectancy. On the other hand, they are confronted with a chronic medical condition that often distinguishes them from healthy peers. Perhaps not surprisingly, therefore, a significant minority of adults with CHD experience emotional difficulties while many patients also experience difficulties related to educational and occupational attainment and health behaviors as a result of having CHD. Conceptualization of the psychological experience of living with CHD, however, must not be restricted to the level of the individual. Relationships with peers, parents, romantic partners, and health professionals contribute to the psychological well-being or maladjustment of adults with CHD.

A well-known African proverb states, "It takes a community to raise a child." Children and adults with CHD are alive today because of the care and dedication of a community of health professionals. The adult care community should also provide support to individuals with CHD as they deal with the psychosocial challenges associated with CHD so they can continue to grow and develop to their maximum potential in all areas of their life.

REFERENCES

Aaronson NK. Methodologic issues in assessing the quality of life of cancer patients. *Cancer.* 1991;67:844–850.

Acute Pain Management Guideline Panel. *Acute Pain Management in Infants, Children, and Adolescents: Operative and Medical Procedures. Quick Reference Guide for Clinicians.* AHCPR Pub. No. 92–0020. Rockville, MD: Agency for Health Care Policy and Research, Public Health Service, U.S. Department of Health and Human Services; 1992a.

Acute Pain Management Guideline Panel. *Acute Pain Management: Operative or Medical Procedures and Trauma. Clinical Practice Guideline.* 1st ed. AHCPR Pub. No. 92–0032. Rockville, MD: Agency for Health Care Policy and Research, Public Health Service, U.S. Department of Health and Human Services; 1992b.

Ahern DK, Gorkin L, Anderson JL, et al. Biobehavioral variables and mortality or cardiac arrest in the cardiac arrhythmia pilot study (CAPS). *Am J Cardiol.* 1990;66:59–62.

Alden B, Gilljam T, Gillberg C. Long-term psychological outcome of children after surgery for transposition of the great arteries. *Acta Paediatr.* 1998;87:405–410.

Alderman EM, Lauby JL, Coupey SM. Problem behaviors in inner-city adolescents with chronic illness. *J Dev Behav Pediatr.* 1995;16:339–344.

American Psychiatric Association. *DSM-IV: Diagnostic and Statistical Manual of Mental Disorders.* 4th ed. Washington, DC: American Psychiatric Association; 1994.

Anand KJ. Effects of perinatal pain and stress. *Prog Brain Res.* 2000;122:117–129.

Anand KJ, Sippell WG, Aynsley-Green A. Randomised trial of fentanyl anaesthesia in preterm babies undergoing surgery: effects on the stress response. *Lancet.* 1987;1:62–66.

Anand KJS, Hickey PR. Halothane-morphine compared with high-dose sufentanil for anesthesia and postoperative analgesia in neonatal cardiac surgery. *N Engl J Med.* 1992;326:1–9.

Anand KJS, McGrath PJ. An overview of current issues and their historical background. In: Anand KJS, and McGrath PJ, eds. *Pain in Neonates.* 5th ed. Amsterdam: Elsevier; 1993:1–18.

Barefoot JC, Schroll M. Symptoms of depression, acute myocardial infarction, and total mortality in a community sample. *Circulation.* 1996;93:1976–1980.

Berghammer M, Dellborg M, Ekman I. Young adults experiences of living with congenital heart disease. *Int J Cardiol.* 2006;110:340–347.

Berwick DM, Murphy JM, Goldman PA, Ware JE, Barsky AJ, Weinstein MC. Performance of a five-item mental health screening test. *Medical Care.* 1991;29:169–176.

Bolig R, Weddle KD. Resiliency and hospitalization of children. *Child Health Care.* 1988;16:255–260.

Brandhagen DJ, Feldt RH, Williams DE. Long-term psychologic implications of congenital heart disease: a 25-year follow-up. *Mayo Clinic Proceed.* 1991;66:474–479.

Bromberg JI, Beasley PJ, D'Angelo EJ, Landzberg M, DeMaso DR. Depression and anxiety in adults with congenital heart disease: a pilot study. *Heart Lung.* 2003;32:105–110.

Brown RL, Leonard T, Saunders LA, Papasouliotis O. A two-item screening test for alcohol and other drug problems. *J Fam Pract.* 1997;44:151–160.

Carinci F, Nicolucci A, Ciampi A, et al. Role of interactions between psychological and clinical factors in determining 6-month mortality among patients with acute myocardial infarction: application of recursive partitioning techniques to the GISSI-2 database. *Eur Heart J.* 1997;18:835–845.

Casey FA, Sykes DH, Craig BG, Power R, Mulholland HC. Behavioral adjustment of children with surgically palliated complex congenital heart disease. *J Pediatr Psychol.* 1996;21:335–352.

Cetta F, Warnes CA. Adults with congenital heart disease: patient knowledge of endocarditis prophylaxis. *Mayo Clinic Proceed.* 1995;70:50–54.

Chambless DL, Sanderson WC, Shoham V, et al. An update on empirically validated therapies. *Clin Psychol.* 1996;49:5–18.

Child JS, Collins-Nakai RL, Alpert JS, et al. Task force 3: workforce description and educational requirements for the care of adults with congenital heart disease. *J Am Coll Cardiol.* 2001;37:1183–1187.

Claessens P, Moons P, de Casterle BD, Cannaerts N, Budts W, Gewillig M. What does it mean to live with a congenital heart disease? A qualitative study on the lived experiences of adult patients. *Eur J Cardiovasc Nurs.* 2005;4:3–10.

Clarke CF, Beall MH, Perloff JK. Genetics, epidemiology, counseling, and prevention. In: Perloff JK, Child JS, eds. *Congenital Heart Disease in Adults.* Philadelphia: W.B. Saunders; 1991;141–165.

Connelly M, Webb GD, Somerville J, et al. Recommendations for the management of adults with congenital heart disease: Consensus conference on adult congenital heart disease. *Can J Cardiol.* 1998a;14:395–452.

Connelly MS, Webb GD, Somerville J, et al. Canadian consensus conference on adult congenital heart disease 1996. *Can J Cardiol.* 1998b;14:395–452.

Cox D, Lewis G, Stuart G, Murphy K. A cross-sectional study of the prevalence of psychopathology in adults with congenital heart disease. *J Psychosomat Res.* 2002;52:65–68.

Crossland DS, Jackson SP, Lyall R, Burn J, O'Sullivan JJ. Employment and advice regarding careers for adults with congenital heart disease. *Cardiol Young.* 2005;15:391–395.

Daliento L, Mapelli D, Russo G, et al. Health related quality of life in adults with repaired tetralogy of Fallot: psychosocial and cognitive outcomes. *Heart.* 2005;91:213–218.

Deanfield J, Thaulow E, Warnes C, et al. Management of grown up congenital heart disease. *Eur Heart J.* 2003;24:1035–1084.

DeMaso DR, Beardslee WR, Silbert AR, Fyler DC. Psychological functioning in children with cyanotic heart defects. *Developmental and Behavioral Pediatrics.* 1990;11:289–294.

Denollet J, Brutsaert DL. Personality, disease severity, and the risk of long-term cardiac events in patients with a decreased ejection fraction after myocardial infarction. *Circulation.* 1998;97:167–173.

Devins GM, Bink YM, Yitzahack M. Facilitating coping with chronic physical illness. In: Zeidner M, Endler NS, eds. *Handbook of Coping: Theory Research: Applications.* New York: John Wiley and Sons; 1996;640–696.

Dhont M, De Wit E, Verhaaren H, Matthys D. Quality of life after surgical correction of congenital heart disease: The parents' point of view. In: Walter PJ, ed. *Quality of Life After Open Heart Surgery.* Netherlands: Kluwer Academic Publishers; 1992;347–353.

Doucet SB. The young adult's perception of the effect of congenital heart disease on his life style. *Nursing Papers.* 1981;13:3–16.

Erikson EH. *Childhood and Society.* New York: Norton and Company; 1963.

Fekkes M, Kamphuis RP, Ottenkamp J, et al. Health-related quality of life in young adults with minor congenital heart disease. *Psychol Health.* 2001;16:239–250.

Feldman W. How serious are the adverse outcomes of screening? *J Gen Internal Med.* 1990;5:S50–S53.

Ferencz C, Wiegmann FL, Dunning RE. Medical knowledge of young persons with heart disease. *J School Health*. 1980;50:133–136.

Fonarow GC, Stevenson LW, Walden JA, et al. Impact of a comprehensive heart failure management program on hospital readmission and functional status of patients with advanced heart failure. *J Am Coll Cardiol*. 1997;30:725–732.

Foster E, Graham TP Jr, Driscoll DJ, et al. Task force 2: special health care needs of adults with congenital heart disease. *J Am Coll Cardiol*. 2001;37:1176–1183.

Frasure-Smith N, Lesperance F, Talajic M. Depression and 18-month prognosis after myocardial infarction. *Circulation*. 1995a;91:999–1005.

Frasure-Smith N, Lesperance F, Talajic M. The impact of negative emotions on prognosis following myocardial infarction: is it more than depression? *Health Psychology*. 1995b;14:388–398.

Frasure-Smith N, Prince R. The ischemic heart disease life stress monitoring program: Impact on mortality. *Psychosom Med*. 1985;47:431–445.

Frasure-Smith N, Talajic M, Lesperance F. Depression following myocardial infarction: impact on 6-month survival. *J Am Med Assoc*. 1993;270:1819–1825.

Fredriksen PM, Walker M, Granton JT, Webb GD, Reid GJ, Therrien J. A controlled trial of exercise training in adult patients with repaired Tetralogy of Fallot, 2000.

Gantt LT. Growing up heartsick: the experiences of young women with congenital heart disease. *Health Care Women Int*. 1992;13:241–248.

Geist R, Grdisa V, Otley A. Psychosocial issues in the child with chronic conditions. *Best Pract Res: Clin Gastroenterol*. 2003;17:141–152.

Gersony WM, Hayes CJ, Driscoll DJ, et al. Second natural history study of congenital heart defects. Quality of life of patients with aortic stenosis, pulmonary stenosis, or ventricular septal defects. *Circulation*. 1993;87:I-52–I-65.

Geyer S, Norozi K, Zoege M, Kempa A, Buchhorn R, Wessel A. Psychological symptoms in patients after surgery for congenital cardiac disease. *Cardiol Young*. 2006;16:540–548.

Glassman AH, Shapiro PA. Depression and the course of coronary artery disease. *Am J Psychiatry*. 1998;155:4–11.

Gupta S, Giuffre RM, Crawford S, Waters J. Covert fears, anxiety and depression in congenital heart disease. *Cardiol Young*. 1998;8:491–499.

Hager A, Hess J. Comparison of health related quality of life with cardiopulmonary exercise testing in adolescents and adults with congenital heart disease. *Heart*. 2005;91:517–520.

Hall S, Bobrow M, Marteau TM. Psychological consequences for parents of false negative results on prenatal screening for Down's syndrome: retrospective interview study. *Br Med J*. 2000;320:407–412.

Hart EM, Garson A. Psychosocial concerns of adults with congenital heart disease: employability and insurability. *Cardiol Clinics*. 1993;11:711–715.

Havighurst RJ. *Human Development and Education*. New York: Longmans, Green and Company; 1953.

Horner T, Liberthson R, Jellinek MS. Psychosocial profile of adults with complex congenital heart disease. *Mayo Clinic Proceed*. 2000;75:31–36.

Howard RF. Current status of pain management in children. *JAMA*. 2003;290:2464–2469.

Immer FF, Althaus SM, Berdat PA, Saner H, Carrel TP. Quality of life and specific problems after cardiac surgery in adolescents and adults with congenital heart diseases. *Eur J Cardiovasc Prev Rehab*. 2005;12:138–143.

Irtel TA, Vetter C, Stuber T, et al. Impact of arrhythmias on health-related quality of life in adults with congenital cardiac disease. *Cardiol Young*. 2005;15:627–631.

Irvine J, Ritvo P. Health risk behaviour change and adaptation in cardiac patients. *Clin Psychol Psychother*. 1998;5:86–101.

Irvine MJ. *Predictors of psycho-social and health outcomes?* Paper presented at the International Course on Congenital Heart Disease in the Adult, Toronto, Ontario, June, 1997:5–7.

Irvine MJ, Ritvo PG, Katz J, Shaw BF. Maximizing adherence with non-pharmacological treatment. *Can J Cardiol Pfizer*. 1994;(suppl):6–8.

Janus M, Goldberg S. Treatment characteristics of congenital heart disease and behaviour problems of patients and healthy siblings. *J Paediatri Child Health*. 1997;33:219–225.

Kaemmerer H, Tintner H, Sechtem U, Hopp HW. The psychosocial situation of patients with congenital heart disease. *Padiatric Grenzgeb*. 1994;33:1–10.

Kamarck T, Jennings JR. Biobehavioral factors in sudden cardiac death. *Psycholog Bull*. 1991;109:42–75.

Kamphuis M, Ottenkamp J, Vliegen HW, et al. Health related quality of life and health status in adult survivors with previously operated complex congenital heart disease. *Heart*. 2002a;87:356–362.

Kamphuis M, Verloove-Vanhorick SP, Vogels T, Ottenkamp J, Vliegen HW. Disease-related difficulties and satisfaction with level of knowledge in adults with mild or complex congenital heart disease. *Cardiol Young*. 2002;12:266–271.

Kamphuis M, Vogels T, Ottenkamp J, Van Der Wall EE, Verloove-Vanhorick SP, Vliegen HW. Employment in adults with congenital heart disease. *Arch Pediatr Adolesc Med*. 2002b;156:1143–1148.

Kamphuis M, Zwinderman KH, Vogels T, et al. A cardiac-specific health-related quality of life module for young adults with congenital heart disease: development and validation. *Qual Life Res*. 2004;13:735–745.

Kann L, Warren CW, Harris WA, et al. Youth risk behavior surveillance: United States, 1995. *MMWR*. 1996;45:2–83.

Kantoch MJ, Collins-Nakai RL, Medwid S, Ungstad E, Taylor DA. Adult patients' knowledge about their congenital heart disease. *Can J Cardiol*. 1997;13:641–645.

Kawachi I, Colditz GA, Ascherio A, et al. Prospective study of phobic anxiety and risk of coronary heart disease in men. *Circulation*. 1994;89:1992–1997.

Kennedy CE. Adulthood. In: Thomas RM, ed. *The Encyclopedia of Human Development and Education: Theory Research and Studies*. Oxford: Pergamon Press; 1990:193–196.

Kokkonen J, Paavilainen T. Social adaptation of young adults with congenital heart disease. *Int J Cardiol*. 1992;36:23–29.

Kostanski M, Gullone E. Adolescent body image dissatisfaction: relationships with self-esteem, anxiety, and depression controlling for body mass. *J Child Psychol Psychiatry*. 1998;39:255–262.

Kovacs AH, Harrison J, Colman J, Sermer M, Siu S, Silversides C. Women with congenital heart disease and pregnancy: have we provided adequate education? *Can J Cardiol*. 2006b;22:98D.

Kovacs AH, Sears SF, Saidi AS. Biopsychosocial experiences of adults with congenital heart disease: review of the literature. *Am Heart J*. 2005;150:193–201.

Kovacs AH, Silversides C, Saidi A, Sears SF. The role of the psychologist in adult congenital heart disease. *Cardiol Clin*. 2006a;24:607–618.

Kramer HH, Awiszus D, Sterzel U, van Halteren A, Clafen R. Development of personality and intelligence in children with congenital heart disease. *J Child Psychol Psychiatry*. 1989;30:299–308.

Ladwig KH, Kieser M, Konig J, Breithardt G, Borggrefe M. Affective disorders and survival after acute myocardial infarction: Results from the post-infarction late potential study. *Eur Heart J*. 1991;12:959–964.

Lane D A, Lip GY, Millane TA. Quality of life in adults with congenital heart disease. *Heart.* 2002;88:71–75.

Leon AC, Olfson M, Weissman MM, et al. Brief screens for mental disorders in primary care. *J Gen Internal Med.* 1996;11:426–430.

Lock J. Psychosexual development in adolescents with chronic medical illnesses. *Psychosomatics.* 1998;39:340–349.

Lynch DJ, Birk TJ, Weaver MT, et al. Adherence to exercise interventions in the treatment of hypercholesterolemia. *J Behav Med.* 1992;15:365–377.

Madlon-Kay DJ, Harper PG, Reif CJ. Use of health habits questionnaire to improve health promotion counseling. *Arch Fam Med.* 1995;4:459–462.

McMurray R, Kendall L, Parsons JM, et al. A life less ordinary: growing up and coping with congenital heart disease. *Coron Health Care.* 2001;5:51–57.

Mohr DC, Likosky W, Bertagnolli A, et al. Telephone-administered cognitive-behavioral therapy for the treatment of depressive symptoms in multiple sclerosis. *J Consul Clin Psychol.* 2000;68:356–361.

Moons P, De Volder E, Budts W, et al. What do adult patients with congenital heart disease know about their disease, treatment, and prevention of complications? A call for structured patient education. *Heart.* 2001;86:74–80.

Moons P, De GS, Budts W. Comprehensive care for adults with congenital heart disease: expanding roles for nurses. *Eur J Cardiovasc Nurs.* 2002;1:23–28.

Moons P, Marquet K, Budts W, De GS. Validity, reliability and responsiveness of the "Schedule for the Evaluation of Individual Quality of Life-Direct Weighting" (SEIQoL-DW) in congenital heart disease. *Health Qual Life Outcomes.* 2004;2:27.

Moons P, Van DK, Marquet K, et al. Individual quality of life in adults with congenital heart disease: a paradigm shift. *Eur Heart J.* 2005;26:298–307.

Moser DK, Dracup K. Is anxiety early after myocardial infarction associated with subsequent ischemic and arrhythmic events? *Psychosomat Med.* 1996;58:395–401.

Neumark-Sztainer D, Story M, Resnick M, Garwick A, Blum RW. Body dissatisfaction and unhealthy weight-control practices among adolescents with and without chronic illness: A population-based study. *Arch Pediatr Adolesc Med.* 1995;149:1330–1335.

Nieminen HP, Jokinen EV, Sairanen HI. Late results of pediatric cardiac surgery in Finland: a population-based study with 96% follow-up. *Circulation.* 2001;104:570–575.

Norozi K, Zoege M, Buchhorn R, Wessel A, Geyer S. The influence of congenital heart disease on psychological conditions in adolescents and adults after corrective surgery. *Congent Heart Dis.* 2006;1:282–288.

North TC, McCullagh P, Tran ZV. Effect of exercise on depression. *Exerc Sport Sci Rev.* 1990;18:379–415.

Oates RK, Turnbull JAB, Simpson JM, Cartmill TB. Parent and teacher perceptions of child behaviour following cardiac surgery. *Acta Paediatr.* 1994;83:1303–1307.

Oechslin EN, Harrison DA, Connelly MS, Webb GD, Siu SC. Mode of death in adults with congenital heart disease. *Am J Cardiol.* 2000;86:1111–1116.

Otterstad JE, Tjore I, Sundby P. Social function of adults with isolated ventricular septal defects: possible negative effects of surgical repair? *Scand J Soc Med.* 1986;14:15–23.

Perloff JK. Pregnancy in congenital heart disease. In Perloff JK, Child JS, eds. *Congenital Heart Disease in Adult.* Philadelphia: W.B. Saunders; 1991;124–140.

Perrin EC. Ethical questions about screening. *J Dev Behav Pediatr.* 1998;19:350–352.

Popelova J, Slavik Z, Skovranek J. Are cyanosed adults with congenital cardiac malformations depressed? *Cardiol Young.* 2001;11:379–384.

Porter FL, Grunau RE, Anand KJ. Long-term effects of pain in infants. *J Dev Behav Pediatr.* 1999;20:253–261.

Pratt LA, Ford DE, Crum RM, Armenian HK, Gallo JJ, Eaton WW. Depression, psychotropic medication, and risk of myocardial infarction: prospective data from the Baltimore ECA follow-up. *Circulation.* 1996;94:3123–3129.

Reid GJ, Irvine MJ, McCrindle BW, et al. Prevalence and correlates of successful transfer from pediatric to adult health care among a cohort of young adults with complex congenital heart defects. *Pediatrics.* 2004;113:e197–e205.

Reid GJ, Siu SC, McCrindle BW, Irvine MJ, Webb GD. Sexual behavior and reproductive concerns among adolescents and young adults with congenital heart disease. *Int J Cardiol.* 2008;125:332–338.

Reid GJ, Webb GD, Barzel M, McCrindle BW, Irvine MJ, Siu SC. Estimates of life expectancy by adolescents and young adults with congenital heart disease. *J Am Coll Cardiol.* 2006;48:349–355.

Reid GJ, Webb GD, McCrindle BW, Irvine MJ, Siu SC. Health behaviors among adolescents and young adults with congenital heart defects. *Congent Heart Dis.* 2008b;3:16–25.

Remschmidt H. Psychosocial milestones in normal puberty and adolescence. *Horm Res.* 1994;41:19–29.

Report of the British Cardiac Society Working Part. Grown-up congenital heart (GUCH) disease: current needs and provision of service for adolescents and adults with congenital heart disease in the UK. *Heart.* 2002;88:(suppl 1) i1–14.

Rietveld S, Mulder BJ, van B, et al. Negative thoughts in adults with congenital heart disease. *Int J Cardiol.* 2002;86:19–26.

Rose M, Kohler K, Kohler F, Sawitzky B, Fliege H, Klapp BF. Determinants of the quality of life of patients with congenital heart disease. *Qual Life Res.* 2005;14:35–43.

Rosenquist RW, Rosenberg J. Postoperative pain guidelines. *Reg Anesth Pain Med.* 2003;28:279–288.

Rost K, Burnam MA, Smith GR. Development of screeners for depressive disorders and substance abuse history. *Med Care.* 1993;31:189–200.

Roth A, Fonagy P. *What Works for Whom?—A Critical Review of Treatments for Children and Adolescents.* 2nd ed. New York: Guilford; 2006.

Rozanski A, Blumenthal JA, Kaplan J. Impact of psychological factors on the pathogenesis of cardiovascular disease and implications for therapy. *Circulation.* 1999;99:2192–2217.

Saliba Z, Butera G, Bonnet D, et al. Quality of life and perceived health status in surviving adults with univentricular heart. *Heart.* 2001;86:69–73.

Salzer MU. Highlights of the meeting of the Psychosocial Working Group of the Association for European paediatric Cardiology, Vienna, March 4–6, 2004. *Cardiology in the Young.* 2005;15:111–113.

Schneider MB, Davis JG, Boxer RA, Fisher M, Friedman SB. Marfan syndrome in adolescents and young adults: psychosocial functioning and knowledge. *J Dev Behav Pediatr.* 1990;11:122–127.

Shapiro PA, Lidagoster L, Glassman AH. Depression and heart disease. *Psychiatr Ann.* 1997;27:347–352.

Sherbourne CD, Hays RD, Ordway L, DiMatteo MR, Kravitz RL. Antecedents of adherence to medical recommendations: results from the medical outcomes study. *J Behav Med.* 1992;15:447–468.

Simko LC, McGinnis KA. Quality of life experienced by adults with congenital heart disease. *AACN Clin.* 2003;14:42–53.

Siu SC, Colman JM, Sorensen S, et al. Adverse neonatal and cardiac outcomes are more common in pregnant women with cardiac disease. *Circulation.* 2002;105:2179–2184.

Siu SC, Sermer M, Colman JM, et al. Prospective multicenter study of pregnancy outcomes in women with heart disease. *Circulation.* 2001;104:515–521.

Siu SC, Sermer M, Harrison DA., et al. Risk and predictors for pregnancy-related complications in women with heart disease. *Circulation.* 1997;96:2789–2794.

Sparacino PS, Tong EM, Messias DK, Foote D, Chesla CA, Gilliss CL. The dilemmas of parents of adolescents and young adults with congenital heart disease. *Heart Lung.* 1997;26:187–195.

Suris JC, Resnick M, Cassuto N, Blum RW. Sexual behavior of adolescents with chronic disease and disability. *J Adolesc Health.* 1996;19:124–131.

Swift EE, Balzano J. *Assessment of body image among adolescents with congenital heart disease (CHD).* Poster presented at the Society for Pediatric Psychology National Conference on Child Health Psychology. Charleston South Carolina, April 15–17, 2004.

Taddio A, Goldbach M, Ipp M, Stevens B, Koren G. Effect of neonatal circumcision on pain responses during vaccination in boys. *Lancet.* 1995;345:291–292.

Taddio A, Katz J, Ilersich AL, Koren G. Effect of neonatal circumcision on pain response during subsequent routine vaccination. *Lancet.* 1997;349:599–603.

Ternestedt BM, Wall K, Oddsson H, Riesenfeld T, Groth I, Schollin J. Quality of life 20 and 30 years after surgery in patients operated on for tetralogy of Fallot and for atrial septal defect. *Pediatr Cardiol.* 2001;22:128–132.

Thomas RM. Developmental tasks. In Thomas RM, ed. *The Encyclopedia of Human Development and Education: Theory Research and Studies.* Oxford: Pergamon Press; 1990:118–120.

Tong EM, Sparacino PS, Messias DK, Foote D, Chesla CA, Gilliss CL. Growing up with congenital heart disease: the dilemmas of adolescents and young adults. *Cardiol Young.* 1998;8:303–309.

U.S. Department of Health and Human Service. *Mental Health: A Report of the Surgeon General.* Rockville, MD: U.S. Department of Health and Human Services, Substance Abuse and Mental Health Services Administration, Center for Mental Health Services, National Institutes of Health, National Institute of Mental Health; 1999.

Utens EMWJ, Verhulst FC, Erdman RAM, et al. Psychosocial functioning of young adults after surgical correction for congenital heart disease in childhood: a follow-up study. *J Psychosomat Res.* 1994;38:745–758.

Utens EMWJ, Verhulst FC, Meijboom FJ, et al. Behavioural and emotional problems in children and adolescents with congenital heart disease. *Psychol Med.* 1993;23:415–424.

Utens EMWJ, Versluis-Den Bieman HJ, Verhulst FC, Meijboom FJ, Erdman RA, Hess J. Psychopathology in young adults with congenital heart disease: follow-up results. *Eur Heart J.* 1998;19:647–651.

Uzark K, VonBargen-Mazza P, Messiter E. Health education needs of adolescents with congenital heart disease. *J Ped Health Care.* 1989;3:137–143.

van Rijen EH, Utens EM, Roos-Hesselink JW, et al. Psychosocial functioning of the adult with congenital heart disease: a 20–33 years follow-up. *Eur Heart J.* 2003;24:673–683.

van Rijen EH, Utens EM, Roos-Hesselink JW, et al. Medical predictors for psychopathology in adults with operated congenital heart disease. *Eur Heart J.* 2004;25:1605–1613.

van Rijen EH, Utens EM, Roos-Hesselink JW, et al. Longitudinal development of psychopathology in an adult congenital heart disease cohort. *Int J Cardiol.* 2005;99:315–323.

Van Tongerloo A, De Paepe A. Psychosocial adaptation in adolescents and young adults with Marfan syndrome: an exploratory study. *J Med Genet.* 1998;35:405–409.

Vingilis E, Adlaf E. The structure of problem behaviour among Ontario high school students: a confirmatory-factor analysis. *Health Edu Res Theory Pract.* 1990;5:151–160.

Warnes CA, Liberthson R, Danielson GK, et al. Task force 1: the changing profile of congenital heart disease in adult life. *J Am Coll Cardiol.* 2001;37:1170–1175.

Weinstein MC, Berwick DM, Goldman PA, Murphy JM, Barsky AJ. A comparison of three psychiatric screening tests using receiver operating characteristic (ROC) analysis. *Med Care.* 1989;27:593–607.

Wenninger K, Weiss C, Wahn U, Staab D. Body image in cystic fibrosis—development of a brief diagnostic scale. *J Behav Med.* 2003;26:81–94.

Wernovsky G. Current insights regarding neurological and developmental abnormalities in children and young adults with complex congenital cardiac disease. *Cardiol Young.* 2006;16(suppl 1):92–104.

Wilson KM, Klein JD. Adolescents who use the emergency department as their usual source of care. *Arch Pediatr Adolesc Med.* 2000;154 361–365.

Woodgate RL. Adolescents' perspectives of chronic illness: "it's hard". *J Pediatr Nurs.* 1998;13:210–223.

Wright M, Jarvis S, Wannamaker E, Cook D. Congenital heart disease: functional abilities in young adults. *Arch Physic Med Rehab.* 1985;66:289–293.

22

The Exercise and Rehabilitation Needs of Children and Adolescents with Congenital Heart Defects, and Their Parents

LYNNE KENDALL

INTRODUCTION

The health and well-being benefits and recommendations for regular exercise (physical activity) are clearly documented (Fletcher et al., 1996; Thompson et al., 2003). It is important that children with congenital heart defects (CHDs) are encouraged to take part in regular physical activity within any limitations of their condition.

The focus within the field of pediatric congenital cardiology over the last few decades has been directed toward improving mortality and morbidity rates through the improvement of medical and surgical interventions. The resultant growing population of children, adolescents, and their families' present new challenges to the congenital cardiology services currently provided. Central to these challenges is the need to maximize the health gains afforded by improved medical management and the need to address the wider lifestyle issues caused by the impact of the condition on the children and their families. Identifying the exercise/physical activity and rehabilitation needs of children and adolescents with CHD, and their parents, and how health professionals might meet those needs, is the focus of this chapter.

CHDs have been shown to occur with an incidence of 4–12 children in every 1000 live births—approximately 1% of all live births (Hoffman, 1995). Significant advances in medical and surgical technology within pediatric cardiology have led to increasing numbers of children with CHD surviving into adolescence and adulthood (Perloff, 1991; Warnes, 2005).

The prognosis for many children with CHD has improved greatly in recent years; there remains, however, a wide variation in severity both between and within the various defects. Many with simple cardiac defects show little or no residual physical impairment, while others have severe restrictions including very limited exercise capacity, small stature, and cyanosis at rest. Many have to follow onerous medical regimes and require repeated surgery or other interventions; some develop further life-threatening cardiac problems such as ventricular dysfunction or rhythm disturbances. Medical treatment and follow-up is often lifelong (Deanfield et al., 2003; Engelfriet et al., 2005; Perloff, 1991; Warnes, 2005).

THE FOCUS OF RESEARCH INTO CONGENITAL HEART DEFECTS

Literature Review Relating to Exercise and Health Care Needs

Previous research into CHD has largely concentrated on medical issues such as the hemodynamic effects of medication, surgery, or other invasive procedures. A review of the literature relating to the health care needs and current focus of services in pediatric cardiology reveals five key areas of interest: using exercise testing to evaluate the clinical condition; using exercise training in the management of children with CHD; the views and beliefs of children and their parents about exercise relative to their cardiac condition; neurodevelopmental aspects; and the psychological impact of CHD. The first three topics are reviewed here; the latter two topics are reviewed in Chapters 19 and 20, respectively.

EXERCISE TESTING

Exercise testing is an important tool used by clinicians in the management of children with CHD. An exercise test can be used to evaluate the severity of a condition, to assess changes in condition following surgery or other medical intervention, or to aid diagnosis (Diller et al., 2005; Fredriksen et al., 2001; Thaulow and Fredriksen, 2004; Tomassoni, 1996). The literature concerning exercise testing in the medical management of children with CHD is extensive, particularly in conditions with a long history of surgical repair; for example, tetralogy of Fallot, transposition of the great arteries and the Fontan procedure for single ventricle (Driscoll, 1993; Ensing et al., 1988; Fredriksen et al., 2002; Hechter et al., 2001; Reybrouck et al., 2004; Tomassoni et al., 1991). These studies use cardiopulmonary exercise testing, following standard protocols using either a treadmill or a cycle ergometer. Patients are encouraged to exercise to their maximum ability (point of exhaustion), the main purpose being to assess their cardiac and respiratory response to exercise. The resulting data can provide valuable information about an individual's ventricular and lung function. Research with the growing population of adults with CHD (ACHD) has established that cardiopulmonary exercise testing is a reliable tool for identifying those at risk of developing arrhythmias, for assessing exercise capacity, and ventricular dysfunction. It is recommended that exercise testing should become a routine part of the clinical assessment of ACHD patients to assess risk; inform clinical decisions regarding timing of interventions; provide information regarding safety to exercise; and serve as a useful prognostic tool (Diller et al., 2005; Dimopoulos et al., 2006a, 2006b; Fredriksen et al., 2001; Reybrouck et al., 2004).

Quality of Life

In recent years, researchers have begun to assess the health-related quality of life of children with CHD. When used in a medical context, quality of life is generally conceptualized as a multidimensional construct encompassing several domains (Eiser and Morse, 2001). This follows from the widely accepted definition of health put forward by the World Health Organization (WHO) in 1952 as the state of complete physical, mental, and social well-being and not merely the absence of disease or infirmity. In 1994 the WHO

(WHOQoL Group, 1994) revised the definition to "an individual's perception of his/her position in life in the context of the culture and value systems in which he/she lives, and in relation to his/her goals, expectations, standards and concerns. It is a broad-ranging concept, incorporating in a complex way the person's physical health, psychological state, level of independence, social relationships, and their relationship to salient features of their environment." An important study by Gill and Feinstein (1994) defined quality of life as "a uniquely personal perception, denoting the way individual patients feel about their health status and/or non-medical aspects of their lives." Researchers use the term "health-related quality of life" when attempting to measure the impact of the cardiac condition, but few studies measure all the domains described here and so do not truly measure the quality of life. There is still no consensus regarding the definition or measurement of quality of life used by researchers (Eiser, 2007; Moons, 2004); this can lead to ambiguity and inaccurate conclusions being made. Moons et al. (2004) reviewed 70 studies reporting quality-of-life assessments in CHD; they found that the term "quality of life" was often inappropriately used, with several studies drawing conclusions about patients' quality of life when it had not actually been measured. Studies reporting health-related quality of life have often used physiological measurements of exercise capacity such as treadmill testing or bicycle ergometry combined with various questionnaires, psychological tests, and rating scales. This type of research is very medical in its approach, often measuring functional ability and self-perceived health status, which alone do not equate to health-related quality of life. They also rely heavily on the parent's perspective of the child's condition. For example, a study by Bowyer et al. (1990), studied 20 children aged 6–14 years, who had previously undergone surgery for transposition of the great arteries. Each child performed a graded treadmill test and their parents completed a questionnaire about their child's exercise ability. One of the findings was that the parents were pleased with the result of the surgery, even when that fell short of normality. The parents did not, unless specifically asked, draw attention to any moderate exercise limitation. Other studies (Casey et al., 1994; Meijboom et al., 1995) have used similar combinations of exercise testing and questionnaires to assess health-related quality of life and exercise capacity in patients with CHD. Casey et al. (1994) in their study with 26 children with complex cyanotic heart disease found that a comparison of the results of formal exercise testing with parental estimates of exercise tolerance indicated that parents generally underestimated their child's exercise capability. Other researchers have also reported parental inaccuracy in estimating their child's exercise tolerance (Godfrey, 1987). Meijboom et al. (1995) also concluded that personal health assessment as measured by the questionnaire was not a good indicator for the objective clinical condition of the patient as measured by exercise capacity.

Summary. The consensus of opinion in these studies is that formal exercise testing can contribute useful information to decision making about further clinical interventions, but subjective (parental) estimates of exercise tolerance may be unreliable in children with CHD. Quality-of-life research plays an important role in the evaluation of CHD but its measurement is complex, and as stated by Moons et al. (2004) there is a need "for more conceptual and methodological rigor with respect to future quality of life studies in this group of patients."

EXERCISE TRAINING AND PHYSICAL ACTIVITY IN CONGENITAL HEART DEFECTS

Benefits of Physical Activity

It is widely accepted that regular physical activity positively influences general health and well-being (Department of Health, 2004; Fletcher et al., 1996; Marcus et al., 2006; Maron and Zipes, 2005; Thompson et al., 2003). Various public health guidelines have been published that recommend the frequency, volume, and intensity of physical activity for healthy adults and children (e.g., Cavill et al., 2001; Department of Health, 2004; Fletcher et al., 1996; Pate et al., 1995). Most recommend 30 minutes of at least moderate intensity physical activity on 5 days, and preferably every day, of the week for adults. For children the recommendation is for 60 minutes per day. There is growing support for the benefits of accumulating the daily physical activity requirements in shorter bouts of 10–15 minutes of activity taken throughout the day (Department of Health, 2004; Fletcher et al., 1996; Marcus et al., 2006; Pate et al., 1995). This approach may help people to reach their recommended targets by incorporating activity into their daily lifestyle and help them to become more active in the long term (Department of Health, 2004; Marcus et al., 2006).

Clinicians have long advocated that children with CHD should be encouraged to take part in regular exercise within the limits imposed by their cardiovascular defect (Deanfield et al., 2003; Gutgesell et al., 1986; Hirth et al., 2006; Kitchiner, 1996; Koster, 1994; Maron et al., 2004; Maron and Zipes, 2005; Moons et al., 2006; Soni and Deanfield, 1997).

Summary. Specific advice about physical activity should be regularly discussed with children, adolescents, and ACHD, and their families, and regular

exercise promoted (Dua et al., 2007; Dimopoulos et al., 2006b, 2006a; Hirth et al., 2006; Kendall et al., 2007; Lunt et al., 2003; Massin et al., 2006; Moons et al., 2001; Saidi et al., 2007; Swan and Hillis, 2000; Thaulow and Fredriksen, 2004). Detailed recommendations are in place for participation in sports and recreational activities in patients with CHD (see Physical Activity Guidelines section).

Reduced Exercise Tolerance

There is increasing evidence that a reduced exercise capacity in children, adolescents, and adults with a broad range of congenital cardiac conditions, including asymptomatic patients with simple lesions, is a common finding (Diller et al., 2005; Dimopoulos et al., 2006b; Driscoll et al., 1992; Dua et al., 2007; Engelfriet et al., 2005; Fredriksen et al., 1999, 2001; Massin et al., 2006; Wessel and Paul, 1999), with many patients failing to meet public health guidelines for activity. It may not always be meaningful to compare exercise capacity in patients with CHD to that of a healthy population (Fredriksen et al., 2001). As described previously, exercise testing in the various CHD groups provides useful reference data against which individual patient's with comparable circulation and physiology can be compared (Diller et al., 2005; Dimopoulos et al., 2006b; Fredriksen et al., 2001). Limitations in exercise capacity in CHD patients are often attributable to the abnormal hemodynamics and physiology associated with their condition. However, an important contributing factor includes a low level of daily physical activity (Dimopoulos et al., 2006a; Dua et al., 2007; Fredriksen et al., 2001; Lunt et al., 2003; Reybrouck and Mertens, 2005). This is often the result of overprotection of children with CHD by parents and teachers (Hirth et al., 2006; Reybrouck and Mertens, 2005). Other researchers, however, have not found overprotection by parents to be a significant problem (Lunt et al., 2003; Swan and Hillis, 2000). In addition, physicians have been reluctant to encourage physical activity in the CHD population and have either neglected to give specific advice or imposed unnecessary restrictions to activities even in those with mild CHD and belonging to a good functional class (Fekkes et al., 2001; Swan and Hillis, 2000; Therrien et al., 2003).

Summary. Applying excessive and unnecessary restrictions, especially in young children, may have a negative impact both physically and psychologically (Maron and Zipes, 2005).

Misconceptions and a lack of specific recommendations regarding physical activity may result in a lack of confidence and/or incentive to exercise in patients with CHD, further reducing their exercise capacity.

Physical Activity Misconceptions

Misconceptions regarding exercise in patients with CHD are a recurring theme in research. A poor knowledge base about physical activity in CHD may lead to needless restriction of activity by parents, teachers, or the patient themselves (Bowyer et al., 1990; Casey et al., 1994; Rogers et al., 1994). Conversely, some patients may be oblivious to the risks of exercising at potentially dangerous levels (Cheuk et al., 2004; Falk et al., 2006; Kamphuis et al., 2002; Kendall et al., 2003, 2007; Maron et al., 2004; Swan and Hillis, 2000). A questionnaire survey of 99 ACHD demonstrated that the majority had never received any appropriate help in understanding their exercise needs or capacity (Swan and Hillis, 2000). The authors concluded that there was "room for a significant improvement in the understanding of safe and effective exercise, even in patients who attend paediatric and adult specialist services."

Summary. It appears that despite all the recommendations, and the efforts of medical staff to promote physical activity, evidence indicates that many patients still present with limited understanding of their CHD and the implications for safe, effective exercise (Cheuk et al., 2004; Kendall et al., 2007; Lunt et al., 2003; Moons et al., 2001, 2006b; Swan and Hillis, 2000).

It is essential, therefore, that health professionals provide ongoing patient and parent education regarding exercise, and other lifestyle issues, with specific individual recommendations made. This concept is further explored in the Views and Beliefs of Children and Parents section.

Risks of Physical Inactivity

A sedentary lifestyle results in the loss of the health benefits associated with regular physical activity. Additional risk factors of physical inactivity include weight gain and an increased risk of development of coronary artery disease (Fletcher et al., 1996). Pediatric obesity is becoming a significant problem throughout Europe and North America (Pate et al., 2006). Children and adolescents with CHD may be restricted from taking part in physical activity, sometimes inappropriately, which may incur additional health risks. A recent study in the United States by Pinto et al. (2006) compared a cohort of 1055 pediatric CHD outpatients to the national prevalence of obesity data. The results indicated that, excluding the Fontan population, the pediatric CHD population is at no less risk for obesity and the associated risks for acquired heart disease than the national population.

Summary. These findings further support the importance of giving children with CHD detailed information and advice regarding exercise and the risks associated with a sedentary lifestyle.

Exercise Training and Rehabilitation Interventions

For many years, researchers have reported the benefits of exercise training for children with CHD (e.g., Goldberg et al., 1981; Ruttenberg et al., 1983; Tomassoni et al., 1990). In addition, several studies have reported the positive effects of cardiac rehabilitation programs for these children (e.g., Balfour et al., 1991; Calzolari et al., 1997; Galioto and Tomassoni, 1993; Longmuir et al., 1985). However, many studies were mainly small-scale, uncontrolled trials measuring the effects of supervised exercise programs on exercise capacity. Although the researchers reported improvements in physical work capacity and cardiopulmonary function after undertaking exercise training, the results should be viewed within the limitations of the studies. These include a small sample size, a significant dropout rate, incomplete description of methodology, and inadequate research design (Galioto and Tomassoni, 1993; Tomassoni, 1996; Washington, 1992).

More recently a study by Fredriksen et al. (2000) using exercise tests, questionnaires, and activity monitors to test the effect of systematic, supervised exercise training in 55 children and adolescents with a wide range of CHD, found the recruitment and retention of patients to be a major problem with poor parental compliance. However, the results indicated that those patients participating in the study did demonstrate significantly increased physical activity levels. Parents also reported a marked increase in social effect, suggesting that participation in the study itself had a positive effect. The authors concluded that "the increase in physical activity level indicates that participation in a study, involving exercise test and information, makes parents and patients aware that exercise may be harmless, and perhaps also lowers the threshold for participating in physical activity."

Studies with adult patients with CHD confirm that exercise training programs are safe and can improve exercise capacity (Thaulow and Fredriksen, 2004; Therrien et al., 2003).

A recent study (Rhodes et al., 2005) of 16 children with complex CHD concluded that a 12-week cardiac rehabilitation exercise program significantly improved their exercise performance. The children attended rehabilitation sessions for 1 hour twice a week for 12 weeks. The sessions were conducted in a room in a suburban satellite clinic. The children were divided by age into two groups for their exercise sessions, 8–13 years and 13–17 years. The sessions included 5–10 minutes warm-up, 45 minutes aerobic exercises and games, and 5–10 minutes cool-down. In addition, they were encouraged to exercise at home on at least two more occasions each week. Patients completed cycle ergometer exercise testing before and after the 12-week exercise program.

Their results showed an increased exercise function (improved peak oxygen consumption [VO_2] and peak work rate) in 15 of the 16 patients. The authors concluded that "routine use of formal cardiac rehabilitation may reduce the morbidity of complex CHD" but recommended further research was needed to establish whether any short-term benefits are maintained over time, and whether an improvement in activity levels and lifestyle can be demonstrated.

Most of the work relating to cardiac rehabilitation in the field of pediatric cardiology has been undertaken in Europe and the United States where practice may be different to that in the United Kingdom; for example, Tomassoni's (1996) definition of cardiac rehabilitation as "supervised, progressive exercise training to improve aerobic fitness" In adult cardiac rehabilitation for acquired heart disease, the American Heart Association and the American Association of Cardiovascular and Pulmonary Rehabilitation (Balady et al., 2007) recognize that all cardiac rehabilitation/secondary prevention programs should contain specific core components "that aim to optimize cardiovascular risk reduction, foster healthy behaviors and compliance to these behaviors, reduce disability, and promote an active lifestyle for patients with cardiovascular disease." Similarly, in the United Kingdom exercise is just one component of an interdisciplinary cardiac rehabilitation team that aims to address the physical, educational, and psychosocial needs of cardiac patients. However, currently there is no provision for such services within pediatric cardiology in the United Kingdom (Lewin et al., 2002).

A recent study in North America by McCrindle et al. (2006) observed that clinicians need to be more aware of the nonmedical impact of CHD on their patients. The questionnaire study with 537 Fontan patients aged 6–18 years found that they had important deficits in many domains of health status, mainly related to physical functioning. The authors recommended that assessment of patients should include health status, especially psychosocial issues, for clinicians to better understand the impact of nonmedical, as well as medical, morbidities and to identify specific areas of unmet need. They conclude "opportunities and aspects of rehabilitation have, to date, received little attention in survivors of CHD; our study clearly points to a potential need."

Alternative approaches to hospital-based programs may encourage young people to participate in cardiac rehabilitation, for example, by using home-based activities in combination with a specialized center (Fredriksen et al., 2000; Kendall et al., 2007; Longmuir et al., 1985; Moalla et al., 2006; Rhodes et al., 2006; Therrien et al., 2003). Close follow-up of patients after a period of exercise training, advice, or rehabilitation is recommended to ensure that activity levels are maintained and motivation encouraged,

for example, by personal contact, telephone, or e-mail follow-up between the specialized center and patients, parents, teachers, sports coaches, and local authorities (Fredriksen et al., 2000; Lunt et al., 2003; Kendall et al., 2007). Liaison with school is especially important to communicate individual information regarding physical activity levels for children with CHD (Lightfoot et al., 1998; Kendall et al., 2007).

Moons et al. (2006) assessed the changes in self-perceived health of 31 children with CHD attending a special 3-day multisports camp. Their results indicated that after attending the camp (which included a variety of recreational sports activities but excluded intense sports), the children's perception of their physical functioning had improved significantly, as had their self-esteem and other dimensions of subjective health status. A follow-up study (Moons et al., 2006a) found that the improvement in perceived health status was still evident 3 months after the sports camp. The authors suggest that further research is needed to assess the benefits of using this type of intervention in children with CHD.

A comprehensive overview of physical activity intervention studies (Marcus et al., 2006) identified some key points; it is clear that exercise training programs can and do increase exercise performance in most individuals; however, there are often problems with recruitment, retention, and sustained motivation once the program has finished. Whilst structured exercise programs may be appropriate for some patient groups, it is recommended that health professionals should promote the increase of moderate to vigorous physical activity in daily life. The use of alternative modes of patient contact, other than face-to-face, using, for example, a telephone or Internet sites is suggested. Further research is needed, however, to test the efficacy of such methods.

Summary. Despite the abundance of research indicating that exercise rehabilitation is both beneficial and safe in the majority of patients with CHD, the review of the literature clearly identifies weaknesses in the existing evidence regarding the provision of comprehensive rehabilitation services for young people with CHD. The gaps in service identified suggest that health professionals need to be much more proactive in providing specific, individual, exercise advice in order to meet current recommendations and guidelines.

Physical Activity Guidelines

Competitive Sports. Comprehensive North American guidelines for competitive sports participation in athletes with an identified cardiovascular abnormality have been available for more than two decades in the 16th and 26th Bethesda conference reports of 1985 and

1994 (Graham et al., 1994; McNamara et al., 1985); these guidelines were further updated in 2005 in the report of the 36th Bethesda conference (Graham et al., 2005). The recommendations made in the reports are the consensus of an expert panel, with several task forces considering the different aspects of cardiovascular abnormalities. These recommendations apply to the competitive athlete defined as "one who participates in an organized team or individual sport that requires regular competition against others as a central component, places a high premium on excellence and achievement, and requires some form of systematic (and usually intense) training." This definition applies to those taking part in any competitive sporting discipline, and covers all age-groups or levels of participation including schoolchildren, college, professional, and master's sports (Maron and Zipes, 2005). Whilst the recommendations are not specifically designed for noncompetitive sports activities, the panel recognizes that they may be used appropriately in some selected recreational sports and/or occupations that involve vigorous physical exertion. The panel emphasizes that the recommendations "should not be regarded as an injunction against physical activity in general...."; indeed they advise regular physical activity in patients with CHD and recognize the health benefits of regular exercise.

Similar recommendations for competitive sports participation for athletes with cardiovascular disease were published in Europe in 2005 (Pelliccia et al.), representing the consensus of an international panel of experts appointed by the European Society of Cardiology. Both the European and American guidelines stress that caution is needed when applying the recommendations and an individual assessment must always be used to determine the relative risk of participation in sports. Individual patients vary a great deal in their cardiovascular function, making it impossible to apply the recommendations in all cases; detailed cardiovascular assessment in each patient, plus an assessment of the individual's personality and competitive spirit, the effect of emotional stress during competition, the potential effect of environmental factors, and the level/intensity of training regimens (which may be more intense than the competition itself), is essential (Mitchell et al., 2005).

Classification of Sports. Some sporting activities create more intense cardiac stress than others do either directly or through changes in autonomic tone, dehydration, or electrolyte balance (Heidbüchel et al., 2006; Mitchell et al., 2005). A classification of the different type of sports—the two main types are dynamic (isotonic) and static (isometric)—and the relative intensity—high, moderate, and low—of each, are provided in a table in the American guidelines (Mitchell et al., 2005) and in an adapted table in the European guidelines (Pelliccia et al., 2005). This classification indicates the relative cardiovascular demands associated with different sports; in addition, sports with a high risk of bodily collision, and those associated with additional risk in the case of syncope, are highlighted. Dynamic exercise is generally more suitable for patients with cardiovascular disease; this is because dynamic exercise imposes a volume load on the ventricles, whereas static exercise causes mainly a pressure load on the heart, which can be difficult to control (Dent, 2003; Mitchell et al., 2005).

Recreational Sports. Until recently, recommendations for recreational physical activity were limited to the American Heart Association statement published in 1986 (Gutgesell et al., 1986).

This lack of detailed recommendations for the many patients with CHD taking part in recreational sports and activities prompted the development of further guidelines, again using the consensus of expert panels. In North America, recommendations for recreational sports participation in young patients with genetic cardiovascular diseases was published in 2004 (Maron et al.). In Europe, a series of consensus documents have been produced with recommendations for participation in leisure-time physical activity and competitive sports in patients with CHD (Hirth et al., 2006); patients with arrhythmias and potentially arrhythmogenic conditions, part 1: supraventricular arrhythmias and pacemakers (Heidbüchel et al., 2006) and part 2: ventricular arrhythmias, channelopathies, and implantable defibrillators (Heidbüchel et al., 2006a); and patients with cardiomyopathies, myocarditis, and pericarditis (Pelliccia et al., 2006). The recommendations again stress that they must be individualized to each patient's current cardiovascular status, as well as taking account of the intensity and level of participation in their physical activities. As Maron et al. (2004) observe, the application of these recommendations are only the starting point for clinical judgments, and the weighing of perceived risk with respect to benefit must be assessed for every patient.

Summary. It is essential, therefore, to assess and advise children, adolescents, and young ACHD on an individual basis and to review them regularly, with respect to physical activity and sports participation (Gardner and Angelini, 1995; Hirth et al., 2006; Kendall et al., 2007; Soni and Deanfield, 1997; Swan and Hillis, 2000), using the recommendations now available.

VIEWS AND BELIEFS OF CHILDREN AND PARENTS

Exercise and Congenital Heart Disease

Concerns regarding exercise, lack of knowledge and/or misconceptions about exercise, and a need for detailed information about physical activity relative to their cardiac condition have been identified in a number of studies.

A study by Cheuk et al. (2004) used a questionnaire survey to assess parents' understanding of their child's CHD. They found that parents had important knowledge gaps about their child's condition. Particular areas of concern were poor knowledge regarding appropriate exercise, risks of infective endocarditis, and the effects of cardiac medications. With regard to exercise capacity, 59% of parents were correct in indicating the appropriate level of exercise for their child's heart condition. However, the majority of the remaining parents tended to impose excessive exercise restriction. The study concluded that parental education about their child's CHD needs to be improved; parents may then pass on accurate knowledge to their children. Similar significant gaps in parental knowledge were identified more recently (Chessa et al., 2005; Van Deyk et al., 2004). In the Chessa study, 148 families returned a knowledge questionnaire about their child's CHD. Again, the responses identify that parents have poor knowledge of the risks for appropriate physical activities for their child. About 40% of parents were correct in their knowledge of appropriate levels of competitive sport for their child, 15% were incorrect, and 45% did not know what level of sport was appropriate. Wray and Maynard (2006) in their questionnaire evaluation of the needs of 209 families of children with CHD found that, even for a medically stable population, more than half of the families had one or more unmet needs. The greatest area of perceived need was the provision of information. Kendall et al. (2003a) interviewed 17 parents of children and adolescents with CHD to ascertain their views about the need for, and shape of, services for rehabilitation. The main areas of need concerned detailed guidance about physical activity; the quantity, timing, and content of information provided to parents; and information provided to school. The parents often felt less than adequately informed or supported in managing their child's condition and welcomed a partnership between the child, parents, and health professional. A parallel study (Kendall et al., 2003) aimed to identify the rehabilitation or support needs of young people with CHD and to explore how services may be provided to help meet those needs. Interviews with 16 children (8–18 years) with CHD identified two key areas of need: constructive support from others, including health professionals, and specific information on how their condition could affect lifestyle issues. This research showed a wide variation in how much young people wanted to know, and when they wanted to know. Health professionals cannot assume that having a cardiac condition necessarily means the young person wants to know everything about the medical condition and its management, as research with other chronic childhood illness has shown (Beresford and Sloper, 1999; Phipps and Srivastava, 1997). What most young people did want to know about was exactly how the condition would affect their daily life; that is, the lifestyle issues, often related to physical activity, that they face as a consequence of having CHD. Uzark (1992) discussed the need to provide adolescents with CHD with individual information about their condition and any lifestyle implications. She identified recreational and vocational physical activity as particular topics to address, along with preventative health care needs, pregnancy, contraception, and psychosocial stresses.

Other researchers have also identified the need to provide accurate information regarding lifestyle issues such as education, career choices, and family planning (Crossland et al., 2005; Reid et al., 2006; Wray and Maynard, 2006). A study by Lightfoot et al. (1999) investigated the views of 33 mainstream secondary school pupils with a variety of illnesses and disabilities, including some children with CHD, regarding the impact of their condition on school life. One recommendation was that all health professionals need to take a holistic approach to caring for children, including consulting them about their own needs, since their views are not necessarily the same as adult proxies.

Other studies with parents of children with CHD (Sparacino et al., 1997; Utens et al., 2000; Van Horn et al., 2001; Walker et al., 2004) show that they experience raised levels of psychological distress and less adequate coping strategies, in comparison with normative reference groups. Similar findings were noted in the United Kingdom's Bristol Heart Surgery inquiry report (Kennedy, 2001). Van Horn et al. (2001) commented that the overall improved status of CHD patients may result in health professionals underestimating the level of concern and stress experienced by their families. Parents may experience stress during busy outpatient visits and be unable to ask questions or express concerns, especially when they receive new information regarding their child's condition. This may result in missed opportunities to discuss, for example, their child's physical activity levels and/or sports participation, and other important lifestyle issues.

Poor understanding and/or a lack of knowledge about the child's CHD and the effect on lifestyle are prevalent. A study by Falk et al. (2006) with 100 young people aged 12–18 years examined the concordance between the cardiologist's definition of the severity of the CHD and recommendations for physical activity, and the patient's perceptions of their condition. The young people had a range of conditions, 38% with trivial CHD, 21% mild, and 41% moderate.

Thirty-one percent of patients rated their condition as less severe than their cardiologist's rating, whilst 15% rated it more severe. Most young people had an appropriate level of participation in physical activity for their condition, but a "noteworthy percentage" took part in activities more intense than those recommended by their cardiologist. A questionnaire survey with 253 children and adolescents aged 7–17 years, and their parents, to assess a method for determining risk and providing advice about activity relative to their congenital cardiac condition, found that 47% showed incorrect responses in their belief about their advised level of exercise (Kendall et al., 2007). The study compared the patient's belief about safe levels of activity with that recommended by the pediatric cardiologist. Of the group that showed incorrect beliefs: more than 60% believed they could exercise at a level above that advised by the cardiologist, with a small number unknowingly putting themselves at risk of sudden death by taking part in competitive sports; almost 40% believed they needed to restrict their activity levels more than that advised by the cardiologist, with more than two-thirds applying restrictions when none were necessary.

Research with adult patients with CHD confirms that there are significant gaps in their knowledge about the effects of their condition (Dore et al., 2002; Moons et al., 2001; Reid et al., 2006; Swan and Hillis, 2000). The researchers conclude that structured patient education is needed to overcome the lack of knowledge and improve the outcome in the CHD population. Dua et al. (2007) in a study with 61 ACHD patients found that most patients showed a willingness to take part in exercise but did not because of uncertainty of the safety or benefit.

A qualitative study in New Zealand compared 64 ACHD with 48 (nonpatient) matched controls (Prapavessis et al., 2005) using psychological measures (theory of planned behavior) and a physical activity questionnaire (self-report) to look at their beliefs toward physical activity and to determine whether their beliefs might affect physical activity behavior. The results indicated that CHD patients did not differ from the control group in their beliefs about exercise or in the amount of exercise they perform. The authors queried whether the subnormal exercise tolerance in ACHD was due to their beliefs toward physical activity being a limiting factor in their exercise participation. Their data suggest this is not the case, but the authors recommend further detailed research using more objective measures of exercise behavior, larger sample size, and more detailed assessment of exercise behavior before any definitive conclusions can be made.

Summary. These studies indicate that future services should include both physical and psychosocial rehabilitation based on the individual assessment needs of the family. The research evidence clearly indicates that there are gaps in many patients' knowledge and understanding of appropriate physical activity levels and highlights the gaps in the current provision of services within the field of CHD.

Gaps in Service Provision

Others studies have commented on deficiencies in support, communication, lack of partnership in decision-making, and services that are available to patients with CHD and their families (Children's Heart Federation, 2001; Department of Health, 2003; Knowles et al., 2005; Spall, 2003).

A recent study (Moons et al., 2006b) as part of the Euro Heart Survey on ACHD (Engelfriet et al., 2006) found that the provision of care for ACHD patients in Europe is suboptimal. Their survey of 79 health care centers in Europe to determine the type of care, and type of health professionals involved in delivering the care, found that the majority did not comply with the recommendations for optimal ACHD care (Deanfield et al., 2003; Department of Health, 2006; Foster et al., 2001; Warnes et al., 2001).

Summary. As long ago as 1993 (Galioto and Tomassoni) clinicians were advocating cardiac (exercise) rehabilitation for children as "a new and evolving service intended to integrate the child with a significant cardiovascular impairment into a lifestyle of normal physical activity." The same authors observed that whilst many children with less complex, or successfully treated, CHD do not need structured cardiac rehabilitation, they should not be restricted from full participation in mainstream sports. They advised that "for these children, rehabilitation requires only the advice and encouragement of their physician to enjoy unrestricted, normal activities, including competitive sports." Unfortunately, the data from the studies reviewed here suggest that these recommendations are not being met in many patients; clearly, a far more proactive approach is needed to ensure that young people and their families DO receive the appropriate intervention regarding physical activity.

IMPLICATIONS FOR HEALTH PROFESSIONALS

Addressing the Gaps in Service Provision

It is evident from the literature review that although the medical world has recognized the need for services to develop to complement the advances in the medical management of children with CHD, there are still gaps in service provision, some children and their families do have unmet needs, and recommendations for physical activity and/or cardiac rehabilitation are not fully met. The challenge to health professionals is how to address those needs. Health professionals need to take account of a wide range of issues when considering rehabilitation for young people with CHD. Key areas to develop should include specific exercise and physical activity advice or intervention, and interdisciplinary team working to address the wider education and information needs.

Meeting Rehabilitation and Physical Activity Needs

The evidence shows that patient and family needs are complex and multifactorial. An individual, nonprescriptive approach should be used throughout childhood, adolescence, and transition to adult care, to identify exercise/physical activity needs and, in consultation with the young person and their parents, plan appropriate methods of intervention. Provision of information and advice need not always require face-to-face contact, other methods, for example, telephone, e-mail, and Web sites, may be appropriate and indeed preferable to some young people. Exercise rehabilitation should be targeted at those with greater need, for example, to improve fitness levels following medical intervention, to increase physical activity levels to meet public health guidelines, to aid weight loss, and promote a healthier less sedentary lifestyle. Some patients may require or prefer a structured exercise program, but alternative methods of improving daily activity should be actively promoted, especially for those patients who dislike, or are unable to participate in, sports activities.

Families should be proactively followed up and accurate, age-appropriate verbal and written information offered regarding physical activity at regular intervals. Times of particular need are likely to include starting, changing, and leaving school, college, or employment, and during any change in cardiac status. It is important that health professionals give detailed, individual exercise information with the emphasis on what children and adolescents with CHD *can* do. Teachers, for example, should be encouraged to adapt physical activities to include, rather than exclude, these young people (Kendall et al., 2007; Lightfoot et al., 1999; Maron et al., 2004).

All young people with CHD should know the extent, and the type, of physical activity that is appropriate and recommended for them—including what, if anything, they should avoid—to enable them to make informed choices about exercise. The use of individual patient held records or patient passports may help patients in keeping their information updated and accessible.

Interdisciplinary Teams

Researchers now frequently recommend that children with CHD and their families have the support of an interdisciplinary team that has appropriate expertise in their care (Chessa et al., 2005; Department of Health, 2003; Gardner and Angelini, 1995; Kendall et al., 2003a; Kennedy, 2001; McCrindle et al., 2006). In the United Kingdom the report of the Paediatric and Congenital Cardiac Services Review Group (Department of Health, 2003) provided comprehensive standards for the optimum care of patients with CHD and their families, with standard 1 stating that "the congenital heart service should function as a team."

There has been an increase in the number of pediatric cardiac liaison nurses in the United Kingdom following on from the recommendations of the Kennedy Report (2001) and the Paediatric and Congenital Cardiac Services Review Group (Department of Health, 2003). These specialist cardiac nurses have an essential role to play and the development and impact of their role needs careful evaluation (Killey and Flynn, 2006). However, a survey of all United Kingdom pediatric cardiac centers indicated that whilst the health professionals agreed that interdisciplinary rehabilitation services were needed in this patient population, only one center reported having a formal rehabilitation program (Lewin et al., 2002).

The growing numbers of adult patients with CHD requiring specialist care has resulted in a number of European and North American expert panels and task forces being formed to develop recommendations for management and standards of care in ACHD. The ACHD guidelines also recommend the interdisciplinary approach with patients receiving care from a multispecialty team experienced in the management of CHD (British Cardiac Society, 2002; Deanfield et al., 2003; Department of Health, 2006; Foster et al., 2001; Moons et al., 2006b; Warnes et al., 2001).

It is evident that in order to optimize care, young people with CHD should have access to a range of specialized health professionals (interdisciplinary team) experienced in the management of CHD such as, for example, physicians, cardiac liaison nurses, psychologists, cardiac physiotherapists, dieticians, and social workers.

The development of such services will have resource and training implications for health care providers. It is essential that such services are structured, evidence based, and evaluated to assess their impact on patient care.

Further development of a working interdisciplinary team would enable cross-referral within the team in order for the most appropriate team member to provide care, education, and information to patients with CHD on a structured, repetitive basis.

Education and Information

The research literature review identifies the need for structured patient information and suggests that health professionals need to consider a more holistic view of the young person's life. Rehabilitation services should encompass all aspects of the young person's condition. When giving information, it is important that health professionals discuss with the young person and their parents what their individual needs and requirements are, taking account of the wider lifestyle issues that young persons may face as a consequence of their condition, in addition to the specific medical details. In the United Kingdom the findings of the Kennedy Report (2001) indicate that parents themselves do not always feel fully informed about their child's condition. One of the key recommendations of the Kennedy report was that patients should be involved, where possible, in decisions about their treatment and care.

Given that children mainly rely on their parents for information regarding their condition, especially the younger children, it is essential that parents are fully informed at all stages of care so that they can effectively take part in making decisions. The ultimate aim is to enable the child to take responsibility for managing their CHD in order to make informed decisions and choices about lifestyle issues, and to maximize their potential in life. Recommendations for the management of ACHD emphasize that preparation for transition from pediatric to adult care should begin with patient education in childhood and continue throughout adolescence (Foster et al., 2001; Reid et al., 2006; Saidi et al., 2007).

Depending on the age of the patient, topics should include details of the cardiac condition, any surgeries and interventions, medication effects and side effects, physical activity and exercise prescription, endocarditis risks and prevention, importance and frequency of outpatient visits, career planning, transition to adult care, genetic counseling, contraception and family planning, insurance, symptoms to look for, and when to contact their health professional service.

It is important that families are made aware of how to make contact with health professionals, given that the status of their CHD and information needs may change over time.

OUTCOME MEASURES IN CONGENITAL HEART DEFECTS

Identifying which families have unmet needs requiring intervention can be difficult when targeting scarce resources. It is known that severity of CHD is not a predictor of quality of life or level of stress associated with the condition (Majnemer et al., 2006; McCrindle et al., 1995; Ternestedt et al., 2001; Walker et al., 2004; Wray and Maynard, 2005) and mild CHD or indeed innocent murmurs may have a significant adverse impact on some families. Patients, parents, and health professionals may have differing opinions on the relative importance of specific outcome measures (Kennedy, 2001; Knowles et al., 2005; Van Rijen et al., 2004; Verrips et al., 2000; Verrips et al., 2000). It is essential, therefore, that health professionals continue to explore the needs and values of children, adolescents, and their parents, and adults with CHD, and to assess outcomes, in order to inform and develop appropriate methods of providing treatment (Knowles et al., chapter 8, 2005; Mussato, 2006). There is a need, however, for more rigorous research to measure outcomes in CHD (Moons et al., 2004). This is a complex field to measure but only good-quality research with large patient populations can enhance the existing body of knowledge.

Disease-Specific Measurement Tools

Validated measures of health-related quality of life in children, adolescents, and young ACHD are now being developed. Such measures include the TAAQOL, Netherlands Organisation for Applied Scientific Research-Academic Medical Centre (TNO/AZL) Adult Quality of Life, a questionnaire for use with ACHD (Kamphuis et al., 2002); the PedsQL, a generic measure with an added cardiac module, comprising a self-report for children and young people aged 2–18 plus a parent-proxy report (Varni et al., 2002); the ConQol, a disease-specific measure for use with children aged 8–11 and 12–16 years (Macran et al., 2006); and the Pediatric Cardiac Quality of Life Inventory (PCQLI), a disease-specific instrument for children aged 8–12 and adolescents aged 13–18, with supplementary parent-proxy reporting (Marino et al., 2006, 2008).

It is anticipated that such measures may be used by clinicians and researchers to determine individual patient needs for care provision, for example, to identify those needing physical activity interventions, to assess whether their needs had been met, or to assess the effects of rehabilitation/exercise programs. This would allow for more specific targeting of resources to those patients with the most urgent need.

FURTHER RESEARCH

There is a need for future research using rigorous methodology and large-scale, multicenter studies, as used in ACHD with the Euro Heart Survey, for example, to assess the efficacy of interventions in young people with CHD. The evidence suggests that there is a place for structured exercise rehabilitation in some patients and regular promotion of increased daily activity in all patients. More work needs to done to ensure this happens in the clinical situation, with careful evaluation and assessment of outcomes.

Key areas for future research should include:

- The potential benefits of actively promoting regular, low-to-moderate-intensity physical activity in *all* patients with CHD should be assessed, irrespective of their exercise capacity or function.
- Methods of motivating young people with CHD to increase their daily, habitual physical activity levels, and sustaining increased levels, should be addressed—possibly in comparison with structured exercise training/rehabilitation programs.
- The potential benefits of using interdisciplinary teams and rehabilitation programs in the management of patients with CHD should be assessed and evaluated.
- Further research to refine the use of measurement tools to assess the need for, and measure the outcome following, exercise rehabilitation or other lifestyle interventions should be supported.

CONCLUSIONS

The ultimate aim of caring for children and adolescents with CHD and their parents is to enable each of them to maximize their potential in life within the constraints of their condition. Consideration of the psychosocial issues that young persons may face because of their condition should be given equal importance as medical issues. Health professionals must not underestimate the impact of CHD on the functioning of some young people and their families and the depth of information, counseling, and physical activity advice needed; some young people will require specific exercise or rehabilitation interventions. There is a need for increased awareness among health professionals, public, schools, and families themselves about safe appropriate exercise and physical activity in CHD, the consequences of living with CHD, and optimal standards of care.

The goal of enabling children and adolescents with CHD to enter the world of ACHD as young people with the ability to make informed decisions, and choices, about their life will only be achieved by listening to the needs of families, and targeting resources to those areas of need.

REFERENCES

Balady GJ, Williams MA, Ades PA, et al. Core components of cardiac rehabilitation/secondary prevention programs. A scientific statement from the American Heart Association exercise, cardiac rehabilitation, and prevention committee, the council on clinical cardiology; the councils on cardiovascular nursing, epidemiology and prevention, and nutrition, physical activity, and metabolism; and the American association of cardiovascular and pulmonary rehabilitation. *Circulation.* 2007;115:2675–2682.

Balfour IC, Drimmer AM, Nouri S, Pennington DG, Hemkens CL, Harvey LL. Pediatric cardiac rehabilitation. *Am J Dis Child.* 1991;145:627–630.

Beresford B, Sloper T. The information needs of chronically ill or physically disabled children and adolescents. NHS 1639 (3.99). Full research report. Social Policy Research Unit, University of York, York; 1999.

Bowyer JJ, Busst CM, Till JA, Lincoln C. Shinebourne EA. Exercise ability after mustard's operation. *Arch Dis Child.* 1990;65:865–870.

British Cardiac Society. Grown-up congenital heart (GUCH) disease: current needs and provision of service for adolescents and adults with congenital heart disease in the UK. Report of the British Cardiac Society Working Party. *Heart.* 2002;88(suppl 1):i1–i14.

Calzolari A, Pastore E, Biondi G. Cardiac rehabilitation in children. Interdisciplinary approach. *Minerva Pediatr.* 1997;49:559–565.

Casey FA, Craig BG, Mulholland HC. Quality of life in surgically palliated complex congenital heart disease. *Arch Dis Child.* 1994;70:382–386.

Cavill N, Biddle S, Sallis JF. Health enhancing physical activity for young people: statement of the United Kingdom Expert Consensus conference. *Pediatr Exerc Sci.* 2001;13:12–25.

Chessa M, De Rosa G, Pardeo M, et al. What do parents know about the malformations afflicting the hearts of their children? *Cardiol Young.* 2005;15:125–129.

Cheuk DKL, Wong SMY, Choi YP, Chau AKT, Cheung YF. Parents' understanding of their child's congenital heart disease. *Heart.* 2004;90:435–439.

Children's Heart Federation. *Report of the findings from the Children's Heart Federation Conference: Children's Heart Services—Into the Future: A guide to care standards.* London, September 2001.

Crossland DS, Jackson SP, Lyall R, Burn J, O'Sullivan. Employment and advice regarding careers for adults with congenital heart disease. *Cardiol Young.* 2005;15:391–395.

Deanfield J, Thaulow E, Warnes C, et al. Management of grown up congenital heart disease: the task force on the management of grown up congenital heart disease of the European Society of Cardiology. *Eur Heart J.* 2003;24:1035–1084.

Dent JM. Congenital heart disease and exercise. *Clin Sports Med.* 2003;22:81–99.

Department of Health. Report of the paediatric and congenital cardiac services review group. Department of Health, London 2003/0519:1–49. www.dh.gov.uk/; 2003.

Department of Health, Physical Activity, Health Improvement, and Prevention. At least five a week. Evidence on the impact of physical activity and its relationship to health. A report from the Chief Medical Officer: Department of Health, London 2004/2389:1–128. www. dh.gov.uk/; 2004.

Department of Health. Adult congenital heart disease—A commissioning guide for services for young people and grown ups with congenital heart disease (GUCH). Department of Health, London 2006/6397:1–40. www.dh.gov.uk/; 2006.

Diller GP, Dimopoulos K, Okonko D, et al. Exercise intolerance in adult congenital heart disease: comparative severity, correlates, and prognostic implication. *Circulation.* 2005;112:828–835.

Dimopoulos K, Diller GP, Piepoli MF, Gatzoulis MA. Exercise intolerance in adults with congenital heart disease. *Cardiol Clin.* 2006;24:641–660.

Dimopoulos K, Okonko DO, Diller GP, et al. Abnormal ventilatory response to exercise in adults with congenital heart disease relates to cyanosis and predicts survival. *Circulation.* 2006a;113:2796–2802.

Dore A, De Guise P, Mercier LM. Transition of care to adult congenital heart centres: What do patients know about their heart condition? *Can J Cardiol.* 2002;18:141–146.

Driscoll DJ, Offord KP, Feldt RH, Schaff HV, Puga FJ, Danielson GK. Five to fifteen year follow up after Fontan operation. *Circulation.* 1992;85:469–496.

Driscoll D. Exercise responses in functional single ventricle before and after Fontan operation. *Prog Pediatr Cardiol.* 1993;2:44–49.

Dua JS, Cooper AR, Fox KR, Stuart AG. Physical activity levels in adults with congenital heart disease. *Eur J Cardiovasc Prev Rehab.* 2007;14:287–293.

Eiser C, Morse R. A review of measures of quality of life for children with chronic illness. *Arch Dis Child.* 2001;84:205–211.

Eiser C. No pain, no gain? Integrating QoL assessment in paediatrics. *Arch Dis Child.* 2007;92:379–380.

Engelfriet P, Boersma E, Oechslin E, et al. The spectrum of adult congenital heart disease in Europe: morbidity and mortality in a 5 year follow-up period. The Euro Heart Survey on adult congenital heart disease. *Eur Heart J.* 2005;26:2325–2333.

Engelfriet P, Tijssen J, Kaemmerer H, et al. Adherence to guidelines in the clinical care for adults with congenital heart disease: the Euro Heart Survey on adult congenital heart disease. *Eur Heart J.* 2006;27:737–745.

Ensing G, Heise C, Driscoll D. Cardiovascular response to exercise after the mustard operation for simple and complex transposition of the great vessels. *Am J Cardiol.* 1988;62:617–622.

Falk B, Bar-Mor G, Zigel L, Yaaron M, Beniamini Y, Zeevvi B. Daily physical activity and perception of condition severity among male and female adolescents with congenital heart malformation. *J Pediatr Nurs.* 2006;21:244–249.

Fekkes M, Kamphuis RP, Ottenkamp J, et al. Health-related quality of life in young adults with minor congenital heart disease. *Psychol Health.* 2001;16:239–250.

Fisher HR. The needs of parents with chronically sick children: a literature review. *J Adv Nurs.* 2001;36:600–607.

Fletcher GF, Balady G, Blair SN, et al. Statement on exercise: benefits and recommendations for physical activity programs for all Americans: a statement for health professionals by the committee on exercise and cardiac rehabilitation of the council on clinical cardiology, American Heart Association. *Circulation.* 1996;94:857–862.

Foster E, Graham TP, Driscoll DJ, et al. 32nd Bethesda Conference: Care of the adult with congenital heart disease. Task force 2: Special health care needs of adults with congenital heart disease; 2001.

Fredriksen PM, Ingjer F, Nystad W, Thaulow E. A comparison of VO2 peak between patients with CHD and healthy subjects, all aged 8–17 years. *Eur J Appl Physiol.* 1999;80:409–416.

Fredriksen PM, Kahrs N, Blaasvaer S, et al. Effect of physical training in children and adolescents with congenital heart disease. *Cardiol Young.* 2000;10:107–114.

Fredriksen PM, Veldtman G, Hechter S, et al. Aerobic capacity in adults with various congenital heart diseases. *Am J Cardiol.* 2001;87:310–314.

Fredriksen PM, Therrien J, Veldtman G, et al. Aerobic capacity in adults with tetralogy of fallot. *Cardiol Young.* 2002;12:554–559.

Galioto FM, Tomassoni TL. Exercise rehabilitation in congenital heart disease. *Prog Pediatr Cardiol.* 1993;2:50–54.

Gardner FV, Angelini GD. Psychological aspects of congenital heart disease. *Cardiol Young.* 1995;5:302–309.

Gill TM, Feinstein AR. A critical appraisal of the quality of quality of life measurements. *JAMA.* 1994;272:619–626.

Godfrey S. Exercise and pulmonary function. In: Anderson R, Macartney F, Shinebourne EA, Tynan M, eds. *Paediatric Cardiology.* Edinburgh: Churchill Livingstone; 1987;395–417.

Goldberg B, Fripp RR, Lister G, Loke J, Nicholas JA, Tainer NS. Effect of physical training on exercise performance of children following surgical repair of congenital heart disease. *Pediatrics.* 1981;68:691–699.

Graham TP Jr, Bricker JT, James FW, Strong WB. 26th Bethesda conference: recommendations for determining eligibility for competition in athletes with cardiovascular abnormalities. Task force 1: congenital heart disease. *J Am Coll Cardiol.* 1994;24:867–873.

Graham TP, Driscoll DJ, Gersony WM, Newburger JW, Rocchini A, Towbin JA. 36th Bethesda Conference: eligibility recommendations for competitive athletes with cardiovascular abnormalities. Task force 2: Congenital heart disease. *J Am Coll Cardiol.* 2005;45:1326–1333.

Gutgesell HP, Gessner IH, Vetter VL, Yabeck SM, Norton JB. Recreational and occupational recommendations for young patients with heart disease. *Circulation.* 1986;74:1195A–1198A.

Hechter SJ, Webb G, Fredriksen PM, et al. Cardiopulmonary exercise performance in adult survivors of the Mustard procedure. *Cardiol Young.* 2001;11:407–414.

Heidbüchel H, Panhuyzen-Goedkoop N, Corrado D, et al. Recommendations for participation in leisure-time physical activity and competitive sports in patients with arrhythmias and potentially arrhythmogenic conditions: Part 1: supraventricular arrhythmias and pacemakers. *Eur J Cardiovasc Prev Rehab.* 2006;13:475–484.

Heidbüchel H, Corrado D, Biffi A, et al. Recommendations for participation in leisure-time physical activity and competitive sports in patients with arrhythmias and potentially arrhythmogenic conditions: part 2: ventricular arrhythmias, channelopathies and implantable defibrillators. *Eur J Cardiovasc Prev Rehab.* 2006a ;13:676–686.

Hirth A, Reybrouck T, Bjarnason-Wehrens B, Lawrenz W, Hoffman A. Recommendations for participation in competitive and leisure sports in patients with congenital heart disease: a consensus document. *Eur J Cardiovasc Prev Rehab.* 2006;13:293–299.

Hoffman J. Incidence of congenital heart disease: I. Postnatal incidence. *Pediatric Cardiol.* 1995;16:103–113.

Kamphuis M, Ottenkamp J, Vliegen HW, et al. Health related quality of life and health status in adult survivors with previously operated complex congenital heart disease. *Heart.* 2002;87:356–362.

Kendall L, Sloper P, Lewin RJP, Parsons JM. The views of young people with congenital cardiac disease on designing the services for their treatment. *Cardiol Young.* 2003;13:11–19.

Kendall L, Sloper P, Lewin RJP, Parsons JM. The views of parents concerning the planning of services for rehabilitation of families of children with congenital cardiac disease. *Cardiol Young.* 2003a;13:20–27.

Kendall L, Parsons JM, Sloper P, Lewin RJP. A simple screening method for determining knowledge of the appropriate levels of activity and risk behaviour in young people with congenital cardiac conditions. *Cardiol Young.* 2007;17(2):151–157.

Kennedy I. Learning from Bristol: The report of the public inquiry into children's heart surgery at the Bristol Royal Infirmary 1984–1995. The Stationery Office, London Cm:5207-I. www.bristol-inquiry.org.uk; 2001.

Killey M, Flynn M. Hearts and minds: developing and expanding the role of the paediatric cardiac liaison nurse. *Br J Cardiac Nurs.* 2006;1:198–202.

Kitchiner D. Physical activities in patients with congenital heart disease. *Heart.* 1996;76:6–7.

Knowles R, Griebsch I, Dezateux C, Brown J, Bull C, Wren C. Newborn screening for congenital heart defects: a systematic review and cost-effectiveness analysis. *Health Technol Assess.* 2005;9(44):1–176. www.hta.ac.uk/project/1207.asp.

Koster NK. Physical activity and congenital heart disease. *Nurs Clinic North Am.* 1994;29:345–356.

Lewin RJP, Kendall L, Sloper P. Provision of services for rehabilitation of children and adolescents with congenital cardiac disease: a survey of centres for paediatric cardiology in the United Kingdom. *Cardiol Young.* 2002;12:412–414.

Lightfoot J, Wright S, Sloper P. *Service support for children with a chronic illness or physical disability attending mainstream schools.* NHS 1576 (10.98). Full research report. Social Policy Research Unit, University of York, York; 1998.

Lightfoot J, Wright S, Sloper P. Supporting pupils in mainstream school with an illness or disability: young people's views. *Child Care Health Dev.* 1999;25:267–283.

Longmuir PE, Turner JA, Rowe RD, Olley PM. Post-operative exercise rehabilitation benefits children with congenital heart disease. *Clin Invest Med.* 1985;8:232–238.

Lunt D, Briffa T, Briffa NK, Ramsay J. Physical activity levels of adolescents with congenital heart disease. *Aust J Physiother.* 2003;49:43–50.

Macran S, Birks Y, Parsons J, Sloper P, et al. The development of a new measure of quality of life for children with congenital cardiac disease. *Cardiol Young.* 2006;16:165–172. www.cardiacrehabilitation.org.uk/conqol.htm.

Majnemer A, Limperopoulos C, Shevell M, Rohlicek C, Rosenblatt B, Tchervenkov C. Health and well-being of children with congenital cardiac malformations, and their families, following open-heart surgery. *Cardiol Young.* 2006;16:157–164.

Marcus BH, Williams DM, Dubbert PM, et al. Physical activity intervention studies: what we know and what we need to know. A scientific statement from the American Heart Association council on nutrition, physical activity, and metabolism (subcommittee on physical activity); council on cardiovascular disease in the young; and the interdisciplinary working group on quality of care and outcomes research. *Circulation.* 2006;114:2739–2752.

Marino BS, Shera D, Shea JA, et al. *The pediatric cardiac quality of life inventory (PCQLI) testing trial: reliability and validity data.* Paper presented at Psychosocial Care in Congenital Heart Disease: Biannual Meeting of the Association for European Paediatric Cardiology Working Group in Psychosocial Problems in Congenital Heart Disease. Belfast, March 8, 2006.

Marino BS, Shera D, Wernovsky G, et al. The development of the pediatric cardiac quality of life inventory: a quality of life measure for children and adolescents with heart disease. *Qual Life Res.* 2008;17:613–626.

Maron BJ, Chaitman BR, Ackerman MJ, et al. Working groups of the American Heart Association committee on exercise, cardiac rehabilitation, and prevention; Councils on clinical cardiology and cardiovascular disease in the young. Recommendations for physical activity and recreational sports participation for young patients with genetic cardiovascular diseases. *Circulation.* 2004;109:2807–2816.

Maron BJ, Zipes DP. 36th Bethesda conference: introduction: eligibility recommendations for competitive athletes with cardiovascular abnormalities—general considerations. *J Am Coll Cardiol.* 2005;45:1318–1321.

Massin MM, Hövels-Gürich HH, Gérard P, Seghaye MC. Physical activity patterns of children after neonatal arterial switch operation. *Ann Thorac Surg.* 2006;81:665–670.

McCrindle BW, Shaffer KM, Kan JS, Zahka KG, Rowe SA, Kidd L. An evaluation of parental concerns and misperceptions about heart murmurs. *Clin Pediatr (Phila).* 1995;34:25–31.

McCrindle BW, Williams RV, Mitchell PD, et al. Relationship of patient and medical characteristics to health status in children and adolescents after the Fontan procedure. *Circulation.* 2006;113:1123–1129.

McNamara DG, Bricker JT, Galioto FM, Graham TP Jr, James FW, Rosenthal A. 16th Bethesda conference: cardiovascular abnormalities in the athlete: recommendations regarding eligibility for competition: task force 1: congenital heart disease. *J Am Coll Cardiol.* 1985;6:1200–1208.

Meijboom F, Szatmari A, Deckers JW, et al. Cardiac status and health related quality of life in the long term after surgical repair of tetralogy of fallot in infancy and childhood. *J Thorac Cardiovasc Surg.* 1995;110:883–891.

Mitchell JH, Haskell W, Snell P, Van Camp SP. 36th Bethesda conference: task force 8: classification of sports. *J Am Coll Cardiol.* 2005;45:1364–1367.

Moalla W, Maingourd Y, Gauthier R, Cahalin LP, Tabka Z, Ahmaidi S. Effect of exercise training on respiratory muscle oxygenation in children with congenital heart disease. *Eur J Cardiovasc Prev Rehab.* 2006;13:604–611.

Moons P, De Volder E, Budts W, et al. What do adult patients with congenital heart disease know about their disease, treatment, and prevention of complications? A call for structured patient education. *Heart.* 2001;86:74–80.

Moons P, Van Deyk K, Budts W, De Geest S. Caliber of quality of life assessments in congenital heart disease: a plea for more conceptual and methodological rigor. *Arch Pediatr Adolesc Med.* 2004;158:1062–1069.

Moons P, Barrea C, De Wolf D, et al. Changes in perceived health of children with congenital heart disease after attending a special sports camp. *Pediatric Cardiol.* 2006;27:67–72.

Moons P, Barrea C, Suys B, et al. Improved perceived health status persists three months after a special sports camp for children with congenital heart disease. *Eur J Pediatr.* 2006a;165:767–772.

Moons P, Engelfriet P, Kaemmerer H, Meijboom FJ, Oechslin E, Mulder BJM. On behalf of the expert committee of Euro Heart Survey on adult congenital heart disease. Delivery of care for adult patients with congenital heart disease in Europe: results from the Euro Heart Survey. *Eur Heart J.* 2006b;27:1324–1330.

Mussato KA. Beyond survival: what are the outcomes that really matter to our patients? *Cardiol Young.* 2006;16:125–127.

Pate RR, Pratt M, Blair SN, et al. Physical activity and public health: a recommendation from the centers for disease control and prevention and the American College of Sports Medicine. *JAMA.* 1995;273:402–407.

Pate RR, Davis MG, Robinson TN, Stone EJ, McKenzie TL, Young JC. Promoting physical activity in children and youth: a leadership role of schools: a scientific statement from the American Heart Association council on nutrition, physical activity, and metabolism (physical activity committee) in collaboration with the councils on cardiovascular disease in the young and cardiovascular nursing. *Circulation.* 2006;114:1214–1224.

Pelliccia A, Fagard R, Bjornstad HH, et al. Recommendations for competitive sports participation in athletes with cardiovascular disease: a consensus document from the study group of **sports** cardiology of the working group of cardiac rehabilitation and exercise physiology and the working group of myocardial and pericardial diseases of the **European** Society of Cardiology. *Eur Heart J.* 2005;26:1422–1445.

Pelliccia A, Corrado D, Bjornstad HH, et al. Recommendations for participation in competitive sport and leisure-time physical activity in individuals with cardiomyopathies, myocarditis and pericarditis. *Eur J Cardiovasc Prev Rehab.* 2006;13:876–875.

Perloff, J. Congenital heart disease in adults: a new cardiovascular subspecialty. *Circulation.* 1991;84:1881–1890.

Phipps S, Srivastava DK. Repressive adaptation in children with cancer: it may be better not to know. *J Pediatrics.* 1997;130:257–265.

Pinto NM, Marino BS, Wernovsky G, et al. *Obesity is prevalent, and is a significant additional comorbidity in children with congenital and acquired heart disease.* Atlanta, March 14, 2006.

Pinto NM, Marino BS, Wernovsky G, et al. Obesity is a common comorbidity in children with congenital and acquired heart disease. *Pediatrics.* 2007;120:e1157–1164.

Prapavessis H, Maddison R, Ruygrok PN, Bassett S, Harper T, Gillanders L. Using theory of planned behavior to understand exercise motivation in patients with congenital heart disease. *Psychol Health Med.* 2005;10:335–343.

Reid GJ, Webb GD, Barzel M, McCrindle BW, Irvine MJ, Siu SC. Estimates of life expectancy by adolescents and young adults with congenital heart disease. *J Am Coll Cardiol.* 2006;48:349–355.

Reybrouck T, Boshoff D, Vanhees L, Defoor J, Gewillig M. Ventilatory response to exercise in patients after correction of cyanotic congenital heart disease: relation with clinical outcome after surgery. *Heart.* 2004;90:215–216.

Reybrouck T, Mertens L. Physical performance and physical activity in grown-up congenital heart disease. *Eur J Cardiovasc Prev Rehab.* 2005;12:498–502.

Rhodes J, Curran TJ, Camil L, et al. Impact of cardiac rehabilitation on the exercise function of children with serious congenital heart disease. *Pediatrics.* 2005;116:1339–1345.

Rogers R, Reybrouck T, Weymans M, Dumoulin M, Van Der HL, Gewillig M. Reliability of subjective estimates of exercise capacity after total repair of tetralogy of fallot. *Acta Paediatrica.* 1994;83:866–869.

Ruttenberg HD, Adams TD, Orsmond GS, Conlee RK, Fisher AG. Effects of exercise training on aerobic fitness in children after open heart surgery. *Pediatric Cardiol.* 1983;4:19–24.

Saidi AS, Paolillo J, Fricker FJ, Sears SF, Kovacs AH. Biomedical and psychosocial evaluation of "cured" adults with congenital heart disease. *Congenit Heart Dis.* 2007;2:44–54.

Soni NR, Deanfield JE. Assessment of cardiovascular fitness for competitive sport in high risk groups. *Arch Dis Child.* 1997;77:386–389.

Spall JA. Patient-centred services. *Cardiol Young.* 2003;13:3–6.

Sparacino PS, Tong EM, Messias DK, Foote D, Chesla CA, Gillis CL. The dilemmas of parents of adolescents and young adults with congenital heart disease. *Heart Lung J Acute Crit Care.* 1997;26:187–195.

Swan L, Hillis WS. Exercise prescription in adults with congenital heart disease: a long way to go. *Heart.* 2000;83:685–687.

Ternestedt BM, Wall K, Oddsson H, Riesenfeld T, Groth I, Schollin J. Quality of life 20 and 30 years after surgery in patients operated on for tetralogy of fallot and for atrial septal defect. *Pediatr Cardiol.* 2001;22:128–132.

Thaulow E, Fredriksen PM. Exercise and training in adults with congenital heart disease. *Int J Cardiol.* 2004;97(suppl 1):35–38.

Therrien J, Fredriksen PM, Walker M, Granton J, Reid GJ, Webb G. A pilot study of exercise training in adult patients with repaired tetralogy of Fallot. *Can J Cardiol.* 2003;19:685–689.

Thompson PD, Buchner D, Piña IL, et al. Exercise and physical activity in the prevention and treatment of atherosclerotic cardiovascular disease: a statement from the council on clinical cardiology (subcommittee on exercise, rehabilitation, and prevention) and the council on nutrition, physical activity, and metabolism (subcommittee on physical activity). *Circulation.* 2003;107:3109–3116.

Tomassoni T, Galioto F, Vaccaro P, Vaccaro J. Effect of exercise training on exercise tolerance and cardiac output in children after repair of congenital heart disease. *Sports Train Med Rehab.* 1990;2:57–62.

Tomassoni TL, Galioto FM Jr, Vaccaro P. Cardiopulmonary exercise testing in children following surgery for Tetralogy of Fallot. *Am J Dis Child.* 1991;145:1290–1293.

Tomassoni TL. Role of exercise in the management of cardiovascular disease in children and youth. *Med Sci Sports Exerc.* 1996;28:406–413.

Utens EM, Bieman HJ, Verhulst FC, Witsenburg M, Bogers AJ, Hess J. Psychological distress and styles of coping in parents of children awaiting elective cardiac surgery. *Cardiol Young.* 2000;10:239–244.

Uzark K. Counselling adolescents with congenital heart disease. *J Cardiovasc Nurs.* 1992;6:65–73.

Van Deyk K, Moons P, Gewillig M, Budts W. Educational and behavioral issues in transitioning from pediatric cardiology to adult-centered health care. *Nurs Clin North Am.* 2004;39:755–768.

Van Horn M, DeMaso DR, Gonzalez-Heydrich J, Erickson JD. Illness-related concerns of mothers of children with congenital heart disease. *J Am Acad Child Adolesc Psychiatry.* 2001;40:847–854.

Van Rijen EHM, Utens EMWJ, Roos-Hesselink JW, et al. Medical predictors for psychopathology in adults with operated congenital heart disease. *Eur Heart J.* 2004;25:1605–1613.

Varni JW, Seid M, Smith T, Uzark K, Szer IS. The PedsQL 4.0 Generic core scales: sensitivity, responsiveness, and impact on clinical decision-making. *J Behav Med.* 2002;25:175–193.

Verrips G, Vogels A, Den Ouden A, Paneth N, Verloove-Vanhorick S. Measuring health-related quality of life in adolescents: agreement between raters and between methods of administration. *Child Care Health Dev.* 2000;26:457–469.

Walker RE, Gauvreau K, Jenkins KJ. Health-related quality of life in children attending a cardiology clinic. *Pediatr Cardiol.* 2004;25:40–48.

Warnes CA, Liberthson R, Danielson GK, et al. Task force 1: the changing profile of congenital heart disease in adult life. *J Am Coll Cardiol.* 2001;37:1170–1175.

Warnes CA. The adult with congenital heart disease. Born to be bad? *J Am Coll Cardiol.* 2005;46:1–8.

Washington RL. Cardiac rehabilitation programmes in children. *Sports Med.* 1992;14:164–170.

Wessel HU, Paul MH. Exercise studies in tetralogy of fallot: a review. *Pediatr Cardiol.* 1999;20:39–47.

WHOQoL Group. The development of the World Health Organization Quality of Life Assessment Instrument (the WHOQoL). In: Orley J, Kuyken W, eds. *Quality of Life Assessment: International Perspectives.* Heidleberg: Springer-Verlag; 1994.

Wray J, Maynard L. Living with congenital or acquired cardiac disease in childhood: maternal perceptions of the impact on the child and family. *Cardiol Young.* 2005;15:133–140.

Wray J, Maynard L. The needs of families of children with heart disease. *J Dev Behav Pediatr.* 2006;27:11–17.

23

Frequency of Congenital Heart Defects in Various Regions of the World

DIEGO F. WYSZYNSKI

There are several reasons to study the incidence and prevalence at birth of congenital heart defect (CHD). Knowing the relative frequencies of different lesions may aid diagnosis because common lesions should be considered before rarer lesions. The frequency of occurrence of various types of CHD—no matter their intensity, their clustering in time or place, or their association with certain external agents—may ultimately lead to understanding what caused them. Finally, information about the frequency of occurrence of clinically important CHDs is needed to assess their economic effect and to plan for effective medical services (Hoffman, 1995).

Major CHDs are usually apparent in the neonatal period, but minor defects may not be detected until adulthood. Thus, true measures of *incidence* for CHDs would need to record new cases of defects presenting anytime in fetal life through adulthood. However, estimates are largely available for new cases detected after birth, known as *prevalence at birth*. Both of these are typically reported as cases per 1000 live births per year and do not distinguish between minor defects that resolve without treatment and major malformations. To differentiate the more serious defects, some studies report new cases of sufficient severity to undergo an invasive procedure or to result in death within the first year of life.

Reported total rates of CHDs differ, in part because of changes in diagnostic and registration criteria and the degree to which prenatally diagnosed conditions are included (Pradat et al., 2003). Although the total prevalence of cardiac defects at birth has been estimated at 7 to 10 per 1000 births (Carlgren, 1959; Carlgren et al., 1987; Hanna et al., 1994; Mitchell et al., 1971; Romano-Zelekha et al., 2001), the exact figure depends on ascertainment of cases, the inclusion criteria used, and the duration of follow-up review

during the neonatal period, when the diagnosis may be indefinite (Pradat et al., 2003). A review by Hoffman and Kaplan (2002) reported the interquartile range of prevalence estimates across 44 international studies for the common forms of CHD. For all types of CHD combined, the interquartile range was 60 to 105 CHDs per 10,000 births (Hoffman and Kaplan, 2002), and CHDs comprise approximately in 40% of all congenital defects (Romano-Zelekha et al., 2001).

Reller et al. (2008b) has also shown that another important source of variation is the nomenclature and classification systems used in the prevalence studies. The most widely referenced sources are the *International Classification of Disease, 9th Revision* (ICD-9), the modified version of the British Paediatric Association system, and the crossmapping of existing classification lists by the International Working Group for the Mapping and Coding of Nomenclatures for Paediatric and Congenital Heart Disease. A recent development that should help reduce this variation is the creation of a standard CHD nomenclature, the International Paediatric and Congenital Cardiac Code (http://www.IPCCC.net), developed by members of the Society of Thoracic Surgeons (STS) and the European Association for Cardio-Thoracic Surgery (Beland et al., 2004; Mavroudis and Jacobs, 2000; STS, 2008). At the National Birth Defects Prevention Study in Atlanta, GA, Botto et al. (2007) developed a classification scheme of cardiac defects according to heart anatomy and fetal heart development stages. The authors reviewed all available information on infants with CHDs registered in their hospital surveillance system and categorized the infants into less than 70 detailed cardiac phenotypes. Their procedure also contained a "mapping system" that allowed the detailed phenotypes to be grouped together into broader categories. In a similar approach using individual-level ICD codes,

Oyen et al. (2009) constructed an algorithm to group certain combinations of ICD codes using a hierarchical procedure, yielding 17 cardiac phenotypes.

Maternal ethnicity, exposures to potential teratogens, comorbidities, and positive family history of CHD are additional factors that deserve careful consideration when evaluating frequency data. Some maternal illnesses such as phenylketonuria (PKU), diabetes, rubella, maternal febrile illnesses, and influenza increase the risk of a CHD-affected pregnancy. Reported increased risks range from an odds ratio (OR) of 1.6 (febrile illness and conotruncal defects) to an OR of 27.2 (maternal diabetes and d-transposition of the great arteries [d-TGA]) (Jenkins et al., 2007; Wren et al., 2003). High vitamin A intake and use of certain therapeutic drugs during pregnancy, specifically, anticonvulsants, thalidomide, sulfasalazine, and vitamin A congeners/retinoids, also increases risk of CHD. While the results of studies investigating the effect of environmental exposures on CHD risk are inconclusive, organic solvents are associated with increased risk of CHD (Jenkins et al., 2007). In contrast, the association between sociodemographic factors, such as maternal and paternal age; socioeconomic status; and prenatal maternal stress is inconsistent (Jenkins et al., 2007).

Nembhard et al. (2009) determined the prevalence of CHDs and specific types of CHDs for non-Hispanic (NH)-white, NH-black, and Hispanic infants. The authors found that the prevalence of CHDs was similar for all racial/ethnic groups but varied for a few specific types of CHDs and by number of defects. Hispanics had the highest prevalence of CHDs overall (80.09 per 10,000 live births) and for infants with isolated and multiple heart defects, followed by NH-whites (79.11 per 10,000 live births) and NH-blacks (77.67 per 10,000 live births). The racial/ethnic observed differences may be the result of differential loss of CHD-affected pregnancies during the gestational period rather than true differences in the incidence of CHDs and/or due to racial/ethnic differences in CHD diagnosis after birth.

PREVALENCE OF CONGENITAL HEART DEFECT IN SPONTANEOUS ABORTUSES

A considerable proportion of human pregnancies end in spontaneous abortion: prospective studies using very sensitive early pregnancy tests have found that 25% of pregnancies are miscarried by the sixth week LMP (i.e., since the woman's last menstrual period) (Wang et al., 2003; Wilcox et al., 1999). Approximately half of the aborted fetuses have serious malformations (Byrne and Warburton, 1986; Creasy and Alberman, 1976; Dejmek et al., 1992), and chromosomal rearrangements

are present in 3.5% of the progenitors, according to a recent study by Iyer et al. (2007). Indeed, spontaneous abortion has been regarded as a natural mechanism for the disposal of defective fetuses (Janerich, 1975), a process which has been called "terathanasia" (Warkany, 1978).

Relatively little information has been published concerning CHD in spontaneous abortuses, particularly those abortuses in the late second trimester, and these studies vary widely in their scope and methods. The first publication aimed at assessing the prevalence and nature of cardiac lesions in spontaneous abortuses was by Gerlis (1985), who examined 247 spontaneously aborted fetuses, under the age of 24 weeks' gestation and found 38 instances of cardiac malformation (15.4%). Ursell et al. (1985) investigated the impact of CHD on the developing human fetus by examining 412 hearts from consecutive spontaneous abortuses of developmental ages 8–28 weeks. In each case, the cardiac morphology was correlated with the autopsy findings and the karyotype (unavailable in 115 hearts not successfully cultured). Of the 412 hearts, 10 (2.4%) contained structural defects (six ventricular septal defects [VSDs], one atrial septal defect [ASD] with VSD, and one each coarctation, atrioventricular septal defect [AVSD], and tetralogy of Fallot [TOF]). As stated by the authors, a direct comparison of their series to that of Gerlis may be impossible for several reasons. First, although "unselected," the series of hearts studied by Gerlis may not have been derived from consecutive spontaneous abortions, as the one of Ursell was. In any epidemiological study, careful control over inclusion of specimens (preferably at one institution) is critical to ensure an unbiased sample. Second, although cardiac malformation is not specifically defined, the Gerlis series included hearts with several minor malformations, such as bilateral superior caval veins and pericardial defects, which were excluded in the series of Ursell. On the other hand, there was a preponderance of relatively complex cardiac defects, such as valve atresias, transpositions, and double-outlet ventricles in the Gerlis series. It is unlikely that histological analysis would have yielded many more cardiac malformations in the Gerlis series, since these structural defects are readily identifiable grossly under the dissecting microscope. By not examining tissue histologically, Ursell may have missed abnormal ductus tissue, a precursor for patent ductus arteriosus (PDA). However, from the report it appears that ductus tissue was not examined in the Gerlis study either, and so this cannot explain the discrepancy in prevalence rates found in the two studies.

Chinn et al. (1989) studied the prevalence, range, and associations of CHD among 400 spontaneous abortuses between 9 and 40 weeks' gestation. Fifty-two (13.0%)

cases of CHD were detected. To minimize selection bias, the specimens were grouped by external appearance and the prevalence expressed accordingly. CHD was detected in 21 (7.3%) of 289 externally normal and 31 (27.9%) of 111 externally abnormal fetuses. VSD was the most frequent CHD found in isolation, as well as in combination with extracardiac malformations. Seventy-five percent of isolated CHD was VSD. Forty (69.2%) of the 52 cases of CHD were associated with extracardiac malformations. Chromosomal syndromes were responsible for a minimum of 19.2% of the cases and suspected in up to 36.5%. The most frequent associations involved the musculoskeletal system, central nervous system, abdominal wall, and kidneys. In contrast, studies of live born infants have reported 70% of CHD as isolated defects, including many CHD infrequently seen among spontaneous abortuses. This suggests that fetuses with isolated CHD often survive to term, and CHD does not significantly affect the survival of the fetus in utero. Ventricular septum formation may be particularly susceptible to hemodynamic changes and may be indicative of an underlying pathological condition that also leads to a spontaneous abortion.

Tennstedt et al. (1999) performed necropsies on 815 fetuses—448 induced abortions (55%), 220 spontaneous abortions (27%), and 147 stillbirths (18%)—during a 7-year period (1991–1997) in the department of pathology of the Charité Medical Center in Berlin. A CHD was identified in 129 cases (16%). CHDs were present in 22% of induced abortions (99 cases), 9% of spontaneous abortions (20 cases), and 7% of stillbirths (10 cases). The heart malformations were classified into 13 categories. A fetus with more than one defect was included only in the category of the most serious defect. The malformations in order of frequency were VSD (28%), AVSD (16%), left hypoplastic heart (LHH) (16%), double-outlet right ventricle (DORV) (12%), coarctation of the aorta (AoCo) (6%), TGA (4%), aortic valve stenosis (AoVS) (4%), TOF (3%), truncus arteriosus communis (TAC) (3%), pulmonary valve stenosis/pulmonary valve atresia (PaVS/PaVA) (3%), tricuspid atresia (TA) (3%), single ventricle (SV) (1.5%), and ASD (0.5%). The most common CHDs were VSD, AVSD, LHH, and DORV, which made up to 72% of all the cases. In 11 cases (8.5%), the heart defect was isolated (no other cardiovascular or extracardiac malformations present), in 85 cases (66%) additional cardiac malformations were present, in 85 cases (66%) extracardiac malformations were present, and in 43 cases (33%) chromosome anomalies were detected. The authors noted that VSD has been reported to be the most frequent cardiac defect in various other necropsy studies of live births and stillbirths (Hyett et al., 1997; Samanek et al., 1985; Tennstedt et al., 1983), and in those studies the proportion was higher than

in theirs (between 32% and 42%); this difference may reflect the composition of the case population, as the studies cited included not only stillbirths but also live born infants, among whom VSD mainly occurs as an isolated lesion that may allow the infant to survive the first few days after birth. In prenatal ultrasound investigations by Hanna et al. (1996), VSD was diagnosed in 35% of the cases (21/60). In the Baltimore-Washington Infant Study (BWIS) (Ferencz et al., 1993), which was a 9-year (1981–1989) epidemiological study of CHD in 4390 live births up to the end of the first year of life, VSD made up a higher proportion of the defects (32%) than in the Tennstedt et al. (1999) study, with 81% of the cases occurring in isolation.

Hoffman (1995) showed how the incidence of CHD is greatly increased if abortuses and stillborn infants were included in the estimation. In his example, spontaneous abortion occurred in as many as 22%–43% of pregnancies, and the incidence of stillbirths was about 2% (Bierman et al., 1965; Miller et al., 1980; Wilcox et al., 1988). Thus, among 100,000 pregnancies that last at least 4 weeks, there are likely to be about 21,800 spontaneous abortions, 1900 stillbirths, and 76,000 live births (Bierman et al., 1965). If the incidence of CHD in each group, respectively, is 20% (assumed), 10%, and 1% (the latter incidences from Hoffman and Christianson [1978]), the total incidence of CHD is 4360 + 190 + 763 = 5313. Consequently, adding the increased incidence of CHD in abortuses and stillborn children gives a total CHD incidence that could be about five times the incidence of CHD in live born children alone. By ignoring the incidence of CHD in prenatal deaths, the potential importance of genetic and chromosomal factors is grossly underestimated, and even the importance of environmental teratogens may be incorrectly assessed (Stein et al., 1975).

Although this has not been specifically evaluated in South America, a Brazilian population study performed to screen fetal cardiac abnormalities through prenatal echocardiography in low-risk pregnancies showed some interesting data (Hagemann and Zielinsky, 2004). From July 1996 to November 2000, 3980 fetuses of pregnant women with no obstetrical or cardiological risk were studied in the municipality of Porto Alegre. Forty seven cases were diagnosed with morphological and functional fetal cardiovascular abnormalities, corresponding to an overall prevalence of 11.8/1000 (47/3980). Three false-negative and no false-positive results increased the overall prevalence to 12.5/1000 (50/3980). Given these figures, the authors went on to conclude that the inclusion of cardiovascular malformation screening into the routine care assessment of obstetrical ultrasonography would be justified. Probably, cardiovascular screening of fetuses in high-risk mothers would yield even higher rates.

INTERNATIONAL PREVALENCE AT BIRTH OF CONGENITAL HEART DEFECT

Prevalence at Birth of Congenital Heart Defect in the United States

As of 2002, the prevalence of congenital cardiovascular defects in the United States was estimated to range from 650,000 to 1.3 million (Hoffman et al., 2004). Almost as many people with CHD are younger than 25 years as they are older, but the proportions differ among disease types. Some defects occur more commonly in males or females, or in whites or blacks (Botto et al., 2001). Nine defects per 1000 live births are expected, or 36,000 babies per year in the United States. Of these, several studies suggest that 9200, or 2.3 per 1000 live births, require invasive treatment or result in death in the first year of life (Moller, 1998). Estimates are also available for bicuspid aortic valves, occurring in 13.7 per 1000 people (Hoffman and Kaplan, 2002; Larson and Edwards, 1984). Some studies suggest that as many as 5% of newborns, or 200,000 per year, are born with tiny muscular VSDs, almost all of which close spontaneously (Roguin et al., 1995; Sands et al., 1999).

Using available data to estimate the expected numbers of infants with each type of congenital cardiovascular defect at birth, Hoffman et al. (2004) estimated their prevalence assuming no treatment (the low estimate) and full treatment (the high estimate). Of the 1.3 million infants with CHDs, 750,000 would be simple lesions, 400,000 would be moderate, and 180,000 would be complex. There are an estimated 3 million more people with bicuspid aortic valve: 2 million adults and 1 million children. Assuming that prevalence is two thirds of the way between the estimated high and low ranges, representing a total of about 1 million persons with CHD, the most common types would be VSD, 199,000 people; ASD, 187,000 people; PDA, 144,000 people; and valvular pulmonary stenosis, 134,000 people (Hoffman et al., 2004).

Based on a review of published studies, Hoffman and Kaplan (2002) reported that the mean prevalence per million live births of selected CHDs was as follows (number of studies in parentheses): VSDs, 3570 (43); PDA, 799 (40); ASD, 941 (43); AVSD, 348 (40); pulmonic stenosis, 729 (39); aortic stenosis (AoSt), 401 (37); AoCo, 409 (39); TOF, 421 (41); complete TGA, 315 (41); hypoplastic right heart, 222 (32); TA, 79 (11); Ebstein's anomaly, 114 (5); pulmonary atresia (PulAtr), 132 (11); LHH, 266 (36); truncus arteriosus, 107 (30); DORV, 157 (16); SV, 106 (23); total anomalous pulmonary venous connection, 94 (25); all cyanotic lesions, 1391 (37); all CHD (excluding bicuspid nonstenotic aortic valves, isolated partial anomalous pulmonary venous connection, and silent ductus arteriosus), 9596

(43); and bicuspid aortic valve, 13,556 (10). The authors speculate that variations in the reported prevalence at birth of CHDs are primarily due to variations in the ability to detect trivial lesions, notably small muscular VSDs that usually close in infancy. The prevalence at birth of severe CHDs that will require expert cardiological care is quite stable at about 2.5–3 per 1000 live births. The moderately severe forms of CHD probably account for another 3 per 1000 live births, although another 13 per 1000 live births have bicuspid aortic valves that will also eventually need cardiological care (Hoffman and Kaplan, 2002).

Reller et al. (2008b) used the STS classification described in Table 23–1 for the Metropolitan Atlanta Congenital Defects Program (MACDP) data from the years 1998 to 2005 to estimate the prevalence of CHD in Atlanta. MACDP is a population-based surveillance system established in 1967 by the Centers for Disease Control and Prevention (CDC), Emory University, and the Georgia Mental Health Institute (Correa et al., 2007) for major structural birth defects, chromosomal abnormalities, and clinical syndromes. The authors identified 3240 infants with CHD and 398,140 live births in metropolitan Atlanta. The overall prevalence of CHD was 81.4 infants/10,000 births. The left-to-right shunt lesions were the most prevalent group of defects, comprising over half of the total number of CHDs. The most common defect was muscular VSD occurring at a prevalence of 27.5/10,000 births. This prevalence was over twice that of the next two most common cardiac defects (perimembranous VSD at 10.6 and secundum ASD [ASD II] at 10.3/10,000 births). As a group, the prevalence of ASDs was somewhat higher than the range published by Hoffman and Kaplan (2002). Conversely, the prevalence of PDA was on the lower end of predicted at 2.9/10,000. As a group, the full spectrum of AVSD occurred at a prevalence of 4.1/10,000, with complete AVSD comprising roughly half of the total group (2.2/10,000). Of the 88 children with complete AVSD (excluding those with heterotaxy syndrome), 70 (80%) had Down syndrome.

Methodological aspects of the MACDP data should be mentioned here, as this resource is often quoted as a reference by many authors. First, the MACDP includes CHD cases among live births and stillbirths; however, the data do not include pregnancy losses less than 20 weeks of age, stillbirths without autopsies, infant deaths with undiagnosed CHD, and cases of CHD first diagnosed beyond 6 years of age (i.e., ASD or AoVS associated with bicuspid aortic valve). Because some prenatally diagnosed cases may result in pregnancy termination, the possibility of underreporting should be evaluated. Second, the classification approach in the study by Reller et al. (2008b) does not distinguish infants with isolated cardiac defects from those with

TABLE 23–1. *Definitions of Congenital Heart Defects with Inclusion and Exclusion Criteria*

Defect Group	Definition
Left-to-Right Shunts	
Ventricular septal defect (VSD)	Includes type 2 (perimembranous), type 4 (muscular), type 1 (subarterial (conoseptal, infundibular, supracristal), and unspecified types of VSD; excludes VSD with interrupted aortic arch type B or cyanotic defects
Atrial septal defect (ASD)	Includes secundum, sinus venosus, and unspecified types of ASDt > 4 mm in size; excludes patent foramen ovale and obligatory shunts
Atrioventricular septal defect (AVSD)	Includes complete, intermediate, and unbalanced AVSD and those associated with TOF, ostium primum ASD, and type 3 (inlet) VSD
Complete AVSD	Includes complete AVSD
Patent ductus arteriosus (PDA)	Includes term infants (≥36 weeks' gestation) with patent ductus arteriosus persisting for ≥ 6 weeks after delivery; excludes obligatory shunt lesions or if maintained by prostaglandin infusion
Cyanotic Congenital Heart Defects	
TOF	Includes typical TOF, TOF with absent pulmonary valve, pulmonary atresia with VSD, pulmonary atresia with major aortopulmonary collateral arteries, and TOF-type double outlet right ventricle
Transposition of the great arteries (TGA)	Includes concordant atrioventricular connections and discordant ventricular arterial connections, with or without VSD or left ventricular outflow tract obstruction; also includes double-outlet right ventricle with malpositioned great arteries
Discordant atrioventricular connections	Includes discordant atrioventricular and ventriculoarterial connections (congenitally corrected TGA), with or without VSD or outflow tract obstruction; and discordant atrioventricular with concordant ventriculoarterial connections
Truncus arteriosus	Includes all truncus arteriosus subtypes; excludes hemitruncus and pseudotruncus
Total anomalous pulmonary venous return	Includes all types of total anomalous pulmonary venous return
Tricuspid atresia	Includes tricuspid valve atresia with normally related great arteries
Ebstein's anomaly	Includes Ebstein's anomaly of the right heart with atrioventricular concordance
Single ventricle complex	Includes double-inlet left or right ventricle, mitral or tricuspid valve atresia with aortic malposition, or other specified or unspecified types of single ventricle
Heterotaxy syndrome	Includes atrial situs abnormalities, situs inversus with or without dextrocardia, situs ambiguous, isolated dextrocardia, and unspecified heterotaxy; cases with other heart defects and heterotaxy syndrome are only considered in the heterotaxy group, and excluded from the other heart defect groups
Left-Heart Obstructive Defects	
Coarctation of the aorta	Includes coarctation of the aorta with or without aortic valve stenosis, aortic arch hypoplasia, and interrupted aortic arch type A
Valvar Aortic Stenosis	Includes valvar or unspecified aortic valve stenosis, dysplasia, or atresia Excludes isolated bicuspid aortic valve, and aortic stenosis with coarctation
Interrupted aortic arch type B	Includes type B and unspecified type of interrupted aortic arch
Hypoplastic left heart syndrome (HLHS)	Includes HLHS with or without VSD
Right-Heart Obstructive Defects	
Valvar pulmonic stenosis	Includes valvar and unspecified pulmonary stenosis, or valvar dysplasia
Pulmonary atresia	Includes pulmonary atresia with intact ventricular septum

Source: From Reller et al. (2008b)

cardiac defects and other noncardiac anomalies (i.e., chromosomal disorders, well-known syndromes, and other associations). Also, the STS classification codes do not allow for assessment of severity. Third, the population of the five-county metropolitan Atlanta differs from the population of Georgia and the United States as a whole, particularly with respect to the proportion of residents living in urban areas (Correa et al., 2007); therefore, the results may not be comparable to other populations.

Prevalence at Birth of Congenital Heart Defect in Norway

Meberg et al. (2007) evaluated medical records in the Departments of Paediatrics and Obstetrics, Vestfold Hospital in Tønsberg, Norway. Close to 90% of all births in the region occur in this hospital. Of 57,027 live births during 1982–2005, CHDs were detected in 662 (11.6 per 1000), of whom 146 (22%) had associated anomalies. Of these, 52 (36%) had chromosomal anomalies (exclusive microdeletions), 26 (18%) genetic syndromes/microdeletions, 1 (0.7%) a teratogenous syndrome, and 67 (46%) extracardiac malformations. In perimembraneous VSDs, associated anomalies occurred in 22 of 70 (31%) compared to 27 of 298 (9%) in VSDs located in the muscular part of the septum (p <0.0001). The prevalence of CHDs with associated disorders increased significantly from the cohort born during 1982–1993 to those born during 1994–2005 (2.0 vs. 3.1 per 1000, respectively; p < 0.0001), mainly caused by an increase of chromosomal trisomies (0.5 vs. 1.1 per 1000;

p = 0.026). The percentage of women giving live birth at 35 years of age or more was 7.6% for the period 1982–1993 compared to 13.4% for 1994–2005 (p = 0.001).

Prevalence at Birth of Congenital Heart Defect in the United Kingdom

The current sources of heart defect prevalence within the United Kingdom include the National Congenital Anomaly System (NCAS), the European Surveillance of Congenital Anomalies EUROCAT (acronym derived from its original name "European Concerted Action on Congenital Anomalies and Twins"), and the General Practice Research Database (GPRD). The NCAS is a surveillance system that began around 1964 and is operated by the Office for National Statistics. It records congenital anomalies for both live and still-births in England and Wales. NCAS is a two-tier system consisting of both voluntary notifications from child health information units and notifications from congenital anomaly registers (Misra et al., 2006). The NCAS uses the defect exclusion list developed by EUROCAT in 1990. Spontaneous and induced abortions are not included in the system (Misra et al., 2006). In 1999, the NCAS system covered all births in Wales and 23% of births in England (Boyd et al., 2005). The EUROCAT began in 1979 and is a European network of population-based registries for the epidemiological surveillance of congenital anomalies (http://www.eurocat.ulster.ac.uk/pubdata/index. html). It records congenital anomalies for live births, fetal deaths, and induced abortions. There are six registries that make up the EUROCAT system in the United Kingdom, contributing data to the 2001–2003 prevalence: North Thames, Northern Congenital Anomaly Survey (NorCAS), Oxford, Wessex, Trent, and Wales Congenital Anomaly Register and Information Service (CARIS). Merseyside/Cheshire registry and Glasgow registry also contribute UK data to the EUROCAT system, but these registries did not provide data for 2001–2003. The EUROCAT covers approximately 35.2% of the United Kingdom (Dolk, 2005). The GPRD is a medical records database in which events are recorded in the medical record for the purpose of patient care. The database was established in June 1987, at which time participating general practitioners received practice computers and a text-based practice management system in return for undertaking data quality training and submitting anonymous patient data for research purposes. The GPRD contains information on 3,000,000 patients in the United Kingdom (a geographical and demographically representative sample of 4.6% of the UK population) and covers 30,000 births per year. There are 350 general practices contributing to the GPRD, all members of the National Health Service (NHS) in England (Charlton et al., 2008). Wurst et al. (2007) examined whether the rates of all, and specific types of, CHDs obtained from the GPRD are similar to those obtained from UK national systems. For 2001, 2002, and 2003, the prevalence of all heart defects in the GPRD was 54 per 10,000, 53 per 10,000, and 45 per 10,000, respectively (the difference in prevalence rates among years was not statistically significant). The overall prevalence in the GPRD was higher than that in either the NCAS or EUROCAT: more than twice as high in the GPRD than in the NCAS and slightly higher in the GPRD than in EUROCAT. The rates of specific heart defects also varied across the GPRD, NCAS, and EUROCAT in 2001, 2002, and 2003. For brevity, results for only 2001 will be described (the rates for 2002 and 2003 showed similar variation across specific heart defects). In 2001, the GPRD showed a prevalence rate of malformations of cardiac septal almost four times higher than NCAS (relative risk [RR] = 3.7; 95% confidence interval [CI] = 3.1–4.5) and nearly twice as high as EUROCAT (RR = 1.8; 95% CI = 1.5–2.2). The rate of VSD within the GPRD was six times higher than that in NCAS (RR = 5.9; 95% CI = 4.8–7.2) and over two times higher than that in EUROCAT (RR = 2.4; 95% CI = 2.0–3.0). VSD prevalence was also significantly lower in infants up to age 1 compared to children up to age 6 (RR = 0.61; 95% CI = 0.48–0.77). The rate of TOF in the GPRD was more than four times higher than that in NCAS (RR = 4.3; 95% CI = 2.4–7.8) and more than twice as high as that in EUROCAT (RR = 2.4; 95% CI = 1.3–4.4). The GPRD did not include any cases of very rare defects such as SV, TA, or Ebstein's anomaly during 2001–2003. The EUROCAT rates of malformations of the great arteries and veins and AoCo were significantly higher than those in both the GPRD and NCAS. Rates from NCAS and the GPRD had overlapping CIs for these defects (Wurst et al., 2007).

The British Paediatric Cardiac Association (BPCA) undertook a national collaborative study of fetal cardiac screening to assess the effect of fetal diagnosis of CHD on the pattern of serious CHD at term (Bull, 1999). Members of the BPCA submitted lists of all infants with serious CHD seen at the centers between 1993 and 1995. The frequency of serious CHD per 1000 live births was reported as follows: England and Wales, 1.7; Scotland, 1.8; Northern Ireland, 2.0; total, 1.7. Nationally, and with the author's stringent definition of serious CHD, the estimates give a rate of 2.12 affected pregnancies per 1000 live births and 1.74 affected livebirths per 1000 live births. The inclusion criteria reflect an interest in major abnormalities with demands on emergency and inpatient pediatric cardiology services. By this definition, the results show that an obstetric center with 3000 deliveries per year would expect to deal each year with 6.3 pregnancies affected by such disorders. Many of the published studies on the incidence of CHD suggest a higher incidence at term than that documented in the current study, but published figures can be inflated by the definition of CHD chosen and can also reflect the method of ascertainment (Bull, 1999).

Tanner et al. (2005) determined the prevalence and spectrum of cardiovascular malformations in a preterm population and the prevalence of prematurity among infants with cardiovascular malformations. The study was based on the population of the former Northern Health Region of England. All infants with suspected cardiovascular malformations are referred to a single pediatric cardiology center. The population of about 3 million is stable and geographically well defined. The recent average annual live birth rate has been about 35,000 births per year. In common with most previous epidemiological studies, the authors defined a cardiovascular malformation as "a gross structural abnormality of the heart or intrathoracic great vessels that is actually or potentially of functional importance." They limited ascertainment to malformations diagnosed by the age of 12 months. Of 521,619 live births in the study population in 1987–2001, 2964 infants were recognized as having a cardiovascular malformation (excluding ASD and PDA) in infancy. This gives a prevalence of 5.7 cases per 1000 live births. With the assumption that 7.3% of all live births are preterm, the prevalence at live birth of cardiovascular malformations among preterm infants was 12.5 cases per 1000 live births. In comparison, cardiovascular malformations were present in 5.1 cases per 1000 term infants, giving an OR for cardiovascular malformations in prematurity of 2.4. The distribution of live births by gestational age was reported as follows, with the prevalence of cardiovascular malformations in parentheses: less than 28 weeks, 0.4% (0.62%); 28–31 weeks, 0.9% (1.28%); 32–36 weeks, 6.0% (1.28%); 37 or more weeks, 92.7% (0.51%); total, 100% (0.57%). More infants were born preterm with diagnoses of PulAtr with VSD (23%), complete AVSD (22%), and AoCo, TOF, and PaVS (each 20%). Fewer were born preterm with diagnoses of PulAtr and intact ventricular septum (7%), TGA (8%), and SV (9%) (Tanner et al., 2005).

Prevalence at Birth of Congenital Heart Defect in Italy

In Italy, several general birth defects registries, especially those in the north and center of the country, have monitored CHD since the late 1970s. Data suggest a CHD birth prevalence of around 4.5% of live births (Calzolari et al., 2003). The Italian Multicentric Study on Epidemiology of Congenital Heart Disease (IMS-

CHD), performed between 1992 and 1993, suggests an average CHD prevalence varying from 3.2% in Southern to 6% in Northern Italy (Bosi et al., 1999). Bosi et al. (2003) examined the temporal variability in the prevalence of CHD during a 21-year period of registration (1980–2000) using the Emilia-Romagna birth defects registry (IMER). Consecutive live births (480,793 total) and stillbirths were surveyed with a mean of 22,894 per year. In the 21 years of the study, 2456 CHD cases were registered; among these, 2442 cases were detected in live births, with a birth prevalence ranging from 3.1% to 7.5%, the average being 5.1%. Isolated VSD occurred with an average prevalence of 19.7 per 10,000 live births. Isolated ASD II had a prevalence of 3.4 per 10,000 live births. AVSD and TGA formed a cluster with a prevalence of about 2.7 per 10,000 live births. A second cluster, including TOF, left hypoplastic heart syndrome (LHHS), pulmonary valvar stenosis (PulSt), and isolated AoCo, had prevalence from 1.6 to 2.2 per 10,000 live births. PDA in mature infants had a prevalence of 1.2 and AoSt 0.7 per 10,000 live births. Miscellaneous CHDs represent a significant proportion of all cardiovascular malformations, with a prevalence of about 4.4 per 10,000 live births. Among the complex CHDs, which represent 11.7% of all the cardiovascular malformations, double-inlet ventricle (DIV) and PulAtr (with and without VSD) had a prevalence of about 1.2 per 10,000 live births each. DORV, common arterial trunk (CAT), and tricuspid valve atresia had a prevalence of 0.5 to 1.2 per 10,000 live births. Total anomalous pulmonary venous return and Ebstein's malformation varied from 0.2 to 0.3 per 10,000 live births. In this study, the average birth prevalence of CHD, as registered during the period of the study, is 5.1%, with a range from 3.1% to 7.5%. The observed average CHD birth prevalence is similar to that in other epidemiological studies covering a similar period. Nevertheless, there was a significant difference in CHD prevalence from earlier to later periods of the study, demonstrating a higher prevalence in the second decade of the study. In other words, a significant time-related variation in the birth prevalence of CHD has been confirmed. The main reason for this variation is probably related to an increasing recognition of minor cardiac lesions among the simple CHD.

Additional prevalence studies are presented in Table 23–2.

SURVIVAL OF INDIVIDUALS WITH CONGENITAL HEART DEFECTS

Without Surgery

Although outcomes for infants with CHDs have improved, primarily due to advances in clinical care

TABLE 23–2. *Selected Prevalence Studies around the World*

Author (year)	Location	Prevalence per 10,000 births
Boneva et al. (2001)	US national health statistics	5.6
Boneva et al. (2001)	US national health statistics	9.2
Baltaxe and Zarante (2006)	Colombia	12
Dastgiri et al. (2002)	Glasgow, UK	50
Pradat et al. (1992)	Sweden	28
Borman et al. (1987)	New Zealand	35
Sever et al. (1988)	Washington state, US	35.2
Wren and O'Sullivan (2001)	Several counties in the UK	52
Guitti (2000)	Londrina, Brazil	54.9
Chen et al. (2008)	Tibet	72.1
Garne (2004)	Denmark	79
Reller et al. (2008a)	Metropolitan Atlanta	81.4
Tagliabue et al. (2007)	Northern Italy	90.8
Amorim et al. (2008)	Brazil	95.8
Oyen et al. (2009)	Denmark	103
Marelli et al. (2007)	Quebec	118.9
Forrester et al. (2004)	Hawaii	177.1

Note: Sorted from lowest to highest prevalence.

and new technologies in pediatric cardiology and cardiothoracic surgery, CHDs remain among the most prevalent and fatal of all birth defects. According to the final 1999 National Vital Statistics report, of the 5473 infants who died as a result of congenital malformation (CM) and chromosomal abnormalities in the United States, 1598 (29.2%) deaths were attributed to CHDs (Hoyert et al., 2001). Surviving infants with CHDs often require repeated surgeries and lengthy hospitalizations. Many will have a lifetime of disability, imposing a significant burden on families, caregivers, and society (Kecskes and Cartwright, 2002; Limperopoulos et al., 2001; Mahle and Wernovsky, 2001; Tilford et al., 2001).

Cleves et al. (2003) carried out a population study from the state of Arkansas linking birth and death certificate records to the birth defects registry for infants born with CHD in Arkansas. A total of 1983 infants with CHD were included in this study. The neonatal survival probability for this cohort was 94.0% (95% CI: 93.0–95.1%), and the first-year survival probability was 88.2% (95% CI: 86.8%–89.6%). The presence of LHHS conferred the greatest reduction in survival, whereas infants with PVS and infants with VSD had the highest first-year survival. Infants with multiple CHD had decreased survival compared to those with isolated heart defects.

Following are selected results from clinical reports:

PulAtr associated with VSD is a serious anomaly, with such patients rarely reaching adulthood, with or without previous surgery. It has been estimated that around 16% of patients reach the third decade of life (Bull et al., 1995).

Among AoCo patients, more than 75% of the non-operated patients died at around 50 years of age from systemic arterial hypertension-dependent cardiovascular alterations, for example, cerebral hemorrhage, aortic rupture or dissecting aneurysm, coronary obstruction, and secondary myocardiopathy with cardiac insufficiency (Campbell, 1970).

In PaVS, the most common cause was right ventricular insufficiency, usually appearing during the fourth decade of life. Half of these patients die before reaching 27 years of age (Atik and Atik, 2001).

ASD is the second most common congenital anomaly in adults, approximately 40% of patients survive beyond the age of 40 (Atik and Atik, 2001).

TOF has an unfavorable prognosis, with 50% of the patients dying during the first 3 years of life and 75% before reaching 10 years of age. About 11% of the patients reach the age of 20 years, 6% attain 30 years, and only 3% reach 40 years (Atik and Atik, 2001).

In Ebstein anomaly, half of the patients reach the third decade of life, but rarely reach 50 years of age (5%). Death is due to cardiac failure, thromboembolism, arrhythmia, and hypoxia (Atik and Atik, 2001).

Natural occurrence of other cyanotic cardiopathies is extremely rare in adults, and no predominance of one over the other have been noted (Atik and Atik, 2001).

Table 23–3 summarizes selected studies on the survival of individuals with CHD who have not undergone surgery.

With Surgery

Population study from a county in Denmark. Using data from the EUROCAT Registry of Congenital Malformations for Funen County, Denmark, between 1986 and 1998, Garne (2004) identified that 32% of all infants and children had an intervention (surgery or

TABLE 23–3. *Selected Survival Rates in Patients with CHD without Surgery in Studies around the World*

Author (Year)	Defect	Survival Rates without Surgical Intervention
Wren and O'Sullivan (2001)	Congenital heart defects	82% survival at 1 year
Cleves et al. (2003)	Congenital heart defects	88.2% survival at 1 year
Campbell et al. (1970)	Coarctation of the aorta	25% survival at 50 years
Cumming (1999)	Pulmonary valve stenosis	50% survival at 27 years
Zaver and Nadas (1965)	Atrial septal defects	40% survival at 40 years
Atik and Atik (2001)	Tetralogy of Fallot	50% survival at 3 years
Atik and Atik (2001)	Ebstein anomaly	5% survival at 50 years
Bull et al. (1995)	Pulmonary atresia with ventricular septal defect	16% survival at 30 years

catheter treatment) performed. Eighteen percent died within the first 5 years, with the majority of deaths within the first year of life. For 74% of all deaths, surgery had not been performed.

Following are selected results from clinical reports:

With major advances to treatment over the past decade, babies born today with the more serious heart defects are likely to have much higher 1-year survival rates than these data suggest. For example, today, around 50% of babies born with LHH survive infancy (Andrews et al., 2001).

Combining data on observed infant survival with estimates of the likely childhood survival rates (from 1 year to 16 years), it is predicted that overall 78% of babies diagnosed with CHD will survive to adulthood. This prediction is based on published survival rates in patients who mostly had operations 15 or more years ago when they were in infancy. Marked improvements in care in the last 15 years mean that this prediction is likely to be an underestimate of the true survival rate into adulthood. Data from the United States suggest this is likely to be around 85% (Perloff and Warnes, 2001).

When AoCo is corrected in infancy, long-term survival occurs in 92% of the cases (Kirklin et al., 1993). With the current practice of repair at younger than 5 years, long-term survival will probably improve (Cumming, 1999).

The Mayo Clinic (Kopecky et al., 1988) reported their 25-year follow-up of patients having surgery for valvular pulmonary stenosis. Standard mortality is assigned a value of 100%, twice normal mortality 200%, and so on. Mortality ratio is the observed mortality divided by the expected mortality times 100. With surgery occurring in patients younger than 5 years, the mortality ratio was 350%. However, this series included sick infants at a time when these patients that were not as well managed as they are today.

VSD is the second most frequent congenital anomaly. About 50% to 75% of small defects spontaneously close during the first 2 years of life. The Natural History Study (Kidd et al., 1993) was a multicenter study, with 25 years of follow-up of patients treated medically or surgically for three congenital lesions. Patients classified as having Eisenmenger syndrome (based on pulmonary to systemic resistance ratios exceeding 0.7) had a mortality ratio during the 25 years of follow-up of more than 1500%. Patients with large VSDs labeled as severe, with pulmonary artery systolic pressures of 70% or more of systemic pressure and pulmonary/systemic flow ratios of 1.2 or greater, had a mortality ratio of 1100% in 25-year follow-up.

At the time of the Natural History Study-II study, surgery was also performed in occasional patients with trivial VSD, 45% of patients with mild VSD, and 52% of those with moderate VSD, with a near-zero late mortality (Kidd et al., 1993).

Moller et al. (1991) reported on the 30-year survival of 296 survivors of VSDs surgery between 1954 and 1960. The overall mortality ratio for the entire series was about 750%. Increased pulmonary vascular resistance was an important determinant of high mortality, and if pulmonary vascular resistance was over 7 units, the 30-year-mortality was 44%. Complete atrioventricular block and even transitory atrioventricular block postoperatively was associated with a high mortality. The excess mortality persisted with each decade of follow-up. Eleven percent of patients died in the first 9 years, 5% in the next 10 years, and 6% in the last 10 years of follow-up. Five sudden deaths occurred in patients without pulmonary vascular disease 3, 8, 22, 29, and 33 years after surgery.

The data from the Mayo Clinic series (Murphy et al., 1990) of 191 VSD patients having surgery between 1956 and 1959 were analyzed at intervals of 5 years after surgery. The mortality ratio was 1500% for the first 5 years. It was still 1000% for 11–15 years, but decreased to around 100% (standard mortality rate) after 20 years.

In the Oregon series (Morris and Menashe, 1991), 312 patients with VSD repair followed for 25 years had a mortality ratio of about 333%.

Those with TOF operated on during the first decade of their lives have an average survival rate of 32 years (Hu et al., 1985; Murphy et al., 1993).

Currently, most centers advise repair for tetralogy patients in the first 2 years of life. The late results (mean

TABLE 23–4. *Number of Cases, Observed Survival in Infancy and Predicted Survival throughout Childhood by Diagnostic Category of CHD, 1985–1999, Northern England*

Diagnostic Category	Number of Cases*	Observed Survival to 1 Year (%)	Predicted Survival to 16 Years (%)
Hypoplastic left heart	54	0	0
Truncus arteriosus	35	34	31
Pulmonary atresia with intact ventricular septum	21	43	31
Aortic stenosis with intervention or death in infancy	36	47	37
Tricuspid atresia	23	56	31
Complete atrioventricular septal defect	104	56	54
Mitral regurgitation	7	57	54
Double-inlet ventricle	30	60	43
Ventricular septal defect with intervention or death in infancy	182	66	64
Pulmonary atresia with ventricular septal defect	39	72	48
Total anomalous pulmonary venous connection	33	73	71
Transposition of the great arteries	113	77	67
Partial atrioventricular septal defect	29	79	72
Mitral atresia	10	80	32
Pulmonary stenosis with intervention or death in infancy	46	83	81
Miscellaneous	69	83	79
Atrial septal defect	84	87	84
Coarctation of aorta	90	88	86
Tetralogy of Fallot	113	89	84
Patent ductus arteriosus	95	94	93
Congenitally corrected transposition of the great arteries	17	100	96
Ventricular septal defect with no intervention	577	100	100
Aortic stenosis with no intervention	38	100	94
Pulmonary stenosis with no intervention	97	100	97
Total	**1942**	**82**	**78**

*Number of live born diagnosed with congenital heart defect by the age of 12 months.

Source: Wren and O'Sullivan (2001)

follow-up 5 years) for 184 survivors operated on at Children's Hospital, Boston (Walsh et al., 1988), indicated a need for reoperation in 17%, and a 1.6% death rate. This calculates out to a mortality ratio of more than 500% but later follow-up results are expected to be considerably better than those in patients operated on between 1955 and 1975.

Sudden death several years after successful repair of TOF occurs less often than in the past, but it remains a disturbing feature of long-term follow-up in these patients. Kirklin et al. (1992) showed that the probability was 0.9% with surgery before 2 years of age, 1.3% at 10 years of age, and 2.4% at 20 years of age.

AoVS is an anomaly requiring attention as it progresses with the age of the patient, that is, valve degeneration, appearance of aortic insufficiency, and infectious endocarditis. Long-term survival times for this disease are estimated at 82% 20 years after the operation and 77% 22 years after the operation (Hsieh et al., 1986). The need for reoperation increases with time, with the percentage being 2% after 5 years, 8% after 10 years, 19% after 15 years, 35% after 20 years, and 44% after 22 years (Presbitero et al., 1982). Sudden

death is the main long-term cause of death occurring in 37% of all cases, 26% of which are related to the reoperation, 18% to endocarditis, and 4% to cardiac and aortic insufficiency (Presbitero et al., 1982).

Morris and Menashe (1991) followed a large population with various degrees of severity of AoSt for 25 years. Twenty-one percent of those with initial gradients of less than 25 mmHg required surgery by 25 years because of deterioration. In subjects with gradients of less than 50 mmHg at the entry to the study, the 25-year mortality was about 200%. In subjects with initial peak gradients greater than 50 mmHg the mortality ratio after 25 years was 530%. The mortality ratio of those having surgery for congenital AoSt followed for 25 years was 525%.

In the Minnesota series with 30-year follow-up the mortality ratio of those having AoSt classified as simple was 150% and for complex it was 300% (Moller and Anderson, 1992). These values did not include patients with extremely severe AoSt requiring intervention in infancy, in whom the long-term mortality ratio was more than 1000% (Cumming, 1999).

In aortic supravalvar stenosis, mostly associated with Williams syndrome, a 94% favorable outcome after 10 years and 91% after 20 years following operation have been observed (van Son et al., 1994).

Operation for congenital mitral stenosis shows a more unfavorable evolution in cases where the patient achieves a survival times of 30%–60% over a 10-year period (Kirklin et al., 1992).

In the TGA, Jatene's anatomical correction carries a 2% risk of sudden death (Kirklin et al., 1992). When the correction is aimed at redirecting intra-atrial redirecting of blood flow by means of the Senning and Mustard operations, a survival index of up to 85% by the first technique and of 80% by the second has been reported during a 20-year period (Williams et al., 1988).

Patients having ligation of PDA are expected to have a normal subsequent long-term mortality unless there are some other underlying health problems. The actual mortality with more than 25 years of follow-up by Morris and Menashe (1991) was 133% and the extra deaths were due to associated non-cardiac disorders.

Medium-term results after the arterial switch operation for TGA are available for 470 patients operated on at the Children's Hospital of Boston (Wernovsky et al., 1995). Survival was 93% at 30 days, 92% at 1 year, 91% at 5 years, and 91% at 8 years, so there were no deaths after 5 years. Six percent of patients required second procedures to correct pulmonary artery stenosis. The 1.1% mortality difference between 1 and 5 years represents a mortality ratio of more than 500%.

Table 23–4 presents the 1- and 16-year survival of individuals with CHD (combined with and without surgery) in Northern England by diagnostic category.

REFERENCES

Amorim LF, Pires CA, Lana AM, et al. Presentation of congenital heart disease diagnosed at birth: analysis of 29,770 newborn infants. *J Pediatr (Rio J)*. 2008;84:83–90.

Andrews R, Tulloh R, Sharland G, et al. Outcome of staged reconstructive surgery for hypoplastic left heart syndrome following antenatal diagnosis. *Arch Dis Child*. 2001;85:474–477.

Atik E, Atik FA. Congenital heart disease in adults. Considerations about its natural evolution and in operated patients. *Arq Bras Cardiol*. 2001;76:423–436.

Baltaxe E, Zarante I. Prevalence of congenital heart disease in 44,985 newborns in Colombia. *Arch Cardiol Mex*. 2006;76:263–268.

Beland MJ, Franklin RC, Jacobs JP, et al. Update from the International Working Group for mapping and coding of nomenclatures for paediatric and congenital heart disease. *Cardiol Young*. 2004;14:225–229.

Bierman JM, Siegel E, French FE, Simonian K. Analysis of the outcome of all pregnancies in a community. Kauai Pregnancy Study. *Am J Obstet Gynecol*. 1965;91:37–45.

Boneva RS, Botto LD, Moore CA, Yang Q, Correa A, Erickson JD. Mortality associated with congenital heart defects in the United States: trends and racial disparities, 1979–1997. *Circulation*. 2001;103:2376–2381.

Borman B, Chapman C, Howard K, Buckfield P, Findlay J. Using a national register for the epidemiological study of congenital heart defects. *N Z Med J*. 1987;100:404–406.

Bosi G, Garani G, Scorrano M, Calzolari E. Temporal variability in birth prevalence of congenital heart defects as recorded by a general birth defects registry. *J Pediatr*. 2003;142:690–698.

Bosi G, Scorrano M, Tosato G, Forini E, Chakrokh R. The Italian multicentric study on epidemiology of congenital heart disease: first step of the analysis. Working Party of the Italian Society of Pediatric Cardiology. *Cardiol Young*. 1999;9:291–299.

Botto LD, Correa A, Erickson JD. Racial and temporal variations in the prevalence of heart defects. *Pediatrics*. 2001;107:E32.

Botto LD, Lin AE, Riehle-Colarusso T, Malik S, Correa A. Seeking causes: Classifying and evaluating congenital heart defects in etiologic studies. *Birth Defects Res A Clin Mol Teratol*. 2007;79:714–727.

Boyd PA, Armstrong B, Dolk H, et al. Congenital anomaly surveillance in England—ascertainment deficiencies in the national system. *BMJ*. 2005;330:27.

Bull C. Current and potential impact of fetal diagnosis on prevalence and spectrum of serious congenital heart disease at term in the UK. British Paediatric Cardiac Association. *Lancet*. 1999;354:1242–1247.

Bull K, Somerville J, Ty E, Spiegelhalter D. Presentation and attrition in complex pulmonary atresia. *J Am Coll Cardiol*. 1995;25:491–499.

Byrne J, Warburton D. Neural tube defects in spontaneous abortions. *Am J Med Genet*. 1986;25:327–333.

Calzolari E, Garani G, Cocchi G, et al. Congenital heart defects: 15 years of experience of the Emilia-Romagna Registry (Italy). *Eur J Epidemiol*. 2003;18:773–780.

Campbell M. Natural history of atrial septal defect. *Br Heart J* 32:820–826.

Carlgren LE. The incidence of congenital heart disease in children born in Gothenburg 1941–1950. *Br Heart J*. 1959;21:40–50.

Carlgren LE, Ericson A, Kallen B. Monitoring of congenital cardiac defects. *Pediatr Cardiol*. 8:247–256.

Charlton RA, Cunnington MC, de Vries CS, Weil JG. Data resources for investigating drug exposure during pregnancy and associated outcomes: the General Practice Research Database (GPRD) as an alternative to pregnancy registries. *Drug Saf*. 2008;31:39–51.

Chen QH, Wang XQ, Qi SG. Cross-sectional study of congenital heart disease among Tibetan children aged from 4 to 18 years at different altitudes in Qinghai Province. *Chin Med J (Engl)*. 2008;121:2469–2472.

Chinn A, Fitzsimmons J, Shepard TH, Fantel AG. Congenital heart disease among spontaneous abortuses and stillborn fetuses: prevalence and associations. *Teratology*. 1989;40:475–482.

Cleves MA, Ghaffar S, Zhao W, Mosley BS, Hobbs CA. First-year survival of infants born with congenital heart defects in Arkansas (1993–1998): a survival analysis using registry data. *Birth Defects Res A Clin Mol Teratol*. 2003;67:662–668.

Correa A, Cragan JD, Kucik ME, et al. Reporting birth defects surveillance data 1968–2003. *Birth Defects Res A Clin Mol Teratol*. 2007;79:65–186.

Creasy MR, Alberman ED. Congenital malformations of the central nervous system in spontaneous abortions. *J Med Genet* 13:9–16

Cumming GR. Life insurance implications of mortality for up to 40 years after repair of congenital heart defects in childhood. *J R Soc Med*. 1999;92:73–79.

Dastgiri S, Stone DH, Le-Ha C, Gilmour WH. Prevalence and secular trend of congenital anomalies in Glasgow, UK. *Arch Dis Child*. 2002;86:257–263.

Dejmek J, Vojtassak J, Malova J. Cytogenetic analysis of 1508 spontaneous abortions originating from south Slovakia. *Eur J Obstet Gynecol Reprod Biol*. 1992;46:129–136.

Dolk H. EUROCAT: 25 years of European surveillance of congenital anomalies. *Arch Dis Child Fetal Neonatal Ed*. 2005;90:F355–358.

Ferencz C, Rubin JD, Loffredo CA. Epidemiology of congenital heart disease: the Baltimore–Washington Infant Study 1981–1989. Mount Kisko: Futura; 1993.

Forrester MB, Merz RD. Descriptive epidemiology of selected congenital heart defects, Hawaii, 1986–1999. *Paediatr Perinat Epidemiol.* 2004;18:415–424

Garne E. Congenital heart defects—occurrence, surgery and prognosis in a Danish County. *Scand Cardiovasc J.* 2004;38:357–362.

Gerlis LM. Cardiac malformations in spontaneous abortions. *Int J Cardiol.* 1985;7:29–46.

Guitti JC. Epidemiological characteristics of congenital heart diseases in Londrina, Parana south Brazil. *Arq Bras Cardiol.* 2000;74:395–404.

Hagemann LL, Zielinsky P. Population screening of fetal cardiac abnormalities through prenatal echocardiography in low-risk pregnancies in the municipality of Porto Alegre. *Arq Bras Cardiol.* 2004;82:313–326

Hanna EJ, Nevin NC, Nelson J. Genetic study of congenital heart defects in Northern Ireland (1974–1978). *J Med Genet.* 1994;31:858–863.

Hanna JS, Neu RL, Lockwood DH. Prenatal cytogenetic results from cases referred for 44 different types of abnormal ultrasound findings. *Prenat Diagn.* 1996;16:109–115.

Hoffman JI. Incidence of congenital heart disease: II. Prenatal incidence. *Pediatr Cardiol.* 1995;16:155–165.

Hoffman JI, Christianson R. Congenital heart disease in a cohort of 19,502 births with long-term follow-up. *Am J Cardiol.* 1978;42:641–647.

Hoffman JI, Kaplan S. The incidence of congenital heart disease. *J Am Coll Cardiol.* 2002;39:1890–1900.

Hoffman JI, Kaplan S, Liberthson RR. Prevalence of congenital heart disease. *Am Heart J.* 2004;147:425–439.

Hoyert DL, Arias E, Smith BL, Murphy SL, Kochanek KD. Deaths: final data for 1999. *Natl Vital Stat Rep.* 2001;49:1–113.

Hsieh KS, Keane JF, Nadas AS, Bernhard WF, Castaneda AR. Long-term follow-up of valvotomy before 1968 for congenital aortic stenosis. *Am J Cardiol.* 1986;58:338–341.

Hu DC, Seward JB, Puga FJ, Fuster V, Tajik AJ. Total correction of tetralogy of Fallot at age 40 years and older: long-term follow-up. *J Am Coll Cardiol.* 1985;5:40–44.

Hyett J, Moscoso G, Nicolaides K. Abnormalities of the heart and great arteries in first trimester chromosomally abnormal fetuses. *Am J Med Genet.* 1997;69:207–216.

Iyer P, Wani L, Joshi S, et al. Cytogenetic investigations in couples with repeated miscarriages and malformed children: report of a novel insertion. *Reprod Biomed Online.* 2007;14:314–321.

Janerich DT. Letter: epidemiology of birth defects. *Lancet.* 1975;2:1304.

Jenkins KJ, Correa A, Feinstein JA, et al. Noninherited risk factors and congenital cardiovascular defects: current knowledge: a scientific statement from the American Heart Association Council on Cardiovascular Disease in the Young: endorsed by the American Academy of Pediatrics. *Circulation.* 2007;115:2995–3014.

Kecskes Z, Cartwright DW. Poor outcome of very low birthweight babies with serious congenital heart disease. *Arch Dis Child Fetal Neonatal Ed.* 2002;87:F31–33.

Kidd L, Driscoll DJ, Gersony WM, et al. Second natural history study of congenital heart defects. Results of treatment of patients with ventricular septal defects. *Circulation.* 1993;87:I38–51.

Kirklin JW, Barratt-Boyes BG. *Cardiac Surgery.* 2nd ed. New York: Churchill Livingstone, Inc.; 1993:1263–1325.

Kirklin JW, Blackstone EH, Tchervenkov CI, Castaneda AR. Clinical outcomes after the arterial switch operation for transposition. Patient, support, procedural, and institutional risk factors. Congenital Heart Surgeons Society. *Circulation.* 1992;86:1501–1515.

Kopecky SL, Gersh BJ, McGoon MD, et al. Long-term outcome of patients undergoing surgical repair of isolated pulmonary valve stenosis. Follow-up at 20–30 years. *Circulation.* 1988;78:1150–1156.

Larson EW, Edwards WD. Risk factors for aortic dissection: a necropsy study of 161 cases. *Am J Cardiol.* 1984;53:849–855.

Limperopoulos C, Majnemer A, Shevell MI, et al. Functional limitations in young children with congenital heart defects after cardiac surgery. *Pediatrics.* 2001;108:1325–1331.

Mahle WT, Wernovsky G. Long-term developmental outcome of children with complex congenital heart disease. *Clin Perinatol.* 2001;28:235–247.

Marelli AJ, Mackie AS, Ionescu-Ittu R, Rahme E, Pilote L. Congenital heart disease in the general population: changing prevalence and age distribution. *Circulation.* 2007;115:163–172.

Mavroudis C, Jacobs JP. Congenital Heart Surgery Nomenclature and Database Project: overview and minimum dataset. *Ann Thorac Surg.* 2000;69:S2–17.

Meberg A, Hals J, Thaulow E. Congenital heart defects—chromosomal anomalies, syndromes and extracardiac malformations. *Acta Paediatr.* 2007;96:1142–1145.

Miller JF, Williamson E, Glue J, Gordon YB, Grudzinskas JG, Sykes A. Fetal loss after implantation. A prospective study. *Lancet.* 1980;2:554–556.

Misra T, Dattani N, Majeed A. Congenital anomaly surveillance in England and Wales. *Public Health.* 2006;120:256–264.

Mitchell SC, Korones SB, Berendes HW. Congenital heart disease in 56,109 births. Incidence and natural history. *Circulation.* 1971;43:323–332.

Moller JH. Prevalence and incidence of cardiac malformations. Armonk, NY; Futura Publishing Co; 1998.

Moller JH, Anderson RC. 1,000 consecutive children with a cardiac malformation with 26- to 37-year follow-up. *Am J Cardiol.* 1992;70:661–667.

Moller JH, Patton C, Varco RL, Lillehei CW. Late results (30 to 35 years) after operative closure of isolated ventricular septal defect from 1954 to 1960. *Am J Cardiol.* 1991;68:1491–1497.

Morris CD, Menashe VD. 25-year mortality after surgical repair of congenital heart defect in childhood. A population-based cohort study. *JAMA.* 1991;266:3447–3452.

Murphy JG, Gersh BJ, Mair DD, et al. Long-term outcome in patients undergoing surgical repair of tetralogy of Fallot. *N Engl J Med.* 1993;329:593–599

Murphy JG, Gersh BJ, McGoon MD, et al. Long-term outcome after surgical repair of isolated atrial septal defect. Follow-up at 27 to 32 years. *N Engl J Med.* 1990;323:1645–1650.

Nembhard WN, Salemi JL, Wang T, Loscalzo ML, Hauser KW. Is the prevalence of specific types of congenital heart defects different for non-Hispanic white, non-Hispanic black and Hispanic infants? *Matern Child Health J.* 2009.

Oyen N, Poulsen G, Boyd HA, Wohlfahrt J, Jensen PK, Melbye M. National time trends in congenital heart defects, Denmark, 1977–2005. *Am Heart J.* 2009;157:467–473, e461.

Perloff JK, Warnes CA. Challenges posed by adults with repaired congenital heart disease. *Circulation.* 2001;103:2637–2643.

Pradat P. Epidemiology of major congenital heart defects in Sweden, 1981–1986. *J Epidemiol Community Health.* 1992;46:211–215.

Pradat P, Francannet C, Harris JA, Robert E. The epidemiology of cardiovascular defects, part I: a study based on data from three large registries of congenital malformations. *Pediatr Cardiol.* 2003;24:195–221.

Presbitero P, Somerville J, Revel-Chion R, Ross D. Open aortic valvotomy for congenital aortic stenosis. Late results. *Br Heart J.* 1982;47:26–34.

Reller MD, Strickland MJ, Riehle-Colarusso T, Mahle WT, Correa A. Prevalence of congenital heart defects in metropolitan Atlanta, 1998–2005. *J Pediatr.* 2008;153:807–813.

Roguin N, Du ZD, Barak M, Nasser N, Hershkowitz S, Milgram E. High prevalence of muscular ventricular septal defect in neonates. *J Am Coll Cardiol.* 1995;26:1545–1548.

Romano-Zelekha O, Hirsh R, Blieden L, Green M, Shohat T. The risk for congenital heart defects in offspring of individuals with congenital heart defects. *Clin Genet.* 2001;59:325–329.

Samanek M, Goetzova J, Benesova D. Distribution of congenital heart malformations in an autopsied child population. *Int J Cardiol.* 1985;8:235–250.

Sands AJ, Casey FA, Craig BG, Dornan JC, Rogers J, Mulholland HC. Incidence and risk factors for ventricular septal defect in "low risk" neonates. *Arch Dis Child Fetal Neonatal Ed.* 1991;81:F61–63.

Sever LE, Hessol NA, Gilbert ES, McIntyre JM. The prevalence at birth of congenital malformations in communities near the Hanford site. *Am J Epidemiol.* 1988;127:243–254.

Stein Z, Susser M, Warburton D, Wittes J, Kline J. Spontaneous abortion as a screening device. The effect of fetal survival on the incidence of birth defects. *Am J Epidemiol.* 1975;102:275–290.

STS. Society of Thoracic Surgeons Congenital Heart Surgery Database. 2008. http://wwwstsorg/sections/stsnationaldatabase/datamanagers/congenitalheartsurgerydb/datacollection/indexhtml

Tagliabue G, Tessandori R, Caramaschi F, et al. Descriptive epidemiology of selected birth defects, areas of Lombardy, Italy, 1999. *Popul Health Metr.* 2007;5:4.

Tanner K, Sabrine N, Wren C. Cardiovascular malformations among preterm infants. *Pediatrics.* 2005;116:e833–838.

Tennstedt A, Gutermann M, Schreiber D. [Malformations of the heart and vascular system in autopsy material of children]. *Zentralbl Allg Pathol.* 1983;128:127–132.

Tennstedt C, Chaoui R, Korner H, Dietel M. Spectrum of congenital heart defects and extracardiac malformations associated with chromosomal abnormalities: results of a seven year necropsy study. *Heart.* 1999;82:34–39.

Tilford JM, Robbins JM, Hobbs CA. Improving estimates of caregiver time cost and family impact associated with birth defects. *Teratology.* 2001;64(suppl 1):S37–41.

Ursell PC, Byrne JM, Strobino BA. Significance of cardiac defects in the developing fetus: a study of spontaneous abortuses. *Circulation.* 1985;72:1232–1236.

van Son JA, Danielson GK, Puga FJ, et al. Supravalvular aortic stenosis. Long-term results of surgical treatment. *J Thorac Cardiovasc Surg.* 1994;107:103–114; discussion 114–105.

Walsh EP, Rockenmacher S, Keane JF, Hougen TJ, Lock JE, Castaneda AR. Late results in patients with tetralogy of Fallot repaired during infancy. *Circulation.* 1988;77:1062–1067.

Wang X, Chen C, Wang L, Chen D, Guang W, French J. Conception, early pregnancy loss, and time to clinical pregnancy: a population-based prospective study. *Fertil Steril.* 2003;79:577–584.

Warkany J. Terathanasia. *Teratology.* 1978;17:187–192.

Wernovsky G, Mayer JE Jr, Jonas RA, et al. Factors influencing early and late outcome of the arterial switch operation for transposition of the great arteries. *J Thorac Cardiovasc Surg.* 1995;109:289–301; discussion 301–282.

Wilcox AJ, Baird DD, Weinberg CR. Time of implantation of the conceptus and loss of pregnancy. *N Engl J Med.* 1999;340:1796–1799.

Wilcox AJ, Weinberg CR, O'Connor JF, et al. Incidence of early loss of pregnancy. *N Engl J Med.* 1988;319:189–194.

Williams WG, Trusler GA, Kirklin JW, et al. Early and late results of a protocol for simple transposition leading to an atrial switch (Mustard) repair. *J Thorac Cardiovasc Surg.* 1988;95:717–726.

Wren C, Birrell G, Hawthorne G. Cardiovascular malformations in infants of diabetic mothers. *Heart.* 2003;89:1217–1220

Wren C, O'Sullivan JJ. Survival with congenital heart disease and need for follow up in adult life. *Heart.* 2001;85:438–443

Wurst KE, Ephross SA, Loehr J, Clark DW, Guess HA. Evaluation of the general practice research database congenital heart defects prevalence: comparison to United Kingdom national systems. *Birth Defects Res A Clin Mol Teratol.* 2007;79:309–316.

Zaver AG, Nadas AS. Atrial septal defect—secundum type. *Circulation.* 1965;32:III24–32.

IV

Epidemiology of Congenital Heart Defects

24

Epidemiological Studies of Congenital Heart Defects: Challenges and Opportunities

MARGARET A. HONEIN

SONJA A. RASMUSSEN

A major goal in the study of congenital heart defects (CHDs) is to better understand their etiology. Improved understanding of causes allows for provision of more accurate recurrence risk information following the birth of a child with a CHD and raises the possibility of primary prevention of these relatively common defects. While genetic (e.g., chromosome abnormalities and single-gene disorders) and environmental (e.g., maternal infections, diabetes, and medications) causes of CHDs are well recognized, their etiology is unknown in most infants. Current evidence suggests that most CHDs are of multifactorial etiology, with both genetic and environmental risk factors playing a role (Garg, 2006; Gelb, 2004).

Previous epidemiological studies have provided important insights into the genetic and environmental factors contributing to CHDs. Large epidemiological studies of CHDs have collected clinical information on infants and demographic information on families (e.g., maternal and paternal age and education, race-ethnicity, income, etc.). They have also collected information on exposures during pregnancy, usually from maternal interviews. Exposures assessed have included maternal medical conditions and pregnancy complications, medication use, nutrition, occupation and occupational exposures, and other lifestyle exposures (e.g., smoking, alcohol, and illicit drug use); some studies have also assessed selected paternal exposures.

A brief review of selected previous large epidemiological studies demonstrates their potential for identifying risk factors for CHDs (Table 24–1). The Atlanta Birth Defects Case-Control Study (ABDCCS) was a population-based study conducted by the Centers for Disease Control and Prevention to assess whether children of Vietnam veterans were at increased risk of any major birth defects and to identify other maternal and paternal exposures associated with major birth defects (Erickson et al., 1984; & Erickson et al., 1985). Case-infants were ascertained from population-based birth defects surveillance in the five counties of metropolitan Atlanta for births from 1968 to 1980 and control-infants were a random sample of live births for the same years, frequency matched to case-infants on race, birth hospital, and time period. While all major structural birth defects were included, mothers of 1012 infants with major heart defects were interviewed for this study. The ABDCCS identified numerous environmental exposures associated with CHDs (Adams et al., 1989; Becerra et al., 1990; Boneva et al., 1999; Botto et al., 2000, 2001c; Watkins and Botto, 2001).

In 1976, the Slone Epidemiology Center at Boston University began the Birth Defects Study (BDS), an ongoing study of major birth defects, including CHDs (Hernandez-Diaz et al., 2000; Werler et al., 1999). Infants are ascertained from hospitals in multiple sites across the United States. Slone's BDS completed interviews with 3870 mothers of infants with CHDs from 1976 to 1998, and data collection has continued for more recent births. Many environmental risk factors have been assessed using data from this study

The findings and conclusions in this chapter are those of the authors and do not necessarily represent the official position of the Centers for Disease Control and Prevention.

TABLE 24–1. *Summary of Selected Large Epidemiological Studies of Congenital Heart Defects*

Study	Location and Time Period	Method of Case Ascertainment	Method of Exposure Ascertainment	Number of Infants with Heart Defects with Completed Exposure Assessment
Atlanta Birth Defects Case-Control Study (Erickson et al., 1984)	Five counties of metropolitan Atlanta Births from 1968 to 1980	Population-based birth defects surveillance system with active case-finding	Detailed maternal and paternal telephone interviews completed in 1981–1982	1012 infants with congenital heart defects
Slone Epidemiology Center's Birth Defects Study (Hernandez-Diaz et al., 2000; Werler et al., 1999)	Metropolitan areas of the following cities: Boston (MA) 1976–present Philadelphia (PA) 1977–present Toronto (Canada) 1978–present San Diego 2001–present	Hospital-based birth defects surveillance with active case-finding at major referral hospitals and clinics and newborn nurseries in community hospitals	Detailed maternal in-person or telephone interview completed within 6 months of delivery	3870 infants with congenital heart defects among infants born 1976–1998; data collection is ongoing to the present
Hungarian Case-Control Surveillance of Congenital Abnormalities (Czeizel et al., 2001a)	1980–1996 with cases selected from the Hungarian Congenital Abnormalities Registry	Population-based birth defects surveillance	Medical records, antenatal logbook, and maternal questionnaire (self-administered)	4479 infants with isolated congenital heart defects
Baltimore-Washington Infant Study (Ferencz et al., 1997; Ferencz et al., 1993; Loffredo 2000)	Maryland, District of Columbia, and six adjacent counties in Virginia 1981–1989	Population-based ascertainment from multiple sources	Detailed in-person maternal interviews; all mothers of infants with severe heart defects and a random sample of those with mild defects were eligible for interview	3377 infants with congenital heart defects
International Database on Maternal Drug Exposure (MADRE) (Botto et al., 2006)	12 registries from European countries 1990–present	Case-only study of infants with major birth defects whose mother took medication in the first trimester		More than 15,000 infants with birth defects including an unspecified number of infants with congenital heart defects
Swedish Medical Birth Registry (Kallen and Otterblad Olausson, 2003)	1 July 1995–2001, Sweden	Cases identified from Swedish health registries; comparison group is all infants born in Sweden	Maternal medication use and other exposures are abstracted from antenatal care records	5015 infants with congenital heart defects
National Birth Defects Prevention Study (Botto et al., 2007; Caton et al., 2009; Yoon et al., 2001)	Arkansas (1998–present) California* (1997–present) Georgia* (1997–present) Iowa (1997–present) Massachusetts* (1997–present) New Jersey (1998–2002) New York* (1998–present) North Carolina* (2003–present) Texas* (1997–present) Utah (2003–present)	Population-based birth defects surveillance systems	Detailed maternal telephone interviews completed between 6 weeks and 24 months after the estimated date of delivery; buccal cell samples collected for DNA	5608 infants with congenital heart defects born on/after October 1997 and with an estimated date of delivery prior to January 1, 2004; data collection is ongoing for 2004 to the present

Note: *Study conducted in a defined geographic region of the state based on maternal residence at delivery.

(Hernandez-Diaz et al., 2000; Mitchell et al., 1981; Werler et al., 1989, 1990, 1991, 1999).

The Hungarian case-control study of congenital abnormalities began in 1980 and continued through 1996. The study included 4479 infants with isolated CHDs with completed exposure information. Exposures were ascertained using a maternal questionnaire, antenatal logbooks, and birth hospitalization summaries (Czeizel et al., 2001a), and data from this

study have been used to assess the effects of maternal illnesses and medication use on the risk for birth defects (Czeizel et al., 2001b, 2004; Czeizel and Rockenbauer, 2000; Nielsen et al., 2005).

The Baltimore-Washington Infant Study (BWIS) was a case-control study of infants with CHDs from 1981 to 1989 (Ferencz et al., 1993, 1997; Loffredo, 2000). The study sought to ascertain all cases in the birth cohort born in Maryland, the District of Columbia, and the northern part of Virginia. CHDs were ascertained up to 12 months of age, and in-person interviews were conducted to ascertain the effects of a large number of risk factors for CHDs (Botto et al., 2001b; Correa-Villasenor et al., 1991; Ewing et al., 1997; Ferencz et al., 1993, 1997; Loffredo et al., 2001a, 2001b; Rosenthal et al., 1991; Steinberger et al., 2002).

The Maternal Drug Exposure (MADRE) project is an ongoing collaborative project of 12 birth defects registries coordinated by the International Clearinghouse for Birth Defects Surveillance and Research (Botto et al., 2006). The MADRE project enrolls infants with major birth defects with reported maternal medication exposure in the first trimester. Neither control-infants nor case-infants without a maternal medication exposure are included in the study. More than 15,000 infants with major birth defects and a maternal medication exposure were enrolled as of 2006, but the distribution of infants by type of defect has not been published. The MADRE project data have been used to assess the association between maternal exposure to antiepileptic drugs and major structural defects, including CHDs, with a positive association identified between several of the antiepileptic medications and CHDs (Arpino et al., 2000).

The Swedish health registers have been used to conduct a large epidemiological study of risk factors for CHDs (Kallen and Otterblad Olausson, 2003) for births from July 1, 1995, through the end of 2001, using data abstracted from antenatal medical records on medication use and other exposures. The study includes 5015 infants with CHDs, and the comparison group is all infants born in Sweden during this period (N = 577,730).

The National Birth Defects Prevention Study (NBDPS) is an ongoing, multi-site case-control study of major birth defects including CHDs (Yoon et al., 2001). Data collection for the NBDPS began in 1997, and data are included from 10 different sites in the United States: Arkansas, California, Georgia, Iowa, Massachusetts, New Jersey, New York, North Carolina, Texas, and Utah. Infants with major birth defects, including most types of CHDs, are ascertained by population-based birth defects surveillance systems at each site, and mothers of infants are asked to participate in a telephone interview. To allow study of genetic risk factors and gene–environment interactions, mothers are mailed a buccal cell collection kit following the interview and asked to collect samples from themselves, the infant, and the infant's father (Rasmussen et al., 2002). A total of 5608 mothers of infants with CHDs who were born on or after October 1, 1997, and had an estimated date of delivery (EDD) on or before December 31, 2003, have been interviewed (Botto et al., 2007; Caton et al., 2009); maternal interviews for infants with an EDD

in 2004, 2005, and 2006 have also been completed, and maternal interviews are ongoing for infants with an EDD in 2007 or later.

Large epidemiological studies of CHDs also provide the opportunity to explore mortality due to CHDs, particularly infant mortality or mortality in early childhood. These studies could help identify causal factors that might contribute to the racial/ethnic disparities in mortality identified in previous studies (Boneva et al., 2001). The studies could also determine whether infant mortality from specific types of heart defects varies by environmental exposures during heart development (e.g., maternal smoking or maternal medication use) or by identified genetic risk factors.

A recent comprehensive review article summarized the evidence for a wide range of environmental exposures that are associated with either an increased or a decreased risk of CHDs (Jenkins et al., 2007). A decreased risk of CHDs with exposure to multivitamins containing folic acid has been suggested by some studies. Exposures associated with a possible increased risk of CHDs included maternal phenylketonuria, diabetes, rubella infection, influenza, febrile illness, and epilepsy. Maternal medication exposures that were suggested to increase the risk of CHDs included vitamin A, anticonvulsants, nonsteroidal anti-inflammatory medications, sulfasalazine, thalidomide, and trimethoprim-sulfonamide. Other exposures associated with increased CHD risk in some studies included maternal marijuana use and exposure to organic solvents (Jenkins et al., 2007).

Although large epidemiological studies hold considerable promise for identifying genetic and environmental risk factors for birth defects, several issues must be considered to optimize a study's potential for success. These main challenges fall into three categories: (1) case ascertainment and phenotype characterization; (2) epidemiological challenges including exposure assessment, statistical power, and overcoming barriers to study participation; and (3) collection of biological specimens (including types, quality control, and optimization of participation rates) and methods of analysis of genetic risk factors and gene–environment interactions.

CASE ASCERTAINMENT AND PHENOTYPE CHARACTERIZATION

A key consideration in designing an epidemiological study of CHDs is establishing case definitions for the study. CHDs, as with other birth defects, can be considered major (those of medical, surgical, or cosmetic importance) or minor (Rasmussen and Moore, 2001). Typically, epidemiological studies have focused on major defects, but sometimes what is considered to be a major CHD might not be readily apparent. For example, ventricular septal defects, one of the most common types of CHDs (Ferencz et al., 1997; Hoffman and Kaplan, 2002), clearly meet the definition of a major birth defect, given that they sometimes require surgical intervention (Turner et al., 2002). Also, because of their frequent occurrence (Botto et al., 2001a), these defects are of public health significance (Boneva et al., 2001). However, ventricular septal defects are phenotypically heterogeneous, with a significant proportion closing spontaneously; the rate of spontaneous closure in previous studies has varied from 11% to 71% (Axt-Fliedner et al., 2006). Ascertainment of defects that later close spontaneously is likely to be variable and possibly associated with certain demographic factors. Thus, risk factors identified for these phenotypes could actually be risk factors for ascertainment, rather than for occurrence, supporting their exclusion from studies. However, at the time of diagnosis, prediction of ventricular septal defects that will eventually close spontaneously versus those that will require surgical repair is challenging; to distinguish these cases would require long-term follow-up (Garne, 2006; Turner et al., 1999, 2002), which may be cumbersome in epidemiological studies.

Some CHDs are observed much more frequently among preterm infants. For example, the ductus arteriosus plays an important role in fetal circulation, shunting blood from the high-resistance pulmonary circulation to the systemic circulation (Hermes-DeSantis and Clyman, 2006). Whereas the ductus arteriosus closes by 96 hours in more than 95% of infants weighing 1500 g or more at birth, spontaneous permanent closure occurs in only about 34% of infants weighing 1000 g or less (Koch et al., 2006). For this reason, most birth defects surveillance programs exclude these prematurity-related anomalies, based either on the infant's gestational age or birth weight (e.g., patent ductus arteriosus is not considered a defect among infants born preterm). It should also be noted that infants with certain cyanotic CHDs depend on patency of the ductus arteriosus for survival (Alwi et al., 2004; Talosi et al., 2004) until more definitive surgical intervention can be performed; in these situations, the patent ductus arteriosus should also not be considered to be a birth defect.

Another consideration is whether rare CHDs should be included. Large numbers of eligible cases are necessary to allow for consideration of confounding factors and examination of infrequent exposures and genetic risk factors, as well as of gene–environment interactions. Unless the study population is very large, case numbers are unlikely to be sufficient for analysis of very rare types of defects, unless they are combined for analysis with other types of defects presumed to

be pathogenetically and etiologically similar (Martin et al., 1992). Unfortunately, lack of knowledge about the etiology of CHDs limits the degree to which smaller categories can be grouped together with confidence.

It is also important to consider what type of diagnostic modality will be considered adequate for case inclusion in the study. Advances in cardiac imaging have resulted in improved accuracy of CHD diagnosis, when compared with clinical examination alone (Danford et al., 1999, 1997, 2002). Increased availability of color Doppler echocardiography is believed to be the primary reason for the increased prevalence of CHDs observed in recent years (Bosi et al., 2003). Thus, a case definition needs to explicitly state what diagnostic modality is sufficient for study inclusion. For example, for the NBDPS, the diagnosis of a CHD by physical examination is insufficient; the diagnosis must be confirmed by echocardiography, catheterization, surgical evaluation, or autopsy for the defect to be included in the study (Yoon et al., 2001). Case definitions for epidemiological studies need to be responsive to changes in clinical knowledge and practices. For example, recent studies have suggested that magnetic resonance imaging studies are highly accurate in the diagnosis of partial anomalous pulmonary venous return, a diagnosis previously made by cardiac catheterization (Festa et al., 2006). Therefore, for the NBDPS, the case definition was recently modified to include magnetic resonance imaging as an acceptable modality for the diagnosis of anomalous pulmonary venous return. These differences in diagnostic modality and technical advances across studies and over time can make comparison of results from different studies difficult.

CHDs are now often diagnosed prenatally (Montana et al., 1996), and in some cases, pregnancies with more severe defects (e.g., hypoplastic left heart syndrome) are terminated (Brackley et al., 2000; Lin et al., 1999). Whether to include prenatally diagnosed cases for which postnatal confirmation is not available is another important issue in epidemiological studies of CHDs. Although the accuracy of prenatal diagnosis of CHDs has improved substantially in recent years (Sivanandam, et al., 2006), diagnoses made prenatally are often not as accurate as those made postnatally, and some structural heart defects may evolve during the course of fetal development (Trines and Hornberger, 2004). In addition, in some instances, prenatal diagnosis might miss accompanying defects or genetic conditions, resulting in inappropriate classification of cases. However, exclusion of cases that are prenatally diagnosed and not confirmed postnatally is also problematic. In recent years, a significant proportion of cases with certain cardiovascular malformations has been prenatally diagnosed and electively terminated (Lin et al., 1999); thus, their exclusion would result in a substantial decrease in the number of eligible cases. In addition, given that demographic factors (e.g., race-ethnicity) (and likely other risk factors) have been shown to differ among women who undergo prenatal diagnosis and elective pregnancy termination after diagnosis of an abnormality when compared with women who continue their pregnancy (Forrester and Merz, 1999; Siffel et al., 2004), exclusion of these cases could present a selection bias in epidemiological analyses.

Another important topic for discussion related to ascertainment of CHDs is that most surveillance systems exclude diagnoses made among spontaneous abortions occurring at less than 20 weeks' gestation because of concern for incomplete ascertainment. Given that the prevalence of CHDs has been shown to be higher among spontaneous abortions (Hoffman, 1990, 1995) than among live births, excluding these cases could result in a significant underascertainment of CHDs and could have an effect on the study of risk factors for CHDs as well.

Consideration must also be given to whether to include infants with CHDs associated with a syndrome of known etiology (e.g., single-gene disorder or chromosome abnormality) in an epidemiological study. The pathogenesis of and risk factors for CHDs in a child with a chromosome abnormality (e.g., for atrioventricular septal defect in a child with Down syndrome) are likely to be different from those in a child without a chromosome abnormality. Some studies have considered infants with a syndrome to be a highly susceptible population that could provide insight into the risk factors for heart defects (Kerstann et al., 2004; Khoury and Erickson, 1992). Other studies have excluded these infants to increase the homogeneity of case-groups (Yoon et al., 2001).

All of the aforementioned issues emphasize the importance of establishing careful case definitions, with precise inclusion and exclusion criteria, when designing an epidemiological study of CHDs. Without careful case definitions, the likelihood of valid risk factors being identified by the study will be diminished.

Another important consideration is how infants with CHDs will be ascertained. Several different methods have been used in different studies of birth defects, including ascertainment from birth certificates, from hospital discharge data, and from birth defects surveillance systems using multiple sources of ascertainment. Birth certificate data have been shown to be unreliable for ascertainment of birth defects: in one study, only 14% of birth defects reported by the Metropolitan Atlanta Congenital Defects Program, a population-based birth defects surveillance system, were ascertained using birth certificates (Watkins et al., 1996). Concerns have also been raised about the reliability of hospital discharge data (Frohnert et al., 2005).

Although *International Classification of Diseases, 9th Revision, Clinical Modification (ICD-9-CM)* codes from hospital discharge data were able to identify most infants with CHDs (sensitivity of 0.857), many cases identified were false positives (positive predictive value was 0.364) (Frohnert et al., 2005). Birth defects surveillance systems differ with regard to their methods (e.g., whether they are hospital- or population-based and whether they use active or passive case ascertainment methods), and these differences affect data quality. Hospital-based systems are dependent on the catchment area covered by the hospital and whether the hospital provides primary or specialty care. Non–population-based sources of ascertainment can lead to incomplete and biased ascertainment of certain conditions (Parkes et al., 2006). Prevalence of certain birth defects has been shown to differ between states that use passive (i.e., methods that rely on reports from other sources) versus active (i.e., programs that actively review records to ascertain cases of birth defects) methods (Hobbs et al., 2001). In addition, different types of ascertainment sources (e.g., hospital discharge and specialty clinic records) vary in their ability to ascertain cases, emphasizing the importance of using multiple sources of ascertainment (Cronk et al., 2003; Feldkamp et al., 2005). However, even in the Metropolitan Atlanta Congenital Defects Program, which uses multiple ascertainment sources and active ascertainment methods and has served as a model for some other birth defects surveillance systems, the sensitivity of ascertainment of birth defects was not 100% (Honein and Paulozzi, 1999). Further, in a study by Kuehl et al. (1999), nearly 10% of infants with CHDs who died in the first year of life did not have the diagnosis made before the infant's death and were instead ascertained through a search of autopsy records. This study emphasizes the importance of including autopsy records as an ascertainment source, as well as the difficulty in making the diagnosis of some CHDs in infancy. All of these issues affecting case ascertainment for an epidemiological study of CHDs need to be considered in the study design, and ascertainment of all infants meeting the case definition needs to be maximized.

Another important consideration is how to classify CHDs for analysis. Some epidemiological studies have combined all CHDs together into a single category for analysis. The finding that certain risk factors, such as maternal pregestational diabetes (Jenkins et al., 2007) and mutations in the cardiac transcription factor *NKX2.5* (Benson et al., 1999), affect diverse cardiac developmental pathways provides some support for this approach. However, several lines of evidence suggest that CHDs are etiologically heterogeneous. First, conditions of known genetic etiology that often present with CHDs are usually associated with a specific type of malformation. For example, CHDs observed in children with 22q11.2 deletions typically involve the outflow tract or aortic arch (Botto et al., 2003) and the most commonly observed heart defects in children with Down syndrome are atrioventricular septal defects (Freeman et al., 1998). Similar effects of single-gene conditions (Bossert et al., 2002) and cardiac teratogens (Hastreiter et al., 1967; Lammer et al., 1985) are also observed. Information from embryological studies of the developing heart also supports the idea that CHDs are pathogenetically and etiologically heterogeneous (Clark, 1996). And, finally, different types of heart defects have been shown to have different epidemiological characteristics, suggesting that they are etiologically distinct (Ferencz et al., 1997; Harris et al., 2003).

Because CHDs are likely to be etiologically heterogeneous, many investigators have attempted to define subcategories of CHDs for analysis (Botto et al., 2007; Clark, 1996). However, the definition of appropriate subcategories of CHDs has been challenging. Because of the lack of consensus on methods of classification, different studies have used various strategies to classify heart defects. Some studies have used an anatomical classification system, others have used an embryologically based morphogenetic hierarchical system, and still others have divided groups by the ICD-9 or they have used a combination of these systems (Botto et al., 2007; Ferencz et al., 1997; Harris et al., 2003; Pradat, 1993). This lack of consistency and lack of use of standardized nomenclature across different epidemiological studies of CHDs might have contributed to the difficulty in replicating study findings. Infants with complex heart defects (e.g., those with multiple CHDs with no apparent underlying morphogenetic mechanism) are particularly challenging to classify. These phenotypes have not been consistently addressed in previous epidemiological studies and are an important area for future etiologic research.

Another important clinical issue is how to deal with infants who have additional major defects unrelated to the heart or those with conditions of known etiology. Guidelines for classification of infants with birth defects into more etiologically homogeneous categories have been developed for the NBDPS (Rasmussen et al., 2003). These guidelines classify infants as having an isolated defect (including those with sequences), multiple major defects, or a syndrome (single-gene condition or chromosome abnormality) and might be helpful for other studies of CHDs.

EPIDEMIOLOGICAL CHALLENGES

Several challenges also need to be considered when designing epidemiological studies of CHDs or interpreting results from these studies. The study design is key, but the options are somewhat limited given the rarity of the outcome under consideration. Given that CHDs have affected about 9 per 1000 live births in the United States in recent years (Botto et al., 2001a), the case-control design is by far the most practical approach to epidemiological research of CHDs. While prospective cohort studies would likely improve the capacity to completely ascertain maternal exposures during pregnancy, they are unlikely to result in a sufficient number of cases of CHDs to adequately address environmental exposures and genetic risk factors, which often are also somewhat uncommon exposures. For example, the planned National Children's Study will use a cohort design to identify 100,000 births and follow the infants for up to 21 years. While this study will provide an extremely rich data source for evaluating many outcomes, the potential to identify risk factors for birth defects is more limited. In a cohort of 100,000 births, approximately 900–1000 infants with CHDs would be expected, which would then be further subdivided into the different types of CHDs. In contrast, the NBDPS interviewed nearly 5000 mothers of infants with CHDs during the first 5 years of the study (Botto et al., 2007). A cohort study such as the National Children's Study is well suited to evaluating a hypothesis regarding one exposure such as maternal diabetes in relation to an outcome such as CHDs or a specific type of CHD. However, our limited knowledge about the causes of CHDs necessitates an approach that assesses a wider range of exposures for these specific outcomes.

It is also important to balance the homogeneity of case-groups with concerns related to statistical power. The classification scheme chosen to create categories of infants (isolated, multiple, or syndrome), as well as the classification of the heart defect itself, will affect the assessment of exposure-outcome analyses. While creation of the most homogeneous etiologic groups possible should enhance the capacity to identify potential risk factors for specific types of CHDs, division of CHDs into smaller and presumably more homogeneous subgroups will severely limit the power to detect weak associations between risk factors and smaller subgroups of CHDs. A balance will need to be struck between strength of association (which should be increased if groups are more homogeneous) and sample size (which will decrease as more homogeneous groups are created). For example, to detect an odds ratio of 2 between a particular CHD and a maternal exposure that occurs in 1% of mothers (e.g., use of a particular medication or of assisted reproductive technology), assuming a case-control study with two controls for every case, 1866 cases of the particular CHD of interest will need to be included in the defect group being assessed (Schieve et al., 2005). It is also important to note that the current state of knowledge on how to create homogeneous case-groups is quite limited, and case-control studies might help us to determine how best to create these case-groups.

Multiple comparisons are a challenge faced by essentially all large epidemiological studies. To maximize their utility, large studies are designed to address a very wide range of exposures, and often also large number of outcome groups, because it is very important to assess associations between exposures and specific types of CHDs. If 20 different exposures are assessed for 10 different specific types of CHDs, 200 comparisons are made. At an alpha level of 0.05, a statistically significant finding would be expected by chance alone for 10 of these comparisons—even if there are no true associations. And, the reality of large studies is that we are often assessing far more than 20 exposures. Unfortunately, available adjustment techniques for multiple exposures are as likely to eliminate true associations as those due to chance. However, given our awareness of problems related to multiple comparisons, it is extremely important that novel findings be replicated before gaining acceptance as true risk factors for CHDs.

For most epidemiological studies of CHDs, maternal interviews are one source of assessment of exposures during pregnancy. While maternal report can be imperfect, it is likely the best source of pregnancy exposure information available postnatally (and after diagnosis of the CHD) for certain exposures, such as use of over-the-counter medications, use of alcohol and tobacco during pregnancy, symptomatic infections or illnesses that did not result in a visit to a health care provider, and maternal vitamin use. While the quality of data from maternal interviews is often criticized, this method of exposure assessment has improved the understanding of birth defects etiology. As an example, data from maternal interviews were used to initially detect an inverse association between consumption of multivitamins containing folic acid and neural tube defects (Mulinare et al., 1988), a finding that was later validated in randomized controlled trials (Czeizel and Dudas, 1992; MRC Vitamin Study Research Group, 1991) and a community intervention study (Berry et al., 1999). Some exposures might be underreported by maternal interviews after pregnancy when compared to medical records or interviews during pregnancy, but there is also considerable variation depending on the exposure of interest (Bryant et al., 1989; Tilley et al., 1985; Yawn et al., 1998). Methodological studies have also demonstrated that the quality of the exposure data obtained during maternal interview can be improved with the use of detailed questions and probes (Mitchell et al., 1986) and that reported exposure information is valid and reproducible for many exposures of interest (Paganini-Hill and Ross, 1982; Tomeo et al., 1999). To maximize the utility of the interview, questions should be targeted to the most critical periods of exposure for development of CHDs. However, the capacity to do this is limited by our understanding of the critical timing for some defects and the likelihood that the critical period varies by type of defect, and perhaps even has variability within one type of defect. It is also critical to ensure that the maternal interview includes those exposures most strongly suspected to have a role in the etiology of CHDs.

Data quality can also be affected by the length and setting of the maternal interview. Maternal interviews need to be somewhat limited in length due to practical barriers of the period that women recruited to the study will be willing to spend answering detailed questions about their pregnancy, particularly given that case-mothers are often caring for a young infant with significant health problems at the time they are asked to participate in an interview. Participants can be allowed to complete the interview in multiple, shorter time segments; however, many participants who complete only part of the interview and ask to be recontacted later might never complete the interview. The interview should be focused on those exposures most likely to have a role in the etiology of CHDs and should be as convenient as possible for the mother. Telephone interviews might be the most practical for the mother and the researcher, particularly in a geographically large study area. And, some sensitive exposures might be more accurately reported in a telephone interview than in an in-person interview, although comparisons have been somewhat inconclusive on this point, with some suggesting no difference in reporting by location of interviewer (Rosenbaum et al., 2006). Mailed survey forms can provide more detailed information on certain types of exposures, such as family history (that can be aided by contacting other family members) (Romitti et al., 1997) and dietary intake questionnaires that benefit from careful thought (Caan et al., 1991), or for some sensitive exposures, such as alcohol use (Kraus and Augustin, 2001). However, mailed survey forms typically suffer from lower participation than can be obtained for a telephone interview (Duncan et al., 2005). In-person interviews might create a better rapport between the interviewer and the participant, and can provide an opportunity to request additional information such as biological samples, access to medical records, or photographs. However, an in-person interview requires that either the participant or the interviewer travel to a different location, and interviews in a participant's home can lack the necessary privacy for obtaining accurate data on a range of exposures including some that are quite sensitive in nature such as use of illicit substances, history of sexually transmitted diseases, and other exposures.

The timing of the maternal interview relative to the pregnancy might affect participation rates, recall bias, and selection bias. Interviews conducted at the time of prenatal diagnosis of a CHD will be done much nearer in time to the critical periods of exposure and might result in more complete recall of the maternal exposures. However, conducting the interview during pregnancy might increase the stress and anxiety of the mother and will be possible only for the subset of infants whose CHD is prenatally diagnosed. This group might be substantially different from those infants with a CHD that is not prenatally diagnosed, in terms of both the type and severity of the defect, and the education and socioeconomic level of the mother. It is also problematic to determine an appropriate comparison group of infants not affected by a CHD whose mothers could also be interviewed prenatally. Participation rates could be positively affected by use of prenatal interviews if a major issue for participation is tracking and tracing in a mobile society. The rates also could be potentially negatively affected if women are not comfortable participating in an interview prior to fully understanding the magnitude of the infant's health problems. Interviews conducted shortly after delivery might also result in improved participation and more complete recall, but this likely will vary by the medical issues the family is facing. The early postnatal months might include multiple hospitalizations for case-infants and almost certainly will include parental fatigue. Interviews conducted a little later (6–12 months after delivery) might benefit from more complete ascertainment of all cases in a population-based setting and thus minimize selection bias of who is included in the study. However, such interviews will likely suffer from less complete ascertainment of exposures, which might contribute to recall bias. Interviews in early childhood (1–5 years) would make it possible to ask about both exposures and some longer-term outcomes of the child but likely would be hampered by major obstacles in tracking and tracing the potential participants, depending on the mobility of the study population.

Finally, appropriate incentives are increasingly necessary to ensure adequate participation in epidemiological studies and to minimize selection bias (Brealey et al., 2007; Crider et al., 2006; Olshan et al., 2006, 2007; Whiteman et al., 2003). It is increasingly difficult to contact potential participants because of a number of factors, including increased use of cellular telephones as the primary household line, use of caller ID (identification) to screen calls, and use of a single telephone line for both telephone service and internet access (Blumberg et al., 2006; Kempf and Remington, 2006, 2007; Tuckel and O'Neill, 2001). Studies relying on random-digit dialing for ascertainment of a control population will be particularly affected by the changes in telephone-related behavior, but other studies that rely on telephones for initial contact or for completion of a telephone interview are also affected (Galesic et al., 2006; Stone et al., 2007). For example, potential participants who use a cellular telephone for their sole telephone line would have to use a substantial number of their allotted minutes to complete a lengthy telephone interview. Addressing this issue will likely require the use of an appropriate incentive, whether monetary, a calling card, or provision of a disposable cellular telephone. Study sites might also need to adapt to cellular telephone company policies such as by ensuring that each study site has an available cellular telephone from each major cellular provider in the area so that the call to conduct the interview can be done "in network" and thus become more acceptable or less costly to the participant.

The addition of a monetary incentive has been shown to increase participation for both telephone and mail surveys (Edwards et al., 2002; Kropf and Blair, 2005), and personalizing the initial contact letter with the potential participant's name also improves participation (Scott and Edwards, 2006). However, one study suggested that control participation might be affected more than case participation by monetary incentives and that some participants might actually interpret the offer of an incentive in a negative manner (Coogan and Rosenberg, 2004). When considering the use of monetary incentives, it is important that the incentive be reasonable in terms of the time or effort being requested from the participant, but not at a level that could coerce participation from someone who actually did not want to participate in the research (Singer and Bossarte, 2006).

Although no ideal approach regarding maternal interview setting, timing, and incentives has been identified, it is extremely important for investigators launching epidemiological studies of CHDs to carefully consider these study design issues. Investigators should consider conducting a pilot study or focus group research to determine the best approach for the intended study population.

Information on some key exposures (e.g., maternal infections, occupational exposures, nutritional exposures, and early pregnancy exposure levels to certain environmental factors) is not likely to be well measured by maternal interview, and alternative measures of exposure assessment are needed. Epidemiological studies should consider alternative means of ascertaining these exposure levels using available samples such as newborn blood spots (Olney et al., 2006) or stored midpregnancy serum samples (Iovannisci et al., 2006). Retention of such samples in a manner that can be linked to outcomes can expand the potential of epidemiological studies of CHDs. Studies should also consider accessing samples that can be collected postnatally, such as hair samples that might be used to assess levels of pregnancy exposure to certain factors (Ozkaynak et al., 2005).

BIOLOGICS ISSUES

Current evidence supports the inclusion of an evaluation of genetic risk factors and gene–environment interaction in studies of the etiology of CHDs. Nevertheless, most previous studies have not included these factors in epidemiological investigations because technological advances to allow consideration of these factors have only become available recently. Several issues are raised by including genetic risk factors in large epidemiological investigations. A critical issue is to determine the optimal types of specimens to be collected from case- and control-infants. Although venous blood specimens allow the greatest versatility in the types of analyses that can be done (both DNA and RNA can be evaluated, as well as measures of exposures, to complement questionnaire responses) (Bernert et al., 1997) and the largest amount of DNA, these specimens might not be optimal for maximizing participation rates, given that many parents are reluctant to have their child's blood drawn for research purposes. Collection of other types of samples can be considered to maximize participation rates (Dlugos et al., 2005). One option is dried newborn blood spots, specimens that are routinely collected from more than 95% of newborns born in the United States as part of newborn screening programs to test for inborn errors of metabolism, endocrinopathies, and other disorders. Residual dried blood spots provide a valuable, population-based resource to study the prevalence of certain factors among newborns and their mothers (Henderson et al., 1997). Although policies regarding storage of residual dried blood spots vary by state, a recent survey demonstrated that approximately half of states store residual spots, often for use in epidemiological studies (Olney et al., 2006). DNA obtained from previously collected newborn blood spots has been used to study susceptibility genes for childhood leukemia (Klotz et al., 2006) and genetic factors for birth defects (Shaw et al., 2005).

Buccal (cheek) cell collection is another option. Buccal cell collection is less invasive than phlebotomy and thus might be more acceptable to participants. Buccal cells can be collected using mouthwash or cytobrush methods. Mouthwash samples appear to provide a higher quality and quantity of DNA sample than those collected by cytobrush but are not practical for studies that include young infants (Garcia-Closas et al., 2001;

Lum and Le Marchand, 1998). Buccal samples can be collected from young infants using cytobrush (Garcia-Closas et al., 2001; Rasmussen et al., 2002). Although use of buccal cell collection is cheaper and less invasive, the quality and quantity of DNA collected is not optimal. Methods that allow the amplification of DNA, such as whole genome amplification, might be useful in increasing the number of analyses that can be done using buccal specimens (Thompson et al., 2005). Saliva might be another reasonable alternative, in terms of DNA quantity and quality (Ng et al., 2006). Collection methods, such as the use of foam swabs (Rogers et al., 2007), make collection of saliva from infants an option. Other possible methods include using chemically treated paper cards (e.g., IsoCode Cards or FTA Cards) for collection of buccal specimens (Lema et al., 2006; Milne et al., 2006; Vidal-Taboada et al., 2006).

Regardless of the specimen collection method used, some families will be hesitant to participate in a study of genetic risk factors. Participation rates in biologics sampling have been shown to vary by demographic factors, such as race-ethnicity and maternal age (Crider et al., 2006). Some studies have suggested that inclusion of genetic risk factors in an epidemiological study might decrease the overall study participation rate (Matsui et al., 2005). While low interview participation introduces the likelihood of selection bias, this is less of a concern for biologics specimen collection because in this case participation is less likely to vary by any specific genetic risk factors. However, low participation rates for biologics specimen collection will severely limit the power to identify genetic risk factors, particularly when appropriate analyses include stratifying by race-ethnicity, and will limit a study's generalizability.

Incorporating analyses of genetic risk factors into epidemiological studies also raises several human subjects–related issues (Jenkins et al., 2008). Given the rapid advancement in genetics knowledge, the specific genetic studies to be performed and their significance to participants might not be known at the time that informed consent is obtained. Thus, participants are sometimes asked to consent to genetic studies without knowing the risks and benefits associated with the specific genetic test results. Two options, periodic reconsent and "blanket consent," have been considered to deal with this situation (Burke and Diekema, 2006). When the periodic reconsent approach is used, the participant is updated regarding uses of the data and given the opportunity to reconsent. Under the "blanket consent" approach, a participant consents to unspecified future use of the biological specimen. In some cases, the types of research for which the specimens can be used might be stipulated (e.g., the informed consent might specify that specimens will be used only for research related to birth defects).

Another issue is whether and when individual research results should be provided to participants. At this time, there are no federal regulations regarding disclosure of individual research results (Burke and Diekema, 2006). Both the National Bioethics Advisory Commission and a recent National Heart, Lung, and Blood Institute Working Group on Reporting Genetic Results in Research Studies recognized that genetic results should be shared with individuals under certain circumstances (Bookman et al., 2006; National Bioethics Advisory Commission, 1999). The working group recommended that results of genetics tests should be provided to individuals if the following criteria are met: (1) the risk for the disease is significant, (2) the disease has important health implications, and (3) proven interventions to treat or prevent the disease are available (Bookman et al., 2006). However, other authors have disagreed with this restrictive perspective, noting that these recommendations emphasize protecting research participants from harm but overlook the need for respecting research participants, and they argue for making individual research results available to participants on request (Shalowitz and Miller, 2005).

Issues related to disclosure of genetic testing results from a study of children are even more complex. Policy statements of the American Society of Human Genetics and American Academy of Pediatrics both propose that genetic testing of children for clinical purposes occur only when required for medical care during childhood (Burke and Diekema, 2006). Although guidelines are not clear, it is apparent that issues of when and how individual results will be provided need to be carefully considered by the researcher and the institutional review board during the design phase of a study (Shalowitz and Miller, 2005) and included in the informed consent process (Burke and Diekema, 2006).

Another critical issue that needs to be addressed is data protection to ensure that confidentiality is maintained. When large datasets that include genome sequence data linked to clinical and demographic data and interview responses are created, the methods to ensure confidentiality need to be specifically addressed and communicated to potential participants (Austin et al., 2003; Burke and Diekema, 2006).

Another consideration for those working to better understand genetic contributions to CHDs is which genes to study. For most previous studies, a candidate gene approach has been used, with knowledge from genes involved with known syndromes, other identified environmental risk factors (e.g., folic acid suggesting studies of the methylenetetrahydrofolate reductase gene and other genes involved in folate metabolism), or developmental studies, to guide assessment of genes to be studied. Approaches for identification of possible candidate genes for birth defects were recently summarized (Green and Moore, 2006). Development of

high-throughput genotyping techniques have made possible genome-wide association studies, and these, along with the availability of key resources including the Human Genome Project and the International HapMap Project (Collins et al., 2003; Pe'er et al., 2006), have advanced the potential to identify novel genetic risk factors for CHDs (Lidral and Moreno, 2005). Each of these approaches has advantages and disadvantages that will need to be weighed by study investigators. Although genome-wide association studies have the ability to detect new risk factors not previously suspected of being associated with CHDs, the cost, amount of DNA, and large sample size needed for these studies can limit their use (Green and Moore, 2006). In addition, these studies often present statistical challenges, given the large number of tests performed (Altmuller et al., 2001; Dudbridge et al., 2006). While these very exploratory approaches can yield important clues to genetic etiology, it is critical that the findings be replicated in separate studies (Moonesinghe et al., 2007). In addition, meta-analyses techniques can be employed to help guide interpretation of results from studies attempting to replicate findings on genetic risk factors (Evangelou et al., 2007; Khoury et al., 2006).

Studies of gene–gene and gene–environment interactions require even larger numbers than those needed to study single genetic risk factors when using a case-control study design. Other approaches, such as the case-only design, may be more efficient for the study of these interactions (Weinberg and Umbach, 2000; Yang et al., 1997, 1999).

CONCLUSIONS

Large epidemiological studies of CHDs hold tremendous promise for the identification of environmental risk factors that are amenable to prevention and for the identification of genetic risk factors that might interact with environmental exposures. CHDs affect nearly 1% of infants in the United States and are a major contributor to infant mortality. Thus, identifying strategies to prevent CHDs will have a major effect on the morbidity and mortality associated with these serious disorders. However, in designing such studies or interpreting results from these studies in the literature, it is critical to consider clinical, epidemiologic, and biological issues that can affect results.

REFERENCES

Adams MM, Mulinare J, Dooley K. Risk factors for conotruncal cardiac defects in Atlanta. *J Am Coll Cardiol.* 1989;14:432–442.

Altmuller J, Palmer LJ, Fischer G, Scherb H, Wjst M. Genomewide scans of complex human diseases: true linkage is hard to find. *Am J Hum Genet.* 69:936–950.

Alwi M, Choo KK, Latiff HA, Kandavello G, Samion H, Mulyadi MD. Initial results and medium-term follow-up of stent implantation of patent ductus arteriosus in duct-dependent pulmonary circulation. *J Am Coll Cardiol.* 2004;44:438–445.

Arpino C, Brescianini S, Robert E, et al. Teratogenic effects of antiepileptic drugs: use of an International Database on Malformations and Drug Exposure (MADRE). *Epilepsia.* 2000;41:1436–1443.

Austin MA, Harding SE, McElroy CE. Monitoring ethical, legal, and social issues in developing population genetic databases. *Genet Med.* 2003;5:451–457.

Axt-Fliedner R, Schwarze A, Smrcek J, Germer U, Krapp M, Gembruch U. Isolated ventricular septal defects detected by color Doppler imaging: evolution during fetal and first year of postnatal life. *Ultrasound Obstet Gynecol.* 2006;27:266–273.

Becerra JE, Khoury MJ, Cordero JF, Erickson JD. Diabetes mellitus during pregnancy and the risks for specific birth defects: a population-based case-control study. *Pediatrics.* 1990;85:1–9.

Benson DW, Silberbach GM, Kavanaugh-McHugh A, et al. Mutations in the cardiac transcription factor NKX2.5 affect diverse cardiac developmental pathways. *J Clin Invest.* 1999;104:1567–1573.

Bernert JT Jr, Turner WE, Pirkle JL, et al. Development and validation of sensitive method for determination of serum cotinine in smokers and nonsmokers by liquid chromatography/atmospheric pressure ionization tandem mass spectrometry. *Clin Chem.* 1997;43:2281–2291.

Berry RJ, Li Z, Erickson JD, et al. Prevention of neural-tube defects with folic acid in China. China-U.S. Collaborative Project for Neural Tube Defect Prevention. *N Engl J Med.* 1999;341:1485–1490.

Blumberg SJ, Luke JV, Cynamon ML. Telephone coverage and health survey estimates: evaluating the need for concern about wireless substitution. *Am J Public Health.* 2006;96:926–931.

Boneva RS, Botto LD, Moore CA, Yang Q, Correa A, Erickso. Mortality associated with congenital heart defects in the United States: trends and racial disparities, 1979–1997. *Circulation.* 2001;103:2376–2381.

Boneva RS, Moore CA, Botto L, Wong LY, Erickson JD. Nausea during pregnancy and congenital heart defects: a population-based case-control study. *Am J Epidemiol.* 1999;149:717–725.

Bookman EB, Langehorne AA, Eckfeldt JH, et al. Reporting genetic results in research studies: summary and recommendations of an NHLBI working group. *Am J Med Genet A.* 2006;140:1033–1040.

Bosi G, Garani G, Scorrano M, Calzolari E. Temporal variability in birth prevalence of congenital heart defects as recorded by a general birth defects registry. *J Pediatr.* 2003;142:690–698.

Bossert T, Walther T, Gummert J, Hubald R, Kostelka M, Mohr FW. Cardiac malformations associated with the Holt-Oram syndrome—report on a family and review of the literature. *Thorac Cardiovasc Surg.* 2002;50:312–314.

Botto LD, Correa A, Erickson JD. Racial and temporal variations in the prevalence of heart defects. *Pediatrics.* 2001a;107:E32.

Botto LD, Lin AE, Riehle-Colarusso T, Malik S, Correa A. Seeking causes: classifying and evaluating congenital heart defects in etiologic studies. *Birth Defects Res A Clin Mol Teratol.* 2007;79:714–727.

Botto LD, Loffredo C, Scanlon KS, et al. Vitamin A and cardiac outflow tract defects. *Epidemiology.* 2001b;12:491–496.

Botto LD, Lynberg MC, Erickson JD. Congenital heart defects, maternal febrile illness, and multivitamin use: a population-based study. *Epidemiology.* 2001c;12:485–490.

Botto LD, May K, Fernhoff PM, et al. A population-based study of the 22q11.2 deletion: phenotype, incidence, and contribution to major birth defects in the population. *Pediatrics.* 2003;112:101–107.

Botto LD, Mulinare J, Erickson JD. Occurrence of congenital heart defects in relation to maternal multivitamin use. *Am J Epidemiol.* 2000;151:878–884.

Botto LD, Robert-Gnansia E, Siffel C, Harris J, Borman B, Mastroiacovo P. Fostering international collaboration in birth defects research and prevention: a perspective from the International Clearinghouse for Birth Defects Surveillance and Research. *Am J Public Health.* 2006;96:774–780.

Brackley KJ, Kilby MD, Wright JG, et al. Outcome after prenatal diagnosis of hypoplastic left-heart syndrome: a case series. *Lancet.* 2000;356:1143–1147.

Brealey SD, Atwell C, Bryan S, et al. Improving response rates using a monetary incentive for patient completion of questionnaires: an observational study. *BMC Med Res Methodol.* 2007;7:12.

Bryant HE, Visser N, Love EJ. Records, recall loss, and recall bias in pregnancy: a comparison of interview and medical records data of pregnant and postnatal women. *Am J Public Health.* 1989;79:78–80.

Burke W, Diekema DS. Ethical issues arising from the participation of children in genetic research. *J Pediatr.* 2006;149:S34–38.

Caan B, Hiatt RA, Owen AM. Mailed dietary surveys: response rates, error rates, and the effect of omitted food items on nutrient values. *Epidemiology.* 1991;2:430–436.

Caton AR, Bell EM, Druschel CD, et al. Antihypertensive medication use during pregnancy and the risk of cardiovascular malformations. *Hypertension.* 2009; published online ahead of print.

Clark EB. Pathogenetic mechanisms of congenital cardiovascular malformations revisited. *Semin Perinatol.* 1996;20:465–472.

Collins FS, Morgan M, Patrinos A. The Human Genome Project: lessons from large-scale biology. *Science.* 2003;300:286–290.

Coogan PF, Rosenberg L. Impact of a financial incentive on case and control participation in a telephone interview. *Am J Epidemiol.* 2004;160:295–298.

Correa-Villasenor A, McCarter R, Downing J, Ferencz C. White-black differences in cardiovascular malformations in infancy and socioeconomic factors. The Baltimore-Washington Infant Study Group. *Am J Epidemiol.* 1991;134:393–402.

Crider KS, Reefhuis J, Woomert A, Honein MA. Racial and ethnic disparity in participation in DNA collection at the Atlanta site of the National Birth Defects Prevention Study. *Am J Epidemiol.* 2006;164:805–812.

Cronk CE, Malloy ME, Pelech AN, et al. Completeness of state administrative databases for surveillance of congenital heart disease. *Birth Defects Res A Clin Mol Teratol.* 2003;67:597–603.

Czeizel AE, Dudas I. Prevention of the first occurrence of neural-tube defects by periconceptional vitamin supplementation. *N Engl J Med.* 1992;327:1832–1835.

Czeizel AE, Rockenbau. A population-based case-control teratologic study of oral oxytetracycline treatment during pregnancy. *Eur J Obstet Gynecol Reprod Biol.* 2000;88:27–33.

Czeizel AE, Puho E, Sorensen HT, Olsen J. Possible association between different congenital abnormalities and use of different sulfonamides during pregnancy. *Congenit Anom (Kyoto).* 2004;44:79–86.

Czeizel AE, Rockenbauer M, Siffel C, Varga E. Description and mission evaluation of the Hungarian case-control surveillance of congenital abnormalities, 1980–1996. *Teratology.* 2001a;63:176–185.

Czeizel AE, Rockenbauer M, Sorensen HT, Olsen J. Augmentin treatment during pregnancy and the prevalence of congenital abnormalities: a population-based case-control teratologic study. *Eur J Obstet Gynecol Reprod Biol.* 2001b;97:188–192.

Danford DA, Martin AB, Fletcher SE, Gumbiner CH. Echocardiographic yield in children when innocent murmur seems likely but doubts linger. *Pediatr Cardiol.* 2002;23:410–414.

Danford DA, Martin AB, Fletcher SE, et al. Children with heart murmurs: can ventricular septal defect be diagnosed reliably without an echocardiogram? *J Am Coll Cardiol.* 1997;30:243–246.

Danford DA, Salaymeh KJ, Martin AB, Fletcher SE, Gumbiner CH. Pulmonary stenosis: defect-specific diagnostic accuracy of heart murmurs in children. *J Pediatr.* 1999;134:76–81.

Dlugos DJ, Scattergood TM, Ferraro TN, Berrettinni WH, Buono RJ. Recruitment rates and fear of phlebotomy in pediatric patients in a genetic study of epilepsy. *Epilepsy Behav.* 2005;6:444–446.

Dudbridge F, Gusnanto A, Koeleman BP. Detecting multiple associations in genome-wide studies. *Hum Genomics.* 2006;2:310–317.

Duncan P, Reker D, Kwon S, et al. Measuring stroke impact with the stroke impact scale: telephone versus mail administration in veterans with stroke. *Med Care.* 2005;43:507–515.

Edwards P, Roberts I, Clarke M, et al. Increasing response rates to postal questionnaires: systematic review. *BMJ.* 2002;324:1183.

Erickson JD, Mulinare J, James LM, Fitch TG. Design and execution of a very large birth-defects case-control study. *Prog Clin Biol Res.* 1985;163B:273–277.

Erickson JD, Mulinare J, McClain PW, et al. Vietnam veterans' risks for fathering babies with birth defects. *JAMA.* 1984;252:903–912.

Evangelou E, Maraganore DM, Ioannidis JP. Meta-analysis in genome-wide association datasets: strategies and application in Parkinson disease. *PLoS One.* 2007;2:e196.

Ewing CK, Loffredo CA, Beaty TH. Paternal risk factors for isolated membranous ventricular septal defects. *Am J Med Genet.* 1997;71:42–46.

Feldkamp M, Macleod L, Young L, Lecheminant K, Carey JC. The methodology of the Utah Birth Defect Network: congenital heart defects as an illustration. *Birth Defects Res A Clin Mol Teratol.* 2005;73:693–699.

Ferencz C, Loffredo CA, Correa-Villasenor A, Wilson PD. Genetics and environmental risk factors of major cardiovascular malformations: the Baltimore-Washington Infant Study: 1981–1989. Armonk, NY :Futura Publishing Co. Inc; 1997.

Ferencz C, Rubin JD, Loffredo CA, Magee CM. The Epidemiology of Congenital Heart Disease, The Baltimore-Washington Infant Study (1981–1989). Mount Kisco, NY: Futura Publishing Co. Inc; 1993.

Festa P, Ait-Ali L, Cerillo AG, De Marchi D, Murzi B. Magnetic resonance imaging is the diagnostic tool of choice in the preoperative evaluation of patients with partial anomalous pulmonary venous return. *Int J Cardiovasc Imaging.* 2006;22:685–693.

Forrester MB, Merz RD. Prenatal diagnosis and elective termination of Down syndrome in a racially mixed population in Hawaii, 1987–1996. *Prenat Diagn.* 1999;19:136–141.

Freeman SB, Taft LF, Dooley KJ, et al. Population-based study of congenital heart defects in Down syndrome. *Am J Med Genet.* 1998;80:213–217.

Frohnert BK, Lussky RC, Alms MA, Mendelsohn NJ, Symonik DM, Falken MC. Validity of hospital discharge data for identifying infants with cardiac defects. *J Perinatol.* 2005;25:737–742.

Galesic M, Tourangeau R, Couper MP. Complementing random-digit-dial telephone surveys with other approaches to collecting sensitive data. *Am J Prev Med.* 2006;31:437–443.

Garcia-Closas M, Egan KM, Abruzzo J, et al. Collection of genomic DNA from adults in epidemiological studies by buccal cytobrush and mouthwash. *Cancer Epidemiol Biomarkers Prev.* 2001;10:687–696.

Garg V. Insights into the genetic basis of congenital heart disease. *Cell Mol Life Sci.* 2006;63:1141–1148.

Garne E. Atrial and ventricular septal defects—epidemiology and spontaneous closure. *J Matern Fetal Neonatal Med.* 2006;19:271–276.

Gelb BD. Genetic basis of congenital heart disease. *Curr Opin Cardiol.* 2004;19:110–115.

Green RF, Moore C. Incorporating genetic analyses into birth defects cluster investigations: strategies for identifying candidate genes. *Birth Defects Res A Clin Mol Teratol.* 2006;76:798–810.

Harris JA, Francannet C, Pradat P, Robert E. The epidemiology of cardiovascular defects, part 2: a study based on data from three large registries of congenital malformations. *Pediatr Cardiol.* 2003;24:222–235.

Hastreiter AR, Joorabchi B, Pujatti G, van der Horst RL, Patacsil G, Sever JL. Cardiovascular lesions associated with congenital rubella. *J Pediatr.* 1967;71:59–65.

Henderson LO, Powell MK, Hannon WH, et al. An evaluation of the use of dried blood spots from newborn screening for monitoring the prevalence of cocaine use among childbearing women. *Biochem Mol Med.* 1997;61:143–151.

Hermes-DeSantis ER, Clyman RI. Patent ductus arteriosus: pathophysiology and management. *J Perinatol.* 2006;26(suppl 1):S14–18; discussion S22–23.

Hernandez-Diaz S, Werler MM, Walker AM, Mitchell AA. Folic acid antagonists during pregnancy and the risk of birth defects. *N Engl J Med.* 2000;343:1608–1614.

Hobbs CA, Hopkins SE, Simmons CJ. Sources of variability in birth defects prevalence rates. *Teratology.* 2001;64(suppl 1):S8–13.

Hoffman JI. Congenital heart disease: incidence and inheritance. *Pediatr Clin North Am.* 1990;37:25–43.

Hoffman JI. Incidence of congenital heart disease: II. Prenatal incidence. *Pediatr Cardiol.* 1995;16:155–165.

Hoffman JI, Kaplan S. The incidence of congenital heart disease. *J Am Coll Cardiol.* 2002;39:1890–1900.

Honein MA, Paulozzi LJ. Birth defects surveillance: assessing the "gold standard". *Am J Public Health.* 1999;89:1238–1240.

Iovannisci DM, Ha TT, Shaw GM. Recovery of genomic DNA from residual frozen archival blood clots suitable for amplification and use in genotyping assays. *Genet Test.* 2006;10:44–49.

Jenkins KJ, Correa A, Feinstein JA, et al. Noninherited risk factors and congenital cardiovascular defects: current knowledge: a scientific statement from the American Heart Association Council on Cardiovascular Disease in the Young: endorsed by the American Academy of Pediatrics. *Circulation.* 2007;115:2995–3014.

Jenkins MM, Rasmussen SA, Moore CA, Honein MA. Ethical issues raised by incorporation of genetics into the National Birth Defects Prevention Study. *Am J Med Genet C Semin Med Genet.* 2008;148:40–46.

Kallen BA, Otterblad Olausson P. Maternal drug use in early pregnancy and infant cardiovascular defect. *Reprod Toxicol.* 2003;17:255–261.

Kempf AM, Remington PL. *New Challenges for Telephone Survey Research in the Twenty-First Century.* Annu Rev Public Health; 2006.

Kempf AM, Remington PL. New challenges for telephone survey research in the twenty-first century. *Annu Rev Public Health.* 2007;28:113–126.

Kerstann KF, Feingold E, Freeman SB, et al. Linkage disequilibrium mapping in trisomic populations: analytical approaches and an application to congenital heart defects in Down syndrome. *Genet Epidemiol.* 2004;27:240–251.

Khoury MJ, Erickson JD. Can maternal risk factors influence the presence of major birth defects in infants with Down syndrome? *Am J Med Genet.* 1992;43:1016–1022.

Khoury MJ, Little J, Gwinn M, Ioannidis JP. On the synthesis and interpretation of consistent but weak gene-disease associations in the era of genome-wide association studies. *Int J Epidemiol.* 2006.

Klotz J, Bryant P, Wilcox HB, Dillon M, Wolf B, Fagliano J. Population-based retrieval of newborn dried blood spots for researching paediatric cancer susceptibility genes. *Paediatr Perinat Epidemiol.* 2006;20:449–452.

Koch J, Hensley G, Roy L, Brown S, Ramaciotti C, Rosenfeld CR. Prevalence of spontaneous closure of the ductus arteriosus in neonates at a birth weight of 1000 grams or less. *Pediatrics.* 2006;117:1113–1121.

Kraus L, Augustin R. Measuring alcohol consumption and alcohol-related problems: comparison of responses from self-administered questionnaires and telephone interviews. *Addiction.* 2001;96:459–471.

Kropf ME, Blair J. Eliciting survey cooperation: incentives, self-interest, and norms of cooperation. *Eval Rev.* 2005;29:559–575.

Kuehl KS, Loffredo CA, Ferencz C. Failure to diagnose congenital heart disease in infancy. *Pediatrics.* 1999;103:743–747.

Lammer EJ, Chen DT, Hoar RM, et al. Retinoic acid embryopathy. *N Engl J Med.* 1985;313:837–841.

Lema C, Kohl-White K, Lewis LR, Dao DD. Optimized pH method for DNA elution from buccal cells collected in Whatman FTA cards. *Genet Test.* 2006;10:126–130.

Lidral AC, Moreno LM. Progress toward discerning the genetics of cleft lip. *Curr Opin Pediatr.* 2005;17:731–739.

Lin AE, Herring AH, Amstutz KS, et al. Cardiovascular malformations: changes in prevalence and birth status, 1972–1990. *Am J Med Genet.* 1999;84:102–110.

Loffredo CA. Epidemiology of cardiovascular malformations: prevalence and risk factors. *Am J Med Genet.* 2000;97:319–325.

Loffredo CA, Hirata J, Wilson PD, Ferencz C, Lurie IW. Atrioventricular septal defects: possible etiologic differences between complete and partial defects. *Teratology.* 2001a;63:87–93.

Loffredo CA, Silbergeld EK, Ferencz C, Zhang J. Association of transposition of the great arteries in infants with maternal exposures to herbicides and rodenticides. *Am J Epidemiol.* 2001b;153:529–536.

Lum A, Le Marchand L. A simple mouthwash method for obtaining genomic DNA in molecular epidemiological studies. *Cancer Epidemiol Biomarkers Prev.* 1998;7:719–724.

Martin ML, Khoury MJ, Cordero JF, Waters GD. Trends in rates of multiple vascular disruption defects, Atlanta, 1968–1989: is there evidence of a cocaine teratogenic epidemic? *Teratology.* 1992;45:647–653.

Matsui K, Kita Y, Ueshima H. Informed consent, participation in, and withdrawal from a population based cohort study involving genetic analysis. *J Med Ethics.* 2005;31:385–392.

Milne E, van Bockxmeer FM, Robertson L, et al. Buccal DNA collection: comparison of buccal swabs with FTA cards. *Cancer Epidemiol Biomarkers Prev.* 2006;15:816–819.

Mitchell AA, Cottler LB, Shapiro S. Effect of questionnaire design on recall of drug exposure in pregnancy. *Am J Epidemiol.* 1986;123:670–676.

Mitchell AA, Rosenberg L, Shapiro S, Slone D. Birth defects related to bendectin use in pregnancy. I. Oral clefts and cardiac defects. *JAMA.* 1981;245:2311–2314.

Montana E, Khoury MJ, Cragan JD, Sharma S, Dhar P, Fyfe D. Trends and outcomes after prenatal diagnosis of congenital cardiac malformations by fetal echocardiography in a well defined birth population, Atlanta, Georgia, 1990–1994. *J Am Coll Cardiol.* 1996;28:1805–1809.

Moonesinghe R, Khoury MJ, Janssens AC. Most published research findings are false-but a little replication goes a long way. *PLoS Med.* 2007;4:e28.

MRC Vitamin Study Research Group. Prevention of neural tube defects: results of the Medical Research Council Vitamin Study. *Lancet.* 1991;338:131–137.

Mulinare J, Cordero JF, Erickson JD, Berry RJ. Periconceptional use of multivitamins and the occurrence of neural tube defects. *JAMA.* 1988;260:3141–3145.

National Bioethics Advisory Commission. *Research Involving Human Biological Materials.* Vol. 1. Rockville, MD: National Bioethics Advisory Commission; 1999.

Ng DP, Koh D, Choo S, Chia KS. Saliva as a viable alternative source of human genomic DNA in genetic epidemiology. *Clin Chim Acta.* 2006;367:81–85.

Nielsen GL, Norgard B, Puho E, Rothman KJ, Sorensen HT, Czeizel AE. Risk of specific congenital abnormalities in offspring of women with diabetes. *Diabet Med.* 2005;22:693–696.

Olney RS, Moore CA, Ojodu JA, Lindegren ML, Hannon WH. Storage and use of residual dried blood spots from state newborn screening programs. *J Pediatr.* 2006;148:618–622.

Olshan AF, Perreault SD, Bradley L, et al. The healthy men study: design and recruitment considerations for environmental epidemiologic studies in male reproductive health. *Fertil Steril.* 2007;87:554–564.

Ozkaynak H, Whyatt RM, Needham LL, Akland G, Quackenboss J. Exposure assessment implications for the design and implementation of the National Children's Study. *Environ Health Perspect.* 2005;113:1108–1015.

Paganini-Hill A, Ross RK. Reliability of recall of drug usage and other health-related information. *Am J Epidemiol.* 1982;116:114–122.

Parkes J, Kerr C, McDowell BC, Cosgrove AP. Recruitment bias in a population-based study of children with cerebral palsy. *Pediatrics.* 2006;118:1616–1622.

Pe'er I, de Bakker PI, Maller J, Yelensky R, Altshuler D, Daly MJ. Evaluating and improving power in whole-genome association studies using fixed marker sets. *Nat Genet.* 2006;38:663–667.

Pradat P. Maternal occupation and congenital heart defects: a case-control study. *Int Arch Occup Environ Health.* 1993;65:13–18.

Rasmussen SA, Lammer EJ, Shaw GM, et al. Integration of DNA sample collection into a multi-site birth defects case-control study. *Teratology.* 2002;66:177–184.

Rasmussen SA, Moore CA. Effective coding in birth defects surveillance. *Teratology.* 2001;64 (suppl 1):S3–7.

Rasmussen SA, Olney RS, Holmes LB, Lin AE, Keppler-Noreuil KM, Moore CA. Guidelines for case classification for the National Birth Defects Prevention Study. *Birth Defects Res A Clin Mol Teratol.* 2003;67:193–201.

Rogers NL, Cole SA, Lan HC, Crossa A, Demerath EW. New saliva DNA collection method compared to buccal cell collection techniques for epidemiological studies. *Am J Hum Biol.* 2007;19:319–326.

Romitti PA, Burns TL, Murray JC. Maternal interview reports of family history of birth defects: evaluation from a population-based case-control study of orofacial clefts. *Am J Med Genet.* 1997;72:422–429.

Rosenbaum A, Rabenhorst MM, Reddy MK, Fleming MT, Howells NL. A comparison of methods for collecting self-report data on sensitive topics. *Violence Vict.* 2006;21:461–471.

Rosenthal GL, Wilson PD, Permutt T, Boughman JA, Ferencz C. Birth weight and cardiovascular malformations: a population-based study. The Baltimore-Washington Infant Study. *Am J Epidemiol.* 1991;133:1273–1281.

Schieve LA, Rasmussen SA, Reefhuis J. Risk of birth defects among children conceived with assisted reproductive technology: providing an epidemiologic context to the data. *Fertil Steril.* 2005;84:1320–1324; discussion 7.

Scott P, Edwards P. Personally addressed hand-signed letters increase questionnaire response: a meta-analysis of randomised controlled trials. *BMC Health Serv Res.* 2006;6:111.

Shalowitz DI, Miller FG. Disclosing individual results of clinical research: implications of respect for participants. *JAMA.* 2005;294:737–740.

Shaw GM, Iovannisci DM, Yang W, et al. Risks of human conotruncal heart defects associated with 32 single nucleotide polymorphisms of selected cardiovascular disease-related genes. *Am J Med Genet A.* 2005;138:21–26.

Siffel C, Correa A, Cragan J, Alverson CJ. Prenatal diagnosis, pregnancy terminations and prevalence of Down syndrome in Atlanta. *Birth Defects Res A Clin Mol Teratol.* 2004;70:565–571.

Singer E, Bossarte RM. Incentives for survey participation when are they "coercive"? *Am J Prev Med.* 2006;31:411–418.

Sivanandam S, Glickstein JS, Printz BF, et al. Prenatal diagnosis of conotruncal malformations: diagnostic accuracy, outcome, chromosomal abnormalities, and extracardiac anomalies. *Am J Perinatol.* 2006;23:241–245.

Steinberger EK, Ferencz C, Loffredo CA. Infants with single ventricle: a population-based epidemiological study. *Teratology.* 2002;65:106–115.

Stone MB, Lyon JL, Simonsen SE, White GL Jr, Alder SC. An internet-based method of selecting control populations for epidemiologic studies. *Am J Epidemiol.* 2007;165:109–112.

Talosi G, Katona M, Racz K, Kertesz E, Onozo B, Turi S. Prostaglandin E1 treatment in patent ductus arteriosus dependent congenital heart defects. *J Perinat Med.* 2004;32:368–374.

Thompson MD, Bowen RA, Wong BY, et al. Whole genome amplification of buccal cell DNA: genotyping concordance before and after multiple displacement amplification. *Clin Chem Lab Med.* 2005;43:157–162.

Tilley BC, Barnes AB, Bergstralh E, et al. A comparison of pregnancy history recall and medical records. Implications for retrospective studies. *Am J Epidemiol.* 1985;121:269–281.

Tomeo CA, Rich-Edwards JW, Michels KB, et al. Reproducibility and validity of maternal recall of pregnancy-related events. *Epidemiology.* 1999;10:774–747.

Trines J, Hornberger LK. Evolution of heart disease in utero. *Pediatr Cardiol.* 2004;25:287–298.

Tuckel P, O'Neill H. *The Vanishing Respondent in Telephone Surveys.* Proceedings of the Annual Meeting of the American Statistical Association; 2001.

Turner SW, Hornung T, Hunter S. Closure of ventricular septal defects: a study of factors influencing spontaneous and surgical closure. *Cardiol Young.* 2002;12:357–363.

Turner SW, Hunter S, Wyllie JP. The natural history of ventricular septal defects. *Arch Dis Child.* 1999;81:413–416.

Vidal-Taboada JM, Cucala M, Mas Herrero S, Lafuente A, Cobos A. Satisfaction survey with DNA cards method to collect genetic samples for pharmacogenetics studies. *BMC Med Genet.* 2006;7:45.

Watkins ML, Botto LD. Maternal prepregnancy weight and congenital heart defects in offspring. *Epidemiology.* 2001;12:439–446.

Watkins ML, Edmonds L, McClearn A, Mullins L, Mulinare J, Khoury M. The surveillance of birth defects: the usefulness of the revised US standard birth certificate. *Am J Public Health.* 1996;86:731–734.

Weinberg CR, Umbach DM. Choosing a retrospective design to assess joint genetic and environmental contributions to risk. *Am J Epidemiol.* 2000;152:197–203.

Werler MM, Hayes C, Louik C, Shapiro S, Mitchell AA. Multivitamin supplementation and risk of birth defects. *Am J Epidemiol.* 1999;150:675–682.

Werler MM, Lammer EJ, Rosenberg L, Mitchell AA. Maternal vitamin A supplementation in relation to selected birth defects. *Teratology.* 1990;42:497–503.

Werler MM, Lammer EJ, Rosenberg L, Mitchell AA. Maternal alcohol use in relation to selected birth defects. *Am J Epidemiol.* 1991;134:691–698.

Werler MM, Mitchell AA, Shapiro S. The relation of aspirin use during the first trimester of pregnancy to congenital cardiac defects. *N Engl J Med.* 1989;321:1639–42.

Whiteman MK, Langenberg P, Kjerulff K, McCarter R, Flaws JA. A randomized trial of incentives to improve response rates to a mailed women's health questionnaire. *J Womens Health (Larchmt).* 2003;12:821–828.

Yang Q, Khoury MJ, Flanders WD. Sample size requirements in case-only designs to detect gene-environment interaction. *Am J Epidemiol.* 1997;146:713–720.

Yang Q, Khoury MJ, Sun F, Flanders WD. Case-only design to measure gene-gene interaction. *Epidemiology.* 1999;10:167–170.

Yawn BP, Suman VJ, Jacobsen SJ. Maternal recall of distant pregnancy events. *J Clin Epidemiol.* 1998;51:399–405.

Yoon PW, Rasmussen SA, Lynberg MC, et al. The National Birth Defects Prevention Study. *Public Health Rep.* 2001;116 (suppl 1):32–40.

25

Congenital Heart Defects Associated with Genetic Syndromes

MARIA CRISTINA DIGILIO

ANNA SARKOZY

BRUNO DALLAPICCOLA

BRUNO MARINO

Epidemiological studies, clinical observations, and recent advances in molecular genetics all contribute to the comprehension of the etiology of an increasing number of congenital heart defects (CHDs). In general, one third of all CHDs is associated with extracardiac anomalies, in the setting of chromosomal anomalies, and Mendelian syndromes or associations (Ferencz et al., 1997). Some types of CHDs are more frequently diagnosed in association with genetic syndromes, such as atrioventricular canal defect (AVCD) and interrupted aortic arch (IAA), whereas other types are prevalently isolated defects.

In the following review of cardiac defects and syndromes, CHDs are listed according to the pathogenetic classification by Clark (1986). This classification, grouping CHDs according to possible morphogenetic pathways instead of anatomical or clinical criteria, is particularly appropriate for the identification of a link among causes, mechanisms, and defects, creating a connection between genetic defects and cardiac malformations (Table 25–1).

CONOTRUNCAL DEFECTS

Conotruncal defects represent an anatomically heterogeneous group of CHDs affecting the outflow tract of the ventricles and the arterial pole of the heart.

Classic Tetralogy of Fallot and Pulmonary Atresia with Ventricular Septal Defect

Extracardiac malformations in the setting of chromosomal or Mendelian syndromes are found in 25%–35% of the patients with classic tetralogy of Fallot (TOF) and with pulmonary atresia with ventricular septal defect (PA-VSD) (Digilio et al., 1996; Ferencz et al., 1993, 1997; Marino et al., 1996a). Chromosomal anomalies are involved in 12% of the total cases, Mendelian syndromes or non-Mendelian associations in 7%, and nonclassified multiple anomalies defects in 13% (Ferencz et al., 1993). The association of classic TOF with chromosomal anomalies is well known (Marino, 1996b; Musewe et al., 1990). The most frequently diagnosed chromosomal syndromes are trisomy 13 (Patau syndrome), trisomy 18 (Edwards syndrome), and trisomy 21 (Down syndrome) (MIM 190685).

Trisomy 13 is a malformation syndrome characterized by orofacial clefts, microphthalmia/anophthalmia, cutis aplasia of the occipital region, postaxial polydactyly of hands and feet, and significant mental retardation, with a predisposition to increased neonatal and infant death (Carey, 2005).

Trisomy 18 is characterized by prenatal growth deficiency, facial anomalies, distinctive hand posture of overriding fingers, visceral anomalies, and mental retardation (Baty et al., 1994; Carey, 2005). About

TABLE 25–1. *Listing of Congenital Heart Defects According to the Pathogenetic Classification by Clark (1986) and Associated Genetic Syndromes*

Congenital Heart Defect	Syndrome	Genetic Defect	Anatomical Subtype
Conotruncal Defects			
Classic tetralogy of Fallot	Patau	Trisomy 13	
	Edwards	Trisomy 18	
	Down	Trisomy 21	Large ventricular septal defect
			With atrioventricular canal defect
	DiGeorge/velocardiofacial	22q11.2 microdeletion	With right aortic arch
			With cervical aortic arch
			Hypoplasia or absence of infundibular septum
			Absence of pulmonary valve
			Discontinuity/hypoplasia of pulmonary arteries
	Alagille	*JAG1* mutations	
		NOTCH2 mutations	
	CHARGE	*CHD7* mutations	
		SEMA3E mutations	
	VACTERL	Unknown	
	Oculoauriculovertebral spectrum	Unknown	
Pulmonary atresia with ventricular septal defect	DiGeorge/velocardiofacial	22q11.2 microdeletion	Major aortopulmonary collateral arteries
Truncus arteriosus	DiGeorge/velocardiofacial	22q11.2 microdeletion	Type A3
			Discontinuity of the pulmonary arteries
			With aortic arch anomalies
			Severe dysplasia of the truncal valve
	Duplication 8q	Duplication 8q22qter	
	CHARGE	*CHD7* mutations	
		SEMA3E mutations	
Interrupted aortic arch	DiGeorge/velocardiofacial	22q11.2 microdeletion	Type B
			With aberrant right subclavian artery
			Hypoplasia or absence of infundibular septum
Atrioventricular Canal Defects			
	Down syndrome	Trisomy 21	Complete atrioventricular canal defect
	Deletion 8p	Deletion 8p23	Complete atrioventricular canal defect
			With pulmonary valve stenosis
	Deletion 3p	Deletion 3p25	
	Noonan/LEOPARD	*PTPN11* mutations	Partial atrioventricular canal defect
			With mitral valve anomalies causing subaortic obstruction
	Ellis-van Creveld	*EVC1, EVC2* mutations	Partial atrioventricular canal defect
			With common atrium
			With persistent left superior vena cava
	Oral-facial-digital	*Ofd1* mutations	Partial atrioventricular canal defect
		Other unknown genes	With common atrium
	Bardet-Biedl	*BBS1-BBS12* mutations	Partial atrioventricular canal defect
	Smith-Lemli-Opitz	*DHCR7* mutations	Partial atrioventricular canal defect
			With anomalous pulmonary venous return
Right-Sided Obstructive Lesions			
Pulmonary valve stenosis	Noonan syndrome	*PTPN11* mutations	With dysplastic valvular leaflets
			With supravalvular pulmonary stenosis
			With atrial septal defect
		SOS1 mutations	With dysplastic valvular leaflets
			With supravalvular pulmonary stenosis
			With atrial septal defect
		KRAS mutations	With hypertrophic cardiomyopathy
		RAF1 mutations	With hypertrophic cardiomyopathy
	LEOPARD	*PTPN11* mutations	With hypertrophic cardiomyopathy
		RAF1 mutations	With hypertrophic cardiomyopathy
	Cardiofaciocutaneous	*BRAF, KRAS, MEK1, MEK2* mutations	With dysplastic valvular leaflets
			With hypertrophic cardiomyopathy
			With atrial septal defect

(Continued)

TABLE 25–1. *Continued*

Congenital Heart Defect	Syndrome	Genetic Defect	Anatomical Subtype
	Costello	*HRAS* mutations	With hypertrophic cardiomyopathy
			With atrial arrhythmias
	Wolf-Hirschhorn	Deletion 4p	With/without atrial septal defect
Pulmonary artery stenosis	Weill-Marchesani	*ADAMTS10* mutations	
	Robinow	*ROR2* mutations	
	Alagille	*JAG1* mutations	
		NOTCH2 mutations	
	Williams	Microdeletion 7q11.23	With supravalvular aortic stenosis
Left-Sided Obstructive Lesions			
Supravalvular aortic stenosis	Williams	Microdeletion 7q11.23	With pulmonary artery stenosis
Aortic coarctation	Turner	Monosomy X	
		Deletion X	
		Ring X	
	Kabuki	Unknown	
Hypoplastic left ventricle	Jacobsen syndrome	Deletion 11q	
	Turner	Monosomy X	
Ventricular Septal Defects			
Perimembranous	Down	Trisomy 21	
	Edwards	Trisomy 18	
	Cri-du-chat	Deletion 5	
Muscular	Holt-Oram	*Tbx5* mutations	With atrioventricular block
			With atrial septal defect
Posterior	Down	Trisomy 21	With cleft of mitral valve
Subarterial	DiGeorge/Velocardiofacial	22q11.2 microdeletion	With right or cervical aortic arch
			With aberrant subclavian artery
	Edwards	Trisomy 18	
Targeted Growth Anomalies			
Anomalous pulmonary venous return	Cat-eye	Inv dup(22)(q11)	
	Turner	Monosomy X	
	Smith-Lemli-Opitz	*DHCR7* mutations	With partial atrioventricular canal defect
	Oculoauriculovertebral spectrum	Unknown	With hypoplastic right pulmonary artery (Scimitar syndrome)

90% of patients with trisomy 18 die before the second year of life.

CHDs are present in about 80% of patients with trisomy 13 and 90% of children with trisomy 18. Anatomical types include classic TOF, VSD with polyvalvular dysplasia, atrial septal defect (ASD), and double-outlet right ventricle (Musewe et al., 1990; Van Praagh et al., 1989).

Trisomy 21 (Down syndrome) is the most common identifiable cause of mental retardation, with a prevalence of 1:700 live births. The clinical diagnosis is based on the characteristic facial appearance with upslanted palpebral fissures, epicanthal folds, low nasal bridge with short nose, downturned mouth with protruding tongue, small ears, redundant skin on the neck, short hands with a high frequency of single palmar crease, neonatal hypotonia, gastrointestinal malformations, prevalently duodenal stenosis and Hirschsprung disease, and cardiovascular malformations (Hunter, 2005). AVCD is the commonest CHD in Down

syndrome, while TOF is the only conotruncal anomaly described, occurring in 8% of the cases (Marino et al., 1990a, 1993, 1996b). As a distinctive anatomical characteristic, the VSD in patients with TOF and Down syndrome is particularly large. Additionally, the only cardiac anomaly associated with TOF in trisomy 21 is the complete AVCD type C, sometimes with hypoplastic right ventricle (Marino et al., 1993; Vergara et al., 2006). Interestingly, cardiac defects sometimes associated with TOF in nonsyndromic patients or in those with different syndromes, like pulmonary atresia, absent pulmonary valve, discontinuity of pulmonary arteries, and absent infundibular septum, are very rare in Down syndrome (Marino, 1993, 1996b).

Advances in molecular/cytogenetic techniques led to the identification of chromosomal syndromes due to submicroscopic anomalies, such as the **22q11.2 deletion syndrome** causing the DiGeorge/velocardiofacial syndrome (MIM 192430). The 22q11.2 deletion syndrome is one of the most common genetic disorders in humans,

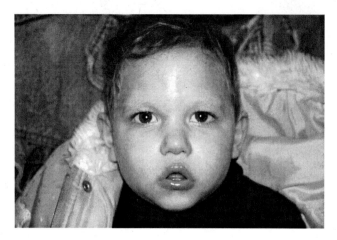

FIGURE 25-1. Facial appearance of a male patient with 22q11.2 microdeletion (DiGeorge/Velo-Cardio-Facial syndrome) at 1 year of age.

with an estimated prevalence of approximately 1:4000 live births (Devriendt et al., 1998). Clinical characteristics include CHD, palatal anomalies, facial dysmorphisms, neonatal hypocalcemia, immune deficit, and speech and learning disabilities (McDonald-McGinn et al., 1999; Ryan et al., 1997). Characteristic facial features include periorbital fulness, upslanting palpebral fissures, prominent nose, carp-shaped mouth, and small dysmorphic ears (Figure 25-1). There is wide variability in the clinical expression of the syndrome, and the spectrum of associated anomalies is becoming wider (Digilio et al., 2003a; Shprintzen, 2005). CHD is present in 75% of patients with 22q11.2 deletion syndrome (McDonald-McGinn et al., 1999; Ryan et al., 1997). The most frequent cardiac malformations are conotruncal defects, with classic TOF accounting for about 25% of CHDs in 22q11.2 deletion syndrome, and TOF with PA-VSD for an additional 25% (Marino et al., 2001). On the contrary, 22q11.2 deletion syndrome is diagnosed in about 10% of patients with classic TOF (Marino et al., 1996c; Goldmuntz et al., 1998) and in about 35% of patients with PA-VSD (Digilio et al., 1996).

Patients with TOF and 22q11.2 deletion syndrome often have additional CHDs as a distinctive recognizable pattern. In fact, additional cardiac defects are found in the half of the patients with classic TOF and 22q11.2 deletion syndrome (Marino et al., 2001). The associated defects include (1) right or cervical aortic arch with or without aberrant left subclavian artery; (2) hypoplasia or absence of the infundibular septum; (3) absence of the pulmonary valve; and (4) discontinuity and diffuse hypoplasia of the pulmonary arteries (Johnson et al., 1995; Maeda et al., 2000; Marino et al., 1996a; Momma et al., 1995).

In regard to PA-VSD, major aortopulmonary collateral arteries, sometimes with discontinuity of the pulmonary arteries, are commonly present in patients with

22q11.2 deletion syndrome (Anaclerio et al., 2001; Chessa et al., 1998; Digilio et al., 1996; Hofbeck et al., 1998; Momma et al., 1996a). On the contrary, major intracardiac anomalies and ductus-dependent pulmonary circulation are prevalent in patients with PA-VSD without 22q11.2 deletion (Anaclerio et al., 2001).

The typical 3-megabase deletion found in patients with 22q11.2 deletion syndrome contains just over 30 genes. It is still unknown whether all clinical features are caused by different genes or whether the majority of phenotypical signs are caused by a single gene in the chromosomal region. TBX1 gene is mapping in the 22q11.2 "critical region," and experimental animal studies have demonstrated that TBX1 is likely to be responsible for many heart and vascular anomalies in 22q11.2 deletion syndrome (Lindsay et al., 2001; Yagi et al., 2003). Interestingly, TBX1 mutations have been rarely detected also in humans manifesting the DiGeorge/velocardiofacial syndrome phenotype (Torres-Juan et al., 2007; Yagi et al., 2003; Zweier et al., 2007).

Among monogenic syndromes, **Alagille syndrome** (MIM 118450) is known to be frequently associated with TOF. The syndrome is clinically characterized by paucity of the interlobular bile ducts, CHD, butterfly vertebrae, anterior chamber of the eye with posterior embryotoxon, and a characteristic facial phenotype (Emerick et al., 1999; Krantz et al., 1997). CHD has been reported in up to 90% of patients with Alagille syndrome, the most frequent finding being peripheral pulmonary stenosis. TOF is the most common complex cardiac malformation associated with pulmonary involvement in those patients (Krantz et al., 1997). It has been first recognized that mutations in the JAG1 gene, a ligand in the Notch signaling pathway, are responsible for Alagille syndrome in more than 90% of the cases (Li et al., 1997b; Oda et al., 1997). The study of the expression pattern of JAG1 in the murine and human embryonic heart and vascular system demonstrated a correlation with the anatomical types of CHDs observed in Alagille syndrome (Loomes et al., 1999). Recently, mutations in the gene for the Notch2 receptor (NOTCH2) have been identified in two families segregating Alagille syndrome (McDaniell et al., 2006).

Additional conditions known to be associated with TOF include **CHARGE syndrome** (C: Coloboma of the eye, H: Heart defect, A: Atresia choanae, R: Retarded growth and development, G: genital hypoplasia, E: Ear anomalies) (MIM 214800) (Pagon et al., 1981; Wyse et al., 1993), related to mutations in the CHD7 and SEMA3E genes (Lalani et al., 2004; Vissers et al., 2004); **VACTERL association** (V: Vertebral defects, A: Anal atresia, C: Cardiac defect, TE: Tracheoesophageal fistula/esophageal atresia, R: Renal anomalies, L: Limb malformations) (Botto et al., 1997) (MIM 192350); and the **oculoauriculo-vertebral spectrum** (MIM 164210), characterized by microtia, hemifacial microsomia with mandibular hypoplasia, ocular epibulbar dermoid, and cervical vertebral malformations (Kumar et al., 1993).

Nonsyndromic TOF is genetically heterogeneous, the number of identified genes is low, and molecular analysis of large series of patients has shown that each single gene defect is detectable in a few cases. Up to now, *NKX2.5* gene mutations have been detected in 4% of nonsyndromic TOF (Goldmuntz et al., 2001), *FOG2* gene mutations in an additional 4% (Pizzuti et al., 2003), and *CFC1* gene mutations in singular patients (Goldmuntz et al., 2002).

Patients with TOF and an associated genetic syndrome represent a challenge to the cardiac surgeon, due to the possible need of extracardiac surgery for associated malformations, to the presence of immunodeficiency or altered compliance of the pulmonary vasculature. The study of the outcome of surgical correction of classic TOF in syndromic and nonsyndromic patients, including several different syndromic conditions, shows that genetic syndromes different from 22q11.2 deletion and Down syndromes have an important negative impact on the surgical outcome of CHD (Michielon et al., 2006). Particularly, risk factors for mortality in this group of patients included pulmonary artery hypoplasia and surgical repair of extracardiac anomalies, possibly leading to secondary changes in pulmonary compliance and pulmonary mechanics, and to an increased incidence of gram-negative infections (Michielon et al., 2006).

Truncus Arteriosus

Truncus arteriosus (TA) is a rare cardiac defect associated with genetic syndromes in about 40% of the cases (Ferencz et al., 1997). The **22q11.2 deletion syndrome (DiGeorge/Velocardiofacial syndrome)** is detectable in 30% of patients with TA (Goldmuntz et al., 1998; Marino et al., 1998, 2001; Momma et al., 1997). The role of neural crest abnormalities in the pathogenesis of TA due to deletion 22 is well established (Nishibatake et al., 1987; Kirby and Waldo, 1990). Considering the specific subtypes of TA, the type A1 and A2 of Van Praagh (Van Praagh and Van Praagh, 1965) are the most frequent types in general and are also common in patients with 22q11.2 deletion syndrome. Nevertheless, a specific association of 22q11.2 deletion syndrome with the rare type A3 TA with discontinuity of the pulmonary arteries and aortic arch anomalies (interruption type B, right-sided or double aortic arch) has been documented (Marino et al., 1998, 2001; Momma et al., 1997). Severe dysplasia with stenosis of the truncal valve should also be present (Marino et al., 1998).

Additional genetic conditions associated with TA are **duplication 8q22-qter syndrome** (and other chromosomal defects involving 8q, such as mosaic trisomy 8 and recombinant [8] syndrome) (Gelb et al., 1991; Digilio et al., 2003b; Sujansky et al., 1993) and **CHARGE syndrome** (Koletzko and Majewski, 1984; Lin et al., 1987; Tellier et al., 1998).

Genetic basis of nonsyndromic TA is at present unknown, but a mutation of NKX2.6 gene has been pathogenetically related to TA type A1 in a large pedigree with six affected individuals (Heathcote et al., 2005).

Interrupted Aortic Arch

IAA is one of the CHDs most frequently associated with extracardiac anomalies (40%–50% of the cases) (Ferencz et al., 1997). The **22q11.2 deletion syndrome (DiGeorge/velocardiofacial syndrome)** is the more frequent genetic condition also associated with this type of CHD. Particularly, IAA type B, between left carotid and left subclavian arteries, is associated with 22q11.2 deletion in 40%–80% of the cases (Loffredo et al., 2000; Marino et al., 1999a). In addition, patients with IAA type B and 22q11.2 deletion have frequently additional cardiac defects, including aberrant right subclavian artery and subarterial VSD with hypoplasia of infundibular septum (Marino et al., 1999a). On the contrary, IAA type A (distal to the left subclavian artery) is rarely associated with 22q11.2 deletion syndrome and often presents with complex intracardiac anomalies (Marino et al., 1999a).

ATRIOVENTRICULAR CANAL DEFECTS

AVCD include a spectrum of anomalies of the atrioventricular valves and the atrial and ventricular septa. In the complete form there is a single common atrioventricular valve, an ASD (ostium primum), and a confluent posterior ventricular septal defect in the inlet portion of the ventricular septum. In the partial form, there are two separate right and left atrioventricular valves with a "cleft" of the mitral valve, an ASD (ostium primum), and no ventricular septum communication. From the pathogenetic point of view, this malformation is classified in the group of defects of the extracellular matrix (Clark et al., 1986).

The AVCD is associated with extracardiac malformations in about 75% of the cases (Digilio et al., 1999a ; Ferencz et al., 1997). Four groups can be distinguished, including patients with Down syndrome (45%), heterotaxia (15%), other syndromes (15%), and nonsyndromic AVCD (25%).

The genetic syndrome more frequently associated with AVCD is **Down syndrome**, due to trisomy 21.

Clinical manifestations of the syndrome include facial anomalies, mental retardation, CHD, and gastrointestinal malformations (Hunter, 2005). The prevalence of CHD is 40%–50%, and AVCD and VSDs are the most common ones. The anatomical patterns and the associated cardiac malformations are specific in Down syndrome, since the complete form of AVCD is prevalent, affecting about 75% of the cases, and left-sided obstructive lesions are rare, in contrast to that occurring in patients with AVCD without Down syndrome (Carmi et al., 1992; De Biase et al., 1986; Digilio et al., 1999a; Marino et al., 1989, 1990a, 1996b). Interestingly, some types of CHD such as l-loop of the ventricles, atresia of the atrioventricular valves, and transposition of the great arteries are virtually absent in patients with Down syndrome (Marino, 1996b), suggesting that the overexpression of genes located on chromosome 21 may represent a "protective factor" in regard to these malformations. Molecular studies have identified a critical region for CHD on chromosome 21. Inside this region are located several genes that could be pathogenetically related with AVCD, including *DSCAM* (Korenberg et al., 2000), the collagen type VI gene (Jongewaard et al., 2002), and *DSCR1* (Arron et al., 2006).

It is interesting to outline the impact of specific genetic syndromes and related cardiac characteristics on the surgical outcome of CHD. In patients with Down syndrome, the presence of peculiar cardiac anatomical features has a positive impact on medical and surgical management. In fact, the comparison of surgical results among patients affected by AVCD with and without Down syndrome showed lower mortality and morbidity in children with trisomy 21 (Formigari et al., 2004).

The AVCD is complete also in the additional chromosomal anomalies, the most frequent being **deletion 8p23 syndrome**, clinically characterized by CHD, microcephaly, mental retardation, hypospadia, and facial anomalies (Digilio et al., 1998a). In this syndrome, the AVCD is often associated with pulmonary valve stenosis (PVS). The short arm of chromosome 8 also contains a critical region for CHD, and a candidate gene is the *GATA4* gene (Devriendt et al., 1999; Giglio et al., 2000). Additionally, **deletion 3p25-pter syndrome** is also associated with AVCD (Green et al., 2000). Interestingly, a gene causing nonsyndromic AVCD, *CRELD1*, is mapping on the short arm of chromosome 3 (Rupp et al., 2002), and is found to be mutated in about 6% of the cases in a studied series (Robinson et al., 2003).

Several Mendelian syndromes are included among monogenic conditions presenting with AVCD. In patients with **Noonan** (MIM 163950) **or LEOPARD** (151100) **syndrome** the AVCD is usually partial and may be associated with mitral valve anomalies causing subaortic stenosis (Marino et al., 1999b). Mutations in *PTPN11* gene have been detected in these patients (Digilio et al., 2002; Sarkozy et al., 2003a, 2006). Additional clinical and molecular details about Noonan and LEOPARD syndromes are included in the section on PVS.

Also a group of syndromes with postaxial polydactyly are significantly associated with AVCD. For example, **Ellis-van Creveld syndrome** (MIM 225500) is characterized by partial AVCD with common atrium and persistent left superior vena cava with unroofed coronary sinus, postaxial polydactyly of hands and feet, skeletal dysplasia with short limbs, and ectodermal defects. The cardiac phenotype of this syndrome resembles that of CHD in heterotaxia syndrome with left isomerism (Digilio et al., 1999b). The Ellis-van Creveld syndrome is due to mutations in *EVC1* and *EVC2* genes (Ruiz-Perez et al., 2000, 2003).

Additional syndromes with postaxial polydactyly presenting with AVCD include the **oral-facial-digital syndromes** (MIM 252100), **the Bardet-Biedl** (MIM 209900) **and Kaufmann-McKusick** (MIM 236700) **syndromes, the Smith-Lemli-Opitz syndrome** (MIM 270400) (Digilio et al., 1999b, 2006a; Lin et al., 1997). It is interesting to note that the pathogenetic Sonic Hedgehog pathway may be involved in some of these anomalies (Digilio et al., 2003c). Additionally, recent experimental evidences have demonstrated that several Bardet-Biedl proteins (Ansley et al., 2003; Fan et al., 2004; Kim et al., 2004; Li et al., 2004) and the product of oral-facial-digital type 1 (*Ofd1*) gene in mice (Ferrante et al., 2006) have an important role in regulating ciliary function. The finding of AVCD as a partial manifestation of heterotaxia in patients with these syndromes is in agreement with the involvement of the causative genes in ciliary function, since dysfunction of the nodal cilium is known to be related with left–right axis defects in vertebrates (Supp et al., 1997; Okada et al., 1999).

RIGHT-SIDED OBSTRUCTIVE LESIONS

Pulmonary Valve Stenosis

PVS consists of a dome-shaped pulmonary valve formed by the fusion of pulmonary semilunar valve, with poststenotic dilatation of the main pulmonary artery. Associated genetic syndromes are found in about 9% of the patients (Ferencz et al., 1997). Noonan syndrome and Noonan-like phenotypes are the predominant associated conditions, being diagnosed in one third of syndromic patients.

Noonan syndrome (MIM 163950) is an autosomal dominant disorder characterized by short stature, pterygium colli, thoracic anomalies, CHD, and facial anomalies including hypertelorism with down-slanting fissures; palpebral ptosis; a deeply grooved philtrum with high, wide peaks to the vermillion border of the upper lip; and low-set, posteriorly rotated ears with a thickened helix (Figure 25-2) (Allanson, 1987, 2005). Mutations in *PTPN11*, a gene encoding the protein tyrosine phosphatase SHP-2 located at chromosome 12q22-qter, are detected in 40%–50% of patients with Noonan syndrome (Musante et al., 2003; Sarkozy et al., 2003a; Tartaglia et al., 2001, 2002). *PTPN11* was considered a candidate gene for Noonan syndrome because of its chromosome location (van der Burgt et al., 1994) and because its protein product, SHP-2, is a component of several signal transduction pathways that control protean developmental processes, particularly cardiac semilunar valvulogenesis (Chen et al., 2000).

PVS in Noonan syndrome is frequently characterized by dysplastic pulmonary valve with fibrous thickening of the annulus and of the leaflets (Burch et al. 1993; Marino et al., 1999b; Narayanswami et al., 1994; Van der Hauwaert et al., 1978). In some cases the stenosis is in effect "supravalvular" and is caused by a fusion of the cusps with the wall of the pulmonary artery. Histological examination shows a marked thickening of the spongiosa layer of the valve leaflets due to stellate and fusiform cells resembling embryonic connective tissue (Koretzki et al., 1969; Neill, 1987). The transcatheter valvuloplasty is frequently ineffective in patients with Noonan syndrome because of these peculiar anatomical characteristics, and surgical valvotomy is often required.

Severe dysplasia of the pulmonary leaflets is a distinct marker of Noonan syndrome, and nonsyndromic pulmonary stenosis without valvular thickening is not related to *PTPN11* mutations (Sarkozy et al., 2003b), suggesting that a different genetic background causes distinct pulmonary stenosis subtypes. Nevertheless, the spectrum of cardiac anomalies associated with Noonan syndrome is wide (Marino et al., 1999b), including also hypertrophic cardiomyopathy and AVCD, so that the pathogenesis of cardiac defects in Noonan syndrome may be related to anomalies of cardiac jelly and extracellular matrix (Clark, 1986; Neill, 1987; Marino and Digilio, 2000). In this regard, Krenz et al. (2005) modeled the effect of Noonan syndrome–related *PTPN11* mutations through expression in valve primordia using the chick explant culture system, documenting that mutations induce increased cell proliferation during endocardial cushion development because of increased signaling via the Ras-MAPK pathway.

Additional genes causing Noonan syndrome have been recently identified. These included *KRAS* gene (Carta et al., 2006; Schubert et al., 2006), *SOS1* gene

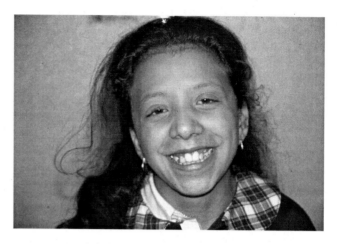

FIGURE 25-2. Facial appearance of a female patient with Noonan syndrome at 11 years of age.

(Roberts et al., 2007; Tartaglia et al., 2007; Zenker et al., 2007), and *RAF1* gene (Pandit et al., 2007; Razzaque et al., 2007).

KRAS gene mutations are related to a severe Noonan syndrome phenotype (Carta et al., 2006; Schubert et al., 2006). Clinical features of patients with *SOS1* gene mutations are distinctive, with a high prevalence of ectodermal anomalies, PVS, normal mental development, and linear growth (Tartaglia et al., 2007). On the contrary, *RAF1* mutations are associated with a classic Noonan syndrome phenotype with a high frequency of hypertrophic cardiomyopathy (Pandit et al., 2007; Razzaque et al., 2007).

Interestingly, hypertrophic cardiomyopathy is less common in patients with Noonan syndrome and *PTPN11* and *SOS1* gene mutations, while it is the predominant cardiac manifestation of **LEOPARD syndrome** patients with *PTPN11* and *RAF1* mutations (Digilio et al., 2002, 2006b, 2006c; Limongelli et al., 2007; Pandit et al., 2007; Sarkozy et al., 2003a, 2004). Noonan and LEOPARD syndromes are genetic conditions with overlapping features, related to different mutations in *PTPN11* gene (Digilio et al., 2002) and to mutations in *RAF1* gene (Pandit et al., 2007). Diagnostic clues of LEOPARD syndrome are cutaneous manifestations, including café-au-lait spots and multiple lentigines developing during childhood, and deafness (Figure 25–3) (Coppin and Temple, 1997; Digilio et al., 2006b). *PTPN11* mutations associated with Noonan syndrome cluster mainly in exons 3 and 8, while two recurrent mutations in exons 7 and 12 are specific for LEOPARD syndrome (Digilio et al., 2002, Sarkozy et al., 2004). Interestingly, *PTPN11* mutations causing LEOPARD syndrome appear to dysregulate Ras-Mapk pathway in a different manner from those of Noonan syndrome. In fact, LEOPARD syndrome–related mutations seem to have a negative effect on catalytic activity, implying a

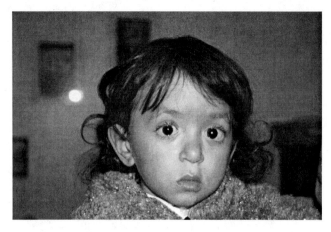

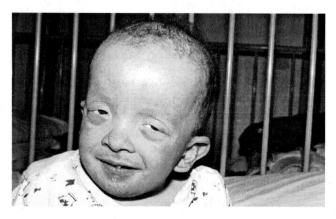

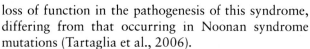

FIGURE 25–3. Facial appearance of a female patient with LEOPARD syndrome at 3 years of age.

FIGURE 25–4. Facial appearance of a male patient with cardio-facio-cutaneous (CFC) syndrome at 2 years of age.

loss of function in the pathogenesis of this syndrome, differing from that occurring in Noonan syndrome mutations (Tartaglia et al., 2006).

It has been demonstrated that clinical conditions considered as variants of Noonan syndrome, including **cardiofaciocutaneous (CFC)** (MIM 115150) **and Costello** (MIM 218040) **syndromes**, are caused by gain-of-function of several different genes, all belonging to the same Ras-Mapk pathway. Particularly, mutations in *BRAF, KRAS, MEK1,* and *MEK2* genes have been found in patients with CFC syndrome (Figure 25–4) (Gripp et al., 2007; Niihori et al., 2006; Rodriguez-Viciana et al., 2006; Schubbert et al., 2006), while mutations in *HRAS* gene have been detected in Costello syndrome (Figure 25–5) (Aoki et al., 2005; Digilio et al., 2007; Gripp et al., 2006).

CHDs in CFC and Costello syndrome include PVS with dysplastic leaflets and hypertrophic cardiomyopathy (Lin et al., 2002; Roberts et al., 2006). Atrial tachycardias or other arrhythmias are characteristic of Costello syndrome (Lin et al., 2002).

Patients with chromosomal **deletion 4p** (Wolf-Hirschhorn syndrome) have CHD in about 30% of the cases, frequently PVS with or without ASD (Battaglia et al., 1999).

The genetically heterogeneous **Weill-Marchesani syndrome** (MIM 608328, 277600) can be associated with PVS, particularly the autosomal recessive form due to mutations in the *ADAMTS10* gene (Faivre et al., 2003), and so is the autosomal recessive **Robinow syndrome** (MIM 268310) associated with mutations in the *ROR2* gene (Al-Ata et al., 1998).

Pulmonary Artery Stenosis

Anatomical stenosis of the pulmonary arteries is rare in patients without other types of CHD. A specific association with two syndromic conditions is known, including

Alagille syndrome (Krantz et al., 1997) and **Williams syndrome** (MIM 194050) (Brand et al., 1989; Giddings et al., 1989; Hallidie-Smith and Karas, 1988).

Williams syndrome is characterized by specific facial anomalies, developmental delay with a unique cognitive profile and typical personality, CHD, short stature, and connective tissue abnormality. Specific facial features include bitemporal narrowing, periorbital fullness, stellate iris pattern, strabismus, malar flattening, long philtrum, full lips, wide mouth, and small widely spaced teeth (Burn, 1986; Morris et al., 1988). Williams syndrome is caused by a submicroscopic deletion of chromosome 7q11.23, as evidenced by fluorescent in situ hybridization (FISH) (Ewart et al., 1993). The commonly deleted region spans approximately 1.5 megabases, and more than 20 genes have been mapped within this region (Perez-Jurado et al., 1996). Many of the clinical features of Williams syndrome are caused by the deletion of the elastin (*ELN*) gene (Ewart et al., 1993). In fact, the connective tissue anomalies, including

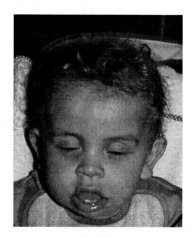

FIGURE 25–5. Facial appearance of a male patient with Costello syndrome at 20 months of age.

elastin arteriopathy, hoarse voice, facial anomalies, and hernias, are all the result of abnormal elastin protein production. In patients with Williams syndrome, peripheral pulmonary artery stenosis is usually associated with supravalvular aortic stenosis, representing the most severe cardiac defect in this syndrome.

LEFT-SIDED OBSTRUCTIVE LESIONS

Supravalvular Aortic Stenosis

Supravalvular aortic stenosis is also specific for **Williams syndrome**, alone or in association with pulmonary artery stenosis (Brand et al., 1989; Giddings et al., 1989; Hallidie-Smith and Karas, 1988). In fact, both CHDs are pathogenetically related to disruption of the *ELN* gene. Supravalvular aortic stenosis consists of a narrowing of the ascending aorta immediately above the valve, presenting as an "hourglass" constriction or as a diffuse narrowing extending to the ascending aorta (Brand et al., 1989; Giddings et al., 1989; Hallidie-Smith and Karas, 1988; Wessel et al., 1994). This arterial malformation can also be present in nonsyndromic patients, in absence of chromosomal 7q11.23 microdeletion, related to a point mutation of the *ELN* gene (Li et al., 1997a).

Aortic Coarctation

Aortic coarctation is associated with extracardiac anomalies in about 10% of the cases (Ferencz et al., 1997). This CHD is characteristically associated with **Turner syndrome** (Mazzanti and Cacciari, 1998), a genetic disorder, in which there is absence or a structural anomaly of one of the X chromosomes. Clinical features include short stature, gonadal dysgenesis, CHD, renal malformation, facial anomalies, and pterygium colli (Sybert et al., 2005). CHDs are present in half of the cases, aortic coarctation being the most frequent one. Nevertheless, the entire spectrum of left-sided obstructive lesions may also be found, including hypoplastic left heart syndrome, aortic stenosis, and bicuspid aortic valve (Gotzsche et al., 1993; Mazzanti and Cacciari, 1998; Sybert, 2005). Patients with "mosaic" chromosome anomaly often present with milder types of CHD, such as bicuspid aortic valve.

A subgroup of patients with **Noonan syndrome** can also have aortic coarctation (Digilio et al., 1998b; Hasegawa et al., 1996). It has been suggested that a Turner-Noonan phenotype could be a malformation sequence initiated by lymphatic hypoplasia and that the haploinsufficiency of a putative lymphogenic gene(s) located on Xp chromosome could cause aortic coarctation and the somatic anomalies in Turner and Noonan syndromes (Hasegawa et al., 1996).

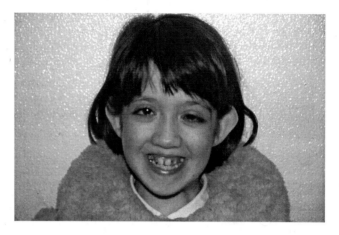

FIGURE 25–6. Facial appearance of a female patient with Kabuki syndrome at 5 years of age.

An additional syndrome frequently associated with aortic coarctation is **Kabuki syndrome** (MIM 147920) (Digilio et al., 2001). This syndrome is characterized by psychomotor delay and learning disability, CHD, renal malformations, skeletal anomalies, and typical facial appearance with long palpebral fissures, eversion of the lower lateral eyelid, depressed nasal tip, dental anomalies, and large everted ears (Figure 25–6) (Kawame et al., 1999; Matsumoto and Niikawa, 2003; Philip et al., 1992). The finding of sex chromosome anomalies in several reports of Kabuki syndrome, and the observation of male preponderance in patients with Kabuki syndrome and aortic coarctation, suggest the involvement of X-linked factors in determining the cardiac defect in some patients with Kabuki syndrome. (Digilio et al., 2001). Nevertheless, the genetic basis of Kabuki syndrome is at present still unknown.

Hypoplastic Left Heart

Hypoplastic left heart is included among left-sided obstructive cardiac lesions found in **Turner syndrome** (Sybert, 2005). Additionally, patients with terminal **deletion of chromosome 11q** (Jacobsen syndrome) may have hypoplastic left heart in 5%–10% of the cases, a frequency significantly higher in comparison to the general population (Grossfeld et al., 2004). A candidate gene (*JAM3*) expressed during cardiogenesis has been identified inside the "11q critical region" (Phillips et al., 2002).

VENTRICULAR SEPTAL DEFECTS

Perimembranous Ventricular Septal Defect

This is the most frequent type of VSD, and it is associated with extracardiac anomalies in about 20% of the cases (Ferencz et al., 1997). Chromosomal anomalies include

Down syndrome (Hunter, 2005), trisomy 18 (Baty et al., 1994), and deletion 5p (cri-du-chat syndrome) (Hills et al., 2006). Also several types of Mendelian syndromes are diagnosed. Moderate- and large-sized defects are more often syndromic in comparison to small defects (Lewis et al., 1996). Nevertheless, this type of defect is not specifically associated with a particular syndrome.

Muscular Ventricular Septal Defect

Muscular VSD is associated with extracardiac anomalies in about 10% of the cases (Ferencz et al., 1997). Several chromosomal anomalies may be diagnosed in patients with this type of CHD, but it must be considered that the specific association of muscular VSD with Holt-Oram syndrome (MIM 142900) is well known. This syndrome is an autosomal dominant disorder that causes anomalies of the upper limbs and the heart. Upper limb anomalies may be unilateral or bilateral and involve structures derived from the embryonic radial ray, typically the radial, carpal, and thenar bones. A wide spectrum of skeletal phenotypes may be present, including triphalangeal or absent thumbs, foreshortened arms, and phocomelia (Basson et al., 1994; Newbury-Ecob et al., 1996). The most common cardiac anomaly is muscular VSD, which may be in the setting of multiple VSDs and may be associated with atrioventricular block. Additional CHDs found in Holt-Oram syndrome are ASD and AVCD (Bruneau et al., 1999; Kumar et al., 1994; Sletten and Pierpont, 1996). Holt-Oram syndrome is genetically heterogeneous but is frequently due to mutations in *Tbx5* gene (Basson et al., 1997). In animal models, *Tbx5* is expressed particularly at the atrial level and in the left-sided endocardium of the ventricular septum (Bruneau et al., 1999).

Posterior Inlet Ventricular Septal Defect

Posterior inlet VSD is rare as an isolated malformation but is usually associated with a common atrioventricular valve and an ostium primum ASD in the setting of complete AVCD. In patients with Down syndrome a posterior VSD can be associated with the cleft of the mitral valve, being considered as a variant of AVCD (Marino et al., 1990, 1991).

Subarterial Ventricular Septal Defect

Subarterial VSD is quite rare in the white population (Ferencz et al., 1997) and significantly more common in the Asian population (Momma et al., 1984). This type of VSD can be associated with del22 (DiGeorge/velocardiofacial syndrome) (Goldmuntz et al., 1998; Momma et al., 1996b; Toscano et al., 2002) and with trisomy 18 (Musewe et al., 1990). The pathogenesis of VSD in del22 may be related to abnormal neural crest/secondary heart field development, since the infundibular septum involved in this type of VSD is formed by the contribution of neural crest cells (Waldo et al., 1998). Subarterial VSD in del22 is frequently associated with right or cervical aortic arch with aberrant subclavian artery (Toscano et al., 2002).

TARGETED GROWTH ANOMALIES

Anomalous Pulmonary Venous Return

Extracardiac malformations are detected in one fourth of patients with anomalous pulmonary venous return (Ferencs et al., 1997). Among chromosomal anomalies, a specific association has been described with inv dup(22)(q11)(cat eye syndrome)(MIM 115470)(Ferencz et al., 1997). Additionally, it has also been reported in patients with Turner syndrome (van Wassanaer et al., 1988). Anomalous pulmonary venous return with or without hypoplastic right pulmonary artery (Scimitar syndrome) has been detected in patients with oculoauriculovertebral spectrum (Bustamante et al., 1989; Shiono et al., 1990; personal observation). The Smith-Lemli-Opitz syndrome is a monogenic condition in which anomalous pulmonary venous return can be specifically found, alone or in association with AVCD (Lin et al., 1997).

CONCLUSIONS

It is undoubted that, in the last years, the improvement of molecular genetic technologies has led to the identification of several genes implicated in the etiology of syndromes with CHD. Nevertheless, it is important to point out the relevant contribution of clinical and molecular studies on phenotype–genotype correlation, since several results are suggesting that specific morphogenetic mechanisms put in motion by genes can result in a specific cardiac phenotype (Marino and Digilio, 2000). In this regard, the peculiar anatomical subtypes of conotruncal heart defect in del22 or the different anatomical subtypes of AVCD in various genetic conditions may be cited, and so can PVS with dysplastic valve characteristic of Noonan syndrome.

The phenotype–genotype correlations have several clinical implications. First, the particular attention to the cardiac anatomical subtype may help in correlation with a specific genetic cause, so that the right molecular test for a particular disease can be used. Genetic counseling to families is then more precise and detailed. Secondly, in several instances it has been demonstrated that the presence of peculiar anatomical cardiac features can be correlated with a positive or negative surgical outcome (Formigari et al., 2004, Michielon et al., 2006). These notions make possible the use of specific surgical techniques in different cases, and the arrangement of pre- and postsurgical protocols. Third, the utility of the multidisciplinary approach in the follow-up and treatment of patients assessed the presence of risk factors related to specific genetic syndromes is becoming clear. Earlier, children with CHDs were examined only by cardiologists, whereas the present trend aims at a multidisciplinary clinical management of patients with syndromes (Cassidy and Allanson, 2005).

REFERENCES

Al-Ata J, Paquet M, Teebi AS. Congenital heart disease in Robinow syndrome. *Am J Med Genet.* 1998;77:332–333.

Allanson J. Noonan syndrome. *J Med Genet.* 1987;24:9–13.

Allanson JE. Noonan syndrome. In: Cassidy SB, Allanson JE, eds. *Management of Genetic Syndromes.* Hoboken, New Jersey: John Wiley & Sons, Inc; 2005:385–397.

Anaclerio S, Marino B, Carotti A, et al. Pulmonary atresia with ventricular septal defect: prevalence of deletion 22q11 in the different anatomic patterns. *Ital Heart J.* 2001;2:384–387.

Ansley SJ, Badano JL, Blacque OE, et al. Basal body dysfunction is a likely cause of pleiotropic Bardet-Biedl syndrome. *Nature.* 2003;425:628–633.

Aoki Y, Niihori T, Kawame H, et al. Germline mutations in *HRAS* proto-oncogene cause Costello syndrome. *Nat Genet.* 2005;37:1038–1040.

Arron JR, Winslow MM, Polleri A, et al. *NFAT* dysregulation by increased dosage of *DSCR1* and *DYRK1A* on chromosome 21. *Nature.* 2006;441:595–600.

Basson CT, Coeley GS, Solomon SD, et al. The clinical and genetic spectrum of the Holt-Oram syndrome (Heart-Hand syndrome). *N Engl J Med.* 1994;330:885–891.

Basson CT, Bachinsky DR, Lin RC, et al. Mutations in human TBX5 cause limb and cardiac malformation in Holt-Oram syndrome. *Nat Genet.* 1997;15:30–35.

Battaglia A, Carey JC, Cederholm P, Viskochil DH, Brothman AR, Galasso C. Natural history of Wolf-Hirschhorn syndrome: experience with 15 cases. *Pediatrics.* 1999;103:830–836.

Baty BJ, Blackburn BL, Carey JC. Natural history of trisomy 18 and trisomy 13. I. Growth, physical assessment, medical histories, survival and recurrence risk. *Am J Med Genet.* 1994;49:175–188.

Botto L, Khoury MJ, Mastroiacovo P, et al. The spectrum of congenital anomalies of the VATER association: an international study. *Am J Med Genet.* 1997;71:8–15.

Brand A, Karen A, Reifen RM, Gross-Kieselstein echocardiographic and Doppler findings in the Williams syndrome. *Am J Cardiol.* 1989;63:633–635.

Bruneau BG, Logan M, Davis N, et al. Chamber-specific cardiac expression of Tbx5 and heart defects in Holt-Oram syndrome. *Devel Biol.* 1999;211:100–108.

Burch M, Sharland M, Shinebourne E, Smith G, Patton M, McKenna. Cardiologic abnormalities in Noonan syndrome: phenotypic diagnosis and echocardiographic assessment in 118 patients. *J Am Coll Cardiol.* 1993;22:1189–1192.

Burn J. Williams syndrome. *J Med Genet.* 1986;23:389–395.

Bustamante LNP, de Guerra IV, Iwahashi ER, Ebaid. Sindrome de Goldenhar, relato de cinco casos em associacao com malformacoes cardiacas. *Arq Bras Cardiol.* 1989;53:287–290.

Carey J. Trisomy 18 and trisomy 13 syndromes. In: Cassidy SB, Allanson JE, eds. *Management of Genetic Syndromes.* Hoboken, New Jersey: John Wiley & Sons, Inc; 2005:555–568.

Carmi R, Boughman JA, Ferencz . Endocardial cushion defect: further studies of "isolated" versus "syndromic" occurrence. *Am J Med Genet.* 1992;43:569–575.

Carta C, Pantaleoni F, Bocchinfuso G, et al. Germline missense mutations affecting KRAS isoform B are associated with a severe Noonan syndrome phenotype. *Am J Hum Genet.* 2006;79:129–135.

Cassidy SB, Allanson JE, eds. *Management of Genetic Syndromes.* Hoboken, New Jersey: John Wiley & Sons; 2005.

Chen B, Bronson RT, Klaman RD, et al. Mice mutant for Egfr and Shp2 have defective cardiac semilunar valvulogenesis. *Nat Genet.* 2000;24:296–299.

Chessa M, Butera G, Bonhoeffer P, et al. Relation of genotype 22q11 deletion to phenotype of pulmonary vessels in tetralogy of Fallot and pulmonary atresia-ventricular septal defect. *Heart.* 1998;79:186–190.

Clark E. Mechanisms in the pathogenesis of congenital heart defects. In: Pierpont ME, Moller J, eds. *The Genetics of Cardiovascular Disease.* Boston: Martinus-Nijoff; 1986:3–11.

Coppin BD, Temple I. Multiple lentigines syndrome (LEOPARD syndrome or progressive cardiomyopathic lentiginosis). *J Med Genet.* 1997;34:582–586.

De Biase L, Di Ciommo V, Ballerini L, Bevilacqua M, Marcelletti C, Marino. Prevalence of left-sided obstructive lesions in patients with atrioventricular canal without Down's syndrome. *J Thorac Cardiovasc Surg.* 1986;91:467–469.

Devriendt K, Fryns J-P, Mortier G. The annual incidence of DiGeorge/velocardiofacial syndrome. *J Med Genet.* 1998;35:789–790.

Devriendt K, Matthijs G, Van Dael R, et al. Delineation of the critical deletion region for congenital heart defects, on chromosome 8p23.1. *Am J Hum Genet.* 1999;64:1119–1126.

Digilio MC, Marino B, Grazioli S, Agostino D, Giannotti A, Dallapiccola. Comparison of occurrence of genetic syndromes in ventricular septal defect with pulmonic stenosis (classic tetralogy of Fallot) versus ventricular septal defect with pulmonic atresia. *Am J Cardiol.* 1996;77:1375–1376.

Digilio MC, Marino B, Guccione P, Giannotti A, Mingarelli R, Dallapiccola B. Deletion 8p syndrome. *Am J Med Genet.* 1998a;75:534–536.

Digilio MC, Marino B, Picchio F, et al. Noonan syndrome and aortic coarctation. *Am J Med Genet.* 1998b;80:160–162.

Digilio MC, Marino B, Toscano A, Giannotti A, Dallapiccola B. Atrioventricular canal defect without Down syndrome: a heterogeneous malformation. *Am J Med Genet.* 1999a;85:140–146.

Digilio MC, Marino B, Ammirati A, Borzaga U, Giannotti A, Dallapiccola B. Cardiac malformations in patients with oral-facial-skeletal syndromes: clinical similarities with heterotaxia. *Am J Med Genet* .1999b;84:350–356.

Digilio MC, Marino B, Toscano A, Giannotti A, Dallapiccola B. Congenital heart defects in Kabuki syndrome. *Am J Med Genet.* 2001;100:269–274.

Digilio MC, Conti E, Sarkozy A, et al. Grouping of multiple-lentigines/LEOPARD and Noonan syndromes on the *PTPN11* gene. *Am J Hum Genet.* 2002;71:389–394.

Digilio MC, Angioni A, De Santis M, et al. Spectrum of clinical variability in familial deletion 22q11.2: from full manifestation to extremely mild clinical anomalies. *Clin Genet.* 2003a;63:308–313.

Digilio MC, Angioni A, Giannotti A, Dallapiccola B, Marino B. Truncus arteriosus and duplication 8q. *Am J Med Genet.* 2003b; 121A:79–81.

Digilio MC, Marino B, Giannotti A, Dallapiccola B, Opitz JM. Specific congenital heart defects in RSH/Smith-Lemli-Opitz sindrome: postulated involvement of the Sonic Hedgehog pathway in syndromes with postaxial polydactyly or heterotaxia. *Birth Defects Res A Clin Mol Teratol.* 2003c;67:149–153.

Digilio MC, Dallapiccola B, Marino B. Atrioventricular canal defect in Bardet-Biedl syndrome: clinical evidence supporting the link between atrioventricular canal defect and polydactyly syndromes with ciliary dysfunction. *Genet Med.* 2006a;8:536–538.

Digilio MC, Sarkozy A, de Zorzi A, et al. LEOPARD syndrome: clinical diagnosis in the first year of life. *Am J Med Genet.* 2006b;140A:740–746.

Digilio MC, Sarkozy A, Pacileo G, Limongelli G, Marino B, Dallapiccola B. *PTPN11* gene mutations: linking the Gln510Glu mutation to the "LEOPARD syndrome phenotype". *Eur J Pediatr.* 2006c;165:803–805.

Digilio MC, Sarkozy A, Capolino R, et al. Costello syndrome: clinical diagnosis in the first year of life. *Eur J Pediatr.* 2007. (online publication, Aug 29 PMID:17726614).

Emerick KM, Rand EB, Goldmuntz E, Krantz ID, Spinner NB, Piccoli D. Features of Alagille syndrome in 92 patients: frequency and relation to prognosis. *Hepatology.* 1999;29:822–829.

Ewart AK, Morris CA, Atkinson D, et al. Hemizygosity at the elastin locus in developmental disorder, Williams syndrome. *Nat Genet.* 1993;5:11–16.

Faivre L, Dollfus H, Lyonnet S, et al. Clinical homogeneity and genetic heterogeneity in Weill-Marchesani syndrome. *J Med Genet.* 2003;40:34–36.

Fan Y, Esmail MA, Ansley SJ, et al. Mutations in a member of the Ras superfamily of small GPT-binding proteins causes Bardet-Biedl syndrome. *Nat Genet.* 2004;36:989–993.

Ferencz C, Rubin JD, Loffredo CA, Magee CA, eds. *Epidemiology of Congenital Heart Disease.* The Baltimore-Washington Infant Study. 1981–1989. Mount Kisco, New York: Futura Publishing Company Inc; 1993.

Ferencz C, Loffredo CA, Correa-Villasenor A, Wilson PD, eds. *Genetic and Environmental Risk Factors of Major Cardiovascular Malformations.* The Baltimore-Washington Infant Study 1981–1989. Armonk, New York: Futura Publishing Company Inc; 1997.

Ferrante MI, Zullo A, Barra A, et al. Oral-facial-digital type I protein is required for primary cilia formation and left-right axis specification. *Nat Genet.* 2006;38:112–117.

Formigari R, Di Donato RM, Gargiulo G, et al. Better surgical prognosis for patients with complete atrioventricular septal defect and Down's syndrome. *Ann Thorac Surg.* 2004;78:666–672.

Gelb BD, Towbin JA, McCabe ERB, Sujanski E. San Luis Valley recombinant chromosome 8 and tetralogy of Fallot: a review of chromosome 8 anomalies and congenital heart disease. *Am J Med Genet.* 1991;40:471–476.

Giddings NG, Finley JP, Nanton MA, Douglas L. The natural course of supravalvar aortic stenosis and peripheral pulmonary artery stenosis in William's syndrome. *Br Heart J.* 1989;62:315–319.

Giglio S, Graw SL, Gimelli G, et al. Deletion of a 5-cM region at chromosome 8p23 is associated with a spectrum of congenital heart defects. *Circulation.* 2000;102:432–437.

Goldmuntz E, Clark BJ, Mitchell LE, et al. Frequency of 22q11 deletions in patients with conotruncal defects. *J Am Coll Cardiol.* 1998;32:492–498.

Goldmuntz E, Geiger E, Benson W. *NKX2.5* mutations in patients with tetralogy of Fallot. *Circulation.* 2001;104:2565–2568.

Goldmuntz E, Bamford R, Karkera JD, dela Cruz J, Roessler E, Muenke M. CFC1 mutations in patients with transposition of the great arteries and double-outlet right ventricle. *Am J Hum Genet.* 2002;70:776–780.

Gotzsche CO, Krag-Olsen B, Nielsen J, Sorensen KE, Kristensen BO. Prevalence of cardiovascular malformations and association with karyotypes in Turner's syndrome. *Arch Dis Child.* 1994;71:433–436.

Green EK, Priestley MD, Waters J, Maliszewska C, Latif F, Maher ER. Detailed mapping of a congenital heart disease gene in chromosome 3p25. *J Med Genet.* 2000;37:581–587.

Gripp KW, Lin AE, Stabley DL, et al. *HRAS* mutation analysis in Costello syndrome. *Am J Med Genet.* 2006;140A:1–7.

Gripp KW, Lin AE, Nicholson L, et al. Further delineation of the phenotype resulting from *BRAF* or *MEK1* germline mutations helps differentiate Cardio-Facio-Cutaneous syndrome from Costello syndrome. *Am J Med Genet.* 2007;143A:1472–1480.

Grossfeld PD, Mattina T, Lai Z, et al. The 11q terminal deletion disorder: a prospective study of 110 cases. *Am J Med Genet.* 2004;129A:51–61.

Hallidie-Smith KA, Karas S. Cardiac anomalies in Williams-Beuren syndrome. *Arch Dis Child.* 1988;63:809–813.

Hasegawa T, Ogata T, Hasegawa T, et al. Coarctation of the aorta and renal hypoplasia in a boy with Turner-Noonan surface anomalies and a 46,XY karyotype: clinical model for the possible impairment of a putative lymphogenic gene(s) for Turner somatic stigmata. *Hum Genet.* 1996;97:564–567.

Heathcote K, Braybrook C, Abushaban L, et al. Common arterial trunk associated with a homeodomain mutation of *NKX2.6. Hum Molec Genet.* 2005;14:585–593.

Hills C, Moller JH, Finkelstein M, Lohr J, Schimmenti L. Cri du chat syndrome and congenital heart disease: a review of previously reported cases and presentation of an additional 21 cases from the Pediatric Cardiac Care Consortium. *Pediatrics.* 2006;117:e924–e927.

Hofbeck M, Rauch A, Buheitel G, et al. Monosomy 22q11 in patients with pulmonary atresia, ventricular septal defect, and major aortopulmonary collateral arteries. *Heart.* 1998;79:180–185.

Hunter AGW. Down syndrome. In: Cassidy SB, Allanson JE, eds. *Management of Genetic Syndromes.* Hoboken, New Jersey: John Wiley & Sons, Inc; 2005:191–210.

Jongewaard IN, Lauer RM, Behrendt DA, Patil S, Klewer S. Beta 1 integrin activation mediates adhesive differences between trisomy 21 on non-trisomic fibroblasts on type VI collagen. *Am J Med Genet.* 2002;109:298–305.

Johnson MC, Strauss AW, Dowton SB, et al. Deletion within chromosome 22 is common in patients with absent pulmonary valve. *Am J Cardiol.* 1995;76:66–69.

Kawame H, Hannibal MC, Hudgins L, Pagon RA. Phenotypic spectrum and management issues in Kabuki syndrome. *J Pediatr.* 1999;134:480–485.

Kim JC, Badano JL, Sibold S, et al. The Bardet-Biedl protein BBS4 targets cargo to the pericentriolar region and is required for microtubule anchoring and cell cycle progression. *Nat Genet.* 2004;36:462–470.

Kirby ML, Waldo K. Role of neural crest in congenital heart disease. *Circulation.* 1990;82:332–340.

Koletzko B, Majewski F. Congenital anomalies in patients with choanal atresia: CHARGE association. *Eur J Pediatr.* 1984;142:271–275.

Korenberg JR, Barlow GM, Chen X-N, et al. Down syndrome congenital heart disease: narrowed region and DSCAM as a candidate gene. In: Clark EB, Nakazawa M, Takao A, eds. *Etiology and Morphogenesis of Congenital Heart Disease: Twenty Years of Progress in Genetics and Developmental Biology.* Armonk, New York: Futura Publishing Co, Inc; 2000:365–370.

Koretzki ED, Moller JH, Korus ME, Schwartz CJ, Eduards JE. Congenital pulmonary stenosis resulting from dysplasia of valve. *Circulation.* 1969;40:43–45.

Krantz ID, Piccoli DA, Spinner NB. Alagille syndrome. *J Med Genet.* 1997;34:152–157.

Krenz M, Yutzey KE, Robbins J. Noonan syndrome mutation Q79R in Shp2 increases proliferation of valve primordia mesenchymal cells via extracellular signal regulated kinase 1/2 signaling. *Circ Res.* 2005;97:813–820.

Kumar A, Friedman JM, Taylor GP, Patterson MW. Pattern of cardiac malformation in oculoauriculovertebral spectrum. *Am J Med Genet.* 1993;46:423–426.

Kumar A, Van Mierop LHS, Epstein ML. Pathogenetic implications of muscular ventricular septal defect in Holt-Oram syndrome. *Am J Cardiol.* 1994;73:993–995.

Lalani SR, Safiullah AM, Molinari LM, Fernbach SD, Martin DM, Belmont JW. *SEMA3E* mutation in a patient with CHARGE syndrome. *J Med Genet.* 2004;41:e94.

Lewis DA, Loffredo CA, Correa-Villasenor A, Wilson D, Martin GR. Descriptive epidemiology of membranous and muscular ventricular septal defects in the Baltimore-Washington Infant Study. *Cardiol Young.* 1996;6:281–290.

Li DY, Toland AE, Bak BB, et al. Elastin point mutations cause an obstructive vascular disease, suoravalvular aortic stenosis. *Hum Mol Genet.* 1997a;6:1021–1028.

Li L, Krantz ID, Deng Y, et al. Alagille syndrome is caused by mutations in human *Jagged1*, which encodes a ligand for Notch1. *Nat Genet.* 1997b;16:243–251.

Li JB, Gerdes JM, Haycraft CJ, et al. Comparative genomics identifies a flagellar and basal body proteome that includes the *BBS5* human disease gene. *Cell.* 2004;117:541–552.

Limongelli G, Pacileo G, Marino B, et al. Prevalence and clinical significance of cardiovascular abnormalities in patients with the LEOPARD syndrome. *Am J Cardiol.* 2007;100:736–741.

Lin AE, Chin AJ, Devine W, Park SC, Zackai E. The pattern of cardiovascular malformation in the CHARGE association. *Am J Dis Child.* 1987;141:1010–1013.

Lin AE, Ardiger HH, Ardiger RHJr, Cunniff C, Kelley RI. Cardiovascular malformations in Smith-Lemli-Opitz syndrome. *Am J Med Genet.* 1997;69:270–278.

Lin AE, Grossfeld PD, Hamilton RM, et al. Further delineation of cardiac abnormalities in Costello syndrome. *Am J Med Genet.* 2002;111:115–129.

Lindsay EA, Vitelli F, Su H, et al. *Tbx1* haploinsufficiency in the DiGeorge syndrome region causes aortic arch defects in mice. *Nature.* 2001;410:97–101.

Loffredo CA, Ferencz C, Wilson PD, Lurie IW. Interrupted aortic arch: an epidemiologic study. *Teratology.* 2000;61:368–375.

Loomes KM, Underkoffler LA, Morabito J, et al. The expression of *JAGGED1* in the developing mammalian heart correlates with cardiovascular disease in Alagille syndrome. *Hum Molec Genet.* 1999;8:2443–2449.

Maeda J, Yamagishi H, Matsuoka R, et al. Frequent association of 22q11.2 deletion with tetralogy of Fallot. *Am J Med Genet.* 2000;92:269–272.

Marino B. Left-sided cardiac obstruction in patients with Down syndrome. *J Pediatr.* 1989;115:834–835.

Marino B, Vairo U, Corno A, et al. Atrioventricular canal in Down syndrome. Prevalence of associated cardiac malformations compared with patients without Down syndrome. *Am J Dis Child.* 1990a;144:1120–1122.

Marino B, Papa M, Guccione P, Corno A, Morosini M, Calabrò R. Ventricular septal defect in Down syndrome. Anatomic types and associated malformations. *Am J Dis Child.* 1990b;44:544–545.

Marino B, Corno A, Guccione P, Marcelletti C. Ventricular septal defect and Down syndrome. *Lancet.* 1991;337:245–246.

Marino B. Congenital heart disease in patients with Down's syndrome: anatomic and genetic aspects. *Biomed & Pharmacother.* 1993;47:197–200.

Marino B, Digilio MC, Grazioli S, et al. Associated cardiac anomalies in isolated and syndromic patients with tetralogy of Fallot. *Am J Cardiol.*1996a;77:505–508.

Marino B. Patterns of congenital heart disease and associated cardiac anomalies in children with Down syndrome. In: Marino B, Pueschel SM, eds. *Heart Disease in Persons with Down Syndrome.* Brookes; 1996b:33–140.

Marino B, Digilio MC, Dallapiccola B. Severe truncal valve dysplasia: Association with DiGeorge syndrome ? *Ann Thorac Surg.* 1998;66:980.

Marino B, Digilio MC, Persiani M, et al. Deletion 22q11 in patients with interrupted aortic arch. *Am J Cardiol.* 1999a;84:360–361.

Marino B, Digilio MC, Toscano A, Giannotti A, Dallapiccola B. Congenital heart diseases in children with Noonan syndrome: an expanded cardiac spectrum with high prevalence of atrioventricular canal. *J Pediatr.*1999b;135:703–706.

Marino B, Digilio MC. Congenital heart disease and genetic syndromes: correlation between cardiac phenotype and genotype. *Cardiovasc Pathol.* 2000;9:303–315.

Marino B, Digilio MC, Toscano A, et al. Anatomic patterns of conotruncal defects associated with deletion 22q11. *Genet Med.* 2001;3:45–48.

Matsumoto N, Niikawa N. Kabuki syndrome: a review. *Am J Med Genet.* 2003;117C:57–65.

Mazzanti L, Cacciari E. Congenital heart disease in Turner's syndrome. *J Pediatr.* 1998;133:688–692.

McDaniell R, Warthen DM, Sanchez-Lara PA, et al. *NOTCH2* mutations cause Alagille syndrome, a heterogeneous disorder of the Notch signaling pathway. *Am J Hum Genet.* 2006;79:169–173.

McDonald-McGinn DM, Kirschner R, Goldmuntz E, et al. The Philadelphia story. The 22q11.2 deletion: report on 250 patients. *Genet Couns.* 1999;10:11–24.

Michielon G, Marino B, Formigari R, et al. Genetic syndromes and outcome after surgical correction of tetralogy of Fallot. *Ann Thorac Surg.* 2006;81:968–975.

Momma K, Tayama K, Takao A, et al. Natural history of subarterial infundibular ventricular septal defect. *Am Heart J.* 1984;108:1312–1317.

Momma K, Kondo C, Ando M, Matsuoka R, Takao A. Tetralogy of Fallot associated with chromosome 22q11 deletion. *Am J Cardiol.* 1995;76:618–621.

Momma K, Kondo C, Matsuoka R. Tetralogy of Fallot with pulmonary atresia associated with chromosome 22q11 deletion. *J Am Coll Cardiol.*1996a ;27:198–202.

Momma K, Kondo C, Matsuoka R, Takao A. Cardiac anomalies associated with a chromosome 22q11 deletion in patients with conotruncal anomaly face syndrome. *Am J Cardiol.* 1996b;78:591–594.

Momma K, Ando M, Matsuoka R. Truncus arteriosus communis associated with chromosome 22q11 deletion. *J Am Coll Cardiol.* 1997;30:1067–1071.

Morris CA, Dilts C, Dempsey SA, Leonard CO, Blakburn B. The natural history of Williams syndrome: Physical characteristics. *J Pediatr.* 1988;113:318–326.

Musante L, Kehl HG, Majewski F, et al. Spectrum of mutations in *PTPN11* and genotype-phenotype correlation in 96 patients with Noonan syndrome and five patients with cardio-facio-cutaneous syndrome. *Eur J Hum Genet.* 2003;11:201–206.

Musewe NN, Alexander DJ, Teshima I, Smalhorn JF, Freedom RM. Echocardiographic evaluation of the spectrum of cardiac anomalies associated with trisomy 18 and 13. *J Am Coll Cardiol.* 1990;15:673–677.

Narayanswami S, Kitchiner D, Smith A. Spectrum of valvar abnormalities in Noonan's syndrome. A pathologic study. *Cardiol Young.* 1994;4:62–66.

Neill CA. Congenital cardiac malformations and syndromes. In: Pierpont MEM, Moller JH, eds. *Genetics of Cardiovascular Disease*. Boston: Martinus-Nijoff Publishing; 1987:95–112.

Newbury-Ecob RA, Leanage R, Raeburn JA, Young ID. Holt-Oram syndrome: a clinical genetic study. *J Med Genet*. 1996;33:300–307.

Niihori T, Aoki Y, Narumi Y, et al. Germline KRAS and BRAF mutations in cardio-facio-cutaneous syndrome. *Nat Genet*. 2006;38:294–296.

Nishibatake M, Kirby ML, Van Mierop LHS. Pathogenesis of persistent truncus arteriosus and dextroposed aorta in the chick embryo after neural crest ablation. *Circulation*. 1987;75:255–264.

Oda T, Elkahloun AG, Pike BL, et al. Mutations in the human *JAGGED1* gene are responsible for Alagille syndrome. *Nat Genet*. 1997;16:235–242.

Okada Y, Nonaka S, Tanaka Y, Saijoh Y, Hamada H, Hirokawa N. Abnormal nodal flow precedes situs inversus in *iv* and *inv* mice. *Mol Cell*. 1999;4:459–468.

Ondine Mendelian Inheritance in Man (OMIM): http://www.ncbi.nlm.nih.gov/omim.

Pagon RA, Graham JM, Zonana J, Yong S-L. Coloboma, congenital heart disease, and choanal atresia with multiple anomalies: CHARGE association. *J Pediatr*. 1981;99:223–227.

Pandit B, Sarkozy A, Pennacchio LA, et al. Gain-of-function *RAF1* mutations cause Noonan and LEOPARD syndromes with hypertrophic cardiomyopathy. *Nat Genet*. 2007;39:1007–1012.

Perez-Jurado LA, Peoples R, Kaplan P, Hamel B, Francke U. Molecular definition of the chromosome 7 deletion in Williams syndrome and parent-of-origin on growth. *Am J Hum Genet*. 1996;59:781–792.

Philip N, Meinecke P, David A, et al. Kabuki syndrome (Niikawa-Kuroki) syndrome: a study of 16 non-Japanese cases. *Clin Dysmorphol*. 1992;1:63–77.

Phillips HM, Renforth GL, Spalluto G, et al. Narrowing the critical region within 11q24-qter for hypoplastic left heart and identification of a candidate gene, *JAM3*, expressed during cardiogenesis. *Genomics*. 2002;79:475–478.

Pizzuti A, Sarkozy A, Newton AL, et al. Mutations in ZFPM2/FOG2 gene in sporadic cases of tetralogy of Fallot. *Hum Genet*. 2003;22:372–377.

Razzaque MA, Nishizawa T, Komoike Y, et al. Germline gain-of-function mutations in *RAF1* cause Noonan syndrome. *Nat Genet*. 2007;39:1013–1017.

Roberts A, Allanson J, Jadico SK, et al. The Cardio-Facio-Cutaneous syndrome: a review. *J Med Genet*. 2006. Online publication.

Roberts AE, Araki T, Swanson KD, et al. Germline gain-of-function mutations in *SOS1* cause Noonan syndrome. *Nat Genet*. 2007;39:70–74.

Robinson SW, Morris CD, Goldmuntz E, et al. Missense mutations in *CRELD1* are associated with cardiac atrioventricular septal defects. *Am J Hum Genet*. 2003;72:1047–1052.

Rodriguez-Viciana P, Tetsu O, Tidyman WE, et al. Germline mutations in genes within the MAPK pathway cause cardio-facio-cutaneous syndrome. *Nat Genet*. 2006.Online publication.

Ruiz-Perez VL, Ide SE, Strom TM, et al. Mutations in a new gene in Ellis-van Creveld syndrome and Weyers acrodental dysostosis. *Nat Genet*. 2000;24:283–286.

Ruiz-Perez VL, Tompson SWJ, Blair HJ, et al. Mutations in two non-homologous genes in a head-to-head configuration cause Ellis-van Creveld syndrome. *Am J Hum Genet*. 2003;72:728–732.

Rupp PA, Fouad GT, Egelston CA, et al. Identification, genomic organization and m-RNA expression of *CRELD1*, the founding member of a unique family of matricellular proteins. *Gene*. 2002;293:47–57.

Ryan AK, Goodship JA, Wilson DI, et al. Spectrum of clinical features associated with interstitial chromosome 22q11 deletions: a European collaborative study. *J Med Genet*. 1997;34:798–804.

Sarkozy A, Conti E, Digilio MC, et al. Clinical and molecular analysis of 30 patients with multiple lentigines LEOPARD syndrome. *J Med Genet*. 2004;41:e68.

Sarkozy A, Conti E, Seripa D, et al. Correlation between *PTPN11* gene mutations and congenital heart defects in Noonan and LEOPARD syndromes. *J Med Genet* .2003a;40:704–708.

Sarkozy A, Conti E, Esposito G, et al. Nonsyndromic pulmonary valve stenosis and the *PTPN11* gene. *Am J Med Genet*. 2003b;116A:389–390.

Sarkozy A, Lepri F, Marino B, Pizzuti A, Digilio MC, Dallapiccola B. Additional evidence that PTPN11 mutations play only a minor role in the pathogenesis of non-syndromic atrioventricular canal defect. *Am J Med Genet*. 2006;140:1970–1972.

Schubert S, Zenker M, Rowe SL, et al. Germline *KRAS* mutations cause Noonan syndrome. *Nat Genet*. 2006;38:331–336.

Shiono N, Takanashi Y, Yoshihara K, Tokuhiro K, Komatsu H, Matsuo N. A successful surgical repair of anomalous right pulmonary venous connection with Goldenhar syndrome. *Nippon Kyobu Geka Gakkai Zasshi*. 1990;38;135–139.

Shprintzen RJ. Velo-cardio-facial syndrome. In: Cassidy SB, Allanson JE, eds. *Management of Genetic Syndromes*. Hoboken, New Jersey: John Wiley & Sons, Inc; 2005:615–631.

Sletten LJ, Pierpont MEM. Variation in severity of cardiac disease in Holt-Oram syndrome. *Am J Med Genet*. 1996;65:128–132.

Sujanski E, Smith ACM, Prescott KE, Freehauf CL, Clericuzio C, Robinson A. Natural history of the recombinant (8) syndrome. *Am J Med Genet*. 1993;47:512–525.

Supp DM, Wite DP, Potter SS, Brueckner M. Mutation in an axonemal dynein affects left-right asimmetry in *inversus viscerum* mice. *Nature*. 1997;389–966.

Sybert VP. Turner syndrome. In: Cassidy SB, Allanson JE, eds. *Management of Genetic Syndromes*. Hoboken, New Jersey: John Wiley & Sons, Inc; 2005:589–605.

Tartaglia M, Mehler EL, Goldberg R, et al. Mutations in *PTPN11*, encoding the protein tyrosine phosphatase SHP-2, cause Noonan syndrome. *Nat Genet*. 2001;29:465–468.

Tartaglia M, Kalidas K, Shaw A, et al. *PTPN11* mutations in Noonan syndrome: molecular spectrum, genotype, phenotype correlation, and phenotypic heterogeneity. *Am J Hum Genet*. 2002;70:1555–1563.

Tartaglia M, Martinelli S, Stella L, et al. Diversity of functional consequences of germline and somatic *PTPN11* mutations in human disease. *Am J Hum Genet*. 2006;78:279–290.

Tartaglia M, Pennacchio LA, Zhao C, et al. Gain-of-function *SOS1* mutations cause a distinctive form of Noonan syndrome. *Nat Genet*. 2007;39:75–79.

Tellier AL, Cormier-Daire V, Abadie V, et al. The CHARGE syndrome: report of 47 cases and review. *Am J Med Genet*. 1998;76:402–409.

Torres-Juan L, Rosell J, Morla M, et al. Mutations in *TBX1* genocopy the 22q11.2 deletion and duplication syndromes: a new susceptibility factor for mental retardation. *Eur J Hum Genet*. 2007;15:658–663.

Toscano A, Anaclerio S, Digilio MC, Giannotti A, Fariello G, Dallapiccola B, Marino B. Ventricular septal defect and deletion of chromosome 22q11: anatomical types and aortic arch anomalies. *Eur J Pediatr*. 2002;161:116–117.

van der Burgt I, Berends E, Lommen E, van Beersum S, Hamel B, Mariman E. Clinical and molecular studies in a large Dutch family with Noonan syndrome. *Am J Med Genet*. 1994;53:187–191.

Van der Hauwaert LG, Fryns JP, Dumoulin M, Logghe. Cardiovascular malformations in Turner's and Noonan's syndrome. *Br Heart J*. 1978;40:500–509.

Van Praagh S, Truman T, Firpo A, et al. Cardiac malformations in trisomy 18: A study of 41 postmortem cases. *J Am Coll Cardiol.* 1989;13:1586–1597.

van Wassanaer AG, Lubbers LJ, Losekoot G. Partial abnormal pulmonary venous return in Turner syndrome. *Eur J Pediatr.* 1988;148:101–103.

Vergara P, Digilio MC, De Zorzi A, et al. Genetic heterogeneity and phenotypic anomalies in children with atrioventricular canal defect and tetralogy of Fallot. *Clin Dysmorphol.* 2006;15:65–70.

Vissers LELM, van Ravenswaaij CMA, Admiraal R, et al. Mutations in a new member of the chromodomain gene family cause CHARGE syndrome. *Nat Genet.* 2004;36:955–957.

Waldo K, Miyagawa-Tomita S, Kumiski D, Kirby ML. Cardiac neural crest cells provide new insight into septation of the cardiac outflow tract: aortic sac to ventricular septal closure. *Devel Biol.* 1998;196:129–144.

Wessel A, Pankau R, Kegecioglu D, Ruschewsh W, Brusch JH. Three decades of follow-up of aortic and pulmonary vascular lesions in the Williams-Beuren syndrome. *Am J Med Genet.* 1994;52:297–301.

Wyse RKH, Al-Mahdawi S, Burn J, Blake. Congenital heart disease in CHARGE association. *Pediatr Cardiol.* 1993;14:75–81.

Yagi H, Furutani Y, Hamada H, et al. Role of TBX1 in human del22q11.2 syndrome. *Lancet.* 2003;362:1366–1373.

Zenker M, Horn D, Wieczorek D, et al. *SOS1* is the second most common Noonan gene but plays no major role in cardio-facio-cutaneous syndrome. *J Med Genet.* 2007;44:651–656.

Zweier C, Sticht H, Aydin-Yaylagül, Campbell CE, Rauch A. Human *TBX1* missense mutations cause gain of function resulting in the same phenotype as 22q11.2 deletions. *Am J Hum Genet.* 2007;80:510–517.

V

Genetics of Congenital Heart Defects

26

The Genetic Basis of Nonsyndromic Cardiovascular Malformations

JOHN W. BELMONT

INTRODUCTION

The estimated frequency of severe cardiovascular malformation (CVM) is 0.6% of live born infants (Hoffman, 1995, 2004; Hoffman and Kaplan, 2002; Pradat et al., 2003). If less serious and clinically mild defects are included, the incidence is near 0.9% (Hoffman et al., 2004; Hoffman and Kaplan, 2002; Tutar et al., 2005). Adding bicuspid aortic valve (BAV), which often goes undetected until late middle age, the incidence is near 2% (Movahed et al., 2006; Nistri et al., 2005; Tutar et al., 2005). If one includes infants ascertained in unbiased newborn echocardiography screening, up to 1 in 20 infants may be born with a CVM such as atrial septal defect (ASD) or small muscular ventricular septal defect (VSD) (Roguin et al., 1995).

The estimated rate of severe CVM has not varied much from study to study over the last 50 years (Hoffman and Kaplan, 2002; Scott and Niebuhr, 2007). Apparent increases in the frequency of cardiac defects over the last 15–20 years can largely be attributed to the increased use of echocardiography and the consequent observation of mild anomalies that might otherwise have gone undetected and most often resolved without intervention (Hoffman and Kaplan, 2002). Given the manifest differences in environmental exposures comparing geographic locations and time, the stable prevalence rate for severe CVM is most consistent with a prominent role for fixed factors that are most likely genetic. There is a 10-fold higher rate of CVMs in fetuses compared to live born infants (Freire-Maia and Arce-Gomez, 1971; Hoffman, 1995a, 1995b; Nora and Nora, 1976; Salvador et al., 2005). This indicates that severe CVMs are a common cause of miscarriage and intrauterine fetal demise. It also suggests

that there may be many familial occurrences that are unaccounted for in typical epidemiological studies. This effect tends to lead to an underestimation of the role of genetic factors.

In this review, nonsyndromic congenital CVMs refer to the cases in which there is heart defect but no other birth defect, dysmorphism, or neurodevelopmental disability. Approximately 25%–35% of CVMs are accompanied by another birth defect. There are less data regarding neurodevelopmental problems associated with heart defects, and the problem is confounded by the possible occurrence of postnatal brain injuries resulting from hypoxia in the cyanotic lesions, or perioperative complications. Chromosomal abnormalities that can be detected by karyotype virtually always have associated features even if the individual does not have mental retardation. The other genetic mechanisms known to contribute to CVMs—genomic imbalances, single gene mutations, and complex inheritance—may play also important roles in nonsyndromic CVM. Based on available data at present, one can define a genetic basis for <10% of nonsyndromic CVM.

CARDIOVASCULAR MALFORMATIONS AS INBORN ERRORS OF DEVELOPMENT

Inborn errors of development are genetic disorders causing defects in embryonic patterning and organogenesis that lead to structural malformations present at birth. These disorders may involve many different types of gene functions—transcription factors, receptors and their signaling components, metabolic defects, structural proteins, and so on. There are more than 660 entries in the Online Mendelian Inheritance in

Man (OMIM, http://www.ncbi.nlm.nih.gov/sites/entrez?db=omim) associated with congenital malformations involving more than 500 genes. Many genetic mechanisms are at work in causing congenital anomalies. Cytogenetic abnormalities, submicroscopic chromosomal aberrations, and Mendelian disorders have most often been identified first because they are generally easier to study. Together these simpler forms of genetic abnormality account for only 10%–20% of cases. In a few notable cases recent research has established that common genetic variants can also play a role in the inborn errors of development just as they do in common adult-onset diseases.

CARDIOVASCULAR MALFORMATIONS EXHIBIT HIGH HERITABILITY IN FAMILIES AND POPULATIONS

One of the largest and most consistent risk factors for CVM in epidemiological studies is a positive family history of a heart defect (Romano-Zelekha et al., 2001; Wollins et al., 2001; Zavala et al., 1992). There have also been numerous studies that document much higher rates of occurrence of CVMs in the close relatives of affected individuals (Abushaban et al., 2003; Allan et al., 1986; Boon and Roberts, 1976; Calcagni et al., 2007; Clementi et al., 1996; Corone et al., 1983; Cripe et al., 2004; Czeizel and Meszaros, 1981; Digilio et al., 2001; Ehlers and Engle, 1966; Ferencz et al., 1989; Hinton et al., 2007; Kumar et al., 1994; Kwiatkowska et al., 2007; Loffredo et al., 2004; Maestri et al., 1989; Nicolae et al., 2007; Nora and Meyer, 1966; Pacileo et al., 1992; Piacentini et al., 2005; Udwadia et al., 1996; Wulfsberg et al., 1991; Yunis et al., 2006). Sibling recurrence risk is usually estimated at 2%–4% across all CVMs. When the mother or father is affected with a heart defect the risk to offspring may range from 2% to %13%. The very high offspring risk for affected mothers may be an example of the "Carter effect" in which the risk to offspring is greater for the less frequently affected sex.

The word heritability has a formal meaning in genetics in that it refers to a feature of certain statistical models of causation. Although the concept of heritability does not allow one to make an inference about a particular person, it does give a useful summary of the effect of genes in the population. Because of the difficulty in making estimates of heritability there have been only a few studies of CVMs. These studies have been consistent with heritability of 50%–90% for the CVM studied (Hinton et al., 2007; McBride et al., 2005). If we estimate that a trait has 90% heritability then this indicates that genetic variation among individuals in the population is probably playing a very large

role in the overall frequency of the trait. Several factors cause heritability to be underestimated in CVM: (1) heart defects are approximately 10-fold more common in miscarried pregnancies and so many affected offspring may not be counted in population surveys; (2) affected individuals have fewer children than people without heart defects; and (3) families whose first born is affected may decide against having further offspring. These factors systematically reduce the number of sibling recurrences that we use to make the estimate of heritability.

PATTERNS OF INHERITANCE

There are rare families that exhibit Mendelian segregation of isolated CVMs. These families generally have autosomal dominant inheritance with incomplete penetrance (Ching et al., 2005; Garg et al., 2005; Hosoda et al., 1999; Maslen, 2004; Sheffield et al., 1997). The disorder X-linked heterotaxy demonstrates the single known example of X-linked inheritance of nonsyndromic CVMs (Gebbia et al., 1997; Mathias et al., 1987; Megarbane et al., 2000). Several publications have argued for autosomal recessive inheritance based on the observation of affected siblings of both sexes born to unaffected parents (Abushaban et al., 2003; Kumar et al., 1994; Piacentini et al., 2005). In addition, there are several genetic epidemiology studies that demonstrate an excess occurrence of CVM in consanguineous families or in inbred populations (Becker et al., 2001; Nabulsi et al., 2003; Ramegowda and Ramachandra, 2006). A striking demonstration of recessive inheritance of persistent truncus arteriosus is given by a pedigree with six affected individuals and multiple first cousin matings (Heathcote et al., 2005). Heathcote et al., showed that the gene involved in this family is the transcription factor NKX2.6. However, the interpretation that inbreeding and consanguinity equate to autosomal recessive inheritance should be viewed with caution. Oligogenic inheritance (gene interaction through variants at 2 or more loci) could be enhanced in inbred populations. Inbreeding reduces the effective population size and increases the variance of allele frequencies. In such populations, rare weakly deleterious variants may become more common due to drift.

SINGLE GENE DISORDERS

There is increasing awareness that the anatomical spectrum of CVMs due to mutations in specific genes can vary surprisingly within and among families. Two general conclusions have emerged in studies of the genetic factors underlying common CVMs: specific genetic loci can play a causal role in anatomically disparate anomalies (variable expression) and anatomically similar anomalies can be caused by defects in multiple genes in distinct biochemical pathways (locus heterogeneity). More than 200 syndromes and single gene disorders have been associated with cardiac malformations. A small number of genomic disorders are consistently associated with CVMs and the heart defect can be specifically ascribed to aberrant expression of a single gene. Examples include 22q11del (DiGeorge/velocardiofacial syndrome) and *TBX1*, 7q11.23del (Williams syndrome) and *ELN*, and 8p23del and *GATA4*. Mutations in more than 100 single genes that are involved in causing multiple congenital anomalies with heart defects have been identified. Most of these conditions cause complex phenotypes or syndromes such that the cardiac component is the only somewhat variable component. Examples include Noonan (*PTPN11*, *KRAS*, *RAF1*, *SOS1*), Holt-Oram (*TBX5*), CHARGE (*CHD7*), and Char (*TFAP2B*) syndromes (Pandit et al., 2007; Razzaque et al., 2007; Satoda et al., 2000; Schubbert et al., 2006; Stennard and Harvey, 2005; Tartaglia et al., 2007; Tartaglia and Gelb, 2005; Vissers et al., 2004). A less common scenario, so far, is the identification of Mendelian genetic disorders in which the cardiac phenotype is either isolated or defining. Examples include familial ASD caused by mutation in *NKX2.5* (Elliott et al., 2003; McElhinney et al., 2003; Schott et al., 1998), *GATA4* (Garg et al., 2003), and *MYH6* (Ching et al., 2005), as well as familial calcific BAV caused by *NOTCH1* mutation (Garg, 2006; Garg et al., 2005). A third category are genes that were initially identified as causing syndromic CVM but have also been shown to play a role in patients with isolated heart defects. Examples include *JAG1*, originally identified in Alagille syndrome (Oda et al., 1997) but also found in subjects with apparently isolated tetralogy of Fallot (TOF) (Eldadah et al., 2001), and *ZIC3*, which causes X-linked heterotaxy (Gebbia et al., 1997; Ware et al., 2004) but has also been observed in familial isolated transposition of the great arteries (TGA) (Megarbane et al., 2000) and in sporadic isolated heart defects (Ware et al., 2004).

In many reviews over the past decade there have been attempts to illustrate the role of each gene within a single step in cardiac morphogenesis. While it is true that certain lesions seem to predominate in the few examples of Mendelian segregation of cardiac developmental traits, even within those families there can be remarkable phenotypic heterogeneity (Brassington et al., 2003). To reflect the essential change in view from a linear developmental program to a systems biology perspective where the emphasis is on networks of gene activity, one can examine the genes known to cause CVMs for mutual protein and transcription

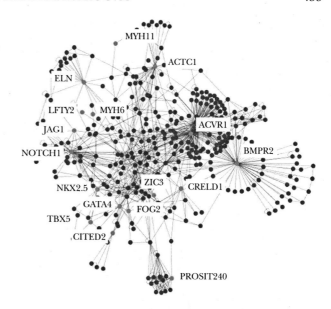

FIGURE 26–1. Network representation of gene and gene product interaction among loci known to cause cardiovascular malformations (highlighted in light gray). Many other known components of these networks (shown in black) are candidates for playing a causal role.

interactions. As shown in Figure 26–1, most of these genes are already known to interact at the molecular level. Future work may profitably focus on the potential role of the other components of these networks in CVMs.

TRANSCRIPTION FACTORS

NKX2.5

NKX2.5 was isolated as a mammalian homolog of tinman, a homeodomain-containing protein that controls heart formation in Drosophila. *Nkx2.5* is expressed in early cardiac mesoderm and in heart muscle lineage throughout life (Lints et al., 1993). At the molecular level, *NKX2.5* binds to DNA and participates in protein interaction with at least two other important cardiac transcription factors, GATA4 and TBX5 (Chen and Schwartz, 1995; Durocher et al., 1997). Mutation in mice leads to failure of cardiac development at the linear heart tube stage (Lyons et al., 1995). Loss of *NKX2.5* revealed essential roles in the establishment of a ventricular gene expression program, septal morphogenesis, and maintenance of the conduction system. In rare families with multiple occurrences of ASDs, mutations of *NKX2.5* are associated with heart malformations and arrhythmias (Hirayama-Yamada et al., 2005; Konig et al., 2006; Sarkozy et al., 2005; Schott et al., 1998). Two independent cases of dextrocardia associated with sporadic rare mutations in *NKX2.5* have been reported (Hirayama-Yamada et al., 2005; Watanabe et al., 2002). This may be explained in part by a necessary role for *NKX2.5* in the left–right patterning of the dHand transcription factor during ventricular development (Biben and Harvey, 1997). *NKX2.5* mutations have also been observed in case-control studies in which rare variants were found in (TOF) (Goldmuntz et al., 2001), anomalous pulmonary venous return (Gutierrez-Roelens et al., 2002), and other sporadic congenital heart defects (CHDs) (Elliott et al., 2003; McElhinney et al., 2003). Heart failure due to dilated cardiomyopathy (DCM) has been observed in some individuals with *NKX2.5* mutations (Benson et al., 1999; Schott et al., 1999). Cardiomyopathy, as evidenced by severe pericardial effusion, occurs in mouse *Nkx2.5* homozygous null mutants.

NKX2.6

Mouse *Nkx2.6* is expressed in the caudal pharyngeal arches and at opposite poles of the developing heart and it is expressed in the developing outflow tract. Although mutation of *Nkx2.6* does not result in heart defects, overlapping functions of *Nkx2.5* and *Nkx2.6* are demonstrated in double knockout mouse embryos (Tanaka et al., 2001). These animals lack pharyngeal pouches because of reduced proliferation and survival of pharyngeal endodermal cells. Homozygous mutation in *NKX2.6* as a probable mechanism for persistent truncus arteriosus has been observed in a single consanguineous pedigree (Heathcote et al., 2005). Homozygosity mapping placed the gene within a 6-Mb region on chromosome 8. A missense variant, F151L, which was absent from controls, was shown to segregate with the heart defect.

GATA4

The GATA family belongs to the zinc finger superfamily of transcription factors that bind a common consensus 6 base pair RGATAW DNA sequence. Of the six GATA genes three are expressed in the heart—*GATA4*, *GATA5*, and *GATA6*. *GATA4* is expressed in cardiac precursors at all developmental stages and in mature cardiomyocytes. *GATA5* is restricted to endocardial cells and *GATA6* is in myocardial and vascular smooth muscle cells. More than 30 direct gene targets of GATA4 transcriptional regulation have been identified. GATA4 contains two class IV zinc finger domains. However, null mutations in the Drosophila Gata4 ortholog, *pannier*; Zebrafish *gata*; or mouse *Gata4* result in early defects in cardiogenesis. Although mice heterozygous for *Gata4* do not have obvious cardiac anomalies, further reduction in *Gata4* dosage from a hypomorphic *Gata4* allele causes cardiac septal and other CHDs.

Mutations in human GATA4 underlie autosomal dominant transmission of ASD in rare families (Garg et al., 2003). One of the mutations was shown to specifically disrupt GATA4 protein interaction with TBX5, the transcription factor mutated in Holt-Oram syndrome. *GATA4* mutations are also associated with a small percentage of isolated heart defects (Nemer et al., 2006; Posch et al., 2008; Rajagopal et al., 2007; Schluterman et al., 2007; Sarkozy et al., 2005b; Zhang et al., 2006). The *GATA4* gene is located in 8p23.1 near the defensin gene cluster. Within and flanking that cluster there are segmental duplications that probably underlie the DNA copy number variation observed in population samples. Deletions and, more recently, duplications have been observed in patients with complex birth defects including cardiac malformations (Paez et al., 2008; Pehlivan et al., 2008). The 8p23 duplication disorder apparently may be very subtle and so it may be involved in cases that are currently classified as nonsyndromic (Barber et al., 2008).

ZIC3

The mouse *Zic* gene family was first identified by its similarity to the Drosophila pair-rule gene, *odd-paired* (Aruga et al., 1996). *Zic3* contains five highly conserved C2H2-type zinc finger motifs and belongs to the GLI transcription factor superfamily. It can bind to the GLI-consensus DNA binding site and function as a weak transcriptional coactivator (Mizugishi et al., 2001). Both human clinical studies and Zic3 deficiency mouse models establish Zic3 as an important regulator of left–right patterning during embryonic development (Purandare et al., 2002). Its deficiency is also associated with CVMs both in human and in mouse. It is unclear whether heart defects are the sole consequence of abnormal left–right patterning or whether there is an additional function of Zic3 in heart development. Zhu et al., showed that Zic3 is expressed in the embryonic heart and that its deficiency is associated with decreased expression of cardiac-specific genes, including *Nkx2.5*, *Tbx5* and ANF, which are not known to be directly involved in left–right patterning (Zhu et al., 2007). Defective myocardial development, as evidenced by the absence of cardiac ANF expression, thin myocardium, and decreased trabeculation, was observed in Zic3 null embryos without heart looping defects. Decreased expression of ANF observed in the developing heart of Zic3 null embryos could result from a direct effect of ZIC3 interaction with serum response factor (SRF) interaction. Mutations in the zinc finger transcription factor ZIC3 cause X-linked heterotaxy (Gebbia et al., 1997) and have also been identified in patients with isolated CHD (Megarbane et al., 2000).

Ware et al., screened the coding region of ZIC3 in 194 unrelated patients with either classic or related heart defect (Ware et al., 2004). In addition to classic heterotaxy, mutations associated with sporadic ASD and pulmonic stenosis were identified.

TBX20

TBX20 is a member of the T-box family of transcription factors, several of which have important roles in cardiac development (Kraus et al., 2001). T-box transcription factors are characterized by the presence of a highly conserved, 180–amino acid DNA-binding domain (Plageman and Yutzey, 2005). These factors act as transcriptional activators and repressors and are known to function in a combinatorial and hierarchical fashion in many developmental processes. At least seven members of the T-box gene family are expressed in the developing heart in humans and vertebrate model organisms. Mutations in TBX5 cause Holt-Oram syndrome, an autosomal dominant disorder characterized by radial ray hand and heart malformations. The cardiac malformations associated with TBX5 mutation are typically ASD and VSD, but other diverse defects including TOF, hypoplastic left heart, and anomalous pulmonary venous return have also been recorded. Animal models demonstrate roles for Tbx2, Tbx3, and Tbx18 in cardiac development, but no mutations in humans have been reported. In mice Tbx20 is expressed in the developing myocardium of the endocardial cushions (a precursor structure for the atrioventricular septum) (Kraus et al., 2001). TBX20 interacts with Nkx2–5, Gata4, Gata5, and Tbx5 (Stennard et al., 2003). Mouse Tbx20 null mutants lack ventricular myocardium and have severe embryonic lethal cardiac malformations (Singh et al., 2005). Adult heterozygous Tbx20-knockout mice show mild atrial septal abnormalities, including an increased prevalence of patent foramen ovale (PFO) and aneurysmal atrial septum primum, as well as mild DCM and a genetic predisposition to frank ASD. The essential roles of Tbx20 in heart development and adult heart function in mice raise the possibility that mutations in human TBX20. Recently, two mutations were found in two families in a screen of 352 individuals with cardiac malformations (Kirk et al., 2007). Both mutations occurred in the T-box DNA-binding domain. DCM was present with structural heart malformation in two individuals with a TBX20 truncating mutation. While this could indicate decompensation due to flow abnormalities caused by the structural defects, cardiomyopathy is also observed in Tbx20 null mice. It is more likely TBX20 has a continuing role in cardiomyocyte maintenance and that this is compromised in some individuals with the mutation.

CITED2

CITED2 is a transcriptional cofactor that coactivates TFAP2, a regulator of Pitx2c, in the embryonic heart. Mice homozygous for Cited2 mutations exhibit ASDASD and VSDs, as well as common outflow tract abnormalities like double-outlet right ventricle (DORV). A case-control study of the CITED2 gene in a cohort of patients with well-characterized phenotypes of sporadic nonsyndromic CHD demonstrated several mutations Previous reports of mice lacking Cited2 suggested that it plays a direct role in the development of the atrioventricular canal and cardiac septa, and that it is required for the normal establishment of the left–right axis. Seven potential disease-causing mutations in 8 of nearly 400 patients were discovered. These mutations were exclusively observed in the patient cohort and not found in 192 control individuals. Further analysis of these mutations using reporter-gene assays revealed significant loss in the HIF1A transcriptional repressive capacity of CITED2 and diminished TFAP2C coactivation.

FOG2

As noted in the earlier section, GATA4 is essential in the normal development of the heart. Mice harboring a hypomorphic mutation in Gata4 that impairs its physical interaction with its cofactor FOG2 demonstrate malformations of the semilunar cardiac valves, DORV, and TOF. These data identified FOG2 as the likely mediator of GATA4 cardiac developmental defects. A splice donor site mutation in Fog2 induced by N-ethyl-N-nitrosourea in mice also led to pulmonary hypoplasia and abnormal diaphragmatic development. Subsequently, a single de novo mutation in human FOG2 was found in a child who died on the first day of life secondary to severe bilateral pulmonary hypoplasia and an abnormally muscularized diaphragm. Two out of 47 patients with sporadic TOF, the most common cyanotic conotruncal heart defect (CTD), showed heterozygous missense mutations of the ZFPM2/FOG2 gene, but no mutations were found in children with tricuspid atresia (Ackerman et al., 2005; Bleyl et al., 2007; Crispino et al., 2001; Kantarci and Donahoe, 2007; Pizzuti et al., 2003; Sarkozy et al., 2005a).

PROSIT240

A gene related to the thyroid hormone receptor–associated protein (TRAP) gene on 12q24 was disrupted by a translocation breakpoint in a single patient with d-TGA and mental retardation. The gene was named PROSIT240 (protein similar to TRAP240). Mutational screening of 97 additional patients with d-TGA revealed several sequence variants, including three missense mutations, which were not detected in controls. *PROSIT240* is strongly expressed in the heart and brain. Three missense mutations (Glu251Gly, Arg1872His, and Asp2023Gly) found in the patient cohort could not be identified in 400 control chromosomes. Finding the mutation in a healthy parent can also be explained by incomplete penetrance, which has been previously reported in CHD (e.g., in ZIC3; see earlier section). Detecting three missense mutations and one gene interruption (leading to haploinsufficiency) in d-TGA patients strongly suggests a contribution of *PROSIT240* to heart development. The putative relatedness of *PROSIT240* to *TRAP240* could point to an involvement of the TRAP complex. The *Drosophila* homologs of *TRAP240* and *TRAP230* were shown to act together to control cell affinity to establish cell boundaries, a process that might also be relevant to our observation relating *PROSIT240* malfunction to d-TGA. Pitx2 and Dvl mutant mice present with outflow tract abnormalities, including TGA and laterality defects. Both genes are part of the Wnt/Dvl/catenin/Pitx2 pathway, which was shown to recruit TRAP components. Ablation of murine *TRAP220*, for example, has been shown to result in impaired heart and nervous system development. Thyroid hormone and its receptor TR, for example, play key roles in the development of the central nervous system. An important role for related nuclear receptors in cardiac morphogenesis is clearly demonstrated by RXR α and RXR/RAR double mutants, which display outflow tract malformations and abnormalities of the great arteries.

TBX1

TBX1 is deleted in 22q11 deletion syndrome, the most common genetic deletion syndrome in humans. *TBX1* is required for proper development of the anterior heart progenitor population (the anterior second heart field) that contributes cardiomyocytes, smooth muscle, and endothelial cells to the outflow tract and the right ventricle. *TBX1* is a member of a phylogenetically conserved family of genes that share a common DNA-binding domain, the T-box. Like the related Xenopus T protein (Xbra), *TBX1* was shown to bind a palindromic T oligonucleotide as a dimer. Deletion 22q11.2 is a major cause of CVMs, accounting for about 3% of all heart defects. Since only about 70% of patients with 22q11 deletion have a heart defect, Rauch et al. (2004). investigated whether mutations, variants, or common haplotypes within the remaining *TBX1* gene could play a role in the heart phenotype in patients with 22q11.2 deletion. They detected nine rare variants within the remaining *TBX1* copy in 174 patients with the deletion—in deletion patients

both with and without CHDs. Mutational analysis of a total of 162 patients without deletion initially failed to identify pathogenically significant alterations in the human homolog *TBX1* (Conti et al., 2003). Only in 2003, by the screening of tenten patients with DGS/VCFS without deletion, Yagi et al. (2003) identified missense mutations in two patients with sporadic disease and one truncation mutation segregating in a family with the characteristic 22q11.2 deletion phenotype. The truncation mutation was shown to result in loss of function due to the deletion of a C-terminal nuclear localization signal of *TBX1*. This mutation and a novel C-terminal truncating mutation identified in another family with the DGS/VCFS phenotype were also shown to result in lack of activation in a transcriptional chloramphenicol acetyltransferase–reporter assay. To date only five mutations in *TBX1* have been identified in children with features of velocardiofacial syndrome and no deletion of 22q11 (Gong et al., 2001; Kantarci and Donahoe, 2007; Yagi et al., 2003; Zweier et al., 2007). Functional analyses suggest that several of these mutations may lead to increased transcriptional activity of *TBX1* (Zweier et al., 2007). If these mutations do lead to misregulation of *TBX1* expression in the early embryo it would support the concept already emerging from the mouse model, that any imbalance of TBX1 activity (i.e., dosage sensitivity) will lead to similar phenotypic manifestations. Although the question has not been extensively investigated, there is no definitive evidence for *TBX1* mutations in nonsyndromic forms of common outflow tract malformations (Cabuk et al., 2007; Gong et al., 2001).

NOTCH SIGNALING

NOTCH1

Notch signaling is a conserved molecular network that controls cell-fate decisions in the axial skeleton, immune system, muscle, central nervous system, and vasculature. *NOTCH1* encodes a transmembrane protein that functions as a receptor and transcriptional cofactor to activate or repress specific downstream target genes. After binding to a delta-like (Dll1, Dll3 and Dll4) or serrate (Jag1, Jag2) ligand, the Notch transmembrane receptor undergoes a complex cleavage process, which releases its intracellular domain (NICD). The NICD then translocates into the nucleus, where it activates a transcription factor called RBPJk (also known as CBF1 or Su[H]) (Hansson et al., 2004). Using expression patterns as the guide, Notch is mainly active in the endocardium and outflow tract in the developing heart.

In the heart, *NOTCH1* controls the migration of cells from the endocardial cushions into the conotruncal cushions from which the aortic and pulmonary valves are formed. *NOTCH1* is highly expressed during the development of aortic valve where it probably influences the epithelial to mesenchymal transition. In addition to its role in cardiogenesis and valvulogenesis, the *NOTCH1* signaling pathway has a role in the development and maintenance of the aorta and other vessels. The mechanisms by which imbalance of NOTCH signaling causes CVMs are poorly understood. *Hes* and *Hey* transcription factor gene families are known targets of NOTCH signaling. *Hes* genes are mammalian homologs of the *Drosophila* genes *hairy* and *Enhancer of split* [*E(spl)*]. There are seven members in the Hes family (*Hes1–7*), although *Hes4* is absent in the mouse genome. During cardiogenesis *HeyL* cooperates with *Hey1* to permit epithelial to mesenchymal transition of endocardial cells to promote endocardial cushion development. As a consequence, a combined *Hey1/L* loss causes CHDs leading to cardiac failure shortly after birth (Fischer et al., 2007).

Garg et al. (2005) described a multiplex family affected with BAV and aortic valve calcification and stenosis. Linkage was demonstrated with a single locus on chromosome 9q34–35. DNA sequencing of *NOTCH1* revealed a heterozygous mutation that predicts a premature stop codon at amino acid position 1108 (p.R1108X). They also described a second family bearing a different NOTCH1 mutation that cosegregated with BAV but without independent evidence of linkage. Two other reports have associated rare NOTCH1 missense variants with BAV with or without late-onset aortic aneurysm (McKellar et al., 2007; Mohamed et al., 2006). Although BAV with aortic aneurysm is a well-recognized clinical disorder it has not been typically included in the category of CVMs. However, BAV is the most common congenital cardiac malformation, occurring in 1%–2% of the population. BAV shows familial clustering and occasional autosomal dominant inheritance pattern. Mohamed et al. (2006) reported two mutations in *NOTCH1* in 48 patients with sporadic BAV. Both mutation-positive subjects were affected with aortic aneurysm. McKellear et al. (2004) examined only four exons of *NOTCH1* in 24 individuals with BAV plus thoracic aortic aneurysm. They observed rare NOTCH1 missense variants in 5 of 48 BAV plus aortic aneurysm cases. When analyzed together, these studies can lead one to the conclusion that there is significant overrepresentation of *NOTCH1* missense mutations in BAV/TAA.

JAG1

The Notch ligand JAGGED1 (encoded *JAG1* in 20p) encodes a highly conserved protein that is expressed in the developing mammalian heart. Targeted disruption of *JAG1* in mice results in common outflow tract anomalies of cardiovascular development. JAG1 is a relatively large 1218 amino acid protein with an N-terminal "DSL" motif also found in the *delta and serrate*, Notch ligands, 16 epidermal growth factor (EGF)-like repeats; and a transmembrane region. The transmembrane domain anchors JAGGED1 protein such that Notch signaling takes place as a cell–cell interaction.

Mutations of the Notch ligand JAGGED1 (*JAG1*) are responsible for most cases of Alagille syndrome (Li et al., 1997; Oda et al., 1997), an autosomal dominant condition that causes biliary atresia, growth retardation, butterfly vertebra, posterior embryotoxon, and right-sided heart defects. Both hemizygosity for *JAG1* by chromosomal deletion and point mutations that create premature termination codons typically result in the full complex phenotype of Alagille syndrome. These observations demonstrate that haploinsufficiency with resulting imbalances of Notch signaling is the most likely mechanism.

Isolated right-sided heart lesions may also be caused by JAG1 mutation. TOF, with a birth prevalence rate of about 3 per 10,000, is the most common complex CVM. Rare families affected with isolated TOF have also been found to have mutations in *JAG1*. A *JAG1* missense mutation (G274D) was observed in 13 members of a single large kindred segregating TOF as an autosomal dominant trait with reduced penetrance. This particular mutation retains residual function given the lack of noncardiac phenotypes typical of Alagille syndrome.

TGF/BMP/NODAL SIGNALING

The transforming growth factor (TGF) superfamily is composed of a diverse group of growth and differentiation factors including TGFβ, activins, inhibins, and bone morphogenetic proteins (BMPs). TGFβ ligands bind to type I and type II receptors, which are transmembrane serine-threonine kinases, and their interaction leads to activation of cytoplasmic and nuclear Smad proteins. The type II receptors include BMPRII, ActRIIA, and ActRIIB. The type I receptor family has seven members—called activin-like kinases (ALKs) 1–7. Ligand binding to type II receptors induces phosphorylation and activation of the type I receptors. The activated forms of the type I receptors phosphorylate either Smad2,-3 or Smad1,-5,-8 depending on the ligand and receptor specificity. Altogether, there are eight Smad proteins: (a) receptor-activated Smads (R-Smads) including Smad1,-2,-3,-5, and -8; (b) the Smad nuclear co-activator, Smad4; and (c) inhibitory Smad (I-Smads) consisting of Smad6 and -7. TGFβ binding to type II receptors results in phosphorylation of Smad2 and -3, whereas BMP signaling affects Smad1,-5, and -8. Once activated, R-Smads the ratio of nuclear to cytoplasmic location increases. R-Smad/Smad4 complexes together with cotranscription factors such as FoxH1 in the nucleus where they directly regulate gene transcription.

This pathway integrates signaling not only from TGFβs and BMPs but also Nodal, which plays an essential role in early embryonic axis formation. In particular, Nodal is required in the left lateral plate mesoderm as an effector of left–right patterning. The EGF-CFC gene family, of which CFC1/CRYPTIC is a member, codes for extracellular proteins that are Nodal coreceptors. CFC1 is known to be essential in Nodal signaling in the lateral plate mesoderm. The Lefty proteins are additional members of the TGFβ family of cell-signaling molecules. Lefty1 and Lefty2 are asymmetrically expressed on the left side of the embryo in the floor-plate and in the lateral-plate mesoderm, respectively. Lefty1 and Lefty2 expression is controlled by Nodal and they, in turn, act as inhibitors of Nodal to limit its domain of activation. GDF1 is another member of the activin subclass of TGFβ signaling molecules, which has been shown to play a role upstream of the left signaling cascade. Members of the TGFβ/BMP signaling pathway are particularly important in vasculogenesis and embryonic heart development. After binding BMPs, heterodimers of BMPR2 form a heterotetrameric complex with the type-1 receptors, ALK3 and ALK6. Mouse mutants of virtually all of these TGFβ class receptors and signaling molecule exhibit complex cardiac malformations that are highly similar to those observed in humans.

CFC1

Several patients with heterotaxy syndrome exhibited heterozygous CFC1 mutations, all of whom had congenital cardiac malformations (Bamford et al., 2000). The clinical phenotype of these subjects included dextrocardia, d-TGA, common atrioventricular canal, and venous anomalies. In another mutation study, a total of three heterozygous sequence alterations were identified in d-TGA and DORV patients (Goldmuntz et al., 2002). A single-base-pair deletion (G174 del1) was identified in one subject with sporadic DORV. This mutation had previously been reported in two patients with heterotaxy syndrome but was not identified in 200 normal chromosomes. These examples demonstrate that isolated TGA or DORV can be part of the same phenotypic spectrum that includes heterotaxy. Thus, some patients with isolated TGA or DORV may have a forme fruste of a laterality disorder confined to malpositioning of the great vessels, without overt noncardiac laterality defects. Because high-level Nodal

expression in the lateral plate mesoderm is dependent on amplification through a positive feedback loop, Nodal signaling may be particularly sensitive to gene dosage effects.

LEFTY-A

Human LEFTY-A and LEFTY-B are more closely related to each other than to either of the mouse homologs, Lefty1 and Lefty2, suggesting that some mechanism such as recent duplication or gene conversion acted after the divergence of the mouse and human common ancestor. Two mutations in LEFTY-A were identified in patients with left–right patterning defects. One mutation led to a premature termination codon and would be predicted to be null for protein expression. The S342K missense substitution occurred in the cysteine-knot region, a portion of the secreted protein thought to be directly involved in receptor binding. The phenotypes of the two individuals with LEFTY-A mutations were similar to those seen in the Lefty1-deficient mice, that is, left pulmonary isomerism, cardiac malformations characterized by complete atrioventricular canal defect and hypoplastic left ventricle, and interrupted inferior vena cava. This constellation of findings is most typically associated with polysplenia and is interpreted as indicating failure of right side patterning or failure to restrict the left side patterning signal at the midline.

ACVR2B

Several patients with mutations in the NODAL type II receptor ACVR2B have also been reported. Although the study did not include functional analyses, the mutations occurred in highly conserved positions within the ligand-binding domain and were not found in a large number of matched controls. Unlike the LEFTY-A patients, there was no obvious genotype–phenotype correlation. Rather than right side or left side dominance, each of the three affected patients had malformations suggesting randomized left–right axis specification. One patient had l-TGA, a lesion that strongly implies defective looping of the cardiac tube during ventricular development. This resulted in discordance of both the atrioventricular and ventriculoarterial relationships.

NODAL

Mutations in NODAL itself were suspected to cause heterotaxy or related isolated CHDs. A more extensive study has recently demonstrated that NODAL mutations likely play a role in isolated TOF, as well (Roessler et al., 2008). In a case-control study a large excess of NODAL missense substitutions were observed in both TOF patients and patients with laterality defects compared to controls. This study also demonstrated functional variants in the NODAL signaling pathway coactivator, FOXH1. A recent study of NODAL missense variants found in subjects with heterotaxy confirmed that the mutated forms of NODAL have reduced signaling activity (Mohapatra et al., 2009), further confirming a role for the NODAL pathway albeit with complex inheritance.

GDF-1

Gdf1 requires the coreceptor Cfc1 to activate the type II receptor ActRIIB making GDF1 a strong candidate gene for human mutation in complex CVMs. Karkera et al., demonstrate mutations in patients with isolated CHDs. The phenotypes observed with the GDF1 loss-of-function mutations are consistent with a model of disturbed left-right patterning, with incomplete establishment of left-sided identity. Patients with TGA, DORV, stenosis of the left pulmonary artery, atrioventricular canal defect, and TOF were observed. These findings are consistent with the emerging picture of overlap between conotruncal malformations, such as d-TGA, DORV, and TOF, and lesions that are more typical of cardiac looping defect, such as complex atrioventricular canal and l-TGA.

BMPR2

BMP2R mutations have recently been found to underlie rare dominant forms of primary pulmonary hypertension. Five percent to ten percent of idiopathic pulmonary hypertension can be attributed to BMPR2 mutation. Because pulmonary hypertension may complicate a variety of CVMs, BMP2R mutation analysis was undertaken in patients with such combined disorders. Forty adults and 66 children with combined disease were tested. Six percent of these patients had a missense variant that was not observed in controls. Three adults with atrioventricular canal, one of whom had Down syndrome, were found to have a mutation. Children were observed with ASD, patent ductus arteriosus (PDA), and partial anomalous pulmonary venous return.

SMOOTH MUSCLE CELL FUNCTION AND CELL ADHESION

MYH6

A genome-wide linkage screen in a large family with dominantly inherited ASDASD and no other cardiac abnormalities demonstrated linkage to MYH6.

Sequencing identified a single nucleotide change in all affected family members. This mutation causes the missense substitution I820N in the MYH6 protein. Amino acid 820 is conserved in type II myosins across all species examined.

MYH11

One American and one French kindred were identified in which aneurysm of the ascending aorta was associated with PDA. Genetic analysis of six members of the American kindred confirmed cosegregation with region including the MYH11 locus. Mutation screening in both families showed two heterozygous mutations affecting the same allele in the French kindred (Figure 26–1). The first was a substitution at the splice-donor site of intron 32 (IVS32+1GT). The second was a missense mutation in exon 37 (G5361A), resulting in a charged amino acid, arginine, being replaced by an uncharged amino acid, glutamine (R1758Q). Both mutations were identified in all subjects carrying the disease haplotype, but neither was found in 340 normal chromosomes. A similar search for mutations in the American kindred detected a 72-nucleotide deletion within exon 28 of the MYH11 gene (3810_3881del). The MYH11 mutations may affect its coiled-coil structure and the assembly of myosin thick filaments. The question of whether the MYH11 gene was a susceptibility gene for sporadic occurrence of isolated persistent patency of the arterial duct was then investigated. The entire coding sequence of the MYH11 gene was sequenced in 60 white children with PDA. Two possible functional missense mutations were found in two affected individuals. One of the seven major MYH11 haplotypes was significantly less frequent among cases than among controls (7% vs. 22%; odds ratio [OR] 0.23; confidence interval [CI] 0.08–0.27). This observation has not yet been confirmed in an independent sample.

ACTC1

Linkage analysis in two large families segregating autosomal-dominant isolated ASD identified a chromosome 15q13–q21 locus (Matsson et al., 2008). Mutations in alpha-cardiac actin (ACTC1), which is the predominant actin in embryonic heart, were detected in each family. There was marked clinical variability from an asymptomatic shunt to a severe heart failure, but none of the affected were diagnosed with cardiomyopathy. Another study by Monserrat et al., however, identified septal defects in some individuals with cardiomyopathy and ACTC1 mutations.

ACTC1 is the only actin in the embryonic heart muscle. ACTC1 is the major component of the sarcomeric thin filaments where it interacts with two actin monomers along the cardiac filament structure (F-actin). Mice lacking cardiac actin do not survive more than 2 weeks. Hearts are apparently normal at the level of gross morphology, but increased apoptosis was found in the atrial and ventricular walls at fetal day 17. In BALB/c mice, a duplication of the promoter and three first exons result in a reduced cardiac actin expression and abnormally high accumulation of the skeletal actin transcripts.

Elastin (ELN)

One of the first genes associated with any form of nonsyndromic CVM was reported in 1993. A translocation t(6;7)(p21.1;q11.23) that cosegregated with autosomal dominant supravalvular aortic stenosis (SVAS) was found to disrupt the elastin gene. The breakpoint was localized to exon 28 of the gene. Metcalfe et al., described 35 unrelated patients with SVAS who also had mutations in the elastin gene but obvious genotype–phenotype correlation was detected. Missense or splicing mutations were as likely to have severe SVAS as cases with truncating mutations, indicating that imbalanced elastin expression either through haploinsufficiency or through abnormal protein interactions could lead to progressive aortic stenosis in these patients.

CRELD1

One large family has been characterized in which atrioventricular canal type septal defects map to chromosome 1p31-p21. This locus has been named AVSD1, but the gene responsible has not yet been identified. AVSD1 segregates as a typical autosomal dominant trait with incomplete penetrance. A second locus, termed AVSD2, has been attributed to a position in 3p25. In a survey of 12 patients with 3p25 deletion syndrome, CRELD1 gene was deleted in all five patients with a CVM. Based on these observations, Robinson et al., chose CRELD1 as a candidate gene for this class of CVMs. They found heterozygous mutations in CRELD1 gene in 3/50 patients. One mutation, R329C, occurs in the second cb-EGF domain and is predicted to disrupt the disulfide-bonding pattern. Another mutation, T311I, affects the second cb-EGF domain, perhaps emphasizing the functional importance of these units.

A third heterozygous missense mutation occurred in a patient with heart defects suggestive of disrupted left–right patterning—dextrocardia, right ventricle aorta with pulmonary atresia, and a right aortic arch. Zatyka et al., identified four missense variants in the CRELD1 gene among 49 subjects but three were also identified in normal controls. However, Posch et al., (2008) excluded mutation of CRELD1 in 170 subjects with secundum ASD.

MULTIFACTORIAL INHERITANCE

Genetic epidemiology studies and modeling have strongly suggested multifactorial inheritance as a cause of CVMs. Many studies have shown statistical association of nonsyndromic cardiac defects with common variants in various genes. Several studies have implicated gene–environment interactions and a potential role for folate metabolism through methylenetetrahydrofolate reductase (MTHFR) polymorphisms. Other studies of MTHFR have given negative results. All of these studies have been quite small and would have had very low power to detect true associations. None of the positive associations has been replicated. At this time the field awaits well-powered studies with adequate attention to the increased probability of false positives introduced by multiple testing and with replication of potentially positive findings.

WHY ARE CARDIOVASCULAR MALFORMATIONS SO COMMON?

A major problem for the field is to explain why severe CVMs are so common. The frequency of these conditions seems to run counter to our intuition that variation in such a crucial developmental process would not be tolerated. There are several potential explanations.

Dosage Sensitivity

Developmental pathways are exquisitely sensitive to the amount of gene product available at specific times and in very specific locations in the embryo. Even mild increases or decreases can lead to a cascade of problems that result in a birth defect. Many other gene pathways not directly involved in organ development are much more tolerant of deficiencies or other variation.

Large Mutation Target

Another potential explanation is that there could be many genes that when mutated result in a heart malformation. We know from the study of animal models that more than 300 genes are required for normal heart development. Because heart development is so complex, it may be that mutations in a large number of different genes could potentially cause a heart malformation. Even though mutations in each individual gene might be quite rare, the large number of potential genetic faults might make defects very common.

Genetic Loci with High Mutation Rates

We know of a few examples of parts of the genetic material that experience much *higher mutation rates* than the average across the genome. The frequent loss of one copy of the *TBX1* gene (which causes the velocardiofacial syndrome in about 1 in 4000 live born children) is an example of this mechanism. If there are more such genomic regions that have yet to be uncovered, they might be contributing to a substantial fraction of total cases.

The Frequency of Gene Variants that Contribute to Cardiovascular Malformation

Finally, we have to consider the frequency of gene variants that contribute to CVMs. Common genetic variants may have a weak effect in raising the individual's chance of having a heart malformation. The fraction of individuals who have a specific trait when they carry a particular gene variant is called the *penetrance*. Common variants can contribute to a trait but have very low penetrance values. But because such variants are common they can account for a large number of cases. This is called the *attributable fraction* and it is a function both of the magnitude of the risk increase (i.e., the penetrance), which can be quite small, and of the frequency of the variant, which could occur in 5%–95% of the population.

REFERENCES

Abushaban L, Uthaman B, Kumar AR, Selvan J. Familial truncus arteriosus: a possible autosomal-recessive trait. *Pediatr Cardiol.* 2003;24:64–66.

Ackerman KG, Herron BJ, Vargas SO, et al. Fog2 is required for normal diaphragm and lung development in mice and humans. *PLoS Genet.* 2005;1:58–65.

Allan LD, Crawford DC, Chita SK, Anderson RH, Tynan MJ. Familial recurrence of congenital heart disease in a prospective series of mothers referred for fetal echocardiography. *Am J Cardiol.* 1986;58:334–337.

Aruga J, Nagai T, Tokuyama T, et al. The mouse zic gene family. Homologues of the Drosophila pair-rule gene odd-paired. *J Biol Chem.* 1996;271:1043–1047.

Bamford RN, Roessler E, Burdine RD, et al. Loss-of-function mutations in the EGF-CFC gene CFC1 are associated with human left-right laterality defects. *Nat Genet.* 2000;26:365–369.

Barber JC, Maloney VK, Huang S, et al. 8p23.1 duplication syndrome; a novel genomic condition with unexpected complexity revealed by array CGH. *Eur J Hum Genet.* 2008;16:18–27.

Becker SM, Al Halees Z, Molina C, Paterson RM. Consanguinity and congenital heart disease in Saudi Arabia. *Am J Med Genet.* 2001;99:8–13.

Benson DW, Silberbach GM, Kavanaugh-McHugh A, et al. Mutations in the cardiac transcription factor NKX2.5 affect diverse cardiac developmental pathways. *J Clin Invest.* 1999;104:1567–1573.

Biben C, Harvey RP. Homeodomain factor Nkx2-5 controls left/right asymmetric expression of bHLH gene eHand during murine heart development. *Genes Dev.* 1997;11:1357–1369.

Bleyl SB, Moshrefi A, Shaw GM, et al. Candidate genes for congenital diaphragmatic hernia from animal models: sequencing of FOG2 and PDGFRalpha reveals rare variants in diaphragmatic hernia patients. *Eur J Hum Genet.* 2007;15:950–958.

Boon AR, Roberts DF. A family study of coarctation of the aorta. *J Med Genet.* 1976;13:420–433.

Brassington AM, Sung SS, Toydemir RM, et al. Expressivity of Holt-Oram syndrome is not predicted by TBX5 genotype. *Am J Hum Genet.* 2003;73:74–85.

Cabuk F, Karabulut HG, Tuncali T, Karademir S, Bozdayi M, Tukun A. TBX1 gene mutation screening in patients with nonsyndromic Fallot tetralogy. *Turk J Pediatr.* 2007;49:61–68.

Calcagni G, Digilio MC, Sarkozy A, Dallapiccola B, Marino B. Familial recurrence of congenital heart disease: an overview and review of the literature. *Eur J Pediatr.* 2007;166:111–116.

Chen CY, Schwartz RJ. Identification of novel DNA binding targets and regulatory domains of a murine tinman homeodomain factor, nkx-2.5. *J Biol Chem.* 1995;270:15628–15633.

Ching YH, Ghosh TK, Cross SJ, et al. Mutation in myosin heavy chain 6 causes atrial septal defect. *Nat Genet.* 2005;37:423–428.

Clementi M, Notari L, Borghi A, Tenconi R. Familial congenital bicuspid aortic valve: a disorder of uncertain inheritance. *Am J Med Genet.* 1996;62:336–338.

Conti E, Grifone N, Sarkozy A, et al. DiGeorge subtypes of nonsyndromic conotruncal defects: evidence against a major role of TBX1 gene. *Eur J Hum Genet.* 2003;11:349–351.

Corone P, Bonaiti C, Feingold J, Fromont S, Berthet-Bondet D. Familial congenital heart disease: how are the various types related? *Am J Cardiol.* 1983;51:942–945.

Cripe L, Andelfinger G, Martin LJ, Shooner K, Benson DW. Bicuspid aortic valve is heritable. *J Am Coll Cardiol.* 2004;44:138–143.

Crispino JD, Lodish MB, Thurberg BL, et al. Proper coronary vascular development and heart morphogenesis depend on interaction of GATA-4 with FOG cofactors. *Genes Dev.* 2001;15:839–844.

Czeizel A, Meszaros M. Two family studies of children with ventricular septal defect. *Eur J Pediatr.* 1981;136:81–85.

Digilio MC, Casey B, Toscano A, et al. Complete transposition of the great arteries: patterns of congenital heart disease in familial precurrence. *Circulation.* 2001;104:2809–2814.

Durocher D, Charron F, Warren R, Schwartz RJ, Nemer M. The cardiac transcription factors Nkx2-5 and GATA-4 are mutual cofactors. *Embo J.* 1997;16:5687–5696.

Ehlers KH, Engle MA. Familial congenital heart disease. I. Genetic and environmental factors. *Circulation.* 1966;34:503–516.

Eldadah ZA, Hamosh A, Biery NJ, Montgomery RA, Duke M, Elkins R, Dietz HC. Familial Tetralogy of Fallot caused by mutation in the jagged1 gene. *Hum Mol Genet.* 2001;10:163–169.

Elliott DA, Kirk EP, Yeoh T, et al. Cardiac homeobox gene NKX2-5 mutations and congenital heart disease: associations with atrial septal defect and hypoplastic left heart syndrome. *J Am Coll Cardiol.* 2003;41:2072–2076.

Ferencz C, Boughman JA, Neill CA, Brenner JI, Perry LW. Congenital cardiovascular malformations: questions on inheritance. Baltimore-Washington Infant Study Group. *J Am Coll Cardiol.* 1989;14:756–763.

Fischer A, Steidl C, Wagner TU, et al. Combined loss of Hey1 and HeyL causes congenital heart defects because of impaired epithelial to mesenchymal transition. *Circ Res.* 2007;100:856–863.

Freire-Maia N, Arce-Gomez B. The epidemiology of congenital cardiovascular malformations. *Hum Hered.* 1971;21:209–215.

Garg V. Molecular genetics of aortic valve disease. *Curr Opin Cardiol.* 2006;21:180–184.

Garg V, Kathiriya IS, Barnes R, et al. GATA4 mutations cause human congenital heart defects and reveal an interaction with TBX5. *Nature.* 2003;424:443–447.

Garg V, Muth AN, Ransom JF, Schluterman MK, Barnes R, King IN, Grossfeld PD, et al. Mutations in NOTCH1 cause aortic valve disease. *Nature.* 2005;437:270–274.

Gebbia M, Ferrero GB, Pilia G, et al. X-linked situs abnormalities result from mutations in ZIC3. *Nat Genet.* 1997;17:305–308.

Goldmuntz E, Bamford R, Karkera JD, dela Cruz J, Roessler E, Muenke M. CFC1 mutations in patients with transposition of the great arteries and double-outlet right ventricle. *Am J Hum Genet.* 2002;70:776–780.

Goldmuntz E, Geiger E, Benson DW. NKX2.5 mutations in patients with tetralogy of fallot. *Circulation.* 2001;104:2565–2568.

Gong W, Gottlieb S, Collins J, et al. Mutation analysis of TBX1 in non-deleted patients with features of DGS/VCFS or isolated cardiovascular defects. *J Med Genet.* 2001;38:E45.

Gutierrez-Roelens I, Sluysmans T, Gewillig M, Devriendt K, Vikkula M. Progressive AV-block and anomalous venous return among cardiac anomalies associated with two novel missense mutations in the CSX/NKX2-5 gene. *Hum Mutat.* 2002;20: 75–76.

Hansson EM, Lendahl U, Chapman G. Notch signaling in development and disease. *Semin Cancer Biol.* 2004;14:320–328.

Heathcote K, Braybrook C, Abushaban L, et al. Common arterial trunk associated with a homeodomain mutation of NKX2.6. *Hum Mol Genet.* 2005;14:585–593.

Hinton RB, Jr., Martin LJ, Tabangin ME, Mazwi ML, Cripe LH, Benson DW. Hypoplastic left heart syndrome is heritable. *J Am Coll Cardiol.* 2007;50:1590–1595.

Hirayama-Yamada K, Kamisago M, et al. Phenotypes with GATA4 or NKX2.5 mutations in familial atrial septal defect. *Am J Med Genet.* A 2005;135:47–52.

Hoffman JI. Incidence of congenital heart disease: I. Postnatal incidence. *Pediatr Cardiol* 1995a;16:103–113.

Hoffman JI. Incidence of congenital heart disease: II. Prenatal incidence. *Pediatr Cardiol* 1995b;16:155–165.

Hoffman JI, Kaplan S. The incidence of congenital heart disease. *J Am Coll Cardiol.* 2002;39:1890–1900.

Hoffman JI, Kaplan S, Liberthson RR. Prevalence of congenital heart disease. *Am Heart J.* 2004;147:425–439.

Hosoda T, Komuro I, Shiojima I, et al. Familial atrial septal defect and atrioventricular conduction disturbance associated with a point mutation in the cardiac homeobox gene CSX/NKX2-5 in a Japanese patient. *Jpn Circ J.* 1999;63:425–426.

Kantarci S, Donahoe PK. Congenital diaphragmatic hernia (CDH) etiology as revealed by pathway genetics. *Am J Med Genet.* C Semin Med Genet 2007;145C:217–226.

Karkera JD, Lee JS, Roessler E. Loss-of-function mutations in growth differentiation factor-1 (GDF1) are associated with congenital heart defects in humans. *Am J Hum Genet.* 2007;81: 987–994.

Kirk EP, Sunde M, Costa MW, et al. Mutations in cardiac T-box factor gene TBX20 are associated with diverse cardiac pathologies, including defects of septation and valvulogenesis and cardiomyopathy. *Am J Hum Genet.* 2007;81:280–291.

Konig K, Will JC, Berger F, Muller D, Benson DW. Familial congenital heart disease, progressive atrioventricular block and the cardiac homeobox transcription factor gene NKX2.5: identification of a novel mutation. *Clin Res Cardiol.* 2006;95:499–503.

Kraus F, Haenig B, Kispert A. Cloning and expression analysis of the mouse T-box gene tbx20. *Mech Dev.* 2001;100:87–91.

Kumar A, Williams CA, Victorica BE. Familial atrioventricular septal defect: possible genetic mechanisms. *Br Heart J.* 1994;71:79–81.

Kwiatkowska J, Wierzba J, Aleszewicz-Baranowska J, Erecinski J. Genetic background of congenital conotruncal heart defects – a study of 45 families. *Kardiol Pol.* 2007;65:32–37; discussion 38–39.

Li L, Krantz ID, Deng Y, et al. Alagille syndrome is caused by mutations in human Jagged1, which encodes a ligand for Notch1. *Nat Genet.* 1997;16:243–251.

Lints TJ, Parsons LM, Hartley L, Lyons I, Harvey RP. Nkx-2.5: a novel murine homeobox gene expressed in early heart progenitor cells and their myogenic descendants. *Development.* 1993;119:969.

Loffredo CA, Chokkalingam A, Sill AM, et al. Prevalence of congenital cardiovascular malformations among relatives of infants with hypoplastic left heart, coarctation of the aorta, and d-transposition of the great arteries. *Am J Med Genet.* A 2004;124:225–230.

Lyons I, Parsons LM, Hartley L, Li R, Andrews JE, Robb L, Harvey RP. Myogenic and morphogenetic defects in the heart tubes of murine embryos lacking the homeo box gene Nkx2-5. *Genes Dev.* 1995;9:1654–1666.

Maestri NE, Beaty TH, Boughman JA. Etiologic heterogeneity in the familial aggregation of congenital cardiovascular malformations. *Am J Hum Genet.* 1989;45:556–564.

Maslen CL. Molecular genetics of atrioventricular septal defects. *Curr Opin Cardiol.* 2004;19:205–210.

Matsson H, Eason J, Bookwalter CS, et al. Alpha-cardiac actin mutations produce atrial septal defects. *Hum Mol Genet.* 2008;17:256–265.

Mathias RS, Lacro RV, Jones KL. X-linked laterality sequence: situs inversus, complex cardiac defects, splenic defects. *Am J Med Genet.* 1987;28:111–116.

McBride KL, Pignatelli R, Lewin M, et al. Inheritance analysis of congenital left ventricular outflow tract obstruction malformations: Segregation, multiplex relative risk, and heritability. *Am J Med Genet.* A 2005;134:180–186.

McElhinney DB, Geiger E, Blinder J, Benson DW, Goldmuntz E. NKX2.5 mutations in patients with congenital heart disease. *J Am Coll Cardiol.* 2003;42:1650–1655.

McKellar SH, Tester DJ, Yagubyan M, Majumdar R, Ackerman MJ, Sundt TM, 3rd. Novel NOTCH1 mutations in patients with bicuspid aortic valve disease and thoracic aortic aneurysms. *J Thorac Cardiovasc Surg.* 2007;134:290–296.

Megarbane A, Salem N, Stephan E, et al. X-linked transposition of the great arteries and incomplete penetrance among males with a nonsense mutation in ZIC3. *Eur J Hum Genet.* 2000;8:704–708.

Metcalfe K, Rucka AK, Smoot L, Hofstadler G, et al. Elastin: mutational spectrum in supravalvular aortic stenosis. *Eur J Hum Gene.t* 2000;8(12):955–963.

Mizugishi K, Aruga J, Nakata K, Mikoshiba K. Molecular properties of Zic proteins as transcriptional regulators and their relationship to GLI proteins. *J Biol Chem.* 2001;276:2180–2188.

Mohamed SA, Aherrahrou Z, Liptau H, et al. Novel missense mutations (p.T596M and p.P1797H) in NOTCH1 in patients with bicuspid aortic valve. *Biochem Biophys Res Commun.* 2006;345:1460–1465.

Mohapatra B, Casey B, Li H, et al. Identification and functional characterization of NODAL rare variants in heterotaxy and isolated cardiovascular malformations. *Hum Mol Genet.* 2009;18:861–871.

Monserrat L, Hermida-Prieto M, Fernandez X, et al. Mutation in the alpha-cardiac actin gene associated with apical hypertrophic cardiomyopathy, left ventricular non-compaction, and septal defects. *Eur Heart J.* 2007;28(16):1953–1961.

Movahed MR, Hepner AD, Ahmadi-Kashani M. Echocardiographic prevalence of bicuspid aortic valve in the population. *Heart Lung Circ.* 2006;15:297–299.

Nabulsi MM, Tamim H, Sabbagh M, Obeid MY, Yunis KA, Bitar FF. Parental consanguinity and congenital heart malformations in a developing country. *Am J Med Genet.* A 2003;116A:342–347.

Nemer G, Fadlalah F, Usta J, et al. A novel mutation in the GATA4 gene in patients with Tetralogy of Fallot. *Hum Mutat.* 2006;27:293–294.

Nicolae MI, Summers KM, Radford DJ. Familial muscular ventricular septal defects and aneurysms of the muscular interventricular septum. *Cardiol Young.* 2007;17:523–527.

Nistri S, Basso C, Marzari C, Mormino P, Thiene G. Frequency of bicuspid aortic valve in young male conscripts by echocardiogram. *Am J Cardiol.* 2005;96:718–721.

Nora JJ, Meyer TC. Familial nature of congenital heart diseases. *Pediatrics.* 1966;37:329–334.

Nora JJ, Nora AH. Genetic and environmental factors in the etiology of congenital heart diseases. *South Med J.* 1976;69:919–926.

Oda T, Elkahloun AG, Pike BL, et al. Mutations in the human Jagged1 gene are responsible for Alagille syndrome. *Nat Genet.* 1997;16:235–242.

Pacileo G, Musewe NN, Calabro R. Tetralogy of Fallot in three siblings: a familial study and review of the literature. *Eur J Pediatr.* 1992;151:726–727.

Paez MT, Yamamoto T, Hayashi K, et al. Two patients with atypical interstitial deletions of 8p23.1: mapping of phenotypical traits. *Am J Med Genet.* A 2008;146A:1158–1165.

Pandit B, Sarkozy A, Pennacchio LA, et al. Gain-of-function RAF1 mutations cause Noonan and LEOPARD syndromes with hypertrophic cardiomyopathy. *Nat Genet.* 2007;39:1007–1012.

Pehlivan T, Pober BR, Brueckner M, et al. GATA4 haploinsufficiency in patients with interstitial deletion of chromosome region 8p23.1 and congenital heart disease. *Am J Med Genet.* 1999;83:201–206.

Piacentini G, Digilio MC, Capolino R, et al. Familial recurrence of heart defects in subjects with congenitally corrected transposition of the great arteries. *Am J Med Genet.* A 2005;137:176–180.

Pizzuti A, Sarkozy A, Newton AL, et al. Mutations of ZFPM2/FOG2 gene in sporadic cases of tetralogy of Fallot. *Hum Mutat.* 2003;22:372–377.

Plageman TF, Jr., Yutzey KE. T-box genes and heart development: putting the "T" in heart. *Dev Dyn.* 2005;232:11–20.

Posch MG, Perrot A, Schmitt K, et al. Mutations in GATA4, NKX2.5, CRELD1, and BMP4 are infrequently found in patients with congenital cardiac septal defects. *Am J Med Genet.* A 2008;146A:251–253.

Pradat P, Francannet C, Harris JA, Robert E. The epidemiology of cardiovascular defects, part I: a study based on data from three large registries of congenital malformations. *Pediatr Cardiol* 2003;24:195–221.

Purandare SM, Ware SM, Kwan KM, et al. A complex syndrome of left-right axis, central nervous system and axial skeleton defects in Zic3 mutant mice. *Development.* 2002;129:2293–2302.

Rajagopal SK, Ma Q, Obler D, et al. Spectrum of heart disease associated with murine and human GATA4 mutation. *J Mol Cell Cardiol.* 2007;43:677–685.

Ramegowda S, Ramachandra NB. Parental consanguinity increases congenital heart diseases in South India. *Ann Hum Biol.* 2006;33:519–528.

Rauch A, Devriendt K, Koch A, et al. Assessment of association between variants and haplotypes of the remaining TBX1 gene and manifestations of congenital heart defects in 22q11.2 deletion patients. *J Med Genet.* 2004;41(4):e40.

Razzaque MA, Nishizawa T, Komoike Y, et al. Germline gain-of-function mutations in RAF1 cause Noonan syndrome. *Nat Genet.* 2007;39:1013–1017.

Robinson SW, Morris CD, Goldmuntz E, et al. Missense mutations in CRELD1 are associated with cardiac atrioventricular septal defects. *Am J Hum Genet.* 2003;72(4):1047–1052.

Roessler E, Ouspenskaia MV, Karkera JD, et al. Reduced NODAL signaling strength via mutation of several pathway members including FOXH1 is linked to human heart defects and holoprosencephaly. *Am J Hum Genet.* 2008;83:18–29.

Roguin N, Du ZD, Barak M, Nasser N, Hershkowitz S, Milgram E. High prevalence of muscular ventricular septal defect in neonates. *J Am Coll Cardiol.* 1995;26:1545–1548.

Romano-Zelekha O, Hirsh R, Blieden L, Green M, Shohat T. The risk for congenital heart defects in offspring of individuals with congenital heart defects. *Clin Genet.* 2001;59:325–329.

Salvador J, Borrell A, Lladonosa A. Increasing detection rates of birth defects by prenatal ultrasound leading to apparent increasing prevalence. Lessons learned from the population-based registry of birth defects of Barcelona. *Prenat Diagn.* 2005;25:991–996.

Sarkozy A, Conti E, D'Agostino R, et al. ZFPM2/FOG2 and HEY2 genes analysis in nonsyndromic tricuspid atresia. *Am J Med Genet.* A 2005a;133A:68–70.

Sarkozy A, Conti E, Neri C, et al. Spectrum of atrial septal defects associated with mutations of NKX2.5 and GATA4 transcription factors. *J Med Genet.* 2005b;42:e16.

Sarkozy A, Esposito G, Conti E, et al. CRELD1 and GATA4 gene analysis in patients with nonsyndromic atrioventricular canal defects. *Am J Med Genet.* A 2005c;139:236–238.

Satoda M, Zhao F, Diaz GA, et al. Mutations in TFAP2B cause Char syndrome, a familial form of patent ductus arteriosus. *Nat Genet.* 2000;25:42–46.

Schluterman MK, Krysiak AE, Kathiriya IS, et al. Screening and biochemical analysis of GATA4 sequence variations identified in patients with congenital heart disease. *Am J Med Genet.* A 2007;143A:817–823.

Schott JJ, Benson DW, Basson CT, et al. Congenital heart disease caused by mutations in the transcription factor NKX2–5. *Science* 1998;281:108–111.

Schubbert S, Zenker M, Rowe SL, et al. Germline KRAS mutations cause Noonan syndrome. *Nat Genet.* 2006;38:331–336.

Scott JS, Niebuhr DW. Hypoplastic left heart syndrome in US military family members: trends in intervention, survival, and prevalence. *Congenit Heart Dis.* 2007;2:19–26.

Sheffield VC, Pierpont ME, Nishimura D, et al. Identification of a complex congenital heart defect susceptibility locus by using DNA pooling and shared segment analysis. *Hum Mol Genet.* 1997;6:117–121.

Singh MK, Christoffels VM, Dias JM, et al. Tbx20 is essential for cardiac chamber differentiation and repression of Tbx2. *Development.* 2005;132:2697–2707.

Stennard FA, Costa MW, Elliott DA, et al. Cardiac T-box factor Tbx20 directly interacts with Nkx2–5, GATA4, and GATA5 in regulation of gene expression in the developing heart. *Dev Biol* 2003;262:206–224.

Stennard FA, Harvey RP. T-box transcription factors and their roles in regulatory hierarchies in the developing heart. *Development.* 2005;132:4897–4910.

Tanaka M, Schinke M, Liao HS, Yamasaki N, Izumo S. Nkx2.5 and Nkx2.6, homologs of Drosophila tinman, are required for development of the pharynx. *Mol Cell Biol.* 2001;21:4391–4398.

Tartaglia M, Gelb BD. Noonan syndrome and related disorders: genetics and pathogenesis. *Annu Rev Genomics Hum Genet.* 2005;6:45–68.

Tartaglia M, Pennacchio LA, Zhao C, et al. Gain-of-function SOS1 mutations cause a distinctive form of Noonan syndrome. *Nat Genet.* 2007;39:75–79.

Torres-Juan L, Rosell J, Morla M, Vidal-Pou C, Garcia-Algas F, de la Fuente MA, Juan M, et al. Mutations in TBX1 genocopy the 22q11.2 deletion and duplication syndromes: a new susceptibility factor for mental retardation. *Eur J Hum Genet.* 2007;15:658–663.

Tutar E, Ekici F, Atalay S, Nacar N. The prevalence of bicuspid aortic valve in newborns by echocardiographic screening. *Am Heart J.* 2005;150:513–515.

Udwadia AD, Khambadkone S, Bharucha BA, Lokhandwala Y, Irani SF. Familial congenital valvar pulmonary stenosis: autosomal dominant inheritance. *Pediatr Cardiol* 1996;17: 407–409.

Vissers LE, van Ravenswaaij CM, Admiraal R, et al. Mutations in a new member of the chromodomain gene family cause CHARGE syndrome. *Nat Genet.* 2004;36:955–957.

Ware SM, Peng J, Zhu L, et al. Identification and functional analysis of ZIC3 mutations in heterotaxy and related congenital heart defects. *Am J Hum Genet.* 2004;74:93–105.

Watanabe Y, Benson DW, Yano S, Akagi T, Yoshino M, Murray JC. Two novel frameshift mutations in NKX2.5 result in novel features including visceral inversus and sinus venosus type ASD. *J Med Genet* 2002;39:807–811.

Wollins DS, Ferencz C, Boughman JA, Loffredo CA. A population-based study of coarctation of the aorta: comparisons of infants with and without associated ventricular septal defect. *Teratology.* 2001;64:229–236.

Wulfsberg EA, Zintz EJ, Moore JW. The inheritance of conotruncal malformations: a review and report of two siblings with tetralogy of Fallot with pulmonary atresia. *Clin Genet.* 1991;40: 12–16.

Yagi H, Furutani Y, Hamada H, et al. Role of TBX1 in human del22q11.2 syndrome. *Lancet.* 2003;362:1366–1373.

Yunis K, Mumtaz G, Bitar F, et al. Consanguineous marriage and congenital heart defects: a case-control study in the neonatal period. *Am J Med Genet.* A 2006;140:1524–1530.

Zatyka M, Priestley M, Ladusans EJ, et al. Analysis of CRELD1 as a candidate 3p25 atrioventricular septal defect locus (AVSD2). *Clin Genet.* 2005;67(6):526–528.

Zavala C, Jimenez D, Rubio R, Castillo-Sosa ML, Diaz-Arauzo A, Salamanca F. Isolated congenital heart defects in first degree relatives of 185 affected children. Prospective study in Mexico City. *Arch Med Res* 1992;23:177–182.

Zhang L, Tumer Z, Jacobsen JR, Andersen PS, Tommerup N, Larsen LA. Screening of 99 Danish patients with congenital heart disease for GATA4 mutations. *Genet Test.* 2006;10:277–280.

Zhu L, Harutyunyan KG, Peng JL, Wang J, Schwartz RJ, Belmont JW. Identification of a novel role of ZIC3 in regulating cardiac development. *Hum Mol Genet.* 2007;16:1649–1660.

Zweier C, Sticht H, Aydin-Yaylagul I, Campbell CE, Rauch A. Human TBX1 missense mutations cause gain of function resulting in the same phenotype as 22q11.2 deletions. *Am J Hum Genet.* 2007;80:510–517.

27

Gene–Environment Interactions in the Complex Etiology of Congenital Heart Defects

MARIO A. CLEVES

CHARLOTTE A. HOBBS

Evidence from familial aggregation studies, twin studies, adoption studies, chromosomal evaluations, and animal studies indicates that the etiology of nonsyndromic congenital heart defects (CHDs) is multifactorial and results from interactions of genetic and environmental factors (Botto and Correa, 2003; Chien, 1999; Chien, 2000; Gruber et al., 1999; Mark, 1999; Nora, 1968). It is estimated that more than 85% of CHDs result from a complex interaction between maternal_fetal exposures and genetic susceptibilities (Botto and Correa, 2003). Even in families with multiple affected individuals, environmental factors may be needed for the development of CHDs, and it has been postulated that the type and level of environmental exposure controls the development of specific CHD subphenotypes in these families (Sheffield et al., 1997).

We define environmental factors broadly to include all factors external to the genetic architecture of the mother and the developing fetus. These factors may act directly on the fetus or indirectly through the mother. Potential environmental factors include maternal and fetal infections; chemical and pharmacological exposures; physical factors, such as radiation and hyperthermia; and maternal nutrition and behavioral exposures, such as smoking and alcohol consumption. We also define genetic factors broadly to include entire genes, coding and noncoding regions, single nucleotide polymorphisms (SNPs), haplotypes or extended DNA segments, or any other measureable genetic character.

The presence of a gene–environment (GxE) interaction implies either that environmental effects on phenotypes vary according to a person's genetic makeup or that genotype–phenotype relationships vary according to environmental stressors. Seldom is the presence of either a genetic factor or an environmental factor alone sufficient to cause a CHD (Botto and Correa, 2003; Sheffield et al., 1997). Rather, the combined influence of several genetic factors and environmental exposures is often required to cause CHDs. Additionally, depending on the maternal or fetal genotype, the effect of an environmental exposure may differently affect heart development. For example, two different genotypes might result in the same CHD phenotype if the mother is exposed to a certain level of an environmental factor (genetic heterogeneity) or may result in different phenotypes if the mother is exposed to a different level of the same environmental factor (phenotypic heterogeneity). It is also likely that some genetic polymorphisms are more environmentally sensitive than others, resulting in phenotypic heterogeneity at similar level of an environmental exposure.

The recognition that most nonsyndromic CHDs are caused by a complex interplay between genetic and environmental factors predates the current era of molecular genetics. In 1968, Dr. James Nora, in eloquent prose, defended his assertion that most nonsyndromic CHDs result from an interplay between genetic susceptibilities and environmental factors. He suggested that during a critical period of cardiac development, genetic susceptibilities acting in concert with environmental influences could push an individual over a threshold separating normal cardiac development from abnormal development, resulting in a cardiac malformation (Nora, 1968).

Over the past several years, conditions once considered multifactorial are now referred to as complex diseases or conditions. Although the term "complex" frequently replaces "multifactorial," the construct underlying these two terms is identical. With the completion of the Human Genome Project in 2002 and the release of Phase II data from the International HapMap Project in 2005, we have an unprecedented opportunity to investigate the simultaneous impact of environmental factors and common genetic variations in the development of CHDs. The completion of these two endeavors has led to the development of new study designs and analytical techniques. Prior to the completion of these national projects, most investigations were limited to testing the genetic component of CHDs in isolation from environmental components. In epidemiological studies, such as the Baltimore-Washington Infant Study, information about the occurrence of CHDs in family members of probands was obtained by questionnaires in a similar manner to the environmental exposure data. No biologic specimens were collected. Studies that did collect DNA samples most typically focused on CHDs associated with syndromes (Ferencz et al., 1998; Schneider et al., 1989), on single gene disorders, or on candidate genes without considering environmental factors (Boughman et al., 1987; Ferencz et al., 1985; Kuehl and Loffredo, 2002; Maestri et al., 1989).

Untangling the complex interplay between genetic and environmental factors is perhaps the single most important and challenging aspect in understanding the etiology and pathophysiology of CHDs. Rigorous investigations of the combined impact of genetic and environmental factors on CHD risk will enhance our ability to identify high-risk individuals and pregnancies that may, in turn, lead to the development of targeted prevention modalities and better therapeutic intervention strategies.

Before examining the combined effect of genetic and environmental factors on the developing heart, it is vital that CHD phenotypes be classified accurately and environmental exposures and genetic factors be measured accurately. Unfortunately, environmental exposures are often difficult to define and measure without error. For example, measuring exposure to certain air pollutants and environmental toxins during embryogenesis may be problematic without direct observation and sophisticated measuring equipment. Similarly, behavioral exposures, such as alcohol consumption during pregnancy, may be influenced by recall bias or underreporting because of societal pressures or stigma.

INTERACTION DEFINED

The vast majority of CHDs result from the interaction of genetic susceptibility factors and environmental factors. However, interaction usually means different things to statisticians and biologists. Biologic interactions often refer to causal relationships in disease pathways. This implies that the interdependence of genetic and environmental factors is linked to or produces the disease, requiring that these factors act on the same metabolic or causal pathway. On the other hand, interaction in the statistical sense has a clear mathematical meaning that makes no assumption about the physical or metabolic relationship of the factors. Thus, it is possible to find statistical interactions that make little or no biological sense. However, care must be taken not to hastily dismiss such findings without a thorough evaluation. Statistical interactions could lead to the discovery of previously unknown or unexplored biologic mechanisms, pathways, or relationships.

Statistical interactions are classified as being either multiplicative or additive depending on the statistical model assumed (Ottman, 1996). Multiplicative interaction exists when the joint effect of the genetic factor and environmental factor differs from the product of individual risks (Table 27-1). Additive interaction exists when the joint effect of the genetic factor and environmental factor differs from the sum of individual risks. The resulting interaction can be greater or less than the product (multiplicative) or sum (additive) of the individual components.

The following simplified example illustrates the difference between multiplicative and additive interactions. Suppose there is a genetic factor, G, that takes two values, 0 and 1. When $G = 1$ the individual carries the genetic factor of interest, and when $G = 0$ the individual does not. Similarly, assume that there is an environmental factor, E. When $E = 1$ the individual has been exposed to the environmental factor, and when $E = 0$ the individual has not. In this scenario, there are four possible GxE combinations, as depicted in Table 27-1 (Yang et al., 1997).

Using the individuals without the genetic factor of interest and without the environmental exposure as the reference group ($G = 0$, $E = 0$), we can define three odds ratios (ORs). First, from those individuals

TABLE 27-1. *The Four Possible Combinations of Gene and Environment When Each Takes Two Possible Values*

Susceptibility Genotype	Environmental Exposure	# of Case	# of Controls	Odds Ratios
0	0	A	B	Reference
1	0	C	D	$OR_G = BC/AD$
0	1	E	F	$OR_E = BE/AF$
1	1	G	H	$OR_{EG} = BG/AH$

Multiplicative interaction odds ratio $OR_{int} = OR_{EG} / (OR_E \times OR_G)$
Additive interaction odds ratio $OR_{int} = OR_{EG}/(OR_E + OR_G - 1)$

without environment exposure but carrying the genetic risk factor ($G = 1$, $E = 0$), the OR due to genetic factor (OR_G) can be computed as shown in Table 27–1. Similarly, the OR due to environmental exposure alone (OR_E) can be computed using individuals exposed to the environmental factor but not carrying the genetic risk factor ($G = 0$, $E = 1$). Lastly, individuals exposed to the environmental factor and having the genetic risk factor ($G = 1$, $E = 1$) are used to compute the OR associated with the combined effect of the environmental factor and genetic factor (OR_{EG}).

From the computed ORs, the multiplicative interaction OR is defined as $OR_{int} = OR_{EG}/(OR_E \times OR_G)$. Note that the interaction OR (OR_{int}) will be greater than 1 if the risk afforded by having both the genetic factor and the environmental factor (OR_{EG}) is greater than the product of the risks associated with having each factor alone, while the OR_{int} will be less than 1 if the OR_{EG} is less than the product of the risks associated with having each factor alone. Similarly, the additive interaction OR is defined as $OR_{int} = OR_{EG}/(OR_E + OR_G - 1)$. If the OR_{int} in either the multiplicative or the additive model differs significantly from 1, then there is evidence supporting the existence of a GxE interaction. Traditional linear logistic regression, a modeling method well suited and popular for the analysis of dichotomous outcomes in case-control epidemiological studies, can be used to compute multiplicative interaction directly by including interaction terms into regression models.

STUDY DESIGNS

Several study designs have been proposed to test for GxE interactions, including case-control studies with unrelated controls, family-based studies, case-only studies, matched case-control studies, studies using counter-matching, and cohort studies (Hobbs et al., 2002, 2006).

Case-control studies with unrelated controls are common in epidemiology and have gained popularity in the genetic epidemiology of common diseases. In these studies, CHD cases are compared with unrelated healthy controls or unrelated controls without CHDs. In the ongoing National Birth Defects Prevention Study (NBDPS), covering annual births of approximately 482,000 infants, CHD cases are identified from birth defect surveillance registries at nine participating study sites; controls, on the other hand, are infants without congenital malformations born during the same period and randomly selected from birth certificates or birth hospital records from the same study sites as the cases (Yoon et al., 2001). Because subjects are enrolled on the basis of their CHD status (affected or unaffected),

case-control studies of CHDs are more effective and efficient than cohort studies for collecting CHD cases. However, case-control studies are subject to several methodological issues and biases that may distort study findings if they are not addressed. For example, in case-control studies such as the NBDPS, women are asked to recall multiple environmental exposures they may have had before conception or during pregnancy. The ability to identify environmental risk factors is highly dependent on the participants' ability to accurately recall their exposure history.

Case-control studies require large sample sizes to detect even modest interactions when genetic and environmental factors are rare. Several investigators have examined the power of case-control studies to detect GxE interactions under different assumptions; regardless of assumptions made or methods used, the power to detect interactions requires substantially more subjects than those needed to detect similar magnitudes of either genetic or environmental factors individually (Foppa and Spiegelman, 1997; Garcia-Closas et al., 1999; Gauderman, 2002; Hunter, 2005; Hwang et al., 1999).

Another challenge associated with case-control studies is the possibility of drawing incorrect conclusions due to spurious associations resulting from undetected population stratification, for example, resulting from the incomplete mixture of ethnically different populations. This incomplete mixture can produce a population in which the disease prevalence differs between subpopulations (heterogeneity in rates of disease) and in which the allele frequencies at the candidate genetic locus vary between subpopulations (heterogeneity in allele frequencies). If sampling and subsequent analysis is performed without regard to ethnicity, this population stratification can lead to false-positive results (Ewens and Spielman, 1995; Lander and Schork, 1994).

Khoury and Flanders proposed an innovative study design to test for GxE interactions using only cases (Khoury and Flanders, 1996). For this case-only design, only CHD-affected individuals are needed for analysis, and consequently, these studies require fewer resources than case-control studies. Inherent in the case-only design is the assumption that genetic factors and environmental exposures are independent in the study population. That is, this design assumes that the candidate genetic factor does not influence the environmental factor of interest. When this assumption is not met, serious spurious conclusions may result (Albert et al., 2001). However, if the assumption of independence of genes and exposure is met, case-only studies are more powerful than case-control studies for detecting gene–environment interactions (Albert et al., 2001; Hamajima et al., 1999; Khoury and Flanders, 1996).

Case-only studies can only be used to estimate and test interactive effects, not main effects of genes and/or environmental factors. It is worth noting that interaction parameters computed from case-only analyses differ from those computed from case-control analyses (Schmidt and Schaid, 1999). In case-control analyses, multiplicative interaction ORs are estimated, whereas in case-only analyses, multiplicative interaction relative risk ratios are estimated under the assumption of genotype and environmental exposure independence. ORs and relative risks are approximately equal, provided that the disease is rare in the population. Similar to case-control studies, case-only studies can also be subject to confounding caused by admixture and population stratification.

Family-based studies avoid complications due to admixture and population stratification by controlling for genetic background. These studies use family members, such as unaffected siblings, as controls. Two popular family-based designs are case-parental and case-sib (or case-cousin designs). In the former, parents are used as controls; whereas in the latter, unaffected siblings and/or cousins are used as controls. The resulting cases and controls are more closely matched on race, ethnicity, and cultural factors than when using unrelated controls.

Family-based studies are only more powerful than case-control studies when genetic and environmental factors are rare; furthermore, they cannot be used to estimate the independent effect of environmental exposures. If common genetic variants are responsible for the development of CHD, family-based studies have less statistical power than case-control studies to detect GxE interactions. Family-based studies may be less efficient than case-control studies due to overmatching of environmental and genetic factors. This overmatching can result in attenuation of results toward the null hypothesis (Hobbs et al., 2002). In the presence of population stratification, however, family-based studies may be preferred in order to reduce spurious associations and false-positive results due to population stratification.

Family-based studies of CHD may be more difficult to conduct than case-control studies because suitable family members to serve as controls may be unavailable. Although typically one or both parents are available if probands are infants or neonates, siblings or age-matched cousins are not always available.

Recently, various investigators have proposed using prospective cohort studies to evaluate GxE interactions. The most compelling rationale for this proposal is the increased accuracy and precision of measuring environmental exposures prior to the diagnosis of disease, which eliminates recall bias and errors of retrospective exposure assessment (Manolio et al., 2006). The resources required to conduct prospective cohort studies, however, may be substantial. In such studies, women would be enrolled prior to conception and followed until the end of pregnancy. For example, assuming a liberal 50% pregnancy rate and a population incidence of eight CHD cases per 1000 pregnancies, 250 women would need to be enrolled for every expected case of CHD. To ascertain 1000 CHD cases, 250,000 women would need to be enrolled, interviewed, and followed at considerable effort and expense. Unfortunately, 1000 CHD cases would still be too few to test for many GxE interactions, and enrolling a million or more women would be necessary to begin to have sufficient statistical power to detect modest interactive effects (Manolio et al., 2006).

Countermatching, a sampling method that increases statistical power without the need to increase sample size (Andrieu et al., 2001), has been proposed to test for GxE. Compared to simple random sampling, countermatching is designed to increase differences between cases and controls by matching them on exposures. With countermatching, a case that has a particular risk factor is matched to a control that does not have the risk factor or has the opposite risk factor. For example, if cigarette smoking is a risk factor, an exposed case is matched to an unexposed control. This is the opposite of traditional matching schemes in which controls and cases are matched on specific attributes, such as sex or race. The goal of countermatching is to maximize the difference between cases and controls on genetic or environmental factors.

These traditional study designs and, more specifically, traditional analysis methods are becoming outdated in testing for gene–environment interactions as the ability to quickly and efficiently genotype large numbers of polymorphisms has increased dramatically over the last several years. While the development of new statistical methods for analyzing GxE interactions with large sets of genetic markers has lagged behind these genotyping technologies, several statistical methods that show promise for dealing with multidimensional data have been proposed to explore and identify GxE interactions. These include classification and regression trees (CART) methods based on the recursive partitioning of the sample space (Breiman, 1984), multivariate adaptive regression splines (MARS) methods (Friedman, 1991), and multifactor dimensionality reduction (MDR) methods (Moore and Williams, 2002; Ritchie et al., 2001). Although CART and MARS methods are not new, they are only now gaining popularity and being used to investigate GxE interactions. These methods have advantages over traditional logistic regression modeling in that they may detect interactions whose factors do not display strong main effects.

STUDIES OF GENE-ENVIRONMENT INTERACTION IN CONGENITAL HEART DEFECTS

Until recently, most epidemiological studies investigating the etiology of CHDs focused on either genetic or environmental determinants, but not both. In some studies, such as the Baltimore-Washington Infant Study, biological samples were not collected from participants, limiting the study of genetic factors, but information about occurrence of CHDs in extended families was collected.

To date, only a few studies have reported on the effect of GxE interactions on the development CHDs. Most of these investigate the role of folic acid supplementation in the prevention of CHDs. The effect of folic acid in the prevention of neural tube defects, specifically spina bifida, is well known and documented. However, the impact of folic acid supplementation in cardiac development had not received as much attention.

In 2003, Shaw et al. (2003) examined the association between the SNP 80A>G in the transport-reduced folate carrier-1 gene (*RFC1*) and the occurrence of conotruncal defects. They compared 163 infants with conotruncal heart defects and 364 nonmalformed controls. They found evidence suggestive of an interaction between the infant G80/G80 genotype and maternal supplemental vitamin use in the development of conotruncal defects.

Three additional studies conducted in the past few years have reported GxE interactions associated with CHDs (Hobbs et al., 2006; Shaw et al., 2005; van Beynum et al., 2006). In 2006, van Beyum published a case-control and family-based study investigating the association between nonsyndromic CHDs and the MTHFR 677 C>T polymorphism. No association was found between infants' genotypes and CHDs among 158 women who had offspring with CHD. However, women who carried the MTHFR 677 CT or TT genotype, and who did not take folate supplements, had an increased risk of having a fetus with conotruncal heart defect (OR for MTHFR 677 CT: 3.3 95% CI: 1.5–7.3 and OR MTHFR 677 TT: 6.3 95% CI: 2.3–17.3). More recently, van Beynum and colleagues conducted a relatively small meta-analysis and concluded that among women who did not take periconceptional folate supplements, the risk for conotruncal heart defects was increased among those who carried one or two copies of the T allele in the *MTHFR* 677 CT polymorphism (3.3. 95% CI 1.5–7.3) (van Beynum et al., 2007).

In 2006, we reported a GxE interaction between maternal homocysteine levels, smoking status, and maternal MTHFR 677 C>T polymorphism (Hobbs et al., 2006). In our study, women who had a child affected by CHD were more likely to have elevated homocysteine levels than women with unaffected offspring. However, women with normal homocysteine levels who smoked and carried the CT/TT genotype had an increased risk of having a child affected by CHD, compared to women with normal homocysteine levels who either smoked and were homozygous CC or did not smoke and were heterozygous CT/TT. This suggests the existence of an interaction between smoking, the MTHFR 677 polymorphism, and homocysteine.

Shaw et al. (2005) extended the exploration of candidate genes to those involved in one of five pathways: homocysteine metabolism, coagulation, cell–cell interaction, inflammatory response, and blood pressure regulation. DNA samples were available from infants with conotruncal heart defects, but not from their mothers. In this study, GxE interactions between periconceptional folic acid use and the infant's MTHFR 677 CT genotype, and between maternal smoking and the infant's polymorphisms were evaluated. No significant interaction was found between the infant's MTHFR 677 C>T polymorphism and maternal periconceptional supplement use; however, they did find evidence suggesting an interaction between fetal NOS3 922 A>G, 298 G>T polymorphisms, and maternal smoking. Women who smoked and whose infant carried the NOS3 298 GT genotype were approximately 2.2 times more likely than control women to have an affected infant (OR: 2.2 95% CI 1.2–4.0). The OR for women who smoked and whose infant was heterozygous or homozygous for the 922 AG genotype was 1.9 (95% CI 1.1–3.4).

NATIONAL BIRTH DEFECTS PREVENTION STUDY

The Centers for Disease Control and Prevention (CDC)-funded NBDPS is the largest ongoing population-based, case-control study of birth defects, including CHDs, in the United States. By the fall of 2006, over 7676 nuclear families affected by CHDs have been enrolled and interviewed in the NBDPS. DNA samples from approximately 3378 case-parental triads (mother, father, and offspring) have been collected. The NBDPS is conducted at nine different sites, representing nine US state populations. As such, the NBDPS provides an unprecedented opportunity to examine the complex etiology of nonsyndromic CHDs. With the completion and release of Phase II data from the International HapMap Project, NBDPS DNA samples will provide a valuable resource to examine the impact of common genetic variants on the occurrence of CHDs. At the time of publication, intensive efforts are underway by several laboratories to examine GxE interactions that may lead to CHDs. Such efforts will strengthen the knowledge base needed to develop primary prevention strategies.

REFERENCES

Albert PS, Ratnasinghe D, Tangrea J, Wacholder S. Limitations of the case-only design for identifying gene-environment interactions. *Am J Epidemiol.* 2001;154:687–693.

Andrieu N, Goldstein AM, Thomas DC, Langholz B. Counter-Matching in Studies of Gene-Environment Interaction: Efficiency and Feasibility. *Am J Epidemiol.* 2001;153:265–274.

Botto LD, Correa A. Decreasing the burden of congenital heart anomalies: an epidemiologic evaluation of risk factors and survival. *Prog Pediatr Cardiol.* 2003;18(2):111–121.

Boughman J, Berg K, Astemborski J, et al. Familial risks of congential heart defect assessed in a population-based epidemiologic study. *Am J Med Genet.* 1987;26:839–849.

Breiman L, Friedman JH, Olshen RA, Stone CJ. *Classification and regression trees.* Belmont, CA: Wadsworth; 1984.

Chien KR. Stress pathways and heart failure. *Cell.* 1999;98:555–558.

Chien KR. Genomic circuits and the integrative biology of cardiac diseases. *Nature.* 2000;407:227–232.

Ewens WJ, Spielman RS. The transmission/disequilibrium test: history, subdivision, and admixture. *Am J Hum Genet.* 1995;57:455–464.

Ferencz C, Boughman JA, Neill CA, Brenner JI, Perry LW. Congenital cardiovascular malformations: questions on inheritance. Baltimore-Washington Infant Study Group. *J Am Coll Cardiol.* 1989;14:756–763.

Ferencz C, Rubin JD, McCarter RJ, et al. Congenital heart disease: prevalence at livebirth. The Baltimore-Washington Infant Study. *Am J Epidemiol.* 1985;121:31–36.

Foppa I, Spiegelman D. Power and sample size calculations for case-control studies of gene-environment interactions with a polytomous exposure variable. *Am J Epidemiol.* 1997;146:596–603.

Friedman JH. Multivariate adaptive splines. *Annals of Statistics.* 1991;19:1–66.

Garcia-Closas M, Lubin J. Power and sample size calculations in case control studies of gene-environment interactions: Comments on different approaches. *Am J Epidemiol.* 1999;149:689–692.

Gauderman WJ. Sample size requirements for association studies of gene-gene interaction. *Am J Epidemiol.* 2002;155:478–484.

Gruber PJ, Kubalak SW, Pexieder T, Sucov HM, Evans RM, Chien KR. RXR alpha deficiency confers genetic susceptibility for aortic sac, conotruncal, atrioventricular cushion, and ventricular muscle defects in mice. *J Clin Invest.* 1996;98:1332–1343.

Hamajima N, Yuasa H, Matsuo K, Kurobe Y. Detection of gene-environment interaction by case-only studies. *Jpn J Clin Oncol.* 1999;29:490–493.

Hobbs CA, Cleves MA, Lauer RM, Burns TL, James SJ. Preferential transmission of the MTHFR 677 T allele to infants with down syndrome: implications for a survival advantage. *Am J Med Gene.t* 2002;113:9–14.

Hobbs CA, James SJ, Jernigan S, Melnyk S, Lu Y, Malilk S, Cleves MA. Congenital heart defects, maternal homocysteine, smoking, and the 677 C>T polymorphism in the methylenetetrahydrofolate reductase gene: Evaluating gene-environment interactions. *Am J Obstet Gynecol.* 2006;194:218–224.

Hunter DJ. Gene-environment interactions in human diseases. *Nat Rev Genet.* 2005;6:287–298.

Hwang S-J, Beaty TH, Liang K-Y, Coresh J, Khoury MJ. Minimum sample size estimation to detect gene-environment interaction in case-control designs. *Am J Epidemiol.* 1999;140:1029–1037.

Khoury MJ, Flanders WD. Nontraditional epidemiologic approaches in the analysis of gene-environment interaction: Case-control studies with no controls. *Am J Epidemiol.* 1996;144:207–213.

Kuehl KS, Loffredo C. Risk factors for heart disease associated with abnormal sidedness. *Teratology.* 2002;66:242–248.

Lander ES, Schork NJ. Genetic dissection of complex traits. *Science* 1994;265:2037–2048.

Maestri NE, Beaty TH, Boughman JA. Etiologic heterogeneity in the familial aggregation of congenital cardiovascular malformations. *Am J Hum Genet.* 1989;45:556–564.

Manolio TA, Bailey-Wilson JE, Collins FS. Genes, environment and the value of prospective cohort studies. *Nat Rev Genet.* 2006;7:812–820.

Mark M, Ghyselinck NB, Wendling O, et al. A genetic dissection of the retinoid signalling pathway in the mouse. *Proc Nutr Soc.* 1999;58:609–613.

Moore JH, Williams SM. New strategies for identifying gene-gene interactions in hypertension. *Ann Med.* 2002;34:88–95.

Nora JJ. Multifactorial inheritance hypothesis for the etiology of congenital heart diseases. The genetic-environmental interaction. *Circulation.* 1968;38:604–17.

Ottman R. Gene-environment interaction: definitions and study designs. *Prev Med.* 1996;25:764–770.

Ritchie MD, Hahn LW, Roodi N, et al. Multifactor-dimensionality reduction reveals high-order interactions among estrogen-metabolism genes in sporadic breast cancer. *Am J Hum Genet.* 2001;69:138–147.

Schmidt S, Schaid DJ. Potential misinterpretation of the case-only study to assess gene-environment interaction. *Am J Epidemiol.* 1999;150:878–885.

Schneider DS, Zahka KG, Clark EB, Neill CA. Patterns of cardiac care in infants with Down syndrome. *Am J Dis Child.* 1989;143:363–365.

Shaw GM, Iovannisci DM, Yang W, et al. Risks of human conotruncal heart defects associated with 32 single nucleotide polymorphisms of selected cardiovascular disease-related genes. *Am J Med Genet. A* 2005;138:21–26.

Shaw GM, Zhu H, Lammer EJ, Yang W, Finnell RH. Genetic variation of infant reduced folate carrier (A80G) and risk of orofacial and conotruncal heart defects. *Am J Epidemiol.* 2003;158:747–752.

Sheffield VC, Pierpont ME, Nishimura D, et al. Identification of a complex congenital heart defect susceptibility locus by using DNA pooling and shared segment analysis. *Hum Mol Genet.* 1997;6:117–121.

Van Beynum IM, Den Heijer M, Blom HJ, Kapusta L. The MTHFR 677C>T polymorphism and the risk of congenital heart defects: a literature review and meta-analysis. *QJMed,* 2007;100:743–753.

van Beynum IM, Kapusta L, den Heijer M, et al. Maternal MTHFR 677C>T is a risk factor for congenital heart defects: effect modification by periconceptional folate supplementation. *Eur Heart J.* 2006;27:981–987.

Yang Q, Khoury MJ, Flanders WD. Sample size requirements in case-only designs to detect gene-environment interaction. *Am J Epidemiol.* 1997;146:713–720.

Yoon PW, Rasmussen SA, Lynberg MC, et al. The National Birth Defects Prevention Study. *Public Health Rep.* 2001;116 (suppl 1): 32–40.

28

Genetic Counseling for Congenital Heart Defects

ANGELA E. LIN

MARY ELLA PIERPONT

Congenital heart defects (CHDs) are a group of birth defects that are familiar to primary care practitioners, specialists, allied health care professionals, and families, alike. They are common, with a birth prevalence ranging from approximately 5 to 15 per 1000 depending on study design, contributing significantly to infant morbidity and mortality (Botto et al., 2007). Despite the obvious impact of CHDs on personal and public health, enormous strides in medical care and surgical treatment have resulted in better outcomes. For an increasing number of individuals and families affected by a CHD, reproduction and recurrence risk assessment are issues that are discussed at more than one point in the lifespan. This chapter discusses the role of genetic counseling in providing information and assisting families whether the dialogue is preconceptual, prenatal, neonatal, or with an adolescent. The maturation from patient with a CHD to a potential parent completes a medical, psychological, and social "circle of life" for discussion.

A recent update by the National Society of Genetic Counselors defines genetic counseling as the process that helps people "understand and adapt to the medical, psychological, and familial implications of the genetic contributions to disease" (Resta et al., 2006). As a profession, genetic counseling refers to the practice carried out by a genetic counselor, a professional with a master's degree. For this chapter, the term "genetic health provider" will refer to either a trained genetic counselor or a medical geneticist who may provide genetic counseling for an individual with a CHD as part of a genetics evaluation. Some pediatric cardiologists with training in genetics will also have the ability to provide genetic counseling.

Although clinicians may view genetic counseling as one of the final consultations in the care of a child with a CHD, most parents are thinking about the relevant issues soon after their child's birth. Whether or not they verbalize the questions, they may wonder "how did this happen?" and "will it happen again?" Even in the neonatal period, many parents are asking, "if we have another child, can we prevent the occurrence of a CHD, or can it be diagnosed in a future pregnancy?" In the short term, families are dealing with a medical condition that will impact their life to some degree. Those who "take the long view" question whether the CHD could occur in their child's own offspring or extended family. Parents will have coping needs whether the CHD is detected in a 16-week-gestation fetus, 16-month-old toddler, or 16-year-old young adult.

The exact manner in which a family or individual with a CHD participates in genetic counseling depends on the time of diagnosis, and whether a diagnostic genetic evaluation precedes the counseling. An official genetic counseling discussion may be one of the last consultations for the family following an arduous period of diagnostic tests and hospital admissions. Ideally, the family and genetic health provider meet to review past events, discuss genetic topics, explore ongoing psychological and coping issues, and look ahead to the future. In reality, the routine history taking and initial discussion at the time of the diagnostic investigation of a newborn or child is misconstrued as genetic counseling. If the knowledge base is incomplete or consultation time is insufficient, the complete counseling experience for the family cannot be developed.

This chapter updates a 20-year-old review on this topic (Lin and Garver, 1988), which discussed the process of genetic counseling for a family or an individual with a CHD. We encourage readers to integrate this topic with information found elsewhere in this book.

GUIDING PRINCIPLES FOR GENETIC COUNSELING FOR CONGENITAL HEART DEFECTS

Several recent review articles and chapters have discussed the clinical situations in which genetic counseling can be provided (Goldmuntz and Lin, 2007; Hoess et al., 2002; Lacro, 2006; Pierpont et al., 2007; Salbert, 2003). Whether genetic counseling is provided by a genetic counselor or genetic physician is partly influenced by the patient's age at presentation and additional medical history, for example, a fetus/pregnant woman, child, or adult (Table 28–1). Logistics and referral patterns also probably play a role. As medical and genetic issues arise, the roles of the genetic health providers evolve. For example, a pregnant woman who is evaluated in a prenatal diagnostic center is usually provided genetic counseling by a genetic counselor with support from a medical geneticist. A parent may meet a pediatric cardiologist when a fetal (or subsequent postnatal) echocardiogram is performed, and the information about the fetal heart anatomy and potential for cardiac surgery is integrated into the genetic counseling. Depending on availability, an individual with a CHD may be referred to a medical geneticist or a pediatric cardiologist with expertise in genetics, and to a few cardiovascular clinics where a geneticist and genetic counselor is a member of a cardiology department, to provide genetic assessment as patients are being diagnosed (Lin et al., 2004). When the focus in these medical settings is a diagnostic evaluation, genetic counseling awaits the conclusion of the testing.

Importance of Understanding Cardiac Anatomy

The genetic health provider should have a sufficient knowledge of cardiac anatomy to lead the consultation with a reasonable degree of confidence. Consider the difference between two types of atrial septal defect, secundum and primum, in which the latter belongs to the atrioventricular canal family of defects, which will not close spontaneously, and typically has associated valve abnormalities. The genetic health provider should have a sense of whether the cardiac anatomy had been sufficiently defined, ideally, after discussion with the relevant medical personnel such as the fetal

echocardiographer, pediatric cardiologist, maternal–fetal medicine specialist, or neonatologist. The genetic health provider is not expected to understand every detail of a complex echocardiography report, but should be aware that a vague diagnosis stating "possible septal defect" would not allow precise counseling. Beyond reading the description of the CHD in a diagnostic report, discussion with a pediatric cardiologist may be needed to thoroughly understand certain complex defects. A genetic health provider should know whether "pulmonary atresia" was associated with tetralogy of Fallot and collateral aortopulmonary vessels rather than intact ventricular septum since the former has a strong association with deletion 22q11.2 syndrome. Likewise, pulmonary "atresia" differs from the "absent pulmonary valve syndrome" despite apparent linguistic similarity. Although a key element of genetic counseling is establishing a firm knowledge base for patient and provider so that decisions will be based on accurate facts, it is not the responsibility of the genetic health provider to provide a cardiology tutorial, which should be deferred to the cardiologist.

Review of Family and Medical History, Diagnostic Tests

The cornerstone of a genetic counseling consultation is a careful family and medical history. Rather than recording simple yes or no responses about the presence or absence of CHDs, the intake history should note the verbatim responses. A parent may not be able to articulate "truncus arteriosus," but may report that there was "one big artery coming out of the heart." However, nonspecific information such as a self-reported "blue baby" cannot be viewed reliably as a CHD without documentation. Maternal history about exposures and risk factors (e.g., maternal fevers, over-the-counter medications, poorly controlled maternal diabetes, cigarette/drug/alcohol use) is less reliable when it is obtained many years after the child's birth.

When important diagnoses, procedures, or lab test results are reported, the supportive medical record or report should be requested. Complex terms and results can be reviewed at a subsequent counseling session visit with the individual. For an adult with a CHD, the genetic counseling session might be the rare opportunity to learn about their own childhood medical events.

From Patient Phenotype to Counseling Strategy

CHDs can be classified as "isolated" (no additional major malformations) or "complex" (additional malformations, variable minor anomalies, dysmorphic facial features), which can be further subdivided into

TABLE 28–1. *Examples of Congenital Heart Defects and Genetic Counseling Scenarios*

Affected Individual	Type of CHD	History, Additional Defects	Issues: the Exact Role of the Geneticist, Genetic Counselor and/or Pediatric Cardiologist Varies
18-week female fetus	CAVC	Down syndrome (trisomy 21) diagnosed at 16 weeks by amniocentesis; CAVC detected on screening ultrasonography, confirmed by higher resolution fetal echocardiography	Assuming that a genetic counselor or geneticist established a relationship with the mother at the initial prenatal genetics visit was explained, the discussion would continue after the chromosome and cardiac diagnoses were made; discussion would include information about CHDs, chromosome abnormalities, Down syndrome manifestations, etc.; additional topics would include options for pregnancy termination/continuation; emotional and psychosocial support would be provided (Pierpont et al., 2007)
Newborn male	HLHS	Proband recently had Stage I of the Norwood procedure; female sibling died 3 years ago in Honduras in the first week of life with "half a heart"; father takes penicillin whenever he has dental work because of "tight valve problem"; 5-year-old brother has systolic murmur	Family history suggests autosomal dominant LVOTO, but should be confirmed with imaging (documenting sibling's history by medical records if possible); the father and brother need an echocardiogram to confirm suspicion of aortic stenosis with or without BAV; a culturally appropriate discussion about inheritance and recurrence risk would be provided; if a clear distinction between clinical testing and research was understood, family could be offered the opportunity to participate in research studies searching for possible predisposing genes (Cripe et al., 2004; Lewin et al., 2004; Loffredo et al., 2004; McBride et al., 2005)
6-year-old male	Small muscular VSD, PDA	VSD closed in infancy; echocardiogram performed for persistence of systolic murmur shows PDA; family history reveals that mother and maternal uncle had surgical ligation of PDA in infancy	Family history suggests autosomal dominant PDA; when photographs of the mother are examined, there are facial features to support the diagnosis of Char syndrome; molecular diagnostic testing is not available, and discussion about inheritance is provided (Satoda and Gelb, 2004)
16-year-old female	TOF	TOF repaired in childhood, excellent result; has received special education for mild learning disability, functions well otherwise; at well-child care visit prior to cheerleading camp, new pediatrician noticed long fingers and square nasal root	The type of CHD, learning disability and physical features suggest deletion 22q11.2 syndrome; because the individual was being followed at a pediatric tertiary care center, the diagnostic evaluation should proceed prior to genetic counseling; assuming deletion 22q11.2 is detected, calcium studies, immunologic testing, formal psychology support, and testing should be considered; reproductive risks should be discussed, and other family members, especially parents, may need testing (McDonald-McGinn et al., 2005; Pierpont et al., 2007)
22-year-old female	BAV	Turner syndrome (45,X) diagnosed during evaluation for infertility; patient had baseline echocardiogram that noted a BAV; MRI showed normal aortic root and arch; received extensive counseling about pregnancy and potential cardiac risk; pregnancy conceived with IVF, now at 16-week gestation; screening ultrasonography on fetus is reassuring	This woman's relationship with the genetic health providers dramatically shifts to include an adult cardiologist with expertise in managing aortic dissection; this patient had appropriate prenatal cardiac care and should continue during and after pregnancy; the main issue is monitoring the BAV and blood pressure as possible risk factors for aortic dissection (Bondy et al., 2007)
25-year-old male	ASD2	ASD2 repaired in childhood; patient maintained regular followup at major CHD surgery center; no hemodynamic or electrophysiologic residua; referred for prenatal counseling	If extended family history is negative, a low recurrence risk can be discussed (Calcagni et al., 2007).
25-year-old male	ASD2	Known to have had a murmur in childhood, and a "small hole which closed"; recently diagnosed with ASD2 following mild stroke; noted by adult cardiologist to have finger-like thumb and first degree heart block, but viewed as insignificant; proband's mother had heart murmur and "little thumb"; referred for prenatal counseling	Strong suspicion of Holt-Oram syndrome, indicating need for careful examination; proband's mother should have cardiology evaluation with echocardiogram, and radiograph of the hand; proband should be offered testing for *TBX5*; depending on referral pattern, geneticist can perform complete examination, order tests, complete prenatal testing, or genetic counselor can initiate the counseling, followed by examination and testing (McDermott and Basson, 2006; Pierpont et al., 2007)

Abbreviations: ASD2, secundum-type atrial septal defect; BAV, bicuspid aortic valve; CAVC, complete atrioventricular canal; CHD, congenital heart defect; HLHS, hypoplastic left heart syndrome; IVF, *in vitro* fertilization; LVOTO, left ventricular outflow tract obstruction; PDA, patent ductus arteriosus; TOF, tetralogy of Fallot; VSD, ventricular septal defect.
See also review by Lin et al., 2008.

those who have a recognizable syndrome and those who remain as unspecified malformation complexes. Optimal genetic counseling should be guided by a similar understanding of whether an individual has an isolated CHD or whether it is associated with other malformations, and of course, whether the etiology is known or unknown (Goldmuntz and Lin, 2007; Lacro, 2006). Although this type of classification has been used for epidemiological and clinical genetic research (Botto et al., 2007; Browne et al., 2007; Rasmussen et al., 2003), it also provides a pragmatic basis for genetic counseling. Of all the possible combinations based on phenotype and etiology, they can be distilled to three major categories, which include: (1) isolated CHD, unknown cause; (2) complex, known cause; (3) complex, unknown cause. The syndromes of known cause may be due to a chromosome or gene abnormality, or maternal exposure. It is important to note that some of the terminologies used to describe a heart with many component defects ("complex heart" and "complex single ventricle") may cause confusion since it overlaps the same term, which is used to describe the heart and its relationship to other malformations. Thus, a heart with a double inlet left ventricle with l-transposed great arteries, mitral atresia, and pulmonary atresia is viewed as a single CHD, albeit anatomically complex CHD. It is classified as "isolated" if there are no other malformations, and classified as "complex" if it occurs in a child with cleft palate, omphalocele, low-set ears, and short fingers.

Genetic research and counseling can be enhanced when CHDs are viewed not as individual defects due to unique errors of morphogenesis, but as members of pathogenetic families in which there are patterns of embryological errors (Ferencz et al., 1993; Goldmuntz and Lin, 2007; Lacro, 2006). Irrespective of hypothetical developmental mechanisms, CHDs can be grouped pragmatically according to similar hemodynamics, for example, left ventricular outflow tract obstruction. This approach has been supported by echocardiographic studies of extended family members (Cripe et al., 2004; Lewin et al., 2004; Loffredo et al., 2004; McBride et al., 2005).

RISK ASSESSMENT

It is generally agreed that it is inappropriate to use a single all-purpose empiric recurrence risk for all individuals with CHDs. The authors feel that there is insufficient data to provide a comprehensive table listing the risks for siblings and parents for major CHDs using current reports since most studies have been unable to exclude the growing number of chromosome and gene syndromes. In the past, the vast majority of CHDs were

attributed to a multifactorial etiology with a recurrence risk of 2%–4% based on population-based studies, which did not exclude syndromic and familial causes (Nora, 1968). However, a substantial genetic contribution in the etiology of CHDs was demonstrated by the innovative family studies of the Baltimore-Washington Infant Study (Boughman et al., 1987; Ferencz et al., 1993; Loffredo et al., 2004). Probands with chromosome and mendelian gene syndromes were excluded, and CHD "families" were studied.

In the past 20 years, the proportion of CHD cases with an identifiable etiology has increased from 13% (Kramer et al., 1987) to approximately 20% (Table 9.1 Ferencz et al., 1993; summarized in Botto et al., 2007). Increasingly sophisticated diagnostic testing and greater attention to syndrome diagnosis likely contribute (Pierpont et al., 2007). The trend to identify causes among live births with a CHD may be balanced by an increase in the number of terminated fetuses with chromosome abnormalities (Lin et al., 1999). The increased ability to identify the underlying cause of a CHD means that a customized risk assessment is preferred rather than using empiric population-based figures. An individualized risk approach integrates multiple levels of data including genetic inheritance assumptions, current understanding of the spectrum of findings, and severity associated with a specific diagnosis, the impact of potential genetic and/or environmental influencers (protective or increasing risk), possible epigenetic factors, and epidemiological data.

Risk assessment addresses the chance that another offspring or relative would be affected with a CHD, or whether an affected parent could transmit the CHD to his or her child. Most genetic epidemiology studies had been designed to obtain *recurrence* risk frequencies by monitoring the number of pregnancies after the birth of an affected child. Because future childbearing can be influenced by the birth of a child with a birth defect, *precurrence* figures may be more reliable (Burn and Goodship, 2002). The optimally designed study of CHD risk occurrence would have a sufficiently large cohort, rigorous CHD definition, careful screening of offspring, analyses looking at concordance of CHD classes between proband and sibling or parent, and exclusion of cases with known syndromes, which may require aggressive dysmorphology examinations, chromosome, and gene testing.

As noted, we have refrained from publishing a summary table of available familial risks although we acknowledge the challenges faced by genetic health providers who seek risk figures for real-life counseling situations. Several publications are noteworthy for size or study design. Burn and Goodship (2002) masterfully summarized the major recurrence risk studies published prior to the 1980s. The important role of precurrence in familial risk assessment of CHDs was delineated by the landmark studies of Baltimore-Washington Infant Study (Boughman et al., 1987; Ferencz et al., 1993) in which the precurrence risk of having a (previous) sibling with any CHD was 3.1%, but a much higher rate was observed when the proband had either bicuspid aortic valve (8.8%), hypoplastic left heart syndrome (8.0%), or coarctation of the aorta (6.3%).

Precurrence was also measured by Calzolari et al. (2003) who noted a 2.3% sibling risk for any CHD; among affected parents, mothers were more commonly affected. Digilio et al. (2001) and Piacentini et al. (2005) studied d-transposition of the great arteries and congenitally corrected transposition of the great arteries, respectively, noting a precurrence sibling risk of 1.8% and 5.2%. Because the cases were classified, they were able to show familial segregation of both looping abnormalities in sibs indicating a pathogenetic link in some families. Calcagni et al. (2007) have provided what is probably a "state of the art" review of familial risks for major CHDs, which they have grouped as nonsyndromic "multifactorial" CHDs and those with likely genetic etiology.

An alternative cohort ascertainment was used by Gill et al. (2003) who found a 2.7% recurrence risk of CHDs using fetal echocardiography in 6640 consecutive pregnancies in which a first degree relative had a CHD. Concordance for the exact type of CHD was noted in 37%, and for the same CHD family in 44%, increasing further to 55% in families with two or more affected siblings. Two defects, isolated atrioventricular canal and laterality defects, showed the highest concordance at 80% and 64%, respectively.

In the largest study of recurrence risks using a population-based registry of adult survivors with significant CHDs, the recurrence risk among offspring (4.1%) was significantly greater than among siblings (2.1%) (Burn et al., 1998). Despite the strength of this large study, there was inconsistent testing for deletion 22q11.2 and other chromosome abnormalities, and thus, the proportion in the general population was not estimated. A recent review reported that among all patients with a CHD, deletion 22q11.2 occurred in 50%–89% with interrupted aortic arch type B, 34%–41% with truncus arteriosus, 8%–35% with tetralogy of Fallot and 10% with various ventricular septal defect types (Table 28–1. in Pierpont et al., 2007), and in 6%–28% of parents of affected individuals. From a population perspective, 1.5% of all CHDs in the general population surveyed by Botto et al. (2003b) were associated with deletion 22q11.2.

Practically speaking, in most counseling situations, geneticists, cardiologists, and genetic counselors will encounter patients in which the CHD under consideration is either a hemodynamically mild or a repaired atrial or ventricular septal defect, or left or right ventricular outflow tract obstructive defect. With increased improvements in surgical repair and treatment, patients with more complex CHDs are encountered.

Isolated Congenital Heart Defect, Unknown Cause

Most (approximately 75%) of the CHDs are isolated (without major extracardiac defects) (Botto et al., 2007). Clinicians unfamiliar with the importance of genetic counseling may neglect to refer affected individuals and families for formal consultation. The most important element of their evaluation is to ensure that what is presumed as "isolated" is not accompanied by an overlooked associated extracardiac defect, developmental delay, psychological abnormality, unusual facial appearance, or related family history, which may be a clue to an underlying disorder and indicate a formal genetics evaluation. Diagnostic tests such as high-resolution chromosome analysis, fluorescence in situ hybridization (FISH) testing, and gene mutation analysis may be required (Pierpont et al., 2007).

Complex (Congenital Heart Defect, Additional Extracardiac Defects), Known Cause

In almost 25% of patients with multiple defects, defined as a CHD and with at least one extracardiac defect, almost half (8%–17% of all patients) will have a recognized syndrome (Botto et al., 2007). Recognizing a genetic syndrome depends not only on astute diagnostic skills applied to the individual patient with a CHD with variable dysmorphic facial features and multiple congenital anomalies, but also on having a high level of awareness of distinctive CHD patterns. For example, the familiar association of Turner syndrome and left-sided obstructive defects imply that all newborn females with this type of CHD should be carefully scrutinized for subtle dysmorphic features. It is generally advised that all newborns with truncus arteriosus, interrupted aortic arch, type B, or tetralogy of Fallot have chromosome analysis and FISH analysis to check for a deletion 22q11.2, although the presence of facial anomalies, absent thymus, abnormal calcium levels, and other conditions would strengthen the suspicion of DiGeorge syndrome. In many ways, this group of patients comprises the most straightforward genetic counseling. Patients with a chromosome abnormality such as Down syndrome can be provided genetic counseling based on whether the abnormality is a complete trisomy occurring in a mother of advanced maternal age, or a de novo rearrangement, familial translocation, or mosaicism. The general principles of genetic counseling should be followed (Tolmie, 2002).

Likewise, individuals with a CHD associated with mendelian gene syndrome should receive genetic counseling based on the mode of inheritance. The dramatic progress in discovering disease-causing genes allows diagnostic testing, more accurate family screening and prenatal testing. For example, when counseling the family of an affected child with Alagille syndrome in which one parent is mildly affected, discussion about the 50% risk of recurrence extends beyond performing a physical examination, radiographs, and eye examination. The parents can now be offered molecular testing to determine if one of them is a carrier of a *JAG1* mutation (Goldmuntz and Lin, 2007; Pierpont et al., 2007). Genetic testing benefits the individual and the immediate family in the short term by firmly establishing a diagnosis, and allowing more accurate counseling for cardiac and noncardiac clinical outcomes.

Complex (Congenital Heart Defect with Additional Extracardiac Defects), Unknown Cause

In almost 25% of patients with multiple defects, approximately half will lack a specific syndrome diagnosis. Long-term follow-up is essential, since improved testing, and greater awareness of new syndromes may permit diagnosis. An example of evolved understanding of risks associated with a specific diagnosis would be the risk of systemic vasculopathy associated with Alagille syndrome. Providing a recurrence risk for the families of these individuals is challenging. If the constellation of defects represents a possible sporadic single-gene mutation, a very low recurrence risk can be provided. If, however, the multiple defects represent an autosomal recessive syndrome, either a new syndrome or one that has not been recognized, then the recurrence risk is potentially 25%. The genetics health provider can discuss a range of risks, citing both the lowest empiric recurrence risk and the highest risk for autosomal recessive disease. It is ill-advised to render an opinion about an unseen or inadequately evaluated individual or their relative, unless specifically seeing a family as a group upon the request of the family member; providers do not share information about relatives.

PRENATAL DIAGNOSIS AND TREATMENT

It is beyond the scope of this chapter to discuss the details of fetal cardiac imaging, but a brief review of this extremely important diagnostic technique highlights the relevance to genetic counseling for CHDs. A fetus may be imaged during a routine (level I) prenatal ultrasound designed to check pregnancy dates, examine the placenta, and conduct a general survey for birth defects. The targeted exam (level II) requires more time (30 minutes to several hours) and greater expertise to further investigate a fetal abnormality. Fetal echocardiography implies a detailed ultrasonographic examination of the fetal heart by a pediatric cardiologist. There has been a steady increase in the frequency and accuracy, and earlier use of fetal cardiac diagnosis (Mohan et al., 2005; Rasiah et al., 2006). Prenatal diagnosis of the CHD was obtained in 57% of infants who had cardiac surgery in one survey (Mohan et al., 2005). First-trimester ultrasound examination for nuchal thickness has resulted in an increased detection of CHDs (Allan, 2006; Rasiah et al., 2006). Parents should be reminded, however, that a few types of CHDs, such as aortic or pulmonic stenosis, and coarctation of the aorta, may develop or progress in severity later in gestation.

The detection of a CHD in a fetus may appear on the screening ultrasound as the result of prenatal testing for a general maternal genetic concern, for example, advanced maternal age, recurrent miscarriages. The ultrasonographic examination, which detects the fetal CHD, will often be followed by fetal echocardiography by a pediatric cardiologist. Alternatively, the primary indication for imaging the fetal heart may be a specific cardiac issue such as a family history of a prior CHD or a malformation syndrome with a risk of having an associated CHD. If a parent has an autosomal dominant disorder, there is a 50% recurrence risk that a fetus will inherit the genetic change. Depending on the specific syndrome, there may be variable penetrance and expressivity in terms of cardiac and noncardiac features.

A general appreciation of the surgical treatment of a CHD should be part of the knowledge base for the genetic health provider. Needless to say, it is usually the responsibility of the pediatric cardiologist, and in some circumstances, the cardiac surgeon, to explain details to the parents of an affected child and fetus. The parents of a fetus with a CHD who are contemplating pregnancy continuation may be influenced by the prognosis of the CHD based on surgical outcome. In broad terms, the genetic health professional can help the patient and/or family distinguish the difference between cardiac surgical palliation, repair, and cure. As appropriate, they would need to learn that transplantation becomes an exchange of one chronic disease for another. Patients and parents should be encouraged to appreciate the notion of an ongoing relationship with the cardiology and cardiac surgical team, the importance of cardiac and noncardiac data, and a look to the future with regard to lifetime outcomes. Beyond a discussion about hemodynamic or surgical outcome, the parents should be informed of the possibility of neurodevelopmental challenges, which may accompany more complex CHDs or undiagnosed syndromes (Mahle et al., 2006).

In recent years, in utero procedures have been performed on a small number of fetuses with hypoplastic left heart syndrome and/or evolving critical aortic stenosis. Selected pregnancies may be candidates for fetal aortic valve dilation and/or atrial septectomy (Tworetzy et al., 2004; Wilkins-Haug et al., 2006)

PREVENTION

In general, mothers are advised to eat a healthy diet, to refrain from risk factors (e.g., alcohol, retinoic acid) prior to and during a pregnancy, and to have medical conditions treated appropriately (e.g., diabetes, obesity, maternal phenylketonuria, seizure disorder) (reviewed by Botto et al., 2007). Prudent reproductive health care applicable to all women of childbearing age includes the recommendation to consume folic acid supplementation (0.4 mg daily) since data clearly support the reduction in risk of having a pregnancy affected by a neural tube defect (Czeizel and Dudas, 1992). Folic acid's protective effect in preventing CHDs has not been conclusively demonstrated (Botto et al., 2003a, 2004), but there is evidence that a reduction in the frequency of CHDs may be gained as an additional benefit. When a genetic health provider is leading a genetic counseling discussion, the woman will probably have been informed of the importance of periconceptional folate supplementation by her prenatal care provider, but reinforcement or clarification at the time of the genetic counseling visit may be helpful. The role of methylenetetrahydrofolate reductase (MTHFR) variants and CHD risk is promising research, which may provide insight into the possible protective action of folate, but currently has no specific role in genetic counseling for CHDs (Botto et al., 2007; van Beynum et al., 2006).

SUPPORT AND COUNSELING

Part of the role of a genetic health provider is emotional support for the individual, and/or parents of a fetus or child with a CHD. Because a CHD is often an isolated internal malformation, unlike an externally visible facial defect, there may be a tendency to underestimate the impact on the family. Nevertheless, families are deeply affected by the diagnosis of a CHD in a fetus, newborn, or child of any age and may be experiencing various stages of grieving. Depending on the genetic health provider's assessment of whether the family is dealing adequately with the diagnosis of the CHD and variable associated minor or major defects, more professional psychosocial support may be considered. Some parents of some affected fetuses may contemplate possible termination of pregnancy, a very complex, intensely personal decision. Regardless of the family's decision-making strategy (and final decision), the counseling team should offer assistance and access to additional counseling as needed.

High-quality information, often peer-reviewed, is increasingly available to professionals and consumers through the internet. In particular, the pediatric cardiology departments of most children's hospitals sponsor site, which provide information about CHDs. These can be reached through the individual hospital's Web site and typically provide text description, images and links to local and national support groups. For example, the Congenital Cardiovascular Genetics Program at the Children's Hospital of Boston has a specific Web site with links to information about treatment, genetic resources, anatomical explanations and illustrations (/http://www.childrenshospital.org/clinicalservices/Site457/mainpageS457P0.html, accessed May 1, 2009). Another source of readily available genetic information is GeneReviews (http://genereviews.org/, accessed May 11, 2009), and OMIM (Online Inheritance in Man). These are useful for well-characterized genetic syndromes and conditions, which is not as helpful for isolated CHDs.

Disease-specific advocacy groups, also known as peer support groups, play a growing role in providing information, psychosocial support, and networking resources for consumers and professionals. Individuals and families with a CHD might take advantage of a group which focuses on CHDs, such as the Congenital Heart Information Network (CHINs, http://tchin.org/, accessed May 1, 2009), and Little Hearts (http://www.littlehearts.net/, accessed May 1, 2009). Several advocacy groups are available to families of a child with a syndrome-associated CHD, for example, Down syndrome, Noonan syndrome, Costello syndrome, and Marfan syndrome. Using a standard Web browser will access the Web sites of these support groups. The online database of the Genetic Alliance can be searched for an extensive list of genetic related groups and resources (www.geneticalliance.org).

In summary, this chapter utilized genetic counseling concepts, which are established for genetic disorders, in general, and tried to adapt them to CHDs, in particular. Genetic health care providers are encouraged to have a broad-based knowledge about the medical and genetic aspects of CHDs. Emphasis was placed on distinguishing the CHD phenotype based on pattern and etiology, which should assist the genetic counseling strategy. Despite several decades of research analyzing the risk of occurrence of CHDs, there is no study that combines the ideal elements of both precurrence and recurrence, large cohort size, aggressive testing, and genetic evaluation of probands to exclude identifiable chromosome and gene syndromes, and comparing cases or population-based controls. Genetic counseling for CHDs includes assisting families to gain access to the language, information, tools, emotional support, and peer support to become empowered care team members with an important place in the decision-making conversation.

REFERENCES

Allan L. Screening the fetal heart. *Ultrasound Obstet Gynecol.* 2006;28:5–7.

Bondy CA. Writing for the Turner Syndrome Consensus Group Clinical Practice Guideline. Care of Girls and Women with Turner Syndrome: A Guideline of the Turner Syndrome Study Group. *J Clin Endocrinol Metab.* 2007;92:10–25.

Botto LD, Mulinare J, Erickson JD. Do multivitamin or folic acid supplements reduce the risk for congenital heart defects? Evidence and gaps. *Am J Med Genet A.* 2003a;121:95–101.

Botto LD, May K, Fernhoff PM, et al. A population-based study of the 22q11.2 deletion: phenotype, incidence, and contribution to major birth defects in the population. *Pediatrics.* 2003b;112:101–107.

Botto LD, Olney RS, Erickson JD. Vitamin supplements and the risk for congenital anomalies other than neural tube defects. *Am J Med Genet C Semin Med Genet.* 2004;125:12–21.

Botto L, Goldmuntz E, Lin A. Epidemiology and prevention of congenital heart defects. In: Moss and Adams' Heart Disease in Infants, Children, and Adolescents, including the Fetus and Young Adult (7th edition). Williams and Wilkins, Baltimore; 2007.

Boughman JA, Berg KA, Astemborski JA, et al. Familial risks of congenital heart defect assessed in a population-based epidemiologic study. *Am J Med Genet.* 1987;26:839–849.

Browne ML, Bell EM, Druschel CM, et al. Maternal caffeine consumption and the risk of cardiovascular malformations. *Birth Defects Res A Clin Mol Teratol.* 2007;79:533–543.

Burn J, Goodship J. Congenital Heart Disease In: Rimoin D, Connor J, Pyeritz R, et al., (eds.) Emery and Rimoin's Principles and Practice of Medical Genetics. London: Churchill Livingstone; 2002:1239–1326.

Burn J, Brennan P, Little H, et al. Recurrence risks in offspring of adults with major heart defects: results from first cohort of British collaborative study. *Lancet.* 1998;351:311–316.

Calcagni G, Digilio MC, Sarkozy A, Dallapiccola B, Marino B. Familial recurrence of congenital heart disease: an overview and review of the literature. *Eur J Pediatr.* 2007;166:111–116.

Calzolari E, Garani G, Cocchi G, et al. Congenital heart defects: 15 years of experience of the Emilia-Romagna Registry (Italy). *Eur J Epidemiol.* 2003;18:773–780.

Cripe L, Andelfinger D, Martin LJ, Shooner K, Benwon DW. Bicuspid aortic valve is heritable. *J Am Coll Cardiol.* 2004;44:138–143.

Czeizel AE, Dudas I. Prevention of the first occurrence of neural-tube defects by periconceptional vitamin supplementation. *N Engl J Med.* 1992;327:1832–1835.

Digilio MC, Casey B, Toscano A, et al. Complete transposition of the great arteries. Patterns of congenital heart disease in familial precurrence. *Circulation.* 2001;104:2809–2814.

Ferencz C, Loffredo CA, Rubin JD, Loffredo CA, Magee CA. Epidemiology of congenital heart disease: the Baltimore-Washington Infant Study 1981–1989. Mount Kisco, NY: Futura Publishing Company, Inc.; 1993.

Gill JK, Splitt M, Sharland GK, Simpson JM. Patterns of recurrence of congenital heart disease. an analysis of 6,640 consecutive pregnancies evaluated by detailed fetal echocardiography *J Am Coll Cardiol.* 2003;42:923–929.

Goldmuntz E, Lin A. Genetics of congenital heart defects. In: Moss and Adams' Heart Disease in Infants, Children, and Adolescents, including the Fetus and Young Adult (7th edition). Baltimore: Williams and Wilkins; 2007

Hoess K, Goldmuntz E, Pyeritz R. Genetic counseling for congenital heart disease: new approaches for a new decade. *Curr Cardiol Rep.* 2002;4:68–75.

Jenkins KJ, Correa A, Feinstein JA, et al. Non-inherited risk factors and congenital cardiovascular defects: Current knowledge. A scientific statement from the American Heart Association Council on Cardiovascular Disease in the Young. *Circulation.* 2007;115: 2995–3014.

Kramer HH, Majewski F, Trampisch HJ, Rammos S, Bourgeois M. Malformation patterns in children with congenital heart disease. *Am J Dis Child.* 1987;141:789–795.

Lacro R. Genetic counseling for cardiovascular malformations. In: Keane JF, Lock JE, Fyler DC (eds). Nadas' Pediatric Cardiology (Second Edition). Saunders: Elsevier, Philadelphia; 2006:57–61.

Lewin MB, McBride KL, Pignatelli R, et al. Echocardiographic evaluation of asymptomatic parental and sibling cardiovascular anomalies associated with congenital left ventricular outflow tract lesions. *Pediatrics.* 2004;114:691–696.

Lin AE, Garver KL. Genetic counseling for congenital heart defects. *J Pediatr.* 1988;113:1105–1109.

Lin AE, Herring AH, Scharenberg KS, et al. Changes in hospital-based birth prevalence of cardiovascular malformations. *Am J Med Genet.* 1999;84:102–110.

Lin AE, Salbert B, Belmont J, Smoot L. The whole is greater than the sum of the parts: Phenotyping the heart in cardiovascular genetics clinics. *Am J Med Genet.* 2004;131A:111–114

Lin AE, Basson CT, Goldmuntz E, et al. Adults with genetic syndromes and cardiovascular abnormalities: Clinical history and management. *Genet Med* 2008;10:469–494.

Loffredo CA, Chokkalingam A, Sill AM, et al. Prevalence of congenital cardiovascular malformations among relatives of infants with hypoplastic left heart, coarctation of the aorta, and d-transposition of the great arteries. *Am J Med Genet.* 2004;124A:225–230.

Mahle WT, Visconti KJ, Freier C, et al. Relationship of surgical approach to neurodevelopmental outcomes in hypoplastic left heart syndrome. *Pediatrics.* 2006;117;90–97.

Marshall AC, van der Velde ME, Tworetzky W, et al. Creation of an atrial septal defect in utero for fetuses with hypoplastic left heart syndrome and intact or highly restrictive atrial septum. *Circulation.* 2004;20;110:253–258.

McBride KL, Pignatelli R, Lewin M, et al. Inheritance analysis of congenital left ventricular outflow tract obstruction malformations: Segregation, multiplex relative risk, and heritability. *Am J Med Genet A.* 2005;134:180–186.

McDermott DA, Basson CT. Holt-Oram syndrome. GeneReviews. http://www.genetests.org. Updated November 22, 2006. Accessed February 27, 2007.

McDonald-McGinn DM, Emanuel BS, Zackai EH. 22q11.2 deletion syndrome. GeneReviews. http://www.genetests.org. Updated December 12, 2005. Accessed February 27, 2007.

Mohan UR, Kleinman CS, Kern JH. Fetal echocardiography and its evolving impact 1992 to 2002. *Am J Cardiol.* 2005;96:134–136.

Nora JJ. Multifactorial inheritance hypothesis for the etiology of congenital heart diseases. The genetic-environmental interaction. *Circulation.* 1968;38:604–617.

Piacentini G, Digilio MC, Capolino R, et al. Familial recurrence of heart defects in subjects with congenitally corrected transposition of the great arteries *Am J Med Genet A.* 2005;137:176–80.

Pierpont ME, Basson CT, Benson DW, et al. The genetic basis for congenital heart defects: Current knowledge. A scientific statement from the American Heart Association Council on Cardiovascular Disease in the Young. endorsed by the American Academy of Pediatrics *Circulation*. 2007;115:3015–3058.

Rasiah SV, Publicover M, Ewer AK, Khan KS, Kilby MD, Zamora J. A systematic review of the accuracy of first-trimester ultrasound examination for detecting major congenital heart disease. *Ultrasound Obstet Gynecol*. 2006;28:110–116.

Rasmussen SA, Olney RS, Holmes LB, Lin AE, Keppler-Noreuil, Moore CA and the National Birth Defects Prevention Study. Guidelines for case classification for the National Birth Defects Study. Birth Defects Research (Part A). 2003;67:193–201.

Resta R, Biesecker BB, Bennett RL, et al. Defining and redefining the scope and goals of genetic counseling. *J Genet Counseling*. 2006;15:77–83.

Salbert BA. Cardiovascular genetics—redefining the role of the clinical geneticist. *Prog Pediatr Cardiol*. 2003;8:105–110.

Satoda M, Gelb BD. *TFAP2B* and the Char syndrome. In:Epstein CJ, Erickson RP Wynshaw-Boris A, (eds). *Inborn Errors of Development: The Molecular Basis of Clinical Disorders of Morphogenesis*. New York: Oxford University Press; 2004:798–803.

Tolmie J. Down syndrome and other autosomal trisomies. In: Rimoin DL, Connor JM.

Tworetzky W, Wilkins-Haug L, Jennings RW, et al. Balloon dilation of severe aortic stenosis in the fetus: potential of prevention of hypoplastic left heart syndrome: candidate selection, technique, and results of successful intervention. *Circulation*. 2004;110:2125–2131.

Van Beynum IM, Kapusta L, Den Heijer M, et al. Maternal MTHFR 677C>T is a risk factor for congenital heart defects: effect modification by periconceptional folate supplementation. *Eur Heart J*. 2006;27:981–987.

Wilkins-Haug L, Tworetzky W, Benson CB, Marshall AC, Jennings RW, Lock JC Factors affecting technical success of fetal aortic valve dilation. *Ultrasound Obstet Gynecol*. 2006;28:47–52.

29

Primary Prevention of Congenital Heart Defects

LORENZO D. BOTTO

PRIMARY PREVENTION IN PEDIATRIC CARDIOLOGY

"Will it happen again?" Parents of affected children often ask this question, if not immediately, certainly at some point after the diagnosis of a congenital heart defect. For many years, this question related mainly to measuring risk rather than reducing it. Typically, medical professionals would evaluate clinical findings, family history, and pregnancy exposures to provide counseling, recurrence figures, and perhaps advice for clinical monitoring of subsequent pregnancies.

The more satisfactory answer, however, is to lower such risk of heart defects, that is, to achieve primary prevention. Unlike pregnancy termination, which reduces disease by reducing the birth of affected children, primary prevention prevents disease by ensuring that a child is born healthy. Primary prevention aims at preventing the recurrence or occurrence of congenital heart defects, much like childhood immunizations prevent infection by reducing disease susceptibility in the population, or safety measures (e.g., head helmets or harnesses) reduce workplace injuries.

But what is meant today by prevention in pediatric cardiology? By most measures, it appears to include many issues, but only in small part the primary prevention of congenital heart defects. Searching the Internet for "prevention" and "pediatric cardiology," both in the general domain (using www.google.com) and in the medical literature (using www.PubMed.gov), provides an instructive example. Most search results relate to issues such as the prevention of hyperlipidemia, hypertension, and obesity in children and adolescents, and the prevention of clinical complications of congenital heart defects or related surgery. A few more documents discuss the prevention of rheumatic fever. However, the primary prevention of congenital heart defects is dealt with in a small fraction of documents and mainly in the context of experimental or epidemiologic studies.

Such low visibility of primary prevention may be related to several factors, some of which are explored in this chapter. First, for many heart defects, the scientific evidence for effective primary prevention is limited, compared, for example, to the prevention of adult cardiovascular disease. Second, interest and public funding appears to favor research on genetic rather than modifiable risk factors. However, futuristic visions of gene therapy notwithstanding, identifying modifiable (environmental) risk factors appears to be more realistic basis for primary prevention than gene-based interventions. This is particularly true in the global context. Most births occur today in developing countries, so that the primary prevention strategies aimed at must be widely available, simple, and inexpensive, if they are to bring global benefits. Third, the impact of congenital heart defects, not only at birth but throughout life, may not be well known. This implies that the full benefits of primary prevention are probably underestimated, and for this reason the arguments for investing in primary prevention may be less convincing to the community and policy makers than they should be.

In this chapter, primary prevention of congenital heart defects is discussed through three themes: potential benefits, best evidence, and suggested strategies. The potential benefits provide the personal and community incentives for making prevention happen—by reducing or controlling exposures to risk factors, as discussed under the section Estimating the Benefits of Prevention: Incentive for Action. Second, the evidence related to risk factors and protective factors is summarized with a focus on their potential impact on disease occurrence (e.g., by their potential attributable fraction). Such evidence provides the opportunity to translate science into action or change in practice. Finally, based on these concepts, a framework for prevention will be suggested that can form the basis for a (tentative) plan for action. The focus throughout is on primary prevention, as the most desirable form of prevention for individuals and society, and on the crucial need for new and better data so that prevention strategies can be safe and effective.

ESTIMATING THE BENEFITS OF PREVENTION: INCENTIVE FOR ACTION

To properly estimate the benefits of prevention, a person-centered, a lifespan perspective can be helpful (Botto et al., 2008). Such perspective strives to assess the impact of heart defects on the affected person, family, and society; furthermore it expands beyond the weeks or months surrounding birth or diagnosis to encompass the lifespan of the individual within the society, and thus can help establish a comprehensive benchmark for discussing the benefits of prevention.

Historically, the impact of heart defects has been discussed in terms of morbidity and mortality related to diagnosis, and medical and surgical treatments. While these are crucial elements, it is important to also incorporate the individual long-term outcomes and societal issues. The list of such issues is long and includes developmental disabilities, quality of life, insurability, employment, impact on caregivers, costs (to families and society), societal integration, and health disparities. These elements allow one to evaluate the impact of prevention not only as the number of cases averted but also as years of life or quality-adjusted years of life saved, and cost savings. Although the comprehensive assessment of impact is not entirely available yet, data are becoming increasingly available from scientific reports. As these results are discussed, it will be important to monitor changes over time. Because survival, treatment, costs, and the health care system changes over time, so will the estimates of impact that depend on them. Finally, from an epidemiologic perspective, it is crucial to promote population-based evaluations, to understand the issues more completely, and to reduce biases that could be associated with the exclusive reliance on selected samples.

Reducing Occurrence

A key benchmark in assessing the potential impact of prevention is the occurrence of heart defects. For example, this information helps to translate estimates of relative risks of established risk factors into absolute numbers of cases potentially averted in a given population.

Occurrence can be evaluated using incidence and prevalence. Incidence measures the number of new cases among an initially disease-free cohort of at-risk individuals within a specific time frame. Although a good indicator of the absolute risk of disease in a population, incidence is a difficult measure for heart defects. For example, the disease-free cohort is formed, strictly, by conceptuses, whose number cannot be estimated with any accuracy because of the many unrecognized early pregnancy losses (Mason et al., 2005). Prevalence, on the other hand, reflects the occurrence of disease at a point in time in a defined population. Prevalence, therefore, can be estimated for fetuses at a certain gestational age, stillbirths, newborns, infants, or a combination of these. Excluding pregnancy losses (unrecognized and recognized) from prevalence calculations results in an underestimation of the overall occurrence of heart defects among conceptuses. However, because it is easier to measure operationally, prevalence is commonly used in epidemiologic studies of heart defect occurrence (Mason et al., 2005).

Even so, estimating prevalence correctly is challenging. Prevalence at birth has been assessed in many reports, even in recent decades (Abu-Harb et al., 1994; Chinn et al., 1989; Eichhorn et al., 1990; Fixler et al., 1990; Fyler et al., 1980; Grabitz et al., 1988; Kidd et al., 1993; Roy et al., 1994; Samanek 1994; Stoll et al., 1989; Tanner et al., 2005; Ursell et al., 1985). When interpreting these data, one crucial question is how much of this variation is real (related perhaps to variations in risk factors for disease), and how much depends on how the information is obtained. For example, local prevalence estimates could be influenced by diagnostic practices, case definitions, case classification, inclusion of pregnancy terminations, timing of diagnosis (fetal, birth, or childhood), length of follow-up from birth to potential diagnosis, and reporting procedures (Hoffman and Kaplan, 2002; Lin et al., 1999; McCrindle, 2004; Rosenthal, 1998). Estimates of the birth prevalence of heart defects are available in other chapters and in several reviews (Botto et al., 2008; Hoffman and Kaplan, 2002; McCrindle, 2004; Rosenthal, 1998). Overall, these estimates suggest a prevalence of approximately 3 per 1000 for clinically severe conditions, 6 per 1000 when also including moderately serious conditions (Hoffman and Kaplan, 2002), and 9 per 1000 to 15–20 per 1000 when further including smaller septal defects and milder valvar stenoses (Hiraishi et al., 1992; Tegnander et al., 2006).

Generalizing these findings from relatively small sample areas to countries or continents requires considerable caution. Nevertheless, some extrapolation is necessary since there are few data from large areas of the world (Hoffman, 1995; Hoffman and Kaplan, 2002; Lopez and Mathers, 2006; Murray and Lopez, 1998). For example, based on the overall estimate of 9 per 1000 for all heart defects, and 3 per 1000 for severe heart defects, it can be estimated that every year roughly 1.2 affected million babies are born worldwide with heart defects (36,000 in the United States), and of these, 400,000 babies have severe heart defects (12,000 in the United States). As high as they may appear, these numbers may be conservative, if the rates in developing countries are higher than those in developed countries because of greater exposure to nutritional, maternal, or environmental risk factors. Moreover, these numbers underscore the importance of promoting simple and inexpensive prevention measures that can be implemented with limited resources.

Heart defect prevalence among children and adults is less known. The American Heart Association estimates that approximately 1 million adults (or approximately 1 in 300 people) live in the United States with a congenital heart defect. Such figures are estimates, typically computed by estimating the birth prevalence of specific conditions combined with estimated survival rates (Hoffman et al., 2004; McCrindle, 2004). More detailed data and additional validation are urgently needed so that the actual number of affected adults can be more accurately assessed (Warnes et al., 2001; Williams et al., 2006). At issue is that certain conditions may be more significant for adults than for children, and vice versa. For example, certain septal defects may become smaller or close over time; surgery may modify the effects on daily life; and certain conditions that are asymptomatic at birth, such as bicuspid aortic valve, may evolve into clinically significant lesions in adults (Cecconi et al., 2006; Chambers, 2005; Ward, 2000).

Reducing Mortality

Preventing heart defects has a significant potential for decreasing infant deaths. Worldwide, congenital heart defects are the leading cause of infant deaths due to congenital anomalies (Lopez and Mathers, 2006; Rosano et al., 2000). In North America, according to one estimate, congenital heart defects contribute to one third of infant deaths due to congenital anomalies, and, overall, to approximately one tenth of all infant deaths (Lopez and Mathers, 2006; Rosano et al., 2000). In developing countries, the impact is likely even higher, because of the fewer resources available to treat affected babies. In fact, in one study based on international vital records data from the World Health Organization, the infant mortality due to birth defects was inversely correlated to a country's per capita gross domestic product (Rosano et al., 2000).

In the United States, at least two studies documented a decline of mortality from congenital heart defects in recent decades (Boneva et al., 2001; Gillum, 1994). In the more recent study (Boneva et al., 2001) this mortality declined from 80% to 40% from 1979 through 1997, yet in the last years of the study (1995–1997) heart defects still caused approximately 6000 deaths per year. The extent to which these deaths are averted is one measurable potential benefit of prevention.

Reducing Developmental Disabilities

In estimating the impact of prevention on the life of people with heart defects, it is important to consider neurodevelopmental outcomes. In fact, in one study, clinicians and parents alike rated neurologic disability a greater concern than cardiac disability when considering quality of life for children with congenital heart defects (Knowles et al., 2006). With improving survival, these outcomes are of increasing importance (Brown et al., 2005; Mahle, 2006; Wernovsky, 2005; Williams, 2005).

Neurodevelopmental challenges are common in children whose congenital heart defect is a component of an underlying genetic syndrome or multiple congenital anomaly complex. However, recent data suggest that children without obvious extracardiac involvement may still be at increased risk for unrecognized or secondary neurodevelopmental disability (Wernovsky, 2005). For example, with improvements in brain imaging, children with apparently isolated heart defects are now increasingly found to have also subtle brain anomalies such as neuronal migration defects and Chiari I malformation (Limperopoulos et al., 2000). In addition, their brain may be affected by altered hemodynamics related to the heart defect or to the surgery, resulting in seizures, intraventricular hemorrhage, and periventricular leukomalacia (Limperopoulos et al., 2002; Mahle, 2006; Mahle et al., 2000). Finally, neuropsychiatric conditions, including attention deficit and hyperactivity disorders, anxiety, and depression, are being increasingly diagnosed in older children and adults with congenital heart defects. Although it is unclear what can be done to reduce these adverse outcomes, it is reasonable to expect that at least the developmental disabilities secondary to surgery or altered hemodynamics could be eliminated by the primary prevention of heart defects.

Improving Quality Of Life

There is an increased recognition of the need for long-term studies of quality of life (Schultz and Wernovsky, 2005; Williams, 2005), which include school functioning, social functioning, independent living, and social integration (Brown et al., 2005). Importantly, quality-of-life studies emphasize the perspective of the people with a heart defect and their families. Evaluating quality of life, however, is challenging. It is a relatively new area of investigation and its methods and tools are still being developed (Eiser and Morse, 2001a, 2001b, 2001c; Goldbeck and Melches, 2005).

This relative novelty may be one reason why the current evidence from quality-of-life studies is not always consistent. In addition, quality of life is inherently a complex concept, as it depends on many interdependent medical, personal, and social factors such as disease severity, medical and surgical interventions, health care coverage and quality, income, personal attitude, and societal attitudes toward chronic illness (Culbert et al., 2003; Goldbeck and Melches, 2006; McCrindle et al., 2006; Moons et al., 2005; Rose et al., 2005; Williams, 2005).

For example, one population-based study in Finland found reasonably good outcomes in a group of individuals with heart defects (mainly mild to moderate conditions such as septal defects), including educational attainment, employment level, and frequency of steady relationship, compared to individuals without heart defects (Sairanen et al., 2005). By contrast, several studies in North America and Europe reported worse health-related quality of life in people with heart defects compared to unaffected controls or normative data (Green, 2004; Lane et al., 2002; Spijkerboer et al., 2006). Quality of life seemed to be influenced not only by the type of heart defect and of surgery (Culbert et al., 2003) (Moons et al., 2004) but also by family income (McCrindle et al., 2006) and a person's age (Claessens et al., 2005; Lip et al., 2003; Rietveld et al., 2002). In the United States, the difficulty in obtaining employment, health insurance, and mortgages was also reported to considerably influence the quality of life of adults with heart defects in the United States (Jefferies et al., 2004), even among people with relatively mild conditions (Crossland et al., 2004).

Even though the evidence is preliminary and incomplete, it clearly indicates deficits in quality of life among many individuals with heart defects and their families. Evaluations of the benefits of primary prevention should incorporate as much as possible this new and increasing body of literature on the quality of life of people with heart defects and their families.

Reducing Disparities

Reducing health disparities is a primary consideration in prevention. Health disparities include differences in the occurrence, mortality, and burden of disease among groups of people. Disparities are a particular concern when they arise because of the unequal distribution in the population of modifiable risk factors, such as environmental exposures, low socioeconomic status, and access to care. Identifying and eradicating health disparities are also critical components of the path to achieving social justice in the community at large (Johnson et al., 2006).

One obvious example of disparity is the excess burden of morbidity and mortality related to heart defects in developing compared to developed countries, which was discussed previously as being related, broadly, to differences in a nation's gross income and infrastructure. Subtler but important disparities also exist within developed countries, but may go unrecognized or untreated. In the United States, some evidence suggests that children of African American or Hispanic ethnicity with heart defects may have higher mortality rates compared to similarly affected white children (Benavidez et al., 2006; Boneva et al., 2001; Gillum, 1994). The factors determining this excess risk of death are unclear. There is an urgent need to identify and eliminate these factors.

The implications for primary prevention are twofold. By reducing occurrence, primary prevention may serve as one way to eliminate health disparities. To do so, however, primary prevention activities need to be implemented so that the benefits accrue to the entire population. This goal will likely require activities aimed at decreasing the root causes of disparities and targeted at those groups in which such disparities are found.

Reducing Cost

Congenital heart defects are costly, even based on current data that typically are partial and, in some instances, antiquated (a reassessment of cost issues is presented in another section of this book). One study published over a decade ago estimated that lifetime cost of illness for babies born each year in the United States with a few selected heart defects (Table 29–1) exceeded 500 million dollars in medical costs and 1.2 billion dollars in total costs (in 1992 dollars) (Centers for Disease Control and Prevention et al., 1995; Waitzman et al., 1996). These figures included estimates of direct costs (medical, developmental, and special education services) and some indirect costs (costs of lost work and household productivity). A large fraction of the direct costs was related to surgery and a larger fraction of indirect costs was related to lost productivity due to death in infancy.

The real costs today are likely even higher, for several reasons. In-hospital charges were recently estimated for 2003 in the United States for selected major heart defects (Centers for Disease Control and Prevention, 2007), but there is much more work to be done. For example, there are many more heart defects than those

TABLE 29-1. *Lifetime Costs for Selected Birth Defects for Babies Born in One Year in the United States. All Cost Estimates Are in 1992 US Dollars*

	Medical Costs	Total Cost	Cost/Case
Congenital Heart Defect			
Single ventricle	61,659,000	172,631,000	344,000
Truncus arteriosus	107,578,000	209,676,000	505,000
Tetralogy of Fallot	185,122,000	360,486,000	262,000
Transposition of great arteries	166,334,000	514,529,000	267,000
Total	520,693,000	1,257,322,000	
Other Congenital Anomalies			
Spina bifida	204,512,000	489,289,000	294,000
Down syndrome	278,696,000	1,847,752,000	451,000
Cerebral palsy	851,809,000	2,425,781,000	503,000

Rate: cases per 1,000 live births (for cerebral palsy, rate per 1,000 3-year olds)

Source: Waitzman et al.,1996 references 86–87.

included in the published cost analysis. Also, some heart defects that are seldom considered in childhood, such as bicuspid aortic valve, can evolve into serious conditions requiring surgery in the adult, adding to lifetime costs. The actual costs of management and intervention have likely increased since the time of the published estimates. Time spent and loss of productivity by family members for provision of care typically has not been included in cost estimates (Centers for Disease Control and Prevention et al., 1995). Finally, the costs related to neurodevelopmental disabilities may have been underestimated in previous studies.

Having valid and recent estimates of costs is crucial as an impetus and rationale for prevention. For example, underscoring that preventing one case of d-transposition of the great arteries through preconceptional treatment of a diabetic woman saves at least 277,000 US dollars (in 1992 dollars) may help strengthen the currently low investment in preventive services (Centers for Disease Control and Prevention et al., 1995; Waitzman et al., 1996).

CHARACTERIZING RISK FACTORS: SCIENCE FOR ACTION

For effective primary prevention, risk factors must be reduced and protective factors must be increased. For heart defects, characterizing such factors has been challenging, and the current evidence for many exposures is limited or inconsistent (Jenkins et al., 2007). When discussing primary prevention, it is helpful to focus on environmental risk factors, which can be modified, rather than on genetic factors alone. Genetic risk

factors for heart defects are reviewed regularly in the literature (Garg, 2006; Gruber, 2005; Pierpont et al., 2007) and will not be explored here in any detail.

Selected findings are discussed here, mainly from the perspective of prevention. A more extensive review of the data is available and includes extensive tables and references (Jenkins et al., 2007). Additional resources include other chapters of this book, online databases such as Reprotox and TERIS (2006a; 2006b), and, for the practicing professional with specific queries, the staff at Teratogen Information Services (TIS), which are present in several countries.

From Epidemiology to Prevention: Concepts of Risk and Attributable Fraction

Because much of the evidence on risk factors comes from epidemiologic studies, it can be helpful to discuss briefly their strengths and limitations, and how to best use their data to guide action (Jenkins et al., 2007). Two key issues are how to characterize and interpret risk estimates in epidemiologic studies and how to translate risk into metrics, such as attributable fraction, that can help assess the benefits of prevention strategies that reduce such risks.

Ideally, risk estimates in epidemiologic studies provide valid and precise information on items such as the magnitude of the risk, the specific outcome associated with the exposure, the risk by type of exposure, and potential interactions (the changes in risk by gender, race, age, or other factors). As an example, for maternal diabetes, one should like to validly assess the relative and absolute risk for each major heart defect, ideally by type or severity of diabetes. A major challenge is evaluating risk so that estimates are valid (e.g., unbiased) and precise (e.g., with tight confidence intervals). This can be difficult and likely explains in part the often different or inconsistent findings across epidemiologic studies.

For example, finding in one study that smoking is associated with a certain heart defect does not imply that smoking is a cause or even a risk factor. Such association may be due to a confounder (e.g., alcohol use, if alcohol causes heart defects and is more common among smokers compared to non-smokers), or to bias (e.g., recall bias, if mothers of affected babies are more likely than mothers of controls to remember or report smoking during pregnancy), or perhaps to chance, if the excess of smokers among case-mothers in a case-control study is randomly due to sampling. Even good studies can generate spurious findings, if only by chance. Thus, reasonable indicators of a finding's validity are not only the epidemiologic quality of the single study but also the reproducibility of that finding across several well-designed studies in different settings.

Another source of variation in studies of environmental exposures or maternal illnesses is the limited use of biomarkers of exposures. In many etiologic studies of heart defects, exposure assessment relies on maternal reports (e.g., of fever, chronic illnesses, medication use), usually with limited validation. Susceptibility genotypes, which may play a major role in the causal web, are typically unknown or unmeasured.

Even well-characterized risk factors may not be necessarily causal. Causality is a complex concept and difficult to infer from epidemiological studies alone. An understanding of causality, of its logical underpinnings, and of the likely complexity of most causal factors (better characterized as causal webs than as individual factors) is crucial when trying to move from information on risk factors to models of causality for intervention and prevention (Rothman, 2002).

Let us assume that a risk factor has been validly and precisely characterized, preferably through replicated studies, and that a convincing argument can be made for causality. Then, by factoring the frequency of the exposure in the population, an estimate can be made of attributable fraction.

Attributable fraction, or attributable risk, is a helpful concept in prevention, because it provides an estimate of the potential impact of the risk factors in the population (attributable fraction). Because of its role in planning prevention, and because of the potential pitfalls in its use, a brief discussion can be helpful. The concept of attributable fraction is being increasingly used as a way to evaluate the impact at the population level of an association between an exposure and a disease. Attributable fraction is defined as the proportion of disease cases that can be attributed to exposure (Rothman, 2002).

Unlike measures of association like the relative risk, attributable fraction depends both on the strength of the association between exposure and disease and the prevalence of exposure in the population. Whereas in its simplest form attributable fraction is a straightforward concept (Hanley, 2001), in many practical settings it can have subtleties that need to be appreciated and incorporated in the estimations. In particular, many epidemiologic studies use multivariate techniques to obtain risk estimates for one factor adjusted for other factors or confounders, or examine factors across multiple (more than two) levels of exposure. Estimating attributable fraction in these common situations requires additional considerations, lest the results be invalid (Benichou, 2001; Rockhill et al., 1998). Although the literature on attributable fraction in relation to congenital heart defect is scarce, one systematic assessment has been conducted on data from a large epidemiologic study of heart defects (Wilson et al., 1998).

Candidates for Prevention: Selected Risk Factors

The following section focuses on selected exposures (Table 29-2), chosen either because they are established risk factors for heart defects (e.g., diabetes, retinoic acid) or because they are so common in many populations (e.g., smoking, obesity) that they may be of concern even if associated with mildly increased risks for heart defects. The examination of these risk factors is not exhaustive. Rather, it focuses on specific aspects relevant to primary prevention, such as the strength of the evidence, the specific outcomes related to the factor, the preventability of the risk factor, and its frequency in the population. As noted, a recent review with additional discussion and references has been published (Jenkins et al., 2007).

Diabetes. Maternal diabetes is an established teratogen that causes multiple congenital anomalies, including heart defects (Becerra et al., 1990; Correa et al., 2003; Ferencz et al., 1997; Kousseff, 1999; Loffredo, 2000; Moore et al., 2000; Ray et al., 2001; Wren et al., 2003). Separate risk estimates associated with type 1 and type 2 diabetes are rarely available. Specific heart defects consistently associated with maternal diabetes include laterality defects (heterotaxy), several conotruncal defects, and, less consistently, some left ventricular outflow obstructive defects and septal defects (Becerra et al., 1990; Correa et al., 2003; Ferencz et al., 1997; Loffredo, 2000; Rowland et al., 1973; Wren et al., 2003). Obstructive hypertrophic cardiomyopathy also occurs but typically resolves. Estimates of relative risks for heart defects in the aggregate are approximately 4–5, though they can be higher for some types of heart defects, especially when associated with extracardiac anomalies (Table 29-3) (Becerra et al., 1990; Ferencz et al., 1997; Loffredo, 2000; Ray et al., 2001; Wren et al., 2003) Studies examining risks associated with gestational diabetes are inconsistent (Aberg et al., 2001; Martinez-Frias et al., 1998; Sheffield et al., 2002).

Studies have shown that the teratogenic risk associated with maternal diabetes can be reduced considerably by careful glycemic control before conception, thus providing an important opportunity for primary prevention (Cousins, 1991; Johnson et al., 2006). However, this finding has yet to be fully implemented in practice, and many affected pregnancies continue to occur (Holing et al., 1998; Johnson et al., 2006; Ray et al., 2001). The frequency of diabetes among women of childbearing age varies by country, age, and other factors. One recent report estimates that diabetes affects approximately 2% or 1.85 million women of childbearing age in the United States and states that preconceptional diabetes management could decrease the risk for pregnancy loss and congenital malformation for approximately 113,000 births

TABLE 29-2. *Selected Exposures and Risk for Congenital Heart Defects: Estimated Risk, Phenotypes, Exposure Frequency*

Factor	Congenital Heart Defect	Estimated Risk	Exposure Type, and Frequency	Comments
Diabetes	Laterality defects, conotruncal defects, septal defects	OR usually 4 to 5, higher for some phenotypes	Pregestational diabetes reported in 1%–2% of women of childbearing age in United States	Established teratogen; diabetes increasing in many countries; preventable by glycemic control before conception
Febrile illness, influenza	Left-sided defects, including coarctation of the aorta; tricuspid atresia, dTGA and other conotruncal malformations, VSD, possibly others.	Relative risk of 1.5–3, possibly higher for tricuspid atresia and other defects	First trimester febrile illness reported in approximately 6%–8% of pregnancies (usually in context of respiratory illness)	Established teratogen in animals and for some human malformations; risk for heart defects may be higher with flu associated with high fever
Folic acid deficiency	Conotruncal defects, septal defects, possibly others	Doubling of risk among nonusers of supplements in clinical trial, but wide confidence interval	In many countries at most half and usually many fewer women conceive while on folic acid supplements	Possible risk factor; data are suggestive that not taking a folic acid-containing supplement can increase the risk for certain heart defects, but the data are not definitive, compared for example to those on neural tube defects
Maternal phenylketonuria	Tetralogy of Fallot, VSD, PDA, left-sided defects (including hypoplastic left heart syndrome)	With high phenylalanine levels in pregnancy, relative risk up to 6	Frequency of PKU is approximately 1 in 20,000 newborn girls among whites	Established teratogen; rare but preventable with strict dietary compliance from before conception
Retinoic acid	Conotruncal defects	High relative and absolute risk	Oral therapy teratogenic, topical unlikely; accurate data on frequency of use are not generally available	Established, potent teratogen; concerning because many users are young women; retinoic acid use is subject to rigorous controls in some countries but not others
Obesity	Several heart defects, including conotruncal defects, unclear if specific	Relative risk between 1 and 3, but some studies are negative	Obesity frequent and rising in many countries; risks typically associated with body mass index (BMI) >29, but some studies show risks at BMI 25 to 29	Causality not clear; association possibly due in part to unrecognized diabetes; important individual and public health concern, because obesity is increasing in many countries
Smoking	Septal defects, others	Relative risk between 1 and 3, but some studies are negative	Frequency of smoking among women is high and rising in many countries, including developing countries; in the US in 2003, 11% of pregnant women smoked	Causality for heart defects not clear, but preventable; strong evidence that smoking can cause other adverse pregnancy outcomes (e.g., low birth weight)
Caffeine	No clear association with structural heart defects	No clear indication of increased risk	Coffee use is common, but caffeine also found in many soft drinks (including diet drinks)	No clear indication of teratogenic risk for heart defects; caffeine crosses the placenta and can have cardiovascular effects
Alcohol	Possibly several heart defects, including conotruncal defects	Inconsistent findings, some studies do not find association	Alcohol use common in many cultures; in US, about 15% of newborns exposed in pregnancy	Known teratogen, major effects on central nervous system, association with specific heart defects still unclear

Adapted and modified from Jenkins et al., 2007 *Circulation.* 115(23):2995–3014; and Botto et al. Epidemiology and Prevention of Congenital Heart Defects. In: Allen HD, Driscoll DJ, Shaddy RE, Feltes TF, (eds). Moss and Adams' Heart Disease in Infants, Children, and Adolescents, including the Fetus and Young Adult. Seventh ed. Philadelphia: Lippincott.

per year (Johnson et al., 2006). The high and rising rates of diabetes and diabetes-related risk factors (Harris et al., 1998; Mokdad et al., 2003) underscores the need for a renewed call to action for health providers to help prevent diabetes-related heart defects.

Rubella. The teratogenicity of rubella in pregnancy is well established, and the effectiveness of rubella immunization in decreasing rubella-associated birth defects is testimony to the power of primary prevention worldwide (Forrest et al., 2002). Specific heart defects associated with congenital rubella syndrome include pulmonic stenosis (valvar, supravalvar, or peripheral), patent ductus arteriosus, and, less frequently, other conditions such as tetralogy of Fallot (Reef et al., 2000).

Through sustained immunization campaigns, congenital rubella syndrome has been nearly eliminated in the United States, though continued vigilance is crucial

TABLE 29-3. *Prevention by Vitamin Use: Summary of Studies on Periconceptional Use of Vitamins and Occurrence of Congenital Heart Defects*

Type of Study	Authors and Year	Population-based	Study Participants	Exposure	Relative Risk (95% Confidence Interval)		
					Heart Defects (Overall)	Outflow tract defects	Ventricular Septal Defect
Randomized clinical trial	Czeizel et al., 1998	–	2471 women on MV supplements; 2391 on trace elements	MV pill with 0.8 mg folic acid	0.42 (0.19–0.98)	0.48 (0.04–5.34)	0.24 (0.05–1.14)
Case-control	Shaw et al., 1995	Yes	207 with OTD, 481 controls	MV supplements	–	0.70 (0.46–1.1)	–
Case-control	Scanlon et al., 1997	Yes	126 with OTD, 679 controls	MV supplements with folic acid	–	0.97 (0.6–1.6)	–
Case-control	Botto et al., 1996 & 2000	Yes	958 with heart defects, 3029 controls	MV supplements	0.76 (0.60–0.97)	0.46 (0.24–0.86)	0.61 (0.38–0.99)
Case-control	Werler et al., 1999	No	157 with OTD, 186 with VSD, 521 controls	MV supplements	–	1.00 (0.70–1.50)	1.20 (0.80–1.80)

MV, multivitamin; OTD, outflow tract defects, VSD, ventricular septal defects.
Adapted from Botto et al., *Am J Med Genet* C. 2004, 125(1):12–21.

(Reef et al., 2000; Reef et al., 2006). Worldwide, rubella infection and congenital rubella syndrome remain a significant problem, underscoring the need for global eradication of this preventable condition (Robertson et al., 2003).

Fever and Flu. Fever and hyperthermia are established teratogens in animal models (Edwards et al., 1995; Graham and Edwards 1998; Roulston et al., 1999). However, characterizing the cardiac teratogenicity of febrile illnesses in humans remains difficult. For example, reports of febrile illness in pregnancy are rarely validated, and disentangling the potential effects of infection, fever, or medications is challenging. The bulk of the evidence suggests that first-trimester febrile or flulike illnesses are associated with an increased risk for heart defects in the aggregate (relative risks of approximately 2–3), with higher relative risks for certain conditions such as tricuspid atresia, coarctation of the aorta, aortic stenosis, and perhaps ventricular septal defects (Botto et al., 2002; Graham and Edwards, 1998; Loffredo, 2000; Shaw et al., 2002; Tikkanen and Heinonen, 1991a; Zhang and Cai, 1993).

The frequency in the general population of such illnesses in early pregnancy is unclear, though in several studies approximately 6%–8% of women in the control groups report a respiratory infection or febrile illness (Botto et al., 2002; Shaw et al., 2002; Tikkanen and Heinonen, 1991a; Zhang and Cai, 1993). If these figures are valid, at least 250,000 pregnancies are exposed to such illnesses yearly in the United States. If febrile illnesses cause heart defects, prevention

strategies may include avoidance of ill contacts and possibly preconceptional immunization before flu season. In addition, two studies reported that periconceptional use of multivitamin supplements among women with febrile illness reduced the fever-associated risk for heart defects (Botto et al., 2002; Shaw et al., 2002), suggesting a further benefit of supplement use (for a more extensive discussion on the potential risk reduction associated with the use of folic acid–containing supplements, see section on multivitamins).

Maternal Phenylketonuria. Maternal phenylketonuria (PKU) (women with PKU and high blood phenylalanine levels during pregnancy) is teratogenic, with devastating effects on the brain and sometimes the heart (Levy et al., 2001; Matalon et al., 2003; Rouse and Azen, 2004). Specific heart defects associated with maternal PKU include left-sided defects (coarctation of the aorta to hypoplastic left heart syndrome), tetralogy of Fallot, septal defects, and possibly patent ductus arteriosus (Levy et al., 2001; Matalon et al., 2003; Rouse and Azen, 2004). Estimated relative risk has been high (6–15), and in one study, the absolute risk for heart defects was 14% (34 of 235 pregnancies) among pregnancies exposed to high levels of phenyalanine (Levy et al., 2001). Strict control of phenyalanine levels from before conception considerably reduces the risk for heart defects and other adverse outcomes in the child (Levy et al., 2001; Matalon et al., 2003; Rouse and Azen, 2004).

The frequency of women with PKU is unknown. Assuming a birth prevalence of PKU of 1 in 20,000 female births, an estimated 200 girls with PKU are born yearly in the United States, and will eventually be at risk for having an affected pregnancy if untreated.

Seizures Disorders and Seizure Medications. Most women with seizure disorders have uneventful pregnancies, and seizure medications, rather than seizure disorders per se, are currently thought to be the main determinants of risk (Holmes et al., 2001). Medications associated with teratogenic risk include phenytoin, hydantoin, and valproic acid (American College of Obstetricians and Gynecologists 1997; Barrett and Richens, 2003; Crawford, 2005; Pschirrer, 2004; Samren et al., 1999; Samren et al., 1997), although the risk for specific heart defects has not been well studied.

In the United States, seizure medications are prescribed for an estimated 1 million women (19 per 1,000), potentially affecting an estimated 75,000 pregnancies every year (Johnson et al., 2006). Prevention requires a joint effort by women and physicians. Preconceptional counseling is crucial, as is the strategy, where feasible, of not even beginning therapy with teratogenic medications in young girls (American College of Obstetricians and Gynecologists 1997; Crawford, 2005; Johnson et al., 2006; Pschirrer, 2004). It is unclear whether women on these medications benefit from high doses of folic acid, beyond those recommended to all women of childbearing age.

Thalidomide and Retinoic Acid Congeners. These medications are potent teratogens and cause severe and complex heart defects, including conotruncal anomalies, in addition to other major birth defects (Coberly et al., 1996; Lammer et al., 1985; Smithells and Newman, 1992).

From a prevention perspective, retinoic acid and its congeners, which include isotretinoin and etretinate, are particularly concerning because they may be used by young women for the treatment of acne and other skin conditions (Honein et al., 2001). Although strict regulatory guidelines have been issued in some countries, exposures continue to occur (Honein et al., 2001; Johnson et al., 2006; Perlman et al., 2001).

Vitamin A. Vitamin A is widely available in supplements, including in high-dose formulations. Beta carotene (one form of vitamin A) has not been associated with increased risks for congenital heart defects. Retinol (the other main form of vitamin A) has been associated in some studies with an increased risk for heart defects. In particular, exposure to high doses (>10,000 IU) was associated with an increased risk for conotruncal heart defects, in particular d-transposition of the great arteries (Botto et al., 2001; Rothman et al., 1995; Werler

et al., 1990). Other studies did not find this association (Khoury et al., 1996; Mastroiacovo et al., 1999; Mills et al., 1997; Shaw et al., 1996). Nevertheless, it appears reasonable to avoid high-dose retinol supplements in the periconceptional period, unless they are used to treat severe deficiencies (e.g., in developing countries) and to favor supplements containing beta carotene.

Other Medications. Trimethoprim-sulfonamide and sulfasalazine have been associated with a mild to moderate increase in risk for heart defects (Czeizel et al., 2001; Hernandez-Diaz et al., 2000). In one study, the use of folic acid supplements decreased the excess risk associated with these compounds (Hernandez-Diaz et al., 2000).

Lithium. Recent estimates suggest that the risk associated with lithium is smaller than previously thought (Schou et al., 1973), although small to moderate increases in risk for Ebstein anomaly cannot be excluded (Cohen et al., 1994; Jacobson et al., 1992; Warner, 2000). Women with manic-depressive conditions may benefit from targeted preconceptional counseling and prenatal care as they may be at risk for adverse pregnancy outcomes, other than those potentially related to lithium exposure (Cohen et al., 1994; Jacobson et al., 1992; Kallen and Tandberg, 1983; Warner, 2000).

Common Exposures with Limited or Inconsistent Risk Data

Obesity. It is still unclear whether obesity is associated with an increased risk for heart defects, and whether such an association, when found, is causal. Results are inconsistent for heart defects in aggregate (Ferencz et al., 1997; Mikhail et al., 2002; Watkins and Botto, 2001) and for conotruncal anomalies (Ferencz et al., 1997; Shaw et al., 2000; Waller et al., 1994). Such inconsistency is not surprising because obesity is a complex, heterogeneous exposure and is difficult to examine in epidemiologic studies (Jenkins et al., 2007). However, it is important to exclude even small risks, because of the high and rising frequency of obesity in the United States and other countries (Mokdad et al., 2003).

Caffeine. Although caffeine is frequently consumed and has proven cardiovascular effects, there is no evidence of a cardiac teratogenicity, according to numerous reports from the Baltimore-Washington Infant Study (BWIS) (Ferencz et al., 1997), the Finnish cardiovascular study (Tikkanen and Heinonen, 1990; Tikkanen and Heinonen, 1992b), the National Birth Defects Prevention Study (NBDPS) (Browne et al., 2007), as well as from other studies (Linn et al., 1982; Olsen et al., 1991; Rosenberg et al., 1982) and a systematic review (Browne, 2006).

Alcohol. Alcohol is an established human teratogen and causes a wide range of structural malformations and neurodevelopmental abnormalities (Hoyme et al., 2005; Jones, 2005). The association with heart defects has been less impressive, with inconsistent or negative results in several large studies (Adams et al., 1989; Ferencz et al., 1997; Tikkanen and Heinonen, 1990; Tikkanen and Heinonen, 1991b, 1992a, 1992b). Nevertheless, the overall teratogenic effects of alcohol use make prevention of this exposure an important public health priority (Institute of Medicine, 1996; Johnson et al., 2006). According to one study, approximately 7 million women of childbearing age in the United States are frequent drinkers, and without preconception interventions, alcohol misuse might affect approximately 577,000 births per year (Johnson et al., 2006).

Smoking. Although smoking is an established risk factor for low birth weight, preterm birth, and other adverse outcomes, the evidence for cardiac teratogenicity is unclear. The bulk of the evidence suggest that a small risk may exist (odds ratios approximately between 1 and 2) (Kallen, 1999; Malik et al., 2008; Woods and Raju, 2001), or perhaps slightly higher (odds ratio of approximately 2) for some conotruncal anomalies (Ferencz et al., 1997; Shaw et al., 2002). Although small, such risks are of concern because of the frequency of smoking in women. In 2003, an estimated 11% of pregnant women in the United States smoked during pregnancy (Johnson et al., 2006). Rates of smoking are increasing among women in many countries (Amos and Haglund, 2000).

Potential Protective Factors: Folic acid and Multivitamin Supplements

The role of folic acid and multivitamin supplementation in reducing the risk for some heart defects is increasingly studied (Bailey and Berry, 2005; Botto et al., 2004; Daly et al., 2005; Huhta and Hernandez-Robles, 2005). If confirmed, the impact of this finding would be considerable because the fraction of preventable heart defects may be large, many women of childbearing age may benefit, and vitamins, including folic acid, are inexpensive and easily transportable. Thus prevention through vitamin supplementation could be a viable worldwide strategy.

The evidence for a possible protective effect has been recently reviewed (Bailey and Berry, 2005; Botto et al., 2008; Botto et al., 2004; Daly et al., 2005; Huhta

and Hernandez-Robles 2005; Jenkins et al., 2007). Briefly, the majority of the data (Table 29–3), including the randomized trial (Czeizel, 1998), are consistent with a reduced risk for selected heart defects among women who take multivitamin supplements starting before conception. The findings from the randomized trial (Czeizel, 1998) suggested an approximately 50% reduction of risk for heart defects in the aggregate, with a wide confidence interval (relative risk 0.42, 95% confidence interval 0.19–0.98). The apparent risk reduction was mainly attributable to a lower incidence of conotruncal and septal defects in the treatment group (Czeizel, 1998; Czeizel and Dudas, 1992). Among the population-based case-control studies, findings included a decreased risk for heart defects in the aggregate (Botto et al., 2000) for conotruncal anomalies (Botto et al., 2000; Shaw et al., 1995), for ventricular septal defects (Botto et al., 2000), and perhaps coarctation of the aorta (Botto et al., 2000). However, one study showed no decrease in the risk of ventricular septal defects (Werler et al., 1999), and in another study on conotruncal anomalies, the results were mixed, with a trend of reduced risk for tetralogy of Fallot but not other conotruncal anomalies (Scanlon et al., 1998). As is common with observational, retrospective studies, it is unclear to what extent the findings may be confounded by factors such as preconception care, socioeconomic status, or healthy behaviors, even when indicators for these factors are included in the epidemiologic design and analysis.

In some studies, multivitamin supplement use was associated with a decrease in the teratogenic risk from other exposures, including first-trimester use of certain antibiotics (Hernandez-Diaz et al., 2000) and febrile illness (Botto et al., 2002; Shaw et al., 2002).

Some studies have tried to assess the genetic susceptibility related to folate metabolism and possible gene–environment interactions. Some studies found no evidence of an association of a variant of the folate gene *MTHFR* with conotruncal or other heart defects (Hobbs et al., 2006; McBride et al., 2004; Pereira et al., 2005; Shaw et al., 2005), whereas others found an association (Junker et al., 2001; van Beynum et al., 2006; Wenstrom et al., 2001). In one study, a variant in the reduced folate carrier gene *RFC1* was associated with an increased risk for heart defects (Pei et al., 2006). Suggestive data are also being generated in animal studies (Li et al., 2005; Li and Rozen, 2006; Tang et al., 2004), suggesting that folate metabolism is important in cardiac development, both normal and abnormal.

There has been no clear change in heart defect rates following implementation of flour fortification with folic acid in the United States in 1998 (Canfield et al., 2005). Fortification in the United States can be seen as having increased, by the average consumption of folic

TABLE 29–4. *Suggested Guidelines for Primary Prevention of Congenital Heart Defects*

Step	Comments
Take a daily multivitamin containing folic acid	Start using before conception; prevents neural tube defects and may prevent some CHDs; recommended daily dose of folic acid is 0.4 mg; consider higher dose of folic acid if there was a previously affected pregnancy
Get pre-conceptional assessment of risk factors and maternal conditions	Target diabetes, chronic illness, and medication use, maternal phenylketonuria, smoking, alcohol, rubella immunization
Stop common exposures, including smoking and alcohol use, from before conception	Also avoid second-hand smoke, encourage smoking cessation by other members of the household
Reassess medication use	Target medications with known teratogenic effect, (e.g., modify seizure medications), be aware of others which have not been evaluated sufficiently for their safety; contact Organization of Teratogen Informations Services for resources; reassess over-the-counter medications use
Avoid exposures to heavy metals, herbicides, pesticides, and organic solvents	Assess exposure associated with household activities, work related (self and partner), or environmental
Avoid close contact with ill individuals, especially with febrile illnesses	Discuss safe ways to decrease high fever if it occurs; unclear to what extent risk associated with febrile illness is related to fever or illness

Adapted from review by Jenkins et al., 2007 Circulation 115(23):2995–3014, and sources within, with author's modifications.

acid in the general population. The lack of a major decline in birth prevalence of heart defects suggests that small doses of folic acid are probably not effective in preventing a significant fraction of heart defects.

The positive findings from the randomized clinical trial (Czeizel, 1996, 1998; Czeizel and Dudas, 1992) and the negative findings after fortification suggest that relatively large amounts of folic acid are needed to prevent heart defects. This has been suggested for other birth defects such as orofacial clefts. Also, it could be that multivitamin supplements, which were used in most studies, may be more effective than folic acid alone, which was used in fortification.

In summary, these accumulating findings are encouraging, but not conclusive. Because of the importance of conclusively establishing the preventive potential of vitamin supplements, a large randomized trial of vitamin supplementation (vs. the recommended dose of folic acid alone) would be very helpful. The cost of heart defects is such that such a randomized trial would easily be cost effective.

From a practical perspective, pediatric cardiologists need not wait for such a trial. Because of the established protective effect against neural tube defects, daily periconceptional use of folic acid is recommended for all women of childbearing age. By promoting periconceptional use of a multivitamin supplement containing folic acid (400 μg), pediatric cardiologists would provide all women with the benefits of a reduced risk for a neural tube defects–affected pregnancy, and, at the same time, possibly a lower risk for heart defects.

DEVELOPING PREVENTION: PLAN FOR ACTION

Although current knowledge on risk factors is incomplete, some guidelines can be proposed for the primary prevention of heart defects (Jenkins et al., 2007). As a general strategy, developing approaches to prevent heart defects in the broader context of child health is likely more desirable and practical than approaches targeted to heart defects alone (Johnson et al., 2006). Suggested prevention guidelines are presented in Table 29–4.

These recommendations emphasize preconception care (Johnson et al., 2006). A helpful guiding concept is the 12-month pregnancy, to focus attention also on the trimester *before* conception. This preconceptional period, together with at least the first 2 months of pregnancy, provides a crucial opportunity for promoting healthy cardiac development. Much of cardiac development occurs in the first 7 weeks postconception, at a time when many women may be unaware of the pregnancy, potentially exposed to teratogens, and with limited or no prenatal care.

On an individual basis, crucial areas of preconceptional counseling include identifying and managing chronic illnesses or exposures; avoiding exposures to acute illnesses, alcohol, and smoking; and taking a folic acid–containing supplement daily. On a population basis, effective strategies will have to consider an integrated education campaign for women and providers on common or highly preventable risk factors, increasing access to preconceptional and prenatal care, and reducing disparities in access and care.

Specifically, all women of childbearing age should be encouraged to take a daily vitamin supplement containing 400 μg of folic acid to reduce the occurrence of neural tube defects and possibly also for some congenital heart defects. They should reevaluate and treat chronic conditions from before conception, especially diabetes (the increased prevalence of birth defects among infants of women with type 1 and type 2 diabetes is substantially reduced through proper management of diabetes from before conception throughout the pregnancy). Women diagnosed with PKU as infants should be targeted for interventions aimed at ensuring adherence to a low phenylalanine diet before conception and continue it throughout their pregnancy.

Before conception, women who are on a regimen of potentially teratogenic medications (e.g., valproic acid) and who are contemplating pregnancy should be prescribed, if possible, a lower dosage of these medications or moved to other medications. For medications that are strong teratogens, such as isotretinoins (e.g., Accutane), it is very important to avoid unintended pregnancies while on this medication, for example, with the use of contraception and a screening pregnancy test.

Regarding infections, rubella vaccination very early in childbearing years remains an effective strategy to achieve protective seropositivity and prevent congenital rubella syndrome in future pregnancies. Among lifestyle factors, tobacco and alcohol have been targets of prevention activities internationally. However, because only 20% of women successfully control tobacco dependence during pregnancy, cessation of smoking is recommended before pregnancy (Johnson et al., 2006). In addition to the evidence on risk for congenital heart defects, preterm birth, low birth weight, and other adverse perinatal outcomes associated with maternal smoking in pregnancy can be prevented if women stop smoking before or during early pregnancy. Alcohol misuse is a significant concern. Although the evidence for specific cardiac teratogenicity is mixed, it is sensible to recommend ceasing alcohol intake from before conception to prevent fetal alcohol syndrome and alcohol-related birth defects.

With respect to obesity, the risk associated with cardiovascular anomalies is not convincingly established. However, obesity is associated with several adverse perinatal outcomes, including neural tube defects, preterm delivery, diabetes, and hypertensive and thromboembolic disease. Appropriate weight loss and improving nutritional health before pregnancy reduces these risks. Additional recommendation for preconception care include vaccination for hepatitis B, identification and treatment of HIV/AIDS and sexually transmitted diseases, treatment of hypothyroidism, and reassessment of oral anticoagulant therapy for warfarin users.

These general guidelines can reasonably apply to all women of childbearing age, to prevent the occurrence of heart defects and other congenital anomalies. Pediatric cardiologists, perhaps more than other specialists, will also see and be called to counsel women who have a heart defect or a previously affected child, and who are contemplating (or not actively excluding) another pregnancy. In this group, the search for modifiable risk factors should be especially rigorous. Evaluation for underlying genetic conditions (e.g., deletion 22q11), including referral to an experienced

medical geneticists, may be extremely helpful in defining and managing recurrence risk. In the setting of prevention of recurrence of neural tube defects, data from a randomized trial has shown the efficacy of high dose (4 mg) of folic acid, with no adverse effect. No comparable data are available for heart defects.

CONCLUDING COMMENTS

Although an exhaustive assessment of benefits, science, and strategies for prevention still includes considerable data gaps, available data are sufficient to begin a concerted effort to work toward preventing congenital heart defects. Effective prevention will require a concerted effort by the clinical, research, and public health community. Pregnancies exposed to known teratogens such as diabetes continue to occur and affected children continue to be born. As researchers continue to look for new causes and genetic determinants of heart defects, there are areas of prevention that can and should be implemented. In addition to targeting individual women for preconceptional education and care, it will be crucial to sustain population-wide interventions to ensure fair and equitable opportunities for prevention for all groups in the population, so that the benefits of prevention can accrue to all, regardless of origin, education, or economic means.

REFERENCES

www.entis-org.com. (accessed May 13, 2009).

www.otispregnancy.org. (accessed May 13, 2009).

2006a. REPROTOX - information system on environmental hazards to human reproduction and development. www.reprotox.org. (accessed 13 May 2009)

2006b. TERIS - Teratogen Information Service and online version of Shepard's Catalog of Teratogenic Agents. University of Washington.

Aberg A, Westbom L, Kallen B. Congenital malformations among infants whose mothers had gestational diabetes or preexisting diabetes. *Early Hum Dev.* 2001;61(2):85–95.

Abu-Harb M, Hey E, Wren C. Death in infancy from unrecognised congenital heart disease. *Arch Dis Child.* 1994;71(1):3–7.

Adams MM, Mulinare J, Dooley K. Risk factors for conotruncal cardiac defects in Atlanta. *J Am Coll Cardiol.* 1989;14(2):432–442.

American College of Obstetricians and Gynecologists. Seizure disorders in pregnancy. Number 231, December 1996. Committee on Educational Bulletins of the American College of Obstetricians and Gynecologists. *Int J Gynaecol Obstet.* 1997;56(3):279–286.

Amos A, Haglund M. From social taboo to "torch of freedom": the marketing of cigarettes to women. *Tob Control.* 2000;9(1):3–8.

Bailey LB, Berry RJ. Folic acid supplementation and the occurrence of congenital heart defects, orofacial clefts, multiple births, and miscarriage. *M J Clin Nutr.* 2005;81(5):1213S–1217S.

Barrett C, Richens A. Epilepsy and pregnancy: Report of an Epilepsy Research Foundation Workshop. *Epilepsy Res.* 2003;52(3):147–187.

Becerra JE, Khoury MJ, Cordero JF, Erickson JD. Diabetes mellitus during pregnancy and the risks for specific birth defects: a population-based case-control study. *Pediatrics*. 1990;85(1):1–9.

Benavidez OJ, Gauvreau K, Jenkins KJ. Racial and ethnic disparities in mortality following congenital heart surgery. *Pediatr Cardiol*. 2006;27(3):321–328.

Benichou J. A review of adjusted estimators of attributable risk. *Stat Methods Med Res*. 2001;10(3):195–216.

Boneva RS, Botto LD, Moore CA, Yang Q, Correa A, Erickson JD. Mortality associated with congenital heart defects in the United States: trends and racial disparities, 1979–1997. *Circulation*. 2001;103(19):2376–2381.

Botto LD, Erickson JD, Mulinare J, Lynberg MC, Liu Y. Maternal fever, multivitamin use, and selected birth defects: evidence of interaction? *Epidemiology*. 2002;13(4):485–488.

Botto LD, Lin AE, Goldmuntz E. Epidemiology and Prevention of Congenital Heart Defects. In: Allen HD, Driscoll DJ, Shaddy RE, Feltes TF, editors. Moss and Adams' Heart Disease in Infants, Children, and Adolescents, including the Fetus and Young Adult. Seventh ed. Philadelphia: Lippincott; 2008.

Botto LD, Loffredo C, Scanlon KS, et al. Vitamin A and cardiac outflow tract defects. *Epidemiology*. 2001;12(5):491–496.

Botto LD, Mulinare J, Erickson JD. Occurrence of congenital heart defects in relation to maternal mulitivitamin use. *Am J Epidemiol*. 2000;151(9):878–884.

Botto LD, Olney RS, Erickson JD. Vitamin supplements and the risk for congenital anomalies other than neural tube defects. *Am J Med Genet C Semin Med Genet*. 2004;125(1):12–21.

Brown MD, Wernovsky G, Mussatto KA, Berger S. Long-term and developmental outcomes of children with complex congenital heart disease. *Clin Perinatol*. 2005;32(4):1043–57, xi.

Browne ML. Maternal exposure to caffeine and risk of congenital anomalies: a systematic review. *Epidemiology*. 2006;17(3):324–331.

Browne ML, Bell EM, Druschel CM, et al. Maternal caffeine consumption and risk of cardiovascular malformations. *Birth Defects Res A Clin Mol Teratol*. 2007;79(7):533–43.

Canfield MA, Collins JS, Botto LD, et al. Changes in the birth prevalence of selected birth defects after grain fortification with folic acid in the United States: findings from a multi-state population-based study. *Birth Defects Res A Clin Mol Teratol*. 2005;73(10):679–689.

Cecconi M, Nistri S, Quarti A, et al. Aortic dilatation in patients with bicuspid aortic valve. J *Cardiovasc Med* (Hagerstown). 2006;7(1):11–20.

Centers for Disease Control and Prevention. Hospital Stays, Hospital Charges, and In-Hospital Deaths Among Infants with Selected Birth Defects – United States, 2003. *MMWR Morb Mortal Wkly Rep*. 2007;56(2):25–29

Centers for Disease Control and Prevention, Waitzman NJ, Romano PS, Scheffler RM, Harris JA. Economic Costs of Birth Defects and Cerebral Palsy – United States, 1992. *MMWR Morb Mortal Wkly Rep*. 1995;44(37):694–699

Chambers J. Aortic stenosis. *BMJ*. 2005;330(7495):801–802.

Chinn A, Fitzsimmons J, Shepard TH, Fantel AG. Congenital heart disease among spontaneous abortuses and stillborn fetuses: prevalence and associations. *Teratology*. 1989;40(5):475–482.

Claessens P, Moons P, de Casterle BD, Cannaerts N, Budts W, Gewillig M. What does it mean to live with a congenital heart disease? A qualitative study on the lived experiences of adult patients. *Eur J Cardiovasc Nurs*. 2005;4(1):3–10.

Coberly S, Lammer E, Alashari M. Retinoic acid embryopathy: case report and review of literature. *Pediatr Pathol Lab Med*. 1996;16(5):823–836.

Cohen LS, Friedman JM, Jefferson JW, Johnson EM, Weiner ML. A reevaluation of risk of in utero exposure to lithium. *JAMA*. 1994;271(2):146–150.

Correa A, Botto L, Liu Y, Mulinare J, Erickson JD. Do multivitamin supplements attenuate the risk for diabetes-associated birth defects? *Pediatrics*. 2003;111(5 Part 2):1146–1151.

Cousins L. Etiology and prevention of congenital anomalies among infants of overt diabetic women. *Clin Obstet Gynecol*. 1991;34(3):481–493.

Crawford P. Best practice guidelines for the management of women with epilepsy. *Epilepsia*. 2005;46 (suppl 9):117–124.

Crossland DS, Jackson SP, Lyall R, et al. Life insurance and mortgage application in adults with congenital heart disease. *Eur J Cardiothorac Surg*. 2004;25(6):931–934.

Culbert EL, Ashburn DA, Cullen-Dean G, et al. Quality of life of children after repair of transposition of the great arteries. *Circulation*. 2003;108(7):857–62.

Czeizel AE. Reduction of urinary tract and cardiovascular defects by periconceptional multivitamin supplementation. *American Journal of Medical Genetics*. 1996;62(2):179–183.

Czeizel AE. Periconceptional folic acid containing multivitamin supplementation. *European Journal of Obstetrics, Gynecology, & Reproductive Biology*. 1998;78(2):151–161.

Czeizel AE, Dudas I. Prevention of the first occurrence of neural-tube defects by periconceptional vitamin supplementation. *N Engl J Med*. 1992;327(26):1832–1835.

Czeizel AE, Rockenbauer M, Sorensen HT, Olsen J. The teratogenic risk of trimethoprim-sulfonamides: a population based case-control study. *Reprod Toxicol*. 2001;15(6):637–646.

Daly S, Cotter A, Molloy AE, Scott J. Homocysteine and folic acid: implications for pregnancy. *Semin Vasc Med*. 2005;5(2):190–200.

Edwards MJ, Shiota K, Smith MS, Walsh DA. Hyperthermia and birth defects. *Reprod Toxicol*. 1995;9(5):411–425.

Eichhorn P, Sutsch G, Jenni R. [Congenital heart defects and abnormalities newly detected with echocardiography in adolescents and adults]. *Schweiz Med Wochenschr*. 1990;120(45):1697–700.

Eiser C, Morse R. Can parents rate their child's health-related quality of life? Results of a systematic review. *Qual Life Res*. 2001a;10(4):347–357.

Eiser C, Morse R. The measurement of quality of life in children: past and future perspectives. *J Dev Behav Pediatr*. 2001b;22(4):248–256.

Eiser C, Morse R. A review of measures of quality of life for children with chronic illness. *Arch Dis Child*. 2001b;84(3):205–211.

Ferencz C, Loffredo CA, Correa-Villasenor A, Wilson PD. Genetic and environmental risk factors of major congenital heart disease: the Baltimore-Washington Infant Study 1981–1989. Mount Kisco, NY: Futura Publishing Company, Inc; 1997.

Fixler DE, Pastor P, Chamberlin M, Sigman E, Eifler CW. Trends in congenital heart disease in Dallas County births. 1971–1984. *Circulation*. 1990;81(1):137–42.

Forrest JM, Turnbull FM, Sholler GF, et al. Gregg's congenital rubella patients 60 years later. *Med J Aust*. 2002;177(11–12):664–667.

Fyler DC, Buckley LP, Hellenbrand WE, et al. Report of the New England Regional Infant Cardiac Program. *Pediatrics*. 1980;65 (Suppl):376.

Garg V. Insights into the genetic basis of congenital heart disease. *Cell Mol Life Sci*. 2006;63(10):1141–1148.

Gillum RF. Epidemiology of congenital heart disease in the United States. *Am Heart J*. 1994;127(4 Pt 1):919–927.

Goldbeck L, Melches J. Quality of life in families of children with congenital heart disease. *Qual Life Res*. 2005;14(8):1915–1924.

Goldbeck L, Melches J. The impact of the severity of disease and social disadvantage on quality of life in families with congenital cardiac disease. *Cardiol Young*. 2006;16(1):67–75.

Grabitz RG, Joffres MR, Collins-Nakai RL. Congenital heart disease: incidence in the first year of life. The Alberta Heritage Pediatric Cardiology Program. *Am J Epidemiol*. 1988;128(2):381–388.

Graham JM, Jr., Edwards MJ. Teratogen update: gestational effects of maternal hyperthermia due to febrile illnesses and resultant patterns of defects in humans. *Teratology.* 1998;58(5):209–221.

Green A. Outcomes of congenital heart disease: a review. *Pediatr Nurs.* 2004;30(4):280–284.

Gruber PJ. Cardiac development: new concepts. *Clin Perinatol.* 2005;32(4):845–55, vii.

Hanley JA. A heuristic approach to the formulas for population attributable fraction. *J Epidemiol Community Health.* 2001;55(7):508–514.

Harris MI, Flegal KM, Cowie CC, et al. Prevalence of diabetes, impaired fasting glucose, and impaired glucose tolerance in U.S. adults. The Third National Health and Nutrition Examination Survey, 1988–1994. *Diabetes Care.* 1998;21(4):518–524.

Hernandez-Diaz S, Werler MM, Walker AM, Mitchell AA. Folic acid antagonists during pregnancy and the risk of birth defects. *N Engl J Med.* 2000;343(22):1608–1614.

Hiraishi S, Agata Y, Nowatari M, et al. Incidence and natural course of trabecular ventricular septal defect: two-dimensional echocardiography and color Doppler flow imaging study. *J Pediatr.* 1992;120(3):409–415.

Hobbs CA, James SJ, Jernigan S, Melnyk S, Lu Y, Malik S, Cleves MA. Congenital heart defects, maternal homocysteine, smoking, and the 677 C>T polymorphism in the methylenetetrahydrofolate reductase gene: evaluating gene-environment interactions. *Am J Obstet Gynecol.* 2006;194(1):218–224.

Hoffman JI. Incidence of congenital heart disease: I. Postnatal incidence. *Pediatr Cardiol.* 1995;16(3):103–113.

Hoffman JI, Kaplan S. The incidence of congenital heart disease. *J Am Coll Cardiol.* 2002;39(12):1890–1900.

Hoffman JI, Kaplan S, Liberthson RR. Prevalence of congenital heart disease. *Am Heart J.* 2004;147(3):425–39.

Holing EV, Beyer CS, Brown ZA, Connell FA. Why don't women with diabetes plan their pregnancies? *Diabetes Care.* 1998;21(6):889–895.

Holmes LB, Harvey EA, Coull BA, et al. The teratogenicity of anticonvulsant drugs. *N Engl J Med.* 2001;344(15):1132–8.

Honein MA, Paulozzi LJ, Erickson JD. Continued occurrence of Accutane-exposed pregnancies.. 2001;. 2001;64(3):142–147.

Hoyme HE, May PA, Kalberg WO, et al. A practical clinical approach to diagnosis of fetal alcohol spectrum disorders: clarification of the 1996 institute of medicine criteria. *Pediatrics.* 2005;115(1):39–47.

Huhta JC, Hernandez-Robles JA. Homocysteine, folate, and congenital heart defects. *Fetal Pediatr Pathol.* 2005;24(2):71–79.

Institute of Medicine, editor. Committee to Study Fetal Alcohol Syndrome: fetal alcohol syndrome – diagnosis, epidemiology, prevention and treatment.. Washington, DC: National Academy Press; 1996.

Jacobson SJ, Jones K, Johnson K, Ceolin L, Kaur P, Sahn D, Donnenfeld AE, Rieder M, Santelli R, Smythe J and others. Prospective multicentre study of pregnancy outcome after lithium exposure during first trimester. *Lancet.* 1992; 339(8792):530–533.

Jefferies JL, Noonan JA, Keller BB, Wilson JF, Griffith C, 3rd. Quality of life and social outcomes in adults with congenital heart disease living in rural areas of Kentucky. *Am J Cardiol.* 2004;94(2):263–266.

Jenkins KJ, Correa A, Feinstein JA, et al. Noninherited risk factors and congenital cardiovascular defects: current knowledge: a scientific statement from the American Heart Association Council on Cardiovascular Disease in the Young: endorsed by the American Academy of Pediatrics. *Circulation.* 2007;115(23):2995–3014.

Johnson K, Posner SF, Biermann J, et al. Recommendations to Improve Preconception Health and Health Care – United States. MMWR; 2006:55(RR06):1–23.

Jones KL. Smith's Recognizable Patterns of Human Malformation. Philadelphia: Saunders; 2005.

Junker R, Kotthoff S, Vielhaber H, et al. Infant methylenetetrahydrofolate reductase 677TT genotype is a risk factor for congenital heart disease. *Cardiovasc Res.* 2001;51(2):251–254.

Kallen B, Tandberg A. Lithium and pregnancy. A cohort study on manic-depressive women. *Acta Psychiatr Scand.* 1983;68(2):134–139.

Kallen K. Maternal smoking and congenital heart defects. *Eur J Epidemiol.* 1999;15(8):731–737.

Khoury MJ, Moore CA, Mulinare J. Vitamin A and birth defects. *Lancet.* 1996;347(8997):322.

Kidd SA, Lancaster PA, McCredie RM. The incidence of congenital heart defects in the first year of life. *J Paediatr Child Health.* 1993;29(5):344–349.

Knowles RL, Griebsch I, Bull C, Brown J, Wren C, Dezateux C. Quality-of-life and congenital heart defects: comparing parent and professional values. *Arch Dis Child.* 2006.

Kousseff BG. Diabetic embryopathy. *Curr Opin Pediatr.* 1999;11(4):348–352.

Lammer EJ, Chen DT, Hoar RM, et al. Retinoic acid embryopathy. *N Engl J Med.* 1985;313(14):837–841.

Lane DA, Lip GY, Millane TA. Quality of life in adults with congenital heart disease. *Heart.* 2002;88(1):71–75.

Levy HL, Guldberg P, Guttler F, et al. Congenital heart disease in maternal phenylketonuria: report from the Maternal PKU Collaborative Study. *Pediatr Res.* 2001;49(5):636–642.

Li D, Pickell L, Liu Y, Wu Q, Cohn JS, Rozen R. Maternal methylenetetrahydrofolate reductase deficiency and low dietary folate lead to adverse reproductive outcomes and congenital heart defects in mice. *M J Clin Nutr.* 2005; 82(1):188–195.

Li D, Rozen R. Maternal folate deficiency affects proliferation, but not apoptosis, in embryonic mouse heart. *J Nutr.* 2006;136(7):1774–1778.

Limperopoulos C, Majnemer A, Shevell MI, et al. Predictors of developmental disabilities after open heart surgery in young children with congenital heart defects. *J Pediatr.* 2002;141(1):51–8.

Limperopoulos C, Majnemer A, Shevell MI, Rosenblatt B, Rohlicek C, Tchervenkov C. 2000. Neurodevelopmental status of newborns and infants with congenital heart defects before and after open heart surgery. *J Pediatr* 137(5):638–645.

Lin AE, Herring AH, Amstutz KS, et al. Cardiovascular malformations: changes in prevalence and birth status, 1972–1990. *Am J Med Genet.* 1999;84(2):102–110.

Linn S, Schoenbaum SC, Monson RR, Rosner B, Stubblefield PG, Ryan KJ. No association between coffee consumption and adverse outcomes of pregnancy. *N Engl J Med.* 1982;306(3):141–145.

Lip GY, Lane DA, Millane TA, Tayebjee MH. Psychological interventions for depression in adolescent and adult congenital heart disease. *Cochrane Database Syst Rev.* 2003;(3):CD004394.

Loffredo CA. Epidemiology of cardiovascular malformations: prevalence and risk factors. *Am J Med Genet.* 2000;97(4):319–325.

Lopez AD, Mathers CD. Measuring the global burden of disease and epidemiological transitions: 2002–2030. *Ann Trop Med Parasitol.* 2006;100(5):481–499.

Mahle W. Spectrum of heart disease. In: Rubin I, Crocker A, editors. Medical care for children and adults with developmental disabilities. Baltimore: Paul H Brooks Publishing Co; 2006:379–386.

Mahle WT, Clancy RR, Moss EM, Gerdes M, Jobes DR, Wernovsky G. Neurodevelopmental outcome and lifestyle assessment in school-aged and adolescent children with hypoplastic left heart syndrome. *Pediatrics.* 2000;105(5):1082–1089.

Malik S, Cleves MA, Honein MA, et al. Maternal smoking and congenital heart defects. *Pediatrics.* 2008;121(4):e810–6.

Martinez-Frias ML, Bermejo E, Rodriguez-Pinilla E, Prieto L, Frias JL. Epidemiological analysis of outcomes of pregnancy in gestational diabetic mothers. *Am J Med Genet.* 1998;78(2):140–145.

Mason CA, Kirby RS, Sever LE, Langlois PH. Prevalence is the preferred measure of frequency of birth defects. *Birth Defects Res A Clin Mol Teratol.* 2005;73(10):690–692.

Mastroiacovo P, Mazzone T, Addis A, et al. High vitamin A intake in early pregnancy and major malformations: a multicenter prospective controlled study. *Teratology.* 1999;59(1):7–11.

Matalon KM, Acosta PB, Azen C. Role of nutrition in pregnancy with phenylketonuria and birth defects. *Pediatrics.* 2003;112(6 Pt 2):1534–1536.

McBride KL, Fernbach S, Menesses A, et al. A family-based association study of congenital left-sided heart malformations and 5,10 methylenetetrahydrofolate reductase. *Birth Defects Res A Clin Mol Teratol.* 2004;70(10):825–830.

McCrindle BW. The prevalence of congenital cardiac lesions. In: Freedom RM, Yoo S-J, Mikailian H, Williams WG, editors. The natural and modified history of congenital heart disease. New York: Futura, Blackwell Publishing; 2004.

McCrindle BW, Williams RV, Mitchell PD,.et al. Relationship of patient and medical characteristics to health status in children and adolescents after the Fontan procedure. *Circulation.* 2006;113(8):1123–1129.

Mikhail LN, Walker CK, Mittendorf R. Association between maternal obesity and fetal cardiac malformations in African Americans. *Journal of the National Medical Association.* 2002;94(8):695–700.

Mills JL, Simpson JL, Cunningham GC, Conley MR, Rhoads GG. Vitamin A and birth defects. *Am J Obstet Gynecol.* 1997;177(1):31–36.

Mokdad AH, Ford ES, Bowman BA, et al. Prevalence of obesity, diabetes, and obesity-related health risk factors, 2001. *JAMA.* 2003;289(1):76–79.

Moons P, De Bleser L, Budts W, et al. Health status, functional abilities, and quality of life after the Mustard or Senning operation. *Ann Thorac Surg.* 2004;77(4):1359–1365; discussion 1365.

Moons P, Van Deyk K, De Geest S, Gewillig M, Budts W. Is the severity of congenital heart disease associated with the quality of life and perceived health of adult patients? *Heart.* 2005;91(9):1193–1198.

Moore LL, Singer MR, Bradlee ML, Rothman KJ, Milunsky A. A prospective study of the risk of congenital defects associated with maternal obesity and diabetes mellitus. *Epidemiology.* 2000;11(6):689–694.

Murray CJL, Lopez AD. Health Dimensions of Sex and Reproduction: The Global Burden of Sexually Transmitted Diseases, HIV, Maternal Conditions, Perinatal Disorders, and Congenital Anomalies Boston: Harvard University Press; 1998.

Olsen J, Overvad K, Frische G. Coffee consumption, birthweight, and reproductive failures. *Epidemiology.* 1991;2(5):370–374.

Pei L, Zhu H, Zhu J, Ren A, Finnell RH, Li Z. Genetic variation of infant reduced folate carrier (A80G) and risk of orofacial defects and congenital heart defects in China. *Ann Epidemiol.* 2006;16(5):352–356.

Pereira AC, Xavier-Neto J, Mesquita SM, Mota GF, Lopes AA, Krieger JE. Lack of evidence of association between MTHFR C677T polymorphism and congenital heart disease in a TDT study design. *Int J Cardiol.* 2005;105(1):15–18.

Perlman SE, Rudy SJ, Pinto C, Townsend-Akpan C. Caring for women with childbearing potential taking teratogenic dermatologic drugs. Guidelines for practice. *J Reprod Med.* 2001;46(2 Suppl):153–161.

Pierpont ME, Basson CT, Benson WD, et al. Genetic Basis for Congenital Heart Defects: Current Knowledge: A Scientific Statement From the American Heart Association Congenital Cardiac Defects Committee, Council on Cardiovascular Disease in the Young: Endorsed by the American Academy of Pediatrics. Circulation. 2007;115:3015–38. Epub 2007 May 22. Review. PubMed PMID: 17519398

Pschirrer ER. Seizure disorders in pregnancy. *Obstet Gynecol Clin North Am.* 2004;31(2):373–84, vii.

Ray JG, O'Brien TE, Chan WS. Preconception care and the risk of congenital anomalies in the offspring of women with diabetes mellitus: a meta-analysis. *QJM.* 2001;94(8):435–44.

Reef SE, Plotkin S, Cordero JF, et al. Preparing for elimination of congenital Rubella syndrome (CRS): summary of a workshop on CRS elimination in the United States. *Clin Infect Dis.* 2000;31(1):85–95.

Reef SE, Redd SB, Abernathy E, Zimmerman L, Icenogle JP. The epidemiological profile of rubella and congenital rubella syndrome in the United States, 1998–2004: the evidence for absence of endemic transmission. *Clin Infect Dis.* 2006;43(suppl 3):S126–32.

Rietveld S, Mulder BJ, van Beest I, et al. Negative thoughts in adults with congenital heart disease. *Int J Cardiol.* 2002;86(1):19–26.

Robertson SE, Featherstone DA, Gacic-Dobo M, Hersh BS. Rubella and congenital rubella syndrome: global update. *Rev Panam Salud Publica.* 2003;14(5):306–315.

Rockhill B, Newman B, Weinberg C. Use and misuse of population attributable fractions. *Am J Public Health.* 1998;88(1):15–19.

Rosano A, Botto LD, Botting B, Mastroiacovo P. Infant mortality and congenital anomalies from 1950 to 1994: an international perspective. *J Epidemiol Community Health.* 2000;54(9):660–666.

Rose M, Kohler K, Kohler F, Sawitzky B, Fliege H, Klapp BF. Determinants of the quality of life of patients with congenital heart disease. *Qual Life Res.* 2005;14(1):35–43.

Rosenberg L, Mitchell AA, Shapiro S, Slone D. Selected birth defects in relation to caffeine-containing beverages. *JAMA.* 247(10):1429–1432.

Rosenthal. Prevalence of congenital heart disease. In: Garson AJ, Bricker JT, Fisher DJ, Neish SR, editors. The Science and Practice of Pediatric Cardiology. Baltimore: Williams & Wilkins; 1998: 1098.

Rothman KJ. What is causation? Epidemiology: an introduction. New York: Oxford University Press; 2002.

Rothman KJ, Moore LL, Singer MR, Nguyen US, Mannino S, Milunsky A. Teratogenicity of high vitamin A intake. *N Engl J Med.* 1995;333(21):1369–1373.

Roulston A, Marcellus RC, Branton PE. Viruses and apoptosis. *Ann Rev Microbiol.* 1999;53:577–628.

Rouse B, Azen C. Effect of high maternal blood phenylalanine on offspring congenital anomalies and developmental outcome at ages 4 and 6 years: the importance of strict dietary control preconception and throughout pregnancy. *J Pediatr.* 2004;144(2):235–139.

Rowland TW, Hubbell JP, Jr., Nadas AS. Congenital heart disease in infants of diabetic mothers. *J Pediatr.* 1973;83(5):815–820.

Roy DL, McIntyre L, Human DG, et al. Trends in the prevalence of congenital heart disease: comprehensive observations over a 24-year period in a defined region of Canada. *Can J Cardiol.* 1994;10(8):821–826.

Sairanen HI, Nieminen HP, Jokinen EV. Late results and quality of life after pediatric cardiac surgery in Finland: a population-based study of 6,461 patients with follow-up extending up to 45 years. *Semin Thorac Cardiovasc Surg Pediatr Card Surg Annu.* 2005;168–72.

Samanek M. Boy:girl ratio in children born with different forms of cardiac malformation: a population-based study. *Pediatr Cardiol.* 1994;15(2):53–57.

Samren EB, van Duijn CM, Christiaens GC, Hofman A, Lindhout D. Antiepileptic drug regimens and major congenital abnormalities in the offspring. *Ann Neurol.* 1999;46(5):739–746.

Samren EB, van Duijn CM, Koch S, et al. Maternal use of antiepileptic drugs and the risk of major congenital malformations: a joint European prospective study of human teratogenesis associated with maternal epilepsy. *Epilepsia.* 1997;38(9):981–990.

Scanlon KS, Ferencz C, Loffredo CA, et al. Preconceptional folate intake and malformations of the cardiac outflow tract. Baltimore-Washington Infant Study Group. *Epidemiology.* 1998;9(1):95–98.

Schou M, Goldfield MD, Weinstein MR, Villeneuve A. Lithium and pregnancy. I. Report from the Register of Lithium Babies. *Br Med J.* 1973;2(5859):135–136.

Schultz AH, Wernovsky G. Late outcomes in patients with surgically treated congenital heart disease. *Semin Thorac Cardiovasc Surg Pediatr Card Surg Annu.* 2005;145–156.

Shaw GM, Iovannisci DM, Yang W,.et al. Risks of human conotruncal heart defects associated with 32 single nucleotide polymorphisms of selected cardiovascular disease-related genes. *Am J Med Genet A.* 2000;138(1):21–26.

Shaw GM, Nelson V, Carmichael SL, Lammer EJ, Finnell RH, Rosenquist TH. Maternal periconceptional vitamins: interactions with selected factors and congenital anomalies? *Epidemiology.* 2002;13(6):625–630.

Shaw GM, O'Malley CD, Wasserman CR, Tolarova MM, Lammer EJ. Maternal periconceptional use of multivitamins and reduced risk for conotruncal heart defects and limb deficiencies among offspring. *Am J Med Genet.* 1995;59(4):536–545.

Shaw GM, Todoroff K, Schaffer DM, Selvin S. Maternal height and prepregnancy body mass index as risk factors for selected congenital anomalies. *Paediatr Perinat Epidemiol.* 2000;14(3):234–239.

Shaw GM, Wasserman CR, Block G, Lammer EJ. High maternal vitamin A intake and risk of anomalies of structures with a cranial neural crest cell contribution. *Lancet.* 1996;347(9005):899–900.

Sheffield JS, Butler-Koster EL, Casey BM, McIntire DD, Leveno KJ. Maternal diabetes mellitus and infant malformations. *Obstet Gynecol.* 2002;100(5 Pt 1):925–930.

Smithells RW, Newman CG. Recognition of thalidomide defects. *J Med Genet.* 1992;29(10):716–723.

Spijkerboer AW, Utens EM, De Koning WB, Bogers AJ, Helbing WA, Verhulst FC. Health-related Quality of Life in children and adolescents after invasive treatment for congenital heart disease. *Qual Life Res.* 2006;15(4):663–673.

Stoll C, Alembik Y, Roth MP, Dott B, De Geeter B. Risk factors in congenital heart disease. *Eur J Epidemiol.* 1989;5(3):382–391.

Tang LS, Wlodarczyk BJ, Santillano DR, Miranda RC, Finnell RH. Developmental consequences of abnormal folate transport during murine heart morphogenesis. *Birth Defects Res A Clin Mol Teratol.* 2004;70(7):449–458.

Tanner K, Sabrine N, Wren C. Cardiovascular malformations among preterm infants. *Pediatrics.* 2005;116(6):e833–838.

Tegnander E, Williams W, Johansen OJ, Blaas HG, Eik-Nes SH. Prenatal detection of heart defects in a non-selected population of 30,149 fetuses – detection rates and outcome. *Ultrasound Obstet Gynecol.* 2006;27(3):252–265.

Tikkanen J, Heinonen OP. Risk factors for cardiovascular malformations in Finland. *Eur J Epidemiol.* 1990;6(4):348–356.

Tikkanen J, Heinonen OP. Maternal hyperthermia during pregnancy and cardiovascular malformations in the offspring. *Eur J Epidemiol.*1991a;7(6):628–635.

Tikkanen J, Heinonen OP. Risk factors for ventricular septal defect in Finland. *Public Health.* 1991b;105(2):99–112.

Tikkanen J, Heinonen OP. Risk factors for atrial septal defect. *Eur J Epidemiol.* 1992a;8(4):509–515.

Tikkanen J, Heinonen OP. Risk factors for conal malformations of the heart. *Eur J Epidemiol.* 1992b; 8(1):48–57.

Ursell PC, Byrne JM, Strobino BA. Significance of cardiac defects in the developing fetus: a study of spontaneous abortions. *Circulation.* 1985;72(6):1232–1236.

van Beynum IM, Kapusta L, den Heijer M, et al. Maternal MTHFR 677C>T is a risk factor for congenital heart defects: effect modification by periconceptional folate supplementation. *Eur Heart J.* 2006;27(8):981–987.

Waitzman NJ, Romano PS, Scheffler RM. The cost of birth defects: University Press of America; 1996:276 .

Waller DK, Mills JL, Simpson JL,.et al. Are obese women at higher risk for producing malformed offspring? *American Journal of Obstetrics & Gynecology.* 1994;170(2):541–548.

Ward C. Clinical significance of the bicuspid aortic valve. *Heart.* 2000;83(1):81–85.

Warner JP. Evidence-based psychopharmacology 3. Assessing evidence of harm: what are the teratogenic effects of lithium carbonate? *J Psychopharmacol.* 2000;14(1):77–80.

Warnes CA, Liberthson R, Danielson GK, et al. Task force 1: the changing profile of congenital heart disease in adult life. *J Am Coll Cardiol.* 2001;37(5):1170–1175.

Watkins ML, Botto LD. Maternal prepregnancy weight and congenital heart defects in offspring. *Epidemiology.* 2001;12(4):439–446.

Wenstrom KD, Johanning GL, Johnston KE, DuBard M. Association of the C677T methylenetetrahydrofolate reductase mutation and elevated homocysteine levels with congenital cardiac malformations. *Am J Obstet Gynecol.* 2001;184(5):806–812; discussion 812–7.

Werler MM, Hayes C, Louik C, Shapiro S, Mitchell AA. Multivitamin supplementation and risk of birth defects. *American Journal of Epidemiology.* 1999;150(7):675–682.

Werler MM, Lammer EJ, Rosenberg L, Mitchell AA. Maternal vitamin A supplementation in relation to selected birth defects. *Teratology.* 1990;42(5):497–503.

Wernovsky G. Outcomes regarding the central nervous system in children with complex congenital cardiac malformations. *Cardiol Young.* 2005;15 (suppl 1)132–133.

Williams RG, Pearson GD, Barst RJ, et al. Report of the National Heart, Lung, and Blood Institute Working Group on research in adult congenital heart disease. *J Am Coll Cardiol.* 2006;47(4):701–707.

Williams WG. Surgical outcomes in congenital heart disease: expectations and realities. *Eur J Cardiothorac Surg.* 2005;27(6):937–944.

Wilson PD, Loffredo CA, Correa-Villasenor A, Ferencz C. Attributable fraction for cardiac malformations. *Am J Epidemiol.* 1998;148(5):414–423.

Woods SE, Raju U. Maternal smoking and the risk of congenital birth defects: a cohort study. *J Am Board Fam Pract.* 2001;14(5):330–334.

Wren C, Birrell G, Hawthorne G. Cardiovascular malformations in infants of diabetic mothers. *Heart.* 2003;89(10):1217–1220.

Zhang J, Cai WW. Association of the common cold in the first trimester of pregnancy with birth defects. *Pediatrics.* 1993;92(4):559–563.

VI

Public Health Issues

30

Factors Associated with Increased Resource Utilization for Congenital Heart Disease

JEAN ANNE CONNOR

KATHY J. JENKINS

INTRODUCTION

Over the last two decades, health care organizations and the systems by which they deliver care have changed significantly. These changes have resulted from multiple, concurrent events, including major modifications in reimbursement of hospitals, cost containment efforts of hospitals as a response to reimbursement changes, dramatic advancements in technologies and medical treatment, and changes in the health care workforce (IOM, 2004).

Use of advanced technologies and innovative medical therapies has been cited by the Institute of Medicine (IOM) as one of the four main attributes to increasing health care quality (IOM, 2001). It is the application of these advances and innovations that has dramatically decreased the mortality for children with complex heart disease (Boneva et al., 2001).

Each year approximately 24,000 surgical intervention are performed to treat infants/children born with congenital heart defect (CHD) (Chang and Klitzner, 2003). Care for this surgical pediatric population is associated with numerous hospitalizations, services of a multidisciplinary team of specialists, and use of both advanced and innovative technology (Jenkins et al., 1995). Currently between 75% and 85% of health care resources and costs are consumed by 10% of the population (Greeley, 2003). Children born with CHD are included in this complex population of patients.

The objectives for this chapter are to describe resource use for children born with CHD who require surgical intervention, examine factors associated with resource use for this population, and discuss future directions for consideration.

DEFINING RESOURCE USE, HOSPITAL CHARGES, AND HOSPITAL COSTS

To initiate a discussion of resource utilization for children born with CHD, one must first define resource utilization, which may be put simply as the resources used to deliver health care. The two most common surrogates used by investigators to examine resource utilization are total hospital charges and length of stay (Chang and Klitzner, 2003; Connor, 2004, 2005). Less commonly, others have reported staffing ratios of physicians and nurses, days of intensive care bed and ventilator use, and pharmacy, labs, and operating room usage (Alboliras and Hijazi, 2004; Yount and Mahle, 2004; Zellers et al., 2002).

Total hospital charges and length of stay are most often used because they are easily available in administrative datasets and hospital-based administrative systems. Although both of these surrogates are useful in identifying trends in a population, the general limitation is the lack of detail and the timing during hospital admission when the resources were utilized. One further criticism often cited with using total hospital charges is that they signify the charges generated for each case but not the revenue received or the estimated cost of production associated with providing the care. Cost, on the other hand, reflects the actual expenses paid to obtain resources used to deliver care. The resources could be labor, supplies, or pieces of equipment used in delivering the care. These costs, known as accounting costs, may be fixed or variable. Fixed costs are due to resources consumed that cannot be directly tied to patient care, for example, a building, heating and lighting. Variable costs are those costs that can be directly attributed to patient volume, such as labor, supplies, and materials (Greeley, 2003).

Accounting costs can be direct or indirect as well. Direct costs are associated directly with the patient. Examples of these costs would be nursing hours, diagnostic testing, and medication use. Indirect costs such as administrative costs cannot be directly applied to a patient but are averaged over the number of patients receiving care (Greeley, 2003).

One method that we have used for overcoming the limitation of using total hospital charges is to apply a cost-to-charge ratio (CCR) to convert charges to cost. This can be done at the institution or state level.

DATA SOURCES

A number of data sources are currently available for examination of increased resource use for children with CHD (Jacobs et al., 2004, 2005). However, not all contain charge-to-cost information. One such database specific to pediatrics containing total hospital charges is the Kids' Inpatient Database (KID). The KID database was developed as part of the Healthcare Cost and Utilization Project (HCUP) through a Federal-State-Industry partnership sponsored by the Agency for Healthcare Research and Quality. The goal of this partnership is to use this data to make an informed decision at the national, state, and community levels. The KID dataset is currently available in three years—1997, 2000, and 2003. The latest version of the KID database consists of a stratified random sample of 2,984,129 discharges from 3438 institutions in 36 states. The KID uses the American Hospital Association's definition of hospitals to identify all nonfederal, short-term, general and other specialty hospitals. Pediatric hospitals, academic medical centers, and specialty hospitals are included. The database does not include all admissions from participating institutions, but instead includes a 10% sample of uncomplicated in-hospital births from these institutions, and an 80% sample of other pediatric discharges (patients aged less than 21 years). To obtain information that is nationally representative, the sample is weighted to represent the population of pediatric discharges from all community, nonrehabilitation hospitals in the United States that were open for any part of the calendar year examined. To protect patient confidentiality, the KID database does not contain specific patient or hospital identifiers.

Limitations of Administrative Data Sources

Although the KID datasets are considered to be powerful data sources, one must be aware of the universal limitations of using administrative datasets. Unique patient identifiers or record linkage numbers are generally not available, thereby making it impossible to identify discharges as individual patients or link patient data. Missing data, coding errors, and lack of detailed clinical information are also universal limitations in using large administrative datasets in outcomes research (Iezzoni, 2002). Recent examination of the validity of hospital discharge data in infants with cardiac defects has further identified limitations regarding accurate identification of the type of congenital defect with the use of the *International Classification of Diseases, 9th Revision, Clinical Modification* (ICD-9-CM) codes (Cronk et al., 2003; Frohnert et al., 2005; Riehle-Colarusso et al., 2007). One alternative to overcome the limitation of ICD-9-CM coding identified by the authors included the use of data sources employing standard CHD nomenclature and classification system as used in the Society of Thoracic Surgeons (STS) Congenital Heart Surgery Database (Riehle-Colarusso et al., 2007). Although this database contains detailed clinical elements as well as outcomes such as length of stay and mortality, hospital charges or costs are not included.

FACTORS ASSOCIATED WITH INCREASED RESOURCE UTILIZATION FOR CHILDREN UNDERGOING CONGENITAL HEART SURGERY

United States, Non–Population Based

Overall, there is a lack of published information available describing resource utilization for children undergoing congenital heart surgery. In the United States, previous research in this field has been limited to the investigation of the direct charges-to-costs of a single complex cardiac defect and its surgical management, practice patterns and charge-to-cost variations among eight centers caring for children and adults with CHD, and charge-to-cost of intensive care and postintensive care stay for critically ill children (Chalom et al., 1999; Garson et al., 1994; Jaquiss et al., 2006; Kanter, 2000; Williams et al., 2000). In addition, two previous studies described a single institutional experience with cost of surgical care and examined predictors for higher costs associated with congenital heart repair (Silberbach et al., 1993; Ungerleider et al., 1997). Silberbach et al. found the date of operation, cyanosis, previous thoracic surgery, failure to thrive, associated major extra cardiac anomalies, oxygen requirement, and distance more than 100 miles from home to hospital to be predictive of increased hospital charge. Age at operation alone did not influence the dependent variables (Silberbach et al., 1993). Similarly, Ungerleider et al. (1997) reported that age of child, complexity of defect, presence of other noncardiac anomalies or syndromes, and length of stay were associated with increased financial risk (Ungerleider et al., 1997). Both concluded that it is possible to preoperatively identify factors that predict increased resource utilization for children undergoing congenital heart surgery and that knowledge in this area may facilitate implementation of strategic resource allocation (Silberbach et al., 1993; Ungerleider et al., 1997).

Outside the United States

Outcome assessments for children undergoing congenital heart surgery outside the United States have mainly focused in the areas of survival and or resulting morbidity (Dimmick et al., 2007; Garne, 2004; Immer et al., 2005; Larrazabal et al., 2007). As in the United States, research examining cost of care for children undergoing congenital surgery has emerged from single-institution experiences (Fernandes et al., 2004). More often, these assessments have been made with improvement in surgical techniques or structure of cardiac center, and or with change in pre- and/or postoperative management (Daenen et al., 2003; Kang et al., 2006; Meyns, 2004; Zannini and Borini, 2007).

Resource Use during Nonsurgical Hospitalizations

For children born with CHD, the risk of serious morbidity/mortality from respiratory syncytial virus (RSV) is high. Treatment for this illness often requires hospitalization and increased resource use (Chantepie, 2004; Howard et al., 2000). A number of studies both in and outside the United States have described the treatment/prevention of RSV for children with CHD (Feltes and Sondheimer, 2007; Venkatesh and Weisman, 2006). Most of these studies have focused on the cost-effectiveness of preventative treatment with palivizumab, with researchers finding evidence to both support and not support its use in this population (Howard et al., 2000; Meberg and Bruu, 2006; Nuijten et al., 2007; Yount and Mahle, 2004).

Resource Use for Adults with Congenital Heart Disease

Of note, recent examination of resource utilization for adults with CHD has shown an increasing need for resource allocation under national health care–based systems (Gatzoulis, 2004; Mackie et al., 2007; Moons et al., 2001a, 2001b; Price et al., 2007). These examinations have identified the continued need for surgical and medical intervention into adulthood for not only the patients' underlying CHD but also conditions resulting from their cardiac disease. A call for guidelines supporting the care and resource utilization for adults born with CHD was identified as a need for this rapidly growing population.

United States, Population Based

We have taken a population-based approach in our serial examinations of resource utilization for children undergoing congenital heart surgery in the United States using the KID 2000 database. In this database, a sample of 2,516,833 pediatric discharges from 2784 institutions in 27 states[1] was available for review. To identify cases of congenital heart surgery in patients younger than18 years, we used ICD-9-CM diagnostic and procedure codes (Jenkins et al., 2002). In order to focus on structural repairs only, cases with codes for cardiac transplantation were eliminated, as were premature infants and newborns aged 30 days or younger undergoing ligation of patent ductus arteriosus (PDA) only. Total hospital charges accrued during hospitalization, available for most cases in the KID 2000, were used as a surrogate for resource utilization. The distribution of total hospital charges in US dollars for congenital heart surgery cases was examined. An arbitrary cut point was made at the 90th percentile; cases >90th percentile were labeled as especially high resource utilization (Figure 30–1).

Of the 2,516,833 pediatric discharges, 12,717 cases with codes indicating congenital heart surgery were identified. Of these, 11,381 cases met inclusion criteria (i.e., age more than 18 years, cardiac transplants, and premature infants and newborns aged 30 days or younger with PDA ligation as their only cardiac procedure were eliminated); 10,602 (from 198 institutions) had total hospital charges reported. The number of cases by state ranged from 7 to 2394 (Figure 30–2). The median total hospital charge for this group was $51,125, with a minimum of $195 and a maximum of $1,000,000. The 90th percentile cutpoint defining the especially high resource users was $192,272 (Figure 30–1). Total hospital charges varied among the 27 states; CA ($74,294) had the highest median total hospital charges and Maryland had the lowest ($19,722) (Figure 30–2).

---

[1] Arizona, California, Colorado, Connecticut, Florida, Georgia, Hawaii, Iowa, Kansas, Kentucky, Maine, Maryland, Massachusetts, Missouri, North Carolina, New Jersey, New York, Oregon, Pennsylvania, South Carolina, Tennessee, Texas, Utah, Virginia, Washington, Wisconsin and West Virginia.

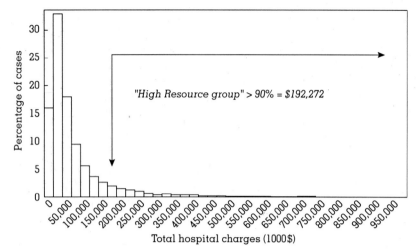

FIGURE 30-1. Distribution of total hospital charges for cases of congenital heart surgery from Kids' Inpatient Database (KID) year 2000. The median total hospital charge for this group was $51,125, with a minimum of $195 and a maximum of $1,000,000. The 90th percentile cutpoint defining the especially high resource users was $192,272.

Using the same data set we then conducted univariate and multivariate analyses to determine demographic descriptors (i.e., age, gender, race, insurance status, and day of admission), clinical indicators (i.e., prematurity and the presence of other noncardiac structural anomalies), and hospital predictors (i.e., hospital bed size, location, teaching status, children's hospital status, and volume of cardiac cases performed by institution) of high-resource-use cases. Geographic variables including region of the United States (Northeast,

South, Midwest, and West) and state (27 states) were also examined.

Case mix severity was approximated using the Risk Adjustment for Congenital Heart Surgery (RACHS-1) risk categories (Jenkins et al., 1998, 2002). The RACHS-1 method was originally developed to adjust for differences in case mix when comparing in-hospital mortality among groups of patients. To apply this method, cases are assigned to one of the six predefined risk categories on the presence or absence of specific

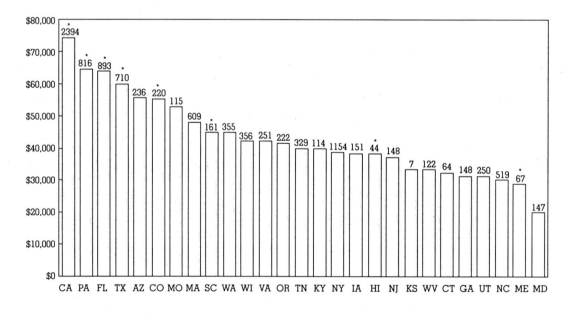

FIGURE 30-2. Median total hospital charges by state. The number of cases by state from Kids' Inpatient Database (KID) year 2000 ranged from 7 to 2394. Total hospital charges varied among the 27 states; CA had the highest median total hospital charges ($74,294) and Maryland had the lowest ($19,722).
*In univariate analysis, 8 states (marked by *) were indentified as having a significantly higher or lower proportion from 7 to 2394. Total hospital charges varied among the 27 states; CA had the highest median total hospital charges ($p < 0.05$) and Maryland had the lowest ($19,722)

TABLE 30–1. *Performance of Final Model for Outcome Increased Resource Utilization*

Predictor		OR	P Value	ROC[†]
State	NY + Other*	1.00	—	
	CA	3.66	<0.001	
	TX	2.34	0.001	
	CO	2.14	0.006	
	HI	2.06	<0.001	
	PA	1.81	0.039	
	FL	1.66	0.011	
	SC	0.60	<0.001	
	ME	0.35	<0.001	0.632
RACHS-1 risk category	1	1.00	—	
	2	1.66	0.005	
	3	3.61	<0.001	
	4	5.10	<0.001	
	5	8.59	0.008	
	6	14.1	<0.001	
	Unassigned	4.95	<0.001	0.759
Age	<1 year	3.81	<0.001	0.810
Prematurity		4.85	<0.001	0.825
Other structural anomaly		2.53	<0.001	0.831
Weekend admission		1.62	<0.001	0.834
Insurance (vs. private)	Medicaid	1.48	<0.001	
	Other	1.25	0.061	0.837

Note: Including in hospital deaths.
*NY, AZ, CT, GA, IA, KS, KY, MD, MA, ME, MO, NC, NJ, OR, TN, UT, VA, WA, WI, WV.
[†]Cumulative area under receiver operating characteristic curve.

diagnosis and procedure ICD-9 codes, where Risk Category 1 has the lowest risk for death and Risk Category 6 the highest (Appendix). Cases with combinations of cardiac surgical procedures (e.g., coarctation of the aorta and ventricular septal defect closure) are placed in the Risk Category corresponding to the single highest risk procedure.

Statewide differences in the proportion of high-resource-use admissions were present; CA, CO, FL, HI, PA, and TX were more likely to have high-resource-use cases and ME and SC to have low-resource-use cases (Figure 30–2). Subsequent analyses were performed adjusting for baseline state effects. Multivariate analyses using generalized estimating equations models identified RACHS-1 risk category (odds ratios [OR] 1.69–14.7), age less than 1 year (OR 3.9), prematurity (OR 4.7), the presence of an other major noncardiac structural anomaly (OR 2.5), Medicaid insurance (OR 1.47), and admission during a weekend (OR 1.64) to be independent predictors of a high-resource-use case (all p < 0.05) (Table 30–1). Although some institutional differences were noted in univariate analyses, gender, race, bed size, teaching and children's hospital status, and hospital volume of cardiac cases were not independently associated with greater odds of high resource utilization.

The results of these population-based analyses of children undergoing surgical repair of CHD using the KID 2000 dataset highlight significant geographic variation in resource utilization. States varied in the frequency of especially high-resource-use cases for congenital heart surgery, with some having a higher and some a lower than average number. It was unclear whether applying risk-adjustment measures for case mix would diminish these differences. Our results also revealed especially high resource utilization to be found within a subset of children undergoing congenital heart repair rather than the population as a whole.

RACHS-1 risk category and younger age were found to be highly predictive of high resource utilization. We also found clinical descriptors such as prematurity, and presence of other noncardiac structural anomalies, to be highly predictive. Although there is a paucity of information with which to compare our findings, the work by Ungelieder et al. (1997), which focused on identification of patients associated with high-cost surgical admissions at a single institution, produced similar findings. Our results would further support their conclusions that there are clinical predictors of financial risk that may facilitate implementation of risk adjustments for payers and for strategic resource allocation within institutions.

Although the timing of hospital admission was noted to be a significant independent predictor of high resource utilization, we do not have a conclusive explanation for this. However, cases admitted on a weekend may possibly be cases that were not diagnosed prenatally, or required emergent surgical intervention, or were stabilized at time of admission and waited for surgery to be performed during a weekday.

Cases reported as Medicaid or other insurance rather than private insurance were found to be independently predictive of high resource utilization. However, this variable added the least to the discrimination between our resource groups in the final model. The structure of the KID database did not specify the timing of recorded status (i.e., admission versus discharge); therefore, it cannot be concluded whether these cases had Medicaid as a primary insurer based on socioeconomic status or whether they became Medicaid cases as a result of accruing significant hospital charges.

DeMone et al. (2003) have previously reported Medicaid as an independent predictor of pediatric cardiac surgical outcomes. Their study examining the effect of insurance type on mortality for congenital heart surgery revealed that not only do Medicaid patients have a higher risk of death as compared with commercial or managed care cases, but differences were present both within and between institutions as well, identified as low, average, and high mortality, suggesting that the adverse effect of Medicaid may be due to both differential referral among patients treated at similar institutions and differential outcomes within institutions. These findings, when combined with our findings regarding resource utilization suggest that differences in care may exist for Medicaid patients, and should become an area of continued study.

Although some institutional differences were noted in univariate analyses, bed size, teaching and children's

hospital status, and hospital volume of cardiac cases were not independently associated with a greater likelihood of being high-resource-use cases. Our findings are not consistent with what has been previously reported on pediatric conditions in teaching facilities (Srivastava et al., 2003) and may be due to the limited number of children's hospital and nonteaching facilities that perform congenital heart repair available in the dataset. As is the current trend, most pediatric cardiac surgical programs exist in teaching facilities with a children's unit, it would be difficult to find an adequate number of nonteaching facilities for examination.

STATEWIDE VARIATION OF RESOURCE UTILIZATION

We felt the finding of significant statewide variation deserved further attention. Using similar inclusion criteria and risk-adjustment methodology, differences between observed and risk-adjusted expected mean charges, which we called the charge differential, were examined for each state. Expected mean charges were derived from a linear regression model with outcome log transformed charges adjusting for RACHS-1 risk category. Predictors of these differences were explored, including ratio of state volume of congenital heart surgery to number of institutions performing congenital heart surgery, state cost of living index, state area wage index, Health Maintenance Organization (HMO) penetration in state, and the proportion of each state's

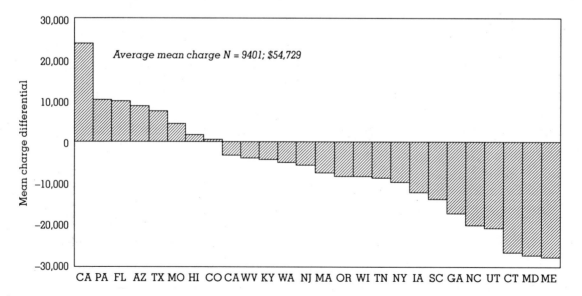

Risk-adjusted charges varied by $51,919.

FIGURE 30–3. Charge differential of states. Among the 26 states examined using the Kids' Inpatient Database (KID) year 2000, risk-adjusted charges varied by $51,919, with a minimum charge differential of −$27,900 and maximum charge differential of $24,019.

TABLE 30-2. *Predictors of State Charge and Cost Differential*

State Characteristics	Change in Charge Differential ($)	P Value	Change in Cost Differential ($)	P Value
≥1 Free-standing children's hospital	14,261	0.003	4582	0.003
≥97% Cases in teaching hospital	–5456	0.37	–1519	0.45
% Caseload with Medicaid insurance (10%↑)	–124	0.95	210	0.75
% Caseload with median income < $25,000 (5%↑)	2452	0.24	795	0.88
Ration volume/institution (↑ of 50)	–535	0.91	915	0.57
Cost of living index (↑ of 10%)	226	0.92	–846	0.24
Wage area index (↑ of 0.1)	1058	0.63	208	0.77
HMO penetration	3282	0.18	294	0.72

caseload at children's and teaching hospitals, and with specific insurance types (i.e., Medicaid, private/HMO, other).

We found that among the 9401 cases of congenital heart surgery for which a RACHS-1 risk category could be assigned, mean charges were $54,729. RACHS-1 risk category, age, prematurity, major noncardiac structural anomaly, multiple surgical procedures, chromosomal abnormality, and weekend admission were associated with higher charges. Among the 26 states examined, risk-adjusted charges varied by $ 51,919, with a minimum charge differential of –$27,900 and a maximum charge differential of $24,019 (Figure 30–3). States with children's hospitals had a $14,261 higher charge differential on average ($p = 0.003$) (Table 30–2). Other state characteristics were not associated with a mean dollar charge differential.

From this second analysis, we concluded that states varied considerably in risk-adjusted hospital charges for congenital heart surgery procedures. States containing one or more children's hospitals were found to have a higher charge differential.

Acknowledging the limitation that total hospital charges is not a direct measure of costs, average state CCR for the 26 states were obtained from the Agency for Health Care Research and Quality (AHRQ). The mean CCR for a state was calculated as a weighted average of the institution-specific CCRs for that state, where each institution's CCR was weighted by the number of pediatric discharges in that hospital. The CCR for a state was assumed to apply for each individual case in that state. For each case, Cost = Charges × CCR.

Repeating the above analysis revealed the average mean cost for the 9401 cases to be $25,295. Risk-adjusted costs varied by $14,764, with a minimum cost differential of –$9305 and a maximum cost differential of $5459 (Figure 30–4). As in the charge analysis, states that contain 1 or more free-standing children's hospital have a higher cost differential; the average increase was $4582 ($p = 0.003$) (Table 30–2). Interestingly, the conversion of hospital charges to hospital costs using the

CCRs dramatically changed the differential ranking of some states and had very little effect on others. These differences may reflect actual differences in resource use or different strategies employed by institutions or states to inflate charges to increase reimbursement from payers. These results suggest that further investigation is needed at the institution level.

Since high-quality care may require additional resources, it is unclear whether the significant variation in charges between states identified high-quality care as costly or whether these findings could be viewed as an opportunity to provide more efficient care. Building on the prior work of developing standardized mortality ratios (SMRs) for children undergoing congenital heart surgery (Jenkins and Gauvreau, 2002), we developed a relative measure of both quality and resource utilization to examine "value" of care and used this measure to examine regional variation.

Relative quality and resource use was examined using the product of the SMR and standardized charge ratio (SCR). This product was termed the *value metric*. For each state, SMR was defined as observed mortality divided by expected mortality. Expected mortality was adjusted for baseline case mix differences using RACHS-1 risk category, age, prematurity, major noncardiac structural anomaly, and multiple surgical procedures. Similarly, the SCR was defined as observed mean charges divided by expected mean charges. Expected mean charges were obtained from a linear regression model predicting log transformed charges and adjusting for the above variables plus chromosomal abnormality and weekend admission. As an example, a state with mortality and charges both equal to expected would have a product equal to one. States were ranked from lowest to highest using this value metric. In addition, the relationship between the SCR and the SMR was examined graphically (Figure 30–5).

With 9401 cases of congenital heart surgery, the mortality rate was 4.1% and the average median charges were $49,722. Mortality rates per state ranged from 0.6% to 6.1%. The SMR ranged from 0.13 to

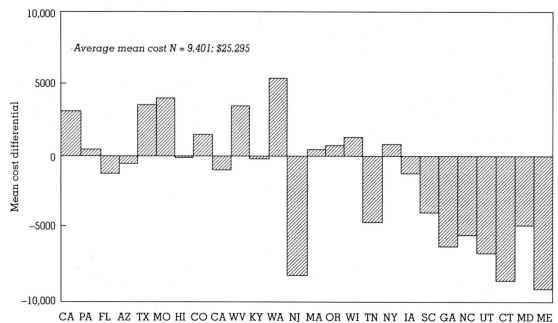

Average mean cost N = 9,401; $25,295

*Risk-adjusted cost varied by $14,764.

FIGURE 30–4. Cost differential of states. Among the 26 states examined using the Kids' Inpatient Database (KID) year 2000, risk-adjusted costs varied by $14,764, with a minimum cost differential of –$9305 and a maximum cost differential of $5459.

1.87 and SCR ranged from 0.47 to 1.4. The product of SMR and SCR (Figure 30–6) ranged from 0.12 to 1.86. CO, MA, ME, MD, OR, and WI had a product <0.50; CT, GA, IA, MO, NC, NY, PA, SC, and UT had a product 0.50–0.99; CA, FL, HI, TN, VA, WA, and WV had a product 1.00–1.49; AZ, KY, NJ, and TX had a product ≥1.50 (Figure 30–6). There was no correlation between the SMR and SCR at the state levels.

We concluded that states varied considerably in a risk-adjusted measure of both quality and resource use for congenital heart surgery procedures. This novel approach may be the first step in identifying the value of care delivered during hospitalizations. Use of this composite measure may be used by health care providers, institutions, payers, and policy makers when formulating interventions and policies to allocate resources for congenital heart surgery.

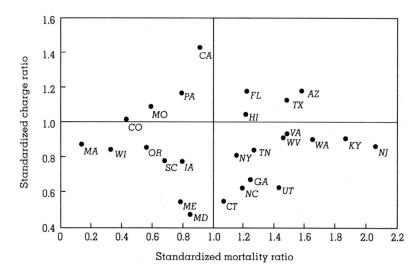

FIGURE 30–5. Relationship of standardized charge ratio (SCR) and standardized mortality ratio (SMR). Among the 26 states examined using the Kids' Inpatient Database (KID) year 2000, the relationship between the SCR and the SMR is displayed graphically. States in the lower left hand quadrant were found to have a SCR and SMR below what was to be expected. States in right upper quadrant were found to have a SCR and SMR above what was to be expected.

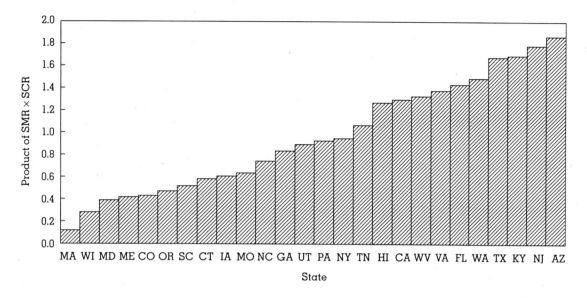

FIGURE 30–6. Product of standardized mortality ratio (SMR) and standardized charge ratio (SCR) by state. The product of SMR and SCR ranged from 0.12 to 1.86. CO, MA, ME, MD, OR, and WI had a product <0.50; CT, GA, IA, MO, NC, NY, PA, SC, and UT had a product 0.50 to 0.99; CA, FL, HI, TN, VA, WA, and WV had a product 1.00 to 1.49; AZ, KY, NJ, and TX had a product ≥ 1.50.

THE CONTRIBUTION OF COMPLICATIONS TO INCREASED RESOURCE UTILIZATION

We have also investigated the role of complications in contributing to increased utilization for children undergoing congenital heart surgery. Recent studies have reported that complications during congenital heart surgery admissions are frequent and are associated with a greater than two-fold increase risk for in-hospital mortality (Benavidez et al., 2007; Benavidez et al., 2006). The Institutes of Medicine estimates that medical errors cost the United States between $17 billion and $29 billion annually (LT et al., 2000).

We utilized a validated method for identifying "medical injury" via *ICD-9-CM* codes recently published by the AHRQ (Layde et al., 2005). We chose this method because of its comprehensive panel of complication diagnoses, its use of *ICD-9-CM* codes to identify complications, and its previous validation and application within a pediatric discharge database (Meurer et al., 2004). This algorithm defines "medical injury" as "untoward harm associated with a therapeutic or diagnostic healthcare intervention" (Layde et al., 2005). Designation of an event as a "medical injury" does not signify that the event was necessarily preventable nor was it due to substandard care. That is, although some of these events may represent preventable or modifiable complications, others may be an unavoidable part of the patient's disease process. These events may occur at any point during the patient's admission (e.g., during anesthesia, catheterization, patient transport, surgery,

intensive care unit care, inpatient ward). This method classifies complications into four broad categories: (1) drug/biologic; (2) procedures; (3) devices, implants, and grafts; and (4) radiation. The list of ICD-9-CM codes used to define complications has been previously published by the AHRQ (Layde et al., 2005).

We added the presence of a complication diagnosis to our prior model predicting the upper decile of hospital charges, to estimate the independent effect of a complication diagnosis on resource use. The added explanatory power attributed to a complication diagnosis was measured by an increase in the area under the receiver operator characteristic (ROC) curve.

Among the complications identified, 71% were procedure-related injuries, 25% were device or implant related and 4% were drug related. Among the 3360 admissions with a complication, 50% had only one, 34% had two, 13% had three, and 3% had four or more complication diagnoses.

Multivariate analysis revealed that admissions with a complications diagnosis were much more likely to be in the upper decile of total hospital charges: OR 3.2 (95% CI 2.8–3.6, p < 0.001). Overall, the addition of the complications variable to the model did not change the statistical significance of the previously identified risk factors for high resource use. The ORs for surgical risk categories remained significant but decreased in magnitude when the complications variable was added to the model. This suggests that part of the risk ascribed to surgical complexity for high resource may be due to an increased risk of complications. With the addition of complication, the area under the ROC curve increased from 0.837 to 0.863.

CONCLUSIONS

A significant portion of our available health care resources is used by a small proportion of the population. Children born with CHD are included in this complex population of patients. Our investigations have revealed significant geographic variations in resource use for children undergoing congenital heart surgery. Further work will determine whether this geographic variation will persist once the effect of individual institutions is considered. Clinical and demographic factors also play a significant role in resource use as does the occurrence of a complication. Although demographic characteristics and disease complexity are fixed and offer no easy solutions for health care reform, further examination of state and institution systems may reflect opportunities for more efficient care to be instituted. In addition, reduction of complications may result in both an economic and clinical benefit.

REFERENCES

Alboliras ET, Hijazi ZM. Comparison of costs of intracardiac echocardiography and transesophageal echocardiography in monitoring percutaneous device closure of atrial septal defect in children and adults. *Am J Cardiol.* 2004;94:690–692.

Benavidez OJ, Gauvreau K, Del Nido P, Bacha E, Jenkins KJ. Complications and risk factors for mortality during congenital heart surgery admissions. *Ann Thorac Surg.* 2007;84:147–155.

Benavidez OJ, Gauvreau K, del Nido P, Bacha E, Jenkins KJ. Medical Injury Diagnoses and Mortality During Congenital Heart Surgery Admissions. *Ann Thorac Surg.* 2006;In Press.

Boneva RS, Botto LD, Moore CA, Yang Q, Correa A, Erickson JD. Mortality associated with congenital heart defects in the United States: trends and racial disparities, 1979–1997. *Circulation.* 2001;103:2376–2381.

Chalom R, Raphaely RC, Costarino AT, Jr. Hospital costs of pediatric intensive care. *Crit Care Med.* 1999;27:2079–2085.

Chang RK, Klitzner TS. Resources, use, and regionalization of pediatric cardiac services. *Curr Opin Cardiol.* 2003;18:98–101.

Chantepie A. [Use of palivizumab for the prevention of respiratory syncytial virus infections in children with congenital heart disease. Recommendations from the French Paediatric Cardiac Society.]. *Arch Pediatr.* 2004;11:1402–1405.

Connor JA, Arons RR, Figueroa M, Gebbie KM. Clinical outcomes and secondary diagnoses for infants born with hypoplastic left heart syndrome. *Pediatrics.* 2004;114:e160–165.

Connor JA, Gauvreau K, Jenkins KJ. Factors associated with increased resource utilization for congenital heart disease. *Pediatrics.* 2005;116:689–695.

Cronk CE, Malloy ME, Pelech AN, et al. Completeness of state administrative databases for surveillance of congenital heart disease. *Birth Defects Res A Clin Mol Teratol.* 2003;67:597–603.

Daenen W, Lacour-Gayet F, Aberg T, et al. Optimal structure of a congenital heart surgery department in Europe. *Eur J Cardiothorac Surg.* 2003;24:343–351.

DeMone JA, Gonzalez PC, Gauvreau K, Piercey GE, Jenkins KJ. Risk of death for Medicaid recipients undergoing congenital heart surgery. *Pediatr Cardiol.* 2003;24:97–102.

Dimmick S, Walker K, Badawi N, et al. Outcomes following surgery for congenital heart disease in low-birthweight infants. *J Paediatr Child Health.* 2007;43:370–375.

Feltes TF, Sondheimer HM. Palivizumab and the prevention of respiratory syncytial virus illness in pediatric patients with congenital heart disease. *Expert Opin Biol Ther.* 2007;7:1471–1480.

Fernandes AM, Mansur AJ, Caneo LF, et al. The reduction in hospital stay and costs in the care of patients with congenital heart diseases undergoing fast-track cardiac surgery. *Arq Bras Cardiol.* 2004;83:27–34;18–26.

Frohnert BK, Lussky RC, Alms MA, Mendelsohn NJ, Symonik DM, Falken MC. Validity of hospital discharge data for identifying infants with cardiac defects. *J Perinatol.* 2005;25:737–742.

Garne E. Congenital heart defects – occurrence, surgery and prognosis in a Danish County. Scand *Cardiovasc J.* 2004;38:357–362.

Garson A, Jr., Allen HD, Gersony WM, et al. The cost of congenital heart disease in children and adults. A model for multicenter assessment of price and practice variation. *Arch Pediatr Adolesc Med.* 1994;148:1039–1045.

Gatzoulis MA. Adult congenital heart disease: a cardiovascular area of growth in urgent need of additional resource allocation. *Int J Cardiol.* 2004;97 9(suppl 1):1–2.

Greeley W, J. Financial Implications in the Care of Complex Congenital Heart Disease. Boston: Kluwer Academic Publishers; 2003.

Howard TS, Hoffman LH, Stang PE, Simoes EA. Respiratory syncytial virus pneumonia in the hospital setting: length of stay, charges, and mortality. *J Pediatr.* 2000;137:227–232.

Iezzoni LI. Using administrative data to study persons with disabilities. *Milbank Q.* 2002;80:347–379.

Immer FF, Althaus SM, Berdat PA, Saner H, Carrel TP. Quality of life and specific problems after cardiac surgery in adolescents and adults with congenital heart diseases. *Eur J Cardiovasc Prev Rehabil.* 2005;12:138–143.

IOM. Crossing the quality chasm a New Health system for the 21st Century. Washington, D.C.: National Academies Press; 2001.

IOM. Keeping patients safe transforming the work enviroment of nurses. Washington, D.C.: National Academies Press; 2004.

Jacobs JP, Jacobs ML, Maruszewski B, et al. Current status of the European Association for Cardio-Thoracic Surgery and the Society of Thoracic Surgeons Congenital Heart Surgery Database. *Ann Thorac Surg* 2005;80:2278–2283; discussion 2283–2274.

Jacobs JP, Mavroudis C, Jacobs ML, et al. Lessons learned from the data analysis of the second harvest (1998–2001) of the Society of Thoracic Surgeons (STS) Congenital Heart Surgery Database. *Eur J Cardiothorac Surg.* 2004;26:18–37.

Jaquiss RD, Siehr SL, Ghanayem NS, et al. Early cavopulmonary anastomosis after Norwood procedure results in excellent Fontan outcome. *Ann Thorac Surg.* 2006;82:1260–1265; discussion 1265–1266.

Jenkins KJ, Gauvreau K, Newburger JW, Kyn LB, Iezzoni LI, Mayer JE. Validation of relative value scale for congenital heart operations. *Ann Thorac Surg.* 1998;66:860–869.

Jenkins KJ, Gauvreau K, Newburger JW, Spray TL, Moller JH, Iezzoni LI. Consensus-based method for risk adjustment for surgery for congenital heart disease. *J Thorac Cardiovasc Surg.* 2002;123:110–118.

Jenkins KJ, Gauvreau K. Center-specific differences in mortality: preliminary analyses using the Risk Adjustment in Congenital Heart Surgery (RACHS-1) method. *J Thorac Cardiovasc Surg.* 2002;124:97–104.

Jenkins KJ, Newburger JW, Lock JE, Davis RB, Coffman GA, Iezzoni LI. In-hospital mortality for surgical repair of congenital heart defects: preliminary observations of variation by hospital caseload. *Pediatrics.* 1995;95:323–330.

Kang N, Tsang VT, Gallivan S, et al. Quality assurance in congenital heart surgery. *Eur J Cardiothorac Surg.* 2006;29:693–697; discussion 697–698.

Kanter RK. Post-intensive care unit pediatric hospital stay and estimated costs. *Crit Care Med.* 2000;28:220–223.

Larrazabal LA, Jenkins KJ, Gauvreau K, et al. Improvement in congenital heart surgery in a developing country: the Guatemalan experience. *Circulation.* 2007;116:1882–1887.

Layde PM, Meurer LN, Guse CE, et al. Patient Safety Monitoring: Identification of Medical Injuries Using Hospital Discharge Data. In: Henricksen K, Battles JB, Marks E, Lewin DI, E. M, (eds). *Advances in patient safety: From research to implementation* Vol 2, Concepts and methodology . Rockville, MD: Agency for Healthcare Research and Quality, 2005;2:119–132.

LT K, JM C, MS D. To Err is Human: Building a Safer Health System. Washington DC: Institute of Medicine, 2000.

Mackie AS, Pilote L, Ionescu-Ittu R, Rahme E, Marelli AJ. Health care resource utilization in adults with congenital heart disease. *Am J Cardiol.* 2007;99:839–843.

Meberg A, Bruu AL. Respiratory syncytial virus infections in congenital heart defects – hospitalizations and costs. *Acta Paediatr.* 2006;95:404–406.

Meurer J, Yang H, Guse C, Scanlon M, Layde PM. Medical Injuries Among Children Hospitalized in Wisconsin. Pediatric Academic Societies' Annual Meeting. San Francisco, California, 2004.

Meyns B. Congenital heart surgery in Belgium. State of the art in 2003. *Acta Cardiol.* 2004;59 9(suppl 1):31–34.

Moons P, De Volder E, Budts W, et al. What do adult patients with congenital heart disease know about their disease, treatment, and prevention of complications? A call for structured patient education. *Heart.* 2001a;86:74–80.

Moons P, Siebens K, De Geest S, Abraham I, Budts W, Gewillig M. A pilot study of expenditures on, and utilization of resources in, health care in adults with congenital heart disease. *Cardiol Young.* 2001b;11:301–313.

Nuijten MJ, Wittenberg W, Lebmeier M. Cost effectiveness of palivizumab for respiratory syncytial virus prophylaxis in high-risk children: a UK analysis. *Pharmacoeconomics.* 2007;25:55–71.

Price S, Jaggar SI, Jordan S, et al. Adult congenital heart disease: intensive care management and outcome prediction. *Intensive Care Med.* 2007;33:652–659.

Riehle-Colarusso T, Strickland MJ, Reller MD, et al. Improving the quality of surveillance data on congenital heart defects in the metropolitan Atlanta congenital defects program. *Birth Defects Res A Clin Mol Teratol.* 2007;79:743–753.

Silberbach M, Shumaker D, Menashe V, Cobanoglu A, Morris C. Predicting hospital charge and length of stay for congenital heart disease surgery. *Am J Cardiol.* 1993;72:958–963.

Srivastava R, Homer CJ. Length of stay for common pediatric conditions: teaching versus nonteaching hospitals. *Pediatrics.* 2003;112:278–281.

Ungerleider RM, Bengur AR, Kessenich AL, et al. Risk factors for higher cost in congenital heart operations. *Ann Thorac Surg.* 1997;64:44–48; discussion 49.

Venkatesh MP, Weisman LE. Prevention and treatment of respiratory syncytial virus infection in infants: an update. *Expert Rev Vaccines.* 2006;5:261–268.

Williams DL, Gelijns AC, Moskowitz AJ, et al. Hypoplastic left heart syndrome: valuing the survival. *J Thorac Cardiovasc Surg.* 2000;119:720–731.

Yount LE, Mahle WT. Economic analysis of palivizumab in infants with congenital heart disease. *Pediatrics.* 2004;114:1606–1611.

Zannini L, Borini I. State of the art of cardiac surgery in patients with congenital heart disease. *J Cardiovasc Med.* (Hagerstown) 2007;8:3–6.

Zellers TM, Dixon K, Moake L, Wright J, Ramaciotti C. Bedside balloon atrial septostomy is safe, efficacious, and cost-effective compared with septostomy performed in the cardiac catheterization laboratory. *Am J Cardiol.* 2002;89:613–615.

APPENDIX

Individual Procedures by Risk Category

RISK CATEGORY 1

- Atrial septal defect surgery (including atrial septal defect secundum, sinus venosus atrial septal defect, patent foramen ovale closure)
- Aortopexy
- Patent ductus arteriosus surgery at age >30 days
- Coarctation repair at age >30 days
- Partially anomalous pulmonary venous connection surgery

RISK CATEGORY 2

- Aortic valvotomy or valvuloplasty at age >30 days
- Subaortic stenosis resection
- Pulmonary valvotomy or valvuloplasty
- Pulmonary valve replacement
- Right ventricular infundibulectomy

- Pulmonary outflow tract augmentation
- Repair of coronary artery fistula
- Atrial septal defect and ventricular septal repair
- Atrial septal defect primum repair
- Ventricular septal defect repair
- Ventricular septal defect closure and pulmonary valvotomy or infundibular resection
- Ventricular septal defect closure and pulmonary artery band removal
- Repair of unspecified septal defect
- Total repair of tetralogy of Fallot
- Repair of total anomalous pulmonary veins at age >30 days
- Glenn shunt
- Vascular ring surgery
- Repair of aortopulmonary window
- Coarctation repair at age ≤30 days
- Repair of pulmonary artery stenosis
- Transection of pulmonary artery
- Common atrium closure
- Left ventricular to right atrial shunt repair

RISK CATEGORY 3

- Aortic valve replacement
- Ross procedure
- Left ventricular outflow tract patch
- Ventriculomyotomy
- Aortoplasty
- Mitral valvotomy or valvuloplasty
- Mitral valve replacement
- Valvectomy of tricuspid valve
- Tricuspid valvotomy or valvuloplasty
- Tricuspid valve replacement
- Tricuspid valve repositioning for Ebstein anomaly at age >30 days
- Repair of anomalous coronary artery without intrapulmonary tunnel
- Repair of anomalous coronary artery with intrapulmonary tunnel (Takeuchi)
- Closure of semilunar valve, aortic or pulmonary
- Right ventricular to pulmonary artery conduit
- Left ventricular to pulmonary artery conduit
- Repair of double outlet right ventricle with or without repair of right ventricular obstruction
- Fontan procedure
- Repair of transitional or complete atrioventricular canal with or without valve replacement
- Pulmonary artery band
- Repair of tetralogy of Fallot with pulmonary atresia
- Repair of cor triatriatum
- Systemic to pulmonary artery shunt
- Atrial switch operation
- Arterial switch operation
- Reimplantation of anomalous pulmonary artery
- Annuloplasty
- Repair of coarctation and ventricular septal defect closure
- Excision of intracardiac tumor

RISK CATEGORY 4

- Aortic valvotomy or valvuloplasty at age ≤30 days
- Konno procedure

- Repair of complex anomaly (single ventricle) by ventricular septal defect enlargement
- Repair of total anomalous pulmonary veins at age ≤30 days
- Atrial septectomy
- Repair of transposition, ventricular septal defect, and subpulmonary stenosis (Rastelli)
- Atrial switch operation with ventricular septal defect closure
- Atrial switch operation with repair of subpulmonary stenosis
- Arterial switch operation with pulmonary artery band removal
- Arterial switch operation with ventricular septal defect closure
- Arterial switch operation with repair of subpulmonary stenosis
- Repair of truncus arteriosus
- Repair of hypoplastic or interrupted arch without ventricular septal defect closure
- Repair of hypoplastic or interrupted aortic arch with ventricular septal defect closure
- Transverse arch graft
- Unifocalization for tetralogy of Fallot and pulmonary atresia
- Double switch

RISK CATEGORY 5

- Tricuspid valve repositioning for neonatal Ebstein anomaly at age ≤30 days
- Repair of truncus arteriosus and interrupted arch

RISK CATEGORY 6

- Stage 1 repair of hypoplastic left heart syndrome (Norwood operation)
- Stage 1 repair of nonhypoplastic left heart syndrome conditions
- Damus-Kaye-Stansel procedure

31

Health Care Costs of Congenital Heart Defects

SHEREE L. BOULET
SCOTT D. GROSSE
TIFFANY RIEHLE-COLARUSSO
ADOLFO CORREA-VILLASEÑOR

INTRODUCTION

Congenital heart defects (CHD) are a diverse group of serious birth defects that contribute to approximately one-half of all infant deaths and one third of all hospitalizations due to congenital anomalies in the United States (Rosano et al., 2000; Russo and Elixhauser, 2007). In particular, severe defects that often require surgical treatment and lengthy hospitalizations presumably account for a disproportionate share of costs associated with CHD. Medical costs associated with specific severe defects often exceed the costs associated with other types of birth defects (Waitzman et al., 1994, 1996; CDC, 1995, 2007). However, no previous analysis has reported the relative contributions of severe CHD to overall health care costs associated with CHD or the costs associated with children who have multiple anomalies compared with those with isolated defects. One analysis has estimated the additional health care costs associated with CHD among children with Down syndrome (Boulet et al., 2008).

Estimates of cost can aid decision makers in understanding the societal impact of illnesses and the potential effects of preventive interventions and changes in incidence. In particular, up-to-date cost estimates are needed to accurately measure the economic impact of effective interventions to prevent birth defects (Grosse et al., 2005). The cost of CHD includes direct costs of providing medical care and other services to affected individuals, as well as the so-called indirect costs of reduced economic productivity among affected individuals (Waitzman et al., 1996); the lost economic productivity of parental caregivers is classified as a direct cost but is only rarely included in birth defects cost studies (Tilford et al., 2009). In this chapter we focus on health care utilization and costs for children with different types of CHD.

SOURCES OF DATA

The term "cost" has multiple meanings. In economic analyses from the societal perspective, cost refers to the consumption of resources in producing and delivering a good or service. Payments or expenditures represent costs from the payer perspective. There are two primary empirical approaches used to estimate the costs of health care services. One is to use average total expenditures for all payers or for a specific group of payers as a proxy for average cost, although reimbursements for specific services are not necessarily equivalent to the resources required to provide those services. Also, average expenditures for private payers typically exceed reimbursements by public payers. The

The findings and conclusions in this report are those of the authors and do not necessarily represent the official position of the Centers for Disease Control and Prevention.

other approach is to multiply list prices or charges (e.g., a bill for hospital services) by cost-to-charge ratios published by the Centers for Medicare & Medicaid Services and the Agency for Healthcare Research and Quality (AHRQ) to convert average hospital charges into cost estimates. In this chapter, the term "cost" is used to encompass both types of cost estimates. Often, cost-to-charge ratios are less than 0.50, meaning that the estimated cost to society for hospital services is less than half the typical bill (Russo and Elixhauser, 2007). Consequently, charges substantially overstate costs and should never be used as a proxy for costs.

Health care costs associated with specific diseases can be studied with different types of data. These include population surveys, clinical datasets for patients seen at particular centers, and administrative databases that contain individual-level records, such as those collected from hospitals, physicians, and insurance or billing firms. The Medical Expenditure Panel Survey (MEPS) collects information from a random sample of the US population on prevalent health conditions and the utilization and expenditures for medical care. Costs associated with common conditions, such as asthma, diabetes, or cardiovascular disease have often been studied with MEPS data (Cohen and Krause, 2003), but the sample size is not sufficient to analyze birth defects. Discharge data from one or multiple clinical centers are often used to study health care utilization and charges, including those for birth defects (Berk and Marzarita, 2002). The advantage of such data is that information from medical records can be used to validate diagnoses and procedures. A disadvantage is that the information is not necessarily representative of individuals with a condition.

The primary sources of information on health care costs associated with birth defects are administrative databases, either hospital discharge or public and private health insurance claims data. Advantages of hospital discharge data are public access and the inclusion of all admissions regardless of payer type. Corresponding limitations of health insurance claims data are that they generally either are proprietary or require complicated permissions from government entities to gain access, and they cover only one type of payer, either public or private. A disadvantage of most hospital discharge datasets is that they treat the discharge as the unit of observation and do not allow one to link different hospitalizations for the same individual. In contrast, health claims databases allow one to cumulatively record health care utilization for individuals over a period, ranging from a single year to multiple years. A further disadvantage of hospital discharge datasets is that they only include facility fees. Physician and other professional fees can add approximately 20% to facility fees (Rogowski, 1998), which means that hospital

cost estimates based on facility fees alone are understated. The chief advantage of claims data is that they include multiple types of medical care, including inpatient and outpatient care and prescription medications. It is worthwhile to note, however, that there is variation across databases in how these components are defined. For example, inpatient claims may be composed of professional fees and facility fees or just facility fees.

For researchers interested in estimating health care expenditures, a few administrative datasets exist and are widely available. State hospital discharge datasets can be directly accessed by researchers with permission from state governments. The Health Care Cost and Utilization Project (HCUP) of the AHRQ pools hospital discharge data supplied by 37 participating states. HCUP has two national databases that provide nationally weighted estimates of hospital facility charges. The Nationwide Inpatient Sample (NIS) is available on an annual basis since 1994 and consists of a 20% sample of community-based hospitals in participating states. The sample is weighted to provide national estimates of hospital discharges. For pediatric admissions, a sample of all nonroutine births and all nonbirth admissions is provided by HCUP through the Kids' Inpatient Database (KID) every 3 years beginning in 1997. The KID contains an 80% sample of all pediatric hospital discharges from 36 participating states, accounting for approximately 90% of US births, weighted to produce national estimates of hospitalizations and costs.

National-level data on the utilization and costs of inpatient hospital care specific to CHDs are available through HCUPNet, the online search tool for all HCUP databases, including both NIS and KID. NIS data in HCUPNet are currently available for each year from 1997 through 2005 and KID data for 1997, 2000, and 2003. Detailed information, including length of stay and charges, is provided for principal diagnoses only. Thus, these data may not be representative of the total costs for a condition because secondary diagnoses are not included. Estimates of hospitalization costs, exclusive of professional fees, can be estimated by applying HCUP hospital-specific cost-to-charge ratios to reported costs based on hospital accounting reports from Centers for Medicare & Medicaid Services.

Health insurance claims databases include both public (Medicare and Medicaid) and private health insurance. Although Medicare is a national program with national databases, Medicaid is a state-based program, and one needs to access state-specific Medicaid databases. Because of differences among states in Medicaid reimbursement practices, cost estimates from state-specific databases may be limited in generalizability. A number of proprietary private health insurance claims databases exist that require licensing agreements to access (e.g., MarketScan commercial claims databases from Thomson Reuters). These databases typically include information on encounters and total payments for each type of covered health service, including inpatient and outpatient care and, depending on the plan and database, prescription medications, home health care, and physical, speech, or occupational therapy. Medicaid databases often include more services than private insurance databases, notably dental services. A limitation is that health care services for which a claim is not submitted are not included. This is particularly an issue for private health insurance plans that may restrict coverage for certain conditions or types of services.

A major challenge to the use of administrative datasets for studying the costs of birth defects is case ascertainment. The ideal approach is to link administrative data with a birth defects registry. That way, one can identify children with a birth defect through validated birth defects surveillance data and use hospital discharge records, state Medicaid data, or both to track health service utilization and charges or expenditures. The pioneering California cost of birth defects study used all of these types of linkages to derive their estimates (Waitzman et al., 1994, 1996). In general, it is not an option to link private insurance databases with vital records or birth defects surveillance data because information identifying individuals is withheld from researchers for reasons of confidentiality.

Case ascertainment through administrative datasets generally uses *International Classification of Disease, Ninth Revision, Clinical Modification* (ICD-9-CM) codes reported for billing purposes. The accuracy of diagnostic codes within these databases is uncertain and appears to be low for certain CHD diagnostic codes. One study in Minnesota assessed the ICD-9-CM codes for cardiac defects in discharge records for 2697 infants born in one hospital during 2001 and compared them with the review of medical records (Frohnert et al., 2005). A total of 66 infants had been discharged with one or more of the ICD-9-CM codes for CHD. Review of medical records confirmed only 24 as having CHD according to birth defect surveillance case definitions, for a positive predictive value of only 0.364. In addition, four CHD cases were identified through chart reviews that were not listed on discharge statistics, for a sensitivity of 0.857. Most false positives were associated with two codes, 747.0 for patent ductus arteriosus (PDA) (n = 36) and 745.5 for atrial septal defects (ASDs) (n = 7), and occurred in infants who were born preterm. These false positives may reflect normal physiological findings in newborns and premature infants and therefore not true defects.

The Metropolitan Atlanta Congenital Defects Program (MACDP) is a population-based birth defect surveillance system that uses a unique six-digit coding system modified from the ICD-9-CM and British Pediatric Association systems. A MACDP study adopted the clinical nomenclature from the Society of Thoracic Surgeons (STS) database for use in recoding and classifying all cases with presumed CHD from 1968 to 2003 (Riehle-Colarusso et al., 2007). Out of 12,639 cases with presumptive CHD, 4890 (38%) were found to have structurally normal hearts. The high percentage of normal hearts largely reflected the elimination of cases with insignificant lesions, such as PDA and patent foramen ovale (PFO), that are related to normal newborn physiology, and vague codes in which a particular defect could not be identified. The application of standard clinical nomenclature and classification improved surveillance data accuracy by eliminating normal variants and obligatory shunt lesions. Not only can ICD-9-CM codes include both normal variants and severe CHD, but they also can make it difficult to distinguish among different CHD. A recent evaluation of the diagnostic accuracy of ICD-9-CM codes relative to the STS system in the MACDP 1968–2003 birth cohort revealed that the sensitivity of ICD-9-CM varied among defects: 83% for tetralogy of Fallot, 100% for transposition of the great arteries, and 95% for hypoplastic left heart syndrome, with false-positive fractions of 2%, 49%, and 11%, respectively (Strickland et al., 2008).

Another challenge in the use of administrative datasets in identifying individuals with birth defects is that many defects are only recorded for billing purposes while they are being actively managed. Children with surgically corrected CHD during the first year or two do not necessarily continue to have an ICD-9 code for their condition recorded during subsequent encounters with the health care system. Analyses that ascertain cases based on current ICD-9 codes would miss such children and the cost estimates for CHD could be biased because of underascertainment. To the extent that administrative datasets are able to track children for several years from infancy this problem can be avoided, but sample attrition due to insurance plan turnover is typically a serious limitation. The direction of bias is likely to differ for average and total costs or expenditures. To the extent that those individuals currently receiving cardiac care would have used more services than individuals with corrected defects, average costs for all CHD would be overstated. On the other hand, total costs for all individuals with CHD would be understated if older children, adolescents, and adults with corrected CHD have elevated rates of health care utilization and expenditures relative to those without CHD but their data are not included because they did not have a CHD code recorded. Finally, certain CHD that are difficult to detect at birth may not be identified during the first 2 years of life, but these are relatively few in number compared with those that are surgically corrected before the age of 2 years.

PREVIOUS CONGENITAL HEART DEFECT COST STUDIES

The most thorough study of costs associated with CHD was conducted in the early 1990s in California using 1988–1989 data (Waitzman et al., 1994; 1996), also summarized in two other publications (CDC, 1995; Harris and James, 1997). That study produced cost estimates for a total of 17 specific birth defects, including four CHD: truncus arteriosus, transposition of great vessels/double-outlet right ventricle (DORV), tetralogy of Fallot, and single ventricle. The investigators linked data from the California Office of Statewide Health Planning and Development (OSHPD) hospital discharge file, the California Medicaid (MediCal) program, and the California Birth Defects Monitoring Program (CBDMP). The latter data were used to identify children with specific birth defects, and the other databases were used to identify medical care utilization for such individuals. The OSHPD data were used to identify inpatient care, regardless of insurance type. Charges from OSHPD were adjusted to equivalent resource costs using a cost-to-charge ratio because hospital charges typically overstate costs, often to compensate for costs not reimbursed by third party payers. The MediCal data were used to assess outpatient costs (expenditures), with the assumption made that the ratio of outpatient to inpatient costs was comparable for children with different plan types.

Waitzman et al. (1994, 1996) calculated the present value at birth of lifetime costs on the basis of synthetic cohorts who were assumed to experience contemporary age-specific costs as they aged and using a 5% discount rate (equivalent to an after-inflation or "real" interest rate) to adjust costs in future years. They subtracted costs for the general population from those with birth defects to estimate "incremental" or net costs. The net medical cost per child, in 1988 dollars, was found to be highest for children with truncus arteriosus ($209,000) followed by tetralogy of Fallot ($109,000), single ventricle ($99,000), and transposition/DORV ($69,000).

Waitzman et al. reported medical care costs for children with CHD and for the general population of US children. During the first 2 years of life, expenditures were 38 times higher for those with truncus arteriosus and 13–17 times higher for the other three defects relative to the general population. At ages 2–4 years, expenditures were 127 times higher for children with truncus arteriosus and 19–23 times higher for the other defects. At 5–17 years of age, medical expenditures were 3–13 times higher for children with the four cardiac defects. The study also included estimates of special education costs, but because only 8% of children with CHD required special education, this added relatively little to the estimates of medical care costs.

The California study was comprehensive and methodologically sophisticated but the estimates are now dated. The estimates are based on surgical procedures and survival rates characteristic of the 1980s. In any case, they need to be updated for inflation in medical costs. Furthermore, lifetime cost estimates are now calculated using a 3% discount rate rather than a 5% rate. Finally, the cost estimates presumed that Medicaid reimbursements and cost-to-charge ratios reflected actual costs of providing care, whereas private expenditures might be higher. Garson et al. (1994) performed the only other US study to attempt to provide comprehensive estimates of charges for medical care for CHD. They collected information on health services utilization and charges for children with CHD up to 21 years of age from hospitals and outpatient clinics in Charleston, SC; Columbus, OH; Detroit, MI; Houston, TX; Los Angeles, CA; and New York, NY. They estimated how many patients would receive different types of interventions and the frequency of follow-up clinical visits, which they combined with charges reported by each of the participating centers to estimate total expected charges. Their highest estimate of total charges through 21 years of age was for hypoplastic left heart syndrome ($120,140), followed by tetralogy of Fallot ($92,933), acyanotic CHD with infant surgery ($72,443), acyanotic CHD with staged surgery ($46,163), and acyanotic CHD with nonsurgical (catheter) intervention ($18,115). These estimates of charges substantially overstated actual costs and were also overstated because the authors did not use discounting to calculate present values.

Russo and Elixhauser (2007) recently analyzed 2004 NIS data for birth defects and reported that as a group these accounted for 139,100 hospitalizations and an estimated $2.6 billion in total costs. Cardiac and circulatory anomalies (ICD-9-CM codes of 745.0–747.9) accounted for 33.5% of all birth defects–specific hospital stays and 53.3% of estimated costs, or $1.4 billion. This is the first-ever estimate of aggregate costs for any component of health care associated with CHD and hence is an important study. A limitation is that this is an underestimate because it excluded professional fees. The authors also reported that total charges for these defects in 2004 were $3.5 billion. Comparing this with their cost estimate, the authors used an average cost-to-charge ratio of 0.396.

Another recent study used the 2002 NIS dataset to examine hospitalization patterns among adults aged 18 and greater who had a diagnosis for "complex congenital heart disease" (CCHD) (Okumura et al., 2006). CCHD was defined as ICD-9-CM codes 745–745.39, 745.6–745.60, 745.69–745.9, 746–746.5, 746.7–746.9, and 747.1–747.49. They excluded individuals for whom the only CHD codes were for ASD or ventricular septal defect (VSD). They calculated a national estimate of 28,072 discharges for adults with CCHD, with a mean patient age of 50.8 years. The mean charge per discharge was $31,740.

Investigators at the University of Arkansas for Medical Sciences and at the Centers for Disease Control and Prevention (CDC) analyzed the 2003 KID dataset to calculate charges associated with hospitalizations that began within the first 10 days of birth and were associated with a birth defect diagnosis (CDC, 2007). Because of concerns about the validity of ICD-9-CM codes alone for accurately identifying cases, PDA, ASD, and VSD were excluded. Two specific types of CHD (hypoplastic left heart syndrome and common truncus arteriosus) were associated with the highest average charges per discharge during 2003 ($199,597 and $192,781, respectively). Two other cardiac defects—coarctation of the aorta and transposition of the great arteries—had average hospital charges in excess of $150,000. In comparison, the average hospital charge for uncomplicated births was $1844 in 2003. Although this study was the first to provide comparative information on hospital admissions and charges for different specific CHD, albeit for newborns only, a limitation was that children with multiple defects were included under each defect type. Consequently, no aggregate estimate of CHD charges, let alone costs, for neonatal hospitalizations could be derived from this study.

This chapter presents in the next two sections two original data analyses. First, we replicated and extended the analysis of NIS hospital discharge data by Russo and Elixhauser (2007) to provide more detail on the distribution of inpatient costs for subsets of CHD across the life span, the only such study that was not restricted to infants or adults. Specifically, our interest was in distinguishing costs for severe and nonsevere CHD. Second, we conducted a detailed analysis of MarketScan claims data on medical expenditures for children with CHDs. An important purpose of this analysis was to compare with comparable estimates of medical costs for children with CHD in the earlier California study.

HCUPNET CONGENITAL HEART DEFECT ANALYSIS

We used HCUPNet to analyze data from the 2004 NIS on principal discharges for CHD for patients of all ages. Using ICD-9-CM codes 745.0–747.9, we classified cardiac and circulatory anomalies into two types, severe and nonsevere for all ages (0–85+ years). As explained in Table 31–1, severe CHD was defined as the sum of the following conditions (with ICD-9-CM codes): truncus arteriosus (745.0), transposition complexes (745.1), tetralogy of Fallot (745.2), univentricular

TABLE 31-1. *Categories and Diagnostic Codes for Congenital Heart Defects*

Category	ICD9-CM Code(s)	Isolated vs. Multiple Heart Defects
Severe Defects		
Truncus arteriosus	745.0	Infants with only one severe heart defect are
Transposition complex/double-outlet right ventricle (DORV)	745.1	defined as isolated, severe; infants with
Tetralogy of Fallot	745.2	more than one severe heart defect are
Pulmonary valve atresia	746.01	defined as multiple, severe, regardless of the
Ebstein's anomaly	746.2	presence of mild defects
Single ventricle/hypoplastic left heart syndrome	745.3, 746.7	
Endocardial cushion defect	745.6	
Total anomalous pulmonary venous return	747.41	
Cor biloculare	745.7	
Mild Defects		
Pulmonary valve anomalies	746.00, 746.02, 746.09	The isolated, mild category included children
Tricuspid valve disease, congenital	746.1	with one mild defect or with one or more of
Aortic stenosis, congenital	746.3	the following specific defect combinations:
Aortic insufficiency, congenital	746.4	(1) aortic insufficiency *plus* aortic stenosis,
Mitral stenosis, congenital	746.5	or coarctation, atresia, or stenosis of aorta,
Mitral insufficiency, congenital	746.6	or other anomalies of aorta; (2) PDA *plus*
Coarctation, atresia, or stenosis of aorta	747.1, 747.22	coarctation, atresia, or stenosis of aorta
Other anomalies of aorta	747.20, 747.21, 747.29	or other anomalies of aorta; and (3) other
Pulmonary artery anomalies	747.3	unspecified anomalies of the heart *plus* any
Anomalies of great veins	747.40, 747.42, 747.49	mild defect; the multiple, mild category
Ventricular septal defect	745.4	included children with two or more mild
Atrial septal defect	745.5	defects only
Other specified defect of septal closure	745.8	
Unspecified defect of septal closure	745.9	
Patent ductus arteriosus	747.0	
Other specified anomalies of heart	746.8	
Other unspecified anomalies of heart	746.9	

heart (745.3), endocardial cushion defects (745.6), cor biloculare (745.7), pulmonary valve atresia (746.01), Ebstein's anomaly (746.01), and hypoplastic left heart syndrome (746.7). The 2004 NIS data reveal that severe CHD accounted for 10,155 or 21.8% of all CHD discharges for all ages. They accounted for $511 million in estimated costs, which was 37.3% of all costs associated with CHD discharges. Severe CHD codes also accounted for 48.4% of all in-hospital deaths in CHD hospital stays.

Hospital discharges associated with severe and other CHD differed markedly in their age distribution. Almost all (94.7%) severe CHD discharges were among children younger than 18 years, compared with less than half (43.0%) of the remaining CHD codes. Severe CHD accounted for 39.9% of all CHD hospital stays among infants (<1 year of age), 22.0% among other children (1–17 years of age), and 3.0% among adults (18+ years of age) with a CHD principal diagnosis.

Our analysis of NIS data using HCUPNet has both strengths and limitations. A strength, as with that of Russo and Elixhauser (2007), is that because each discharge is associated with only one principal diagnosis, it is possible to aggregate estimates without worrying about double-counting (i.e., including a case in more than one category). On the other hand, hospitalizations associated with a different diagnosis for which CHD might be a complicating factor are excluded, potentially resulting in an understatement of hospital costs attributable to CHD. Another limitation is that the specificity of ICD-9 codes for reporting specific CHD likely diminishes with age. We suspect underreporting of specific ICD-9 codes among adult survivors of CHD who are hospitalized because of cardiac issues, including those with severe CHD.

HEALTH CLAIMS CONGENITAL HEART DEFECT ANALYSIS

To estimate health care expenditures for a privately insured population of children 0–3 years of age with CHD in comparison with unaffected children of the same age, we analyzed data for individuals enrolled in employer-sponsored health plans during 2005 using the MarketScan Commercial Claims and Encounters database. This database has been used in previous analyses of health care costs associated with birth defects (Ouyang et al., 2007; Boulet et al., 2009). As mentioned earlier, these data cannot be linked to birth defects surveillance databases because although each individual has a unique ID variable, identifying information is not made available to researchers. These data include information on inpatient admissions and outpatient services and outpatient prescription drugs for

employees of over 100 large self-insured corporations and their dependents located across the United States. Outpatient services included office visits, emergency department visits, and physical, speech, and occupational therapy. Data from 2002 through 2005 were used to identify children younger than 3 years with CHD in order to increase the likelihood of ascertaining a greater proportion of children with CHD; only expenditures during 2005 were evaluated.

Children with CHD were identified by the presence of an ICD-9-CM code of 745.0–747.9 as the primary or secondary diagnosis for an outpatient claim or as any diagnosis code in an inpatient claim during 2002 through 2005. To separate cases of true CHD from those with newborn and prematurity-associated cardiac conditions or isolated minor defects, we excluded (1) premature infants with isolated ASD or PDA; (2) all CHD cases with isolated pulmonary artery anomalies, isolated PDA, or isolated mitral insufficiency; and (3) CHD cases with selected defects in isolation *and* without a Current Procedural Terminology (CPT) code related to treatment of CHD (i.e., VSD, ASD, other specified or unspecified defect of septal closure, or other specified or unspecified anomalies of heart). The ICD-9-CM codes were categorized into severe and mild CHD by a pediatric cardiologist (Table 31–1) and children with CHD were assigned into one of four mutually exclusive severity categories (isolated severe, multiple severe, isolated mild, and multiple mild).

Administrative prevalence, defined as the prevalence of a condition within the administrative population, was calculated by dividing the number of all children with CHD by the total number of children in the plans. Analysis of costs was restricted to children who were enrolled in a fee-for-service plan in 2005 and for whom data on pharmaceutical claims were available (approximately 85% of the total sample). The final sample included 264,464 children 0–3 years of age, of whom 1530 had CHD. Children aged 1–2 years were included only if they were continuously enrolled for 12 months in 2005 whereas all infants (<1 year of age) were included because a significant proportion of infants with CHD die during the first year of life (Rosano et al., 2000). Enrollees with and without claims were included in the study population. Costs associated with inpatient admissions, outpatient services, and prescription drug claims, and mean and median costs and cost ratios (costs for children with the condition divided by costs for children without the condition) were calculated for children with and without CHD.

The administrative prevalence of CHD among children younger than 3 years was 58 per 10,000. For children 1–2 years of age with CHD, mean medical care costs were 9–12 times greater than those for children without CHD; median costs were 4 times greater (Table 31–2).

TABLE 31-2. *Health Care Expenditures for Infants and Children Less than 3 Years Old with Congenital Heart Defects in a Privately Insured Population, MarketScan Research Database—United States, 2005*

Age and Heart Defect Category	Number of Children	Prevalence* (per 10,000)	Mean Costs (Dollars)	Mean Cost Ratio[†]	Median Costs (Dollars)	Median Cost Ratio[†]	% of Costs Attributable to Inpatient Admissions
No CHD							
<1 year	114,561		3844		1572		67
1 year	71,029		2462		1293		15
2 years	77,344		1583		687		14
Multiple Severe							
<1 year	72	6.3	241,219	63	148,758	95	93
1 year	46	6.4	79,763	32	43,422	34	72
2 years	35	4.5	49,479	31	8951	13	72
Isolated Severe							
<1 year	222	19.3	120,813	31	47,343	30	90
1 year	129	18.1	30,723	12	9317	7	61
2 years	118	15.2	16,503	10	5770	8	44
Multiple Mild							
<1 year	201	17.5	83,379	22	25,190	16	89
1 year	137	19.2	22,902	9	4525	3	56
2 years	134	17.2	13,160	8	2389	3	20
Isolated Mild							
<1 year	168	14.6	23,551	6	4753	3	80
1 year	122	17.1	15,697	6	2813	2	59
2 years	146	18.8	3559	2	1750	3	7
Any CHD							
<1 year	663	57.5	97,894	25	23,438	15	90
1 year	434	60.7	29,228	12	5251	4	63
2 years	433	55.7	13,769	9	2532	4	42

* Administrative prevalence was calculated by dividing the number of all children with CHD by the total number of children in the plans.

[†] Cost ratios were calculated by dividing costs for children with CHD by costs for those without CHD.

The difference in mean costs between those with CHD and those without CHD was $26,766 for 1-year-olds and $12,186 for 2-year-olds. Mean and median costs for infants younger than 1 year with CHD were 25 and 15 times greater, respectively, than costs for infants without CHD; the difference in mean costs was $94,050. Mean costs were 2–3 times higher for children with multiple severe defects than for those with isolated severe defects, 5–15 times higher than for those with isolated mild defects, and approximately 3 times higher than for those with multiple mild defects.

The findings suggest that medical expenditures for children younger than 3 years with CHD are substantially greater than those for children without CHD, with greatest disparities noted among infants younger than 1 year. Infants with CHD who died during the first year of life were included in the sample, which is likely to lower estimated costs since deaths are concentrated in the first month of life (Rogowski, 1998). Mean expenditures were similar to previously reported MarketScan data for 420 children 0–4 years of age with Down syndrome, $86,448 for infants younger than 1 year, and $27,992 for children 1–2 years of age (Boulet et al., 2008). However, approximately half of children with Down syndrome had CHD. Among the children with Down syndrome in that study, the difference in mean cost between those with CHD and those without CHD was $104,278 for infants younger than 1 year and $23,032 for children 1–2 years of age, and the mean cost ratios were 5.0 and 2.5, respectively (Boulet et al., 2008). That evidence indicates that CHD substantially increases health care costs for infants and young children, even for children with another major condition.

Rapid technological advances have improved diagnosis and treatment of CHD but have also contributed to the high cost ratio for providing medical care to infants with CHD compared to infants without CHD. Understanding the costs for medical care for children in privately and publicly insured populations can contribute to an understanding of the potential benefits of interventions to prevent CHD.

This analysis used a large, comprehensive database to estimate medical care expenditures for privately insured children. Compared to the California study of costs associated with CHD, the MarketScan analysis encompassed a wider array of defects. It excluded children who had a CHD code but were unlikely to have clinical disease. Furthermore, the use of mutually exclusive categories to identify cases with isolated or multiple defects facilitated the calculation of health care costs for CHD. Through categorization by a clinician, cases with both a major defect and a dependent minor defect were categorized more accurately as isolated rather than multiple. Because several years of data were used for case ascertainment in this study, it is likely that a greater proportion of cases were captured than in analyses of administrative data that relied on a single year of data.

The findings of the MarketScan analysis are subject to a number of limitations. First, a sample of privately insured children with continuous enrollment in fee-for-service health plans is not representative of all children in the United States. For example, average expenditures for individuals in fee-for-service private health plans are reported to be about 30% higher than those for capitated (managed care) private health plans (Cutler et al., 2000). In addition, there may be attrition in private plans as individuals switch to Medicaid or other health plans when their costs reach lifetime limits. The loss of these high-cost cases may bias estimates downward. Secondly, although multiple years of data were used and both diagnostic and procedural codes were assessed, a proportion of cases may have been missed because a diagnosis was not noted during any health care encounter. Furthermore, ICD-9-CM codes are not very specific or accurate for many CHD; often a single code is used for clinically different conditions. Thus, it is likely that some cases were misclassified; however, we were unable to estimate the extent of this misclassification. In addition, data on race and ethnicity, income, or other sociodemographic factors are not available in the dataset but can have important implications for access to and utilization of health care services.

CONCLUSIONS

It is well established that CHDs are associated with elevated health care utilization and expenditures, especially inpatient care. The largest burden of such costs is attributable to severe CHD in infants and children younger than 3 years. Due to ascertainment issues and lack of long-term follow-up in many datasets used for estimating health care costs, there are inadequate data to characterize utilization of health care among adolescents or adults with CHD. Specifically, the occurrence of an incorrect ICD-9 code for a CHD in an adult could reflect a coding error for another cardiac condition and may not necessarily reflect the presence of a true CHD. Conversely, the lack of a CHD code in an older child or adult does not necessarily indicate absence of CHD, because it may not be noted on records after treatment. Clinic- or hospital-based administrative data validated by medical records for the same patients are probably

the most reliable source of information on health care utilization and expenditures by adults with CHD. However, these data lack a population denominator, thereby making it impossible to draw inferences about the population of adult survivors with CHD.

The imprecision of ICD-9 or ICD-9-CM codes to adequately characterize CHD has been a major limitation for much population-based research on CHD in both infants and adult survivors. Utilization of clinically relevant nomenclature and classification of CHD, as in the STS database or the MACDP, could improve CHD surveillance data. Furthermore, accurate analysis of CHD cost would be maximized by the linkage of birth defects surveillance data with hospital discharge and health claims databases, as was done in the California cost of birth defects study for four specific defects in the late 1980s (Waitzman et al., 1996).

Medical costs for CHD represent only a small portion of the total economic burden for health care systems, individuals, families, and society. Other nonmedical costs, such as caregiver time costs, can be substantial and should be evaluated in future research. Additional studies should also assess the extent to which medical care utilization and expenditures by individuals with CHD differ by type of health insurance coverage, including individuals with Medicaid and those covered by capitated plans. Ideally, longitudinal analyses would be conducted to examine the costs associated with repeated hospitalizations over several years and perhaps even over a lifetime. As medical advances in pediatric cardiac care continue to reduce the morbidity and mortality for infants and young children with CHD, longitudinal analyses will be necessary to provide important information on the economic burden associated with tertiary care for a growing population of adolescents and adults with CHD.

REFERENCES

Berk N, Marazita M. The cost of cleft lip and palate: personal and societal implications. In: Wyszynski DF, (ed). *Cleft Lip and Palate: From Origin to Treatment*. New York: Oxford University Press; 2002:458–467.

Boulet SL, Grosse SD, Honein MA, Correa-Villaseñor A. Children with orofacial clefts: healthcare utilization and costs in a privately insured population. *Public Health Rep.* 2009;124:447–453.

Boulet SL, Molinari NA, Grosse SD, Honein MA, Correa-Villaseñor A. Health care expenditures for children with Down syndrome in a privately insured population. *J Pediatr.* 2008;153:241–246.

Centers for Disease Control and Prevention (CDC). Economic costs of birth defects and cerebral palsy—United States, 1992. *MMWR* 1995;44:694–699.

Centers for Disease Control and Prevention (CDC). Hospital stays, hospital charges, and in-hospital deaths among infants with selected birth defects – United States, 2003. *MMWR* 2007;56:25–29.

Cohen JW, Krauss NA. Spending and service use among people with the fifteen most costly medical conditions, 1997. *Health Aff (Millwood).* 2003;22:129–138.

Cutler DM, McClellan M, Newhouse JP. How does managed care do it? *Rand J Econ.* 2000;31:526–548.

Feldkamp M, MacLeod L, Young L, Lecheminant K, Carey JC. The methodology of the Utah Birth Defect Network: congenital heart defects as an illustration. *Birth Def Res Part A.* 2005;73:693–699.

Frohnert BK, Lussky RC, Alms MA, Mendelsohn NJ, Symonik DM, Falken MC. Validity of hospital discharge data for identifying infants with cardiac defects. *J Perinatol.* 2005;25:737–742.

Garson A Jr, Allen HD, Gersony WM, et al. The cost of congenital heart disease in children and adults. A model for multicenter assessment of price and practice variation. *Arch Pediatr Adolesc Med.* 1994;148:1039–1045.

Grosse SD, Waitzman NJ, Romano PS, Mulinare J. Reevaluating the benefits of folic acid fortification in the United States: economic analysis, regulation, and public health. *Am J Public Health.* 2005;95:1917–1922.

Harris JA, James L. State-by-state cost of birth defects—1992. *Teratology.* 1997;56:11–16.

Okumura MJ, Campbell AD, Nasr SZ, Davis MM. Inpatient health care use among adult survivors of chronic childhood illnesses in the United States. *Arch Pediatr Adolesc Med.* 2006;160:1054–1060.

Ouyang L, Grosse SD, Armour BS, Waitzman NJ. Health care expenditures of children and adults with spina bifida in a privately insured U.S. population. *Birth Def Res A Clin Mol Teratol.* 2007;79:552–558.

Riehle-Colarusso T, Strickland MJ, Reller MD, et al. Improving the quality of surveillance data on congenital heart defects in the metropolitan Atlanta congenital defects program. *Birth Defects Res A Clin Mol Teratol.* 2007;79:743–753.

Rogowski J. Cost-effectiveness of care for very low birth weight infants. *Pediatrics.* 1998;102:35–43.

Rosano A, Botto LD, Botting B, Mastroiacovo P. Infant mortality and congenital anomalies from 1950 to 1994: an international perspective. *J Epidemiol Community Health.* 2000;54:660–666.

Russo CA, Elixhauser A. Hospitalizations for Birth Defects, 2004. HCUP Statistical Brief #24. 2007. Rockville, MD, U.S. Agency for Healthcare Research and Quality.

Strickland MJ, Riehle-Colarusso TJ, Jacobs JP, et al. The importance of nomenclature for congenital heart disease: implications for research and evaluation. *Cardiol Young.* 2008;18:92–100

Tilford JM, Grosse SD, Goodman AC, Li K. Labor market productivity costs for caregivers of children with spina bifida: A population-based analysis. *Med Decis Making.* 2009;29:23–32.

Waitzman NJ, Scheffler RM, Romano PS. Estimates of the economic costs of birth defects. *Inquiry* 1994;31:188–205.

Waitzman NJ, Scheffler RM, Romano PS. The Cost of Birth Defects. Lanham, MD: University Press of America; 1996.

32

Insurability and Access to Health Care for Patients with Congenital Heart Defects

RUEY-KANG CHANG
THOMAS S. KLITZNER

HISTORICAL PERSPECTIVE

Historically, efforts to define insurability of children and young adults with congenital heart disease (CHD) were focused in the area of life insurance. Because of the nature of life insurance, these early endeavors sought to develop actuarial statistics related to the presence of heart murmurs, known forms of CHD, and the sequelae of surgery for CHD. In the 1960s and 1970s, four conferences were organized jointly by the Council on Cardiovascular Diseases in the Young of the American Heart Association and the Association of Life Insurance Medical Directors of America (End et al., 1979). Proceedings of three of these conferences have been reported separately (Gubner, 1964; Manning, 1977; Talner, 1988) and the overall findings have been summarized (End et al., 1979). As an example of the nature of these discussions, by the late 1970s a consensus had developed that innocent murmurs could be distinguished by a trained pediatric cardiologist, and guidelines had been developed for the characteristics of murmurs that presented no increased actuarial risk for issuing life insurance. These criteria, developed before the widespread use of echocardiography, suggested that insurance companies would not assume undue risk if they issued standard risk life insurance policies to applicants with "functional" murmurs if (1) intensity was grade II or less on the conventional scale of I–VI; (2) location was lower left sternal border to mid precordium without radiation; (3) frequency was low pitched, vibratory, musical, or buzzing; (4) timing was early and mid-systolic, but not holosystolic or diastolic; and (5) heart sounds were normal with normal splitting and intensity of the second heart sound (End et al., 1979; Manning, 1977). Life insurance issues for patients with repaired congenital heart defects were also considered. For example, it was recommended that patients who had surgical closure of a ventricular septal defect be considered for standard life insurance without cardiac catheterization if (1) they were asymptomatic; (2) auscultation suggested that the defect was completely closed; (3) there was a normal pulmonary closure sound; (4) chest radiograph was normal; and (5) electrocardiogram was normal or showed only right bundle branch block (RBBB) (Talner, 1988).

While interesting, these early discussions have limited relevance in the current era. Many cardiac lesions commonly addressed today, including various forms of single ventricle and even transposition of the great arteries, were considered in these early conferences to seriously impair survival beyond infancy (End et al., 1979). In addition, important developments in the past two decades have changed the practice of determination for insurability, particularly the widespread use of echocardiography, which allows precise and detailed anatomic diagnosis noninvasively. Finally, tremendous improvements in survival and outcomes related to advances in medical therapy, surgery, postoperative care, and follow-up have changed the consideration of "risk" for patients with CHD in all facets of their lives.

In parallel with the efforts to determine actuarial risk for providing life insurance to patients with CHD, programs were developed to provide health insurance to this population. With the era of modern health insurance heralded by the advent of Medicare and Medicaid in 1965 (Klitzner and Chang, 2003), health insurance for children began to depend on the employment, socio-economic, and insurance status of the child's parents. The 1980s saw growth of employer-based health care (Kintner, 1989), further expanding family coverage and insuring more children. By 1988 the total percentage of the uninsured in the United States counting all socioeconomic groups was only 15% and was closer to 12% for children under age 18 (Holahan et al., 1995).

For the disadvantaged, heath care coverage for children, especially those with special health care needs, has long been a part of social policy in the United States. In 1935, Title V of the Social Security Act established a program to extend and improve medical services to children with chronic disease (Ireys and Eichler, 1988). At that time, most of these children were considered "crippled" and thus the program was known for many years as "Crippled Children's Services" (CCS). Of note, a grant for community programs for adult-onset heart disease was established in 1948 by the federal government; however, this grant never became popular with state health agencies (ACIR). In contrast, conditions of the heart in children were included at a very early stage in CCS, with rheumatic fever being one of the few conditions covered in the first 4 years of the program when medical eligibility was left largely to the states (Huse, 1941). The advent of coverage for heart disease through this mechanism heralded a change in the manner in which health care was delivered to this population. Keeping with the principles of the CCS program, coverage required that in addition to medical care, attention be paid to the effect of the diagnosis on the child's emotional life, education, and social environment. In addition, the program promoted geographically defined areas of regional referral (Huse, 1941). These principles are preserved in today's state-administered Title V programs, which are no longer referred to as CCS, but have a variety of titles, definitions, and services that vary from state to state (Beers et al., 2003). In addition, Title V programs may not provide coverage for primary medical issues not related to the child's chronic illness. In 1972, Congress enacted Title XVI of the Social Security Act to aid socioeconomically disadvantaged families raising a child with a disability by providing Supplemental Security Income (SSI). Since that time, this program has provided primary care medical coverage and income supplements under the Federal Social Security Program for children with heart disease who qualify (Beers et al., 2003).

Primary care for children with chronic conditions was enhanced with the adoption of the State Children's Health Insurance Program (SCHIP) in 1997 (Dubay et al., 2007). In general, Medicaid has more generous income eligibility thresholds than SCHIP (Kenney et al., 2007). Compared to Medicaid, SCHIP is much smaller in its program size. In 2006, Medicaid covered 25 million low-income children, compared to 4 million children covered by SCHIP (KCMU, 2006). In addition, coverage for children with heart disease by the SCHIP varies widely from state to state (Davidoff et al., 2005). Moreover, the hope that SCHIP might provide some help to children with CHD has been largely negated by recent issues related to continued funding for this program (Broaddus and Park, 2007). Overall, a myriad of problems have been identified for children with special health care needs who obtain their primary coverage through programs such as SCHIP (Schwalberg et al., 2000; Yu et al., 2006).

CURRENT STATUS OF INSURANCE FOR CHILDREN WITH CHRONIC DISEASES

According to 2007 data from the United States Census Bureau, 64.2% of children (<18 years) in the United States have private insurance, 31.0% are covered by public programs (Medicaid or SCHIP), and 11.0% do not have insurance (DeNavas-Walt et al., 2008). The uninsured rate is slightly lower in children with special health care needs. A 2001 survey of this group showed that 65% had private coverage, 22% had public coverage, 8% had both private and public coverage, and 5% had no insurance (U.S. Department of Health and Human Services, 2001). While the uninsured rate may be lower for children with special needs, one third of those who have insurance reported that the coverage is inadequate. Reported limitations included inadequate coverage of needs, high uncovered costs, and limited access to specialists.

In the United States, insurance for children is dependent primarily on the insurance status of their parents. Once individuals reach an age between 18 and 23 years, they very often lose eligibility for coverage under a parent's policy, whether it is a private or public insurance plan. Therefore, a "transition" period occurs when children with CHD are no longer covered by a parent's insurance and need to seek health insurance coverage independently. Unfortunately, this transition often occurs at the same time that these patients are moving from the care of pediatric specialists to adult medicine providers. Transition of care to adult CHD services is not structured in the United States. In contrast, health care in Canada is federally funded with typical requirements that individuals older than 18 years be seen in adult hospitals. To ensure successful transition of care of adolescents and young adults with CHD in Canada, the Canadian Adult Congenital Heart (CACH) network consisting of 15 specialized adult CHD centers was formed in 1991. The 32nd Bethesda Conference recommended identification of a similar network for American patients with CHD.

HEALTH INSURANCE AND ACCESS TO CARE FOR CHILDREN WITH CONGENITAL HEART DEFECTS

Insurance coverage is an important determinant of access to care and health services utilization. Lack of insurance may be the most important factor accounting for delays in seeking care. Even among individuals who are insured, the type of insurance may play a significant role in care received. Among adults with angina, the type of insurance coverage has been shown to be an important determinant of service utilization (Brown et al., 1998; Every et al., 1998). Studies in children show a similar role for insurance coverage in determining access to needed services (Newacheck et al., 1996, 1998). For children with special health care needs, it is important to ensure access to care provided by qualified subspecialists. Even when access is theoretically available, children without insurance are much less likely to utilize subspecialty services than are children with insurance (Kuhlthau et al., 2004).

For children with congenital heart defects, type of insurance may also affect access to needed services, as well as process and outcome measures of health care. Uninsured or publicly insured (Medicaid) infants with CHD were found to be nearly twice as likely as commercially insured infants to be transferred between hospitals (Durbin et al., 1997). For children with CHD, it has been reported that those who do not have commercial insurance are at risk for delayed referral to pediatric cardiologists (Perlstein et al., 1997). Erickson et al. (2000) reported that in California, children covered by Medicaid and managed care health insurance were less likely to undergo surgery at a target (low mortality) pediatric cardiac center (odds ratios 0.71 and 0.53, respectively) compared to children with commercial insurance. To examine possible delays in referral for surgical repair, we studied the age at operation of atrial septal defect, ventricular septal defect, atrioventricular canal, and tetralogy of Fallot using California hospital discharge data. Patients with Medicaid were consistently the oldest group for repair for all four types of cardiac defects (Chang et al., 2000). Therefore, infants with CHD who are uninsured or covered by public insurance may be at risk for both delayed referral to a cardiologist and later surgical repair.

INSURANCE AND CARDIAC SURGERY OUTCOMES

Obstacles in access to care, decreased service utilization, and delayed referral to quality centers of uninsured or publicly insured patients with CHD can have significant impact on outcomes. Literature on the effect of insurance on outcomes of children with heart disease is limited, probably because of the large number of patients required to demonstrate significant differences. Using a large hospital discharge database of 11,636 pediatric cardiac surgery cases, DeMonte et al. (2003) reported that children on Medicaid have higher risk-adjusted mortality than children with commercial or managed care insurance. These researchers speculated that the higher mortality rate in Medicaid patients might be due to both differential referral patterns and other differences in care afforded to patients with public insurance as compared to their counterparts with private insurance treated at similar institutions. In our recent study examining risk factors for in-hospital mortality, children with public insurance undergoing cardiac surgery have 22% higher in-hospital morality rate than do children with private insurance (Klitzner and Chang, 2006).

It is unclear exactly how insurance coverage affects the outcomes of care but further understanding of the role of insurance coverage may help clinicians to provide better care to children with heart disease and to improve their outcomes. The mechanisms by which insurance status affects outcome directly and indirectly by interaction with other medical and nonmedical variables remain questions for future research.

INSURANCE AND ADULTS WITH CONGENITAL HEART DISEASE

In the 1970s the leading edge of adult survivors of CHD surgery began to appear (Perloff, 1973), and subsequently in the late 1980s and the early 1990s, the issue of insurance for adult patients with CHD came under consideration (Celermajer and Deanfield, 1993; Talner, 1988). By surveying health and life insurance companies, Celermajer and Deanfield confirmed that those with less severe heart disease could get life insurance albeit at increased rates (Celermajer and Deanfield, 1993). However, the study suggested that for those with CHD, health insurance was only available with complete exclusion of benefits related to the cardiac condition (Celermajer and Deanfield, 1993). By 2007, the situation had improved somewhat, as one study evaluating hospitalization patterns of adult survivors of CHD found that 53% of patients admitted had private insurance, 44% had public insurance, and less than 4% were uninsured (Gurvitz et al., 2007). While the best insurance for patients transitioning to adulthood is usually available through one's employer (Cannobbio, 2001), various other sources of insurance may be available including Medicaid, SCHIP, Ticket to Work and Work Incentives Improvement Act, Consolidated Omnibus Budget Reconciliation Act (COBRA), college health services, employer health plans, and individual health plans (Betz, 2004). Recognizing the importance of this topic, the 32nd Bethesda Conference reporting on the care of the adult with CHD recommended formal, regular discussions with insurance companies and other public and private payers and purchasers to provide information on the special problems encountered and the expertise necessary in the care of adolescents and adults with CHD (32nd Bethesda Conference, 2001).

SUMMARY AND POLICY RECOMMENDATIONS

The current situation regarding insurance for children with CHD is the result of many decades of development of health insurance mechanisms for children, both public and private. As health care financing has changed and reshaped in the current era, the lessons of the past can guide policy makers to utilize the history of insurance for children with heart disease to construct a framework for viewing health insurance for all children with special health care needs. The major challenges will be in three general areas. First, the number of uninsured individuals in the United States remains high including a significant number of uninsured children. Those who lack insurance can be predicted to have significantly decreased access to life-saving interventions. The second great challenge is the growth of primary care coverage at the expense of coverage for chronic, life-threatening diseases such as CHD as cited in the earlier section with regard to the SCHIP program. As proposals are made for universal coverage for adults and/or children, it is imperative that pediatric cardiologists and other pediatric subspecialists advocate for concomitant increases in coverage for children with special health care needs. The final challenge will be the increasing number of adults with CHD. One estimate suggests that this population will soon be over 1 million in the United States, including 750,000 with simple lesions, 400,000 with moderate lesions, and 180,000 with complex lesions (Hoffman et al., 2004). The large and rapidly expanding population of adults with CHD threatens to overwhelm not only our insurance system but also our ability to train qualified care providers (Gurvitz et al., 2005). Continued emphasis on these issues by care providers, researchers, and policy makers will be required to provide the data necessary to frame a solution for these important issues.

ACKNOWLEDGMENTS

The authors wish to thank Ms. Christina Pedley for her help in researching issues related to this chapter.

Thomas Klitzner holds the Jack H. Skirball Chair in Pediatric Cardiology and is supported by a grant from the Skirball Foundation and a Health Tomorrows Partnership for Children Grant from the American Academy of Pediatrics and HRSA (H17MC00406).

REFERENCES

Advisory Commission on Intergovermental Relations (ACIR). Modification of Federal Grants-in-aid for public health services 1961Report A-2.

Beers NS, Kemeny A, Sherritt L, Palfrey JS. Variations in state-level definitions: children with special health care needs. *Public Health Reports.* 2003:118:434–447.

Betz, CL. Adolescent in transition of adult care: why the concern. *Nursing Clinics of North America.* 2004:39:681–713.

Broaddus M, Park E. Freezing SCHIP funding in coming years would reverse recent gains in children's health. Center on Budget Policy and Priority February 22, 2007.

Brown DL, Schneider DL, Colbert R, Guss D. Influence of insurance coverage on delays in seeking emergency care in patients with acute chest pain. *Am J Cardiol.* 1998;82:395–398.

Cannobbio, M. Health Care Issues Facing Adolescents with Congenital Heart Disease. *Journal of Pediatric Nursing.* 2001; 16:5:363–370.

Celermajer DS, Deanfield JE. Employment and insurance for young adults with congenital heart disease. *Br Heart J.* 1993;69:539–543.

Chang RK, Chen AY, Klitzner TS. Factors associated with age at operation for children with congenital heart disease. *Pediatrics.* 2000;105:1073–1081.

DeNavas-Walt, Carmen, Bernadette D.Proctor, Jessica C. Smith. U.S. Census Bureau, Income, Poverty, and Health Insurance Coverage in the United States: 2007, U.S. Government Printing Office

Washington, DC, 2008. http://www.census.gov/prod/2008pubs/p60–235.pdf.

Davidoff A, Kenney G, Dubay L. Effects of the State Children's Health Insurance Program Expansions on children with chronic health conditions *Pediatrics.* 2005 Jul;116(1):e34–42.

DeMone JA, Gonzalez PC, Gauvreau K, Piercey GE, Jenkins KJ. Risk of death for Medicaid recipients undergoing congenital heart surgery. *Pediatr Cardiol.* 2003;24:97–102.

Dubay L, Guyer J, Mann C, Odeh M. Medicaid at the ten-year anniversary of SCHIP: looking back and moving forward. *Health Aff* (Millwood). 2007 26(2):370–381.

Durbin DR, Giardino AP, Shaw KN, Harris MC, Silber JH. The effect of insurance status on likelihood of neonatal interhospital transfer. *Pediatrics.* 1997;100(3):E8.

End JA, McCue HM, Jr. Insurability of the major cardiovascular congenital defects. *Trans Assoc Life Insur Med Dir Am.* 1979;62:175–200.

Erickson LC, Wise PH, Cook EF, Beiser A, Newburger JW. The impact of managed care insurance on use of lower-mortality hospitals by children undergoing cardiac surgery in California. *Pediatrics* 2000;105:1271–1278.

Every NR, Cannon CP, Granger C, et al. Influence of insurance type on the use of procedures, medications and hospital outcome in patients with unstable angina: results from the GUARANTEE Registry. *J Am Coll Cardiol.* 1998;32:387–392.

Gubner RS. Long Term Prognosis and Insurability in Patients with Congenital Cardiac Defects Treated Surgically or Untreated. *Am J Cardiol.* 1964;13:645–649.

Gurvitz M, Chang R-KR, Ramos FJ, Allada V, Child JS, Klitzner TS. Variations in congenital heart disease training in adult and pediatric cardiology fellowship programs. *J Am Coll Cardiol.* 2005;46:893–898.

Gurvitz MZ, Inkelas M, Lee M, Stout K, Escarce J, Chang RK. Changes in hospitalization patterns among patients with congenital heart disease during the transition from adolescence to adulthood. *J Am Coll Cardiol.* 2007;49:875–882.

Hoffman JI, Kaplan S, Liberthson RR. Prevalence of congenital heart disease. *Am Heart J.* 2004;147(3):425–439.

Holahan J, Winterbottom C, Rajan S. A shifting picture of health insurance coverage. 1995:12:4:253–264.

Huse B. Care of children with heart disease in the Crippled Children's Program under the Social Security Act. *Am J Public Health.* 1941:31:809–812.

Ireys HT, Eichler RJ. Program priorities of crippled children's agencies: a survey. *Public Health Reports.* 1988:103:1:77–83.

Kenney G, Rubenstein J, Sommers A, Zuckerman S, Blavin F. Medicaid and SCHIP Coverage: Findings from California and North Carolina. *Health Care Financing Review.* 2007;29(1):71–85.

Kintner H. Demographic change in a corporate health benefits population, 1983–87. *Am J Public Health.* 1989:79:12:1655–1656.

Klitzner TS, Chang RK: Regionalization of pediatric cardiac services; from theory to practice. *Progress in Pediatric Cardiology.* 2003;18:43–47.

Klitzner TS, Chang R-KR. Sex related disparity in surgical mortality among pediatric patients. *Congenit Heart Dis.* 2006;1:77–88.

Kuhlthau K, Nyman RM, Ferris TG, Beal AC, Perrin JM. Correlates of use of specialty care. *Pediatrics.* 2004;113(3 Pt 1):e249–55.

Manning JA. Insurability and employability of young cardiac patients. *Pediatrics.* 1977;60:126–129.

Newacheck PW, Hughes DC, Stoddard JJ. Children's access to primary care: differences by race, income, and insurance status. *Pediatrics.* 1996;97:26–32.

Newacheck PW, Stoddard JJ, Hughes DC, Pearl M. Health insurance and access to primary care for children. *N Engl J Med.* 1998;338:513–519.

Perloff, JK Pediatric congenital cardiac becomes a postoperative adult. The changing population of congenital heart disease. *Circulation.* 1973;47(3):606–619.

Perlstein MA, Goldberg SJ, Meaney FJ, Davis MF, Zwerdling Kluger C. Factors influencing age at referral of children with congenital heart disease. *Arch Pediatr Adolesc Med.* 1997;151: 892–7.

Prodceedings of the 32nd Bethesda Conference: care of the adult with congenital heart disease. *J Am Coll Cardiol.* 2001:37:1161–1198.

Schwalberg R, Hill I, Anderson Mathis S. New opportunities, new approaches: serving children with special health care needs under SCHIP. *Health Serv Res.* 2000:35(5 Pt 3):102–111.

Talner NS. Insurability of the pediatric patient with cardiac disease. *Pediatr Rev.* 1988;10:107–110.

Talner. Insurability of the Pediatric Patient with Cardiac Disease. *Pediatrics in Review,* 1988.

The Kaiser Commission on Medicaid and Uninsured (KCMU). Health coverage for low-income populations: a comparison of Medicaid and SCHIP. Released April 2006. http://www.kff.org/medicaid/upload/7488.pdf.

U.S. Department of Health and Human Services, Health Resources and Services Administration, Maternal and Child Health Bureau. *The National Survey of Children with Special Health Care Needs Chartbook 2001.* Rockville, Maryland: U.S. Department of Health and Human Services, 2004.

Yu H, Dick AW, Szilagyi PG. Role of SCHIP in serving children with special health care needs. *Health Care Financ Rev.* 2006:28(2):53–64.

33

Transition of Adults with Congenital Heart Disease into Adult-Oriented Care

KAREN S. KUEHL

AMY VERSTAPPEN

BACKGROUND AND PERSPECTIVE

A large and growing population of adults with congenital heart disease is a welcome phenomenon of the current century. Open heart surgery in adults began 50 years ago. Survival of infants with congenital heart defects was limited in the 1960s, but now at least 90% of infants born with congenital heart disease are anticipated to survive until adulthood. This change in a medical population demands reciprocal changes from medicine. Consistent with the evolution of an adult population with congenital heart disease is the need for a cardiac care system that can provide congenital cardiac care appropriate to adult status Autonomy is a critical feature of adulthood and one that mandates appropriate treatment of adults with chronic health conditions (Bailey and Pearce, 2003). Transition of patients from pediatric to adult care is particularly difficult when the chronic condition is one that does not have a parallel disease model in the adult population. Although nearly a million people with congenital heart disease live in the United States, they still represent a small percentage of the 25 million adults with acquired heart disease in the country. The challenge of transition for congenital heart patients both mirrors and differs from the challenges that many pediatric populations with new chronic disease now face. In considering transition among congenital heart patients, we will survey the data in overall health care transition and the unique factors affecting congenital heart disease patients.

GUIDELINES AND POLICIES

In 2001 a taskforce convened by the American College of Cardiology wrote guidelines for the care of adults with congenital heart defects. The recommendations were to define the characteristics of a specialized center for care of such adults; this is not equivalent to being a center that thinks itself specialized in this care. The configuration of such centers was described, with emphasis on the multidisciplinary nature of the staff and facilities required. Few such centers were extant at the time the guidelines were written (Child et al., 2001; Foster et al., 2001; Landzberg et al., 2001; Skorton et al., 2001; SR, 2001; Warnes et al., 2001).

Internationally, guidelines for the transition of youth in adult care for congenital heart disease have been published as well, perhaps facilitated by universal access to health care in many countries outside the United States (Deanfield et al., 2003; GUCH, 2002; Therrien et al., 2001). All guidelines emphasize the need for this group of patients to receive specialized attention in every facet of their care; for example, magnetic resonance imaging (MRI) should be specific for congenital heart defects. Provision for care for "usual" conditions of adulthood (e.g., pregnancy) should be coordinated with the specialized centers. There is multidisciplinary staffing at the specialized centers, as shown in Table 33–1.

TABLE 33–1. *Regional Adult Congenital Heart Disease Center Staffing, Facilities, Diagnostic Testing Capacity*

Pediatric ACHD cardiologist	One or several; 365 days/year
Adult medical ACHD cardiologist	One or several; 365 days/year
Mid-level practitioner	Two/several
Congenital heart surgeon	Two/several; 365 days/year
Cardiac anesthesia	Several; 365 days/year
Echocardiography	Two/several; 365 days/year
Diagnostic catheterization	Yes; 365 days/year
Noncoronary interventional catheterization	Yes; 365 days/year
Electrophysiology	Yes; 365 days/year
Exercise testing	Echo, radionuclide, metabolic, cardiopulmonary
Transplant	Heart, lung
Cardiac imaging/radiology	CT scan, cardiac MRI with fast pulse sequencing, nuclear medicine
Cardiac pathology	Yes
Information technology	Data collection and database support

Adapted from Landzberg and Murphy (Landzberg et al., 2001).

CURRENT STATE OF PEDIATRIC–ADULT HEALTH CARE TRANSITION

Transition of all young adults with special health care needs into adult medical care has been stated as a goal by all the relevant societies (AAP, 1996; AMA, 1993; AAP, 2002)—American Academy of Pediatrics, American Academy of Family Physicians, and the American Society of Internal Medicine. Healthy People 2010 (www.healthypeople.gov/Document/HTML/Volume1/06Disability.htm) defines as its primary objectives the promotion of the health of people with disabilities, prevention of secondary conditions, and elimination of disparities between people with and without disabilities. One identified action area is the facilitation of transition for those with pediatric-onset disease. Many resource materials to evaluate readiness for transition and to facilitate transition exist; many are available on the Web site Healthy and Ready to Work, *www.hrtw.org.*

While there are relatively few studies of transition of medical care for people with congenital heart disease, there are multiple relevant studies of individuals with other childhood conditions, including arthritis and rheumatic disease (Robertson, 2006; Robertson et al., 2006; Tucker and Cabral, 2005), sickle cell disease (Anie and Telfair, 2005; Telfair et al., 2004a, 2004b; Wojciechowski et al., 2002), pediatric organ recipients (McDonagh and Kelly, 2003; Kaufman, 2006), end-stage renal disease (Braj et al., 1999), cystic fibrosis

(Downes and Boroughs, 2005; Zack et al., 2003), type 1 diabetes mellitus (Tsamasiros and Bartsocas, 2002; Visentin et al., 2006), and other diseases and conditions originating in childhood. For some of these conditions, similar models exist in the adult population, and training programs for adult medical care encompass these conditions; for example, end-stage renal disease, sickle cell disease, and rheumatoid arthritis. For other conditions, such as congenital heart disease and cystic fibrosis, increases in expected survival to adulthood have occurred only in the last third of the twentieth century; thus, there is no large reservoir of these patients in adult medicine teaching programs. The Cystic Fibrosis Foundation, a patient advocacy and research foundation, has been able to mandate appropriate care for adult patients through a clinic certification program.

More than 43 disease-specific studies of transition models have been published and well reviewed in 2004 by Betz (2004). The information on successful transition rates in seven select studies is shown in Table 33–2 (Rettig and Athreya, 1991; Anderson et al., 2002; Appleton, 2001; Kipps et al., 2002; Reid et al., 2004).

Overall, most programs reported successful transition–defined as the successful transfer to adult-oriented care—about half the time, and this also correlates with Reid's findings in the congenital heart population. Reid found that the strongest predictors of successful transition were proximity to one specific affiliated adult congenital heart center and referral to a specific adult congenital heart cardiologist. Less correlated was having a greater number of previous surgeries. Additional predictors of compliance included greater degree of illness (comorbidities, symptoms, activity restrictions, greater risk of complications), greater pre-existing compliance (using subacute bacterial endocarditis prophylaxis), and more independence in keeping appointments (Reid et al., 2004). These positive predictors are listed in Table 33–3. Only the second of these six predictors is under the control of the pediatric cardiologist. Because the study was undertaken in Canada, where health care is universally provided, health insurance was absent as a factor in care, transition rates are negatively impacted because of insurance barriers in the US context. The findings that symptoms correlate with compliance are of concern since many adults with congenital heart disease report few symptoms until late in the course of deterioration. The data on the value of preparation for transfer are equivocal. For a small sample of young adults with sickle cell disease, preparation before transfer did not predict keeping first appointment in the adult clinic or compliance with the medical regimen in the adult clinic (Wojciechowski et al., 2002).

TABLE 33–2. *Successful Transition Rates in Seven Studies*

Study Author	Year	Disease	% in Adult Care at Follow-up	Mean Age at Transition
Anderson	2002	Cystic fibrosis	76%	Not stated
Appleton	1997	Epilepsy	58%	18.2 years
Bywater	1981	Cystic fibrosis	48%	
Kipps	2002	Type 1 diabetes	57%	17.9 years
Rettig & Athreya	1991	Rheumatic diseases	84% after transition program	
Rettig & Athreya	1991	Rheumatic disease	1/144 without transition program	
Reid et al.	2004	Congenital heart disease	47%	Studied age 19 years and more

TABLE 33–3. *Predictors of Successful Transition (Reid et al., 2004)*

Proximity to specific affiliated adult congenital heart center
Referral to a specifically named adult congenital heart cardiologist
Greater number of previous surgeries
Greater severity of illness
Greater compliance with care in youth
Greater independence in attending appointments

CIRCUMSTANCES OF TRANSITION TO ADULT CARE

The definition of transition given (Blum et al., 1993) by the Society for Adolescent Medicine is "*the purposeful, planned movement of adolescents and young adults with chronic physical and medical conditions from child-centered to adult-oriented health-care systems.*" In contrast to such an orderly and temporally sustained transition program, movement of congenital heart patients typically occurs for a variety of unplanned reasons including passing a critical age for use of a pediatric provider or institution, going to the emergency room and being seen by adult-trained care providers or referred to an adult program, and, in some institutions, pregnancy, mandating transfer to an adult-oriented care provider. A normal developmental step is leaving the care of one's pediatric health care providers and establishing new associations with an adult health care team. Young adults need specific instructions to identify a cardiologist trained in congenital heart disease, if that is what they require. Otherwise they may start obtaining care from any "adult" cardiologist at the same time they transfer from pediatric to adult primary care, and see it as a logical developmental "next step." This is particularly likely if they move for school or career, or to establish an independent residence. Most members of the public are unaware of the training differences in congenital disease between adult and pediatric cardiology and specialized care guidelines and may assume that competent care will be available from any trained adult cardiologist. Thus, they may

independently leave pediatric care without having been transferred to a specialized adult congenital heart disease (ACHD) clinic. Many adults with congenital heart disease report having to leave the care of their pediatrician despite the patient expressing willingness or desire for pediatric care to continue. Few report being instructed on how to establish life-long ACHD care or being explicitly cautioned against choosing a nonspecialized "regular" cardiology practice.

Negative health outcomes from transition are documented even when transition occurs to adult care. For example, diabetic patients show increases in HbA1C when transitioned into adult care (Betz, 2004).

BARRIERS TO SUCCESSFUL TRANSITION

Differences in the Culture of Pediatric and Adult-Oriented Medicine

The pediatric health care delivery model is described as family centered and pediatric practitioners rely on families to strengthen the care provided to their pediatric patient. In contrast, the adult health care delivery model focuses on the individual and the disease process (Fleming et al., 2002). These differences are both positive and negative for the adult patient. Adult patients who transitioned from pediatric to adult hemodialysis centers expressed satisfaction in gaining a greater knowledge about their disease and about their dialysis and in the independence of playing a greater role in their own care (Braj et al., 1999). Cystic fibrosis patients desired adult-focused services such as inpatient rooms, discussion groups, and social service support as they enhanced care after transition to an adult facility or adult program (Zack et al., 2003).

Attitudes and Knowledge Base of Adult Providers

Adult providers may have little or no specific training in disorders that originate in childhood. A survey of nephrologists in Virginia demonstrated that

(LoCasale-Crouch and Johnson, 2005) 60% of adult nephrologists were uncomfortable seeing an adult patient with a "pediatric diagnosis." Although formal data is lacking, anecdotal reports suggest that it is not uncommon for transfer to fail because of the adult-oriented cardiologist's discomfort with congenital diagnosis. However, many of the late-onset diseases that ACHD patients develop secondary to their congenital heart disease, such as congestive heart failure and atrial fibrillation, are common in general adult cardiology practice. A study of cardiac surgery in adults with congenital heart disease demonstrated that many congenital heart surgeries in adults occur in various different hospitals, many of which do less than six such surgeries annually (Gurvitz et al., 2007). Thus, despite the Bethesda guidelines, many physicians consider themselves competent to provide surgical, and perhaps other, care in institutions that would not meet these guidelines.

All components of the guidelines written in 2000 by the 32nd Bethesda Conference Care of the Adult with Congenital Heart Disease support transition of patients to adult-oriented care. A survey of adult cardiology training programs showed that adult cardiology fellows receive minimal congenital heart training, with over one third of adult programs having less than four lectures yearly on ACHD (Gurvitz et al., 2005). The Bethesda guidelines propose that all adult cardiology trainees have sufficient training that "at a minimum,...allows the trainee to recognize CHD and attempt to make a preliminary diagnosis, to refer the patient to a regional ACHD center, and to work with that center in the care of these patient." Such cardiologists are designated level 1 (Child et al., 2001). The same task force recommended that adult cardiology trainees planning to care for ACHD patients should have at least 1 year of training in ACHD—level 2. It is apparent that few patients have the opportunity to transition to a level 2 provider or to a specialized center (level 3) within close range of their home.

In sharp contrast to the recommendations for specialized centers, a survey undertaken by the International Society for Adult Congenital Heart Disease and the Adult Congenital Heart Association identified only 63 self-identified specialized centers caring for less than 40,000 patients (www.achaheart.org). There are predicted to be approximately 800,000 patients alive in the United States with ACHD, of whom half would be appropriately seen in programs specializing in ACHD care. Study of barriers to transition to adult care identifies proximity to a specialized center as one significant barrier. In addition, patients may believe they have no need for further cardiac care and may often rely on the judgment of their primary care provider to determine whether or not they need referral for their congenital heart condition. Such primary care providers would be expected, in general, to be relatively unsophisticated in this specialized area.

Attitudes and Knowledge Base of Pediatric Providers

Many papers refer to the unwillingness of pediatric providers to give up their long-term patient relationships to adult-oriented care providers but attitudinal surveys to document this are lacking. Pediatricians in a survey about their role in transition had strong overlap with parents in thinking that the activities were within the providers' role (Geenen et al., 2003). Surveys in the population with sickle cell disease identified pediatric providers as fostering dependency and there being a lack of communication between adult and pediatric providers. About 89% of providers for youth with sickle cell disease said they thought transition programs were necessary but 81% of family practitioners reported that they did nothing to demonstrate transition. Overall 67% did something to further demonstrate transition, from having a family conference to seeing the youth independently of family (Telfair et al., 2004a).

Attitudes and Knowledge of Patients and Families

Flume et al. initially surveyed patients with cystic fibrosis and their physicians, and subsequently, the nonphysician staff of the cystic fibrosis centers. Patients had less concern about transition then either physicians or nonphysician staff. Patient/family resistance (45%), disease severity (34%), and developmental delay (31.3%) were reasons given for transition not being accomplished (Anderson et al., 2002; Flume et al., 2004). Adult patients transitioning to care in adult congenital heart centers had a median lag of 3 years between last cardiology visit and adult center visit. Over a third of patients had no idea what their cardiac diagnosis was (Dore et al., 2002).

Health Insurance Barriers

In the United States, health insurance is linked to employment status or to qualifying as fully disabled. Most states have Medicaid programs for children up to age 18 for families at the federal poverty level but there is no corresponding program for adults. Supplemental security income (SSI) eligibility for children is often a route to Medicaid coverage but at age 18 years, all individuals on SSI must undergo a redetermination of eligibility based on adult criteria, which focus on inability to work. However, 30% of those with SSI in youth will lose it when redetermined by adult criteria (White, 2004).

In general, lack of health insurance is common among young adults in the United States. Among adults aged between 19 and 29 years, 26% and 28% of those with and without disability, respectively, are uninsured. However, 35% of the group with disability do not meet a health care need because of cost compared to 15% of those without disability. A survey of children aged 13–17 years with special health care needs showed that only 5.9% were uninsured. In this survey directed toward whether core goals addressing transition were met, insurance status was not a predictor (Lotstein et al., 2005). Youth with sickle cell disease had insurance status and the ability to pay for adult care as a major component of transition concerns (Telfair et al., 1994). Similarly, insurance status is not assessed in studies of transition in Canada (Reid et al., 2004).

Context of Transition

Psychosocial development of young adults with congenital heart disease may be delayed or modified by chronic illness. In one small study, adults with congenital heart disease had a fair knowledge of their own illness but in other areas they scored less than their age peers with acquired heart disease (Lyon and McCarter, 2006). Studies of adolescents and young adults with congenital heart disease confirm similar delays; there is no correlation with severity of cardiac disease (Tong and Kools, 2004; Tong et al., 1998). In one study of psychosocial development, European patients were entirely comparable to their peers but a similar US cohort was less so (Kovac et al., 2005). Thus, continuing reassessment of the adolescent with respect to readiness for transition is imperative (Fernandes and Landzberg, 2004; Higgins and Tong, 2003). Undue anxiety and hypervigilance are common among young adults with congenital heart disease; this anxiety may lead to miscommunication with new physician providers (Horner and Jellinek, 2000). The consequences of failed transition are all too apparent. Dore's study of patient knowledge showed that 14% of patients presenting to an adult congenital heart clinic had lapsed 10 or more years after last medical care and before presentation (Dore et al., 2002).

Many proposals and studies of transition concepts are focused on individuals with significant neurological and/or motor impairment (Betz, 1999, 2004; Blomquist, 2006; David, 2001; Lotstein et al., 2005; Scal and Ireland, 2005). In contrast, most adults with congenital heart disease are indistinguishable from their peers intellectually and visually in the school and work environment and live independently. Transition is proposed to occur in the context of normal adolescent development, with the timing when adult responsibilities for self-care are initiated and reliably maintained (Higgins and Tong, 2003; Tong and Kools, 2004). However, studies of adults with various diseases that have onset in childhood demonstrate that such adults frequently lag behind their peers in multiple life milestones while moving toward independence, suggesting that skills assessment as well as age will best guide initiating transition (Stam et al., 2006). Development of self-management and self-determination skills should be taught to adolescents with chronic illness (Stewart et al., 2006).

PROPOSED BEST PRACTICES FOR PEDIATRIC CARDIOLOGY PROGRAMS

The following are proposed as best practices, not yet supported by evidence-based trial, but rationally derived from experience and literature.

All children and families should be taught that the child will have, as we best know now, a need for life-long surveillance of their congenital heart condition despite an excellent surgical repair. As a patient moves into adolescence and young adulthood, he/she should be treated as an evolving adult, with the privacy and independence appropriate to that status. This mandates seeing the child without parents, determining, for example, a social history of substance abuse, sexuality, and educational goals. Beginning at age 12–14 it appears reasonable to ask patients to know what their diagnosis name is and what it means physiologically. About age 16 it seems reasonable to have patients report the medications they take and how often. Shortly after this, patients should take the responsibility of communicating the need for prescription refills and making follow-up appointments. In all cases, access to the practitioners in the program should be available to the patient to facilitate his/her growth in the ability to accomplish these tasks. The fact that care will be transferred to an adult program should be communicated to all patients and families right from the patient's childhood.

There is evidence that adolescence is a time of limited compliance with medical regimens in other disorders (Wysocki et al., 1992). Additionally, patients with chronic illness in childhood have delays in maturation that extend beyond the usual adolescent period (Stam et al., 2006). This may suggest that transition occurs first to a transition clinic in adolescence, and then, when developmental goals are met, to an adult program.

MODELS OF TRANSITION

Models of care for adults with congenital heart disease transitioning to care include pediatric medical settings, adult medical settings, blended settings, or dropping out of medical care (Reiss et al., 2005). The 32nd Bethesda recommendations for specialized centers correspond to a blended setting, with both adult and pediatric cardiologists working together. Of six major, established congenital heart centers with over 20,000 registered patients, all but one included both pediatric and adult cardiology (Niwa et al., 2004). Formal assessment of the efficacy of these different models in comparison to one another has not been made.

Helpful qualitative analysis of the process of health care transition in 13–29-year-old people with a variety of chronic health conditions provides a framework for stages of transition (Reiss et al., 2005). The stages are "envisioning a future," "age of responsibility," and "age of transition." Cognitive delay and progressive nature of disability both were important factors in affecting and limiting transition. It is the responsibility of the first providers caring for a child with congenital heart disease to, within reason, identify the child as a person who is expected to grow to adulthood, be independent and competent. The age of responsibility is that time of transition of responsibility within the home and the medical care system when the child can be a primary participant in the visit, answering questions, knowing his/her own medications, and learning the nature of his/her heart defect. These stages occur within childhood and lead to an age of transition, divided into adolescence and young adulthood. At this time the patient gradually assumes responsibility for making appointments and obtaining medications and other components of care. Actual movement to adult-oriented care is the last stage of transition and is dependent on the patient having demonstrated the maturity and skills to function well in the adult environment.

In common with Reiss et al., many scholars of transition recommend that the transition process be a particular structured aspect of medical care with its own staffing that crosses, with the patient, between pediatric and adult care transiently (Michaud et al., 2004).

Viner succinctly describes barriers to patients leaving pediatric care including precipitous or unplanned transfer, structure of adult-oriented care services, lack of trust between adult and pediatric services, and the willingness of youth to drop out of care if feeling well (McDonagh and Viner, 2006; Viner, 1999, 2001).

Viner's recommendations for best practice (Table 33–4) are strikingly similar to those promulgated by the 32nd conference on ACHD. These included setting a policy on timing of transfer, preparation period

TABLE 33–4. *Recommendations for Best Practice*

1. Transition preparation must be seen as an essential component of high-quality health care in adolescence.
2. Every pediatric general and specialty clinic should have a specific transition policy. More formal transition programs are necessary where large numbers of young people are being transferred to adult care.
3. Young people should not be transferred to adult services until they have the necessary skills to function in an adult service and have finished growth and puberty.
4. An identified person within the pediatric and adult teams must be responsible for transition arrangements. The most suitable persons are nurse specialists.
5. Management links must be developed between the two hospitals.
6. Large children's services should develop a "transition map" detailing where and how transfer occurs specialty by specialty.
7. Evaluation of transition arrangements must be undertaken.

Adapted from Viner, 1999.

and education period that begins in adolescence, coordinated transfer process, interested and capable adult specialized unit administrative support, and primary care involvement (Foster et al., 2001). Sadly, 6 years after that conference recommendation, these recommendations are often not in place in the pediatric cardiology program. Speculation as to why transition plans are not part of the pediatric cardiology practice includes lack of adult cardiology programs with expertise in the care of these patients, a failure to perceive the important differences in adult and pediatric medical practice thus compromising the adult's full autonomy, and a lack of support staff to facilitate the transition process.

Having an advanced practice nurse accompany the patient to first visits to the adult clinic has been suggested (Lewis-Gary, 2001) as has finding mentors to help transitioning patients. Nurses and nurse specialists are cited by many reviewers as critical people in educating and implementing transition to adult care (Betz, 2004; Van Deyk et al., 2004). Nearly half of specialized adult congenital heart programs in Europe employ nurse specialists. Their role as educators places them optimally to assist in transition into adult care (Moons et al., 2002; Van Deyk et al., 2004). One model proposes a nurse-managed clinic especially for youth with special health care needs working with both adult and pediatric practitioners. This model is based on the educational model of an individualized education program for individuals with disability in school. The efficacy is not yet demonstrated (Betz and Redcay, 2003).

CONCLUSION/SUMMATION

The need for pediatric patients with chronic illness to transition into adult-oriented medical care has been recognized by multiple advocacy and physician groups. Guidelines for the care of adults with congenital heart disease have been published in the United States, Britain, and European countries for half a decade or more. The process of implementing these guidelines and of transitioning patients fails on many fronts, at least in the United States. This will result in a greater disease burden for these patients over time. Available information suggests that of the 500,000 people with ACHD for whom specialized adult congenital heart care is recommended, well less than one in five is receiving such care. Efforts must continue to be made to develop appropriate specialized centers for the care of adults with congenital heart disease. Patients and community physicians must receive sustained education about the need for patients to receive specialized care. Educational efforts must be vigorous and national in scope. Development of outcomes research that demonstrates superiority of specialized care for the complex disorders may provide an economic wedge toward this movement.

REFERENCES

American Academy of Pediatrics (AAP). Transition of care provided for adolescents with special health care needs. American Academy of Pediatrics Committee on Children with Disabilities and Committee on Adolescence. *Pediatrics.* 1996;98(6 pt 1): 1203–1206.

American Academy of Pediatrics (AAP). A consensus statement on health care transitions for young adults with special health care needs. *Pediatrics.* 2002;110(6 Pt 2):1304–1306.

American Medical Association (AMA). The health care of children and youths with disabilities. Council on Scientific Affairs,. *Arch Fam Med.* 1993;2(3):326–329.

Anderson DL, Flume PA, Hardy KK, Gray S. Transition programs in cystic fibrosis centers: perceptions of patients. *Pediatr Pulmonol.* 2002;33(5):327–331.

Anie KA, Telfair J. Multi-site study of transition in adolescents with sickle cell disease in the United Kingdom and the United States. *Int J Adolesc Med Health.* 2005;17(2):169–178.

Appleton RE. Transition from paediatric clinic to the adult service. *J R Soc Med.* 2001;94(10):554.

Bailey S OCB, Pearce J. The transition from paediatric to adult health care services for young adults with a disability: an ethical perspective. *Australian Health Review.* 2003;26(1):64–69.

Betz CL, Redcay G. Creating Healthy Futures: an innovative nurse-managed transition clinic for adolescents and young adults with special health care needs. *Pediatr Nurs.* 2003;29(1):25–30.

Betz CL. Adolescents with chronic conditions: linkages to adult service systems. *Pediatr Nurs.* 1999;25(5):473–476.

Betz CL. Transition of adolescents with special health care needs: review and analysis of the literature. *Issues Compr Pediatr Nurs.* 2004;27(3):179–241.

Blomquist KB. Health, education, work, and independence of young adults with disabilities. *Orthop Nurs.* 2006;25(3):168–187.

Blum RW GD, Hodgman CH, Jorissen TW, Okinow NA, Orr DP, Slap GB. Transition from child-centered to adult health-care systems for adolescents with chronic conditions. A position paper of the Society for Adolescent Medicine. *J Adolesc Health.* 1993;14(7):570–576.

Braj B, Picone G, Children HF, Cross N, Pearlman L. The lived experience of adolescents who transfer from a pediatric to an adult hemodialysis centre. *Cannt J.* 1999;9(4):41–46.

Child JS C-NR, Alpert JS, Deanfield JE, et al. Task force 3: workforce description and educational requirements for the care of adults with congenital heart disease. *J Am Coll Cardiol.* 2001;37(5):1183–1187.

David TJ. Transition from the paediatric clinic to the adult service. *J R Soc Med.* 2001;94(8):373–374.

Deanfield J, Thaulow E, Warnes C, et al. Management of grown up congenital heart disease. *Eur Heart J.* 2003;24(11):1035–1084.

Dore A, de Guise P, Mercier LA. Transition of care to adult congenital heart centres: what do patients know about their heart condition? *Can J Cardiol.* 2002;18(2):141–146.

Downes JJ, Boroughs DS. The transition to adulthood by adolescents with chronic respiratory failure: a growing challenge. *Caring.* 2005;24(9):62–67.

Fernandes SM, Landzberg MJ. Transitioning the young adult with congenital heart disease for life-long medical care. *Pediatr Clin North Am.* 2004;51(6):1739–48, xi.

Fleming E, Carter B, Gillibrand W. The transition of adolescents with diabetes from the children's health care service into the adult health care service: a review of the literature. *J Clin Nurs.* 2002;11(5):560–567.

Flume PA, Taylor LA, Anderson DL, Gray S, Turner D. Transition programs in cystic fibrosis centers: perceptions of team members. *Pediatr Pulmonol.* 2004;37(1):4–7.

Foster E GTJ, Driscoll DJ, Reid GJ, et al Task force 2: special health care needs of adults with congenital heart disease. *J Am Coll Cardiol.* 2001;37(5):1176–1183.

Geenen SJ, Powers LE, Sells W. Understanding the role of health care providers during the transition of adolescents with disabilities and special health care needs. *J Adolesc Health.* 2003;32(3):225–33.

Grown-up congenital heart (GUCH) disease: current needs and provision of service for adolescents and adults with congenital heart disease in the UK. *Heart.* 2002;88 (suppl 1):i1–14.

Gurvitz MZ CR, Ramos FJ, Allada V, Child JS, Klitzner TS. Variations in adult congenital heart disease training in adult and pediatric cardiology fellowship programs. *J Am Coll Cardiol.* 2005;46(5):893–898.

Gurvitz MZ, Inkelas M, Lee M, Stout K, Escarce J, Chang RK. Changes in hospitalization patterns among patients with congenital heart disease during the transition from adolescence to adulthood. *J Am Coll Cardiol.* 2007;49(8):875–882.

Higgins SS, Tong E. Transitioning adolescents with congenital heart disease into adult health care. *Prog Cardiovasc Nurs.* 2003;18(2):93–98.

Horner T LR, Jellinek MS. Psychosocial profile of adults with complex congenital heart disease. *Mayo Clinic Proceedings.* 2000;75(1):31–36.

Kaufman M. Transition of cognitively delayed adolescent organ transplant recipients to adult care. *Pediatr Transplant.* 2006;10(4):413–417.

Kipps S BT, Ong K, Ackland FM, et al. Current methods of transfer of young people with Type 1 diabetes to adult services. *Diabet Med.* 2002;19(8):649–654.

Kovacs AH, Sears SF, Saidi AS. Biopsychosocial experiences of adults with congenital heart disease: review of the literature. *Am Heart J.* 2005;150(2):193–201.

Landzberg MJ MDJ, Davidson WR Jr, Jarcho JA, et al. Task force 4: organization of delivery systems for adults with congenital heart disease. *J Am Coll Cardiol.* 2001;37(5):1187–1193.

Lewis-Gary MD. Transitioning to adult health care facilities for young adults with a chronic condition. *Pediatr Nurs.* 2001;27(5):521–524.

LoCasale-Crouch J, Johnson B. Transition from pediatric to adult medical care. *Adv Chronic Kidney Dis.* 2005;12(4):412–417.

Lotstein DS, McPherson M, Strickland B, Newacheck PW. Transition planning for youth with special health care needs: results from the National Survey of Children with Special Health Care Needs. *Pediatrics.* 2005;115(6):1562–1568.

Lyon ME KK, McCarter R. Transition to Adulthood in Congenital Heart Disease: Missed Adolescent Milestones. *J Adolesc Health.* 2006;39:121–124.

McDonagh JE, Kelly DA. Transitioning care of the pediatric recipient to adult caregivers. *Pediatr Clin North Am.* 2003;50(6):1561–83, xi–xii.

McDonagh JE, Viner RM. Lost in transition? Between paediatric and adult services. *BMJ.* 2006;332(7539):435–6.

Michaud PA, Suris JC, Viner R. The adolescent with a chronic condition. Part II: healthcare provision. *Arch Dis Child.* 2004;89(10):943–949.

Moons P, De Geest S, Budts W. Comprehensive care for adults with congenital heart disease: expanding roles for nurses. *Eur J Cardiovasc Nurs.* 2002;1(1):23–28.

Niwa K PJ, Webb GD, Murphy D, Liberthson R, Warnes CA, Gatzoulis MA. Survey of specialized tertiary care facilities for adults with congenital heart disease. *Int J Cardiol.* 2004;96(2):211–216.

Reid GJ, Irvine MJ, McCrindle BW, et al. Prevalence and correlates of successful transfer from pediatric to adult health care among a cohort of young adults with complex congenital heart defects. *Pediatrics.* 2004;113(3 Pt 1):e197–205.

Reiss JG, Gibson RW, Walker LR. Health care transition: youth, family, and provider perspectives. *Pediatrics.* 2005;115(1):112–120.

Rettig P, Athreya BH. Adolescents with chronic disease. Transition to adult health care. *Arthritis Care Res.* 1991;4(4):174–180.

Robertson L. When should young people with chronic rheumatic disease move from paediatric to adult-centred care? *Best Pract Res Clin Rheumatol.* 2006;20(2):387–397.

Robertson LP, McDonagh JE, Southwood TR, Shaw KL. Growing up and moving on. A multicentre UK audit of the transfer of adolescents with juvenile idiopathic arthritis from paediatric to adult centred care. *Ann Rheum Dis.* 2006;65(1):74–80.

Scal P, Ireland M. Addressing transition to adult health care for adolescents with special health care needs. *Pediatrics.* 2005;115(6):1607–1612.

Skorton DJ GAJ, Allen HD, Fox JM, Truesdell SC, Webb GD, Williams, RG. Task force 5: adults with congenital heart disease: access to care. *J Am Coll Cardiol.* 2001;37(5):1193–1198.

Stam H, Hartman EE, Deurloo JA, Groothoff J, Grootenhuis MA. Young adult patients with a history of pediatric disease: impact on course of life and transition into adulthood. *J Adolesc Health.* 2006;39(1):4–13.

Stewart D, Stavness C, King G, Antle B, Law M. A critical appraisal of literature reviews about the transition to adulthood for youth with disabilities. *Phys Occup Ther Pediatr.* 2006;26(4):5–24.

Summary of recommendations (SR) – care of the adult with congenital heart disease. *J Am Coll Cardiol.* 2001;37(5):1167–1169.

Telfair J, Alexander LR, Loosier PS, Alleman-Velez PL, Simmons J. Providers' perspectives and beliefs regarding transition to adult care for adolescents with sickle cell disease. *J Health Care Poor Underserved.* 2004a;15(3):443–461.

Telfair J, Ehiri JE, Loosier PS, Baskin ML. Transition to adult care for adolescents with sickle cell disease: results of a national survey. *Int J Adolesc Med Health.* 2004b;16(1):47–64.

Telfair J, Myers J, Drezner S. Transfer as a component of the transition of adolescents with sickle cell disease to adult care: adolescent, adult, and parent perspectives. *J Adolesc Health.* 1994;15(7):558–565.

Therrien J, Gatzoulis M, Graham T, et al. Canadian Cardiovascular Society Consensus Conference 2001 update: Recommendations for the Management of Adults with Congenital Heart Disease – Part II. *Can J Cardiol.* 2001;17(10):1029–1050.

Tong EM SP, Messias DKH, Foote D, Chesla CA, Gilliss CL. Growing up with congenital heart disease: the dilemmas of adolescents and young adults. *Cardiol Young.* 1998;8:303–309.

Tong EM, Kools S. Health care transitions for adolescents with congenital heart disease: patient and family perspectives. *Nurs Clin North Am.* 2004;39(4):727–740.

Tsamasiros J, Bartsocas CS. Transition of the adolescent from the children's to the adults' diabetes clinic. *J Pediatr Endocrinol Metab.* 2002;15(4):363–367.

Tucker LB, Cabral DA. Transition of the adolescent patient with rheumatic disease: issues to consider. *Pediatr Clin North Am.* 2005;52(2):641–52, viii.

Van Deyk K, Moons P, Gewillig M, Budts W. Educational and behavioral issues in transitioning from pediatric cardiology to adult-centered health care. *Nurs Clin North Am.* 2004;39(4):755–768.

Viner R. Barriers and good practice in transition from paediatric to adult care. *J R Soc Med.* 2001;94 (suppl 40):2–4.

Viner R. Effective transition from paediatric to adult services. *Hosp Med.* 2000;61(5):341–343.

Viner R. Transition from paediatric to adult care. Bridging the gaps or passing the buck? *Arch Dis Child.* 1999;81:271–275.

Viner R. Transition from paediatric to adult care. Bridging the gaps or passing the buck? *Arch Dis Child.* 1999;81(3):271–275.

Visentin K, Koch T, Kralik D. Adolescents with Type 1 Diabetes: transition between diabetes services. *J Clin Nurs,* 2006;15(6):761–769.

Warnes CA LR, Danielson GK, Dore A, et al. Task force 1: the changing profile of congenital heart disease in adult life. *J Am Coll Cardiol.* 2001;37(5):1170–1175.

White PH. Access to health care: health insurance considerations for young adults with special health care needs/disabilities. *Pediatrics.* 2002;110(6 Pt 2):1328–1335.

Wojciechowski EA, Hurtig A, Dorn L. A natural history study of adolescents and young adults with sickle cell disease as they transfer to adult care: a need for case management services. *J Pediatr Nurs.* 2002;17(1):18–27.

Wysocki TH BS, Ward KM, Green LS. Diabetes Mellitus in the Transition to Adulthood: Adjustment, Self-Care, and Health Status. *J Dev Behav Pediatr.* 1992;13:194–201.

Zack J, Jacobs CP, Keenan PM, et al. Perspectives of patients with cystic fibrosis on preventive counseling and transition to adult care. *Pediatr Pulmonol.* 2003;36(5):376–383.

34

End-of-Life Issues in Pediatric Cardiac Care

R. SCOTT SIMPSON
PETER N. COX

INTRODUCTION

The management of congenital heart defects (CHD) has the potential to take many patients, their parents and families, and the health professionals who care for them on a journey that reaches the limits of medical, surgical, and technological capabilities. It is inevitable that some children with CHD will die, despite optimal treatment, and this creates challenges for the health care system. In a recent survey of 19 centers the overall mortality following pediatric cardiac surgery was 2.9%, but individual rates are case specific with a range of 0.4% for simple surgeries, up to 47.7% for complex "high-risk" cases (Welke et al., 2006). Perioperative mortality statistics do not include children who succumb without surgery, or those dying of delayed complications. Nor do they address a significant burden of morbidity among survivors.

"End-of-life care" is a term more commonly associated with hospice-style palliation provided for children dying of progressive illnesses such as cancer, neuromuscular disorders, and severe inborn errors of metabolism. In these cases a multidisciplinary palliative care team will have established a clear understanding with the family that the child is terminally ill—a fact that is pivotal. Care decisions are therefore motivated by a desire to ensure that the child's remaining time alive is of optimum quality, with minimal suffering. Older children may be their own primary decision makers in many cases.

By contrast, when children with CHD die, they are usually in the pediatric intensive care unit (PICU), and death occurs either suddenly and unexpectedly, or after a long struggle to survive with an anatomical and physiological burden that could not be overcome. Occasionally, the complications of treatment may be directly contributory. The environment in PICU is radically different from that of the hospice, and the dying process may be significantly accelerated by comparison, so that when a child dies it is not just an unexpected event, but also one that was hitherto unimaginable for most families (Meyer et al., 2006). When all endeavors have been geared toward a child's survival, parents will be ill-prepared and particularly vulnerable to the emotional trauma the death of their child causes (Truog et al., 2006).

In the general PICU population, as many as 60% of children who die do so following a conscious decision to either limit or withdraw life-sustaining therapy (Garros et al., 2003; Meert et al., 2000). These decisions are usually made by agreement between physicians and families (Levy and McBride, 2006). In the cardiac PICU the nature of the treatments, the aspirations of the surgeons and intensivists, and the hopes and expectations of parents and families may influence, or even preclude, such discussions. As technology advances and more sophisticated mechanical supports become available, there is increasing uncertainty creeping in to end-of-life events, a situation that is perhaps at odds with expectations (Quill and Suchman, 1993). Physicians find themselves working with complex probabilities where possible outcomes do not fall into dichotomous categories of life versus death, and may be faced with reconciling the continued use of aggressive treatments and interventions aimed at keeping children with complex problems alive, against the adoption of a more palliative approach that focuses on relief of pain and anxiety, and provision of emotional support. Wherever possible, both strategies should be used concurrently (Back et al., 2003). Too much attention can be given to the former, and not enough on the latter. Finely tuned communication skills, sensitivity, and compassion are essential to handle these apparently conflicting needs simultaneously.

Supporting a child through PICU to discharge and long-term survival rates among the most rewarding experiences any health professional can have and is highly valued by society. Supporting a child in PICU to die in comfort, with respect and dignity, without suffering, is also an extremely important job that appears to be undervalued, even though it often requires more intensive input and expertise to achieve. Done well, it may also be professionally satisfying. This was expressed eloquently over 20 years ago:

> The success of intensive care is not, therefore to be measured only by the statistics of survival, as though each death were a medical failure. It is to be measured by the quality of lives restored, the quality of the dying in those in whose best interests it is to die, and the quality of the human relationships involved in each death (Dunstan, 1985).

This chapter considers ways of achieving this kind of success.

TIMELINE OF CARE: OPPORTUNITIES TO MANAGE DEATH

Before Admission to the Pediatric Intensive Care Unit

The majority of babies with severe CHD are detected in utero by ultrasound in the second trimester of pregnancy, and parents are counseled accordingly. Cardiologists and cardiac surgeons often collaborate to provide information and guidance in this setting, and many parents independently perform extensive Internet searches, or make contact with voluntary support groups and CHD lesion–focused organizations. Therapeutic options, ranging from no intervention, through staged surgical procedures, up to listing for heart transplantation, when appropriate, may have been decided upon prior to birth. Intrauterine surgery may even be considered. For parents of babies that evaded antenatal detection, there is much less time for decisions to be made after the birth, and a great deal of emotional shock. These babies are usually transferred to an intensive care unit, either neonatal or pediatric, for care until an appropriate decision is made. If a family opts for palliation rather than corrective intervention, the period of survival is quite variable, and death may even be managed at home in some cases.

Care in the Pediatric Intensive Care Unit

When following an interventional approach to the congenital defect, children will usually benefit from a period of preoperative stabilization. Whether they undergo a catheter intervention or surgery, or a combination, they are also likely to require postprocedural care in the PICU. Even patients with uncomplicated courses may need advanced levels of PICU care, and if complications arise, their care may become extremely complex. Extracorporeal membrane oxygenation (ECMO), ventricular assist devices (VAD), and cardiac transplantation are increasingly available, although limited to relatively few patients in a select number of centers. Indications and contraindications for these interventions are changing as clinical experience accumulates and approaches to CHD mature. Through the application of these technologies new challenges have been posed, creating a better understanding of the complex interrelationships between physiology, pharmacology, and pathology. Consequently, the frontiers of knowledge are being constantly expanded. An enhanced ability to prolong life brings opportunities to venture into unknown or experimental clinical situations where there are large gaps in existing knowledge and research. End-of-life decisions may be even harder to contemplate when one's attention is fully absorbed by high-tech life-preservation strategies. For most children with significant CHD lesions, the time from diagnosis to definitive intervention is, by necessity, relatively short. At a number of points in the care process decisions need to be made about the veracity of offering complex surgical interventions versus managing an imminent death. In this stressful, often time-constrained setting, there is considerable debate over what constitutes fully informed consent and the validity of the process of clinical decision making. Standard consent processes entail providing information on the potential negative outcomes directly related to the scheduled surgery, mainly for medicolegal reasons. Truly informed consent should include discussions on the potential longer-term consequences of the choices made, but this is made difficult in many instances because long-term outcome data are often preliminary, scant, or nonexistent.

Example—Hypoplastic Left Heart Syndrome. Only a few decades ago, babies born with hypoplastic left heart syndrome (HLHS) were regarded as having a uniformly fatal condition, and palliative comfort care was all that would be offered. The early pioneers of corrective surgery experienced universally dismal outcomes (Cayler et al., 1970; Noonan and Nadas, 1958; Norwood et al., 1980). As years passed and mounting controversy resounded about them, the pioneers who persisted were eventually rewarded by the development of successful therapies (Norwood et al., 1983). With a modern multidisciplinary approach to HLHS, more than 50% of the babies who undergo corrective surgery can now expect to reach puberty (Krasemann et al., 2005; Malec et al., 2000; McGuirk et al., 2006; Pizarro et al., 2002; Sinzobahamvya et al., 2006; Theilen and Shekerdemian, 2005). The whole process, ironically referred to as "palliative surgeries," is a major undertaking involving three or more major surgical operations, weeks to months in PICU and in hospital wards, and numerous outpatient visits, but the dramatic change in mortality outcomes for HLHS stands as an example of how the limits of the possible are changing. It also stands as an example of the ethical dilemmas that can be posed by experimenting in clinical practice, when no evidence basis exists.

Can We? Should We? HLHS surgery is currently acceptable practice, whereas 30 years ago it was viewed as futile. Even so, recently published follow-up studies of HLHS surgery survivors reaching school age and adolescence indicate a high proportion of significant morbidities, manifesting as stunted physical growth, exercise capacity limitation, major neurodevelopmental deficits, medication use, medical system burden, poor self-image, and family disruption, which amount to a significant reduction in the quality of life, and a quantitative burden on the individual and society (Byrne and Murphy, 2005; Krasemann et al., 2005; McGuirk et al., 2006; Sinzobahamvya et al., 2006). Whether or not these are acceptable outcomes become highly individualized value-based judgements. To add to the conundrum, data suggest that cardiac transplantation is possibly a better alternative option, with lower short-term mortality and morbidity (Chrisant et al., 2005). Comparisons, however, are marred by restricted transplant availability and by organ lifespan being finite, necessitating repeat operations later in life. Obviously, HLHS treatment carries many uncertainties and ethical challenges. How parents can be given impartial information on available choices, in order to make informed decisions, defies belief and observation (Byrne and Murphy, 2005). When a treatment is available, the mere ability to provide it does not automatically make it a "right" choice. While a "never-give-up" approach is well supported by the "consumerist" attitudes of patients and their families who frequently demand all that health care has to offer, it is appropriate to ask whether some treatments should be offered in the first place (Cook et al., 2006). And how are decisions of this nature contemplated? This has been appropriately summarized previously:

> To a great extent, the morally demanding questions of bioethics are related to medicine's rapidly evolving technology.... Should life always be extended? Do some burdens

and some costs make life extension immoral or unreasonable? And always, who should make the decision for whom? Sometimes it is extremely difficult to formulate clear answers to such questions. And even when authorities feel confident about their answers, their answers may disagree with those of other authorities. People often feel passionately about their own positions and just as passionately about the stands of those who hold opposing views.

As difficult as it is to arrive at near certainty or even consensus in medical ethics, the level of controversy rises dramatically whenever children are involved (Hirschorn, et al., 2006).

PERSERVERE OR PALLIATE?

All forms of medical progress involve a learning curve for all members of the team. Some variables can be controlled, and others cannot. Even for clinicians with extensive experience there are new learning opportunities constantly arising, sustaining regular mortality and morbidity meetings. When a child undergoes open heart surgery, or a complex catheter laboratory intervention, and his or her recovery is complicated by major adverse events, such as intracerebral hemorrhage, central thromboembolism, or prolonged cardiac arrest, the probability of an imperfect outcome dramatically increases, and the goals of therapy must be reassessed. In trying to prolong a child's life, it is sometimes possible to merely postpone death, and clinicians must be prepared to recognize when treatments have failed. There is no dignity, comfort, or grace to be found in continuing life support when there is no prospect of recovery. Families who are compelled to beg the doctors to stop are placed in an inexpiable situation. Worse, still, such inappropriate treatment may unfairly deny limited resources to other patients (Fisher and Raper, 2005; Sarnaik et al., 2005). These are difficult topics to address without invoking passionate debate, but they are our reality. Where should PICU physicians look for guidance in making these difficult decisions?

CLINICAL DECISION MAKING IN THE PEDIATRIC INTENSIVE CARE UNIT

Largely uncredited, the entity of "common sense" plays a large part in rational health care provision but not surprisingly bears only one published reference (MacLeod, 2001). Common sense is hard to define, easily recognized, and virtually impossible to teach. It may come naturally to some, but for others it can really only be gained and refined by the observation of senior clinicians, or through first-hand experience. As technological advances allow us to create new areas of uncertainty, common sense alone is insufficient in guiding us forward. Sound principles are needed to enable us to make decisions in the complex situations encountered.

Bioethical Principles

Medical paternalism, whereby doctors make all decisions on behalf of their patients and "protect" them from unsavoury news or distressing information, is virtually an historical relic, surpassed over the last three decades, in the Western world, by the "Principlism model," or four ethical principles first espoused by Beauchamp and Childress. These guiding principles are considered judgements that apply, morally, to all cultures (Beauchamp, 2003). They are:

1. Autonomy: allowing patients to make decisions for themselves and respecting their decisions
2. Beneficence: basing decisions on the best interests of patients, balancing benefits against risks
3. Nonmaleficence: doing no harm, nor intending it
4. Justice: treating all patients equally, regardless of their status in society

(Beauchamp and Childress, 1979)

Two other medical obligations, derived from the four principles, are commonly quoted:

1. Fidelity: always telling the truth, maintaining confidentiality, keeping abreast of new developments, and always doing one's best
2. Utility: doing the most good for the most people, achieving the maximum benefit without squandering the resources of a society on an individual, and not burdening or disadvantaging society with the outcome (Oh, 2003).

There are inherent conflicts, or ethical dilemmas, created by assigning equal value to all of the principles when considering an individual case. This deficiency in the Principlism model is arguably overcome if a specified hierarchy, or priority of importance, is attributed to allow one principle to predominate in a given decision (Strong, 2000; Beauchamp, 2000; Baker, 1997; DeGrazia, 1992; Richardson, 1990). Specified Principlism continues to provide an excellent framework for clinicians to work through complex clinical problems. With increasing legal and economic influences on health care, however, the absolute purity of the physician–patient relationship, and fidelity in particular, is in need of review (Bloche, 2000). It is likely that bioethical principles will be supplanted by other models in the future. Indeed, there is an emerging emphasis, or belief, in "truth telling" in end-of-life care in Western societies, which is consistent with demands for change made by parents and families (Glyn-Pickett,

2005; MacDonald, 2003; Meert, 2000). This view is not necessarily shared in Asian or Eastern cultures, and doctors practising in multicultural environments may need to modify their approach, accordingly (Fan and Li, 2004; Turner, 2005).

AUTONOMY VERSUS PATERNALISM

Until recently, few critical care training programs have included structured teaching in medical ethics. Furthermore, the skills required to approach and resolve ethical dilemmas are not innately granted to all intensivists (Hawryluck and Crippen, 2002). An emphasis on patient autonomy can be misunderstood by physicians, leading them to refrain from offering their "paternalistic" professional opinions and thoughts about appropriate directions in management (Quill and Brody, 1996). This ultimately leaves parents to make decisions using a surfeit of information and a paucity of guidance, with the end result tending toward persistence with apparently futile treatments on the basis that "the patient/family want everything done!" Leaving highly complex decisions entirely in the hands of the patients and family, it could be argued, is an abdication of the doctors' responsibilities (Gold, 2004). Enhancing parental autonomy by openly discussing uncertainties, offering speculative predictions about outcomes, and emphasizing the pros and cons of different approaches is a more complete approach for physicians to adopt that in no way detracts from the parents' involvement, provided the parents are listened to and their situation is considered (Quill and Brody, 1996). Without sharing medical expertise and experience, and making recommendations, the physician may as well be a waiter offering a menu. Initiating discussions at the level of treatment goals, rather than debating specific details of alternative techniques, appears to be a more constructive and successful strategy for engaging parent–physician communication (McDonald, 2003; Quill and Brody, 1996; Tulsky, 2005).

Evidence for these conclusions is found in existing research. Solomon et al. surveyed 781 clinicians in multiple sites across the United States, compiling results from attending physicians, house officers, and nurses who care for children with life-threatening conditions, in both PICUs and general wards. The survey responses indicated a limited understanding of fundamental ethical principles, and high levels of moral distress concerning end-of-life decisions (Solomon et al., 2005). A substantial proportion of respondents reported that "At times, I have acted against my conscience in providing treatment to children in my care." These responses were strongly weighted toward distress about overtreatment, rather than undertreatment. In surveys of nurses in intensive care units, the highest levels of moral distress were found in association with providing aggressive care to patients who were not expected to benefit from it (Elphern, 2005, Hamric, 2007). In a survey of adult patients with severe illness, and their families, the most important factors were "to have trust and confidence in the doctors looking after you," and "not to be kept alive on life support when there is little hope of meaningful recovery" (Heyland et al., 2006). These messages are further testimony to the resilience of the pioneers of new and radical treatments who were clearly able to tolerate the moral dilemmas encountered, including possible resistance from within their own teams, yet continue to push the limits of care. Without this commitment the management of CHD would be unlikely to advance or improve. Such enthusiasm must obviously be tempered by staying true to the humanistic factors of care for the individual involved.

GUIDANCE IN TIMES OF CONFLICTING OPINIONS OR PERSONAL DISTRESS

In situations where there is conflict and moral distress either between families and clinicians, or within health care teams, regarding continuation, or discontinuation, of care, consultation with expert ethics committees has been found to be useful (Bourke, 1997; Hawryluck and Crippen, 2002; Schneiderman et al., 2000; Schneiderman et al., 2003; Teres, 1993; White et al., 2006). Ultimately the committee members need to understand the context of the challenges confronted, and need to be familiar with pace of care in the critical care environment. As the ethical models of end-of-life care are still evolving, an ethics committee may not be able to provide comprehensive guidance for all situations (Cook et al., 2006). Occasionally one may need to seek legal guidance. Legal experts are more inclined to use case-based precedent and to draw upon nonmedical resources to guide them. The medical community is increasingly obliged to consider developments in law, and in "live" documents, such as the United Nations Universal Declaration of Human Rights, as their influence on our practice is likely to increase in the future (Fisher and Raper, 2005; Meisel et al., 2000; Snyder, 1996; White and Baldwin, 2002).

Clinical Practice Guidelines For End-Of-Life Care

Expert committees comprising clinicians, lawyers, ethicists, and the lay public have developed practice guidelines for end-of-life care (Hawryluck et al., 2002; Meisel et al., 2000). Other consensus statements on the conduct of end-of-life care in intensive care units

TABLE 34–1. *Common Themes in Guidelines for End-of-Life Care in Intensive Care Unit*

- Treating the patient and the family with respect and compassion
- Preservation of patient dignity
- Patient-centered care, focusing on their values and treatment preferences, striving to address the physical, psychological, social, and spiritual needs of the patient and family, with sensitivity to their personal, cultural, and religious values, goals, beliefs, and practices
- Creating the right environment for good communication, with sufficient privacy and without interruption
- Communicating honestly, completely, and regularly
- Involving substitute decision makers appropriately
- Excellence in symptom management and pain relief
- Grief and bereavement support after death
- Ensuring emotional and practical support for the ICU clinicians

Source: See text for references.

(ICUs) have been published (Ackermann, 2000; Burns and Rushton, 2004; Cist et al., 2001; Hawryluck et al., 2002; Rubenfeld, 2004; Thompson et al., 2004; Truog et al., 2001). Very few of these guidelines or documents refer to the management of children, and none specifically addresses children with CHD. They are generic entities, providing frameworks for a structured approach, rather than the details. They share common themes, outlined in Table 34–1. Palliative care team involvement in ICU care is a relatively new concept that is supported by the Society of Critical Care Medicine, and recommendations for facilitating the collaboration are outlined in Table 34–2.

These guidelines are useful but do not address some of the particular issues faced in dealing with children with CHD. Children are seen as special cases because of three very relevant differences from adults (Hirschhorn et al., 2006):

- Children are inherently vulnerable and unable to care for themselves, and adults have an innate sense of duty to protect them.
- Children are likely to live a long time with the consequences of decisions that are made, whether the outcome is favorable, or adverse.
- Children lack the capacity to make autonomous decisions for themselves, and therefore, need substitute decision makers.

TABLE 34–2. *Society of Critical Care Medicine (SCCM) Recommendations for Integrated Palliative Care in Intensive Care*

- Strong interdisciplinary collaboration between the critical care team and palliative care specialists
- Changing attitudes about end-of-life care in general, and withdrawal of life support in particular
- Initiating qualitative research in this field

Source: Cook et al., 2006.

Truog et al. have recently pointed out that there is no research published on interventions to improve end-of-life care in the PICU. They also recommend exercising caution before assuming that experiences in adult ICUs can be extrapolated to PICUs, as the children's relationship with family members, and their developmental, psychological, and spiritual capacities are different, and these factors can clearly impact on choices made at the end of life. It is also important to recognize that data accumulated outside the PICU in pediatric oncology and hospice care are not necessarily directly transferable to the PICU (Truog et al., 2006).

Who Shares in Shared Decision Making?

In a survey of families attending Canadian hospitals, there was a wide range of opinions about who should be the decision makers in end-of-life situations (Heyland et al., 2003). The majority (90.4%) of respondents favored collaboration between the physicians and families, with 15.6% desiring the physician to make the final decision after considering the family's opinions and 74.8% feeling that decisions should be shared. Only 1.2% thought that the family alone should be responsible for decisions, and 8.4% of families wanted doctors to make all decisions on their own. In a European study, 48% of patients believed that the responsibility for decision making in the ICU should be theirs alone, without the physician, while 31% of nurses and 8% of physicians shared that opinion. For incompetent patients, 61% of physicians thought they should make decisions alone, whereas 73% of the public thought that family and doctors should make decisions together (Sjokvist et al., 1999). Clear demographic, cultural, and individual differences in professional approaches to end-of-life care were confirmed in another recent survey (Yaguchi et al., 2005). The disparities in these statistics, not only between continents but also between health professionals and the public within continents, highlight that there is considerable merit in establishing, upfront, the exact expectations of the families when we communicate with them.

With increasing cultural diversity in our society, the potential for diverging opinions is perhaps likely to increase. There are many cases in the medical and legal literature, and the lay press, of parents, families, and doctors disagreeing on the right course of action for a patient. Interest groups and politicians have been known to become embroiled in the controversies, with opinions often becoming more polarized as the issues are publicly debated (Burt, 2006; Koop, 1989; Reagan, 1986). Although these cases are the exception, rather than the rule, they exemplify the basic fact that end-of-life care relies on good communication between family and health professionals, and agreement on appropriate actions (Kopelman, 2006; Levy and McBride, 2006). A framework is needed in order to guide caregivers through such situations. We believe the solution is based on redefining a common ground between all parties by acknowledging and embracing a new culture around the patient in the ICU.

THE CULTURE OF PEDIATRIC INTENSIVE CARE UNITS

A common expectation, when submitting one's child to a therapeutic intervention, is that the outcome will be perfect. As the care process evolves this expectation may change, so that parents and families may be willing to accept much lesser outcomes. The family who is expertly managed throughout such an ordeal may even come to accept the death of their child, if it occurs, as a natural outcome. Intensive care, by its nature, fosters intense emotions, and strong relationships can form among patients, nurses, physicians, and parents and families. Trust develops, and in most instances personal interactions are consistent and collaborative. A new culture is created, bringing mutual respect and understanding that engenders an outcome that is satisfactory to all.

In trying to define this culture, we identify four elements, or stakeholders. All must harmonize within a common sphere of cultural, religious, and scientific understanding. We have portrayed this model diagrammatically (Figure 34–1).

THE FOUR MAIN ELEMENTS OF THE MODEL

None of the elements of the model exists in strict isolation, in that they all influence the actions of each other in some way.

1. The child
   The child is placed at the core of our model, given that he or she is the focus of all activity. Health professionals concentrate on treating the disease process, applying technology where appropriate, while parents and family try to retain a relationship with their child in an abnormal and artificial environment.
2. Health care professionals
   PICU care is generally provided by an extensive multidisciplinary team.. For CHD patients there are at least one cardiac surgeon, a cardiologist, a general pediatrician, several PICU physicians and many more PICU nurses, respiratory therapists, dieticians, pharmacists, physiotherapists, sonographers, radiographers, and others. Palliative care experts may also be included. All have direct roles

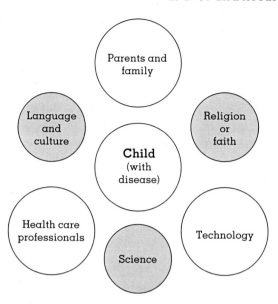

FIGURE 34–1. A model of the culture of care in PICU, as explained in the text. This model may be used to examine the elements, drawn as four white circles (foreground), which strongly influence clinical decision making and reminds us that problems may be perceived differently by different elements. Communication between these elements relies upon common understanding, and the main influences on communication are displayed in gray circles (background).

at one time or another in the care of the patient and have the potential to form a bond with the patient and the family. A team of this nature needs a leader, or principal representative, who, in turn, needs sufficient wisdom and experience to be accepted in that role by other health care team members. PICU physicians usually fulfill this role. Good communication skills are paramount for the dissemination of accurate information to all members of the team, in order that treatment goals are consistently maintained, particularly when tough management decisions need to be made. A secondary relationship between health care professionals, the child, and technology may serve an ulterior purpose, to facilitate research, which is medically gratifying, and potentially assists in further technological development. This may be of no direct benefit to the child.

3. Parents, family, other substitute decision makers
A child "belongs" to his or her parents and family, who, in times of threat to the health or well-being of the child, are expected to act as advocates, sanctioning decisions that will affect their future together, making decisions on their behalf in accordance with the child's place in the world. A threat to the child is a threat to the whole family. Until a child is deemed sufficiently mature and independent, the parents are usually regarded as their substitute decision makers, unless they are incapable of

fulfilling this responsibility. Other family members may be called upon for advice and support. In the absence of any competent and legally acceptable family guardian, children will be represented by an authoritative body, such as a guardianship board. Any given family will hold their own cultural, philosophical, and moral beliefs, but the inclination to apply stereotypes should be resisted. In times of emotional distress families may come to realize that they actually hold personal views that differ from those espoused by their particular ethnic or cultural group.

4. Technology
Technology is an integral part of PICU care, and its availability inevitably influences treatment decisions. Therapies involving highly technical and sophisticated equipment can substitute most bodily functions. Sensitive monitoring techniques also help to mitigate impending complications and adverse events by earlier detection and intervention. The application of highly technological PICU support is expensive, and must be justifiable within the ethical frameworks already outlined. In addition, as each new technological advance permits new frontiers of care to be reached, the ethical and moral obligations to the individual, and to the society they belong to, need to be const antly reassessed, as possible outcomes of particular treatment choices may change dramatically.

THE BACKGROUND CULTURE OF THE MODEL

The four main elements are embedded in an increasingly multifaceted culture, reflecting the global village in which we live and practice. Language, belief systems, and expectations may vary widely within both the providers and the recipients of health care. These differences are often as diverse in the health care team as they are in the patient population. The challenges lie in finding common ground by which meaningful and successful communication can occur. Acknowledging and understanding a family's religious beliefs and cultural needs, especially rituals, can be helpful. For example, reassuring parents that it is possible to make arrangements for prompt burial, should their belief system so require, may relieve considerable anxieties about the impending death of their child. Specific inquiries about particular needs of this nature are usually welcomed. Scientific research is common in PICUs, and patients are often enrolled in trials that dictate certain aspects of treatment. With regulation by research ethics committees, strict enrolment and exclusion criteria, and robust study protocol designs, the impact of research on persistence with futile therapies is likely to be extremely small. Difficult and complex patients may be seen as ideal cases for studying new treatments, but once again, scientific rigour and peer review will prevent wanton experimentation.

Decision Making at End of Life

Parents are comfortable making decisions for their children when they are healthy, but a dying child is not a familiar experience for most parents. The PICU environment, coupled with bombardment of complex information, may be additionally disorienting. Physicians are used to assuming the responsibility for making medical decisions for children under their care, based on their skills, knowledge, and experience, and their intention of restoring them to health (Kopelman, 2006). When reaching the end of life, the prospect of health restoration is lost, and this changes the dynamic between physicians, parents, and the patient. By virtue of their training, doctors are expected to remain scientifically objective and analytical, and to stay emotionally controlled, while parents are expected to experience deeper emotional turmoil, and to need advice, guidance, and support. Ultimately, the parents should not be asked to feel responsible for ending their child's life. End-of-life decisions must be led by the physicians in charge of the patient's care, but may need to be made in stages that are acceptable to those affected. Such strategies include the establishment of "do not resuscitate" (DNR) orders, which allow death to occur peacefully in the event of cardiac arrest. Alternatively, treatment may be "withheld" (for instance, deciding not to use ECMO, or a VAD, or list for transplantation) or "withdrawn" (for instance, by ceasing ventilation and inotropes, and extubating the child for the parents to cuddle him or her for the child's last moments alive, in as natural a state as possible).

Not infrequently, and quite understandably, the initial response of parents and families is to disagree with a recommendation by the health care team that life-sustaining care be withdrawn. With time, clear communication, and understanding of the issues involved, and the assumption that all parties will make decisions in the best interest of the child, this should, theoretically, be only a transient resistance. In reality, however, communications are often not ideal (Meyer et al., 2006).

Five common causes of parental objection to the recommendation of withdrawing therapy have been proposed (Kopelman, 2006); these are shown in Table 34–3.

Communication and the Model Of Care

Although there may be a significant amount of information shared at the bedside, it is common practice

TABLE 34–3. *Common Reasons for Parental Objection to Withdrawing Therapy*

1. Immature, scared, or overwhelmed parents cannot cope with end-of-life discussions, and default to demanding inappropriate care.
2. Religious beliefs, hope for miracles, and the prospect of intolerable shame may confront parents if they weaken their faith.
3. Mistrust of hospitals and doctors because of prior 'bad experiences', or stories of this nature.
4. Using the survival of the child as a solution to a life crisis—keeping the parents together when they would otherwise separate.
5. There are some families who will love and cherish a severely neurologically damaged and totally dependent child as much as any other, and who view any life as a successful outcome.

Source: Kopelman, 2006.

to arrange formal, private family meetings to facilitate communication.

Family Meetings

Well-conducted family meetings are the cornerstone of excellence in palliative care in the PICU (Lautrette et al., 2006). From a purely practical perspective it is preferable to maintain consistency in the members of the health care team conducting these meetings, and to define the roles of all participants (Billings and Keeley, 2006). Physicians usually lead proceedings and may wish to include nurses, social workers, and chaplains, but it can be overwhelming for parents to appear before a panel of experts (Glynn-Pickett, 2005). The family should also nominate its representatives as smaller numbers facilitate greater depth of communication. If time allows, it is better to conduct frequent meetings to address particular issues sequentially, than to attempt to cover all issues in one sitting (Billings and Keeley, 2006). Using the perspectives of the stakeholders in our model we can examine the anatomy of communications in end-of-life care.

1. Needs of Parents and Family

When entering into any discussions about end of life, the perspectives of all the participants need to be understood. For any caregiver, the first task is to acknowledge the sufferer and to legitimize the reality and seriousness of their experience (Counts and Counts, 1991). In other words, the main focus of the first family meeting should be to simply identify the critical nature of the child's condition, including the possibility of death, and then to listen to what the family says in response. When listening, it is important not to be overly judgmental or analytical. Medicalization—the making of the normal social world into abnormalities and foci for treatment—reduces the sense of human life into diagnoses and categories (Fox, 1988). Ordinary unhappiness, sorrow, and bereavement should not be recast as depression, anxiety disorder, and pathological grief, and thus treated as illnesses. It is incumbent on the physician to acknowledge the family's stress, fear, and anxiety to embrace them as normal in these circumstances and to communicate accordingly. Once that level of care and compassion has been displayed, trust develops. From that point forward the family will be more able to receive medical information.

Communication is always bidirectional. Breaking bad news is not difficult to do, but it takes skill to do it well, and the stress this causes leads some clinicians to avoid it wherever possible. Parents and families may sense this and send out signals that they are ready to discuss death, but these indications are also commonly missed or ignored by physicians (Curtis et al., 2001). In a study of recorded interviews, family dissatisfaction correlated as much with "missed opportunities" to discuss sensitive or troubling issues, as with the manner in which the news was delivered (Curtis et al., 2001). With appropriate training there should be diminution of the discomfort felt by physicians when discussing death.

A common way in which physicians fail to meet the needs of the parents and family is by prematurely launching into explaining and deciphering medical technical details, rationalizing the clinical decisions made, and outlining treatment options that might be available. This may be a comfortable platform for the physician; however, it may be neither appropriate nor timely for the parent (Glyn-Pickett, 2005). While there is undoubtedly a need to convey medical information in order to keep the parents informed, this information should only be presented once it is mutually understood exactly how critical their child's condition is and there is agreement about the main goals of therapy (Quill and Brody, 1996). Without a strong frame of reference, parents cannot begin to understand the implications of detailed medical information.

A qualitative, retrospective, questionnaire-based study from Harvard contacted parents of children who died in PICUs following withdrawal of life support and found six themes, or priorities, that parents want in end-of-life care for their children (Meyer et al., 2006). These are displayed in Table 34–4.

TABLE 34–4. *Six Priorities Common to Parents of Children Dying in PICU*

1. Honest and complete information
2. Ready access to staff
3. Communication and care coordination
4. Emotional expression and support by staff
5. Preservation of the integrity of the parent–child relationship
6. Faith

Source: Meyer et al., 2006.

Parents want to be told the truth, even if the truth is likely to be distressing. They want their questions answered, and they want to feel included in the decision making, because there can be intolerable levels of anger and guilt generated by finding out facts after death that could have influenced their decisions earlier (Glyn-Pickett, 2005; McDonald, 2003; Meyer et al., 2006). Continuity of staff communication, by regular interview and by the same person and not a different person each time, helps to foster reassurance, trust, and emotional calm. Communication coordination refers to scheduling meetings at convenient times and to minimizing the number of doctors speaking to parents, as they invariably offer variations on the preceding opinions, which can be disconcerting and disorientating. Lack of communication or brevity of meetings can be interpreted as a lack of caring, or a reluctance to be truthful. Not being afraid to express emotion shows that we are human, compassionate, and caring, and is highly valued by parents (Glyn-Pickett, 2005; McDonald, 2003). Preserving the parent–child relationship involves showing respect for them and for their role in their child's life. Parents often find solace in their religious faith as it provides some foundation by which they can guide their decisions and rationalize their experiences (Meyer et al., 2006). Faith is likely to be both cherished and challenged in PICU.

2. Perspectives of health care professionals

When conducting end-of-life discussions it is important to understand where communications can be misinterpreted or misunderstood. If language difficulties exist, subtle nuances may be missed completely, even when assisted by skilled interpreters. Even with no language barriers, the terminology used in the context of end-of-life care is frequently misleading. "Withdrawal of care" implies abandonment and neglect. "Withdrawing and withholding treatment" is semantically more accurate, but still focuses on the negative. Asking a family, "Do you want everything done?" implies that the alternative is to do nothing (Fisher and Raper, 2005). What should be added is "… that it is appropriate to do" (Worthley, 2004). Fear of abandonment at the end of life is very real for many adults and translates into anxiety for their children. For many, the fear of suffering may be greater than the fear of dying (Fisher and Raper, 2005). Framing discussions in terms of what can be done to meet the physical, psychological, spiritual, and cultural needs of the patient is explaining the essence of palliation. Patient and parent confidence in such a comprehensive, caring approach is unlikely to create conflicts on too many occasions. Differences of opinion within the health care team need to be resolved and consensus should be reached before approaching the family. Conflicts of medical opinion may undermine the family's confidence and trust, with disastrous consequences.

Physicians may also be vulnerable in caring for their dying patients. They may be reminded of their own personal family experiences of death, or have children of similar age and appearance, and emotionally these factors must be acknowledged and dealt with. Physicians may also be sensitive to criticism about their care, whether intended or merely perceived, and find it difficult to deal with negative reactions from parents and family, taking expressions of anger and grief as personal affronts or ingratitude. Peer support and informal debriefing is a strong part of PICU culture, worldwide, that helps physicians to deal with these challenges (personal experience).

3. Influence of technology

The possibilities created by the introduction and application of advanced mechanical supports and highly specialized pharmaceuticals are, in turn, creating new ethical and moral challenges, raising economic questions, and generating geographical inequalities of distribution of health care resources, within and between nations. Some of the moral dilemmas that arise may not be resolvable. By what criteria are successes of that therapy measured? Does the ambition to be the first to do something remove objectivity and pollute the process of informed consent? If a cheaper but older technology is available, that performs statistically less effectively than a newer and more expensive method, is it defensible to apply that older technology? There is inevitably going to be a need for collaborative decision making, including a broader representation of society than medical practitioners alone, to establish guidelines of practice that facilitate appropriate rationing of technology, since resources are not infinite and demand for their use will certainly increase. The cessation, or withdrawal, of technological supports at the end of life must be conducted with skill and compassion, and with particular attention to the concurrent maintenance of appropriate analgesia and sedation to avoid distressing the child, and the parents.

Organ donation is rarely an option following the death of patients with CHD, as a consequence of the patients' young age, the frequency of concurrent multi-organ failure, and the manner in which they die. Tissue donation may give parents some consolation.

PAIN RELIEF AND SEDATION

Parents need to be reassured that their child will not experience pain or discomfort. Opioids are the principal strong analgesics used in ICU. The choice of agent is usually determined by unit protocols, prescriber

familiarity, and the specific indications (Mastronardi and Cafiero, 2001). A "double effect principle" is widely accepted for palliative analgesia. This principle provides legal justification for the moral and medical indications of continuing to administer opioids for patient comfort, acknowledging that some potential side effects, including respiratory depression, may be detrimental or even hasten death (Hawryluck et al., 2002; Hawryluck and Harvey, 2000; Truog et al., 1991). Anxiolytics may also be used to relieve suffering, following the same principle, even if they sedate the patient (Krakauer et al., 2000). Analgesia and sedation should be optimized at the end of life. Consider administering local anesthesia before removing drains, tubes, and lines.

SOME ADDITIONAL POINTS ON PRACTICALITIES OF END-OF-LIFE CARE

Legacy Creation

Legacy creation is the term used to describe a ritual performed in many PICUs for dying children that is often viewed positively by staff and families. It involves making testamentary objects with special meaning that families will keep as mementos of a child's life. Plaster of Paris moulds of the child's hands or feet, often intertwined with the hands of the parents or a sibling, make powerful symbols that are easy to make. Photographs before and after death, with and without attached medical equipment, may be the only photographs parents ever take of their child. Cards, presents, and items of clothing become treasures. For children who have spent longer periods in PICU, journals may have been started with entries written by nursing and medical attendants on a shift-by-shift basis, of how they felt caring for the child at the time. These become surrogate diaries of the child's life, and often allow emotions to be expressed that might otherwise remain unshared. Legacy creation also allows health care staff the opportunity to say goodbye, and to gain some personal closure.

Bereavement Coordinators in the Pediatric Intensive Care Unit

SickKids in Toronto has a full-time bereavement coordinator, a nurse whose primary role is to make contact with parents and families before, during, and after the death of a child in the PICU. Her involvement has far-reaching consequences, providing opportunities for lingering questions to be answered, details of post-mortem findings, and outstanding laboratory results to be shared, and showing support for the family on behalf of the hospital as a whole.

Death

ICU specialists commonly feel competent and experienced enough to manage their own patients, and may be disinclined to recruit the assistance of palliative care teams. At mortality audits it is common to hear references to "good deaths," meaning those which are well managed by all of the criteria discussed in this chapter. But the term is a relative one, especially when children are concerned. As the parents and family leave the hospital without their child the whole process is really just beginning for them. The emptiness, the sorrow, and the hurt are experienced for months and years afterwards (McDonald, 2003). Palliation of the child may have ended, but the family's needs continue. One of the advantages of including a palliative care team in the end-of-life care in the PICU is that these teams often have community outreach and other support networks that can maintain some support of the family after death.

CONCLUSIONS

Society at large is generally in denial of death, and this is no more acutely apparent than with the death of a child (Cook et al., 2006). When a child dies there is an inherent feeling of violation of the natural order of things. With technological advances and wider availability of sophisticated medical care, more children with CHD are likely to have access to life support and complex cardiac surgery. The number of children who survive this is likely to increase, but there will always be a proportion who die. It is incumbent upon us as health professionals to care for all of these children to the utmost of our abilities, following the concepts and principles that we have set out in this chapter, and to rejoice in our successful interventions, but also to actively manage the nonsurvivors through the end of life, ensuring that their respect, comfort, and dignity are preserved, and their families are supported. We hope that the model we have proposed helps clinicians to clarify the issues they confront in these complex situations.

REFERENCES

Ackermann R. Withholding and withdrawing life-sustaining treatment. *Am. Fam. Physician.* 2000;62:7;1555–60, 1562, 1564.

Back AL, Arnold RM, Quill T. Hope for the best, and prepare for the worst. *Ann. Intern. Med.* 2003;138(5):439–443.

Baker A. Assumptions and practice in clinical medical ethics. *Anaesth Int Care.* 1997;Oct 25(5):528–534.

Beauchamp TL. Reply to Strong on principlism and casuistry *J. Med. Philosophy.* 2000;25(3):342–347.

Beauchamp T. Methods and principles in biomedical ethics. *J. Med. Ethics.* 2003;29:269–274.

Beauchamp TL, Childress JF *Principles of biomedical ethics.* Oxford University Press 1st ed.1979.

Billings JA, Keeley. Merging cultures: Palliative care specialists in the medical intensive care unit. *Crit Care Med.* 2006;34:11 Suppl;S388–S393.

Bloche M. Fidelity and deceit at the bedside. *JAMA.* 2000;283(14):1881–84.

Bourke B. Decisions, decisions. *Health. Ala.* 1997;10:1;12–5, 20.

Burns JP, Rushton CH. End-of-life care in the pediatric intensive care unit: research review and recommendations. *Crit Care Clin.* 2004;20:3;467–85, x.

Burt R. Law's effect on the quality of end-of-life care: Lessons from the *Schiavo* case. *Crit Care Med.* 2006;34:11 (suppl);S348–S354.

Byrne PJ, Murphy A. Informed consent and hypoplastic left heart syndrome. *Acta Paediatrica.* 2005;94(9):1171–75.

Cayler GG, Smeloff EA, Miller GE, Jr. Surgical palliation of hypoplastic left side of the heart. *N. Engl. J. Med.* 1970;282:14;780–783.

Chrisant MRK, Naftel DC, Drummond-Webb J, et al and the Pediatric Heart Transplant Study Group. Fate of infants with hypoplastic left heart syndrome listed for cardiac transplantation: a multi-center study. *J. Heart Lung Transplant.* 2005;24:576–8.

Cist AF, Truog RD, Brackett SE, Hurford WE. Practical guidelines on the withdrawal of life-sustaining therapies. *Int. Anesthesiol. Clin.* 2001;39:3;87–10.

Cook D, Rocker G, Giacomini M, Sinuff T, Heyland D. Understanding and changing attitudes toward withdrawal and withholding of life support in the intensive care unit. *Crit Care Med.* 2006;34:11 Suppl;S317–S323.

Counts, D and Counts, D Coping with the final tragedy: cultural variation in dying and grieving. Amityville, NY: Baywood Publishing 1991.

Curtis JR, Patrick DL, Shannon SE, Treece PD, Engelberg RA, Rubenfeld GD. The family conference as a focus to improve communication about end-of-life care in the intensive care unit: opportunities for improvement. *Crit Care Med.* 2001;29:2 Suppl;N26–N33.

DeGrazia D. Moving forward in bioethical theory: theories, cases and specified principlism. *J. Med. Philosophy.* 1992;17:511–539.

Dunstan GR. Hard questions in intensive care. A moralist answers questions put to him at a meeting of the Intensive Care Society, Autumn, 1984. *Anaesthesia.* 1985;40:5;479–482.

Elphern, EH, Covert B, Kleinpell R. Moral distress of staff nurses in a medical intensive care unit. *Am J Crit Care* 2005;14:6;523–530.

Fan R, Li B. Truth telling in medicine: the Confucian view. *J. Med. Philosophy.* 2004;29(2):179–193.

Fisher MM, Raper RF. Courts, doctors and end-of-life care. *Intensive Care Med.* 2005;31:6;762–764.

Fox, R Essays in medical sociology, Piscataway (NJ): Transaction Publishers 1988.

Garros D, Rosychuk RJ, Cox PN. Circumstances surrounding end of life in a pediatric intensive care unit. *Pediatrics.* 2003;112:5;e371.

Glyn-Pickett J. Dialogue, death, and life choices: a parent's perspective. *Arch. Dis. Child.* 2005;90:12;1314–1315.

Gold M. Ethics in medicine. Is honesty always the best policy? Ethics of truth telling. *Intern. Med. J.* 2004;34:574–580.

Hamric AB, Blackhall LJ. Nurse-physician perspectives on the care of dying patients in intensive care units: collaboration, moral distress, and ethical climate. *Crit Care Med* 2007;35:2;641–2.

Hawryluck L, Crippen D. Ethics and critical care in the new millennium. *Crit Care.* 2002;6:1;1–2.

Hawryluck LA, Harvey WR. Analgesia, virtue, and the principle of double effect. *J. Palliat. Care.* 2000;16 suppl:S24–S30.

Hawryluck LA, Harvey WR, Lemieux-Charles L, Singer PA. Consensus guidelines on analgesia and sedation in dying intensive care unit patients. *BMC. Med. Ethics.* August 12, 2002;3:E3.

Heyland DK, Dodek P, Rocker G, et al. What matters most in end-of-life care: perceptions of seriously ill patients and their family members. *CMAJ.* 2006;174:5;627–633.

Heyland DK, Rocker GM, O'Callaghan CJ, Dodek PM, Cook DJ. Dying in the ICU: perspectives of family members. *Chest.* 2003;124:1;392–397.

Hirschhorn K, Holzman I, Moros D, Rhodes R. Introduction.Issues in medical ethics: special challenges in pediatrics. *The Mount Sinai Journal of Medicine.* 2006;73:3;578–589.

Koop EC. The challenge of definition. *Hastings Center Report* 19, 1989; Special supplement; 2–3.

Kopelman AE. Understanding, avoiding, and resolving end-of-life conflicts in the NICU. *Mt. Sinai J. Med.* 2006;73:3;580–586.

Krakauer EL, Penson RT, Truog RD, King LA, Chabner BA, Lynch TJ, Jr. Sedation for intractable distress of a dying patient: acute palliative care and the principle of double effect. *Oncologist.* 2000;5:1;53–62.

Krasemann T, Fenge H, Kehl HG, et al. A decade of staged Norwood palliation in hypoplastic left heart syndrome in a midsized cardiosurgical center. *Pediatr. Cardiol.* 2005;26:6;751–755.

Lautrette A, Ciroldi M, Ksibi H, Azoulay E. End-of-life family conferences: Rooted in the evidence. *Crit Care Med.* 2006;34:11 Suppl;S364–S372.

Levy MM, McBride DL. End-of-life care in the intensive care unit: State of the art in 2006. *Crit Care Med.* 2006;34:11 Suppl;S306–S308.

MacLeod R. Learning from Sir William Osler about the teaching of palliative care. *J. Palliat. Care.* 2001;17:4;265–269.

Malec E, Januszewska K, Kolz J, Pajak J. Factors influencing early outcome of Norwood procedure for hypoplastic left heart syndrome. *Eur. J. Cardiothorac. Surg.* 2000;18:2;202–206.

Mastronardi P, Cafiero T. Rational use of opioids. *Minerva Anestesiol.* 2001;67:4;332–337.

McDonald V. A patchwork of care. *Newsletter of the Canadian Society of Palliative Care Physicians.* 2003;5:1.

McGuirk SP, Stickley J, Griselli M, et al. Risk assessment and early outcome following the Norwood procedure for hypoplastic left heart syndrome. *Eur. J. Cardiothorac. Surg.* 2006; 29:5;675–681.

Meert KL, Thurston CS, Sarnaik AP. End-of-life decision-making and satisfaction with care: parental perspectives. *PediatrCrit Care Med.* 2000;1:2;179–185.

Meisel A, Snyder L, Quill T. Seven legal barriers to end-of-life care: myths, realities, and grains of truth. *JAMA.* 2000;284:19;2495–2501.

Meyer EC, Ritholz MD, Burns JP, Truog RD. Improving the quality of end-of-life care in the pediatric intensive care unit: parents' priorities and recommendations. *Pediatrics.* 2006;117:3;649–657.

Noonan JA and Nadas AS. The hypoplastic left heart syndrome; and analysis of 101 cases. *Pediatr. Clin. North Am.* 1958;5(4):1029–1056.

Norwood WI, Kirklin JK, Sanders SP. Hypoplastic left heart syndrome: experience with palliative surgery. *Am. J. Cardiol.* 1980;45:1;87–91.

Norwood WI, Lang P, Hansen DD. Physiologic repair of aortic atresia-hypoplastic left heart syndrome. *N. Engl. J. Med.* 1983;308:1;23–26.

Oh TE. Ethics in intensive care. Oh's Intensive Care Manual. Bersten A, Soni N, (eds). 5th Ed. Elsevier Ltd. 2003;49–52.

Pizarro C, Davis DA, Galantowicz ME, Munro H, Gidding SS, Norwood WI. Stage I palliation for hypoplastic left heart syndrome in low birth weight neonates: can we justify it? *Eur. J. Cardiothorac. Surg.* 2002;21:4;716–720.

Quill TE, Brody H. Physician recommendations and patient autonomy: finding a balance between physician power and patient choice. *Ann. Intern. Med.* 1996;125(9):763–769.

Quill TE, Suchman AL. Uncertainty and control: learning to live with medicine's limitations. *Humane Medicine.*1993;9:109–120.

Reagan R. Abortion andthe conscience of the nation. 3rd edition.1986;352–358.

Richardson HS. Specifying norms as a way to resolve concrete ethical problems. *Philosophy and Public Affairs.* 1990;19: 279–310.

Rubenfeld GD. Principles and practice of withdrawing life-sustaining treatments. *Crit Care Clin.* 2004;20:3;435–51, ix.

Sarnaik AP, Daphtary K, Sarnaik AA. Ethical issues in pediatric intensive care in developing countries: combining western technology and eastern wisdom. *Indian J. Pediatr.* 2005;72:4;339–342.

Schneiderman LJ, Gilmer T, Teetzel HD. Impact of ethics consultations in the intensive care setting: a randomized, controlled trial. *Crit Care Med.* 2000;28:12;3920–3924.

Schneiderman LJ, Gilmer T, Teetzel HD, et al. Effect of ethics consultations on nonbeneficial life-sustaining treatments in the intensive care setting: a randomized controlled trial. *JAMA.* 2003;290:9;1166–1172.

Sinzobahamvya N, Photiadis J, Kumpikaite D, et al. Comprehensive Aristotle score: implications for the Norwood procedure. *Ann. Thorac. Surg.* 2006;81:5;1794–1800.

Sjokvist P, Nilstun T, Svantesson M, Berggren L. Withdrawal of life support – who should decide? Differences in attitudes among the general public, nurses and physicians. *Intensive Care Med.* 1999;25:9;949–954.

Snyder RD. End of life decisions at the beginning of life. *Med. Law.* 1996;15:2;283–289.

Solomon MZ, Sellers DE, Heller KS, et al. New and lingering controversies in pediatric end-of-life care. *Pediatrics.* 2005;116:4;872–883.

Strong C. Specified principlism: what is it, and does it really resolve cases better than casuistry? *J. Med. Philosophy.* 2000;v25(3):323–341.

Teres D. Trends from the United States with end of life decisions in the intensive care unit. *Intensive Care Med.* 1993;19:6;316–322.

Theilen U, Shekerdemian L. The intensive care of infants with hypoplastic left heart syndrome. *Arch. Dis. Child Fetal Neonatal Ed.* 2005;90:2;F97–F102.

Thompson BT, Cox PN, Antonelli M, et al. Challenges in end-of-life care in the ICU: statement of the 5th International Consensus Conference in Critical Care: Brussels, Belgium, April 2003: executive summary. *Crit Care Med.* 2004;32:8;1781–1784.

Truog RD, Arnold JH, Rockoff MA. Sedation before ventilator withdrawal: medical and ethical considerations. *J. Clin. Ethics.* 1991;2:2;127–129.

Truog RD, Cist AF, Brackett SE, et al. Recommendations for end-of-life care in the intensive care unit: The Ethics Committee of the Society of Critical Care Medicine. *Crit Care Med.* 2001;29:12;2332–2348.

Truog RD, Meyer EC, Burns JP. Toward interventions to improve end-of-life care in the pediatric intensive care unit. *Crit Care Med.* 2006;34:11 Suppl;S373–S379.

Tulsky JA. Interventions to enhance communication among patients, providers, and families. *J. Palliative Med.* 2005;8:suppl:S95–102.

Turner L. From the local to the global: bioethics and the concept of culture. *J. Med. Philosophy.* 2005;30(3):305–320.

Welke KF, Shen I, Ungerleider RM. Current assessment of mortality rates in congenital cardiac surgery. *Ann. Thorac. Surg.* 2006;82:1;164–170.

White DB, Curtis JR, Lo B, Luce JM. Decisions to limit life-sustaining treatment for critically ill patients who lack both decision-making capacity and surrogate decision-makers. *Crit Care Med.* 2006;34:8;2053–2059.

White SM, Baldwin TJ. The Human Rights Act 1998: implications for anaesthesia and intensive care. *Anaesthesia.* 2002;57:9;882–888.

Worthley LI. "While we often manage dying patients, dying is not an indication for admission to an ICU". *Crit Care Resusc.* 2004;6:2;141–142.

Yaguchi A, Truog RD, Curtis JR, et al. International differences in end-of-life attitudes in the intensive care unit: results of a survey. *Arch. Intern. Med.* 2005;165:17;1970–1975.

Index

Note: Page number in *italics* refers to figures, where as **bold** refers to tables